CLINICAL PHARMACOLOGY IN NURSING

CLINICAL PHARMACOLOGY IN NURSING

Morton J. Rodman, B.S., Ph.D.

Professor of Pharmacology and Chairman,
Department of Pharmacology,
College of Pharmacy, Rutgers, The State
University of New Jersey

and

Dorothy W. Smith, R.N., Ed.D.

Professor of Nursing, College of Nursing,
Rutgers, The State University of New Jersey

J. B. Lippincott Company
Philadelphia   **Toronto**

Distributed in Great Britain by
Blackwell Scientific Publications,
London, Oxford, and Edinburgh

ISBN-0-397-54132-5

Library of Congress Catalog Card Number 73-18194

Printed in the United States of America
7 9 8

LIBRARY OF CONGRESS CATALOGING IN PUBLICATION DATA

Rodman, Morton J.
    Clinical pharmacology in nursing.

    Includes bibliographies.
    1. Pharmacology.   I.   Smith, Dorothy W., joint
author.   II.   Title.
RM125.R62   1974   615'.1'024613   73-18194
ISBN 0-397-54132-5

Preface

This book deals with how drugs are used in the management of many medical disorders and other clinical situations such as anesthesia and surgery. Its main aim is to present information about modern medications in a manner relevant to the needs of nurses who are caring for patients in various clinical settings.

Nurses are responsible not only for administering medications but also for making knowledgeable observations of the effects that administered drugs have upon the patient. In addition, the nurse must often teach the patient and his family how to use drugs safely and in a manner that will help to gain their greatest therapeutic benefits.

To do so, she must employ knowledge of both drugs and nursing. However, factual knowledge alone is not enough to assure good patient care. For if knowledge of the technical aspects of drug administration is not accompanied by an understanding of the principles of drug use and of nursing care, the patient may not gain all of the benefits that he otherwise might from his drug therapy.

Thus, the narrative portions of the fifty chapters in this text are devoted, not to presenting detailed data about individual drugs of each class, but rather to showing the reasoning behind the ways in which drugs of different classes are used in treating patients with various disorders. This is intended to foster insights into the fundamental principles of the clinical use of drugs in the context of the nurse's duties and responsibilities.

Nevertheless, nurses often do need to have specific data about such matters as the dosage, administration, and adverse effects of the drugs with which they are dealing. Detailed information of this kind and of the indications and contraindications of important individual drugs is offered in a monograph called *Drug Digest** which is presented in a separate section of most chapters, in order not to interfere with the free flow of the narrative sections and in doing so, possibly obscure the reader's understanding of the basic principles of clinical drug use that are presented in the main body of the text.

Factual data and fundamental principles are, in addition, presented in the form of detailed tables and summaries in the body and at the end of each chapter. Here, the student can quickly find such facts as the dosage of any drug, its clinical indications, and potential adverse effects and the cautions required in its use. The principles that the nurse must apply in her professional use of each drug class are also summarized at the end of each chapter.

Other ways in which the authors have tried to attain the objective of offering material relevant to the practical needs of the nurse are through the presentation of actual clinical nursing situations and by means of a small but selective list of reading references. In each of the clinical situations, a practical problem is presented and the student is challenged to discuss how to handle it, using knowledge and professional judgment acquired in all of her courses. The references are mainly to articles that have appeared in nursing journals in recent years. By reading these articles the interested nursing student can broaden and deepen her knowledge of the management of various medical disorders with more detailed clinical information than can be presented within a general textbook.

---

* A plus sign following the name of any drug discussed in the narrative draws the reader's attention to the fact that detailed information about that drug's actions and uses, adverse effects, cautions and contraindications, and dosage and administration is available at the end of the chapter in a Drug Digest.

Finally, a word about the format of this book: The authors have tried to present both factual knowledge and fundamental principles in a form that would make for easy reading. The various sections and subsections of each chapter are set off by headings in capital letters or boldface type in order to orient the student immediately to the specific subject matter under discussion. Each paragraph is relatively short and specific in its content. Complicated chemical formulas and reactions have been avoided, as have been excessively detailed discussions of the biochemical mechanisms by which drugs exert their effects at the cellular level. This, like everything else in this book, is intended to make it easy for the student to acquire quickly the kind of information most immediately important to her needs as a nurse. The authors hope that this will help her to make a useful contribution to effective patient care through the proper use of medications in practical clinical situations.

Acknowledgments

This book is dedicated to the memory of Beatrice Rodman. She devoted herself for thirty years to the senior author's well-being and thus made it possible for him to find self-fulfillment in scholarly activity. Her constant support helped him to broaden his understanding of biomedical sciences. Beatrice Rodman created an atmosphere which in countless ways facilitated the work of the senior author. Both authors acknowledge her contribution and her encouragement.

David Miller, Managing Editor of the Nursing Department of J. B. Lippincott, originally suggested that the book be written, and that the format emphasize readability and conciseness in presenting essential information. His concern for the success of this project was reflected in his never failing to reply to every communication from the authors. His cheerful outlook helped to strengthen the authors' will and morale whenever they weakened during the travail of writing.

Dr. Roy A. Bowers, Dean of the College of Pharmacy of Rutgers University, helped the senior author find time for research and writing by aiding him in arranging a schedule of maximum flexibility and freedom. Two members of the College staff, Lucille Lear and JoAnn Kulesza, typed the manuscript with great competence and personal concern.

Patricia Blegman contributed useful information on the nursing care of patients with Parkinson's disease.

Carol P. Hanley Germain contributed very effectively to the material dealing with use of drugs in the care of critically ill patients in coronary care and intensive care situations. The enthusiasm of the students at Rutgers University College of Nursing, and their concern about patients, have been a source of encouragement throughout this project.

About the Factual Content of This Textbook

The authors and editors of this book have expended considerable time and effort to insure that the facts and opinions offered in the text and tables of this book are in accordance with official standards and with the consensus of foremost authorities at the time of publication.

However, drug therapy is a very dynamic branch of medicine, marked by the continual marketing of new drugs and the discontinuation and withdrawal (often without notice) of older drug products. In addition, the Food and Drug Administration constantly orders changes in the labeling of even well-established drug products, on the basis of ongoing studies of their safety and efficacy. For this reason, no claims are made that statements made here concerning the current status of these drugs will continue to reflect the stated view or that the data presented in tabular form are, or will remain, complete and correct in every detail.

The most important aspect of this problem lies in the area of dosage recommendations. Every effort has been made to check that statements made in the tables are, within the limits of space, precisely correct. However, dosage schedules are frequently ordered changed in accordance with accumulating clinical experiences.

For this reason, we urge that *before administering any drug, you check the manufacturer's latest dosage recommendations* as presented in the package insert which accompanies each unit of every drug product.

Contents

SECTION 1

General

Principles

of

Pharmacology

Instead of plunging immediately into the study of individual drugs, it is desirable first to gain some understanding of the general principles of pharmacology. Once the student has acquired some insight into the fundamentals of this subject, she can more readily put the many details of drug therapy into their proper perspective. Thus, in this introductory section, we shall introduce certain basic terms and concepts that will make it easier for the student to understand the more detailed material to follow. We shall also make some suggestions about how to study the subject of drugs and their use in patients. We will set the scene with a general orientation to drugs; then, in other chapters of this section, we can take up the principles that apply to various broad subareas such as drug metabolism, drug toxicity, drug dependence, and the administration of drugs.

1.

An Orientation to Drugs

Definition of Terms

The nurse needs to know about drugs mainly because medication plays such an important part in patient care. As a citizen, she should also be concerned with understanding the problem of drug abuse in our society and the effects of potentially toxic chemicals and pollutants on our environment. *Pharmacology,* which in its broadest sense is *the branch of knowledge that deals with every aspect of chemicals that have effects on biological functions,* is therefore a subject of much importance to nurses.

Actually, of course, nurses are not concerned equally with all aspects of pharmacology.* Their chief area of interest is in how drugs are used in the *treatment, prevention, and diagnosis of disease*—the subdivision of pharmacology called *pharmacotherapeutics.* They are often also interested in another aspect of ap-

---

* Included within the scope of pharmacology—in addition to pharmacotherapeutics and toxicology—are such major subdivisions as *pharmacognosy, pharmacy,* and *pharmacodynamics.* Although this book will have relatively little to say about these subjects, we should briefly explain here what aspects of drugs these subareas of pharmacology cover:

Pharmacognosy deals with the study of drugs that come from natural sources—that is, primarily from plants, but also from animal tissues.

Pharmacy has to do with how medicines are prepared, put together, or compounded, and given out or dispensed.

Pharmacodynamics is an experimental science in which the interactions between foreign chemicals and those of living tissues are studied by pharmacologists—scientists who use the techniques of physiology and biochemistry to measure what drugs do and to study the intimate mechanisms by which their effects are brought about.

plied pharmacology—*toxicology*, the study of the *poisonous effects* of chemicals, including drugs.

This book deals mainly with those actions of drugs which are useful in treating patients and with those signs and symptoms of the adverse effects of drugs which the observant nurse should be able to recognize. Before taking up the various classes of medications from this point of view, we shall first present some background material about the nature of drugs and drug therapy.

Ancient and Modern Pharmacology

Pharmacology is one of the most ancient branches of knowledge. Primitive men looking for food soon learned that eating parts of some plants caused diarrhea or other discomforting effects. They then probably used some of these pharmacologically active substances in their religious rites. A cathartic could, for example, have been used to drive a disease-causing evil spirit from a sick person's body, or a psychotropic (mind-affecting) substance might have been taken in order to reach a state of religious ecstasy.

Knowledge about drugs gained by this kind of practical experience through trial and error was handed down from generation to generation. In time, much of this information about medicines was written down in the form of *pharmacopoeias*, books containing recipes for preparations to be used in treating a specific disease. The Ebers papyrus, for instance, is an Egyptian compilation of drug lore dating from about 1500 B.C.

Some of the substances mentioned in that compendium, in the ancient books of the Greeks and Hebrews, and in medieval Arabian and monastic writings are still in use today. Opium, cannabis, colchicum, and belladonna, for example, are drugs of ancient origin that are discussed later in this textbook. The discovery of America added drugs of Indian origin —*Cinchona*, the source of the antimalarial drug quinine, for example, and crude extracts of curare, an arrow poison that is used today in preparing some patients for surgery.

Pharmacology did not, however, become a science until the last century. Advances in pharmaceutical chemistry early in the 19th century made available the *pure active principles* (constituents) of the crude plant and animal drugs. Morphine, the chief constituent of opium, was the first substance extracted in

pure form. The isolation of other potent plant principles—quinine, strychnine, atropine, and others—quickly followed. In this century, *hormones* from animal glands and *vitamins* from foods have also been extracted and purified for use in medical treatment.

The availability of pure, crystalline chemicals brought about two main types of advances in drug therapy. For one, drugs could be standardized so that a given dose of pure drug would produce a relatively predictable effect as compared to what happened when crude plant and animal drugs of variable potency were administered. In addition, organic chemists could synthesize drugs similar in chemical structure to those occurring naturally. Most of today's drugs are synthetic chemicals that found a place in modern treatment only after undergoing extensive trials in several species of animals and in human volunteers and patients.

Pharmacological Evaluation of Drugs

ANIMAL TESTING

New chemicals are tested first in animals to see whether they possess biological activity that may make them useful as medications. *Screening tests* are simple, cheap procedures for detecting the presence of pharmacological actions that might have pharmacotherapeutic applications. Chemicals are constantly being screened, for example, to determine whether they are worth trying in the treatment of cancer, bacterial infections, or other diseases.

Once biological screening has suggested that a new chemical might make a useful drug, it is subjected to more extensive animal testing to determine its safety. In such toxicity testing the drug is administered at several dose levels to groups of two or more animal species to learn how much of the drug is needed to produce its desirable or its toxic effects. The *margin of safety* must be known before any drug is ever administered to humans.

In addition to establishing a drug's varied actions and the doses needed to produce each of its effects, scientists also study how the drug is handled by the body. Such *studies of a drug's metabolism* in animals help to determine the form in which the drug may best be administered to reach effective concentrations in body tissues and how often it has to be given to maintain the desired effects. After such *preclinical studies* in several species of animals have indicated that the trial drug seems safe enough to try in humans for treating disease, it may be cleared for clinical trial.

CLINICAL PHARMACOLOGY STUDIES

Drugs are evaluated in humans in three stages that all have the same purpose—to prove that the drug is reasonably safe and that it is effective for treating a particular clinical condition. The *three phases* of clinical testing differ mainly in the number of patients and doctors involved and in the kind and amount of information that is obtained.

In *phase I*, a single well-qualified clinical investigator may work with just one volunteer at first and then extend the trial to include several other people. If the results of these early trials indicate that the drug can be given to people in doses that are active yet safe, *phase II* studies are started. In this phase, doctors who are recognized as specialists in the management of the particular illness that the drug is designed to treat carry on an expanded study comparing the drug's safety and efficacy with that of standard drugs. Finally, *phase III*, or full scale clinical evaluations, are carried out by many practicing physicians on very large numbers of patients to determine whether the frequency of side effects is low enough to be acceptable.

THE NURSE'S ROLE IN DRUG EVALUATIONS

The nurse who works with doctors in clinical studies can contribute both to the success of the investigation and to the safety of the patient. To do so, she should inform herself fully concerning such facts about the investigational drug as: (1) its usual dosage range; (2) the therapeutically desirable signs of drug-induced improvement that she is to look for; and (3) the signs of side effects and possible toxicity for which she should be particularly observant.

Such information about investigational drugs is often not readily available in the hospital unit. Thus, the nurse should get these facts from the patient's physician and the pharmacist, who have the information in the form of a *clinical investigator's brochure* or *drug package inserts*. In an ideal working relationship, such consultations take place regularly, and the nurse does not have to make hurried queries at the time when she first has to administer the drug. Sometimes, however, the nurse has to insist *firmly* that doctor and pharmacist share all available information about the drug with her, as it is her *legal responsibility* to have these pertinent unpublished data before administering any investigational drug.

The nurse watches the patient for signs of responses to the pharmacological actions of the investigational drug. She records her observations on the patient's chart and tells his doctor about the drug's most important effects on the patient. In doing so, she is not only safeguarding the welfare of the patient himself but also contributing to the safety of all patients who are to receive the drug in future studies.

The nurse should be alert to her patient's attitude toward taking a drug that is being administered during a clinical research study. The doctor, in obtaining the patient's consent, presumably explained the benefits that he hoped to gain. However, it is the nurse who first hears the patient's complaints. She may then advise the patient that he should feel free to express his concerns to the doctor, but she should at the same time encourage the patient to bear the trial drug's discomforts long enough for him to gain its possible benefits.

The nurse should be aware of her own attitude toward the study in order to deal with it in ways that will not effect the patient unfavorably or make the evaluation of the drug's efficacy more difficult. If, for example, the nurse begins to believe that the drug trial is not in the patient's best interests, she should voice her misgivings to the doctor. However, at the same time, she should take care not to communicate her feelings to the patient, even by unconscious, nonverbal means. If the patient or his family ask specific questions about the drug and the testing procedure, she should tell them that she will refer their questions to the physician—and then, of course, do so.

To keep nurses and doctors from unconsciously communicating their attitudes toward the test drug to the patient, techniques have been devised for minimizing bias. In *double-blind studies* neither the patient nor the doctor and nurse who check his responses to medication know whether the patient is receiving the active test drug or a *placebo*, a "blank," or "dummy," medication. This helps to keep medical personnel from giving unintentional suggestions about the drug, to which the patient may respond psychologically rather than to the drug's actual action.

Legal Regulations and Drug Standards

As a result of increasing public awareness of the dangers of uncontrolled traffic in drugs in our society, a large body of federal and state drug laws have been built up during this century. Let us look briefly at the historical background of present-day legislation concerning the development and testing of new drugs for use in medicine, and at the history of laws designed to prevent drug abuse and addiction.

The earliest federal legislation regulating the quality of medicines was the *Pure Food and Drug Act of 1906*, a law intended to stop the marketing of adulterated drugs and to eliminate labeling that made false and misleading claims. Although this pioneer legislation gave the government some control over the marketing of worthless drugs, it really did little to assure the safety of drug products. Passage of such a law did not occur until the next generation, after an untested elixir of sulfanilamide took the lives of a hundred people in 1937.

DRUG TESTING

The Federal Food, Drug and Cosmetic Act of 1938, which was passed as the result of public pressure upon Congress, made it mandatory to test drugs in animals for possible toxicity before marketing them for human use. Although provisions of this law helped to detect grossly dangerous drugs, it did not provide for proper clinical trials in humans. Regulation of drug testing in humans came only after another wave of public alarm and revulsion. This was the result of the notorious thalidomide incident in which a supposedly safe sleep-inducing drug marketed in Europe caused deformities in newborn babies whose mothers had taken the hypnotic during early pregnancy.

Although this tragedy occurred outside the United States, it spurred passage of the *Drug Amendments of 1962* (the *Kefauver-Harris Act*) which empowered the Food and Drug Administration (FDA), an agency of the Department of Health, Education, and Welfare, to regulate procedures for testing drugs in human patients. Today, before any new drug can be tested clinically, the pharmaceutical company must submit all available information about it, including the results of toxicity tests in animals, to the FDA. Only after the filing of such a so-called Investigational New Drug

Exemption, or *IND*, can a company proceed with clinical trials.

The three phases of clinical pharmacology (see p. 5) are carried out under detailed rules intended to protect volunteer subjects and patients. The data obtained in these clinical trials must finally be submitted to the FDA in the form of a New Drug Application, or *NDA*. If the evidence of the drug's safety and effectiveness is considered complete enough, the drug may be approved for marketing; if not, the application is considered incomplete and is returned to the manufacturer who must then provide further evidence that the drug actually does what is claimed for it when administered in safe doses.

Proof of effectiveness is also required for drugs marketed *before* passage of the Drug Amendments of 1962. A *Drug Efficacy Study Implementation* (DESI) carried out for the FDA by panels of scientists appointed by the National Academy of Science–National Research Council (NAS–NRC) resulted in the reevaluation of thousands of older drugs. Products rated as "less than effective" in studies completed by 1968 are in the process of being removed from the market if further evidence proving their effectiveness fails to be found.

The labeling of every remaining product judged only "probably" or "possibly" effective must reveal those ratings of its efficacy in a prominently displayed "box." Such a status will be temporary until additional evidence leads to the drug's being ruled effective or to its being removed from the market. Thus, in time, physicians will finally be assured that every drug they order is one that has been judged effective for the purpose for which it is being prescribed.

DRUG ABUSE PREVENTION LAWS

The first federal act designed to prevent drug addiction was the *Harrison Narcotic Act of 1914*. Later regulations were formulated to control traffic in marihuana and to make certain drugs, including barbiturates and other habit-forming hypnotics, available only on prescription (the *Durham-Humphrey Amendment of 1951*). Continuing abuse of other dangerous drugs, including stimulants, led to the passage of the *Drug Abuse Amendments of 1965*.

Finally, the spread of drug abuse to the point of almost epidemic proportions during the decade of the 1960s caused Congress to enact the *Comprehensive Drug Abuse Prevention and Control Act of 1970*. One section, the *Controlled Substances Act*, replaces all former Federal laws regulating narcotics and dangerous drugs, including the Harrison Act and the 1965 Drug Abuse Amendments. The Federal Bureau of Narcotics and Dangerous Drugs (*BNDD*) of the Department of Justice enforces these regulatory and control measures.

In accordance with regulations issued in 1971, five schedules, or lists, of controlled substances are set up. Drugs are categorized mainly in accordance with their potential for being abused and their status in terms of medical usefulness. Thus, heroin, marihuana, and LSD are included in Schedule I. Schedule II lists methadone, cocaine, and, most recently, the amphetamines, which had at first been included with barbiturates and codeine in Schedule III. Schedules IV and V contain certain tranquilizers and mixtures of narcotics combined in limited quantities with other nonnarcotic drugs. Although the nurse need not know the details of this new law, she should, of course, familiarize herself with those provisions of federal, state, and municipal laws that apply to her professional practice.

OTHER REGULATIONS AND AGENCIES

The *Division of Biological Standards* of the National Institutes of Health regulates the requirements for biological products such as vaccines, antitoxins, and other immunological agents. The advertising of nonprescription drugs is under the jurisdiction of the *Federal Trade Commission (FTC)*. This agency has not had a great deal of influence in protecting the public from being subjected to barrages of drug product advertisements that tend to mislead people as to the true value of many over-the-counter products.

The nurse can try to counteract the effects of such advertising by taking every opportunity to offer people factual information about drug products. She should encourage people to seek diagnosis and treatment by a doctor instead of trying to medicate themselves with remedies that may be misleadingly advertised. Advertisements for arthritis remedies, for example, often suggest that a more expensive product is superior to aspirin, when that substance is actually the most effective drug for most people with arthritic pains.

DRUG STANDARDS

Doctors, pharmacists, and others who prescribe and prepare drug products long ago recognized the importance of setting up standards of quality and purity for drugs. The Pure Food and Drug Act of 1906 (see p. 6) recognized two compendia as official standards. These books, the *United States Pharmacopoeia (U.S.P.)* and the *National Formulary (N.F.)*, still set forth tests for determining the identity and purity of the most important therapeutic agents now in use in the United States.

The *U.S.P.* was first published in 1820, and it has been revised many times since then to reflect scientific advances in the development of chemical methods of drug analysis and in biological assay of the purity of natural products. It is now revised every five years; the current revision, *U.S.P. XVIII*, was issued in 1970. The current *N.F.*, the 13th edition, also became official in that year. The nurse does not ordinarily consult these compendia for drug information as they are intended primarily for use by pharmaceutical scientists and pharmacists. However, she should know that the *U.S.P.* and *N.F.* provide the *official names* of drugs and offer an authoritative guide to information about the *average dosage* and *methods of administration* of drugs.

DRUG NAMES

The fact that a drug usually has a variety of names is often a cause of confusion, not only to nurses trying to learn about drugs, but also to physicians, pharmacists, and the general public. The same drug may be referred to by its chemical name, by the code name given it during its laboratory and clinical evaluation phases, and by the trademark or proprietary name given it by the manufacturer when it is finally marketed. Often, a drug is marketed by several companies, and each advertises it under a different trade name. When the drug is offered in combination with other agents, the mixture has still another trade name.

To avoid confusion, drugs are best referred to by their *nonproprietary names*. These names are now first formulated by a special committee on drug naming, the USAN Council (USAN stands for United States Adopted Name). Later, if a drug becomes recognized by the *U.S.P.* or *N.F.*, the USAN name also becomes the official name. In this book, we shall use *both* the nonproprietary and proprietary names—at least, the first time the drug is mentioned, and in the dosage tables and Drug Digests. This is because doctors often wish to order the drug in the form prepared by a particular company, and when they do, they use the trade name, with or without the nonproprietary name. (The manufacturer's name is capitalized, while the nonproprietary name begins with a lower case letter.)

OTHER REFERENCE SOURCES

Information about drug products is available from several sources. The *Physicians' Desk Reference (P.D.R.)* is an annual publication that offers specific information about many proprietary products. Its monographs are revised during the year of issue in some cases to comply with changes in the drug's labeling required by the FDA. *The American Hospital Formulary Service*, published by the American Society of Hospital Pharmacists, supplies full information about many drugs and their various dosage forms.

Drug Evaluations, the latest in a series of publications by which the Council of Drugs of the American Medical Association has tried to give doctors unbiased information about the drugs they use, is the most complete book of its kind ever published by the A.M.A. In addition to discussing the clinical indications and adverse effects of drugs, it sometimes makes judgments of their effectiveness. *The United States Dispensatory* contains articles dealing both with individual drugs and various pharmacologic classes of drugs. These present detailed information about the actions, indications, dosage and administration, and adverse effects of drugs in a form that is useful for those who order, dispense, and administer these medications.

Studying Pharmacology

You are about to embark on the study of pharmacology, a subject that students often find interesting but also frustrating. Drugs are of great current interest because of the important part they play in present-day society, as well as the sometimes dramatic nature of the benefits they may bring about or the harm they may cause. However, learning about drugs can be difficult because the student may be overwhelmed by the seemingly endless amount of detailed information that is presented.

It would not be correct to suggest that the task of learning the details of drug action is ever an easy one. Memorizing factual data is often tedious and requires concentration and perseverance. However, the nurse is lucky in one important way: she can quickly translate theory into practice, because she functions in a clinical setting. When she sees a patient respond to the effects of a potent drug such as digitalis or morphine, for example, the student is motivated to learn and retain what she then realizes she needs to know in order to use these medications correctly.

PROTOTYPES

To learn what she must know to carry out her professional responsibility relative to drug therapy, the nurse should develop an orderly and systematic approach to the study of pharmacology. One way of systematizing your study is to concentrate first on the best-established and most important drugs of each therapeutic class. Once the prototype compound of each class is thoroughly understood, the many new drugs of the same kind that later appear on the market can be studied more readily in the context of the knowledge acquired earlier about the representative drug.

Thus, it is useful to approach each new drug that is to be administered in terms of finding out how it is similar to and different from the leading drug of the same class. Often, the new drug differs only in a few ways that are of any practical significance. Its advantages, if any, over the other drugs can be quickly learned, as can any points about its dosage and administration that differ from the norm. This way of thinking about drugs can keep the nurse from being swamped in a mass of nonessential detail that keeps her in a constant state of turmoil and breeds distaste for the subject of pharmacology.

TYPES OF DATA

What types of material should the nurse try to retain when studying prototype agents of each major drug class? It is desirable first to learn each drug's *primary* and *secondary* pharmacological effects. When one knows what a drug does to affect normal physiological function, it becomes easier to remember the drug's *clinical indications, side effects*, and *potential toxicity* and to become aware of which patients would be most likely to react adversely to the drug and in whom the drug would be *con-traindicated* or require *special precautions.*

This does not mean that the nurse should ever rely solely on either her reasoning or her memory when she is actually administering drugs to patients. No one has enough knowledge of the vast number and variety of available medications to be sure of all the details of a drug's dosage and actions in any particular case. Thus, an essential rule for even the most experienced nurse should be: *When in doubt, look it up.*

SOURCES OF INFORMATION

To "look it up," the nurse should demand that nursing stations and medicine preparation rooms have available one or more of the sources mentioned above, and that she be given access to similar compendia kept in the hospital's pharmacy. The nurse should also ask to see the insert packaged with each unit of medication, as such package brochures contain detailed information on all important aspects of the drug's dosage, administration, actions, and adverse effects.

The drug data presented in such brochures and in the monographs of various compendia are readily understandable when the nursing student has applied herself to the task of acquiring the fundamental principles of drug action during her student days. Certainly, she should be confident about her ability to administer medications safely on the basis of what she has learned about drugs from lectures, her study of the literature, and her experience in caring for patients. In addition, this background enables her to add to her store of information by talking knowledgeably to the pharmacist and physician in the varied situations involving drugs that arise daily in professional practice.

JOURNALS

To stay abreast of the latest developments in drug therapy all through her professional career the nurse should read various professional journals regularly. The *American Journal of Nursing* and the monthly magazine *RN,* among others, often contain feature articles and data on new drugs and on the changing status of older medical treatments. The biweekly *Medical Letter* is another excellent source of information on the current status of new drugs.

Reading these and certain weekly medical journals such as the *Journal of the American Medical Association* (JAMA) and the *New England Journal of Medicine* helps the nurse to put the advertising claims for various heavily promoted prescription products into better perspective. Nurses who have a need for more detailed knowledge of drugs in carrying out their professional functions—including teaching, for example—may wish to read certain more specialized periodicals such as *Clinical Pharmacology and Therapeutics, Modern Treatment,* and *Medical Clinics of North America.*

CONCLUSION

Before beginning the study of the various classes of drugs, it is best that we first understand some of the general principles that apply to the actions and clinical uses of all drugs. Thus, in the following chapters of this first section, we shall discuss: (1) the factors that influence the actions of all drugs in the body; (2) the prevention and treatment of drug overdosage and other types of toxicity; (3) the factors underlying drug abuse, dependence, and addiction; and (4) the principles involved in the administration of all drugs.

S U M M A R Y of Points for the Nurse to Remember Concerning the Use of Investigational Drugs

1. The nurse is legally responsible for being fully informed about any investigational drug that she is administering to a patient. She should consult with the patient's physician and the pharmacist to obtain all pertinent information that has been made available to them in the form of brochures, package inserts, and so forth.

2. The nurse should watch for signs of the drug's physiological effects upon the patient and record her observations on the patient's chart as well as communicate them orally to his physician. This not only safeguards the patient but also contributes to the safe use of the drug in future clinical investigations.

3. The nurse should listen for complaints that indicate how the patient feels about being part

of an investigational study of a drug. Observing the patient's attitude is an important part of the nurse's responsibility. She should suggest that the patient express his concerns to his physician, but she should also encourage him to take a positive attitude toward taking the investigational drug.

4. The nurse should be aware of her own attitudes toward the study. She should try to remain objective in order to make proper observations and evaluate them with judgment unclouded by personal prejudice. If she develops a negative attitude toward use of an investigational drug, she should take care not to communicate her misgivings to the patient, but instead talk to the doctor about them.

5. It is important for all discussion concerning the drug's purpose and its potentially desirable and adverse effects to be carried out within the framework established by the physician. Thus, after the physician has discussed these matters with the patient and his family, he and the nurse should discuss how information concerning the investigational drug is to be handled. The nurse can then help by reviewing with the patient such matters as the purpose of his treatment, what to expect from it, and how he himself can help to achieve the best possible results.

Discussion Topics: Dealing with Investigational New Drugs

The Situation: Mrs. Brown is a nurse who is caring for Mr. Roberts, a patient with metastatic carcinoma of the prostate. His condition is no longer controlled by administration of female hormones (which caused breast growth), and despite castration, he is still in considerable pain from extensive spread of the cancer to the bones.

Mr. Roberts is about to start treatment with a new drug called Degranol that had received favorable reports in the foreign literature. He is to receive daily parenteral doses of a sample of this new chemotherapeutic agent that his doctor obtained through the National Institutes of Health Cancer Chemotherapy Program.

Mrs. Brown has been unable to find any information about the drug in the reference sources available to her, and the pharmacy has not yet dispensed the drug to the hospital unit, so she hasn't even seen a package insert.

1. Discuss how you might proceed to obtain information about the drug's dosage, method of administration, and potential toxicity, if you were Mrs. Brown.

Mrs. Brown stops in to see and talk with Mr. Roberts while she is making her rounds.

Mrs. Roberts, who is visiting her husband, appears agitated. She asks the nurse to step out into the corridor where she can talk to her without Mr. Roberts overhearing.

Mrs. Roberts is bristling with anger. She says, "My husband tells me that they're going to use him as a guinea pig! Hasn't he suffered enough already? What do they want from him? How much can the man take?" Then she starts to cry.

2. Discuss how you would respond to Mrs. Roberts if you were Mrs. Brown and found yourself in this situation.

During the drug's trial, Mr. Roberts develops purple bruise-like discolorations of the skin all over his body and a severe sore throat and high fever. The drug is discontinued for a while, but the doctor wants to start it again when the patient gets stronger.

3. Discuss what you would do if you were Mrs. Brown and, like her, began to feel misgivings about whether Mr. Roberts's best interests were being served and you wondered whether his doctor might not be inordinately concerned with clinical research.

References

Beckman, H. In defense of tinkers. *New Eng. J. Med.,* 268:72, 1962.

Brown, G.W. Ground rules for physicians who evaluate drugs. *JAMA,* 203:857, 1968.

Burger, A. Approaches to drug discovery. *New Eng. J. Med.,* 270:1098, 1964.

Dowling, H.F. What's in a name? *JAMA,* 173:1580, 1960.

Friend, D.G. One drug-one name. *Clin. Pharmacol. Ther.*, 6:689, 1965.

Gilgore, S.G. Clinical pharmacology. Researching a new drug in man. *Drug and Cosmetic Industry*, May, 1969.

Greiner, T. Subjective bias of the clinical pharmacologist. *JAMA*, 181:92, 1962.

Irwin, S. Drug screening and evaluative procedures. *Science*, 136:123, 1962.

Jerome, J.B. Current status of nonproprietary nomenclature for drugs. *JAMA*, 185:256, 1963.

Modell, W. Safety in new drugs. *JAMA*, 190:141, 1964.

Rodman, M.J. What's behind the new drug drought? *R.N.*, 28:78, 1965 (March).

2.

The Interaction of Drugs and Body Tissues

Drugs and Living Systems

The living body and each of its cells are the site of countless chemical reactions that go on continuously and endlessly. When a drug enters a living system, its millions and millions of molecules immediately begin to react with those of the body's cells. Some of the drug molecules react with those of the living tissues in ways that change the functioning of the cells —that is, they produce pharmacological effects. However, most of the foreign molecules are inactivated by the body's biochemical reactions and are eliminated from the system—the drug is metabolized and excreted.

In this chapter, we shall discuss what happens to drugs after they are administered to patients. In very broad and general terms, we will indicate: (1) how body cells respond to the presence of drugs that are capable of altering their functioning; and (2) how the body handles drugs in order to detoxify and remove them. The nurse who has some understanding of these complex processes is often able to give her patient better care by making more meaningful observations of the patient's responses to drug therapy.

Knowledge of what happens to drugs during their stay in the body helps, for example, to account for the fact that different patients often react very differently to the same dose of a drug. In fact, the same patient may react in quite different ways when he receives the identical dose of a drug at different times. *Individual variation* in the way patients respond to drugs depends upon: (1) differences in the responsiveness of the patient's cells to the drug molecules that reach them; and (2) differences in the ability of the patient's body to metabolize and eliminate the drug.

The Responses of Reactive Cells to Drugs

In order for a drug to produce its pharmacological effects it must reach a certain *critical concentration* in the fluids around the cells that are capable of responding to the drug. When the drug reaches this level in the reactive tissues, it brings about changes in cellular function. The rate of biochemical and physiological activity is altered by the presence of the drug.

Stimulation refers to a drug-induced increase in the activity of the reactive cells. A drug such as digitalis, for example, is a heart stimulant in the sense that its action on cardiac muscle fibers increases the strength of their contractions. Epinephrine increases the rate at which the heart beats as well as the strength of each contraction.

Depression refers to the reduction in cellular activity brought about by drug actions. Barbiturates, for example, reduce the functional activity of groups of cells within the central nervous system. As a result, the wakeful patient becomes drowsy, or—with larger doses—loses consciousness. Toxic doses can depress the activity of brain stem cells that control respiration. As a result, the poisoned person's breathing becomes very slow and shallow.

SITES AND MECHANISMS OF DRUG ACTION

It is often useful to know where and how drugs act to produce the pharmacological effects that account for their therapeutically useful or toxic effects. Some drugs act locally when applied to the patient's skin or mucous membranes. Most drugs must first be absorbed into the systemic circulation and carried to the tissues, which respond by becoming stimulated or depressed.

Systemically acting drugs often bring about changes in a particular physiological state by acting at any of several different sites. For example, one drug may reduce a patient's high blood pressure by depressing the rate of transmission of sympathetic nerve impulses to his blood vessels. Another antihypertensive agent may act directly upon the smooth muscles of the arterioles to reduce their tone, and a third type of drug may reduce the amount of blood that the heart pumps into the circulatory tree. Similarly, drugs can relieve pain by acting at different sites within the central nervous system or peripherally.

The exact mechanisms by which drugs produce their pharmacological effects are not known in most cases. However, as scientists learn more about molecular biology, they become better able to explain just how drug molecules interact with the macromolecules within cells to affect cellular metabolism and function. In this text, we shall discuss the manner of action of various potent drugs, particularly those that affect the functioning of organs which receive impulses from the autonomic nervous system.

The Handling of Drugs by the Body (Drug Metabolism)

In order for a drug to reach the tissues with which it reacts to produce pharmacological effects, its molecules must be able to move from the point at which they enter the body to the site of their action. Similarly, drugs reach the organs responsible for their breakdown and elimination by being able to pass through biological membranes. Since such membranes contain lipids, or fatty substances, most drugs are lipid-soluble substances.

The concentration that the drug reaches in the reactive tissues at any time after it is administered varies from moment to moment. This constantly shifting level depends upon the balance between four processes to which the drug is being subjected during its stay in the body. The ways in which the body handles foreign molecules are: (1) absorption, (2) distribution, (3) biotransformation, and (4) excretion. We shall discuss briefly some practical aspects of each of these processes.

ABSORPTION

The term *absorption* refers to what happens to a drug from the time it enters the body until it enters the circulating fluids. Thus, a drug that is taken by mouth is absorbed into the venous and lymphatic circulation by making its way through the mucous membranes lining the upper part of the gastrointestinal tract. A drug that is injected into a muscle mass or into the layer of fat and connective tissue just beneath the skin must be able to move from these local sites into the bloodstream.

ORAL ABSORPTION. Some orally administered substances such as alcohol and aspirin begin to be absorbed while they are still in the stomach. However, most drugs—including most of any dose of aspirin—are most rapidly absorbed from the upper part of the small intestine. This is because the inner lining of the duodenum contains millions of villi, tiny capillary-filled projections that offer a vast surface area through which the drug molecules can pass into the systemic circulations.

DRUGS AND FOOD. Orally administered drugs are most rapidly and completely absorbed when taken between meals. There are several reasons for this. For one thing, the stomach empties its contents into the duodenum more slowly when filled with food. In addition to delaying the passage of the drug into the intestine, food often binds the drug molecules into complexes that cannot pass through the mucosal lining of the G.I. tract. Also, some drugs may be destroyed by the increased acidity and peptic activity of the gastric contents during digestion of a meal.

The hormones insulin and corticotropin, for example, are protein molecules that are digested when taken orally. Thus, these drugs cannot be absorbed when taken by mouth and must be administered by injection. Oral penicillin products are best given between meals to prevent their destruction in the G.I. tract and to increase the amount that will be absorbed into the systemic circulation and carried to the infected tissues. Other drugs are covered with special enteric coatings to prevent their digestion in the upper G.I. tract or to keep them from causing irritation and possible nausea and vomiting. Often the nurse also gives irritating drugs with a snack to lessen direct contact with the mucosa. Even though this tends to delay the drug's absorption, this is preferable to losing the entire dose through vomiting.

INJECTED DRUGS. Absorption of injected drugs depends mainly upon the blood supply of the tissues into which the drug is deposited. Thus, when a watery solution of a drug is injected into a muscle it is more rapidly absorbed than from the subcutaneous tissues, which do not have as rich a blood supply. On the other hand, subcutaneous injection of drug suspensions results in delayed absorption that may be desired in order to produce a long-lasting effect. (See Chapter 5 for a further discussion of factors involved in the absorption of parenteral dosage forms.)

Intravenous administration provides the most rapid and certain drug action, since the drug enters the bloodstream directly without having to pass any biological membrane barriers. This has both advantages and possible dangers. Administering morphine by vein is preferable to subcutaneous injection when a patient is in shock, as absorption of the drug from under the skin may be very undependable when the patient's peripheral circulation is poor. On the other hand, the instantaneous absorption of a too rapidly administered I.V. dose of morphine may result in deeper depression of the patient's circulation and respiration.

DISTRIBUTION

This term refers to the ways in which drugs are transported by body fluids to their sites of action, metabolism, and excretion. The presence of a drug in the bloodstream does not necessarily mean that it produces immediate effects. Once the drug has been absorbed into the circulation, it must still make its way from the blood into the fluids that bathe the reactive tissues. Many complex physiochemical factors determine whether a particular drug can reach an effective concentration in the tissues and exert its effects on the cells.

Drugs that are absorbed into the bloodstream become attached to the plasma proteins in varying degrees. This drug-protein complex cannot diffuse through the capillary membranes and into the tissues. However, some drug molecules are constantly being freed from their protein binding sites. The free drug then passes from the blood to its sites of action, metabolic breakdown, and excretion.

Once it has reached an effective concentration in the reactive tissues, a drug that is transported with most of its molecules tied tightly to plasma proteins often has a long duration of action. This is because the drug molecules diffuse to the organs of detoxification and excretion (see below) only very slowly. Sometimes, two drugs may compete for the same *plasma binding sites*. If one drug displaces the other, the freed molecules then diffuse into the tissues at an abnormally rapid rate and may thus tend to reach toxic concentrations. (See the section on drug interactions, p. 20.)

The *blood-brain barrier* is made up of biological membranes that bar the entrance of drugs which are poorly soluble in lipids. Such drugs have little or no effect on the functioning of the central nervous system, even when they are present in the blood in large amounts. On the other hand, certain barbiturates, such as secobarbital and thiopental, pass the blood-brain barrier so readily that they enter the brain almost as soon as they get into the blood going to that organ. Thus, I.V. thiopental is employed to produce sleep within seconds.

Drugs do not ordinarily remain in the tissues to which they are first transported. Thus, thiopental, after first piling up in the brain because of that organ's rich blood supply, soon drains out of the brain and is redistributed to other tissues. As the concentration of this anesthetic falls below the level required to keep the patient asleep, he quickly recovers consciousness. This happens even though the barbiturate is still stored in the body in such sites as fat depots, skeletal muscles, connective tissue, skin, and bones. After a while, of course, the drug is transported to the liver and kidneys where it undergoes breakdown and actual elimination from the body.

BIOTRANSFORMATION

Most foreign molecules that enter the body are converted to harmless substances that can be readily excreted. Such detoxifying transformations are brought about by enzyme-catalyzed chemical reactions. Enzyme systems capable of bringing about the breakdown of drugs are present in all body tissues, including the blood.

The liver is the single most important site of drug-detoxifying reactions. Hepatic cells are packed with enzymes capable of catalyzing the oxidation of active drugs to inactive metabolites. People who are born with, or acquire, a high drug-metabolizing capacity are relatively resistant to drugs, while those who lack drug-metabolizing enzymes for any reason may be highly susceptible to the actions of various drugs. (See the discussions of tolerance, pp. 18–19, and of drug interactions, p. 20.)

EXCRETION

Drugs, or their less active or inactive metabolites, are eliminated from the body by many routes, including the kidneys, the lungs, and the sweat, salivary, and mammary glands. Volatile general anesthetics such as ether and nitrous oxide are, for example, excreted largely by the lungs in unchanged form. Alcohol is mainly broken down to small metabolic fragments by reactions that take place in all body cells. However, enough alcohol is excreted intact by the lungs to be measured by chemical methods. This is the basis for so-called breathometer or drunkometer tests designed to determine whether a person is intoxicated.

The *kidneys* play the most important part in eliminating drugs and their metabolites. The molecules of most drugs are filtered through the glomeruli. Some of these filtered molecules may be returned to the bloodstream by tubular reabsorption, while the rest leave the body in the urine. In time, however, after the drug has been passed through the kidneys enough times, all of it is eliminated.

Some drugs are dealt with by still another renal excretory mechanism—tubular secretion, a process in which substances are transported from the blood directly into the tubular fluid. Penicillin, for example, is a rapidly eliminated drug because it is both filtered by the glomeruli and secreted by the tubules without undergoing tubular reabsorption. The reason that most drug metabolites are more readily excreted than the original drug is that the chemically altered molecules are less readily reabsorbed by the tubules after filtration. Thus, the drug metabolites tend to enter the urine more rapidly.

Factors Influencing the Effects of Drugs

The inexperienced nurse, in administering drugs to patients for the first time and in observing how they react, soon learns that the dose that was given does not always produce the desired effect. In some patients the drug's effects are unexpectedly potent while others show little, if any, response to the same dose. In fact, the same patient may react in quite different ways when he receives the identical dose at different times.

In recent years the real reasons for differences in the way patients respond to drugs have begun to be discovered. The nurse should understand some of the underlying factors that account for the variability with which people respond to the so-called usual dose that is listed in such compendia as the U.S.P., N.F., and P.D.R., and in the drug product's labeling and package insert.

The nurse who has some insight into the factors influencing the effects of drugs can make more meaningful observations. Signs that might have seemed unimportant or that might otherwise have escaped her attention entirely are often noted, and take on their true significance when the nurse knows how her patient's own peculiar characteristics can influence his response to the administered drug. This often makes it possible to prevent adverse effects and to bring about therapeutic benefits by adjusting drug dosage more closely to the needs of each individual patient.

Body weight is a well-recognized factor modifying the responses of patients to drugs because there is a definite relationship between the mass of an administered drug and the mass of body tissue in which it is distributed. Generally speaking, the more a person weighs the more diluted the drug becomes in his body and the smaller the amount of the drug that tends to accumulate in the tissues that are the target for its action. The less a person weighs the greater is the amount of drug that concentrates in the reactive tissues and the more powerful is the effect that the drug then produces. The dosage of certain potent drugs is often calculated and administered on the basis of the ratio of milligrams of the drug to pounds or kilograms of the patient's body weight.* Most formulas for adjusting adult dosage of a drug for a child make use of the child's body weight rather than the age of the child. Actually, however, the fraction of the adult dose most suitable for a child is most accurately calculated on the basis of *body surface area* (BSA) and then stated in terms of milligrams or grams per square meter.**

The *age* of a patient will affect his response to drugs. No formula of any kind can be relied upon in calculating dosage for a premature infant or even for a full-term newborn less than a week old. This is because they differ from older infants, children, and adults in their ability to eliminate administered drugs. Because, for example, very young infants lack the liver enzyme system for breaking down the antibiotic chloramphenicol, very small doses of that drug have caused toxicity and death when administered during the first week of life. At

the other extreme of life, the excessive susceptibility of elderly patients to drugs often stems from reduced liver or kidney function. This may cause ordinary doses to reach toxic levels.

Physiological states of a patient's cells and tissues that are related to age, sex, and other factors also often alter the response of patients to drugs. For example, the central nervous system of a child seems sensitive to the stimulating effects of some types of antihistamine agents. Thus, overdoses of these drugs that would cause only drowsiness in adults have caused convulsive seizures when accidentally ingested by young children. Similarly, the cardiovascular system of elderly patients is prone to respond excessively to antihypertensive drugs, presumably because the mechanisms for making reflex adjustments of blood pressure and heart rate are relatively sluggish.

The same patient may respond differently at different times of day because of differences in the level of physiological activity of various body systems. For example, an ordinary bedtime dose of a barbiturate may not be effective for producing sleep during the day, presumably because the patient's nervous system is more resistant to the hypnotic action of depressant drugs in the daytime than at night. Thus, it may be necessary to raise the dose of sedative drugs for patients who must rest and sleep during the day.

The *sex* of a patient sometimes affects the response to a drug. For example, women are said to be more susceptible to the excitatory effects sometimes seen when morphine is administered. Of course, the most important consideration when drugs are ordered for women of child-bearing age is that they may be pregnant and the drug may affect the fetus. The administration of medication to women who may be in the early weeks of pregnancy carries some risk of causing damage to the developing fetus (see *teratogenicity*, p. 28). Also, as pregnancy advances, the uterus becomes increasingly sensitive to drugs that stimulate its muscular contractions. Thus, during the third trimester, care is required to avoid setting off labor prematurely.

Pathological states also often alter the responses of patients to drugs. Damage to the liver and kidneys—the organs most responsible for removing drugs from the body—may cause administered drugs to accumulate to toxic levels. Thus, when a patient's history, or the results of laboratory studies, indicate that these organs lack a normal capacity to handle certain

---

* A kilogram is equal to 2.2 lbs. The drug *dimercaprol*⁺ is administered in a dose ranging from 2.5 to 5.0 mg/kg of body weight. Can you calculate the amount of dimercaprol that would be administered intramuscularly to a child who weighs about 45 lbs?

** Tables called nomograms are now available and simple to use in deriving BSA from the patient's weight and height and for relating surface area to fraction of adult dosage.

drugs, these medications must be administered with extreme caution if at all.

Even small sedative doses of barbiturates, for example, may cause a patient with cirrhosis of the liver to lapse into hepatic coma. Kanamycin and other antibiotics that require renal excretion may cause deafness in patients whose impaired kidneys fail to eliminate them. This happens because, with continued administration of ordinary doses at regular intervals, the drugs accumulate to toxic levels in auditory nerve tissues.

Patients suffering from more than one disorder sometimes prove excessively sensitive to a drug that is administered to treat one of their ailments. A person suffering from hyperthyroidism, for example, is especially sensitive to epinephrine and other adrenergic drugs. Thus, if these drugs are administered for another medical disorder, they may make his heart race excessively. A patient who requires a cholinergic drug to promote postoperative bowel motility may suffer breathing difficulties if he also has a history of bronchial asthma. It is important to be aware of the presence of pathologic processes besides the disease for which the patient is receiving a drug. The patient can then be carefully observed for development of any signs of adverse effects that might make it necessary to discontinue the medication.

Genetic factors sometimes account for differences in the response of patients receiving similar doses of the same drug. People from some families, for example, have a greater ability to break down the antituberculosis drug isoniazid (INH) than do people with a different genetic background. These "rapid inactivators" require higher daily doses of this drug in order to maintain its antiinfective effect. Those who lack the gene for producing the drug-metabolizing enzyme system inactivate isoniazid so slowly that the administration of even ordinary doses at the usual intervals soon causes the drug to accumulate to toxic levels. An inborn lack of various enzymes also accounts for the extreme susceptibility of some people to certain other drugs (see *idiosyncracy*, pp. 26–28, Chapter 3).

Immunologic factors cause some people to react in ways that are totally different from what is known of a drug's pharmacological actions. The presence of drug molecules stimulates the patient's immunity mechanisms to produce protective antibodies. Later, when the person again receives the same drug, an immunity-type reaction occurs that can result in many kinds of changes in physiologic function. The signs and symptoms of illness that result are very varied, ranging from immediate breathing and circulatory difficulties to gradual development of skin, joint, and even blood disorders (see discussion of *drug allergy*, Chapters 3 and 18).

Psychological and emotional factors also play an important part in the way people respond to drugs. We have seen that people often respond even to the administration of a pharmacologically inert material, or *placebo*. A person's response to active drugs is also often influenced by his underlying personality structure and by his hopes, fears, or expectations. This is particularly true of drugs that affect the mood and thought processes, so-called *psychotropic drugs*. Thus, whether a person taking LSD finds the experience pleasurable or panic-provoking (a "bad trip") often depends upon his mental *set*. Patients who are being treated for mental and emotional illnesses should be carefully observed to see how they respond to the tranquilizing and mood-elevating agents with which they are being treated.

Environmental factors also often influence the effects of drugs. For example, the circumstances, or *setting*, in which a person takes a drug is often as important as his mental attitude, or set, in determining his behavioral responses to psychotropic drugs. For instance, a person drinking alcoholic beverages or smoking marihuana may merely get drowsy if he drinks or smokes alone. The same amount of alcohol or "pot" taken when he gets together with a group of friends may make him giddy, gay, and outgoing.

Heat and cold can also affect responses to drugs. For example, it is often desirable to reduce the dose of vasodilator drugs given during hot weather. Patients taking antihypertensive agents may suffer an unexpectedly sharp drop in blood pressure from their usual dose when they take it at the start of a heat wave or following a winter plane trip to a subtropical resort.

Tolerance is another very important factor influencing the effects of drugs. Just as some people have an inherited *hyper*-susceptibility to the actions of certain drugs, others have an inborn resistance, or tolerance, to drugs. Sometimes, such *hypo*susceptibility stems from the ability of reactive cells to function normally even in the presence of relatively high concentrations of the drug. More often, the reason for such *congenital tolerance* is that the person has inherited enzyme systems which function very efficiently in disposing of administered medications; the drug never reaches the blood and tissue levels needed to produce its pharmacological effects or to maintain them.

Tolerance to drugs may also be *acquired*. One reason for resistance developing in this way is that the continued presence of the drug in the body stimulates the synthesis of increased amounts of drug-detoxifying enzymes in the patient's liver. Phenobarbital, for example, induces production of the liver enzymes that catalyze its own destruction. After a while the patient must take higher doses of the barbiturate to become drowsy or calm than he needed when he first began to use the sedative-hypnotic.

Sometimes, however, patients develop tolerance to a drug that does not depend only upon an increased ability to eliminate it. In this type of tolerance, the reactive tissues have somehow learned to adapt to the presence of high concentrations of drugs that had at first been able to affect their functioning when taken in much smaller doses. Heroin addicts who have acquired tolerance of this type can often take many times the amount that would kill a person whose respiratory center cells had not yet had time to develop such resistance.

Patients taking opiate-type analgesics for relief of chronic pain must often keep raising the dose of these drugs to get the desired therapeutic effect. The nurse who is caring for such a patient employs measures that help to delay development of tolerance. The nurse is also aware that alcoholic patients are often resistant to the effects of other depressant drugs, including barbiturates and ether. This is the result of a phenomenon called *cross-tolerance*, in which the patient's body withstands drugs with similar effects.

COMBINED EFFECTS OF DRUGS

The effect that a drug produces when it is given alone is often different from what is seen when it is given together with one or more other drugs. Sometimes the combined effect is greater than when one drug is given alone, but the presence of a second drug can also lessen the effect of the first. The terms used to describe the combined effects of drugs are used in different ways by different writers. In this book the terms are employed in accordance with the following definitions.

Addition or *simple summation* refers to situations in which the combined effect of two drugs is equal to the sum of the effects of each drug administered alone. An example of this is seen in products for pain relief containing aspirin and phenacetin in fractions of the full dose of each that would be needed for producing an analgesic effect. Combining these two drugs in this way does not produce greater pain relief than a full dose of either drug alone.

Synergism refers to situations in which the addition of a second drug tends to increase the intensity or prolong the duration of an effect caused by the first drug. Such *supraadditive* effects are usually brought about in one of two general ways. In one case, two drugs may bring about similar effects by acting at different sites or by different mechanisms. For example, pain may sometimes be more effectively relieved when codeine is combined with aspirin of with a mixture of aspirin and phenacetin because codeine exerts its analgesic action in a different way than the other two pain relievers.

Potentiation is a term sometimes used to describe a second kind of synergism. This is seen when only one of a pair of drugs produces a particular effect, with the presence of the second drug tending to intensify or prolong the effect of the one active agent. This type of drug interaction usually results from the fact that the inactive drug interferes with the way in which an active one is eliminated, or changes some other process by which the body handles the drug. (We shall soon see several examples of such interactions, in which one drug markedly changes the metabolism of another.)

Antagonism is a term employed to describe the combined effect of two drugs that is less than that of either one of them. Examples of how the addition of a second drug decreases or abolishes the effect of the first are seen when antidotes of different kinds are administered to counteract the effects of poisons, or when certain drugs are added to a mixture in order to decrease the side effects of one or more of the other drugs in the combination.

CLINICAL APPLICATIONS

The combined effects of drugs are clinically important in three main ways.

1. Drug products are often offered in the

form of mixtures that are claimed to have various advantages over single drugs in treating some conditions. (Mixtures containing two or more drugs in ratios that are rigidly fixed also have definite disadvantages, however.)

2. As indicated above a drug may be deliberately administered to lessen the toxic effects of a poison or of overdosage with another drug. Some *antidotes* act by combining chemically with the poison to inactivate it; other antidotes act to cancel the effects of an overdose on a particular bodily system. For example, excessive stimulation of the central nervous system by a convulsant poison such as strychnine can be overcome by administering a barbiturate or other central depressant drug as an anticonvulsant.

3. Adverse effects often develop unexpectedly in patients who are taking several drugs at the same time. Sometimes a therapeutically desirable effect of one drug may be reduced or eliminated by the presence of another agent. Recently, as these undesirable reactions have been reported with increasing frequency, doctors, pharmacists, and nurses have been urged to help prevent drug interactions as part of their professional responsibility toward the patient.

Drug Interactions

REASONS FOR DRUG INTERACTIONS

Long lists of potentially dangerous drug interactions are now available in tabular form and in books. The nurse whose patient develops unusual symptoms can use such check lists when she suspects that the unusual reaction stems from an interaction between two or more drugs that the patient may be taking at the same time. It is, however, more helpful to understand the mechanisms by which one drug can alter the effects of another and thus change the effect from what had been expected.

One drug can influence the effects of another by affecting the processes by which the other is absorbed, distributed, biotransformed, or excreted. This happens because it results in a change in the *concentration* of the second drug in the reactive tissue, subsequently leading to pharmacologic effects that may be less intense and long-lasting than expected or markedly more powerful and prolonged than anticipated. Examples of such antagonistic and synergistic actions are listed in Tables 2-1, 2-2, 2-3, and 2-4, and some will be briefly discussed now.

ABSORPTION

Absorption of drugs may be interfered with, not only by food, but also by the presence of certain other drugs. For example, a patient taking antacids for treating peptic ulcer may absorb certain other drugs poorly, including anticoagulant drugs and anti-infective agents that form an unabsorbable complex with the metal ions of the alkalinizers. Tetracycline-type antibiotics should not be administered with antacids or with milk for this reason, as reduced absorption lessens their therapeutic activity against the infectious microorganisms in the tissues.

DISTRIBUTION

Drugs that are transported by the blood with most of their molecules tightly bound to plasma proteins (p. 15) may be made more active by the presence of certain other drugs. For example, the anticoagulant warfarin is carried in the blood with 98 percent of its molecules bound to albumin and only 2 percent free and pharmacologically active. If phenylbutazone is also administered, it can free many more molecules of the anticoagulant from their plasma binding sites. Continued administration of these two drugs in the same doses can lead to unexpected bleeding episodes.

METABOLISM

Biotransformation of drugs by the drug-metabolizing enzymes of the liver (p. 16) can be modified by the presence of other drugs. For example, phenobarbital and other drugs that induce increased synthesis of these enzymes can cause a decrease in the pharmacological response to anticoagulant drugs such as warfarin. This happens because any dose of the anticoagulant is now more rapidly metabolized. Dosage of warfarin must be raised to maintain its desired therapeutic effect. On the other hand, when the barbiturate or other enzyme-inducing drug is discontinued, anticoagulant drug dosage must be reduced. The reason for this is that fewer enzymes will now be available for detoxifying the high dose of anticoagulant, which may then accumulate to toxic levels that cause bleeding.

T A B L E   2 - 1   *Drug Interactions that Result in Altered Absorption from the Gastrointestinal Tract*

Interacting Drugs	Result of Interaction (Synergism or Antagonism)	Effect upon Patient's Treatment
Antacids with anticoagulants such as bishydroxycoumarin and warfarin	Antacids interfere with the absorption of anticoagulants from the G.I. tract, resulting in antagonism of their action	Patient may be made more prone to blood clotting episodes
Antacids with certain anti-infective agents such as sulfonamides, naladixic acid, and nitrofurantoin	Antacids interfere with the absorption of these weakly acid chemotherapeutic agents, resulting in reduction in their systemic activity	Patient's infection may not respond properly to treatment with these antibacterials
Antacids (and milk) with tetracycline-type antibiotics	Calcium, magnesium, and aluminum ions tend to bind tetracycline in poorly absorbable complexes	Patient's infection may fail to respond adequately to antibiotic treatment
Antacids with medications in enteric-coated form (such as the cathartic, bisacodyl)	Alkalinity may cause premature disintegration of the enteric coating while the tablet is still in the stomach	Release of the irritant drug in the stomach may result in nausea and vomiting
Mineral oil with fat-soluble vitamins (A, D, E, K)	Mineral oil may reduce the absorption of fat-soluble vitamins	Patient may be deprived of the desired effects
Mineral oil with fecal softeners such as dioctyl sodium sulfosuccinate, and poloxalkol	Surface active substances may cause systemic absorption of mineral oil through the intestinal mucosa	Mineral oil that is carried to lymph nodes, liver, and spleen may act as a foreign body
Mineral oil and anticoagulants such as bishydroxycoumarin and warfarin	Reduced absorption of vitamin K could potentiate the effect of the anticoagulant, but laxative effect might reduce the amount of anticoagulant that is absorbed and thus lessen the drug's effect	Patient may respond in a variable and unpredictable manner to treatment with anticoagulants
Cholestyramine with vitamins A, D, and K; also anticoagulants, and possibly other weakly acid drugs, including chlorothiazide and phenylbutazone	This anion exchange resin has a strong affinity for acidic substances. Binding of drugs may result in their fecal elimination instead of systemic absorption	Patient may suffer from nutritional deficiencies, or fail to benefit from drug therapy. He should take vitamin supplements and drugs well before the administration of cholestyramine

T A B L E   2 - 2   *Drug Interactions that Are the Result of Changes in a Drug's Distribution or Transport*

Interacting Drugs	Result of Interaction (Synergism or Antagonism)	Effect upon Patient's Treatment
Anticoagulants with certain anti-inflammatory drugs (such as phenylbutazone, oxyphenbutazone, and indomethacin); also with other acidic drugs, including diphenylhydantoin, and clofibrate	Displacement of the anticoagulant from plasma protein binding sites makes more free, active drug available at its site of action in reducing blood clotting components	Patients previously stabilized on individualized dosage of the anticoagulant may suffer a sudden unexpected episode of spontaneous bleeding

TABLE 2-2   *(Continued)*

Interacting Drugs	Result of Interaction (Synergism or Antagonism)	Effect upon Patient's Treatment
Oral hypoglycemic drugs of the sulfonylurea type with such acid drugs as aspirin, sulfonamides, phenylbutazone, and anticoagulants	Displacement of the sulfonylurea-type hypoglycemic drug from bound form makes more of it available at the pancreas for reducing blood sugar	Patient's blood sugar may fall below what was expected. The unexpectedly enhanced hypoglycemic effect may lead to feeling of weakness and fatigue
Methotrexate with acidic drugs such as aspirin, sulfonamides, and possibly sulfonylurea-type hypoglycemic agents, and thiazide-type diuretics	The antineoplastic drug may be displaced from protein binding sites. More of it is then available to poison rapidly proliferating normal cells	Patient may suffer severe toxic effects, including bone marrow depression leading to pancytopenia; also nausea, vomiting, and diarrhea
Trichloroacetic acid, a metabolite of chloral hydrate, with such acid drugs as the oral anticoagulants	Treatment with the sedative drug may increase the concentration of free anticoagulant drug and thus potentiate its effects	Patient's prothrombin time may be lengthened and unexpected bleeding may occur

TABLE 2-3   *Drug Interactions that Are the Result of Changes in Drug Metabolism*

Interacting Drugs	Result of Interaction (Synergism or Antagonism)	Effect upon Patient's Treatment
Anticoagulants such as bishydroxycoumarin with warfarin with various drugs including methylphenidate and phenyramidol	The enzymes responsible for metabolism of the anticoagulants may be inhibited by the presence of the other drugs. This results in an increased anticoagulant action	Patients continuing to take the dose of anticoagulant on which they were stabilized may suffer a severe hemorrhage
Anticoagulants with various drugs including barbiturates glutethimide, meprobamate, and griseofulvin	The presence of other drugs may stimulate production of the enzymes responsible for metabolism of the anticoagulants (that is, enzyme induction). This results in decreased anticoagulant action	Patients get less of the therapeutic effect than desired. However, if they are stabilized on high doses of the anticoagulant, later discontinuance of the other drugs may lead to bleeding
Diphenylhydantoin with various drugs including anticoagulants, para-aminosalicylic acid, isoniazid, phenylbutazone, and disulfiram	The other drugs may interfere with the enzymes responsible for metabolism of diphenylhydantoin. This results in increased toxicity to the nervous system	The patient may suffer toxic effects, including motor incoordination, nystagmus, and lethargy
Oral hypoglycemic drugs of the sulfonylurea type such as tolbutamide and chlorpropamide with certain other drugs such as anticoagulants and phenyramidol	The other drugs may inhibit the enzymes responsible for the metabolism of the oral hypoglycemic drugs. This tends to intensify and prolong their action	The diabetic patient may suffer a severe hypoglycemic reaction, including coma
Mercaptopurine with allopurinol	Allopurinol may inhibit the enzymes responsible for the metabolism of mercaptopurine. This leads to increased toxicity of the anticancer drug	Patients taking mercaptopurine may suffer bone marrow damage, G.I. tract irritation, and other adverse effects, unless its dose is reduced

TABLE 2-4 *Drug Interactions that Result from Interference with Excretion*

Interacting Drugs	Results of Interaction (Synergism or Antagonism)	Effect upon Patient's Treatment
Probenecid with aspirin and other salicylates	Aspirin interferes with the renal tubular secretion of probenecid. This, in turn, interferes with the ability of probenecid to eliminate uric acid and to lower levels of this substance in the plasma of gout patients	Patients with gout may fail to profit from treatment with probenecid. Gout attacks may then occur
Probenecid with indomethacin or with para-aminosalicylic acid (PAS)	Probenecid may interfere with the elimination of PAS and indomethacin by the kidneys, thus raising their level in the blood and tissues	Patients may suffer the adverse effects of overdosage with PAS or indomethacin
Probenecid with thiazide-type diuretics	The thiazide diuretics may act to decrease excretion of uric acid by the kidneys. This tends to antagonize the effectiveness of probenecid	The patient may suffer an attack of gout, unless his dosage of probenecid is increased
Diuretics such as ethacrynic acid, furosemide, and the thiazides with digitalis glycosides	The tendency of the diuretics to remove potassium ions as well as sodium tends to increase the cardiac toxicity of digitalis	Patients may suffer from digitalis toxicity unless they receive potassium supplements
Antacids of the systemic alkalinizer type with various basic drugs including the amphetamines, meperidine, and imipramine	The excretion of the weakly basic drugs may be interfered with by the urinary alkalinizer. This may raise their levels in the plasma and central nervous system	Patients may suffer from excessive stimulation or depression of the nervous system even when taking ordinary doses of these drugs

Some drugs may interfere with the metabolic breakdown of others and as a result increase their pharmacological activity. For example, the antituberculosis drugs isoniazid and PAS inhibit the enzymes responsible for breaking down the antiepileptic drug diphenylhydantoin. If an epileptic patient is also treated for tuberculosis with these drugs, he may develop diphenylhydantoin toxicity because the level of undetoxified drug in the blood and brain rises. To avoid this, the usual dose of the antiepileptic drug must be reduced.

EXCRETION

One drug may interfere with the renal excretion of another and increase the intensity and duration of its action. For example, by preventing the secretion of penicillin through the kidney tubules, probenecid helps to produce higher blood and tissue levels of the antibiotic. Also therapeutically desirable is the administration of urine-alkalinizing drugs to patients poisoned by aspirin or other salicylates, as this increases the rate of excretion of these acidic drugs.

On the other hand, other drug interactions that affect urinary excretion can interfere with desired therapeutic effects. Patients taking probenecid for preventing gout attacks should not also take aspirin, a drug that interferes with the desired effect of probenecid—renal excretion of excess uric acid. Potent diuretics that increase excretion of potassium by the kidneys can potentiate the cardiac toxicity of digitalis.

SIGNIFICANCE OF DRUG INTERACTIONS

The nurse can help to prevent unexpected drug interactions. For example, in talking to patients she often learns things that the patient failed to tell the doctor, such as that he takes certain nonprescription products that may affect the action of a drug ordered by the physician. She also keeps a record of the dates on which patients begin to take various drugs and then stop taking them. The patient should be kept under particularly close observation whenever new drugs are being added to his treatment program or when a drug is being discontinued after long use.

If the nurse then notes a flare-up of either new side effects of drugs or old disease symptoms, she informs the patient's physician. When clinical and laboratory studies indicate that an undesirable drug interaction has in fact occurred, the doses of one or more of the drugs may be adjusted. If necessary, one of the drugs can be discontinued entirely and replaced by an agent that does not produce a toxic effect or one that interferes with a therapeutically desirable pharmacological effect.

References

Berblinger, K.W. The influence of personalities on drug therapy. *Amer. J. Nurs.*, 59:1130, 1959.

Brodie, B.B. Physicochemical and biochemical aspects of pharmacology. *JAMA*, 202:600, 1967.

Burns, J.J. Implications of enzyme induction for drug therapy. *Amer. J. Med.*, 37:327, 1964.

Conney, A.H. Drug metabolism and therapeutics. *New Eng. J. Med.*, 280:653, 1969.

Di Palma, J.R. Drug dosage: the scheduling is what counts. *RN* 28:51, 1965 (April).

———. The way and how of drug interactions. Part 1. *RN* 33:63, 1970 (March).

———. The why and how of drug interactions. Part 2. *RN* 33:67, 1970 (April).

———. The why and how of drug interactions. Part 3. *RN* 33:69, 1970 (May).

Palmer, R.F. Drug interactions. *Med. Clin. N.Amer.*, 55:495, 1971 (March).

Rodman, M.J. What happens to drugs in the body. 1. Absorption, distribution, and termination of action. *RN*, 28:73, 1965 (July).

———. What happens to drugs in the body. 4. Synergism and antagonism. *RN*, 29:72, 1966 (May).

Rosenoer, V.M., and Gill, G.M. Drug interactions in clinical medicine. *Med. Clin. N. Amer.*, 56:585, 1972 (May).

Solomon, H.M., et al. Mechanisms of drug interaction. *JAMA*, 216:1997, 1971.

Williams, R.T. Detoxication mechanisms in man. *Clin. Pharmacol. Ther.*, 4:234, 1963.

3.

The Toxic Effects of Drugs and Chemicals

We have already seen that drugs are tested for toxicity in animals before being evaluated clinically in humans. We have also noted that various circumstances may make an ordinarily safe dose of a drug dangerous for some patients. In this chapter we shall study the main types of drug toxicity in more detail.*

Broadly speaking, the undesirable effects of drugs fall into two classes:

1. Adverse effects that are the result of a drug's known pharmacological effects. Toxic effects of this kind can occur in any patient, provided that he takes a high enough dose of the drug. These *dose-related* effects can be brought about by relatively small doses in the minority of patients who are hypersusceptible to one or another of the drug's primary or secondary pharmacological effects. However, massive overdosage can cause drug poisoning in *all* patients.

2. Adverse effects that are *not* related to a drug's expected pharmacological effects. These effects, which cannot be predicted on the basis of animal and human toxicity tests, are the result of something peculiar to a particular patient's tissue reactivity. *Allergic reactions* come under this category, as does *idiosyncracy*.

Adverse drug reactions of these two kinds that occur during ordinary drug therapy will be discussed next. Acute toxicity caused by accidental or deliberate intake of massive amounts of drugs and other chemicals will be discussed separately later in this chapter.

* One type of chronic toxicity, which occurs in drug abusers and results in drug dependence and drug addiction, is discussed separately in Chapter 4.

Adverse Drug Reactions

Every drug that is used in therapy is capable of causing adverse effects in some patients. Thus, the nurse must be constantly alert so as to detect the signs of drug reactions of different kinds. She often teaches patients and their families what to look for when patients are taking drugs at home. Thus, throughout this book, we shall emphasize the signs and symptoms of toxicity that the nurse should look for with each class of drugs that is being discussed. Here, we shall only state some *general principles* of drug toxicity detection and prevention and give some examples of situations that illustrate various types of toxicity.

PHARMACOLOGICAL TOXICITY

Overdosage is the most common cause of adverse drug effects. Often, this occurs early in treatment before the best dosage level has been established for a particular patient. For example, a patient for whom a sedative or tranquilizer has been prescribed may become excessively drowsy. In this case, the prescribed dose is intended to reduce the patient's anxiety and keep him calm. However, if the patient is unusually responsive to the drug's desired action, the result may be sleepiness, impaired judgment, and poor motor coordination. Thus, patients beginning treatment with barbiturate and *non*barbiturate sedatives and tranquilizers are warned not to drive a car during the first days of drug-induced daytime medication of this kind. Later, when the proper dose of the drug has been determined or the patient develops tolerance to it, these early adverse effects no longer occur.

Pathologic conditions of various kinds must be considered, because they can lead to drug overdosage, adverse effects, and even poisoning. For example, patients taking barbiturates or other drugs that are ordinarily eliminated by the liver and kidneys may suffer toxic effects if these organs fail to perform their functions properly. Thus, these drugs must be administered with caution, or they may even be contraindicated in patients with hepatic or renal insufficiency.

Similarly, patients with emotional and mental disorders may sometimes misuse drugs deliberately that are prescribed for treating their condition. Thus, the doctor may prescribe barbiturates and other psychotropic drugs in only small quantities of capsules, if a patient's history indicates a tendency to abuse drugs, or if he shows symptoms that suggest he is deeply depressed and likely to attempt suicide. Other illnesses that may make some patients particularly susceptible to a drug's primary pharmacological effects include hypothyroidism, hyperthyroidism, hypertension (high blood pressure), and heart disease. In all such cases, caution is required at the start of drug treatment if the doctor decides that the risks of using the drug at all are worth taking because of its potential beneficial effects.

Secondary actions are often responsible for side effects when a drug with several actions is being prescribed. For example, a patient may receive belladonna or atropine (one of its derivatives) to relieve spasm of gastrointestinal smooth muscles. However, atropine has many other effects, including a tendency to cause discomforting mouth dryness and blurring of vision. The nurse often has to encourage the patient with a peptic ulcer to withstand such discomforting side effects in order to gain the benefits of this drug's primary antispasmodic effect.

On the other hand, in patients with pathologic conditions besides the one that is being treated, the doctor proceeds with caution if he decides to use this drug at all. For example, ordinary therapeutic doses of atropine may make it difficult for an elderly man with an enlarged prostate gland to void the urine in his bladder. Atropine is also contraindicated in patients with narrow-angle glaucoma because doses that are safe for most patients may set off an acute attack in people with this eye disease.

The physician must often weigh the risks of using a drug with various pharmacological effects against its benefits. If he decides to prescribe it, he has the obligation to observe the patient closely for possible adverse drug effects. He often depends upon the nurse's ability to recognize and report promptly any signs and symptoms of overdosage or other adverse drug effects.

DRUG ALLERGY AND IDIOSYNCRACY

As we have indicated, some adverse drug reactions have little to do with a drug's ordinary pharmacological effects. They occur as the result of a patient's extreme sensitivity to certain kinds of chemical substances. Reactions that do not develop the first time a patient takes a drug but only upon later exposures to it are usually the result of drug *allergy*. Patients who prove abnormally sensitive to small doses of a drug the very first time it is administered are often said to suffer from drug *idiosyncracy*.

Both types of ill effects have in common the fact that they are not seen in experimental animals during preclinical studies of a drug's potential toxicity. They are also not likely to be detected during the early phases of a drug's clinical evaluation, but only after the drug has been taken by large numbers of people. This is because only a minority of exposed people develop drug allergy; and the number of idiosyncratic individuals is even very much smaller.

DRUG ALLERGY. The nature of allergy is discussed in the introduction to chapter 18, which should be read at this time for a better understanding of what follows here. Allergy to drugs has the same immunologic basis as does allergy to other foreign substances, except that most drugs are *not* proteins. Apparently, however, drugs can combine chemically with body proteins to form a foreign protein called a *hapten*. This then acts like a true *antigen*, a substance that stimulates the production of *antibodies*. Later, when some people who have been exposed to a drug once receive it again, the drug combines with the antibodies in their tissues in ways that do damage to the cells.

In one common kind of allergic reaction— the *immediate*, or *anaphylactoid*, type—the drug antibody reaction results in the release of several chemicals, including histamine. It is these pharmacologically active substances from the person's own tissues that then react with the smooth muscles of his small blood vessels and bronchial tubes, and with other target tissues. The resulting allergic reaction may be relatively mild or severe enough to cause death within a few minutes. The degree of severity does not depend upon the drug that set off the allergic reaction but upon how strongly sensitized the person was when he received the drug on the second, or later, occasion.

Thus, this kind of adverse drug reaction does *not* result from the pharmacological effects of the particular drug that precipitates it. Penicillin and aspirin, for example, both produce the same kinds of allergic signs and symptoms. These and any other drugs to which a person has become hypersensitive through previous exposure cause essentially the same adverse effects. These signs and symptoms may, as we have said, be mild—for example, itchy swellings in the person's skin (urticarial wheals)—or they may be severe enough to cause death from asphyxia or from circulatory collapse (see p. 33 of this chapter and p. 312 in Chapter 24).

Delayed-type reactions differ from the immediate type in the clinical picture that they produce as well as in their relatively slow onset. In cases of this kind, the person's skin breaks out in an inflamed rash rather than in urticarial wheals. Fever and swellings of the joints are other distinguishing features of delayed drug reactions. The patient's bone marrow, liver, and kidneys may also be involved in various ways, just as these organs sometimes are involved in drug reactions that are the result of an idiosyncracy rather than an immunologic response.

DRUG IDIOSYNCRACY. This term is sometimes used to describe the abnormal susceptibility of some people that makes them react to a drug in ways different from most other people. The reason for this inability of the individual to tolerate even small amounts of some drugs is, in many cases, probably genetic. In fact, discoveries in recent years have led to a new field of scientific study called *pharmacogenetics*, which deals with inherited differences in drug responses.

An example of this kind of idiosyncracy is seen in otherwise healthy people who do not have enough of a plasma enzyme called pseudocholinesterase, which breaks down the skeletal muscle relaxant drug *succinylcholine*. When a person with low serum levels of the enzyme or with an abnormal form of it in his blood receives an intravenous injection of succinylcholine, his muscles of respiration may become paralyzed for a long period. The patient's life may depend upon the use of a mechanical breathing apparatus during the prolonged apnea caused by an inherited inability to handle this potent drug.

Other individuals, whose red blood cells lack a dehydrogenating enzyme, may suffer a drug-induced hemolytic anemia. Several kinds of "oxidant" drugs, including aspirin, phenacetin, and other common pain relievers, can cause the erythrocytes of these people to break down. This idiosyncracy was first detected in Negro soldiers who received the antimalarial drug primaquine. The inherited enzyme deficiency has also been found in people of other racial and ethnic groups, including many from Mediterranean countries.

Although several simple tests are available

for diagnosing this disorder, doctors rarely suspect the presence of this genetically-caused condition. Thus, the nurse who notes that a patient passes dark urine and complains of weakness and back pain should report these symptoms to the physician. He will then have the laboratory check the patient's hemoglobin and enzyme levels and, if these are abnormally low, order the offending drug to be withdrawn.

Blood dyscrasias of other kinds may result from the special sensitivity of the bone marrow of some people to certain drugs. The broad spectrum antibiotic *chloramphenicol*, for example, has caused aplastic anemia in a few hundred of the millions of people who have received it. The analgesic drug *aminopyrine* occasionally causes agranulocytosis, a marked reduction in white blood cells. Other drugs cause thrombocytopenia, a deficiency of blood platelets, in susceptible individuals.

These drug-induced blood disorders develop in only a very small minority of patients. Unfortunately, there are no reliable tests to help the doctor learn in advance which patients may react in these ways. Thus, he reserves the use of these drugs for the relatively rare cases in which safer drugs of the same pharmacological classes are not as effective for treating a condition as the drugs that are known to cause dangerous reactions in sensitive patients.

When a doctor decides to put a patient on long-term treatment with a drug that reportedly has caused blood dyscrasias, he has the patient return to the clinic frequently for blood tests. Often, differential blood counts help to detect drops in the various kinds of cells. Discontinuing the drug may then help to keep the patient's bone marrow from being damaged irreversibly. Sometimes, however, clinical signs and symptoms appear in the interval between blood tests. Thus, the nurse often teaches patients with chronic conditions what signs and symptoms to look for.

The nurse may, for example, explain to a patient taking the anti-inflammatory agent, *phenylbutazone*, which can cause agranulocytosis, that the appearance of a severe sore throat and fever may signal the onset of this drug-induced blood disorder. He is told to report such signs of illness to his physician at once. Similarly, the parents of a child receiving the anticonvulsant drug *trimethadione* should be told what signs of illness to watch for during long-term use of this agent for treating petit mal epilepsy.

OTHER KINDS OF DRUG-INDUCED TOXICITY

Other organs such as the liver, kidneys, eyes, and ears are sometimes adversely affected by drug therapy. Often, such ill effects cannot be detected during preclinical toxicity testing in animals. For example, those drugs that directly damage liver cells are not allowed to be used in humans, but other substances that are harmless to hepatic function in animals and in most patients may nevertheless be harmful to the liver function of a few hypersensitive individuals. The antipsychotic chlorpromazine and the antibiotic erythromycin estolate have, for example, occasionally caused jaundice in some patients.

The nurse must be alert for signs that may indicate drug-induced liver involvement such as nausea, vomiting, and abdominal pain, which usually occur even before jaundice appears. Similarly, she observes patients for clinical signs of drug-induced damage to other organs and systems. The doctor, of course, also orders laboratory tests for detecting the development of impairment in renal function. This sometimes occurs during treatment of infections with certain antibiotics and sulfonamides as well as with other drugs.

TERATOGENICITY

Doctors must also consider the possibility of a drug's doing damage to a developing fetus when it is taken by a pregnant woman. The fact that drugs taken by the mother may pass across the placenta to affect the unborn child was brought home most forcibly by the maiming of hundreds of infants whose mothers took *thalidomide*, a seemingly harmless sedative-hypnotic. As a general rule, doctors are now cautious about prescribing any drugs for pregnant women or even women of childbearing age who may have become pregnant and not yet know it. Women should be taught not to treat themselves with nonprescription medicines. Of course, the doctor may decide that the risks of *not* treating a women with a dangerous disorder are greater than the risk to the fetus from drugs that might help to cure her condition. In such casts, the use of most drugs during pregnancy is justified.

Poisoning by Drugs and Chemicals

Poisons are sometimes defined as chemical substances that cause harm, even in very small amounts, to living tissues with which they come in contact. Actually, almost anything may be poisonous if a person takes enough of it. Thus, many medicines that are therapeutically useful in ordinary doses can also cause poisoning when overdoses are administered.

In this book we shall take up aspects of the toxicity of the various drugs that we study which commonly cause poisoning when people accidentally or deliberately take doses much greater than those used in therapeutics. Aspirin, for example, is a very safe drug when people take only a couple of tablets for a headache, yet young children who eat many tablets from a bottle that they find in the medicine cabinet frequently die from the resulting severe salicylate intoxication. Barbiturates are safe drugs when taken in sedative doses but can cause death when a dozen or more capsules are taken at once in a suicide attempt. Other medications, including cold remedies containing antihistamines, have caused accidental poisoning in children, and depressed patients who have ingested all the tablets of tranquilizer or antidepressant drug prescriptions at once have sometimes succeeded in killing themselves with medication that was intended to help them.

Other chemicals not meant to be taken internally as medicines are also a cause of accidental poisoning. These include not only rat poisons, weed destroyers and insecticides, but also many other household products not usually thought of as poisons. Furniture polishes, for example, may contain kerosene and similar toxic petroleum distillates that can cause serious lung damage and death. Other organic solvents in paint thinners, varnish removers, and related products are also dangerous. Disinfectants and drain cleaners containing lye and other caustic substances can cause destruction of the esophagus, stomach perforation, and fatal shock when swallowed. Bleaches, detergents, and even cosmetics often contain chemicals that can be harmful when ingested by youngsters who drink liquids left where they can be easily reached.

DIAGNOSIS AND TREATMENT OF POISONING

DIAGNOSIS. Diagnosis of poisoning is, of course, the doctor's task, and it is often a difficult one. However, the nurse can sometimes help to establish whether a patient's illness is the result of poisoning and what substance was the cause. The emergency room nurse questions the patient or his relatives about what has happened and reports these circumstances to the doctor when he arrives. She also notes various signs and symptoms while observing the patient and reports these to the doctor to supplement his own later observations of the patient. This often aids in early detection of a case of poisoning and results in more rapid and effective treatment.

TREATMENT. The management of poisoning emergencies involves several general steps.

(1) Removing ingested poisons from the gastrointestinal tract or washing chemicals from the skin and eyes before they can do extensive local damage or be absorbed into the bloodstream and tissues

(2) Administering chemical antidotes that combine with the poison in the gastrointestinal tract or occasionally in other body tissues

(3) Applying supportive measures to keep the patient's vital functions operating. This also includes treating complications and speeding the excretion of absorbed poisons

Removal of ingested poisons can be carried out by various means. *Vomiting* is the most rapidly effective way to remove poisons from the stomach soon after they have been swallowed. Thus, no time should be lost in inducing a child to throw up, provided that the ingested poison is not one of those for which the use of emetics is *contraindicated:*

(1) when caustic alkali or corrosive mineral acids have been ingested

(2) when a child has swallowed only a relatively small amount of a light volatile petroleum distillate (kerosene-like substances) and

(3) when the patient is semicomatose or shows signs of impending convulsive seizures.

Sometimes simply encouraging the child to take a glass or two of water or milk and then touching the back of his throat with a finger, spoon-handle, or other blunt object may be enough to set off the gag and vomiting reflexes.

Syrup of ipecac is an effective emetic that the FDA now permits people to buy in one-ounce bottles without a prescription to have available at home. The child or other person who has ingested a toxic substance takes half an ounce with a glass or two of water. This may be repeated if vomiting has not occurred in 15 minutes. However, no more than that should be taken because the alkaloids of ipecac may themselves be toxic if absorbed. (The more concentrated fluidextract of ipecac should *never* be used, as it contains 14 times as much emetine as the syrup and has proved poisonous when taken by mistake.)

Apomorphine, an opium alkaloid, is a rapid-acting emetic that the physician may employ when he finds that the patient has not yet vomited. Injected subcutaneously, 5 mg often causes copious vomiting within five minutes. This clears the stomach completely and sometimes even brings up still unabsorbed material from the upper intestine.

Apomorphine is itself a central depressant so it is not recommended when the patient is already somewhat stuporous. Repeated doses of apomorphine that do not produce the desired vomiting may leave the patient deeply depressed. Narcotic antagonists of the kind that are used to treat opiate overdosage can readily counteract this adverse effect of apomorphine. In fact, some authorities recommend the routine administration of the narcotic antagonist *levallorphan* (Lorfan) following apomorphine administration, even when the patient shows no signs of drowsiness or stupor.

Gastric lavage is often employed in hospital emergency rooms for emptying the stomach. A urethral catheter or a plastic duodenal tube is passed gently down into the patient's stomach by way of the mouth (in young children), or through a nostril (in older children and adults). A syringe is then attached and the stomach contents are withdrawn by suction. The stomach may then be washed out repeatedly with tap water, isotonic saline solution, or fluid to which a chemical antidote has been added. However, gastric lavage can be hazardous and must be carried out skillfully. See other sources for detailed information concerning this technical procedure.

Chemical antidotes (Table 3-1) are various substances that interact chemically with poisons. They may be put into the stomach in order to neutralize them and to prevent their systemic absorption. Some, such as dilute vinegar or citrus fruit juices, act specifically to neutralize alkali just as magnesium oxide neutralizes only acids. Other chemical antidotes antagonize a wide range of organic and inorganic poisonous substances. The most effective material for inactivating most poisons while they are still in the gastrointestinal tract is activated charcoal.

Activated charcoal is a fine black powder which offers a large surface area for the physical adsorption of many substances, ranging from metallic salts such as mercury bichloride through alkaloids such as strychnine to organic acids such as aspirin. One or two tablespoonsful are mixed with water to make a paste, which is then diluted further to make a glassful of a black soupy mixture. The nurse often has to persuade a child to swallow this liquid which looks unappetizing but is actually tasteless and odorless. It is very important to get the patient's cooperation, as early administration of this harmless and effective substance keeps poisons from entering the blood and reaching the tissues. Once within the system, poisons are much more difficult to antagonize with specific chemical antidotes.

Specific antidotes are not available for most poisons. The effects of absorbed poisons can sometimes be counteracted by administering antagonists that produce changes in function that oppose those of the poison. For example, the convulsant effects of strychnine, cocaine, and other nervous system stimulants may be controlled by injecting barbiturates or other depressants (Table 3-1). However, such pharmacological antidotes do not neutralize the poisons themselves.

*Chelating agents** have the ability to bind the molecules of heavy metals and thus prevent these poisons from damaging body cells and tissues. The complex formed in this way is *nontoxic* and can be excreted by the kidneys. *Dimercaprol+* is effective for antagonizing arsenic, mercury, gold, and other poisonous metallic salts. *Calcium disodium edetate+* can be lifesaving when administered intravenously to bind lead in the tissues of a child with acute encephalitis caused by this metal. Other specific antidotes of this kind include the iron-chelating chemical *deferoxamine* and *penicillamine*, a substance capable of combining with copper, lead, mercury, and other metals that may be present in excessive quantities in body tissues. Other systemic antidotes that act chemically to detoxify poisons include the cyanide antidotes listed in Table 3-1, methylene blue, pralidoxime chloride, and protamine sulfate.

Support of the patient's vital functions, including his respiration and circulation, is an

---

* The term is derived from the Greek word *chele*, which means claw. The molecules of a chelating agent grasp (bind) the poisonous metallic ions and carry them out of the body in the form of a nontoxic complex.

TABLE 3-1 *Drugs for Treating Poisoning*

Drugs for Use Against Unabsorbed Poisons

AGENT	USE
Acetic acid (diluted vinegar)	Neutralize alkali
Activated charcoal	Adsorb most chemicals
Ammonium acetate	Neutralize formaldehyde
Ammonium hydroxide	Neutralize formaldehyde
Apomorphine HCl	Emetic
Calcium salts (chloride, gluconate, lactate)	Neutralize fluorides and oxalic acid
Copper sulfate	Neutralize phosphorus
Ipecac syrup	Emetic
Iodine tincture	Neutralize some metals and alkaloids
Magnesium oxide and hydroxide (Milk of Magnesia)	Neutralize acids, including acid from bleach; also demulcent and cathartic
Magnesium sulfate (epsom salt)	Cathartic
Milk, diluted dairy or evaporated	Demulcent, diluent, and precipitant
Olive oil	Demulcent and laxative
Petrolatum, liquid	Demulcent and solvent
Potassium permanganate	Oxidize alkaloids
Sodium bicarbonate	Neutralize ferrous sulfate, and other iron salts; externally only to neutralize acids
Sodium chloride (normal saline solution)	Neutralize silver nitrate
Sodium sulfate	Cathartic
Sodium thiosulfate	Neutralize iodine
Starch solution	Neutralize iodine
Tannic acid	Neutralize metals, alkaloids, and other organic substances
Universal antidote (activated charcoal; magnesium oxide; tannic acid)	Neutralize most poisons (theoretically; practically, activated charcoal alone is preferred)

Drugs for Use Against Systemically Absorbed Poisons

ANTICONVULSANTS AND MUSCLE RELAXANTS

Amobarbital sodium (Amytal)

Benztropine mesylate (Cogentin) (for use against dyskinetic spasms by phenothiazines and other neuroleptic drugs)

Calcium gluconate (for use in hypocalcemic tetany seizures and Black Widow spider bites)

Diazepam (Valium)

Diphenylhydantoin sodium (Dilantin)

Diphenhydramine (Benadryl) for use in drug-induced dystonia)

Methocarbamol (Robaxin)

Methohexital (Brevital)

Orphenadrine citrate (Norflex)

Paraldehyde

Pentobarbital sodium (Nembutal)

Phenobarbital sodium (Luminal)

Succinylcholine chloride (Anectine; Sucostrin)

Thiopental sodium (Pentothal)

CENTRAL NERVOUS SYSTEM STIMULANTS (ANALEPTICS)

Caffeine sodium benzoate

Doxapram (Dopram)

Nikethamide (Coramine)

Pentylenetetrazol (Metrazol)

Picrotoxin

CHELATING AGENTS FOR USE IN HEAVY METAL POISONING

Calcium disodium edetate (Calcium Versenate)

Deferoxamine (Desferal)

Dimercaprol (BAL)

Penicillamine (Cuprimine)

CYANIDE POISON ANTIDOTES

Amyl nitrite

Sodium nitrite

Sodium thoisulfate

NARCOTIC ANTAGONISTS

Levallorphan (Lorfan)

Nalorphine (Nalline)

Naloxone (Narcan)

MISCELLANEOUS SPECIFIC ANTIDOTES

Atropine sulfate—antagonizes anticholinesterase drugs; organic phosphate ester-type insecticides; nerve gases

Chlorpromazine (Thorazine)—antagonizes amphetamine psychosis and LSD "trips"

Ethyl alcohol—antagonizes methyl alcohol

Methylene blue—antagonizes methemoglobinemia caused by nitrites and aniline derivatives

Phytonadione (vitamin K_1)—counteracts bleeding

TABLE 3-1 *(Continued)*

Drugs for Use Against Systemically Absorbed Poisons (continued)

caused by overdosage of oral anticoagulants of the coumarin and indanedione classes

Physostigmine salts—antagonizes central as well as peripheral effects of atropine

Pilocarpine salts—antagonizes peripheral effects of atropine

Pralidoxime chloride (Protopam)—antagonizes organic phosphate ester insecticides

Protamine sulfate — counteracts hemorrhages caused by heparin overdosage

Sodium formaldehyde sulfoxylate—antagonizes mercury salts

Drugs for Supportive Therapy*

CARDIAC DRUGS
Atropine sulfate
Digoxin (Lanoxin and others)
Epinephrine (Adrenalin)
Glyceryl trinitrate (Nitroglycerin)
Isoproterenol HCl (Isuprel)
Lidocaine (Xylocaine)
Procainamide HCl (Pronestyl)
Quinidine HCl

VASOPRESSOR DRUGS
Levarterenol bitartrate (Levophed)
Metaraminol bitartrate (Aramine)
Methoxamine HCl (Vasoxyl)
Phenylephrine HCl (Neosynephrine)

SOLUBLE CORTICOSTEROIDS
Dexamethasone sodium phosphate (Decadron phosphate; Hexadrol phosphate)
Hydrocortisone sodium succinate (Solu-Cortef)
Methylprednisolone sodium succinate (Solu-Medrol)
Prednisolone sodium phosphate (Hydeltrasol)

DIURETIC DRUGS
Ethacrynic acid (Edecrin)
Furosemide (Lasix)
Mannitol (Osmitrol)
Urea (Ureaphil)

ANALGESICS
Codeine sulfate or phosphate

Meperidine (Demerol)
Morphine sulfate

FLUID AND ELECTROLYTE REPLENISHERS
Dextrose injection
Fructose injection
Potassium chloride injection
Sodium chloride injection

SYSTEMIC AND URINARY ALKALINIZERS
Sodium bicarbonate injection
Sodium citrate
Sodium lactate injection
Tromethamine (THAM; Tris buffer)

DIALYSIS SOLUTIONS
Dianeal with dextrose
Impersol with dextrose

PLASMA SUBSTITUTES AND EXPANDERS
Dextran 40 (Gentran 40; LMD 10% Rheomacrodex)
Dextran 75 (Gentran 75; Macrodex)
Normal Human Serum Albumin (Albuminate)
Plasma Protein Fraction (Plasmanate)

MISCELLANEOUS
Antibiotics
Antihistamines
General and local anesthetics
Nutrients
Vitamins

---

* This is only a small sampling of the kinds of substances most commonly employed in poisonings to support vital functions and to counteract complications.

essential part of the management of poisoned patients. Often, the quality of the nursing care that the patient receives determines whether he will survive or develop fatal complications. The actual medical and nursing measures employed in cases of poisoning are the same as those used in caring for other critically ill patients. Thus, we shall review here only briefly some general measures that are relevant to the management of most patients who have been made seriously ill by systemically absorbed poisons.

Respiration must be maintained by every available means, at times including mouth-to-mouth breathing as well as mechanical ventilation of the lungs. The patient's airway is first cleared of secretions. Then an oropharyngeal airway is inserted, or endotracheal intubation is carried out to make suctioning and mechanically assisted ventilation more efficient for longer periods. In some cases the doctor may decide to do a tracheotomy.

The nurse, in addition to assisting the physician with these procedures, is called upon to make careful observations of the patient's response to such measures as positive-pressure oxygenation. She periodically reports changes in the rate, depth, and quality of the poisoned patient's respiration. Patients poisoned by depressant drugs and receiving intravenous fluids must be watched closely for signs of acute pulmonary edema. The semicomatose patient's position is changed often, and he is helped to cough and thus expel secretions. These measures may be more important than antibiotics in preventing such complications as atalectasis and hypostatic pneumonia.

Circulatory function must also be maintained by immediately starting a slow intravenous infusion of saline solution to make up for the loss of salt and water that often occurs in poisoning. If gastrointestinal bleeding from drug-damaged mucosa is present, whole blood transfusion may be needed to prevent shock. In most cases, however, the administration of plasma or a plasma expander such as a dextran solution is adequate for correcting hypovolemia and hypotension. The nurse monitors both the patient's blood pressure and his central venous pressure during the administration of fluids for expanding the blood volume, as abnormalities may lead to reduced cardiac output or even heart failure.

Cases of shock that do not respond to fluid, plasma or blood replacement may require treatment with vasopressor drugs. The nurse must stay with the patient who is receiving an infusion of the potent vasopressors levarterenol or metaraminol and make frequent measurements of his blood pressure to determine how he is responding to the drug. The nurse adjusts the rate of infusion flow to keep the patient's pressure from rising too high, as this can affect cardiac function adversely. She also reports any failure of the patient's pressure to respond, so that the doctor may take measures such as the administration of a soluble corticosteroid drug like hydrocortisone sodium succinate or the correction of acidosis, a condition that sometimes makes shock patients resistant to adrenergic vasopressor drug therapy.

The cardiac complications of poisoning may also require emergency supportive measures. One of the nurse's main responsibilities here is to see that the various kinds of potent drugs for treating heart failure and cardiac irregularities or arrest are available, including epinephrine, atropine, digitalis, and lidocaine. As a member of a hospital's intensive coronary care unit or cardiac resuscitation team the nurse may also be responsible for keeping equipment such as electrical defibrillators in good condition and available for treating poisoning by drugs and chemicals that interfere with cardiac function.

Kidney function may fail either because of damage to renal tubular cells by certain poisons such as mercury or following prolonged circulatory collapse. During the period of recovery of normal kidney function the nurse has many responsibilities in the management of patients with oliguria. She measures the daily urinary output, encourages the patient to sip small amounts of fluid, or supervises the intravenous infusions of fluid and electrolytes that the physician may order.

Often, whether renal failure is present or not, the doctor may make use of an artificial kidney or forced diuresis and other measures to remove certain poisons from the blood and tissues at a greater rate than the patient's kidneys can eliminate them. Hemodialysis and peritoneal dialysis are two of the procedures employed to aid in ridding the body of high concentrations of salicylates (in aspirin and oil of wintergreen poisoning; see Chapter 16) and in poisoning by barbiturates and similar central depressant drugs.

The nurse's observations are often important for the successful management of such patients and of those who must receive diuretic drugs and large amounts of replacement fluids containing potassium, sodium, and other electrolytes for maintaining acid-base balance when acidosis or alkalosis threatens.

Other complications of poisoning in which skilled nursing care is necessary include infection, which must be quickly detected and promptly treated. Fever that may be drug-induced or secondary to infection must be detected by monitoring the patient's temperature and then treated by physical measures and possibly antipyretic drugs. Drug-induced coma, convulsions, pain, and delirium are other possible complications that call upon the nurse's general knowledge of symptomatic and supportive care as well as upon the need to administer appropriate antidotal drug therapy.

PREVENTION OF POISONING

Treatment of a poisoned patient is often difficult, even for experienced and skilled personnel with the most modern equipment and facilities. Thus it is more important to keep poisoning accidents from happening in the first place. Studies carried out in recent years by various medical groups and governmental agencies have gathered information concerning the causes of household poisoning. New federal laws concerning the packaging and labeling of chemical products have helped to reduce the number of cases to some extent. However, the most important preventive measure of all is to educate the public concerning the safe handling and storage of drugs and other chemicals in the home.

The nurse serving in various settings can teach people how to avoid accidents of this kind. Public health and school nurses have an especially important part to play. The school nurse can educate parents through their school-age children. The instructions she gives them about handling and storing potential poisons properly can keep their preschool brothers and sisters from being exposed to this danger. The nurse who makes follow-up visits to homes where poison accidents have occurred will usually still find uncorrected hazards. She can make suggestions to the mother that may keep another accident from happening. In some situations, the visiting nurse may wish to draw upon the services of a medical social worker or even request psychiatric consultation for members of an accident-prone family.

Here are some measures that may be emphasized when nurses teach people about poison prevention:

1. *Keep all drugs and household chemicals out of the reach of children.* All products containing chemicals should be stored in cabinets that can be locked or latched. This applies both to cleaning and polishing materials kept in kitchen cabinets and to drug products kept in bathroom medicine cabinets.

2. *Keep all chemicals in their original containers which now often have special safety closures.* Many accidents occur when a liquid is poured into a measuring cup, soda pop bottle, pitcher, or drinking glass and left where a thirsty child can reach it and take a sip or a swallow. (A single swallow of a caustic alkali in a solution for cleaning clogged drains can severely damage a child's esophagus. A few milliliters of a furniture polish containing a light volatile petroleum distillate liquid can get into a child's lungs and cause a severe chemical pneumonia.)

3. *Read the label before using any medicine or chemical specialty product.* Federal and state laws now require products to be labeled as to their identity and with proper directions for their use. Failure to follow such directions is still a common cause of accidents involving drugs and chemicals.

4. *Take medication only under safe conditions.* For example, do not take any drug in the dark. Elderly patients sometimes go to the bathroom during the night, reach into a medicine cabinet and pour a dose from the wrong bottle. (Sometimes chemicals that are not drugs at all are kept in medicine cabinets next to household remedies.)

Parents should take medications privately, as young children who see them take a drug may later imitate them in their play. In giving medicine to a sick child, never tell him that it is "candy," as he is likely to seek the medication later and take a large amount. (Unfortunately, some manufacturers of medications emphasize the palatability of their products—sometimes even in television promotions that are aimed at the children themselves.)

5. *Destroy all old medications instead of just discarding them.* Drugs should not be simply tossed into trash cans but should, instead, be poured down the sink or flushed down the toilet. (One nurse gave such a good talk to a P.T.A. group about the dangers of retaining the remnants of old prescriptions that the members went home and followed her advice about cleaning out their medicine cabinets. Unfortunately, neighborhood children found some of the discarded drugs and salvaged them for use in their games.)

Thus, the nurse can play an important role in the prevention of poisoning in her community, just as she can contribute to the diagnosis and treatment of poisoning in various professional settings. Neither she nor any other person can know all there is to know about the many aspects of poison accidents prevention and treatment (see Table 3-2) for a discussion of poisoning by common chemicals). However, the nurse should be familiar with the main sources of information about poisons and be able to convey such information to the public (see References at end of this chapter).

TABLE 3-2 *Poisoning by Common Chemicals**

Poison and Sources	Signs and Symptoms	Emergency Treatment
Acids (Corrosive) Hydrochloric, sulfuric, nitric, phosphoric, and other concentrated corrosive acids. *Toilet bowl cleaners* sometimes contain hydrochloric and phosphoric acids, and, more frequently, the less corrosive substance *sodium bisulfate*.	1. Burns about the mouth and throat. 2. Stomach pain, nausea, and vomiting of shreds of mucoid tissue. 3. Circulatory collapse, indicated by weak, rapid pulse, cold clammy pale skin, etc. 4. Death may result rapidly from shock or from asphyxia as a result of respiratory tract edema. 5. Surviving patients may suffer obstructive strictures or stenoses requiring surgical repair.	1. DO *NOT* USE EMETICS OR LAVAGE. 2. Give milk of magnesia, aluminum hydroxide gel, or dilute soap solution. 3. Large quantities of water. 4. Demulcents such as milk, egg whites, olive oil. 5. External skin burns should be flooded with large amounts of water, followed by application of sodium bicarbonate paste. 6. Eye burns should also be flushed with water, possibly after use of topical anesthetic.
Alkali (Caustic) *"Lye"* includes sodium and potassium hydroxides, caustic soda, alkaline carbonates. (Drain pipe cleaners, paint removers, Clini-test urine testing tablets, and stove grease removers contain caustic alkali.)	1. Burns about the mouth and throat edematous, white then turning brown. 2. Burning pain in esophagus and stomach; mucoid, then bloody vomitus. 3. Circulatory collapse indicated by cold, clammy skin and rapid, weak pulse. 4. Death may result rapidly from shock or occur later from this cause as a result of perforation of viscera; early asphyxia, or more slowly developing respiratory tract infections may also prove fatal.	1. DO *NOT* INDUCE EMESIS OR EMPLOY GASTRIC LAVAGE. 2. Give weak acids such as vinegar or lemon juice after having patient drink large quantities of water or milk to dilute the alkali. 3. Demulcents, including olive oil, and egg white, may be given. 4. External burns are washed with large amounts of water or with dilute vinegar. 5. Doctor may order potent analgesics, I.V. fluids and electrolytes, antibiotics, and corticosteroids.
Arsenic Compounds Arsenic trioxide and pentoxide; sodium arsenite and arsenate, and so forth; inorganic and organic forms are found in weed killers, rat killers, insecticides, paints.	1. Burning, cramping pains in G.I. tract; throat constricted; swallowing difficult; severe watery or bloody diarrhea. 2. Dehydration, thirst with sweetish, metallic taste; garlicky odor on breath. 3. Death may result from circulatory collapse following fluid and electrolyte losses and gastrointestinal bleeding. 4. Nervous system toxicity may appear in advanced chronic cases. This is manifested by headache, dizziness, delirium, coma and convulsions.	1. Emetics, gastric lavage, and saline cathartics. 2. Milk, sodium thiosulfate solution, or freshly prepared ferric hydroxide solution may follow the lavage or emesis. 3. *Dimercaprol* (BAL) is administered intramuscularly. 4. I.V. fluids and electrolytes to correct dehydration and deficiencies and to counteract shock.

*Poisoning by these chemicals is not discussed elsewhere in this text. See Index for references to discussions of poisoning by drugs and chemicals not taken up here.

TABLE 3-2 *(Continued)*

Poison and Sources	Signs and Symptoms	Emergency Treatment
Benzene, Toluene, Xylene, and related aromatic hydrocarbons		
These substances are used as solvents for removing paints and lacquers, and as degreasers; they also sometimes serve as the base or vehicle for insecticidal solutions and are often ingredients of glues used by hobbyists and others. Glue sniffers sometimes seek the central effects of such volatile solvents.	1. Local irritation of skin, eyes, and mucous membranes; when swallowed, a burning sensation is felt in the upper G.I. tract, followed by nausea, salivation, and vomiting. 2. Systemic absorption of the inhaled vapors causes effects similar to those of alcoholic intoxication. Continued absorption can result in coma with hyperactive reflexes, and finally respiratory failure. 3. Chronic exposure to benzene can cause bone marrow damage and blood dyscrasias.	1. Skin and eyes should be thoroughly washed; if ingested, the material should be removed by gastric lavage, and mineral oil or a saline cathartic left in the stomach. 2. Supportive measures include artificial respiration, administration of fluids parenterally, and measures for treating pulmonary complications. 3. Epinephrine must *not* be administered, nor should vegetable fats or alcohol be given.
Bleaches (household)		
1. Liquid laundering bleaches commonly contain about 5% sodium hypochlorite (for example, Clorox, and others). These are only mildly alkaline but release irritating hypochlorous acid when they come in contact with acid gastric juice. (When mixed with acid toilet bowl cleaners, chlorine gas may be released.)	1. Vomiting commonly occurs, and there is a burning sensation in the mouth, throat, esophagus, and stomach. However, corrosive burns do *not* occur. Release of chlorine gas may irritate the eyes, nose, and throat and cause tearing, coughing, and choking.	1. Milk may be administered for its diluting and demulcent effects. No further treatment is usually necessary.
2. Solid bleaches contain higher concentrations of sodium, calcium, and lithium hypochlorite or other strongly alkaline substances including sodium carbonate, sodium silicate, sodium tripolyphosphate, or dichlor- and trichlorisocyanurates.	2. Signs and symptoms of severe irritation may resemble those of caustic alkali (see above) and lead to edema of the throat and larynx.	2. See *Alkali (Caustic)* above.
3. Sodium perborate bleaches may be irritating because of their high alkalinity. In addition, their systemic absorption may cause toxicity similar to that of boric acid.	3. In addition to signs of gastrointestinal irritation and hemorrhage, there may be cardiovascular effects including shock, and central effects including confusion, delirium, convulsions, and coma.	3. Supportive measures to counteract shock and convulsions may be required.
Camphor		
An ingredient of the liniment, camphorated oil, which is sometimes mistakenly taken internally instead of castor oil, or otherwise accidentally ingested; camphor moth repellents, balls, and flakes may also be ingested.	1. Nausea, and vomiting following a feeling of warmth in the stomach; vomitus smells of camphor. 2. Headache, dizziness, confusion, restlessness, delirium, and possible hallucinations.	1. Gastric lavage or induction of emesis may be employed immediately after ingestion, but not if signs of central excitement have developed (gavage may be done carefully following sedation).

TABLE 3-2 *(Continued)*

Poison and Sources	Signs and Symptoms	Emergency Treatment
Camphor (continued)	3. Grand mal type seizures followed by postconvulsive depression, and possible coma or respiratory failure.	2. Sedation or light sleep may be induced by administration of barbiturates by slow intravenous infusion.
Carbon Monoxide This gas from automobile exhausts, stoves and heaters causes more cases of poisoning than any other chemical. It acts by combining with hemoglobin in the blood to form carboxyhemoglobin which keeps the blood from picking up oxygen in the lungs and transporting it to the tissues, including the brain.	1. Inhalation of low concentration of CO may cause only mild headache; higher concentrations cause severe throbbing headache. 2. Exposure to very high concentrations can cause loss of consciousness with few symptoms; occasionally, coma may be preceded by confusion and ataxia. 3. The skin often shows a characteristic, cherry-red discoloration.	1. Remove patient to fresh air immediately and apply artificial respiration if breathing has stopped. 2. Inhalation of pure oxygen displaces CO from hemoglobin and restores the oxygen-carrying capacity of the blood; oxygen is then transported more readily to the brain and other body tissues. (Hyperbaric treatment increases the efficiency of this process.)
Carbon Tetrachloride This chlorinated hydrocarbon volatile solvent is used in dry cleaning as a stain remover; as an industrial degreaser; and occasionally in home fire extinguishers.	1. Nausea, vomiting, abdominal pain. 2. Headache, confusion, dizziness, drowsiness, visual disturbances, coma, and possible death from respiratory failure, especially during inhalation of high concentrations of the volatile vapors. 3. Late liver and kidney damage may cause death from acute hepatic necrosis or acute kidney failure. Look for anorexia, nausea, vomiting, jaundice; or oliguria, anuria, albuminuria, edema and weight gain.	1. If inhaled, remove patient to fresh air; if ingested, perform gastric lavage with water or induce emesis; if spilled on skin, remove contaminated clothing and wash skin with water and soap. 2. Oxygen inhalation is desirable after both inhalation and ingestion to protect liver from effects of hypoxia. 3. Prophylactic and supportive measures vs. liver and kidney complications.
Cyanides The gas hydrogen cyanide is used as a fumigant by exterminators of rodents and other vermin in ships' holds, warehouses, greenhouses; the salts such as sodium or potassium cyanide are used in silver and other metal polishes, in photography, metallurgy, and electroplating.	1. Rapid death as a result of respiratory failure can occur from exposure to even small amounts. 2. Less immediately lethal quantities of cyanide cause signs and symptoms of hypoxia which are the result of inability of brain cells and other tissues to utilize oxygen due to inhibition of cellular enzymes, including cytochrome oxidase. 3. Signs and symptoms include headache, dizziness, rapid, difficult breathing; coma followed by generalized muscle tremors and convulsions.	1. Immediate artificial respiration and inhalation of oxygen supplied under positive pressure. 2. Inhalation of amyl nitrite vapors from ampules, followed by intravenous injection of sodium nitrite solution. (This converts part of the blood's hemoglobin to methemoglobin which combines with cyanide.) 3. Injection of sodium thiosulfate solution to convert cyanide to the safer thiocyanate. 4. Whole blood infusion may be necessary.

TABLE 3-2 *(Continued)*

Poison and Sources	Signs and Symptoms	Emergency Treatment
Fluorides		
Sodium fluoride and sodium fluo-silicate are ingredients of certain insecticides such as roach powders; the minute amounts of sodium fluoride in fluoridated water supplies are *not* toxic, neither in the acute sense described here nor chronically.	1. Nausea, salivation, vomiting, abdominal pain and cramps, diarrhea. 2. Dehydration, pallor, cardiac irregularities, cardiovascular collapse. 3. Muscle weakness, tremors, partial paralysis, spasms and, occasionally, convulsions of the tetanic type. 4. Death may occur in a few hours from cardiac or respiratory failure, or circulatory collapse.	1. Neutralize chemically by having the patient drink milk or other fluids containing soluble calcium salts; then do a careful gavage. 2. I.V. injections of calcium salts are used to control muscle spasms. 3. Parenteral fluids are used to control shock.

Petroleum Distillates (Kerosene, Gasoline, Mineral Seal Oil, and others)

These volatile liquids are used not only as fuels for heat, light, and motor vehicles, but also as the solvents for furniture polish waxes, in paint thinners, and in cleaning fluids. They are especially dangerous when aspirated into the lungs; acute bronchopneumonia is a frequently fatal complication.	1. Ingestion may cause a burning sensation in the upper G.I. tract, nausea, and vomiting. Coughing or choking may occur if some of the liquid was inhaled into the lungs while being swallowed. 2. Drowsiness, stupor, and coma may develop. 3. Lung involvement may be indicated by the presence of rales, pulmonary edema with dyspnea, cyanosis, and fever. Death may result from pulmonary edema and cardiac dilatation with irregularities, and finally failure.	1. DO *NOT* INDUCE EMESIS. 2. Very carefully carried out gastric lavage with large amounts of water or sodium bicarbonate solution (3%) may be desirable in some circumstances. 3. This may be followed by olive oil or mineral oil and by a saline cathartic to prevent further absorption. 4. Supportive treatment to overcome or minimize the respiratory tract inflammation may include the use of corticosteroids, antibiotics, and oxygen. Epinephrine is contraindicated.
Nicotine		
This tobacco plant alkaloid is available as Black Leaf 40, a 40% solution of the sulfate salt, which can be rapidly fatal if ingested. Although the nicotine content of tobacco is high, the ingestion of cigarettes or other tobacco products has not proved dangerous, apparently because vomiting occurs and absorption is poor.	1. Small amounts cause salivation, nausea, vomiting, abdominal pain, and diarrhea. 2. Larger amounts at first cause central and cardiovascular effects including headache, dizziness, weakness, visual disturbances and confusion, cardiac irregularities and high blood pressure. 3. Later, in severe poisoning, the blood pressure drops, breathing becomes labored, convulsions are followed by loss of reflex activity; and death may result from respiratory muscle paralysis.	1. Gastric lavage with a solution of potassium permanganate 1:5,000 may be followed by administration of the universal antidote in water to oxidize or precipitate the ingested alkaloid and remove it. 2. If spilled on the skin wash off immediately with water to prevent systemic absorption. 3. Measures for controlling convulsions and supporting the patient's respiration and circulation may be ordered.
Phenol (Carbolic Acid)		
This substance and the related cresols are locally irritating and	1. White burns of the skin and mucous membranes.	1. Delay absorption of ingested phenols by adminis-

TABLE 3-2 *(Continued)*

Poison and Sources	Signs and Symptoms	Emergency Treatment

Phenol (Carbolic Acid) (continued)

destructive and cause severe systemic toxicity when absorbed. Disinfectant solutions containing phenols have sometimes been ingested with suicidal intent; the small amounts (1-2%) in skin lotions is generally safe, but should not be applied frequently to large areas of damaged skin.

2. Burning pain of the mouth, esophagus, and stomach; nausea, vomiting, diarrhea.
3. Pulse weak and irregular, skin pale or cyanotic, breathing shallow indicate shock.
4. Transient stimulation of the nervous system may cause excitement followed by depression.
5. Death may result rapidly from respiratory failure; if patient does not die early, he may suffer late kidney damage. Urine is scanty and turns dark on standing.

tering olive oil or other vegetable oils, which act as solvents. This is followed by gastric lavage, and milk, eggs, or other demulcents.
2. If spilled on skin, remove contaminated clothing immediately and wash with large amounts of running water. Special solvents such as alcohol solutions and fixed oils are unnecessary, although olive oil or castor oil may serve as emollients.

Turpentine

This oil from pine wood is a solvent for paints and varnishes commonly found in the home; its toxicity is similar to that of other volatile oils, including pine oil, which is a common constituent of disinfectant and cleansing solutions.

1. Ingestion is followed by a burning pain in the mouth and throat, pain in the stomach, and nausea, vomiting, and diarrhea.
2. Inhalation into lungs may cause coughing and choking and other respiratory difficulties.
3. Systemic absorption can cause central nervous system stimulation (excitement, delirium, occasional convulsions) followed by depression (stupor, coma, and respiratory failure).
4. Kidney irritation may cause albuminuria and hematuria. The urine has an odor like that of violets.

1. The stomach is lavaged with water or weak sodium bicarbonate solution.
2. Demulcents, including milk or mineral oil, are left in the stomach to allay irritation.
3. Fluids may be forced to produce a copious dilute urine and thus prevent renal irritation.
4. Measures to support respiration may be employed.
5. Relieve pain with codeine rather than with morphine, which may further depress respiration.

SUMMARY of Points for the Nurse to Remember Concerning Poisoning

The nurse has an important role in educating the public about ways to store and handle chemicals safely in the home, in order to avoid poison accidents. She also advises people about the kinds of first aid measures that they should know in order to cope with chemical emergencies.

The nurse should observe patients in the emergency room or at the time of their admission to medical services for signs that may arouse suspicion of poisoning as a possible cause of illness.

The nurse whose duties may involve caring for poison accident victims should request that adequate reference materials be available in the emergency room and other departments. She should learn how to use these and other sources to find required information quickly concerning the chemical contents of various products, their potentially toxic effects, and the recommended antidotes and other treatment measures.

The nurse's role in poison emergencies is a flexible one, in which she cooperates with the physician, the pharmacist, and the family to make the most effective use of community resources, such as poison control centers, in order to treat the patient as quickly and effectively as possible.

In the actual treatment of the poisoned patient the two most important aspects of the nurse's role involve: (1) participating in measures designed to remove the poison from the patient's body as rapidly as possible (such as gastric lavage and emesis) in order to minimize absorp-tion of the poison into the systemic circulation; and (2) aiding in the support of the patient's vital functions (such as: maintaining a patent airway; administering intravenous fluids, and so forth) and offering longer term nursing care aimed at hastening the patient's recovery, reducing his pain, and seeing to his comfort.

Discussion Topics: Clinical Nursing Situation

The Situation: Mrs. Kiernan called the hospital emergency room to ask what she should do for Kevin, her three-year-old son. She had found him looking very ill after vomiting material that looked like medicinal tablets. She found an almost empty bottle that had contained at least 50 5-grain aspirin tablets when she last saw it on her bedside table, and she suspected that Kevin had eaten most of what was gone.

1. Assume that you are the nurse in the emergency room. What would you advise this mother to do? What information would you ask for when she brought the child to the hospital? What observations would you make of the child's condition? What actions would you take in caring for Kevin and his mother?

2. After Kevin's discharge from the hospital, a public health nurse was asked to make a visit to the Kiernan home. Assume that you are that nurse. What observations would you make in the home? What instructions would you give this mother? How would you respond when the mother says, "He could have died, and it would have been all my fault. I never should have left the aspirin in my room"?

DRUG DIGEST

CALCIUM DISODIUM EDETATE U.S.P. (Calcium Disodium Versenate)

Actions and Indications. This chemical combines with lead ions in body tissues to form a nonionized complex, or chelate, that can be excreted by the patient's kidneys. This accounts for its effectiveness as an antidotal treatment in lead poisoning, including acute lead encephalopathy in children. For this purpose, it is administered by vein, but less severe cases are sometimes treated with oral doses.

Side Effects, Cautions, and Contraindications. This drug is used with caution in patients with kidney disease, as it is capable of causing acute tubular necrosis. Its use is contraindicated in patients with severe renal disease and in those with a history of healed or active tuberculosis.

Injection is sometimes followed by fever, chills, malaise, and muscle cramps. Occasionally symptoms of respiratory allergy appear. Oral administration may cause gastrointestinal irritation. It may also result in absorption of lead from the G.I. tract, resulting in a possible increase in toxicity.

Dosage and Administration. The drug is administered intravenously in doses that should not exceed 1 g per 30 lbs of body weight per day in children. Two infusions are administered daily for up to five days. Following a two day rest period, a second course of up to five days may be given, if required. Oral doses of 4 g daily in divided doses may be administered following the injection courses or for patients with abnormally high blood lead levels who show no signs or symptoms of acute lead intoxication.

DIMERCAPROL U.S.P. (BAL; British Anti-Lewisite)

Actions and Indications. This is an effective antidote to poisoning by certain heavy metals including mercury, arsenic, and gold. It combines with the ions of these metals to form a nontoxic complex that is excreted by the kidneys. However, if administered after mercury has already caused kidney damage, it is ineffective and may possibly prove toxic.

BAL has been used to counteract toxicity caused by the gold salts used for treating rheumatoid arthritis and by arsenic compounds used in chemotherapy. It may increase the effectiveness of calcium disodium edetate in treating lead poisoning and of penicillamine in reducing tissue levels of copper in Wilson's disease.

Side Effects, Cautions, and Contraindications. Ordinary doses of BAL do not cause severe toxicity but may produce various discomforting symptoms. Patients may salivate, complain of nausea, and vomit. They may also have a burning sensation in the mouth and transient tingling of the hands and feet, or a feeling of chest tightness.

This drug should not be used after a poison such as mercury has already caused acute kidney damage, as it may then accumulate to cause toxicity, including convulsions and coma. It should not be used in iron poisoning as a complex that is toxic to the kidneys may be formed.

Dosage and Administration: BAL is administered only by deep intramuscular injection in doses of 2.5 mg/kg of body weight. For the first two days, this dose is given every four hours. Later, it is injected only twice daily for 10 days, or until the patient is completely recovered.

References

ADVERSE DRUG REACTIONS

Di Palma, J.R. What to do about adverse drug reactions. *RN* 28:57, 1965 (Oct.).

Done, A.K. Developmental pharmacology. *Clin. Pharmacol. Ther.*, 5:480, 1964.

Friend, D.G. Adverse reactions to drugs. *Clin. Pharmacol. Ther.*, 5:257, 1964.

Modell, W. Hazards of new drugs. *Science*, 139:1180, 1963.

Rodman, M.J. The rising tide of dangerous drug reactions. *Nurs. Forum*, 1:105, 1962.

———. Intolerance, allergy and idiosyncracy. *RN*, 28:51, 1965 (Oct.).

POISONING

Arena, J.M. Poisoning: Toxicology, Symptoms and Treatment, 2nd ed. Springfield, Ill.: Charles C Thomas, 1970.

Coffin, R., et al. Treatment of lead encephalopathy in children. *J. Pediat.* 69:198, 1966.

Done, A.K. Clinical pharmacology of systemic antidotes. *Clin. Pharmacol. Ther.*, 2:750, 1961.

Dreisbach, R.H. Handbook of Poisoning: Diagnosis and Treatment, 6th ed. Los Altos, Cal.: Lange Medical Publishers, 1969.

Gleason, M.N., Gosselin, R.E., and Hodge, H.C. Clinical Toxicology of Commercial Products, 3rd ed. Baltimore: Williams and Wilkins, 1969.

Lawrence, R.A., and Haggerty, R.J. Household agents and their potential toxicity. *Mod. Treatm.*, 8:511, 1971.

Leape, L.L., et al. Hazards to health—liquid lye. *New Eng. J. Med.*, 284:578, 1971.

Matthew, H. Gastric aspiration and lavage. *Clin. Toxic.*, 3:179, 1970.

Press, E. Poison control centers. *Nurs. Outlook*, 5:29, 1957.

Rodman, M.J. Poisoning treatment and prevention. *RN*, 35:51, 1972 (Oct.).

Shirkey, H.C. Ipecac syrup. Its use as an emetic in poison control. *J Pediat.* 69:139, 1966.

Stracener, C.E. and Scherz, R.G. Experiences with safety containers for prevention of accidental childhood poisoning. *Northwest Med.*, 69:334, 1970.

Verhulst, H.L. and Crotty, J.J. Childhood poisoning accidents. *JAMA*, 203:1049, 1968.

Thienes, C.H. and Haley, T.J. Clinical Toxicology, 5th ed. Philadelphia: Lea and Febiger, 1972.

4

Drug Abuse, Dependence, and Addiction

General Considerations

THE DRUG ABUSE PROBLEM

The misuse and abuse of drugs has reached epidemic proportions in American society in the 1970s. Most alarming has been the spread of involvement with drugs among young people, including not only college students but many at the high school and junior high school level.

This indiscriminate use of drugs by youngsters may turn out to be only a passing fad. More probably, however, drug abuse will continue to be a major public health problem. This seems likely because so many people in our society are turning to drugs for escape and for the transient relief of tension that some drugs offer. This has, of course, been true in all times and places. However, no other era has offered such a variety of potent drugs capable of altering people's moods, perceptions, and behavior.

THE NURSE AND DRUG ABUSE

The nurse has an important part to play in helping individuals and communities cope with problems arising from the improper use of drugs. Various ways in which the nurse can help prevent and treat addiction are summarized on page 57. Some nurses have a greater responsibility than others—for example, those involved in specific programs aimed at detoxifying and rehabilitating addicts, and nurses in school and pediatric clinic settings who instruct others about the dangers of drug abuse. However, *all* nurses should know the pharmacological facts and be aware of the social issues that are involved so that they can work with other professionals—physicians, social workers, teachers and clergy—in handling the personal and public health problems that arise from drug abuse.

USEFUL KNOWLEDGE

Drug abuse is an extremely complex problem to which there is no simple solution. Many professional people are concerned with the problems posed by drug misuse. To answer all questions that arise, a person would have to be an authority not only in pharmacology and medicine, but also in the behavioral sciences, such as psychology and sociology, and in such specialties as law and criminology. Often, in fact, the various experts find themselves in violent disagreement when they have to work together. Controversy and disagreement seem to mark most efforts in dealing with the medical, legal, and social aspects of drug abuse.

Nevertheless, the nurse who wants to help people by answering their questions about drug problems has an opportunity to make a valuable contribution. This chapter is intended to furnish a general foundation upon which the student can build and so acquire the detailed knowledge needed in her role of counselor on personal and community drug abuse problems. These are the kinds of abusable drugs which we will discuss:

1. The potent narcotic analgesics—drugs derived from opium, such as heroin and morphine, and synthetic drugs with similar actions

2. The general depressant drugs, including alcohol, the barbiturates and other sedative-hypnotics and tranquilizers, and various inhalable vapors

3. The psychomotor stimulants, including cocaine, the amphetamines and related drugs

4. The hallucinogens or psychotomimetics, such as LSD, mescaline, and others

5. Other drugs that defy easy classification, such as the cannabis derivatives—marihuana and hashish—and belladonna derivatives.

More detailed information will be found elsewhere in this text (see Index) about those of the above mentioned drug classes that have medical applications in drug therapy. Here, however, we shall emphasize the effects of these drugs when they are being misused and abused. For each drug class, the following kinds of information will be furnished:

1. The acute effects—what a person feels when he is under the influence of each of these drugs and how he behaves when intoxicated

2. The chronic effects—the physical and mental changes, including medical and psychiatric complications that may result from long-term misuse of drugs

3. The management of the patient suffering from the acute and chronic intake of excessive amounts of the various types of abuse drugs

The nurse who knows these facts about the effects of the most widely abused drugs will be able to answer most of the questions that concerned parents and other people ask. However, in order to gain perspective on the controversial public issues that arise, the nurse will have to continue to read widely about the many varied aspects of the drug abuse problem. Armed with both basic factual information about the effects of these drugs and an understanding of their social significance, the nurse will feel more confident in her ability to play an important part in health team efforts to help solve the complex problems posed by drug abuse.

Definition of Terms

Before studying the various classes of abused drugs, it is important to know the meanings of the terms that are commonly employed. Unfortunately, the disagreement and controversy that characterize so many aspects of the drug abuse problem extends even to the very meanings of the words that are used to describe the various degrees of involvement with drugs. However, we shall try to clarify the terms by offering explanatory examples.

DRUG USE AND MISUSE

Ours is a drug-taking society. Commercial messages on radio and television tell us to take one drug or another that will make us feel better by eliminating pain and anxiety, or by improving some disordered bodily function. Thus, young and old people become conditioned to the casual use of chemical substances. Drug use of this kind—that is, the self-administration of *non*prescription medications—need not, of course, be harmful. However, some people tend to continue taking drugs even when the need for their effects no longer exists. Drug misuse of this nature *can* lead to harmful consequences of various kinds. For example, people who think that they cannot have a bowel movement unless they take a daily laxative soon become sufferers from chronic constipation that is caused by their misuse of strong cathartic drugs. Chronic misuse of headache remedies has also led to gastrointestinal bleeding and kidney damage.

Substances that are not usually medicines at all are also widely used and *misused*. Alcoholic beverages, for instance, are used by an estimated 75 million Americans. Most people who indulge in social drinking suffer no harm from this drug that is merely a mild sedative or tension-reliever in small doses. Yet even a person who usually takes care to control his intake of alcohol may sometimes misuse this chemical with consequences that are unpleasant (hangover, vomiting) or even dangerous (accidents). Thus, even the occasional use of a chemical for either medicinal or recreational purposes exposes a person to risks resulting from its potential for misuse.

Drug abuse goes well beyond mere misuse. The term is rather hard to define, because its meaning depends in part upon what most people in a particular society think is abusive in another person's pattern of drug-taking behavior. In general, however, people become concerned when they realize that someone is taking too much of a drug, either continually or periodically. A person who drinks alcoholic beverages and shows signs of being even moderately intoxicated at times when most people expect him to be sober (at work, for instance) may be considered a drug abuser. So may someone who goes on frequent sprees or binges, even though he may function more or less normally most of the time.

A person is most likely to be labeled a drug abuser when the substance that he chronically uses to excess is *not* one that most other people use for recreational purposes. Thus, the behavior of a person who drinks too much may be tolerated in our society but another individual who takes several tablets of a prescription-type medication such as a barbiturate to reach the same state of intoxication will commonly be considered a drug abuser.

Drug dependence denotes a further stage in an abuser's involvement with the drug that he has been taking continuously or periodically. Different drugs cause dependence of varying kinds and degrees. In general, however, we can say that the drug-dependent person has lost his ability to keep his drug intake under control. As a result, he finds it hard to function when he is not under the influence of the drug. At the same time, the large doses that he is taking tend to disrupt his mental and physical functioning to a degree that makes it difficult for him to behave in a socially acceptable way. Drugs can cause either *psychological* or *physical* dependence, or dependence of both types together.

Psychological dependence of the most severe kind is marked by a craving for the feeling that the drug produces. The user's compulsive desire to experience the pleasurable state that the drug induces is so great that he gives up all other goals and sources of satisfaction. Some psychiatrists have suggested that people who can become so drug-dependent must be suffering from a personality disorder to begin with. However, no one knows why some emotionally or psychologically disturbed people become drug-dependent, while others do not, and there is reason to think that some drugs may set off dependence-producing behavior in some seemingly stable individuals.

Habituation is a term now often used to denote a much milder degree of psychological dependence. Anyone can form a habit of this kind with one chemical or another—the caffeine in coffee, for example. A person who has such a habit simply feels better when he has taken the chemical than when he has not. However, this in itself need not be harmful personally or socially. Thus, a person habituated to tobacco may miss the effect of nicotine, but he continues to function competently despite his discomfort. Similarly, a person may habitually take a barbiturate-hypnotic, because he thinks that he won't sleep well without it. However, if his doctor decides to discontinue the drug, the patient—if he has a more or less normal personality and average emotional stability—does not show the kind of compulsive drug-seeking behavior that characterizes the truly dependence-prone person.

Physical dependence is a state that develops in people who have been taking certain drugs continuously. It is particularly likely to occur in those who become tolerant to the desired drug effect and take increasingly greater doses to gain the feeling that they seek. Taking the drug in large amounts for varying periods of time tends to bring about biochemical changes, particularly in the tissues of the nervous system. These nerve cells soon seem to require the drug's presence in order to keep functioning normally. When the person is deprived of the drug, and its level in the body begins to drop, the resulting malfunctioning of various systems sets off a series of discomforting signs and symptoms.

The *withdrawal syndromes* that then develop differ depending on: (1) the *type* of drug upon which the person has become physically dependent; and (2) the *amount* of the drug that the drug abuser has been taking continually over a period of time. Thus, as we shall see, an opiate-dependent person suffers a characteristic pattern of ill effects when the drug is withdrawn which is different from the typical abstinence syndrome that develops when a physically dependent barbiturate abuser is deprived of his drug. Also, the discomfort caused by withdrawal of either type of drug is mild in a person who has been steadily taking only relatively low doses; it may be quite severe in a person who has been administering massive amounts of the same drug to himself for a longer time.

Addiction is a term that has been used in so many different ways that it is no longer very meaningful. Some call a drug addicting when it is capable of causing physical dependence. Others consider a drug addicting when people taking it tend to lose control over their intake and become obsessively involved in drug-seeking behavior. Such a compulsive degree of psychological dependence is indeed an important characteristic of addiction. In fact, drug abusers who have undergone drug withdrawal and are no longer physically dependent tend to relapse readily, because they are still psychologically dependent.

Actually, however, in discussing drug abuse of the kind formerly referred to as addiction, it is now thought least confusing to use the general term *dependence*. Because drugs differ in the kinds of dependence they cause, we then specify the type of drug dependence that we mean. Thus, we will speak specifically of drugs that cause *dependence of the opiate type*, or *dependence of the barbiturate type*, or *dependence of the amphetamine type*. Such usage helps us to describe the dependence-producing potential of any *new* drug more specifically than if we were simply to say that it was "addicting."

Narcotic Analgesics

Addiction to the opium derivative *heroin* is commonly considered the most serious form of drug dependence. The recent spread of experimentation with this "hard" drug to younger and younger groups has caused considerable alarm. Many middle-class families now need advice on how to handle the heroin problem of a child who has become dependent on this drug. The nurse should acquire knowledge that will enable her to offer such *counseling*.

PREVENTION

The nurse can also play a part in preventing addiction to other opiates, including *morphine*, and such synthetic analgesics as *meperidine* (Demerol), which are used in medicine for relief of severe pain. She can, for example, help to minimize medically acquired dependence upon these and other narcotic analgesics by using proper precautions whenever administering these drugs to patients (Chapter 13, *Potent Analgesics*).

The nurse, herself, should *never* take a dose of any of these pain relievers, including even *codeine*, unless it has been prescribed for her by a doctor. Such self-medication can lead to *psychic* dependency even in people who do not seem to be suffering from any obvious personality disturbances or emotional disorder. A relatively high proportion of medical personnel—doctors, dentists, pharmacists, and nurses—become addicted to these medications. This is because their occupations expose them to drugs that offer a tempting release from tension and anxiety. (See also *Summary of Nursing Measures in Preventing and Treating Drug Addiction*, p. 57.)

PSYCHIC DEPENDENCE

What effect of heroin accounts for the compulsive craving for it that some people develop? Like the related narcotic analgesics that are used for relief of physical pain, heroin has the ability to make a person indifferent to stressful situations that would ordinarily produce feelings of fear and panic. The drowsy, dreamy state that the drug usually produces makes it hard for a person to stay concerned about any personal problems that may have been worrying him. Some people who are exposed to heroin become dependent on the drug because its effects help them to escape from conflicts in their life situation that they find intolerable. They enjoy the drug-induced feeling of pleasurable relaxation and relief of anxiety. Another kind of euphoric feeling that is sought by those users who inject heroin directly into a vein ("mainlining") is a sudden surge of physical ecstasy (a "jolt," "buzz," or "blast").

PHYSICAL DEPENDENCE AND TOLERANCE

In order to keep getting these highly prized effects, the heroin abuser has to take larger and larger doses as his body becomes increasingly tolerant to the drug. This, in turn, leads to dependence of the physical type, in which the cells of the person's central nervous system actually need to have heroin in order to keep functioning properly. Thus, if he is deprived of the drug, the physically dependent person suffers the typical opiate withdrawal syndrome (see *Summary of Major Drug Withdrawal Symptoms*, pp. 57-58). Avoiding this physical illness, which can be completely relieved only by administering heroin or some similar dependency-producing drug, becomes yet another reason for the dependent person to keep on seeking and taking the drug.

TREATMENT

Detoxification, the process of ridding the patient's body of heroin, is the first step in treatment. It is ordinarily carried out on a hospital ward but may sometimes be done on an ambulatory basis. Depending upon the degree of the patient's physical dependence, his abstinence sickness may be mild or severe (see *Summary of Major Drug Withdrawal Symptoms*, pp. 57-58). In either case, good nursing care is needed to keep the patient comfortable during this "detox" or "drying out" period.

NURSING MEASURES. During withdrawal, the patient is especially sensitive to the attitudes of others. At this time of physical discomfort and psychic distress, he needs emotional support. The nurse can supply this supportive relationship by listening to him, answering his questions, and allaying his fears. The sensitive nurse, who conveys respect rather than condemnation at this trying time, may help the patient in ways that strengthen his determination to stay off drugs during the later stages of his rehabilitation when he is under the care of others.

The nurse makes the patient physically comfortable and lessens his fear of the ordeal by listening to him and answering his questions about what to expect during the "drying out" process. A back rub helps to relax cramped and aching muscles. Chills are counteracted with warm blankets and heating pads set at a safe temperature and observed often to guard against burn damage. Once the patient's early nausea and vomiting has subsided, he should receive frequent, small but nourishing meals.

Keeping these patients from obtaining drugs illicitly while they are under her care is an important nursing responsibility. In following the security measures of the institution, she should be open rather than stealthy. Visitors may have to be observed and packages examined, but this is done in a straightforward, matter-of-fact way that won't humiliate the patient.

Firmness is necessary in dealing with persons who abuse drugs. These patients frequently test the limits set by nurses and other staff members. Thus, an attitude of supportive listening is not to be confused with laxity or indulgence. In many instances patients who abuse drugs have not experienced others' caring about them, and they need a firmness of approach to assist them not only to develop their own self-control but also to show them that someone cares what they do.

Participation of other patients in the treatment program is widely practiced through such measures as group therapy and the group's role in developing rules for the community of patients. An important aspect of the nurse's role involves working not only with individuals but also with groups of patients, through such measures as leading or co-leading group discussions.

DRUG TREATMENT. The doctor may order non-opiate-type drugs to aid relief of symptoms. These include salicylates for muscular pain, sedative-hypnotics such as phenobarbital for anxiety and insomnia, and tranquilizers such as *chlordiazepoxide* (Librium) or *chlorpromazine* (Thorazine) for agitation. If the doctor has ordered these drugs on a p.r.n. basis, the nurse should not hesitate to administer them whenever they seem to be needed. She need not be afraid that giving these drugs with discretion may tend to foster further addiction.

Methadone (Dolophine, and others) is also often used during detoxification in any of several different dosage schedules. Because this drug—unlike the others—is an *opioid*, or *synthetic narcotic* that can itself cause opiate-type dependence, the nurse must administer it exactly as ordered. The drug is used for only a brief period, in order to minimize withdrawal discomfort in moderately dependent patients. Once the patient has been stabilized on a dose of methadone that keeps him comfortable, the dosage is gradually reduced and finally discontinued entirely in a few days.

METHADONE MAINTENANCE. This is an entirely different procedure, in which the administration of methadone is not discontinued. Instead, dosage is gradually increased over a period of four to six weeks. The purpose of this procedure, which is employed along with other rehabilitative measures, is to make the patient tolerant to methadone and cross-tolerant to heroin and other opiates. Once the patient is properly stabilized on methadone, he can take daily doses that do not keep him from functioning normally. That is, once he has acquired tolerance to methadone, the patient on a methadone maintenance program can carry on ordinary activity without showing drowsiness, confusion, euphoria or other effects of the opioid. Most important are the effects of methadone upon the person's responses to heroin.

Administered in this way, methadone has two important effects: (1) it blocks the euphoric effects of heroin, so that patients cannot get "high" on it, and (2) it eliminates the patient's hunger for heroin, the compulsive craving that keeps patients from staying off the drug even after they have been detoxified.

Rehabilitative measures employed together with methadone maintenance include vocational training, education, and various psychosocial services. According to several recently reported studies, patients in these programs have made remarkable progress compared with other addicts. Ordinarily, after detoxification, the addict soon returns to his drug-seeking and drug-taking behavior. He commits crimes continuously to get the large sums of money he needs to support his habit. In time, the addict's round of criminal activities leads to arrest and prison—a pattern repeated again and again. In many cases, the addict ends up in the morgue, a victim of accidental or deliberate overdosage or of hepatitis, endocarditis, tetanus, or other medical complications.

Many hardened addicts with long histories of involvement in crimes related to drug-seeking behavior have made a successful social adjustment when maintained on methadone. Freed from the need to satisfy their craving, these people can stop the vicious cycle of stealing, prostitution, and other types of "hustling" or antisocial behavior. Many are now working, going to school, and rehabilitating themselves in other ways. They *do* have to make almost daily visits to the clinic to take the dose of methadone needed to avoid withdrawal discomfort.

Some authorities disapprove of maintaining addicts on what they call a "chemical crutch." They claim that administration of methadone simply substitutes one addiction for another. This is particularly undesirable for teenage heroin users, who should be weaned away from addicting drugs rather than be maintained on them.

NARCOTIC ANTAGONISTS. Another pharmacological treatment approach, still in experimental stages, involves the use of new *narcotic antagonists*—drugs that do not cause addiction.

Drugs of this kind—for example, *nalorphine* (Nalline) and *levallorphan* (Lorfan)—have previously been used mainly for treating acute opiate overdosage. Two new drugs of this class, *naloxone* (Narcan) and *cyclazocine*, are being tried as part of programs aimed at keeping patients off narcotics. Like methadone, these drugs make it impossible for the addict to experience a heroin "high," but unlike methadone these drugs do not produce physical dependence.

A drawback of the narcotic antagonists is that, unlike methadone, these drugs do not eliminate the patient's craving for heroin. In addition, the duration of action is so short that a patient need miss only one day's dosage, if he desires to begin taking heroin again. Thus, these drugs are effective mainly in addicts whose motivation toward abstinence is high to begin with. It may, of course, prove possible to lengthen the heroin-blocking actions of these drugs by pharmaceutical means, or new longer-acting congener compounds could be developed that would keep the patient resistant to the effects of heroin for several days or more.

General Depressants

Depressant drugs other than the opiates and opioids are also often abused. These drugs, which are classified as general depressants of the central nervous system, include: (1) *ethyl alcohol*; (2) the *barbiturates* and other *sedative-hypnotics* and *minor tranquilizers*, or *anti-*

anxiety agents, and (3) *inhalation anesthetics*, such as ethyl ether and certain volatile solvents that have somewhat similar effects when inhaled.

PATTERN OF DEPRESSANT EFFECTS

As is indicated in more detail in Chapter 6, all of these substances are capable of producing a more or less similar pattern of *depression* of *central nervous system function*. Depending upon the dose and the way it is administered, these drugs cause depression of varying degrees. The progressive central depression produces the following effects:

1. Sedation—a reduction in anxiety, tension, and alertness
2. Drowsiness, lethargy, and sleep
3. Deepening stupor and coma

A fourth effect is often seen before sleep and stupor. This is a period of excitement, confusion, and clouded consciousness. In this stage, the person's behavior becomes unpredictable but is most often boisterous and disorderly, as we all know from observing people inebriated by alcohol. Sometimes, particularly when vapors are being inhaled, the most marked changes are in a person's *sensory perceptions*. As many of us may know from the experience of "going under" after a few whiffs of an anesthetic like ether, vision, hearing, and other sensations may be markedly distorted in this stage.

SEDATIVE-HYPNOTIC TYPE ABUSE AND DEPENDENCE

The barbiturates, particularly those with a relatively rapid onset of action, such as *secobarbital* (Seconal), *pentobarbital* (Nembutal), and *amobarbital* (Amytal), are commonly subjected to abuse. So are such nonbarbiturate sedative-hypnotics as *glutethimide* (Doriden) and methaqualone (Quaalude, Sopor, and others) and antianxiety agents such as *meprobamate* (Equanil, Miltown). See Tables 6-1, 6-2, and 6-3 in Chapter 6 for a complete list of abusable drugs of these classes.)

ABUSE PATTERNS

People take these drugs in excess to get different effects. Some seek the sedation, sleep- and stupor-producing effects to escape from overwhelming anxiety and tension. Others take large doses for the euphoric release they get from feelings of guilt and inadequacy. This is often accompanied by the same sort of uninhibited behavior brought about by alcoholic intoxication. Alcohol is, in fact, often taken in combination with barbiturates, meprobamate, glutethimide, and other drugs of this class to increase the feeling of exhilaration. Occasionally other drugs, such as stimulants of the amphetamine-type, are combined with barbiturates or taken alternately to counteract each others' excessive effects.

Intoxication may—as with alcohol—be both mild and severe. The moderately intoxicated abuser shows signs of impaired mental and motor function (see *Summary of Drug Abuse Signs and Symptoms*, p. 58) that resemble those of alcoholic intoxication. In fact, when you see a person who looks and acts drunk but whose breath has no odor of an alcoholic beverage, you should consider the possibility of his being under the influence of barbiturates or other sedative-hypnotics and tranquilizers.

Poisoning, resulting in coma and death from respiratory and circulatory failure, is a common occurrence in habitual barbiturate abusers. Sometimes this happens when the mentally confused person accidentally takes too many capsules and exceeds his tolerance. Severe toxicity is particularly likely to occur if he has also been drinking heavily. Occasionally, an abuser may, in a fit of depression, deliberately take an overdose of barbiturates. He may not necessarily wish truly to commit suicide, but death may come before a rescuer. (See Chapter 6 for a discussion of the management of barbiturate poisoning.)

LONG-TERM EFFECTS

Like the alcoholic, this type of drug abuser may become unkempt in appearance. If he has been injecting himself with highly alkaline barbiturate salt solutions, his skin may be scarred or abscessed. Often his hands tremble and his reflex responses and eye signs are abnormal. However, because he usually eats better than the alcoholic, he does not ordinarily suffer from malnutrition and show the resulting signs of more severe neurological damage that are so often seen in the chronic alcoholic. The barbiturate abuser's life style and muddled mental state make him especially subject to accidental injury or death from falls, fires, or automobile accidents.

PHYSICAL DEPENDENCE AND WITHDRAWAL

The person who continues to take high doses of barbiturates and related sedative-hypnotic drugs for many weeks or months develops physical dependence. This is manifested by a withdrawal syndrome that is different from the opiate withdrawal pattern and potentially more dangerous. (See *Summary*, pp. 57-58.) This is because the abuser who is abruptly deprived of his drug may suffer from convulsions and delirium. As in the case of the alcoholic with the "D.T.'s," his agitation and restlessness may lead to physical exhaustion and circulatory collapse, if the withdrawal excitement is not brought under control.

TREATMENT OF THE WITHDRAWAL SYNDROME

Patients who, when sobering up, begin to show severe signs of withdrawal from any drug of the sedative-hypnotic-tranquilizer group are given a barbiturate—usually *pentobarbital* (Nembutal) and occasionally *phenobarbital*— in amounts just high enough to make them mildly intoxicated again. Then, after the doctor has determined the dose needed to keep the patient slightly drunk on this barbiturate, he begins to order gradually reduced daily doses. This process often takes several weeks to complete, because too rapid lowering of the dose brings on tremulousness and anxiety, which may be early warning signs of the seizures and delirium that can follow.

PREVENTING SEDATIVE DRUG ABUSE

Most people who receive barbiturates for medical reasons feel no compulsion to raise the daily or nightly dose. However, some people, particularly alcoholics, tend to abuse these and other sedatives, hypnotics and tranquilizers when they are exposed to these drugs. Thus, doctors try to avoid prescribing these agents to addiction-prone patients. If the doctor does choose one of these drugs for controlling the patient's anxiety or sleeplessness, he limits the amounts prescribed and tries to keep the patient under close observation as long as the medication is being employed.

The nurse also plays a part in preventing abuse of these drugs by patients who are prone to become dependent upon them. Such patients, as well as elderly people who are often forgetful, need to be carefully observed when taking sedatives, hypnotics, and tranquilizers. Nonhospitalized patients have to be instructed in how to deal with the problem of preventing dependence on drugs that are readily available to them when they are at home.

Instruction cannot, of course, take the form of coercion and control, as this approach is totally ineffective with these patients and in this setting. Instead, the nurse provides the patient with opportunities to discuss any worries he may have that he could become addicted to a prescribed sedative. She helps him to understand how a drug that is useful for his condition can also be hazardous to him if abused. She encourages him to develop self-control through an awareness of the hazards of drug misuse and also through helping him to find other more healthful ways of coping with his difficulties.

Ordinarily, the nurse deals directly with the patient, as it is better for him to assume the responsibility himself. However, in the case of confused or forgetful elderly patients, the nurse asks a family member to take on the task of administering the medication. She should encourage them to provide such supervision in an open, straightforward manner rather than by sly surveillance.

Volatile Solvent-type Abuse

Nurses are aware that many household products contain organic chemicals that can be hazardous when inhaled. These products should be used only after reading the directions on the label, which often advise that the substance be used only in a well-ventilated place in order to avoid accidental poisoning. Thus, it is astounding to find that teen-agers and others often sniff such organic solvents deliberately just for "kicks."

ORGAN DAMAGE

The volatile solvents used in model airplane glues, plastic cements and other commonly abused products may be any of many different chemical compounds (see Table 4-1). Often these are substances known to be capable of causing damage to the liver, kidneys, and bone marrow under some circumstances. The youngsters who sniff solvents in order to experience certain changes in consciousness have no idea, of course, that they may be subjecting themselves to such organ damage. Yet, some users

TABLE 4-1 *Some Volatile Solvent Chemicals in Products Sniffed for "Kicks"*

Volatile solvents	Where found
Acetone	
Amyl acetate	
Benzene	In tube repair kits
Carbon tetrachloride	In spot removers
Ethylene dichloride	
Fluorocarbons (such as trichlorofluoromethane, dichlorodifluoromethane)	In pressurized aerosol containers
Gasoline	
Methyl cellosolve	
Trichlorethane	In spot removers, and in pressurized aerosol containers
Trichloroethylene	In spot removers
Toluene	In model airplane glues and cements

have suffered blood dyscrasias and abnormalities in liver function that have resulted in jaundice, hepatic coma and kidney failure.

Immediate effects sought by the sniffers are similar to those that people often feel during the early induction phase of the stages of anesthesia. These often include a feeling of floating or dizziness, blurring and doubling of vision, noises and ringing in the ears, or even actual visual and auditory hallucinations. The user is often described as "acting drunk" because he may stagger and his speech may be slurred and his talk incoherent. When even larger amounts are inhaled, he may become drowsy, stuporous, or even unconscious and comatose.

Deaths have occurred as a result of respiratory failure. This may be the result of medullary respiratory center depression by such anesthetic drugs. Sometimes, suffocation has resulted when plastic bags containing the chemicals were placed over the person's face and then cut off his oxygen intake while he was unconscious. More recently, it has been found that many cases of sudden deaths were the result of cardiac arrest caused by the fluoromethane compounds used as carriers in many aerosol sprays. This is similar to what happens occasionally when chloroform or related hydrocarbons cause heart irregularities in patients during induction of anesthesia.

Psychomotor Stimulants

Drugs that stimulate the central nervous system are being very widely misused and abused.

At one time, the most commonly abused drug of this class was *cocaine*, an agent available mainly to members of the criminal subculture. Today the *amphetamines* and related stimulants such as *phenmetrazine* (Preludin) and *methylphenidate* (Ritalin) are commonly used and misused by millions of middle-class Americans, including college students, business executives and housewives.

AMPHETAMINE EFFECTS

As is indicated in more detail in Chapter 9, drugs such as *amphetamine* (Benzedrine), *dextroamphetamine* (Dexedrine) and *methamphetamine* (Methedrine, and others) exert two main effects on the C.N.S.: (1) they cause *increased alertness* and *wakefulness*; and (2) they affect a person's *mood*, making him feel more *confident* and *outgoing* and willing to work. Most of the medical uses of these and related psychomotor stimulants are based on the ability of small doses to produce one or both of these effects in many patients.

The amphetamines also have *sympathomimetic* actions. Thus, they can cause such physical effects as heart palpitations, headache, high blood pressure, dry mouth, and dilated pupils, particularly when large doses are administered.

PATTERNS OF MISUSE AND ABUSE

Federal agencies have recently employed several measures to prevent the diversion into illicit channels of amphetamines produced legitimately by pharmaceutical companies—an amount estimated to be as much as half of their total production. For example, the setting of restrictive quotas on the manufacture of amphetamines in 1972 and 1973 has reduced production, which previously had been over eight billion tablets annually, by more than 50 percent. This control, as well as others, over the availability of prescription products is intended to reduce their widespread use for nonmedical purposes. Patterns of misuse and abuse take several forms, including the following.

OCCASIONAL USE. This may increase the efficiency of a person's performance. Thus, for instance, students cramming for exams, executives trying to complete a big job, truckdrivers on long-distance hauls, and writers racing to meet a deadline may take amphetamines in small doses to ward off fatigue and sleepiness so that they can continue working. Although this does not ordinarily cause harm, some people may push themselves to the point of exhaustion and collapse. These drugs only mask feelings of fatigue; they do not eliminate the body's need for rest.

CONTINUED USE. This may occur to maintain mood elevation or euphoric elation. It is the most prevalent pattern among middle-class adults who may first have received the drug on a doctor's prescription. Thus, for example, a housewife with a weight problem takes the drug in prescribed dosage for depressing her appetite. However, she may so enjoy the feeling of well-being that she begins to self-administer the drug in larger doses and—as tolerance develops—at more frequent intervals. Because these large amounts make her feel irritable, tense and jittery, she may begin to take barbiturates or tranquilizers to reduce these disagreeable feelings. Before long, she may be unable to care for her family, and she may show other signs of social and emotional deterioration from this form of amphetamine abuse.

SPREE-TYPE OF ABUSE. The most dangerous form of abuse involves the continued administration of truly massive doses of amphetamines, usually by the intravenous route. Used in this way by so-called "speed freaks" or "meth-heads"—mainliners of methamphetamine—these drugs can cause severe psychic and physical damage. Although death from overdosage is rare, the life style of the long-term heavy user is extremely hazardous to his health.

❪ *Psychological effects.* The immediate effect of a rapid I.V. injection is the sudden onset of an intensely pleasurable feeling called a "flash" or "rush." This is often followed by a sensation of extreme mental and physical power. The person in this state becomes very active and talkative and stays awake for days without eating. However, as tolerance develops, he has to increase the frequency of injections in order to sustain such "runs." Finally, he "falls out" or "crashes"—that is, he falls into a deep sleep or semicomatose state from which he cannot be readily aroused.

The long-term result of a series of such "runs" and "come-downs" is a marked breakdown in mental and emotional function. When he awakens, the abuser feels extremely lethargic and deeply depressed. (These discomforts may all be part of a withdrawal syndrome, indicating—despite claims to the contrary—that amphetamines may be capable of causing physical dependence.)

Paranoid psychosis occurs sooner or later in individuals who pursue this abuse pattern. The hypomaniac user has visual and auditory hallucinations, and these in turn lead to terrifying delusions. Reacting to his feelings of suspiciousness, the hostile hyperactive amphetamine or cocaine abuser can become violent. Assaults and murders have been committed by stimulant abusers in this mental state. Usually, however, the person's eccentric behavior results in his being hospitalized before he harms anyone. Ordinarily, the patient's psychotic reaction is quickly controlled by treatment with phenothiazine-type tranquilizers.

❪ *Physical complications.* Occasionally, a person who "over-amps" (takes an I.V. overdose) may fall unconscious and awaken hours later temporarily paralyzed and unable to speak. This is thought to result from constriction of brain blood vessels such as occurs in a stroke. Some suffer severe chest pains that are presumably the result of coronary vessel constriction. Deaths following high fever and circulatory collapse have also been reported.

More common, however, in the chronic heavy abuser of amphetamines are signs of physical deterioration that stem from infection and malnutrition. Small skin injuries often fail to heal and become abscessed and ulcerated. Part of this skin damage is done by the patient, who often picks compulsively at his skin, perhaps because he is having the hallucination that insects are crawling under it. As occurs with heroin "mainliners," hepatitis, tetanus and bacterial endocarditis can result from pathogenic microorganisms transmitted through the sharing of unsterilized needles.

REHABILITATION

Amphetamine abuse can, as we have seen, lead to severe psychic and physical deterioration. However, some abusers seem able to make a complete recovery when their life situation is favorable for rehabilitation. Those who have a home and family and a job or profession are most likely to be able to abstain from further drug taking and thus make a complete recovery.

On the other hand, prospects for recovery are poor for those individuals—often suffering from severe personality disturbances, character disorders, or even borderline psychoses—who return to the drug-oriented subcultures of some of our large cities. These people not only fail to stop taking amphetamines but tend to become multiple drug users, involved with many other drugs besides "speed," including various hallucinogens, barbiturates and heroin.

Marihuana and Related Drugs

Marihuana ("pot," "grass," and other terms) is made up of the flowering tops and leaves of the weed *Cannabis sativa*. The dried plant parts are rolled into cigarettes ("joints," "sticks") for smoking. A more potent cannabis product called *hashish* ("hash"), a resin scraped from the flowers, may be smoked in a pipe or mixed into candies and cookies and eaten. The mental effects of these drugs depend upon their content of chemical constituents called cannabinols. One of these—*tetrahydrocannabinol* (THC)—which is believed to be the main psychoactive ingredient, is now available in pure form from natural and synthetic sources.

ACUTE PSYCHIC AND PHYSICAL EFFECTS

THE "HIGH." People differ in what they feel when they smoke "pot" or "hash." In part, this is because samples of marihuana and hashish vary in their content of THC. The effects of the same dose differ, too, depending upon whether it is inhaled or eaten. Also important in determining its effects are such *non*pharma-cological factors as what people of varying personalities and experience expect to feel and the environmental circumstances, or setting, in which they take the drug.

Often, the first drug effect of which a person becomes aware is a feeling of floating and drowsiness. Most marihuana smokers claim to find this "high" feeling pleasurable, but some are more likely to complain of dizziness and sluggishness. Often the novice smoker's throat is made dry and sore and he may become nauseated and vomit. Among other physical effects commonly reported are a rapid pulse rate and reddening eyes.

The emotional effects of marihuana range from euphoria to anxiety and depression. People smoking together may become elated, talkative, and boisterous, while the lone smoker seems, instead, to be more interested in the inner workings of his own mind. Sometimes he claims to see and hear things more clearly. Thus, a painting's colors may appear brighter and its design more intricate, and music may sound more exciting. Other perceptions are disturbed. Time seems to pass slowly, for example, and distances are difficult to judge correctly.

The mild intoxicating effects of one or two marihuana cigarettes usually wear off in a couple of hours without causing any harm. However, a person whose judgment and motor coordination have been adversely affected runs the risk of having an accident if he tries to drive. Higher doses of the drug sometimes set off visual hallucinations, but these do not ordinarily lead to delusions or to psychotic behavior.

Acute panic reactions are the most common type of adverse psychic effects seen in marihuana users. These tend to happen to people who become upset by the strange feelings that cannabis drugs induce. Often, the person feels that he is losing his mind or is dying when he experiences the sense of separation of mind and body that these drugs can cause.

Terminating the panic reaction is best accomplished by calming the patient with simple reassurance. Most often—since marihuana is illegal—this is done by the user's friends, but they may bring him to the hospital emergency ward if they cannot control him. In such situations, the nurse should stay with the patient and tell him repeatedly in a quiet way that his strange feelings are caused by an unusual reaction to the drug that he has taken. She assures him that he will soon be all right and that she will stay with him until he is feeling better.

Acute psychotic reactions are relatively rare but have sometimes required prolonged hospitalization. However, if the patient's temporary agitation and paranoid behavior can be controlled with antipsychotic drugs, and if he can be kept under continuous observation, hospitalization can often be avoided. Individual care is important not only to keep the patient from harming himself and others, but also because care given by a single sensitive professional person is more effective in these cases than is treatment in a hospital ward with the punitive attitudes that sometimes prevail there.

LONG-RANGE PHYSICAL AND PSYCHIC EFFECTS

PHYSICAL. Marihuana does not seem to cause damage to the vital organs of heavy smokers, nor does it bring about biochemical changes of the kind that result in tolerance or physical dependence. However, its safety when taken steadily for long periods has not yet been scientifically proved, and more research will have to be done on the drug's long-term toxicity.

PSYCHIC. Some individuals seem to develop a compulsive need to stay under the influence of marihuana. Such psychological dependence most likely occurs in persons who are already disturbed emotionally. However, marihuana may be particularly hazardous for adolescents because it tends to offer an easy-to-take alternative to the difficult adjustments that have to be made during this period of personality development. Heavy use of the drug may help to make a young person lose interest in pursuing objectives that require concentration and hard work. The pleasure-seeking "pothead," or chronic abuser, may then do poorly in school or be unable to hold a job. Some youngsters may even drop out of ordinary society and become part of a drug subculture dedicated to seeking pleasurable "kicks."

SOCIAL AND LEGAL ASPECTS

The fact that some of those who experiment with marihuana go on to abuse barbiturates, amphetamines, LSD, and heroin does *not* mean that the drug has pharmacological effects that somehow sensitize a user's system, so that he then seeks out and abuses more dangerous drugs. However, the public's failure to differentiate between marihuana and "harder" drugs accounts in part for the harsh penalties imposed for possession of *Cannabis* derivatives. Youngsters arrested and convicted for such offenses can obviously suffer social "side effects" more serious than those of the drug itself.

MISCONCEPTIONS. It is important for nurses to help correct erroneous ideas about this drug. The nurse can play an important part in fostering rational rather than emotional discussion of this important public health issue by taking advantage of opportunities that arise to teach others the facts about marihuana.

Without in any way condoning illegal drug use, the nurse can help to correct misconceptions about marihuana that tend to become codified in the kind of laws that call for unrealistically severe penalties. The following facts concerning the pharmacology of marihuana seem to be most significant, insofar as formulation of social policy is concerned:

1. Marihuana in small doses is a mild intoxicant similar to alcohol in some respects.

2. Much larger doses may induce perceptual changes, but these are weak compared to those induced by LSD and other hallucinogens.

3. Marihuana is not a narcotic, and its use does not induce an opiate-type dependence nor lead directly to heroin addiction.

4. Marihuana intoxication does not cause immoral, violent, or antisocial behavior, even when its use helps to loosen inhibitions, slow down thinking, and impair judgment to some extent.

Lysergic Acid Diethylamide (LSD) and other Hallucinogens

TERMINOLOGY

Certain *psychotropic* (*mind-affecting*) drugs besides those already discussed are also often abused (see Table 4-2). These drugs have been widely publicized, mainly because they can produce dramatic changes in consciousness even when taken in small *nontoxic* amounts. They are commonly called *hallucinogens*, *psychotomimetics*, and *psychedelics*, or are often tagged with other names. None of these terms is entirely satisfactory for describing all that these agents may do, but a brief review of the

TABLE 4-2 *Some Hallucinogenic or Psychotomimetic Drugs*

Belladonna alkaloids (atropine, scopolamine)
Bufotenine (from certain toads and fungi)
Diethyltryptamine (DET)
Dimethyltryptamine (DMT)
Dimethoxymethylamphetamine (DOM, STP)
Ibogaine (from certain African shrubs)
Lysergic acid diethylamide (LSD, "acid")
Mescaline (from peyote)
Morning glory seeds
Myristica (nutmeg)
Peyote (cactus buttons)
Phenylcyclidine (Sernylan)
Psilocybin and Psilocyn (from Mexican mushrooms)

terms may be useful for indicating their various possible actions.

Hallucinogen is a term that indicates the capacity of these drugs to produce changes in perception. LSD and mescaline, for example, are particularly likely to cause visual hallucinations.

Psychotomimetic is a term that suggests the ability of these drugs to cause abnormal thinking, delusions, and behavior such as that which occurs in natural psychoses. However, these drugs rarely precipitate a true psychosis such as schizophrenia.

Psychedelic is a term that means "mind-expanding." Its use is meant to imply that these drugs can open a person's mind to new insights and increase his creativity. Actually, however, this kind of euphoric effect is relatively rare.

Although no one term is adequately descriptive, we can say in summary that these drugs are capable of producing changes in: (1) perception, (2) thought, (3) mood, and (4) behavior.

LYSERGIC ACID DIETHYLAMIDE

LSD, a semisynthetic derivative of the ergot fungus, produces profound psychologic changes when taken in only *microgram* doses. Psychiatrists have tried to use these actions in treating alcoholism and certain types of psychoneuroses. However, the drug's usefulness for any therapeutic purpose has not yet been established.

ILLICIT USE. LSD has been widely misused by people who administer the drug to themselves in order to experience altered states of consciousness. These "kick" seekers often claim that they are trying to gain greater insight into themselves and their place in the cosmic scheme of things. The drug is also said to set free creative powers and to increase sexual drive. None of these claims has been confirmed, and, in fact, objective studies of works of art produced by people under the influence of LSD indicate a marked decrease in quality.

ADVERSE PSYCHOLOGICAL EFFECTS. The mental effects of LSD are highly unpredictable. Sometimes a person may interpret the drug-induced sensory changes in ways that make him feel happy (a "good trip"). However, his next experience may be marked, not by euphoria, but by intensely disagreeable dysphoric feelings (a "bad trip"). The most common psychiatric disability is development of an acute panic reaction. Often a friend is assigned to guide the "bum tripper" through the period of several hours in which the person remains in this state of fear and bewilderment, or he may have to be protected against injuring himself by leaping from a window, running into traffic, or other dangerous behavior.

Hospitalization is, however, often necessary for patients who suffer prolonged panic reactions or even acute psychotic reactions. In such cases, treatment with the antipsychotic agent *chlorpromazine* (Thorazine) is often useful for calming the patient. The nurse reassures the often fearful or depressed patient and tries to establish a psychologically supportive relationship with him. This is necessary not only for minimizing the patient's suffering in the acute phase, but for fostering his rehabilitation following recovery. The nurse can, for example, try to help the patient recognize the adverse effects that continued drug taking can have on his life, and she can put him in touch with clinics and people who can help him with many of his problems.

Dependence of the physical kind does not develop even in those who take LSD regularly. However, some individuals become psychologically dependent upon this drug and continue to take it frequently. Many who do so become unable to study or work, and they often drop out of the larger society and into a drug-oriented subculture. However, the psychic effects of this drug are not so strong as to keep the person from rehabilitating himself. Thus, he can often be convinced that the gap between his personal values and those of society is not so great, and that he can find fulfillment by other means than the drug experience. He may then give up the drug, because he understands that its use keeps him from reaching more important goals.

PHYSICAL EFFECTS. The acute physical effects of LSD are mainly sympathomimetic in nature. The user's pupils dilate, and his heart rate and blood pressure often rise. In addition, LSD may have certain long-term effects. It has, for example, been suggested that the drug can cause breaks in chromosomes. Such damage could result in two types of adverse effects: (1) chromosomal translocation of the kind that has been detected in white blood cells could lead to leukemia; and (2) damage to germ cells (sperm or ovum) or to the cells of the fetus directly could cause birth defects in the children of parents who took LSD before pregnancy, or in the infant of a mother who took the drug during pregnancy.

Scientists, at present, disagree as to whether LSD-induced genetic abnormalities and neoplastic changes have actually occurred in humans. Although the evidence is not conclusive at this time, these reports of rearrangements in genetic material have caused concern in both doctors and in former users of LSD. Nurses talking to youngsters about drugs should discuss the possibility of these adverse effects without, however, employing the kind of scare propaganda that "turns off" today's young people.

OTHER HALLUCINOGENS

Dropouts from society who become part of the drug subculture take the attitude of "I'll try anything once." As a result, they are often hospitalized following intoxication by one or a combination of unknown drugs. Some of these agents, such as those of the belladonna-stramonium type, have been known for centuries; others are newly synthesized chemicals, about which very little information is available. We cannot discuss these drugs in detail here, but a brief description of the effects of a few may serve as examples of the problems created by their abuse.

Mescaline is the psychoactive alkaloid of the cactus plant, peyote. Taken in capsule form or dissolved in a drink, the crystalline powder extracted from the crude cactus causes mainly visual hallucinations, spatial distortions, and intensified color patterns, particularly when the user keeps his eyes closed. This drug does not ordinarily induce disorientation and loss of insight. However, discomforting effects similar to those seen with an overdose of epinephrine or other sympathomimetic drugs often occur. These include anxiety, heart palpitations, sweating and dilated pupils.

Belladonna, *stramonium*, and other drugs of the "nightshade" family have long been known to be capable of causing disorientation, confusion, hallucinations, and delirium. Many synthetic drugs also exert central and peripheral effects similar to those of *atropine* and *scopolamine*, the main alkaloids of these plants. Because proprietary products of this type are being abused, nurses should recognize the typical signs and symptoms of *anticholinergic* drug toxicity as described in Chapter 22 and be prepared to help handle such cases of acute behavioral toxicity.

DOM (dimethoxymethylamphetamine) is a potent hallucinogen that appears periodically on the drug scene. It is also known as *STP*, initials said to stand for "serenity, tranquility, and peace." Actually, the drug, which is a derivative of amphetamine with the effects of LSD and atropine, has often caused prolonged acute panic reactions. The adverse psychological effects and such physical disturbances as the rapid heart rate may be made worse by the administration of the antipsychotic tranquilizer *chlorpromazine* (Thorazine). Instead, such sedatives as *pentobarbital* (Nembutal), *chlordiazepoxide* (Librium) and *chloral hydrate* are recommended for calming the agitated patient and inducing sleep.

S U M M A R Y of Nursing Measures in Preventing and Treating Drug Addiction

1. Nurses play an important part, not only in the management of addicted patients during withdrawal, but also in preventing drug abuse in various ways, including participation in efforts to educate the public. Thus, you must keep your knowledge of both the effects of dependence-producing drugs and of the social issues involved as factually correct and up-to-date as possible.

2. Prevention begins with the nurse herself, who should never take a dose of a prescription drug that has not been specifically ordered for her by a doctor. (The ready availability of dependence-producing drugs is a hazard to many health professionals.)

3. Prevention of medically induced addiction is one of the nurse's responsibilities. Thus, she should employ measures to lessen the likelihood that patients who are in chronic pain will become dependent upon potent analgesics and hypnotics.

4. Prevention also involves measures to keep addicts from obtaining addicting drugs and medical supplies illicitly. Thus, for example, it is necessary to prevent illegal diversion of narcotics by keeping an accurate account of all drugs that are stored and given to patients. Similarly, meticulous technique must be used in destroying disposable syringes and needles before throwing out into the trash.

5. Prevention of drug abuse through education of young people and their parents is part of the nurse's responsibility as a citizen in her community as well as a member of the health team. In accepting the role of adviser to parents and children and as a participant in the projects of professional teams, she should be prepared to work cooperatively with others, including doctors, teachers, social workers, clergy, and ex-addicts.

The school nurse down through the elementary school level has a particularly heavy responsibility for initiating programs and exerting leadership in getting others involved in programs to prevent drug abuse through educational activities.

Pediatric clinic nurses can initiate realistic group discussions involving both children and parents.

6. Establish a supportive relationship with the addict during the detoxification period, as the help that he receives in this phase of treatment may favorably affect his attitudes in the later stages of his rehabilitation.

7. Be sensitively aware of your own attitudes toward drug addiction and abuse. Conveying a feeling of respect for the addict and concern for him and indicating your desire to help him may strengthen his determination to stay off drugs; if he feels that you are condescending or that you condemn him, his motivation may be weakened.

8. Reduce the addict's physical discomfort and psychic distress during withdrawal. Back rubs and warm blankets help to relax cramped and aching muscles; talking to him lessens his anxiety. Be firm in setting limits.

9. Do what is necessary to guard against the patient's obtaining drugs illicitly during detoxification but do so in a straightforward manner, not by stealthy observation that may irritate or humiliate him.

S U M M A R Y of Major Drug Withdrawal Syndromes

Opiate Abstinence Signs and Symptoms

Mild Reaction
Running nose and eyes; sweating; yawning.

Moderate Reaction
Loss of appetite.
Muscular contractions ("kicking the habit").
Dilated pupils.
Gooseflesh ("cold turkey").

*Severe Reaction**
Sleeplessness, or sleep marked by constant restlessness.

Shivering with cold, alternating with hot flashes and fever.
Nausea, retching, vomiting, diarrhea.
Rapid, irregular breathing.
Heart palpitations and high blood pressure.

General Depressant† Abstinence Signs and Symptoms

Minor Manifestations
Restlessness, nervousness, anxiety and insomnia.
Tremulousness, muscular twitching, weakness.
Abdominal cramps, nausea and vomiting.

* This is relatively rare today because: (1) heroin in the highly diluted form generally available does not ordinarily lead to high physical dependence and severe withdrawal sickness and (2) methadone substitution and withdrawal results in a mild, though more prolonged, illness.

† Withdrawals of sedative-hypnotics and minor tranquilizers. (See Chapter 8 for Alcohol Withdrawal Syndrome.)

Major Manifestations
Convulsive seizures of the grand mal type, or status epilepticus occasionally,
Confusion, disorientation, hallucinations.

Delusions and delirium.
Motor agitation, high fever, cardiovascular collapse.

SUMMARY of Drug Abuse Signs and Symptoms

Opiates

Early Effects
Face flushed; skin warm, moist and itchy.
Nausea and vomiting may occur.
Drifts in drowsy, dreamlike state, the "high."
Restlessness and excitement sometimes occur, however.
Pupils constricted to "pinpoint" size.

Late Effects
Overdose may cause coma, pulmonary edema, cardiovascular collapse, or respiratory failure.
Chronic cases have needle marks, scars ("tracks"), sores and abscesses on skin.
Medical complications may include thrombophlebitis, hepatitis, endocarditis, and tetanus.

Barbiturates and Other Sedative-Hypnotics and Tranquilizers

Moderate intoxication
Understanding and judgment impaired.
Speech slurred, slow, and confused.
Difficulty in walking (may stagger).
Appearance often unkempt or untidy.
Irritable, easily upset; may be impulsive in behavior.

Severe intoxication
A period of confusion, excitement, and delirium may be followed by deep sleep, stupor, coma; breathing slow and shallow; blood pressure falls to shock levels.

Solvents (Inhalation of glues, plastic cements, gasoline, lighter fluids, aerosol mixtures, and other such substances)

Effects vary depending upon the actual chemical contents but often resemble intoxication by alcohol: drowsiness, dizziness, confusion, combativeness, motor incoordination; possible perceptual changes and hallucinations; also possible is a brief period of excitement followed by sudden cardiac arrest.

Psychomotor Stimulants (Amphetamines, and others)

Small to moderate overdosage
Nervousness, restlessness, jitteriness, irritability, and insomnia, for all of which the abuser may self-administer barbiturates; also mouth dryness, dilated pupils, heart palpitations.

Spree-type, or chronic use of large overdoses
Intensely active, talkative, and hypomanic.
Increasingly confused and disorganized.
Frightened by perceptual changes and hallucinations; possible development of delusions and paranoid feeling, thinking, and behavior.
Physical effects of failure to eat may include severe weight loss and failure of skin lesions to heal.

LSD, Mescaline, and Other Hallucinogens

Psychopharmacological Effects
Vary considerably but may include perceptual changes, mostly visual; changes in sense of body in relation to environment; emotions ranging from elation to anxiety and fear; thinking confused and disorganized.

Physical Effects
Face may be flushed or pale.
May feel cold, have gooseflesh and shiver.
Pulse rate, blood pressure, and body temperature may all be raised; pupils dilated.

Marihuana and Related Cannabis Products

Small amounts
Feeling of floating, drowsiness and relaxation; thirst, coughing, nausea, and vomiting.

Moderate to high doses
Perceptual changes, particularly distortions in time and space and increased awareness of colors and sounds; possibly visual hallucinations; occasionally confusion, anxiety, and panic; rarely, acute psychosis.

Discussion Topics: Dealing with Drug Abuse

The Situation: You are the nurse in a large pediatric clinic located in the "inner city." Many of the patients are poor and underprivileged, and illicit drugs are widely available in their neighborhoods. Although those in charge of the clinic work hard at meeting the patient's medical needs, little or nothing is being done to prevent drug abuse through education.

The Problem: Discuss

1. How you would go about setting up a drug abuse education program in the clinic
2. How you would get other members of the health team to participate in the program and support it
3. How you would draw up an overall teaching plan and how you would prepare a detailed plan for teaching one particular group, such as the mothers of youngsters between the ages of 10 and 12, or 12 and 14, or older?

The Situation: You are the school nurse in a large high school located in an affluent suburban community. Parents have become alarmed on learning how widespread drug use is among their young people who "have everything"; teachers are disturbed by signs of drug use by students on the school premises.

The Problem: Discuss

1. How you would go about initiating an educational program aimed at the students, parents and teachers of this particular group

2. How such a program of instruction would differ from one aimed at impoverished city people
3. How you would develop an overall teaching plan and how any one unit of it would work out in detail
4. What individuals and groups you would contact and try to involve in the program

The Situation: John is a 15-year-old urban slum dweller who has been taking drugs since he was 12 and has finally become "hooked" on heroin. His mother, who was deserted by John's father before the boy was born, works as an office cleaning woman. Although she says that she is worried about John, she often gets discouraged, drinks excessively, and wastes much of her meager income as well as the little time and energy she has left for John and his problems.

The Problem: Discuss

1. How you would help John to gain admission to a treatment program for young addicts
2. How you would develop a plan of nursing care for John during his first two weeks in the center for detoxication and rehabilitation
3. How you would work with John and his mother in trying to help him rehabilitate himself without the aid of drugs. (Because of John's youth, methadone maintenance therapy is not being considered at this time.)

References

Barbee, E.L. Marihuana—a social problem. *Perspectives in Psychiatric Care*, 9:5:194, 1971.

Dambacher, B. and Hellwig, K. Nursing strategies for young drug users. *Perspectives in Psychiatric Care*, 9:5:200, 1971.

Fink, M., et al. Narcotic antagonists: another approach to addiction therapy. *Amer. J. Nurs.* 71:1359, 1971 (July).

Foreman, N.J. and Zerwekk, J.V. Drug crisis intervention. *Amer. J. Nurs.* 71:1736, 1971 (Sept.).

Grinspoon, L. Marihuana reconsidered, *Harvard Univ. Press*, 1971.

Holmes, D., Appignanesi, L., and Holmes, M. The Language of Trust. New York: Science House, 1971.

Isler, C. Narcotics addicts need nurses. *RN*, 32:36, 1969 (July).

Morgan, A. J. and Moreno, J. Attitudes toward

addiction. *Amer. J. Nurs.*, 73:497, 1973 (March).

Pascarelli, E.F. Methaqualone abuse, the quiet epidemic. *JAMA* 224:1512, 1973.

Poplar, J. Characteristics of nurse addicts. *Amer. J. Nurs.*, 69:117, 1969 (January).

Rodman, M.J. Use and abuse of the amphetamines. *RN*, 33:55, 1970 (August).

———. Drugs used against addiction. *RN*, 33:71, 1970 (October).

———. Marihuana in review, *RN* 34:69, 1971 (Feb.).

Russau, E. Nursing in a narcotic detoxification unit. *Amer. J. Nurs.* 70:1720, 1970 (Aug.).

Smith, D.W., Germain, C.H., and Gips, C.D. Care of the Adult Patient, 3rd ed. Philadelphia: J.B. Lippincott, 1971.

Yolles, S.F. The drug scene. *Nurs. Outlook*, 18:24, 1970 (July).

5.

The Administration of Drugs

The Nurse's Responsibilities in Drug Therapy

The professional nurse has many responsibilities relative to the treatment of patients with drugs. One of the most important of these is the actual administration of the medication that the doctor has ordered. In addition to doing this task efficiently and safely, she must also be able to observe the patient's response to the medication and to understand the significance of what she is observing. The nurse's role also involves instructing patients concerning how to take drugs safely at home and telling them what effects they should watch for.

In this chapter we shall first indicate the sources of the several kinds of drugs administered by the nurse and later we shall discuss some of the various dosage forms that are employed and the methods by which they are administered. Finally, we shall take up some of the specific procedures employed in preparing, distributing, and administering medications in various clinical situations.

In actual practice, of course, the nurse does not follow any textbook-type checklist of things to do and not to do when preparing to administer medication to a patient. Safe practice is based primarily upon the nurse's awareness of the need to stay alert and attentive at all times. She can never simply follow procedures mechanically but must always be prepared to draw upon her knowledge of the nature of the patient's illness and of what the drug that she is administering can do to change the patient's condition for better or worse.

Nevertheless, to assure maximum safety, it does help to learn certain time-tested procedures. Once the nurse has developed effective habit patterns when preparing to administer medications, she will be better able to concentrate upon the total plan of caring for the patient. For while drug administration can never be carried out casually, it is also undesirable to be so concerned with following a detailed routine that you lose sight of the overall purposes of the patient's treatment.

Try not to become so overwhelmed by the legal and ethical responsibilities of administering drugs that tension and fear of making mistakes impair your judgment. This aspect of patient care, like any other, requires a basis of sound factual knowledge. The nurse who has acquired knowledge of the drugs that she is administering and then applies that understanding of drug action with good judgment can proceed with confidence in her ability to carry out the task of drug administration safely.

Sources of Drugs

We have already seen that people have always made use of *natural* substances in treating disease, and that for the past 150 years doctors have also been able to draw upon *synthetic* substances prepared in the laboratory. Now let's look at both these major sources of drugs a bit more closely and at the dosage forms into which they are prepared for administration to patients.

PLANT CONSTITUENTS

Until early in the last century physicians generally used crude botanical drugs or liquid extracts of their active constituents. Preparations of this kind—extracts, fluidextracts, and tinctures, for example—are called *galenicals* (after the Greek physician *Galen*, who practiced in Rome in the second century A.D.). Even though some products of this kind are still available, most doctors now prefer to use the purified crystalline chemicals that modern chemists have succeeded in isolating from the plants.* Among the most important classes of vegetable drug constituents are the alkaloids and glycosides.

* *Digitalis* and *opium tinctures,* containing the active constituents of the plant dissolved in alcohol, and fluidextracts and powdered extracts of *belladonna,* containing the active constituents of that plant in concentrated but not completely pure form, are still sometimes employed by doctors who somehow prefer these preparations rather than the more reliable pure plant principles.

Alkaloids are nitrogenous chemicals that can be extracted from various parts of many plants which are usually quite active pharmacologically. The doctor can depend upon getting a rapid, powerful action when he gives his patient a pure medicinal alkaloid; however, the danger from overdosage is also greater from these constituents than from the galenical preparations or crude drugs that contain them.

The nurse will often know that she is handling an alkaloid because its name ends in "ine"—for example, morphine, atropine, pilocarpine, strychnine. These are not, however, the only drugs with names that end in this suffix. The names of certain other natural and synthetic substances such as the adrenal hormone epinephrine and local anesthetics such as procaine bear this ending. However, despite their potency and their relationship to plant products such as ephedrine and cocaine, these substances cannot be classed correctly as alkaloids.

Glycosides are active plant principles containing a sugar such as glucose in the molecule. Actually, it is the noncarbohydrate portion of the molecule, or aglycone (genin), that accounts for its pharmacological activity. However, in the case of the digitalis glycosides (medically, the most important of the drugs of this class), the sugar portion of the molecule is very important because it permits the aglycone to penetrate into cardiac muscle cells and exert its stimulating effect on myocardial function. The glycoside digitoxin is a thousand times more potent in this respect than the powdered digitalis leaf. Interestingly, it is now cheaper for a heart patient to be maintained on this purified crystalline glycoside than on the crude drug itself. The names of the official glycosides usually end in "in," such as digoxin, digitoxin, strophanthin.

Other types of substances obtained from plants and still used in medicine are:

Fixed oils, such as olive oil and castor oil

Volatile oils, such as peppermint, spearmint, and clove that are used for flavoring

Gums, mucilaginous masses, such as those from agar and psyllium seed that are used as laxatives; or other substances used in soothing skin lotions or as pharmaceutical suspending agents—for example, acacia and tragacanth

Resins, substances like pine tree rosin, some of which act as local irritants when applied to the skin or taken internally (such as podophyllum and others)

Tannins from the bark of trees, including

tannic acid, a substance that antidotes poisons while they are still in the stomach. Tannins precipitate protein to form a protective covering over burn surfaces; they also act as local astringents.

ANIMAL DRUGS

The organs of animals were once used in medicine on a mystical basis. Today, some of our most potent drugs are obtained by extraction from animal tissues, for use as substitutes for human glandular secretions that may be lacking. The hormone insulin, which is used in treating diabetes, is an active principle from animal pancreas; corticotropin (ACTH) is isolated from the pituitary glands of animals that are slaughtered for food. The thyroid glands of animals are dried, defatted, and powdered for use in replacement, or substitution, therapy of hypothyroid patients. Recently, the pituitary glands of human corpses have been employed for extracting the human growth hormone (HGH) which is more effective than animal-derived somatotrophin for treatment of certain types of dwarfism.

INORGANIC CHEMICALS

Some elements such as sulfur and iodine and the salts of metals such as iron have long been used in medicine. The salts of silver and mercury are still employed as antiseptics and disinfectants. Clays such as kaolin and attapulgite are ingredients of certain products for treating diarrhea, and aluminum hydroxide and the phosphate salt of that metal are used for counteracting excessive amounts of hydrochloric acid in the upper gastrointestinal tract. The hydroxide of magnesium also is used for digestive disorders, as both an antacid and laxative, and salts of the same mineral—the sulfate and the citrate—are employed as saline cathartics. Most recently, the radioactive isotopes of inorganic substances such as gold, phosphorus, and iodine have come into use in the diagnosis and treatment of disease.

SYNTHETIC ORGANIC CHEMICALS

Most potent drugs available today originated in the laboratories of synthetic chemists. In most cases these substances never existed before they were prepared in the laboratory. Such chemicals become drugs only after they have undergone intensive study, first in animals and

later in humans, to prove that they are safe and effective enough to be used in modern medical practice.

Other substances that are available in nature can now often be made more cheaply by chemical synthesis. Thus, for example, it is less costly to make the adrenal corticosteroids synthetically from cheap, readily available chemicals than to extract and purify the tiny quantities that must be laboriously extracted from the adrenal glands of animals. Synthetic versions of natural chemicals can also now be prepared that are more pure than the best extracts available. The uterine stimulant *oxytocin* that is now prepared synthetically is, for example, free of impurities found in the preparations of that substance extracted from the posterior pituitary glands of animals.

Routes of Administration of Drugs

The manner in which a drug is administered is one of the most important factors influencing its action. Depending upon how a dose of a drug is given, it may produce a profound effect or none at all. Thus, when a solution of magnesium sulfate (Epsom Salts) is taken by mouth, it acts only within the intestine to exert a cathartic effect; when the same magnesium salt is injected intramuscularly, its molecules reach the central nervous system and produce deep depression.

We shall review briefly the main routes by which drugs are administered so that they can enter the systemic circulation and exert their effects on the distant tissues that have the capacity to react to them. At the same time, we shall offer some information about the *dosage forms* in which drugs are available. However, we will not attempt to take up in detail the techniques for administering medications by various routes, since these are presented in texts on the fundamentals of nursing; nor shall we discuss the ways in which the various solid and liquid dosage forms are put together, since such aspects of pharmaceutical preparations come within the province of the pharmacist rather than the nurse.

ORAL ADMINISTRATION

The best way to give drugs, whenever possible, is by mouth. This is the simplest, safest, and least expensive way to get a drug into the patient's body and on its way into his bloodstream and other tissues. Thus, except for some poorly absorbable substances such as insulin, most drugs are available in dosage forms suitable for oral administration (see below).

Some drugs tend to irritate the lining of the gastrointestinal tract. To avoid nausea and vomiting, these drugs are best administered after meals or with a small amount of food. For example, patients receiving high doses of salicylates for treating acute rheumatic fever should receive milk and crackers or some other snack to lessen salicylate-induced gastrointestinal irritation.

When a patient is already nauseated or vomiting, anything that is given by mouth may make him vomit even more. In such cases, it is desirable to check with the doctor as to whether an ordered dose of oral medication may be omitted. If the patient's vomiting is persistent, the physician may order the drug to be given by injection or rectally in order to avoid its being lost through vomiting or to prevent further irritation of the upper gastrointestinal tract. A discussion with the physician can clarify the issue of route of administration. For instance, if the patient sometimes experiences nausea, the drug may be ordered to be given orally if tolerated, or parenterally, if necessary, thereby facilitating the nurse's use of judgment as situation requires.

Enteric-coated tablets or capsules are intended to delay the release of drugs that might cause nausea or vomiting if they come in contact with the stomach lining in high concentrations. The coating is insoluble in stomach acids, but once the tablet passes into the upper part of the intestine it dissolves in the alkaline secretions there. Occasionally, however, the enteric coating may fail to dissolve, and the drug may then pass out of the intestinal tract without being absorbed.

The absorption of some drugs may be delayed when they are taken with food, or a large part of the dose may even be destroyed by digestive secretions. In such cases, the drug is best administered between meals or even by injection. Most oral penicillin products, for example, are best given before rather than after meals for this reason, in order to be sure that enough will be absorbed to attain therapeutic levels of the antibiotic in the infected tissues. In truly severe infections the oral route is not employed at all; instead, the antibiotic is given by injection.

Prolonged-action tablets and capsules are available for reducing the number of doses the patient has to remember to take. Patients are often more likely to get the benefits of the orally administered drugs prescribed for them when they have to take the medication only twice a day rather than four to six times daily. Thus, doctors sometimes prescribe drugs in the form of Spansules, Gradumets, or other sustained-release medications that need be taken only once every 12 hours or so. An important point for the nurse to remember is that these products—unlike regular tablets that are sometimes crushed and mixed with jelly or jam for children—should never be tampered with in any way. Pouring out the pellets and breaking them up could result in rapid absorption of an overdose.

OTHER ORAL DOSAGE FORMS. Drugs are available for oral administration in many solid and liquid dosage forms. *Tablets* made by compressing powdered or granulated drugs into a compact, readily swallowed form are currently the most common type. A well-made tablet breaks up quickly in the stomach into a finely divided powder that is readily absorbed. In this respect, tablets are much more reliable than pills, which often dry out during storage and then fail to disintegrate in the G.I. tract. (Even though pills are rarely employed today, the term still persists—for example, oral contraceptives are called popularly the "Pill" even though these products all come in tablet form.)

Powders also are relatively rare today and are limited mainly to products for relief of gastrointestinal distress. Perhaps people are impressed by the ritual of pouring a measured amount of a fine powder or rough granules into a quantity of water, stirring as the powder dissolves with effervescence, and then drinking the solution. Such bulky effervescent antacids and laxatives are today being made available more frequently as big tablets that form a bubbling solution, which is apparently just as effective and psychologically satisfying as the older form.

Liquid dosage forms for oral use are popular because they are palatable and easy to take. The vehicles, or solvents for the medication, are usually pleasantly flavored liquids such as syrups or elixirs. *Syrups* are solutions of sugar in water to which various types of flavors are added, such as cherry, licorice, or chocolate. *Elixirs* are hydroalcoholic liquids flavored with volatile oils and slightly sweetened. Adults often prefer these clear liquids—the cough preparation Elixir of Terpin Hydrate and Codeine is an example—to cough mixtures with a heavy viscous syrup base.

Children, on the other hand, do like to take syrupy liquids. It is probably better for the child to enjoy the taste of the syrup in which a bitter or salty substance is dissolved than to have him gag or struggle against efforts to give him undisguised medication. However, advertising that puts too much emphasis on palatability can be dangerous. Children who have been conditioned in this way are likely to take the entire contents of a bottle of medication and become seriously ill. Poisoning from iron-containing antianemia products or cough and cold products containing antihistamines and aspirin has sometimes occurred in this way (Chapter 3).

Emulsions are pharmaceutical mixtures of oil and water that also offer the advantage of palatability. Oily liquids such as mineral oil and cod liver oil lose their unpleasantly bland or fishy taste when the oil is dispersed in water in tiny droplets with the aid of an emulsifying agent. On the other hand, insoluble mineral substances, such as magnesium oxide, are suspended in only a watery liquid as *gels* or *magmas*—for example, Milk (magma) of Magnesia and aluminum hydroxide gel, antacid products that are used in treating peptic ulcer. Such preparations should always be shaken well before use.

PARENTERAL ADMINISTRATION

The term parenteral means by any route other than the enteral, or gastrointestinal, tract. Taken literally, the term includes methods that involve getting a drug into the bloodstream by way of the lungs or through the mucous membranes of the mouth, etc. However, as ordinarily used, parenteral routes refer only to the various ways by which drugs are given as *injections*.

INJECTION OF DRUGS. Injection of drugs is preferred when it is important that all of the drug be absorbed as rapidly and completely as possible or at a steady, controlled rate. However, despite the efficiency with which high blood levels of a drug can be quickly attained and also sometimes be maintained for prolonged periods, parenteral administration has various drawbacks and disadvantages. Injectable medications that come in sterile ampules, vials, or plastic syringes are relatively expensive compared to oral dosage forms; and, of course, the patient usually also has to bear the expense of paying for the skilled person needed to make the injection.

Injection of drugs requires skill and special care, because parenteral administration is more hazardous than the oral dosage form. This is mainly the result of the rapidity and efficiency with which drugs are absorbed from most injection sites. The effect of overdosage resulting from an error in calculating and measuring the dose or in administering it is much more likely to prove disastrous when the drug is given parenterally. Once the drug is injected, it is usually difficult—and, in some situations, impossible—to keep it from being fully absorbed and from producing all of its effects, including adverse ones.

Injections may be painful, cause local tissue damage, or permit the entrance of infectious microorganisms. However, all of these difficulties can be kept to a minimum by the use of proper equipment and procedures. For example, an injection need not hurt if the needle is sharp and is inserted and withdrawn quickly, except, of course, when the injected solution is itself irritating to the tissues. Similarly, infection is unlikely when the medication is furnished in sterile form, the patient's skin is properly cleansed, and the sterility of needles and syringes is assured. The nurse, as she learns the technical details of injection procedures, also learns all the practices and rules that ensure maximum safety. However, we have left to the textbooks of nursing fundamentals the full discussion of all the technical procedures involved in preparing for safe and effective parenteral administration.

Parenteral administration employs various routes. Some—such as the subcutaneous, intramuscular, intraperitoneal, and intravenous routes—are used when a drug's systemic actions are desired; others—for example, intracutaneous and intrasynovial injections—are employed for achieving local effects with minimal generalized activity. Some significant aspects of the more commonly employed parenteral methods of administering drugs will now be discussed.

Subcutaneous, or *hypodermic,* injections are made into the loose connective tissue underneath the skin (both the above Latin and the Greek-derived terms mean exactly that). Soluble drugs deposited at sites such as the outer surface of the arm or the front of the thigh are rapidly absorbed into the blood ordinarily, and the drug's effects come on promptly. However, if the patient is in shock, this route is undesirable because the sluggish circulation slows the drug's absorption. The drug solution is best delivered directly into the bloodstream by intravenous injection ("I.V.") in such situations.

Not all drugs are suited to subcutaneous injection. Since no more than 2 ml can ordinarily be deposited at such sites, the drugs given in this way must be highly soluble and potent enough to be effective in small volume. (Epinephrine, morphine, and insulin are commonly administered in this manner.) The subcutaneous tissues contain nerve endings that transmit pain impulses when the injected solutions are irritating. Sometimes sterile abscesses develop as a result of chemical irritation, and the tissues may become necrotic and slough off. Thus, the I.V. route is preferred for irritating drug solutions, although some are now also administered by deep intramuscular injection.

The rate of absorption from subcutaneous injection sites can sometimes be slowed when a more prolonged action is desired. Addition of the vasoconstrictor epinephrine to local anesthetic solutions, for example, keeps the desired action localized and reduces the likelihood of systemic toxicity from too rapid absorption. Substances such as insulin may be suspended in a protein colloid solution, and heparin and corticotropin may be administered in gelatin solutions, to reduce the rate of absorption and thus prolong their action. Application of an icebag above the site of subcutaneous injection slows absorption still further, as does application of a tourniquet in cases in which a reaction occurs.

Intramuscular injections are made with a longer, heavier needle that penetrates past the subcutaneous tissues and permits the drug solution or suspension to be deposited deep between the layers of muscle masses. Watery drug solutions spread over a larger area than when injected subcutaneously, and absorption is even more rapid than by the latter route. On the other hand, finely divided suspensions of insoluble substances are only very slowly absorbed when deposited in an intramuscular depot. Thus, this route is employed for administering the long-acting esters of sex hormones and corticosteroid drugs or poorly soluble salts, such as benzathine penicillin G and procaine penicillin G, which are absorbed over periods of days or even exert their antibacterial effects for weeks.

The intramuscular injection site contains fewer sensory nerve endings than the subcutaneous sites, so that I.M. injections tend to be less painful. However, with irritating substances, a small amount of the local anesthetics procaine or xylocaine is often added to the injection solution. Irritation is less likely to lead to tissue necrosis deep in the muscle than when irritants are placed under the skin. However, the danger of inadvertent intravenous injection is greater when the needle is placed deep down into these more vascular muscular tissues. Thus, it is essential—especially with oily suspensions of insoluble particles—to ascertain that the needle has not entered a blood vessel by pulling up the plunger after inserting the needle. If blood is aspirated and appears in the syringe, the needle is withdrawn and the injection is given at another site. Care is also taken to avoid injury to the sciatic nerve in making injections into the gluteal muscles. (See texts dealing with the technique of intramuscular injection.)

Intravenous injection bypasses all barriers to drug absorption. As a result, this is the most rapidly effective and, at the same time, the most dangerous route of administration. For, once a drug is placed directly into the bloodstream it cannot be recalled, nor can its action be slowed by tourniquets or other means. Thus, every effort must be made to avoid errors and to detect early signs of adverse reactions. This route is usually reserved for the emergency administration of potent drugs when very rapid action is required, as in the use of epinephrine for anaphylactic shock or norepinephrine for circulatory collapse.

Sometimes substances that would be very irritating to subcutaneous and intramuscular tissues (highly alkaline sulfonamide sodium salt solutions, for example) are given by slow I.V. injection, since they do not harm the inner lining of the veins. Care is taken to avoid leakage of such solutions into the surrounding tissues, because pain, sterile abscesses, and necrotic sloughing can develop if highly irritating substances or potent local vasoconstrictors such as norepinephrine extravasate.

Infusions of large amounts of fluid are often made by venoclysis to overcome dehydration and to supply nutritive substances if patients are unable to take fluids or foods orally. The technique of inserting the needle into the vein under sterile conditions is similar to that used when small quantities of drug solutions are injected. In this case, however, the nurse must adjust the rate of flow and see that it is kept at the speed that the doctor ordered in order to avoid overloading the patient's circulation and, at the same time, to assure an adequately rapid flow of fluids and electrolytes. The nurse now often monitors the patient's central venous pressure (C.V.P.) to avoid the danger of overhydration and pulmonary edema.

Intrathecal or *intraspinal* injections are made by doctors trained in these special techniques. Spinal anesthesia is accomplished by careful placement of a local anesthetic solution in the subarachnoid space. Similarly, antiinfective drugs are sometimes injected intrathecally in the treatment of meningitis to attain a high local concentration of an antibiotic or sulfonamide which does not readily penetrate the subdural and other membranes by way of the bloodstream.

Intradermal or *intracutaneous* injections are made for local rather than systemic effects. Injection of a small amount of solution just below the surface of the skin promptly produces a wheal which delays further absorption into the lymphatics. Local anesthetics are sometimes injected in this way and further deeper injections are then made through the superficially deadened tissues. Tuberculin testing and allergic sensitization tests are also carried out by this method of pricking the skin or by scratching the material into the upper skin surfaces.

Intraarticular and *intralesional* injections are methods employed mainly to attain high local concentrations of corticosteroid drugs within inflamed joints and skin lesions without much danger of causing systemic steroid toxicity. It is important for the physician to employ aseptic procedures to avoid joint infections. Patients must be warned not to overuse the injected joint when their pain is relieved, as this may lead to deterioration of the joint.

APPLICATION TO SKIN AND MUCOUS MEMBRANES. Drugs are often applied to the skin and to the mucous membranes of the mouth and throat, the nose and other parts of the respiratory tract, the eyes, and the genitourinary and gastrointestinal tracts. In the case of the skin, such applications are almost always intended to have only a local effect and any systemic absorption that occurs is only incidental and unintended. On the other hand, drugs are sometimes brought into contact with the mucosa of the mouth and rectum as a means of getting them into the bloodstream

when swallowing the agents is undesirable or impossible. The dosage forms that are administered for both systemic mucosal absorption and local dermatomucosal drug effects will be briefly discussed here.

Sublingual tablets are placed under the tongue and *buccal* tablets between the gums and the cheek in order to attain therapeutic concentrations of certain drugs in distant tissues. The drugs administered in these ways are agents that either tend to be destroyed by the digestive juices (for example, the polypeptide hormone oxytocin) or, even if absorbed, are so rapidly detoxified by liver enzymes that high plasma levels are difficult to attain rapidly by the oral route. Glyceryl trinitrate (nitroglycerin) is a drug of the latter type: when a nitroglycerin tablet is placed under the tongue, it is so rapidly dissolved and absorbed by way of the venous capillaries beneath the tongue that its therapeutic effects on the heart of a person suffering anginal pains are usually felt in one to five minutes.

Patients taking sublingual tablets must be instructed in their proper use. They are told not to chew or swallow the tablet and not to take water with it but simply to place it under the tongue and let it dissolve. Buccal tablets are best placed next to the upper molar teeth, and the patient is instructed to avoid disturbing the dosage form after it is placed in the parabuccal space. As with sublingual tablets, the patient avoids eating, chewing, drinking, or smoking, lest the tablet be swallowed and destroyed instead of being absorbed by way of the mucosa of the buccal pouch between gums and cheek.

The mucous membranes of the mouth and throat are often treated with local applications of antiseptic, anesthetic, and astringent drugs. The public is subjected to a good deal that is obviously nonsense in advertisements for nonprescription mouth washes, gargles, throat lozenges or troches, and medicated chewing gums, and much of the folklore of mouth and throat therapy must be discounted. However, oral hygiene is an important part of patient care. Thus, the nurse should be familiar with the principles of mouth cleaniness.

The throat is sometimes sprayed with local anesthetics during surgical or diagnostic procedures. In this way, sensory receptors are deadened to avoid gagging and thus permit passage of instruments such as endotracheal tubes, laryngoscopes and bronchoscopes. Topically applied anesthetics may be absorbed systemically in amounts that can prove toxic; thus, the doctor may ask the nurse to record the amounts of solution being employed in this way, in order to be sure that, in the administration of the drug, safe amounts are not exceeded.

The nasal mucosa is commonly treated with drug solutions applied as sprays, nose drops, and tampons. Among the drugs applied in this way are decongestants for opening blocked nasal passages and hemostatics to stop nosebleeds. Here, too, the public is often led to expect too much from such topical application, with the result that nonprescription preparations are misused in ways that can prove harmful. The nurse should be familiar with the correct procedure for instilling drops into the nose so that they do not pass wastefully down into the throat. Systemic absorption of the drugs contained in nasal medications can have adverse effects on the cardiovascular and the central nervous systems.

Drugs may also be purposely applied to the nasal mucosa in order to produce systemic effects. The polypeptide hormones of the posterior pituitary gland, *vasopressin* and *oxytocin*, are sometimes administered this way, as they would be digested if taken by mouth. Patients with diabetes insipidus, for example, often take vasopressin in the form of snuff. Similarly, the synthetic form of oxytocin is now also available as a spray that is absorbed into the systemic circulation when applied intranasally. Among drug abusers, "snowbirds" often sniff cocaine and early experimenters with heroin sometimes begin by "snorting" it.

INHALATION. Drugs are also administered by inhalation into the deeper respiratory tract passages both to attain high local concentrations and for their systemic effects. Locally active drugs include the mucolytic detergents, enzymes, and other substances employed to liquefy thick secretions obstructing the bronchi. Drugs that are intended to pass through the thin lining of the lung surfaces include not only oxygen and volatile general anesthetics, such as ether, but also bronchodilator drugs such as epinephrine and isoproterenol. Unfortunately, the systemic actions of these drugs are not limited to the respiratory tract. Isoproterenol can cause serious cardiac irregularities, and epinephrine also has unwanted systemic effects, including a tendency to make patients jittery and tremulous. Other drugs that are occasionally inhaled for the rapid

relief that their systemic actions offer are the coronary vasodilator drug, amyl nitrite, which is used by angina pectoris patients, and ergotamine, which is now sometimes given in this way to abort a migraine headache.

Rectal administration of drugs in the form of enema solutions and glycerinated gelatin or cocoa-butter-based suppositories are commonly employed for local effects as well as a means of getting drugs into the systemic circulation when the oral route cannot or should not be used. The nurse is often responsible for administering medications rectally in a manner that facilitates their absorption from the mucosa of the lower G.I. tract.

The best time for administering drugs rectally is immediately after the patient has moved his bowels. The lower tract may be emptied by administering an evacuant enema or by the use of suppositories that act locally to set off the defecation reflex. After the lower bowel has been cleansed, the suppository or the retention enema containing the dose of the drug for systemic absorption and action is inserted, and the patient is kept lying down for at least 20 minutes in the case of a suppository and about half an hour for an enema. If the patient gets up too soon, the unmelted suppository may be evacuated or the unabsorbed enema fluid may be expelled. The patient should lie still and breathe deeply to help prevent loss of the medication.

One of the drugs commonly administered rectally is aminophylline, a substance that often causes gastric distress when given by mouth. It must be noted, however, that this drug—like the organic mercurial suppositories, which are also given in this way—many cause rectal irritation in some patients. Solutions are less likely to cause local irritation and proctitis because they are absorbed more rapidly and completely than is the material erratically released from suppository bases. On the other hand, the amount of fluid that can be retained is relatively small, and the more rapidly absorbed drug may have too fleeting an action.

Rectal administration of depressant drugs is sometimes employed to put children to sleep prior to general anesthesia with other agents. Thiopental sodium, for example, is available as a rectal suspension for producing preanesthetic hypnosis or basal narcosis and is administered by the use of a disposable plastic syringe and applicator. Antiemetic drugs such as prochlorperazine (Compazine) are commonly administered as rectal suppositories, since the vomiting patient may not be able to retain these drugs when they are given by mouth.

In the *genitourinary tract*, medication is usually intended for local effect, but drugs can reach the systemic circulation by being absorbed from the urethral or vaginal mucosa. Dangerously high plasma concentrations of local anesthetics, for example, have been reached when solutions were instilled into a traumatized urethra prior to passage of a sound or a cystoscope. Urethral suppositories containing soothing substances are sometimes employed after dilatation or other painful procedures. Vaginal suppositories containing estrogens combined with antiinfective drugs are applied in vaginitis, and irrigating solutions, or douches, are sometimes instilled to cleanse and acidify the vaginal mucosa.

The *skin* is treated mainly with liquid lotions and liniments and with semisolid ointments and pastes containing oily bases such as petrolatum or lanolin, or water-miscible bases such as surface-active, or wetting, agents. The dermatologist chooses the dosage form and bases that are best suited for application to the particular area and skin condition which require treatment. The nature of the most common dermatological disorders and the drugs and dosage forms used for relief of skin symptoms are more fully discussed in chapter 46.

Drugs are not ordinarily absorbed through the skin, though poisoning from certain insecticides and by the liquid alkaloid nicotine has occurred in this way. The advertising for some creams that are rubbed on the skin to relieve arthritic pain suggests that their active ingredients are absorbed into the joints. However, whatever effects such products may have (in addition to those that are psychological) are limited mainly to the local skin areas to which they are applied.

The fact that the skin acts as a barrier is an advantage when the corticosteroid drugs are applied to the skin to relieve the symptoms of local inflammation. Applied as ointments, creams, lotions and aerosols, these steroid drugs relieve itching, oozing, and other discomfort without causing their characteristic systemic toxicity. Care is required, however, when corticosteroid preparations are applied to large areas of skin, particularly when occlusive dressings are employed. In such cases, the steroid cream is applied only sparingly before covering the area with the flexible, nonporous plastic film.

Lotions and ointments are best applied in small amounts to avoid both waste and messiness. Applications are made gently, by patting rather than rubbing, in order to avoid damaging irritated, inflamed areas. A firm stroke is desirable, since too lightly dabbing the pruritic skin tends to increase itchiness. If the preparation is one that stains clothing, the patient should be warned about it and advised to avoid having the medication come in contact with his clothing or, if this is not possible, to wear old clothes during the treatment period. Ointments should be removed from jars with a tongue blade and never with the fingers in order to avoid contaminating the remainder of the contents.

Compresses are moist dressings made by soaking sterile towels in plain water or in solutions of chemicals such as potassium permanganate or aluminum acetate that exert astringent and drying effects when the cloths are wrung out and applied to oozing skin lesions. Poultices are mainly home remedies made by mixing absorptive substances such as bread crumbs or linseed meal or kaolin with boiling water or glycerin. The moist mass is then spread on inflamed skin areas to keep constant heat on the affected part.

The Task of Administering Medications

In this section we shall discuss some of the specific procedures involved in carrying out the doctor's orders for medication. This involves obtaining the drug, storing and accounting for it, and, sometimes, preparing dilutions of drug solutions before delivering the medication to the patient and administering it. Thus, to carry out this aspect of patient care efficiently and safely, the nurse needs more than mere technical competence in administering medications. She must also be able to work together with other members of the health team —physicians, pharmacists, and other nursing and allied medical personnel—who share many of the tasks involved in assuring efficient and safe drug treatment for the patient.

MEDICATION ORDERS AND PRESCRIPTIONS

Orders for medication originate with a doctor or other licensed practitioner. In the hospital, orders may be written on the patient's chart or in a special medication book or file. Patients seen by the doctor in his office or at home receive prescriptions that they or their nurse then have filled at a local pharmacy.

No medication should ever be administered without a doctor's order. Ordinarily, all orders are written but, in an emergency, the doctor may order medication by telephone and later sign or initial the order that the nurse has written down. When the doctor is present but wants to hurry away without writing his oral order, it is entirely proper to insist that he write it down and initial it.

Every effort should be made to set up an efficient system for handling medicine orders. A common cause of medication errors is poor communication. Sometimes the doctor simply forgets to write an order on the patient's chart, after telling him that he was going to give him something for pain or some other symptom. Occasionally, a combination of a physician's poor handwriting and a nurse's limited knowledge of drug names or abbreviations

(Table 5-1) leads to the wrong drug's being ordered.

The nurse should be certain that she really understands the physician's directions concerning medication. Illegible and incomplete written orders require the physician's correction before they can be carried out. The best insurance against errors of this kind is for the nurse to have a thorough knowledge of the patient's illness and of the drugs that are ordinarily used in treating it and to insist upon carefully written medication orders.

Prescriptions are written in a traditional form that tells the pharmacist what drug the doctor wants and the amount of the dosage form to be dispensed. The pharmacist is also directed to type the patient's directions for taking the drug on the label. These tell the patient how much of the medication he is to take and at what intervals. Often, however, the directions are quite skimpy so the nurse

---

TABLE 5-1   *Some Abbreviations Commonly Employed in Prescription Orders*

Abbreviation	Latin Derivation	Meaning
aa	ana	of each
a.c.	ante cibos	before meals
ad lib.	ad libitum	as freely, or as often, as is desired
Aq. (dest)	aqua (destillata)	water (distilled)
b.i.d.	bis in die	twice a day
c̄	cum	with
Caps.	capsula	capsule
Chart.	chartula	a medicated powder in a paper wrapping
Comp.	compositus	compound
dil.	dilutus	dilute
d.t.d.	dentur tales doses (no.)	give as many doses as indicated by the number
dis.	dispensa	dispense
elix.	elixir	elixir
ext.	extractum	extract
et	et	and
F, or ft.	Fac. or fiat	make; let be made
Flext.	fluidextractum	fluidextract
Gm.	gramma	gram
gr.	granum	grain
gtt.	gutta	a drop
h.	hora	hour
h.s.	hora somni	at bedtime
M.	misce	mix
non rep.	non repetatur	do not repeat
no.	numerus	number
noct.	nox, noctis	night
o	omnis	every
o.d.	omni die	every day

TABLE 5-1 *(Continued)*

Abbreviation	Latin Derivation	Meaning
o.d.	oculus dexter	right eye
o.h.	omni hora	every hour
o.s.	oculus sinister	left eye
os	os	mouth
pil.	pilula	pill
p.c.	post cibos	after meals
p.r.n.	pro re nata	literally, as the occasion arises; occasionally; when it seems to be desirable or necessary
q. or qq	quaque	every
q.h. or qqh	quaque hora	every hour
q. or qqd.	quaque die	every day
q.i.d.	quater in die	four times a day
q.s.	quantum sufficit	a sufficient amount
℞	recipe	take
s̄	sine	without
s.o.s.	si opus sit	if needed
S. or Sig.	signa	write (on the label)
Sp.	spiritus	spirit
sol.	solutio	solution
ss	semis	half
stat.	statim	immediately
Syr.	syrypus	syrup
tab.	tabella	tablet
t.i.d.	ter in die	three times a day
Tr.	tinctura	tincture
Ung.	unguentum	ointment
ut dict.	ut dictum	as directed
Vin.	vinum	wine

should take every opportunity to discuss this with the patient and be sure that he understands what he is supposed to do.

Today, the doctor often asks the pharmacist to put down the name of the drug on the label. If this is not done, often the patient will request it. In any case, the nurse who has to give a patient his medication should find out exactly what she is administering. When the label indicates only directions for taking the medication, the nurse should telephone the pharmacist for more information. Give him the prescription number and ask him to tell you what drug it contains and what strength it is so that you will know exactly what amount the patient is taking.

Doctors often also indicate whether they want the patient to have a prescription refilled. The pharmacist may refuse to refill a prescription that does not carry such instructions. Some prescriptions cannot be refilled at all. The *Comprehensive Drug Abuse Prevention and Control Act of 1970* (Chapter 1) sets rules that regulate the refilling of prescriptions for drugs in the several different schedules. The doctor has to write a new prescription every time he wants the patient to have potent narcotic analgesic medications.

Computerized systems now coming into use in some medical centers are helping to eliminate the kinds of errors that occur when drug orders are handled by several people. A single legible "print-out" on electronic tape takes the place of the various medication order forms, tickets, and cards that are ordinarily made out and transcribed by hand. Automation of this type clarifies communication and record keeping. The nurse is freed of such tasks as transcribing the order, procuring the drug, storing it, and recording the whole transaction.

In some automated systems, a machine dispenses prepackaged unit doses for each patient. The nurse places the packages on a mobile cabinet tray and wheels the cart to the room where the patient receives the medication. This saves time that the nurse can use for carrying out various other tasks related to patient care. Of course, no automated system can substitute for the nurse's experience and judgment. This is particularly true in any unusual situation in which the regular procedures of a particular institution do not apply. The nurse then does what she thinks is necessary for the well-being of her patient.

In many clinical situations the metric system of measurement is being used exclusively. The practice of converting from apothecary to metric dosage, or vice versa, is not only time-consuming for the nurse; it also presents an additional opportunity for error to occur. Nurses, by insisting upon the use of a single system of measurement, can help to make the administration of drugs safer for patients.

PREPARING MEDICATIONS

In some hospitals nurses still have to prepare dilutions of injectable drug solutions, and they must still make the required calculations. Although the arithmetic is relatively simple, it is easy for mistakes to occur under the pressure of work demands and distractions. Thus, every calculation should be checked by another person. The preparation of medicines should be carried out in a quiet room away from the nurses' station. The nurse should insist on having a private place where preparation can be carried out without interruption. The nurse who bears this responsibility has the duty to point out weaknesses in the way things are done where she works, and she has the duty to demand changes in procedures that might endanger patients. It is highly desirable, for patient safety, to have medications available in the dose ordered by the physician, thus averting the possibility of error through incorrect calculation of the dose.

The *Pharmacy and Therapeutics Committee* (PTC) is a group whose support the nurse should try to enlist when she wants to improve an undesirable situation related to the ordering, storage, preparation, distribution, and administration of drugs. In institutions where this committee exists in name only, the nurse may, instead, try to bring about changes in procedures by planning drug preparation and distribution functions with the chief pharmacist. Today's pharmacist has a broadened concept of his role in various aspects of drug therapy and is often willing to work with the nurse to correct potentially hazardous situations when they are pointed out to him.

CLINICAL PHARMACISTS

Many medical centers are trying to make more effective use of the modern pharmacist's education in all aspects of drug therapy. One way in which some hospitals have done this is by moving pharmacists from a central pharmacy to satellite drug stations located in or near one or several nursing units. Here, they read the doctor's medication orders directly and prepare unit doses of the drugs that each patient is scheduled to receive, including dilutions of solutions for I.V. infusion.

This, of course, relieves the nurse of various duties ranging from drug requisitioning and storage to record keeping. In addition, she can confer with the pharmacist directly about aspects of drug administration, including what to teach patients about the medications that they will continue to take after they leave the hospital. She and the pharmacist can check for possible errors in dosage and help to avoid them. The pharmacist will call the physician if he seems to have ordered a dose that is outside the therapeutic range. All three professional people share a responsibility to help each other avoid medication errors.

Single-unit packages also help to reduce the possibility of errors, particularly in hospitals that do not have 24-hour pharmacy service. The pharmacist stocks an emergency cabinet with individual doses of medication that are prepackaged and labeled. The nursing supervisor or other nursing personnel who have access to this cabinet simply remove the single unit that the patient requires and administer it.

Many frequently employed drugs are now available as strip-packed or blister-packed capsules or tablets, suppository-pack units, or cartridge injection systems. The injectables are dispensed in the form of sterile syringe and needle units that are disposable. In addition to their convenience, these are free of contamination by infectious organisms. Narcotics and barbiturates now come packaged in ways that make it easier to keep stock records. (One such injectable system called Tubex® employs a tamper-resistant package, trade-named Tamp-R-Tel® for such products.) Commercial unit doses are relatively expensive, but many medications can be put up by the pharmacist at a lower cost per unit dose.

THE NURSE AND THE PATIENT

Many psychological factors must be considered when a nurse is administering a patient's medication. The nurse can communicate her own negative feelings toward the treatment without actually saying a word. Medication given in this way may do more harm than good. On the other hand, the nurse may use positive suggestion in ways that increase the effectiveness of many medications or, in any case, make the patient feel better. The act of giving medication is in itself one which conveys the idea that you are concerned with the patient's welfare and want him to get well. Thus, the nurse should offer medication to the patient as a tangible sign that the people charged with his care wish to help him. Most patients want to feel better and are emotionally prepared to expect relief from pain and discomfort when they receive medication. The nurse takes advantage of this belief in the efficacy of drugs and reinforces such expectations by her words and actions. If, for instance, the nurse takes the time to explain that a drug is going to bring about desired rest and relaxation, it is much more likely to do so than if she rushes in and administers an injection with no word of explanation.

The patient's questions about the medication that he is receiving should always be given attention, although the matter of how much the patient should be told about this or any aspect of his treatment must be determined on an individual basis. Certainly, if a patient comments that he "can't take a particular medicine," the nurse should check with the doctor before giving the drug. Generally, the patient's questions about the nature of his drug therapy should be carefully considered, because they sometimes serve as an important safeguard against error.

In general, there is no pat answer to the question of how much the patient should be told about the nature and the purpose of the drug that is being administered. It was once assumed that the patient should know little or nothing about the medicine that he was receiving. However, just as many physicians now have the pharmacist put the name of the medication on the prescription label, they also often explain the drug's expected therapeutic action to the patient and warn him of what side effects to expect.

On the other hand, it is not always necessary or desirable to tell the patient the exact name of the drug that he is receiving. It may not be wise to say "Here is your injection of morphine" to a patient being prepared for an operation or to one who is in temporary pain from trauma. The patient may be so disturbed by the thought of narcotic addiction that he will derive little benefit from the medication. Thus, it is probably better simply to say "The doctor has ordered this medicine to help you rest and relax before you go to the operating room," or something similar.

Listen to the patient and let him ventilate feelings of fear, anxiety, and even anger or frustration. The nurse may not agree with the patient's complaints and doubts but she should give him a chance to voice them, as he then often feels better about his situation and may actually begin to respond to treatment more readily.

Of course, some complaints are entirely legitimate, and the nurse should do what she can to correct the situation. Some medicines do taste bad and should be chilled or otherwise altered to lessen the disagreeable taste or odor. This is particularly true with children but also applies to adults whose medications often leave the mouth uncomfortably dry. Offering the patient a hard candy, mint, or chewing gum often helps.

Children, as well as adults, should be told the truth when they are capable of understanding it. Mentioning a drug's side effects in advance is not undesirable if this is coupled with the honest assurance that they will soon subside. Similarly, if a child asks whether a medicine tastes bad, he should be told the truth, and efforts should then be made to disguise the taste if this is at all possible.

On the other hand, a child in a negative stage of development—the "terrible two," for instance—cannot be reasoned with very well. However, even when it is necessary to go ahead against his wishes, firmness in seeing that the child receives the ordered medication can be tempered by an attitude that conveys the idea that he has not been "bad."

Similarly, mentally ill patients must receive their medication even when they resist its administration. Parenteral administration may have to be employed when a psychiatric patient spits out oral doses of antipsychotic drugs. Later, after the patient becomes less agitated, he will usually respond with less anxiety and take the drug by mouth regularly when it is offered. It is, of course, important always to stay with him to see that he actually swallows it. It is essential that the patient learn about his medication and the ways it can help him. Unfortunately, some psychiatric patients who are fearful about such matters as taking drugs get little help toward understanding the purpose and expected effects of the medicine. It is especially important, if the patient seems fearful of taking the medication, to ask him his views about the purpose of the medication and what it is he fears about taking it.

Reducing the patient's discomfort by nursing measures before and after administering medication is also desirable. Making the patient more comfortable often increases the effectiveness of the drug that is administered. Sometimes the desired response can be achieved with less medication. Thus, a hypnotic drug will often act more rapidly when a patient has received a soothing back rub and has been given a glass of warm milk. Pain-relieving injections seem to work better when the nurse first gives the patient a reassuring explanation and then stays with him for a while, until the pain begins to subside.

Esthetic considerations also have a place in drug administration. In most situations individual disposable containers should be employed. However, if a patient is taking sticky antacid suspensions for treating peptic ulcer, such paper cups should not be permitted to pile up.

Distribution of medication is made easier and the chances of error are reduced by arranging the medications on the cabinet cassettes, or trays, in the order in which patients will be visited. The common practice in an adult medical-surgical or obstetrical unit of pushing a cart of medicine down the corridor is best avoided when distributing drugs to psychiatric patients or to children who might impulsively snatch medication from the cart. In general, medications should not be left unguarded, and it is important to take the medication tray with you when called from any patient's room. Some patients may steal drugs for suicidal purposes; others may hoard medication instead of taking it for the same reason. Thus, it is important to stay with the patient and see that he actually swallows all oral medications.

Identifying the patient properly before administering his medication is, of course, crucial. It may seem unnecessary to go through the ritual of checking a patient's identification band against the name on the medication card when you are caring for only three patients and are well acquainted with each of them. Yet this habit can stand the nurse in good stead later when she may be working under more stressful situations. When the nurse works during the night and may have to give medicines to many sleepy patients, this habit can help to prevent mistakes. Patients often respond affirmatively when addressed by the wrong name; if a patient's identity is at all in doubt, do not give the drug without double checking in various ways, including asking the patient himself to state his name.

Wasting of medication through carelessness can add greatly to the cost of the patient's treatment. It is easy to forget, when dispensing medications on a busy ward, that many modern drugs are quite expensive. Thus, medications should be carefully handled to avoid spilling them or rendering them unfit for use. However, one should not return an unused dose of a drug to a bottle from which medicines are dispensed. When the patient is discharged, any unused medicine should be returned to the pharmacy so that he will receive credit for it and not have to pay for medication never received.

Recording the administration of all medications is, of course, essential. Methods of putting information down on the patient's chart vary from place to place. In general, it is considered necessary to see that each dose and the time of its administration are recorded along with an indication of who gave it. How the patient responded to medication is an important point of information for charting. Various measures are now in use for reducing the amount of time spent in recording medications. If, for example, the same medicine is administered four times daily, only the time of each dose need be charted in some institutions, and the name of the drug need not be entered each time.

Summary

We have tried to take up some of the things that the nurse must consider in carrying out one of her most important patient-care functions—the administration of medicines. The reason for offering so much detailed, step-by-step advice is this: Once the nurse has developed habit patterns based upon safe and efficient ways of administering medicines, she will be able to concentrate on the broader aspects of the patient's total care. Freed of the need to keep myriad details in mind, she can observe the patient's reactions to drugs and integrate her observations into what she knows of the patient's condition and the purpose of treatment with the drug that is being given. This does *not*, of course, mean that she ever acts *mechanically*, for habit can never be relied upon to that degree. Nurses are, for example, often instructed to read the label three times —once when removing the medicine from the cabinet, once when taking the dose of the drug from the bottle, and once when returning the medication to its storage place. It is certainly true that reading the label more than once can help to prevent mistakes—but it is entirely possible to read a label wrong three times when you are really not attending to the task!

Actually, attentiveness is the most significant aspect of safety—attentiveness to the label, attentiveness to the identification band that you are checking. No one is optimally alert at all times. It helps, however, to develop insight into one's own mental processes in this regard. Thus, the nurse who learns to recognize signs of her own inattentiveness and knows that this happens when she is harassed and anxious, can make an extra effort to interrupt such reactions and to concentrate on the task confronting her.

The dispensing of pills and capsules of various colors day after day can become boring. So, for that matter, can the administration of injections, once one's skill has been perfected and even that once challenging procedure becomes a matter of routine. Nevertheless, these tasks can remain interesting to the nurse who looks at them in the total context of how the nurse contributes to effective patient care.

It is thrilling to see a pneumonia patient with a 104° temperature and severe dyspnea respond to penicillin therapy by becoming afebrile and comfortable and begin to breathe normally. A nurse can treasure the experience of seeing a patient in shock, whose pulse and blood pressure were unobtainable, recover in response to an infusion of norepinephrine which she prepared for intravenous administration. Such rewards of nursing are in store for those who acquire the necessary skill and judgment and who make a constant effort to understand the relationships between the actions of drugs and the manner in which the patient's malfunctioning organ systems respond to the presence of pharmacotherapeutic agents.

SUMMARY of Points for the Nurse to Remember About The Administration of Drugs

Timing the administration of drugs is often left to the nurse's judgment. She should consider whether to give the drug with food or between meals, as well as the relationship of administration of the drug to the patient's hours of sleep. When in doubt about when would be preferable to administer a drug, the nurse should confer with the physician or the pharmacist.

The nurse must be alert to the possibility that the route of administration ordered by the physician may not be feasible in a particular situation and be ready to discuss this with the doctor. For example, if the patient is vomiting, administering a previously prescribed oral medication may be unwise.

Be especially alert to avoid any error in administering parenteral dosage forms, since their more rapid and complete absorption makes mistakes particularly hazardous.

Teaching the patient and his family how to take or to administer drugs with the greatest efficiency and safety is often the nurse's responsibility, as is observing and reporting the patient's response to drug therapy.

The individual nurse must assume the responsibility for her own safe practice in administering medication. Such responsibility involves: (1) the habitual employment of measures which lessen the chances of error (such as properly identifying the patient before administering any medication); (2) the acquiring of fundamental knowledge about the medication, such as its therapeutic use, side effects and potential toxicity, and usual dosage range; (3) working toward the establishment of institutional policies and procedures that foster safety and efficiency in the administration of medications.

The nurse's actions and attitudes can increase or impede the effectiveness of drug therapy. Thus, her attitude should be one that conveys positive suggestions that foster realistic expectations of the benefits to be derived from treatment with the drug that is being administered. Her actions (for example, promoting the patient's physical comfort) should also contribute to the total objectives of patient care and treatment.

References

Budd, Ruth. We changed to unit dose system. *Nurs. Outlook*, 19:116, 1971 (Feb.).

Conway, B., et al. The seventh right. *Amer. J. Nurs.*, 70:1040, 1970 (May).

Daylight on prescription prices. *Nurs. Forum*, 11:4:346, 1972.

Di Palma, J.R. Clinical pharmacist: New member of the health team. *RN*, 32:57, 1969 (Aug.).

Donn, R. Intravenous admixture incompatibility. *Amer. J. Nurs.*, 71:325, 1971 (Feb.).

Hecht, A.B. Self-medication, inaccuracy and what can be done. *Nurs. Outlook*, 18:30, 1970 (April).

Kern, M. New ideas about drug systems. *Amer. J. Nurs.*, 68:1251, 1968 (June).

Levine, M.E. Breaking through the medications mystique. *Amer. J. Nurs.*, 70:799, 1970 (April).

Lowenthal, W. Factors affecting drug absorption. *Amer. J. Nurs.*, 73:1391, 1973 (August).

McBride, M.A. The additive to the analgesic. *Amer. J. Nurs.*, 69:974, 1969 (May).

Pitel, M. The subcutaneous injection. *Amer. J. Nurs.*, 71:76, 1971 (Jan.).

Rauffenhart, M. Drug administration by automation. *Nurs. Clinics N. Amer.*, 1(4):611, 1966 (Dec.).

SECTION **2**

Drugs

that

Affect

Mental

and

Emotional

Function

and

Behavior

6.

Sedative-Hypnotics and Other Antianxiety Drugs

In this chapter we shall discuss several classes of drugs that are used mainly for *relief of anxiety*. These drugs are classified as:

1. The *barbiturates*, a class of synthetic chemicals that can be used to produce any degree of depression of the central nervous system. Here we shall take up only those barbiturates (Table 6-1) that are used primarily as sedatives, or drugs that calm nervous patients, and hypnotics, or sleep-producing drugs.

2. The *nonbarbiturate* sedative-hypnotics (Table 6-2), drugs of several other chemical classes that—like the barbiturates—have the ability to reduce nervous tension and help to bring about natural sleep.

3. The *minor tranquilizers*, or *antianxiety agents* (Table 6-3), newer drugs that are used mostly for treating patients with the same kinds of emotional, mental, and physical conditions for which the barbiturates and other classic kinds of sedative-hypnotics have traditionally been employed.

The Nature of Anxiety

Anxiety is an emotion that makes people feel tense and uneasy. Often, when a person becomes anxious, his body reacts just as it does when he is afraid. His heart pounds, his palms sweat, and he may suffer abdominal distress or other discomforting physical symptoms.

There are, however, significant differences between fear and anxiety. People react with fear when they become aware of a dangerous situation. They deal with the situation consciously, and when the emergency is over, the bodily reactions quickly subside. The anxious person, on the other hand, feels threatened by

TABLE 6-1   *Sedative-Hypnotics (Barbiturate Type)* *

Nonproprietary Name	Trade Name	Relative Duration of Action	Usual Daily Oral Dosage Range†
Amobarbital U.S.P.	Amytal	Short to intermediate	50 to 200 mg
Aprobarbital N.F.	Alurate	Short to intermediate	60 to 120 mg
Barbital	Veronal	Long-acting	130 to 400 mg
Butabarbital Sodium N.F.	Butisol	Short to intermediate	45 to 120 mg
Butalbital N.F.	Lotusate	Short to intermediate	30 to 150 mg
Pentobarbital Sodium‡ U.S.P.	Nembutal	Short to intermediate	50 to 200 mg
Phenobarbital§ U.S.P.	Luminal	Long-acting	50 to 200 mg
Secobarbital U.S.P.	Seconal	Short to intermediate	50 to 200 mg
Vinbarbital N.F.	Delvinal	Short to intermediate	100 to 200 mg

  * See Chapter 14 for basal anesthetic barbiturates, the ultra-short-acting type (for example, methohexital, thia-mylal, and thiopental sodium).
  See Chapter 12 for anticonvulsant dosage of phenobarbital and of mephobarbital and metharbital, two other long-acting barbiturates with sedative actions.
  † The smaller dose is administered several times daily to produce daytime sedation; the larger dose represents either the total of daytime sedative doses or the highest single dose administered at bedtime for hypnosis.
  ‡ See *Drug Digest*, this Chapter, p. 90.
  § See *Drug Digest* in Chapter 12, p. 153.

TABLE 6-2   *Nonbarbiturate Sedative-Hypnotics*

Nonproprietary Name	Trade Name	Daily Oral Dosage Range*	Comments
Bromisovalum	Bromural	300–900 mg	Effects last 3 or 4 hours
Carbromal	Adalin; Uradal	300–900 mg	Effects last 3 or 4 hours
Chloral betaine N.F.	Beta-Chlor	870–1740 mg	Tasteless tablet form of chloral hydrate
Chloral hydrate U.S.P.	Noctec; Somnos	250–2000 mg	See *Drug Digest*
Chlorobutanol U.S.P.	Chloretone	300–1000 mg	Also used in dental cavities
Ethchlorvynol N.F.	Placidyl	100–1000 mg	Rapid onset; short duration
Ethinamate N.F.	Valmid	500–1000 mg	Rapid onset; short duration
Flurazepam	Dalmane	15–30 mg	Chemical relative of chlordiazepoxide and diazepam (Table 6-3)
Glutethimide N.F.	Doriden	125–1000 mg	See *Drug Digest*
Methapyrilene HCl	Lullamin	25–100 mg	Sedative antihistamine
Methaqualone	Quaalude; Sopor	150–300 mg	Also has antitussive and antispasmodic effects
Methyprylon N.F.	Noludar	50–400 mg	Similar to secobarbital in onset and duration of action
Paraldehyde U.S.P.	Paral and others	5–30 ml	Also administered rectally and I.M. against acute convulsions
Petrichloral	Perichlor	300–600 mg	Tasteless, less irritating form of chloral hydrate
Scopolamine HBr U.S.P.	Hyoscine	0.3–4 mg	Centrally acting anticholinergic drug

  * The lower dose is usually administered several times daily for daytime sedation; the larger dose represents either the total daily sedative dose or the highest single dose administered at bedtime for hypnosis.

TABLE 6-3 *Minor Tranquilizers (Antianxiety Agents)*

Nonproprietary Name	Trade Name	Usual Single Dosage	Comments
Buclizine HCl	Softran	25–50 mg	Sedative anthihistamine
Chlorazepate	Tranxene	15–60 mg	Similar to chlordiazepoxide
Chlordiazepoxide N.F.	Librium	5–10 mg (orally)	See *Drug Digest*
Chlordiazepoxide HCl U.S.P.		50–100 mg I.M. or I.V.	
Chlormezanone	Trancopal	300–800 mg	Similar to meprobamate
Diazepam N.F.	Valium	2–10 mg	See *Drug Digest* (Chap. 10)
Hydroxyzine HCl N.F.	Atarax	25–100 mg	See *Drug Digest*
Hydroxyzine pamoate N.F.	Vistaril	25–100 mg	See *Drug Digest*
Mephenoxalone	Trepidone	400 mg	Similar to meprobamate
Meprobamate U.S.P.	Equanil; Miltown	400 mg	See *Drug Digest*
Oxanamide	Quiactin	400 mg	Similar to meprobamate
Oxazepam N.F.	Serax	10–30 mg	Similar to chlordiazepoxide
Phenaglycodol	Ultran	300 mg	Similar to meprobamate
Tybamate N.F.	Solacen; Tybatran	250–500 mg	Similar to meprobamate

things of which the sources are rarely recognized. Anxiety that arises from unconscious emotional conflicts is usually long-lasting. Chronic anxiety of this kind can lead to psychosis, psychoneurosis, or many kinds of bodily disorders.

Psychiatrists and other doctors try to get at the underlying causes of the patient's anxiety. While doing so, however, the doctor may employ medications for symptomatic relief of anxiety and for counteracting the ill effects of psychophysiological reactions. The clinical uses for sedative-hypnotics and minor tranquilizers are summarized on p. 86. Details concerning individual drugs of these classes are presented in the *Drug Digests* of the most important prototypes and in Tables 6-1, 6-2, and 6-3. Here we shall discuss only some practical general aspects of these drugs, with emphasis on the nurse's role in relation to patients for whom the doctor orders the administration of sedative-hypnotics and other antianxiety agents.

Management of Anxiety

Anxiety can have adverse effects that require short-term or long-term treatment. Stressful situations can set off transient symptoms ranging from moderate apprehension to severe agitation. To make the patient more comfortable or to control his anxiety level, the doctor may order small oral doses of sedative drugs or the administration of much higher doses parenterally. Once the acute manifestations of anxiety are relieved, the patient may need no further drug therapy. On the other hand, psychoneurotic patients or those with physical illnesses in which chronic anxiety plays a part may require prolonged treatment with sedatives or minor tranquilizers as an adjunct to other forms of therapy for their conditions.

PSYCHOMOTOR IMPAIRMENT

The minor tranquilizers, such as meprobamate+, chlordiazepoxide+, and hydroxyzine+ are claimed to be capable of calming anxious patients without causing the degree of drowsiness seen when barbiturates are employed for the same purpose. Supposedly, these drugs act more specifically on the limbic system, while the chief site of action of the barbiturates is on the reticular activating system.

This is said to account for their ability to reduce the patient's response to emotional stress without making him lethargic or impairing his motor performance. Actually, many authorities doubt that the minor tranquilizers are really superior to the barbiturates in this respect. They suggest that the administration of small oral doses of pentobarbital or phenobarbital+ is just as effective for treating mild to moderate degrees of anxiety and that these barbiturates are no more likely to cause excessive central psychomotor depression than the newer, more expensive minor tranquilizers.

PRECAUTIONS (SUMMARY, p. 87)

Small oral doses of both barbiturates and antianxiety agents are equally safe for most patients with mild to moderate degrees of anxiety. On the other hand, patients taking either kind of sedative drug should be warned that driving a car or doing other tasks that call for complete alertness and motor control may be dangerous, particularly during the first few days of treatment. Similarly, they should be cautioned not to drink alcoholic beverages or take other depressant drugs because of possible hazardous additive effects of combining alcohol with the barbiturates or with meprobamate, chlordiazepoxide, and other minor tranquilizers.

DEPENDENCE ON DEPRESSANT DRUGS

Most patients for whom these drugs are prescribed in small doses do not abuse them. Yet alcoholics and other patients with a history of having once been dependent on opiates or other drugs have to be carefully supervised when taking either barbiturates or other sedative-hypnotics and minor tranquilizers for long periods. This is because these drugs can, when abused, produce a state of euphoria that some people may continue to seek to the point of becoming both psychologically and physically dependent.

Although the drugs most commonly abused by those who want to become inebriated are the rapid-acting barbiturates—secobarbital, pentobarbital, and amobarbital—such nonbarbiturate sedative-hypnotics as glutethimide, methyprylon, ethchlorvynol and the rest (Table 6-2) are also potentially addicting when taken in large daily doses for long periods. Similarly, meprobamate, chlordiazepoxide, and other minor tranquilizers are also sometimes taken in excessive doses—alone or with alcoholic beverages—in order to become intoxicated. (See Chapter 4 and the *Summary of Adverse Effects* in this chapter for further details of the effects of dependence upon these depressant drugs.)

FEAR OF DEPENDENCE

Some patients for whom sedatives are ordered during their hospitalization for an acute illness are afraid of becoming dependent on these drugs. The nurse listens to such a patient and lets him express his apprehension. However, he should be assured that brief exposure to barbiturates and related drugs does not ordinarily produce dependence and that these drugs will, instead, help him to get the rest that he needs to regain his health. Allaying the patient's alarm by explaining that the medication is going to help him relax will also often tend to increase the drug's desired calming effect.

Even when patients must take sedative-hypnotics or minor tranquilizers for long periods, the nurse can help the habituated patient keep from becoming excessively dependent upon these drugs. She can suggest various ways for reducing restlessness without drugs. Patients who learn to relax and reduce their nervousness by reading, listening to music, taking a warm bath, or going for a walk often find that they can gradually give up sedatives and tranquilizers.

SECONDARY EFFECTS

The newer antianxiety agents are sometimes claimed also to produce physical effects that make them better suited for relief of somatic symptoms which result from emotional tension. For example, meprobamate, diazepam, and related compounds (Table 6-3) are said to be better than barbiturates for patients with muscular tension and tremors; these drugs can depress spinal interneurons and thus reduce excessive skeletal muscle tone. However, some authorities argue that this central antispasmodic action develops only when high doses are injected and that ordinary oral doses of these drugs produce only sedative effects.

Other minor tranquilizers are also claimed to possess clinically desirable secondary actions. Actually, however, these actions are so undependable that the sedatives and tranquilizers are usually combined with other drugs which act more specifically to relieve physical symptoms. Thus, for example, hydroxyzine and chlordiazepoxide are often prescribed in combination with: atropinelike antispasmodic drugs for relief of gastrointestinal spasms; nitrites for patients with angina pectoris; estrogens for menopausal women; and salicylates and corticosteroids for rheumatoid arthritis and related musculoskeletal conditions.

MANAGEMENT OF INSOMNIA

Anxiety and discomfort can often keep a patient from getting the rest and sleep that he requires. Barbiturates and other general depressant drugs are often ordered to help the hospitalized patient sleep or to control chronic insomnia in patients who are at home. For this purpose, the same drugs that are used as daytime sedatives are administered as hypnotics at bedtime in several times the sedative dose.

In most cases, hypnotics are effective for producing a period of restful, more or less natural, sleep. The sleep produced by hypnotic doses of these drugs is "natural," or physiologic, in the sense that patients are not narcotized or rendered so stuporous that they cannot be as readily aroused as from ordinary sleep.

The results of recent research in sleep laboratories indicate that the habitual use of barbiturates and most other hypnotics may alter normal sleep patterns. For example, the sleep stage that is marked by rapid eye movements (REM sleep) is reduced in subjects taking pentobarbital, secobarbital, glutethimide, methyprylon, and other such drugs. It has been suggested that this drug-induced sleep pattern alteration may play a part in both (1) the tendency of habitual hypnotic users to sleep poorly and (2) their tendency to develop dependence upon these drugs.

Certain hypnotics including chloral hydrate, methaqualone, and flurazepam did not suppress REM sleep when these drugs were administered in hypnotic doses. Some pharmaceutical manufacturers have exploited these experimental findings to suggest that their nonbarbiturate hypnotic drug products produce a more "natural," or physiologic, sleep.

Actually, it is still uncertain at this time whether REM sleep is necessary for a person's well-being or whether being deprived of REM sleep will result in any psychological harm. Indeed, it has not been fully established that there is any substantial difference in the effects of equivalent doses of different hypnotic drugs upon sleep patterns as measured by electroencephalographic (EEG) and electro-oculographic (EOG) techniques.

However, patients do differ in how they respond to sleep-producing drugs. Thus, to ensure that these drugs prove both effective and safe, the nurse has many responsibilities. Many of the points that she should remember when her duties involve the administration of hypnotics and observation of the patient who has had them are summarized on pp. 84-85, along with comments about her responsibilities in teaching patients how to take these drugs at home in the most beneficial and least dangerous ways.

COMPARISON OF HYPNOTICS

The several types of drugs that are available for inducing sleep are listed in Tables 6-1, 6-2, and 6-3. Although some are claimed more effective and safer than others, all of these drugs share a capacity for producing similar adverse effects (*Summary*, p. 87). Similarly, all require the same kinds of precautions and are generally contraindicated in the same kinds of patients.

Among the advantages often claimed for any new hypnotic are that it is:

1. Less likely to be habit-forming and dependence-producing
2. Less likely to cause "hangover" or residual sedation
3. Less likely to cause "paradoxical excitement" in patients who are prone to react abnormally to depressant drugs
4. Less likely to prove toxic for patients with liver or kidney disease
5. Less likely to cause severe toxicity if taken in massive overdosage

Actually, most of these claimed advantages are not of much practical clinical significance. Patients taking properly administered hypnotic doses of any of these drugs are equally safe from suffering harmful effects. On the other hand, people who abuse any of these drugs or patients for whom these agents are contraindicated are likely to become dependent upon any of them or to suffer their adverse effects. In general, the short- to intermediate-acting barbiturates are still among the most useful hypnotics. The newer nonbarbiturate hypnotics and tranquilizer-type hypnotics are preferred mainly for patients who have developed tolerance or, on the other hand, allergic hypersensitivity to the barbiturates.

ACUTE OVERDOSAGE

One real advantage that some of the newer depressants may have over the barbiturates is that there may be a somewhat wider safety margin between their hypnotic and lethal doses. This is particularly true of the chemical class of minor tranquilizers that includes *flurazepam* (Dalmane) and others (Table 6-2). Patients who accidentally or deliberately take overdoses of these drugs may become stuporous or comatose. However, they rarely die of respiratory or cardiovascular failure as is usually the case when patients ingest heavy doses of barbiturates.

Certain nonprescription or over-the-counter products promoted for "safe sleep," which are weaker than the prescription-type hypnotics, do not produce fatal degrees of central depression when taken in overdoses. This does *not* mean, however, that these products are not capable of causing acute—and even lethal —intoxication of a different kind. Most of these products (for example, Sominex, Compoz, Nytol) contain combinations of the antihistaminic agent, methapyrilene, the anticholinergic compound, scopolamine hydrobromide, and sometimes other substances such as salicylamide. Overdosage with these drugs produces central excitatory effects that tend to counteract their initial depression. This may manifest itself as confusion, disorientation, hallucinations, and bizarre behavior that can in itself endanger the user. In addition, unsupervised patients who overmedicate themselves with these sleep-inducing products can also suffer restlessness, agitation, convulsions, and circulatory collapse.

Physicians often prefer to prescribe bedtime doses of minor tranquilizers rather than barbiturates for patients who they think might attempt suicide. In such cases, even these somewhat safer hypnotics are still prescribed in relatively small amounts. Even though these patients are less likely to succeed in committing suicide, they would require specialized emergency treatment for acute intoxication. (See Chapter 3 for a discussion of the general supportive medical measures, nursing care, and antidotal drugs that are used in the management of patients poisoned by drugs that depress such vital functions as respiration and circulation.)

ADMINISTRATION AND OBSERVATION

Hospitalized patients are often unable to sleep because of physical discomfort or emotional upset. Thus, before administering any ordered hypnotic, the nurse tries to make the patient comfortable by seeing to it that the room is well ventilated and at optimal temperature. It helps, also, to spend some time talking to the patient and letting him voice his concerns about his condition. Often patients respond better to the relaxing effects of these drugs when they are told what to expect and are given a warm drink or a light snack at the time they take the hypnotic.

Deciding what to do when the doctor has left a p.r.n. order is an important professional responsibility. It is necessary to ask yourself *why* the patient has been unable to fall asleep or *why* he has awakened, rather than to administer another hypnotic dose routinely. Patients who are in pain do not respond well to hypnotics alone. Thus, the physician should be notified so that he can combine the barbiturate or other hypnotic with a salicylate such as aspirin. He may even decide that codeine or an even stronger analgesic such as Demerol is needed for the patient whose sleeplessness stems from pain.

It is always important to watch how patients react to hypnotic drugs and to act accordingly. Obviously, if the patient falls into a deep sleep after receiving a drug of supposedly short duration, he should not be awakened for the next scheduled dose. Likewise, if he seems unusually lethargic, the next dose should be withheld until the doctor has been informed. (Patients with respiratory difficulties or with severe liver or kidney disease sometimes become deeply depressed after receiving seemingly safe doses of a barbiturate or a nonbarbiturate hypnotic.)

Elderly patients—particularly those with brain damage secondary to cerebrovascular disease—sometimes tend to become excited, instead of calmed, when they receive hypnotics in the hospital. The night nurse listens for sounds indicating that such a paradoxically excited patient is awake and trying to get up. She may have to help him out of bed or even help him to remember where he is.

It is important to keep the confused patient from falling or otherwise hurting himself. This may require putting up side rails, but other restraints are not usually needed. Instead, it is more desirable to stay with the patient and talk to him. Simply repeating his name and telling him where he is often helps to calm and relax the patient and to reorient him.

INSTRUCTING PATIENTS

People with chronic insomnia who will be taking hypnotics at home for prolonged periods can often profit from advice as to how these drugs should best be taken and stored. Of course, it is the health team's responsibility to try to find and treat the underlying causes of the patient's sleep problems. The nurse can contribute by suggesting ways to induce sleep without medications.

The patient can be taught to control his home environment in much the same way in which the nurse has tried to keep his hospital room free of sleep-disrupting factors. It should, in fact, be easier to ensure quiet and proper temperature and ventilation at home than in the hospital. The nurse can also help the patient work out a bedtime regimen that reduces restlessness and promotes relaxation.

Going for a walk or doing other light exercise followed by a warm bath helps some people fall asleep. Listening to music while reading may also be relaxing. In any case, a patient can be assured that loss of sleep by an otherwise healthy person has no serious physical consequences, according to authorities on sleep. So, it may be best not to be bothered when one occasionally fails to fall asleep and to try, instead, to find constructive ways to use the hours of wakefulness.

SAFE STORAGE

Patients should also be advised not to keep hypnotic capsules or tablets in a place that is readily accessible to children. The brightly colored capsules kept in a bedside table or in an unlocked medicine cabinet can attract toddlers who may then ingest the medication and suffer severe intoxication. The patient himself may, in some circumstances, waken in a dazed or disoriented condition and take an exessive quantity of hypnotic medication if it is within too easy reach.

Miscellaneous Uses of Sedative-Hypnotics and Antianxiety Agents

The effects of drugs that depress the nervous system depend in part upon the excitability of this system. Thus, larger than ordinary doses may be needed to calm patients who are unusually anxious, apprehensive, or agitated. Often such doses are administered parenterally to produce their effects more rapidly and surely. The kinds of clinical situations that often call for parenteral administration of these drugs are summarized on p. 86.

PREOPERATIVE SEDATION

The barbiturates and other drugs of this kind are often ordered for patients who are to undergo surgery. Oral hypnotic doses are administered the night before surgery is scheduled, since the patient comes to the O.R. in better physical and mental condition when he has had a good night's sleep. Listening to the patient and answering his questions about the procedure he is to undergo also helps him to deal more effectively with his anxiety about the next morning's operation.

On the morning of the operation, patients are likely to be particularly apprehensive. To reduce reflex nervous excitability, they usually receive a high hypnotic dose parenterally, alone or combined with morphine, meperidine, and other preanesthetic medications. The nurse should be sure that such medications are given on time so that the patient will arrive at the O.R. in the best condition for undergoing anesthesia induction smoothly. (See Chapter 14 for further discussion of preanesthetic medication and the use of barbiturates for basal anesthesia.)

The patient who has been heavily sedated in this way must be kept from harm while waiting to go to the O.R. for anesthesia and surgery. He should not be allowed to smoke unless someone stays with him. Side rails may also have to be put up to protect the patient. Personal observation and communication are still the best means of making certain that the patient arrives for surgery feeling as relaxed and trusting as possible in this stressful situation. Taking the drug may in itself lead some patients to become fearful, since this step signifies the beginning of a period in which the patient temporarily becomes helpless and thus very dependent on others. If he responds in this way, it is particularly important to stay nearby until he arrives in the operating room.

SEDATION AND AMNESIA DURING LABOR

Although these drugs are themselves not good pain relievers, they are often administered to O.B. patients together with narcotic analgesics such as meperidine and alphaprodine. Because barbiturates combined with narcotics sometimes cause excessive depression of respiration in both mother and baby, some obstetricians do not approve of this use of these depressants.

Recently, some of the minor tranquilizers

that are less likely than barbiturates to depress respiration have been substituted. According to some studies, *diazepam+* and *hydroxyzine+* have been effective in producing pain relief and forgetfulness of the obstetric procedure without causing breathing difficulties in the newborn babies. Use of these drugs permits—and, in fact, requires—reduction in dosage of narcotic analgesics. This may also be a factor in reports that labor was not unduly prolonged when these drugs were used experimentally for this purpose.

ACUTE PSYCHOTIC AND PSYCHONEUROTIC REACTIONS

The injectable forms of such minor tranquilizers as *chlordiazepoxide+* and *diazepam+* are sometimes used for quieting highly agitated patients. These drugs seem safer than the barbiturates for bringing severely excited patients under control. However, the hallucinations and delusions that may underlie a schizophrenic patient's behavior are not relieved. For this purpose, and for long-term therapy of mentally ill patients, the major tranquilizers or antipsychotic agents are preferred.

ACUTE ALCOHOLIC INTOXICATION AND WITHDRAWAL

Paraldehyde+, the barbiturates, and minor tranquilizers still have an important place in the management of combative, disturbed, or delirious alcoholics. Their role when administered alone or combined with phenothiazines is discussed in Chapter 8.

RELIEF OF ACUTE CONVULSIONS AND MUSCLE SPASTICITY

The role of these drugs as anticonvulsants and neurospasmolytics is discussed in Chapter 10.

SUMMARY of Clinical Indications for Sedatives, Hypnotics, and Minor Tranquilizers

Small Oral Doses with Sedative or Antianxiety Effects

1. Calm patients reacting to stressful life situations.

2. Reduce anxiety and tension states in psychoneurosis.

3. Dampen the emotional component in organic and functional disorders in which psychophysiological reactions play a significant psychosomatic or somatopsychic role. For example:

(a) Gastrointestinal (such as hypersecretion and hypermotility in peptic ulcer, pylorospasm, colitis).

(b) Cardiovascular (such as palpitations, tachycardia, chest pains, and high blood pressure in angina pectoris, essential hypertension).

(c) Allergic (such as skin eruptions and pruritus in neurodermatitis; wheezing, cough, dyspnea in bronchial asthma and other obstructive respiratory disorders).

(d) Menopausal (such as nervousness, palpitations, headaches, sweating, "hot flashes," and menstrual disorders, including premenstrual tension, dysmenorrhea).

(e) Arthritis and other chronically painful conditions that are emotionally upsetting, and other musculoskeletal conditions or tension headaches that may be the result of emotional reactions to stressful situations.

Higher Oral Doses with Hypnotic Effects

1. Induce sleep in patients with insomnia who have difficulty in falling asleep.

2. Maintain natural sleep in patients with insomnia who have difficulty in staying asleep.

3. Adjunct to analgesics in patients unable to sleep because of pain.

4. Preoperatively to assure restful sleep on the night before surgery.

Parenterally Administered Doses for Greater Sedation

1. Preoperatively and prior to various anxiety-provoking procedures to reduce the patient's apprehension.

2. During labor to sedate the mother and produce amnesia.

3. In alcoholic intoxication to control combative behavior.

4. In alcoholic withdrawal syndromes to relieve acute anxiety, agitation, and delirium.

5. In acute psychotic and psychoneurotic reactions to reduce agitation and control excessive excitement.

S U M M A R Y of Cautions and Contraindications for Sedatives, Hypnotics, and Minor Tranquilizers

Contraindications

Patients who have had allergic or idiosyncratic reactions when previously exposed to the drug.

Patients with acute intermittent porphyria.

Patients with acute narrow-angle glaucoma (for example, diazepam and other drugs with an anticholinergic component).

Precautions and Warnings

Driving a motor vehicle, operating dangerous machinery, or engaging in other activities requiring complete mental alertness may be hazardous.

Drinking alcoholic beverages or administering narcotics and other depressant drugs may produce additive or supra-additive effects.

Depressed patients with suicidal tendencies should receive only small amounts of these drugs to avoid deliberate ingestion of massive overdoses.

Alcoholics and addiction-prone patients should be carefully supervised to detect any developing tendency toward dependence.

Physically dependent patients who are found to have been taking excessive doses for prolonged periods should have their dosage gradually reduced rather than abruptly stopped.

Epileptic patients should have these drugs added to or withdrawn from their regimens relatively slowly to avoid precipitating seizures.

Hepatic and renal impairment requires careful dosage regulation, as patients often respond to lower doses.

Elderly and debilitated patients require lower dosage initially until tolerance develops and permits gradually increased dosage.

S U M M A R Y of Adverse Effects of Sedatives, Hypnotics, and Minor Tranquilizers

Side Effects of Therapeutic Doses

Central effects. Drowsiness, dizziness, headache, weakness. Occasional paradoxical excitement.

Allergic and idiosyncratic reactions. Skin eruptions, including urticaria and erythematous rash; hematological reactions, including occasional leukopenia, thrombocytopenia and agranulocytosis.

Effects of Continued Excessive Dosage (Chronic Intoxication)

CNS depression. Ataxia, vertigo, slurred speech, impaired thought and judgment; and ocular disturbances, including diplopia, nystagmus, strabismus, and difficulty in accommodation.

Withdrawal Signs and Symptoms in Dependent Persons

Nausea, vomiting, abdominal cramps; anxiety, restlessness, insomnia, confusional states, hallucinations and delirium; muscular twitching, tremors, cramps, and convulsive seizures of the grand mal epileptiform type.

Effects of Massive Overdosage (Acute Intoxication)

Mental confusion, somnolence, stupor, coma; hypotension, shock, circulatory collapse; respiration slow, shallow; transient apnea, or possible respiratory failure.

S U M M A R Y of Points for the Nurse to Remember About Sedative-Hypnotics and Minor Tranquilizers

Remember that administering these drugs is only one way to help the patient relax and rest and thus consider the use of the following nursing measures:

(1) Increase the patient's physical comfort by making certain that the position of his bed is properly adjusted, that the room is well ventilated, and that he feels pleasantly warm.

(2) Help the patient to feel more at ease emotionally if he seems nervous by staying with him for awhile, listening sympathetically to his concerns, and helping him to express his worries.

(3) Advise the patient of the purpose for which the sedative or hypnotic is being administered, as he is more likely to benefit from the relaxing effects of these drugs if he has been given positive suggestions that lead him to expect pleasant drowsiness.

Observe carefully how the patient responds to the administration of these drugs, as your observations can help to increase the safety and effectiveness of their continued use:

(1) For example, elderly patients sometimes tend to become restless, confused, and disoriented, or they become dizzy and faint when they first get out of bed. (Detecting such adverse effects will help you to protect the patient from accidental injury by taking such measures as the use of side rails on his bed, assisting him to get up slowly, and not allowing him to smoke unattended.)

(2) Does the patient become excessively drowsy and difficult to arouse? If so, it is the nurse's responsibility to withhold the next dose until she has conferred with the physician as to whether the drug is having an excessive effect.

(3) Does the patient stay awake or does he awaken during the night? If so, it's important to learn the reason for his wakefulness. He may be in pain and need an analgesic or other measures for relief of pain rather than another dose of a sedative hypnotic.

(4) Is the patient already asleep? If so, the nurse should not awaken him to give him a sleeping pill even if it was ordered for bedtime administration. (In general, she should not insist that patients take ordered sedatives but instead, encourage patients to get along without sleep-producing medications if they can.)

(5) Listen to the patient who expresses fear of becoming dependent upon a sedative or tranquilizer drug that has been ordered. He should be assured that taking such medication for brief periods is unlikely to lead to dependence and

that he will profit from the drug-induced rest and relaxation.

Remember, however, that these drugs can produce dependence when misused, particularly when an addiction-prone person is exposed to these medications over an extended period.

(1) Help the patient who has to use barbiturates and tranquilizers over a long period to find other ways to reduce anxiety and to relax besides taking the prescribed drugs. (Suggest *nondrug ways* of coping with stress-related tension and restlessness, such as exercise and quiet diversions.)

(2) Use discretion in administering sedatives ordered p.r.n. and particularly avoid administering these drugs too readily simply to keep the patient quiet for the convenience of the staff, as such nursing actions could help in fostering dependence.

(3) Be alert for signs that the patient on long-term therapy is becoming dependent in too great a degree on drug-induced relief and discuss your observations and views with his physician.

Remember that an agitated, depressed patient may try to use these drugs in attempting suicide.

(1) Do not leave sedative-hypnotic drugs at the patient's bedside. Stay with him until he has taken the drug. As some patients may pretend to swallow it and instead hoard it in order to attempt suicide with the accumulated medication, observe unobtrusively that he has actually swallowed the drug.

Instruct patients who will be taking drugs of this type at home as to how they are best stored and what other safety precautions to observe.

(1) To prevent accidental ingestion by children or by the patient himself when he is sleepy or confused, the medicine should not be kept at bedside but in the medicine cabinet or in a locked container.

(2) Patients should be warned not to drive or to undertake other activities requiring alertness and motor coordination, until they are sure that the sedative drugs do not have any disabling depressant effects on their mental and motor functions.

Discussion Topics: Dealing with Sedatives, Hypnotics, and Antianxiety Agents

1. *The Situation:* Mr. Ward comes to a community mental health center for weekly psychotherapy. His history indicates that he had first come to the clinic following a three-month period of progressive irritability, insomnia, and depression.

The psychiatrist then ordered Librium 10 mg t.i.d. and at bedtime. He explained to Mr. Ward that this drug would help him to relax. He also suggested that the medication could

help him get the sleep that he complained he had to have but wasn't getting.

The Problem: Discuss how you as the public health nurse who visits Mr. Ward at home once a week would respond to his remark of "I know I need this stuff and that it's helping me to rest, but I'm scared to death of having to keep on taking it."

Discuss the kinds of observations that you

would make concerning Mr. Ward's response to therapy with Librium.

2. *The Situation:* Mrs. Lombard has entered the hospital for a hysterectomy. At bedtime on the night before the surgery is schedule, she received 0.1 Gm. of sodium pentobarbital (Nembutal).

She awakens in an agitated state several hours later, calling for the nurse and saying that she has had a terrifying dream.

The Problem: Discuss the nature of the nursing intervention that you would use in this situation.

3. *The Situation:* Mr. Roberts, a 65-year-old patient recovering from pneumonia, is having difficulty sleeping. You administer the bedtime dose of secobarbital sodium (Seconal) 0.1 Gm. that his physician had ordered (h.s. and p.r.n.).

About an hour later you hear Mr. Roberts shuffling about in his room. When you go in you find that he is looking for his clothes so that you and he—he calls you by his wife's name—can leave the "hotel" and go home.

The Problem: Discuss the kind of nursing intervention that you would use in this situation.

DRUG DIGEST

CHLORAL HYDRATE U.S.P. (Noctec; and others)

Actions and Indications. This is the oldest sedative-hypnotic drug and one which is still considered a relatively cheap, rapidly effective, and safe sleep producer. It is used alone in the management of insomnia or combined with potent analgesics during labor and for pre- and postoperative sedation.

Side Effects, Cautions, and Contraindications. The undiluted liquid occasionally causes nausea and vomiting as a result of gastric irritation. Taken together with alcohol, this drug can cause an excessive degree of depression. Its use is contraindicated in patients with a history of severe hepatic, renal, or cardiac disease. Caution is required when this drug is added to the treatment regimen of patients taking anticoagulant agents, as well as when the sedative is removed from such regimens, since its presence in the body may affect the metabolism of the anticoagulants so as to cause unexpected bleeding episodes.

Dosage and Administration. For daytime sedation oral doses of 250 to 500 mg are administered t.i.d. after meals. For hypnosis 500 mg to 1 Gm. are administered at bedtime in most cases, but some patients may require up to 2 Gm. Capsules are taken with a full glass of fruit juice, ginger ale, or other liquid; syrups are diluted with a half glass of the same fluids. The drug may also be administered rectally in suppository form or by retention enema.

CHLORDIAZEPOXIDE N.F. AND CHLORDIAZEPOXIDE HCl U.S.P. (Librium)

Actions and Indications. This minor tranquilizer is used for relief of anxiety and tension states. Small oral doses help to relieve symptoms of organic and functional disorders of the gastrointestinal tract and cardiovascular system, and may be beneficial in the menopause and in various musculoskeletal and dermatologic disorders. Higher oral and parenteral doses control agitation in alcoholic withdrawal syndromes and reduce preoperative apprehension.

Side Effects, Cautions, and Contraindications. Drowsiness, ataxia, and confusion occur most commonly in elderly and weakened patients. Alcohol, which increases such depressant effects, should be avoided. Patients are cautioned against driving or engaging in other activities that require complete mental alertness.

Addiction-prone and suicidal patients should receive only small supplies of this drug, which can produce dependence if abused and cause coma if taken in massive overdosage. (Danger of respiratory and cardiovascular collapse is, however, less than with barbiturate intoxication.

Dosage and Administration. Mild to moderate anxiety in adults may be managed with 5 to 10 mg t.i.d. or q.i.d. by mouth. Greater excitement may require oral doses up to 25 mg. Agitation in alcoholics and other acutely anxious patients is treated with doses of 50 to 100 mg administered parenterally and repeated every two to four hours. Elderly and debilitated patients receive 10 mg or less daily, until development of tolerance permits a gradual dosage increase.

GLUTETHIMIDE N.F. (Doriden)

Actions and Indications. This nonbarbiturate depressant drug is used for daytime, preoperative, and first stage of labor sedation and in the management of insomnia. It has no advantages over the barbiturates except in patients hypersensitive to the latter hypnotics.

Side Effects, Cautions, and Contraindications. Excessive sedation may occur in sensitive patients, and allergic hypersensitivity may result in skin rashes of several types. Blood dyscrasias and porphyria have also developed on rare occasions. Acute intoxication is similar to that caused by other depressants, but it is sometimes complicated by excitatory effects on motor systems that result in convulsions. Atropinelike effects such as dilated pupils, dry mouth, dysuria, and reduced peristaltic activity are also often seen following ingestion of toxic doses. The drug is used with caution in patients prone to abuse drugs, as it has produced dependence.

Dosage and Administration. Oral doses of 150 to 250 mg are administered t.i.d. after meals for daytime sedation. For hypnotic action 250 to 500 mg may be given at bedtime and repeated during the night if necessary. Doses of 500 mg to 1.0 Gm are administered for preoperative sedation one hour before anesthesia and surgery.

HYDROXYZINE HCl N.F. (Atarax); HYDROXYZINE PAMOATE N.F. (Vistaril)

Actions and Indications. This antianxiety agent is used in conditions marked by nervousness and tension, including psychoneuroses and psychophysiologic reactions. It is claimed to possess a wide spectrum of secondary pharmacological effects, but these are of little clinical significance in the management of organic disorders. In such conditions, this drug is commonly combined with other drugs that have more direct effects on the G.I. and respiratory tracts and other specific peripheral sites.

Side Effects, Cautions, and Contra-indications. Drowsiness occurs commonly early in treatment, so patients are cautioned against driving or drinking alcoholic beverages. Dosage of narcotic analgesics and other central depressant drugs must be reduced up to 50% when administered in combination with parenteral hydroxyzine preoperatively and in management of labor. This drug is contraindicated for use in early pregnancy.

Dosage and Administration. Dosage is individualized in accordance with the individual's response, as it ranges between 25 mg orally t.i.d. to 100 mg q.i.d. by mouth. The drug is also administered intramuscularly in doses of 25 to 100 mg, which may be repeated every four to six hours for control of acute excitement during withdrawal of alcohol and in other emotional emergencies.

MEPROBAMATE U.S.P. (Equanil, Miltown)

Actions and Indications. This drug is used mainly as a minor tranquilizer in anxiety and tension states. It relieves anxiety in alcoholic, neurotic, and some psychotic patients and in medical conditions with an emotional component including, for example, angina pectoris and peptic ulcer. High doses administered parenterally may help to relax painful muscle spasm in tetanus.

Side Effects, Cautions, and Contra-indications. Central depressant effects include drowsiness (in ordinary dosage); ataxia, dizziness, and slurred speech (in higher than recommended doses); and coma, circulatory, and respiratory collapse (in massive overdosage).

Alcohol and other CNS depressants have additive effects so patients are cautioned against drinking and driving, and dosage is carefully controlled in treating patients with a history of alcoholism or addiction.

Acute intermittent porphyria and a history of allergic skin reactions or idiosyncratic blood cell responses on prior administration of the drug constitute contraindications to its further use.

Dosage and Administration. The usual dose administered orally to adults is 400 mg t.i.d. or q.i.d. This dose may also be administered intramuscularly every three or four hours in treating tetanus. Doses above 2400 mg daily are not recommended, despite the experimental clinical administration of higher doses in attempts to control severe skeletal muscle spasm.

PARALDEHYDE U.S.P.

Actions and Indications. This rapid-acting sedative-hypnotic has been used mainly in the management of hospitalized alcoholic patients to prevent or to treat delirium tremens during withdrawal. It has also been employed to control convulsions in tetanus, status epilepticus, and other acute seizure states. It is occasionally used in labor and as a basal anesthetic.

Side Effects, Cautions, and Contra-indications. This liquid's unpleasant taste and odor have not discouraged abuse of the drug by some alcoholics who have become dependent upon it. When deprived of the drug, these addicts suffer the typical depressant drug withdrawal syndrome, including delirium tremens. Accidental overdosage results in deep depression that is sometimes complicated by metabolic acidosis. Decomposed paraldehyde containing high levels of acetaldehyde and acetic acid contaminants should not be used.

Dosage and Administration. The usual oral dose is 5 to 10 ml, but as much as 30 ml may be needed by some patients. The liquid's taste is disguised with flavored syrups or fruit juices and by chilling it. It may be administered rectally for control of convulsions but must be well diluted with olive oil to reduce local irritation. I.M. or I.V. injection has been employed in the past but is now considered inadvisable.

PENTOBARBITAL SODIUM U.S.P. (Nembutal)

Actions and Indications. Oral doses provide daytime sedation and nighttime sleep for emotionally upset patients and for those with various medical conditions that benefit from a reduction in nervous tension. Injections result in rapid sedative, hypnotic, and anticonvulsant effects in acute agitation and convulsive states. Used also preoperatively and during labor for sedation and amnesia.

Side Effects, Cautions, and Contra-indications. Addiction-prone individuals may become psychologically and physically dependent. Liver disease requires caution, as does the simultaneous administration of coumarin-type anticoagulants. Porphyria and a history of hypersensitivity to barbiturates contraindicate use of this drug. Overdose results in depression, ranging from drowsiness to coma, hypotension, and respiratory failure.

Dosage and Administration. For daytime sedation 20 or 30 mg is taken t.i.d. or q.i.d. as a capsule or elixir or in a single 100-mg long-release tablet. A 100-mg capsule or 200-mg suppository is usually capable of producing a hypnotic effect. Intravenous administration of 100-mg doses is made slowly with added increments if required. I.M. injections of 150 to 200 mg are made deep into a large muscle mass.

References

Domino, E.F. Human pharmacology of tranquilizing drugs. *Clin. Pharmacol. Ther.*, 3:599, 1962.

Friend, D.G. Sedative hypnotics. *Clin. Pharmacol. Ther.*, 1:454, 1960.

Kales, A., and Kales, J.D. Sleep laboratory evaluation of psychoactive drugs. *Pharmacol. Physicians*, 4(9):1, 1970.

Kline, N.S. and Davis, J.M. Psychotropic drugs. *Amer. J. Nurs.* 73:54, 1973 (January).

Lasagna, L. The pharmacological basis for the effective use of hypnotics. *Pharmacol. Physicians*, 1(2):1, 1967.

Leff, R., and Bernstein, S. Proprietary hallucinogens. *Dis. Nerv. Sys.*, 29:621, 1968.

Morgan, A.J. Minor tranquilizers, hypnotics, and sedatives. *Amer. J. Nurs.* 73:1220, 1973 (July).

Robinson, R.R., et al. Treatment of acute barbiturate intoxication. *Mod. Treatm.*, 4:679, 1967 (July).

Rodman, M.J. Drugs for treating anxiety. *RN*, 36:57, 1973 (Sept.).

Shideman, F.E. Clinical pharmacology of hypnotics and sedatives. *Clin. Pharmacol. Ther.*, 2:313, 1961.

7

Drugs Used in the Management of Mental Illness

Introduction

Mental and emotional disorders are among the most common of all illnesses. We have seen that even mild to moderate anxiety often leads to psychophysiologic reactions, psychosomatic illnesses, and psychoneurotic restlessness that require treatment with sedative-hypnotics and minor tranquilizers. In this chapter, we shall discuss drugs that are used in the management of more serious psychiatric disorders.

THE NATURE OF PSYCHOSIS

The term "psychosis," like "psychoneurosis," is defined in different ways by doctors of varying schools of thought. One way in which psychotic patients are usually said to differ from psychoneurotic individuals is in the degree to which they are out of contact with reality. Psychosis is usually marked by the presence of hallucinations, delusions, and other thought disturbances. Sometimes the psychotic individual's personality becomes so grossly disorganized that he cannot function adequately and must be hospitalized.

The underlying causes of most psychoses are still not well understood. Sometimes the cause is obviously organic—the result of damage to nerve cells in the brain. Much more commonly, the reason for the patient's illness cannot yet be explained on an organic basis. Such so-called *functional* psychoses are commonly divided into two main groups: (1) the schizophrenias and (2) the affective, or mood, disorders.

PSYCHOTHERAPEUTIC DRUGS

In this chapter, we shall deal mainly with two types of drugs:

1. The major tranquilizers. These drugs, also known as antipsychotic agents and neuroleptics, are used to control the symptoms of schizophrenia and other psychoses that are marked both by agitation and withdrawal

2. The antidepressant drugs. These agents are used to aid depressed patients suffering symptoms of either psychomotor retardation or of agitation and mania. (Methods of treatment other than the use of major tranquilizers or antidepressant drugs will be discussed at the end of this chapter.)

STATUS

Drugs of these kinds have helped to revolutionize the management of mentally ill patients. Although these drugs do not cure psychotic patients, their ability to control symptoms makes it easier for patients to profit from other forms of treatment such as psychotherapy. The tranquilizing drugs have helped to change some mental hospitals from places where patients were merely kept in custody to true treatment facilities. Drug therapy has also been an important factor in enabling patients to be treated in the community, with a brief period of hospitalization, or without admission to the hospital. Antidepressant drugs have reduced the need for electroshock therapy and have made it easier to treat many depressed patients at home rather than in hospitals.

The ability of these newer psychotherapeutic drugs to bring about beneficial changes in the behavior of patients has been one important factor affecting the nurse's role in dealing with psychiatric patients. Instead of spending most of her time keeping disturbed patients in packs, tubs, and other physical restraints, she can now devote more time to therapeutic intervention. This is extremely important, as the patient's recovery really depends upon his ability to establish satisfying interpersonal contacts with others, including a nurse counselor.

Thus, for example, in situations where contacts with patients are often quite limited, the nurse should view the time when she is administering medications as an opportunity to reach out to the patient and show her respect and concern for him. Even brief personal interactions of this kind, made possible by these new drugs that have made it easier to communicate with mental patients, may be quite beneficial.

The nurse can help the outpatient who is taking maintenance doses of the therapeutic drugs. She instructs patients in how to take the drugs and how to observe and report their effects. In checking with patients about their drug therapy on their periodic visits to the psychiatric clinic—or on her own visits to patients' homes—the nurse again has opportunities to interact effectively.

The Major Tranquilizers or Antipsychotic Agents

TERMINOLOGY

The term "tranquilizer" does not adequately describe the effects of drugs of this class. These adjuncts to psychotherapy do more than merely calm patients who are emotionally upset as do the antianxiety agents, or minor tranquilizers. Nor is it only the ability of these drugs to control even severe agitation in psychotic patients that distinguishes these antipsychotic drugs from other psychotropic* agents. The most significant aspect of the action of drugs with potent antipsychotic activity—also called "neuroleptics," "psycholeptics" and "ataractics"—is their ability to favorably influence some of the major characteristics of the psychoses, including hallucinations, delusions and other thought disturbances, and catatonic withdrawal.

Drugs with this kind of antipsychotic activity that are now available for clinical use in this country include chemicals of the following classes (Table 7-1):

1. The phenothiazine derivatives
2. The butyrophenone derivatives
3. The thioxanthine compounds
4. The rauwolfia alkaloids

Here we shall discuss in detail only the drugs of the phenothiazine class, as they are by far the most widely used antipsychotic agents. Certain individual drugs from among the other groups of tranquilizers will also be briefly mentioned together with some miscellaneous agents that are still undergoing clinical trials.

---

* Psychotropic is a broad term that indicates the ability of a drug to affect mental functioning. Not all psychotropic drugs have applications in the treatment of psychiatric disorders. Thus, alcohol is a psychotropic agent, but it is not ordinarily used as a psychopharmacological therapeutic agent.

TABLE 7-1 *Major Tranquilizers (Antipsychotic Agents)*

Nonproprietary or Official Name	Proprietary Name	Usual Daily Dosage Range
Phenothiazines		
ALIPHATIC SUBGROUP		
Chlorpromazine HCl U.S.P.	Thorazine	10 mg–1 gm
Promazine HCl N.F.	Sparine	40–1200 mg
Triflupromazine HCl N.F.	Vesprin	30–150 mg
PIPERAZINE SUBGROUP		
Acetophenazine maleate N.F.	Tindal	40–80 mg
Butaperazine maleate	Repoise	15–100 mg
Carphenazine maleate N.F.	Proketazine	12.5–50 mg
Fluphenazine HCl* N.F.	Permitil; Prolixin	1.5–20 mg
Perphenazine N.F.	Trilafon	6–64 mg
Prochlorperazine edisylate U.S.P. ⎫ Prochlorperazine maleate U.S.P. ⎭	Compazine	5–150 mg
Thiopropazate HCl N.F.	Dartal	15–100 mg
Trifluoperazine HCl N.F.	Stelazine	2–20 mg
PIPERIDYL SUBGROUP		
Mesoridazine	Serentil	30–400 mg
Piperacetazine	Quide	20–160 mg
Thioridazine HCl U.S.P.	Mellaril	20–800 mg
Miscellaneous Non*phenothiazines*		
Chlorprothixene N.F.	Taractan	30–200 mg
Haloperidol N.F.	Haldol	3–15 mg
Reserpine U.S.P.	Serpasil, and others	0.5–10 mg
Thiothixene	Navane	6–60 mg

* Fluphenazine enanthate and decanoate are long-acting forms that may be administered in doses of 25 mg every two weeks.

THE PHENOTHIAZINE-TYPE ANTIPSYCHOTIC AGENTS

HISTORY. One of the first phenothiazine derivatives used in medicine was *promethazine* (Phenergan) which was introduced as an antihistaminic agent for treating allergy symptoms. Later, it was found to possess other properties—such as *sedative* and *antiemetic* effects—which made it useful in preparing patients for surgical and obstetrical procedures.

CHEMISTRY. *Chlorpromazine* (Thorazine), the first drug of this class to be used in psychiatry, was discovered during a search for preoperative sedatives similar to promethazine. When medical scientists accidentally became aware of the then unique effects of this drug on mentally ill patients, they proceeded to prepare many closely related chemical compounds in an attempt to develop drugs that would be safer and more effective than chlorpromazine.

These derivatives can be divided into the following three chemical subgroups (Table 7-1):

1. The *aliphatic* or *dimethylaminoalkyl group* (for example, promazine, chlorpromazine, triflupromazine)

2. The *piperazine* subgroup (for example, fluphenazine, trifluoperazine, perphenazine)

3. The *piperidine* subgroup (for example, thioridazine, mesoridazine, piperacetazine)

Phenothiazines of all three classes are essentially similar to the prototype chemical chlorpromazine in their effectiveness as antipsychotic agents. They differ from one another mainly in their potency and in the types of side effects that they tend to cause. Thus, for example, drugs of the piperazine subclass are as effective in doses of a few milligrams as are hundreds of milligrams of the derivatives of the other two subclasses. These piperazines are, however, much more likely to cause extrapyramidal motor system side effects (see be-

TABLE 7-2 *Signs and Symptoms Often Seen In Depressive Syndromes**

Mood

Sad, dejected, downcast, irritable, tearful, and with loss of ability to find anything pleasurable or enjoyable.

Physiologic

Sleep disturbances—insomnia marked by early morning awakening; anorexia—loss of appetite and weight; loss of libido—decrease in sex drive; headache, abdominal distress, constipation, fatigue or feeling of weakness, and such signs of autonomic imbalance as cardiac palpitations, flushing, sweating.

Thought and Behavior

RETARDED DEPRESSION FEATURES

Signs of psychomotor slowing such as slow speech in a low, weak or whispered voice; apathy or indifference—loss of interest in the environment, family, work, personal appearance; failure to respond to questions; slow, deliberate or dragging gait and movements; unwillingness or inability to get out of bed, and, in severely retarded cases, stupor.

AGITATED DEPRESSION FEATURES

Verbal and motor expressions of anxiety, such as pacing back and forth, wringing the hands, and complaining volubly of the above physical symptons that may be seen as signs of cancer, heart disease, and other serious illnesses; preoccupation with possible tragedy and death; thoughts of personal inadequacy, lack of competence, guilt, hopelessness, worthlessness, hallucinations, delusions, and preoccupation with the idea of suicide.

---

* Depressed patients usually show a half dozen or more of these signs and symptoms but never, of course, all of them.

---

low). Phenothiazines of the other two classes are more prone to produce oversedation and hypotension.

PHARMACOLOGICAL EFFECTS (*Summary,* p. 102). The phenothiazines produce many central and peripheral effects. Some of these effects have been applied clinically in general medicine and in anesthesiology as well as in psychiatry; others are the cause of the adverse effects that often occur when these drugs are used clinically.

❪ *Sedation.* These drugs produce a quieting or calming effect that differs in quality from that which follows administration of the barbiturates, *non*barbiturate sedative-hypnotics, and the minor tranquilizers. Among these differences in their depressant effects are the following:

1. Patients are made apathetic and indifferent to exciting environmental stimuli without suffering severe mental and motor impairment. That is, they can be more readily aroused than patients depressed by drugs such as barbiturates and meprobamate. Thus, they are more alert and responsive, and they can move about with better motor coordination following arousal.

2. Patients do *not* go through any preliminary excitement phase before becoming calm and quiet, as often occurs with alcohol, bar-

biturates, and similar depressants; nor do even very large doses result in severe respiratory depression, stupor, and coma, as occurs with the other depressants.

3. Psychological dependence rarely develops, presumably because patients do not feel the euphoric release of inhibitions often produced by the sedative-hypnotics and minor tranquilizers.

4. Patients show reduced motor activity, as occurs with the general depressants. Unlike the latter, however, the phenothiazines do *not* have good anticonvulsant activity. On the contrary, these drugs may increase susceptibility to seizures in epileptic patients and others, presumably because of their complex effects upon extrapyramidal motor system nerve pathways (see below).

❪ *Antipsychotic effect.* In a schizophrenic patient, these drugs often produce desirable effects in addition to sedation. These may result from a direct effect of the phenothiazines upon the pathogenic processes that are the underlying cause of his psychotic symptoms. At first, the patient may continue to have hallucinations. However, his disordered sensory perceptions do not seem to upset him emotionally as much as before. As his fear and hostility subside, his disturbed thinking and behavior also improve. He is then more responsive to other forms of treatment, including psychotherapy.

❨ *Antiemetic effect.* Most phenothiazines—particularly those of the piperazine subgroup, such as *prochlorperazine+* (Compazine)—depress the nerve cells that relay sensory impulses to the brain's vomiting center. The use of these drugs to prevent or overcome vomiting in many medical conditions and following anesthesia is discussed in Chapter 45.

❨ *Potentiating effect.* The phenothiazines are able to prolong and intensify the effects of other depressant drugs including the narcotic analgesics. This makes them useful in the management of pain and as adjuncts to anesthesia. However, this action may prove dangerous in patients already under the influence of alcohol, barbiturates, or narcotics (see below).

❨ *Autonomic blocking effects.* These effects, which occur more commonly with the aliphatic and piperidine subgroups of phenothiazines, are usually undesired side effects; they are discussed in the section dealing with the adverse effects of these drugs (p. 96).

CLINICAL INDICATIONS (*Summary*, pp. 102-103). The phenothiazines are most dramatically effective when employed for quick control of acute excitement in many psychiatric disorders. However, these drugs also have a place in the long-term management of patients who do *not* show excessive excitement or who may even be deeply withdrawn.

❨ *Control of agitation.* Patients with acute schizophrenic reactions of all types respond rapidly to the sedative effects of the phenothiazines, particularly drugs of the aliphatic subgroup such as *chlorpromazine+*, *promazine*, and *triflupromazine*. These drugs are also useful for quick control of excitement and disturbed behavior in patients disturbed by the effects of drugs such as LSD (toxic psychosis), and in acute alcoholic intoxication.

Alcoholic patients may also profit from phenothiazine administration during withdrawal states such as alcoholic hallucinosis and delirium tremens. Here, however, they are best combined with general depressants such as the barbiturates, paraldehyde, or *chlordiazepoxide* (Librium).

The manic phase of the manic-depressive psychosis can often be brought under control most rapidly with one of the more sedating types of phenothiazines. Slower-acting lithium salts are administered simultaneously, and phenothiazines are now usually discontinued once effective levels of lithium are attained in the brain.

The restlessness, confusion, and excitement seen in patients suffering from chronic brain syndromes are also controlled with phenothiazines. Both elderly patients with organic brain damage due to cerebrovascular atherosclerosis and mentally retarded children are made more calm and quiet with these drugs.

❨ *Activation of withdrawn patients.* The phenothiazines have also proved effective for overcoming states of schizophrenic withdrawal. Drugs of the piperazine subgroup, such as *fluphenazine+* and *trifluoperazine* (Stelazine) are often preferred for counteracting bizarre catatonic posturing and mutism. However, the prototype phenothiazine, *chlorpromazine*, is claimed to be just as effective as the newer drugs for overcoming the seclusiveness and apathy of these and other schizophrenics whose fear and hostility are manifested by such symptoms of psychomotor withdrawal rather than by agitation.

❨ *Depressed patients.* Patients with similar symptoms, such as sluggishness and lethargy, may respond poorly to phenothiazines if their retarded state stems from one of the depressive syndromes (Table 7-2) rather than from schizophrenia. On the other hand, mentally depressed patients who show signs of agitation often profit from the addition of a phenothiazine such as *perphenazine* (Trilafon) to their antidepressant drug medication.

❨ *Mild to moderate anxiety.* Phenothiazine drug therapy is not limited to agitated or withdrawn psychotic patients. Certain selected cases of psychoneurotic excitement are often treated with low oral doses of fluphenazine or other phenothiazines. Chronic alcoholics are often maintained on long-term therapy with *thioridazine+*, or a newer drug of the same subgroup, *mesoridazine* (Serentil). Although low doses of the phenothiazines rarely cause severe side effects, some patients occasionally develop severe hypersensitivity reactions (see below). Thus, many doctors now prefer to use one of the safer minor tranquilizers for control of anxiety and tension in patients with personality disturbances and in patients with conditions that seem to have psychoneurotic or psychosomatic components.

ADVERSE EFFECTS (*Summary*, p. 103).

❲ *Types of toxicity.* The phenothiazines can cause many kinds of ill effects, particularly when these drugs must be administered to hospitalized patients in high doses for long periods. Some of the side effects of phenothiazines are the result of excessive actions on the central nervous system; others are the result of blockade of nerve impulse transmission by way of both divisions of the autonomic nervous system. Endocrine imbalances are occasionally brought about by continued administration of these drugs. Some side effects are the result of allergic hypersensitivity rather than the drugs' direct pharmacological effects.

The observant nurse can help to minimize adverse drug effects of all kinds in mental patients by reporting unusual signs and symptoms to the doctor and discussing the patient's drug reaction problems with him, and by encouraging the patient to discuss these matters with the staff. Thus, for example, patients may complain of drowsiness, dizziness, weakness, and faintness—particularly, early in treatment with aliphatic-type phenothiazines such as chlorpromazine. This should be reported to the doctor who may then reduce the drug's dosage temporarily to counteract the depression and postural hypotension produced by this drug.

The nurse can also often explain to the patient the true significance of drug-induced side effects. Outpatients, for example, are sometimes alarmed by physical feelings that they may think are caused by a return of the perceptual distortions which were part of their illness. The nurse may be able to assure them that visual difficulties or other strange sensations that they may be experiencing are actually the result of temporary central and autonomic side effects of their phenothiazine maintenance medication.

Similarly, the nurse's supportive attitude can help reduce the patient's concern about the sexual function side effects sometimes set off by these. drugs. Reduced sex drive and impotence in the male outpatient are ordinarily only temporary; and women with delayed menstruation, breast enlargement, and a gain in weight can be assured that these are drug-induced effects rather than signs of pregnancy. (Of course, the physician is informed of these side effects so that he can rule out possible pregnancy or the presence of pathology).

The nurse's alertness in listening to the patient's complaints of a sudden severe sore throat has sometimes helped detect the occasional onset of a phenothiazine drug-induced blood dyscrasia such as agranulocytosis. Jaundice may signal liver involvement requiring withdrawal of the drug. In the late spring, patients are warned to avoid exposure to strong sunlight when taking phenothiazine medication in order to prevent severe sunburn and possible skin discoloration resulting from photosensitivity-type drug reactions.

The effects of phenothiazines on the patient's movements may take many forms. In most cases, these drugs diminish motor activity and make hyperactive patients almost immobile. Sometimes patients with such akinesia also show other signs similar to those seen in patients with Parkinson's disease. However, this drug-induced pseudoparkinsonism is reversible when dosage is reduced or the drug is withdrawn.

Other motor reactions are marked by restlessness (*akathisia*) or by sudden contractions of muscle groups that are sometimes so severe that they resemble convulsive seizures (*dyskinesia*). These reactions are usually reversible, but recent reports indicate that abnormal movements may sometimes persist even after these drugs are discontinued. Such persistent dyskinesias have developed most commonly in elderly women with preexisting brain damage who have been maintained on large doses of phenothiazines for long periods.

MISCELLANEOUS ANTIPSYCHOTIC AGENTS

BUTYROPHENONE TYPE. Two drugs of this chemical class are currently available. One of these neuroleptic drugs, *droperidol* (Inapsine) is used mainly as an adjunct to anesthesia. The other, *haloperidol* (Haldol), resembles the piperazine-type phenothiazines in its actions. It is used to control severely agitated manic states in schizophrenia and in manic-depressive psychosis. The drug has also helped reduce hostility and confusion in elderly patients with organic brain damage and to quiet hyperactive, mentally retarded children. It is claimed to be relatively specific for normalizing the behavior of children suffering from Gilles de la Tourette's syndrome.

The most common side effect of haloperidol is the occurrence of extrapyramidal reactions of the parkinsonism type. These are controlled by the administration of antiparkinsonism drugs such as benztropine and trihexyphenidyl. The initially high doses required for control of psychotic symptoms are gradually reduced to lower maintenance levels in order to minimize toxicity in patients who are responding to the drug.

THIOXANTHENE DERIVATIVES. One of the two available drugs of this class, *chlorprothixene* (Taractan) resembles the aliphatic-type phenothiazines chemically and in its pharmacological effects; the other, *thiothixene* (Navane) is chemically and pharmacologically similar to the piperazine phenothiazines. Both drugs are used mainly in the management of acutely and chronically ill schizophrenic patients. The incidence and the severity of side effects are also similar to those of the phenothiazines, as are the precautions that are required in using these drugs (see *Summary of Cautions and Contraindications*, p. 104).

RAUWOLFIA ALKALOIDS. *Reserpine* was one of the first tranquilizers to be employed in psychiatry. However, this and other rauwolfia plant derivatives are less effective and convenient to use than the phenothiazines, and they are today used only for the relatively few patients who are hypersensitive to the several available classes of synthetic antipsychotic chemicals. Reserpine and related drugs are discussed in more detail in Chapter 26 (*Drugs Used in Treating Hypertension*), as their use in the management of high blood pressure is of greater clinical significance today than their use for control of symptoms of schizophrenia.

ON-TRIAL COMPOUNDS

Drugs of several other chemical classes that have antipsychotic activity are currently undergoing clinical trials. None of these newer drugs seems to show significant advantages over the drugs already available for treating mental illness.

Drugs for Treating Affective Disorders: Antidepressant Drugs

In this section we shall study drugs that are used in treating patients who are mentally depressed or who suffer from periods of mania that alternate with periods of depression. Such conditions are included among the *affective disorders*—psychopathological reactions that are marked by disturbances in a patient's mood, thinking and behavior.

Depression, perhaps the most common of all psychiatric disorders, is marked by many different signs and symptoms (Table 7-2). Some depressed patients show mainly signs of retardation, or psychomotor slowing. The condition of other depression sufferers is marked mainly by signs of their anxiety and agitation. Patients of both types often respond to treatment with the modern antidepressant drugs.

The drugs of this category are subdivided into two main classes. The most widely used group is commonly called the *tricyclic type*, a term that refers to their three-ringed chemical structure (Table 7-3). The other group of antidepressant drugs is referred to as the monoamine oxidase (MAO) inhibitor type (Table 7-3) because of their ability to interfere with the function of an enzyme that is thought to play an important part in the metabolism of catecholamines and other amines in the brain and elsewhere in the body.

Both classes of antidepressant drugs are thought to act by helping to overcome a deficiency of monoamines in the brains of severely depressed patients. The MAO inhibitors are believed to do so by interfering with the breakdown of catecholamines such as norepinephrine and dopamine in nerve cells. The tricyclic-type antidepressants are thought to exert their mood elevating effect by increasing the amount of free norepinephrine available for transmitting impulses in nerve pathways involved in emotional activity.

TRICYCLIC-TYPE ANTIDEPRESSANTS (TABLE 7-3)

CLINICAL INDICATIONS AND STATUS. Drugs of this class are usually the first choice for initiating treatment of patients with moderate to severe depression. (See pp. 95 and 100 for a brief discussion of drugs used in management of mild depression and of electroconvulsive and pharmacoconvulsant therapies for dangerously depressed patients.) The tricyclics are less likely to cause dangerous adverse effects than are the MAO inhibitors. If patients fail to respond to treatment with one or more of the drugs in this class, they can be quickly transferred to a course of MAO inhibitor drug treatment. The reverse is not true. If the MAOI-type agents were tried first without success, the patient would have to wait at least two weeks before he could be safely switched to

TABLE 7-3 *Antidepressant Drugs*

Nonproprietary Name	Trade Name	Usual Daily Oral Dosage*	Comments
Tricyclic Type			
Amitriptyline HCl U.S.P.	Elavil	75 mg (25–300 mg)	See *Drug Digest*
Desipramine HCl N.F.	Norpramine, Pertofran	150 mg (25–300 mg)	Relatively rapid onset of action (three to five days)
Doxepin HCl	Sinequan	75 mg (25–300 mg)	Has marked antianxiety as well as antidepressant activity
Imipramine HCl U.S.P.	Tofranil	150 mg (25–300 mg)	See *Drug Digest*
Nortriptyline HCl N.F.	Aventyl	150 mg (25–300 mg)	Claimed useful also for gastrointestinal psychophysiologic disorders and for childhood enuresis
Protriptyline HCl	Vivactil	30 mg (5–60 mg)	Claimed more potent and rapid in onset. Its activating effect may cause increased anxiety in some patients
Monoamine Oxidase Inhibitor Type			
Isocarboxazid N.F.	Marplan	30 mg (10–60 mg)	See *Drug Digest*
Phenelzine sulfate U.S.P.	Nardil	30 mg (15–90 mg)	A potent antidepressant capable of causing all the potential adverse effects of drugs of this class and requiring all the usual precautions
Tranylcypromine sulfate N.F.	Parnate	20 mg (10–60 mg)	See *Drug Digest*

* Dosage range from lowest initial and maintenance dosage to highest doses for hospitalized patients is given in parentheses.

one of the tricyclic compounds. (See below and the *Summary of Cautions and Contraindications.*)

These drugs have proved effective in treating patients with all the main kinds of depression and all types of target symptoms. Among the clinical categories that often respond to these drugs are:

1. The depressed phase of the manic-depressive psychosis

2. Involutional psychotic reactions—the kind of "melancholia" most commonly seen in postmenopausal women and somewhat older men

3. Psychotic depressive reactions of the kind also called severe reactive depressions

4. Miscellaneous other psychotic—for example, schizoaffective—and psychoneurotic depressive states

The prototype drugs of this class, *imipramine+* (Tofranil) and *amitriptyline+* (Elavil), have proved effective for control of all types of depressive target symptoms. However, certain of the more recently introduced related drugs are often claimed to possess advantages in treating particular types of depressed patients. That is, some tricyclics are said to be better for patients presenting with signs of psychomotor retardation, while others are preferred for patients with signs of agitation (Table 7-2).

Nortriptyline (Aventyl), for example, a derivative of amitriptyline, shares with the latter a sedative or tranquilizing component. This action, appearing early in the course of treatment, is said to help overcome states of psychomotor depression. Similarly, another new drug of this class, *doxepin* (Sinequan) is claimed to be particularly effective for patients with symptoms of anxiety as well as of retardation. Actually, however, when the degree of a depressed patient's anxiety or agitation is severe, it is desirable to administer a phenothiazine-type tranquilizer in combination with the tricyclic antidepressant. (*Perphenazine*—Trilafon—is often prescribed in combination with amitriptyline in such cases, as well as for schizophrenics with depressive symptomatology.)

Protriptyline (Vivactil), on the other hand, is a tricyclic compound that has no sedative or tranquilizing effect. Instead, it is said to act more rapidly than most other drugs of this class to overcome the feelings of fatigue and indifference seen in patients whose depression takes the form of psychomotor retardation. As the drug exerts its activating effects, patients often feel a surge of energy and become less withdrawn and more interested in participating in interpersonal relations.

The nurse takes advantage of such signs of recovery to talk with the depressed patient and to listen to what he has to say, when he becomes more willing and able to communicate his thoughts. It is also very important to watch the patient carefully as he becomes more alert and active because some previously apathetic patients also become better able to marshal their energies for a suicide attempt at this time. Patients taking the types of tricyclics that have marked activating effects should also be observed for signs of increasing anxiety and agitation, as the doctor may then order dosage reduced or add a sedative to the patient's regimen.

Adverse Effects of Tricyclic-Type Antidepressants. Although therapeutic doses of these drugs seldom cause the severe toxicity sometimes seen with agents of the MAO inhibitor type, they are capable of producing a wide variety of discomforting side effects. These often are the result of an atropinelike blockade of nerve impulses to the eyes, mouth, and gastrointestinal and genitourinary tract muscles (*Summary*, p. 104). As already indicated, these drugs may also affect the central nervous system to produce symptoms of both excessive excitement and drowsiness of a degree that may be hazardous to patients driving a car or operating machinery.

Precautions with Tricyclic Compounds (*Summary*, p. 105). The autonomic nerve blocking effects of these drugs may make them dangerous for patients with glaucoma or with bladder-voiding difficulties. Particular caution is required in patients with cardiovascular diseases, as drug-induced tachycardia or hypotension aggravate their conditions and even lead to myocardial infarction. These drugs are not administered together with antidepressants of the MAO inhibitor group, which tend to potentiate both the central stimulating and autonomic blocking effects of the tricyclics. This could lead to hyperactive reflexes, muscle rigidity, and even convulsive seizures.

Toxic Overdosage. Actually, the tricyclic drugs are relatively safe when taken alone in ordinary doses. They become dangerous mainly when taken in massive overdosage in a deliberate attempt to commit suicide. Deaths have occurred in patients who hoarded these drugs and then ingested a large quantity of capsules. Most common in such cases are disturbances of cardiac function, including arrhythmias that can result in fatal fibrillations or asystole. Obviously, to avoid such catastrophes, it is important for the nurse to stay with this depressed patient until he has taken the medication that she has brought him.

MONOAMINE OXIDASE INHIBITOR TYPE ANTIDEPRESSANTS (TABLE 7-3)

Clinical Indications and Status. Drugs of this class were the first pharmacological agents to prove effective for treating severe psychotic and psychoneurotic depressions. Today, however, they are largely reserved for treating depressed patients who have failed to respond to one or more courses of the safer tricyclic-type antidepressants. Among the patients who are said to benefit most often from treatment with an MAO inhibitor are those who are classified as suffering from depression of the psychoneurotic, or reactive, type. Some schizophrenic patients with depressive symptoms are also said to do better on combinations of an MAO inhibitor with an antipsychotic phenothiazine-type tranquilizer than they do when treated with the tricyclic compounds.

Adverse Effects of MAOI-type Drugs (*Summary*, pp. 104-105). The first clinically successful drug of this class, iproniazid, was withdrawn from the market when it was found to cause severe liver damage in some patients. Consequently, patients taking other drugs of this class are often subjected to tests of liver function. If abnormalities appear in such hepatic function tests, these drugs are discontinued. Their use is contraindicated in patients with a history of liver disease.

Actually, adverse effects upon cardiovascular function are much more common in patients taking these drugs. Most common are such symptoms of postural hypotension as dizziness, weakness, and feelings of faintness. More dangerous, however, are episodes of hypertension, as these have sometimes resulted in hypertensive crises which have occasionally led to fatal brain hemorrhages. Patients taking these drugs should be observed closely for such signs and symptoms as severe headache, stiff neck, sweating, nausea, and vomiting, as these may be early warning signs of dangerous blood pressure rises.

Because of reactions of this kind, the most potent agent of this class, *tranylcypromine*+ (Parnate), is contraindicated in patients with suspected cerebrovascular disease. It is not in fact ordinarily administered to patients over 60 years old. The latter restriction does not apply to *isocarboxazid*+ (Marplan), *phenelzine* (Nardil), or other drugs of this class. However, their use for treating depressed patients who also have high blood pressure is not recommended. Nurses caring for depressed patients taking MAO inhibitors are often instructed to take frequent blood pressure readings, so that these drugs can be quickly discontinued if hypertension, heart palpitations, or headaches develop.

The nurse should advise patients not to treat themselves with any *non*prescription drug products while they are taking this kind of antidepressant medication. Products for self-medication of colds, certain weight reducing remedies, and other medications containing sympathomimetic drugs are particularly likely to trigger hypertension in such patients. In fact, certain foods that contain the catecholamine, tyramine, may also cause dangerous pressure rises in patients taking MAO inhibitors.

Because drugs of this class can potentiate the actions of central depressants as well as such stimulants as caffeine, amphetamines, and tricyclics, patients should not be treated with narcotics such as *meperidine* (Demerol) and they should be warned against drinking alcoholic beverages. Patients who are also being treated with drugs for managing Parkinson's disease, pheochromocytoma, or essential hypertension may also be subjected to dangerous drug interactions.

Other Types of Treatment for Depression

Psychotherapy is sometimes more effective than drug therapy, particularly for treating so-called reactive or exogenous depressions in psychoneurotic patients. Drugs are, at best, only an adjunct to psychotherapy in such cases.

Electroconvulsive therapy (ECT) is still preferred for acutely suicidal patients, as it is somewhat more rapidly effective than drug therapy and more likely to prove successful in terminating attacks of major endogenous depression in psychotic patients. Administration of drugs during the course of ECT may help to reduce the number of shock treatments needed. On the other hand, the concurrent administration of drugs may increase the dangers of ECT.

Drug therapy of depression is considered safer than ECT, and it is certainly more acceptable to most patients. Patients who are being maintained on antidepressant drugs are often able to continue working, while ECT usually produces too much mental confusion and memory impairment to permit normal activity during the treatment period.

PHARMACOCONVULSANTS

Certain central nervous system stimulant drugs have been employed to produce convulsions in depressed patients. One of these, *pentylenetetrazol* (Metrazol) is administered by rapid intravenous injection; another convulsant, *fluothyl* (Indoklon) is administered by inhalation. Although reports indicate that fluothyl is as safe and effective as ECT, this pharmacoconvulsant has not gained wide acceptance. Similarly, pentylenetetrazol is now rarely used in treating severe depression and other psychiatric disorders.

PSYCHOMOTOR STIMULANTS

The *amphetamines* and *methylphenidate* (Ritalin) are sometimes useful for elevating the mood of mildly depressed patients. However, these drugs are ineffective in patients with moderate to severe degress of depression. The tendency of amphetamines to produce wakefulness and suppress appetite may increase the insomnia and lack of interest in eating that are part of the clinical picture of the serious depressive syndromes.

SEDATIVES AND TRANQUILIZERS

Drugs of this type may be desirable adjuncts in the management of patients who show signs of agitated depression as a result of some stressful event in their life situation, such as the loss of a loved one. People with normal personalities ordinarily recover spontaneously from the relatively mild depression that naturally follows such a bereavement or other losses and disappointments. Small daytime doses of *chlordiazepoxide* (Librium) or of a barbiturate at bedtime often make people more comfortable by reducing restlessness and insomnia. Of course, no drugs at all may be needed for dealing with depression of this degree.

LITHIUM SALTS FOR MANIC DISORDERS

MANIC-DEPRESSIVE PSYCHOSIS. This mood disorder, which is characterized by recurrent swings between episodes of depression and mania, has been one of the most difficult to treat of the affective disturbances. Psychotherapy is difficult to employ successfully in these cases. Electroconvulsive therapy is less effective than in other types of major endogenous depressions and not very useful for managing the manic phase. Phenothiazine-type antipsychotic drugs are often rapidly effective for control of manic behavior, but these depressants tend to produce excessive sedation.

Lithium salts, such as the carbonate, citrate, or acetate, have been recently reported to be effective for ending hypomanic and acute manic episodes without leaving the patient dull and lethargic. Administered orally in relatively low doses, a drug such as *lithium carbonate+* (Eskalith, Lithane, Lithonate) acts gradually over a period of several days to reduce the manic patient's excessive motor activity and erratic thought processes, talk, and behavior (Table 7-4).

Patients can then be maintained on lower doses of lithium to prevent recurrences of acute manic episodes. Such prophylactic use of lithium together with tricyclic-type antidepressants is also claimed to be effective in reducing the relapse rate of depressive episodes in pa-

---

T A B L E   7 - 4 *Signs and Symptoms Often Seen In Manic Syndromes**

Hypomanic State

MOOD
In high good spirits; friendly and warm toward others, but sometimes to a degree not warranted by the circumstances; optimistic, but sometimes too much so in view of the difficulties posed by the reality of the situation.

SPEECH
Talks with great glibness and facility; may move from one topic to another in a nonstop way because of distractibility.

MOTOR ACTIVITY
Appears tireless and full of energy as he moves about in what seems to be inexhaustible physical health and well-being.

Acute Manic State

MOOD
Good spirits become excessive to a degree that may disturb others; his humor may become crude or blasphemous, as he is lacking in discretion and in concern for the feelings of others; if antagonized, he may instantly become viciously angry.

SPEECH
His ideas may be expressed as rapidly as they enter his mind and thus his talk may be marked by flight of ideas and incoherence.

MOTOR ACTIVITY
Extreme mobility, restlessness, and impulsive activity; if real situations pose difficult problems, he may react with tears or aggressive behavior.

Delirious Mania

Pressure of speech to point of complete incoherence; hallucinations and delusions make it difficult to keep contact with the patient and gain his cooperation; constantly in a state of extreme purposeless activity which may lead to high fever and a state of exhaustion; incontinent; this state may end fatally if not controlled.

---

* Manic patients may *not* necessarily progress from minor levels of activity to the most intense degree of delirious mania noted here.

tients with manic-depressive illness. (Lithium does not seem useful in other depressive syndromes, nor for control of mania or depression in schizophrenic patients.)

PREVENTION OF TOXICITY. The use of lithium in medicine is not new. However, deaths in heart patients taking lithium as a salt substitute had given this element a reputation for extreme toxicity that kept it from being used. Actually, acute lithium toxicity (lithium carbonate+) is rare in properly supervised patients. The toxicity of lithium is related to its level in the patient's blood. Serum levels of less than 1.2 mEq lithium/liter—a concentration common in maintenance therapy—cause no serious toxicity. Levels above 2.0 mEq lithium/liter often result in moderate or severe toxic reactions. Thus, laboratory determinations of lithium levels must be made frequently during the period when the individual's daily dosage is being stabilized and periodically during prolonged maintenance therapy.

The nurse should know the early clinical signs of lithium intoxication and should instruct patients and their families to watch for such warning signs. Sudden loss of appetite followed by nausea, vomiting, and diarrhea require discontinuation of the drug. Other early signs of overdosage are drowsiness, muscle weakness, and motor incoordination. Such signs of depression, which are expected with phenothiazines, should not be permitted to develop with lithium, which controls the mania of this disorder by *normalizing* the patient's brain metabolism rather than through sedation.

S U M M A R Y of the Pharmacological Effects of the Phenothiazine-Type Antipsychotic Drugs

1. Sedation (tranquilizing or calming effect)—brings about a reduction in mild to moderate anxiety or in severe agitation.
2. Antipsychotic—at first, reduces the patient's reaction to such symptoms of psychosis as hallucinations and delusions and later helps to improve the patient's disturbed behavior.

3. Potentiation of the effects of narcotic analgesics and of general depressant drugs.
4. Antiemetic—control of nausea and vomiting.
5. Autonomic blockade (*Summary of Adverse Effects*, p. 103.)

S U M M A R Y of Clinical Indications of the Phenothiazine-Type Antipsychotic Drugs

Psychiatric Indications

1. Schizophrenia—acute and chronic
2. Manic phase of the manic depressive psychoses
3. Senile confusional states and psychoses
4. Childhood psychoses and mental retardation
5. Other chronic brain syndromes brought about by organic damage
6. Toxic psychoses caused by LSD, amphetamines, and acute alcoholic intoxication
7. Alcoholic withdrawal syndromes, including alcoholic hallucinosis, impending delirium tremens, and—in combination with general depressants—full-blown delirium tremens
8. Postwithdrawal long-term management of anxious-depressed alcoholics
9. Psychoneurosis (adjunct to psychotherapy)
10. Psychosomatic disorders (adjunct to specific drugs)

Psychiatric Target Symptoms

Psychomotor excitement.
Agitation, mania, tension, anxiety, nervousness, restlessness, and confusion; hyperactive, aggressive, assaultive, destructive behavior.

Psychomotor retardation.

Apathy, withdrawal, seclusiveness, mutism, autism, catatonic posturing, listlessness, lethargy of schizophrenic (not depressive) origin.

Other symptoms of psychosis.

Hallucinations, delusions, and other disturbances in thinking.

Some Medical, Surgical, and Obstetrical Indications

1. Preanesthetic sedation
2. Postoperative vomiting control
3. In labor to reduce dosage of analgesics
4. In management. of cancer patients to potentiate anesthetic and prevent vomiting induced by antineoplastic agents

SUMMARY of Adverse Effects of the Phenothiazine-Type Antipsychotic Drugs

Central Nervous System Side Effects

1. Drowsiness, lethargy, feelings of fatigue and weakness

2. Extrapyramidal motor system reactions:

(a) Pseudoparkinsonism — akinesia, masklike facies, shuffling gait, tremors, rigidity

(b) Akathisia—motor restlessness marked by feelings of inner tension or an inability to sit still or sleep

(c) Acute dyskinesia or dystonia—contractions of small muscle groups resembling tics and of large muscle groups resembling convulsions

(d) Persistent (tardive) dyskinesias—continued movements of the lips, tongue, and jaws may make speech and swallowing difficult. Muscles of upper and lower extremities may twitch and jerk continuously

Cardiovascular and Other Autonomic Reactions

1. Postural (orthostatic) hypotension—dizziness, weakness, fainting can be minimized by keeping the patient lying with head low and legs raised. Development of shocklike state may require administration of vasopressor drugs but *not* epinephrine

2. Cardiac palpitations, changes in the electrocardiogram; possible sudden death due to cardiac arrest

3. Cholinergic blockade type, mouth dryness; blurring of vision; constipation, or possibly obstipation and paralytic ileus; urinary retention; failure of sweating followed by high fever

4. Adrenergic blockage type (in addition to hypotension) include nasal stuffiness; inhibition of ejaculation

Endocrine Disorders

1. Menstrual irregularities, including amenorrhea and false positive pregnancy tests

2. Gynecomastia (breast engorgement) and lactation

3. Reduction in libido (sex drive)

4. Weight gain with increased appetite and edema

5. Hyperglycemia and glycosuria (also hypoglycemia)

Hypersensitivity-type Reactions

1. Hematological: blood dyscrasias reported include leukopenia and agranulocytosis; hemolytic anemia; thrombocytic purpura; and pancytopenia

2. Hepatic: cholestatic jaundice in which laboratory tests of liver function give results resembling extrahepatic obstruction

3. Dermatological: urticaria, contact dermatitis, photosensitivity, erythema, exfoliative dermatitis

Miscellaneous

1. Melanosis: skin pigmentation ranging from mild darkening to deep skin discolorations (slate-gray to violet)

2. Ocular changes: deposits in conjunctiva, lens, and cornea may form star-shaped opacities; rarely, pigmentary retinopathy may impair vision

3. Abrupt withdrawal may be followed by nausea, vomiting, dizziness and tremulousness

4. Pregnant patients should receive this drug only when it is essential, as newborn babies have had hyperreflexia, extrapyramidal signs, and jaundice; offspring of drug-treated animals have shown signs of toxicity, including nervous system damage

SUMMARY of Cautions and Contraindications in the Use of Phenothiazine-Type Antipsychotic Drugs

1. These depressant drugs are contraindicated in patients who are comatose from any cause and particularly from overdoses of other depressant drugs.

2. Dosages of other depressant drugs such as the barbiturates or the narcotic analgesics should be reduced by about one fourth to one half when phenothiazines are added to the patient's regimen. (Phenothiazines tend to prolong and intensify the effects of other depressants, including general anesthetics. They may also have additive effects with atropine.)

3. Patients should be advised against drinking alcohol, the effects of which are potentiated by phenothiazines. (Patients taking phenothiazines should not, in any case, drive or engage in activities which require alertness, such as operating potentially hazardous machinery.)

4. These drugs should be used with caution in patients with cardiovascular diseases such as hypertension or hypotension, and they are contraindicated in patients suffering from cardiovascular collapse.

5. Caution is required in administering these drugs to patients with chronic respiratory tract obstructive disorders, such as emphysema and severe asthma. Their use as antiemetics in children with acute respiratory infections may also be hazardous.

6. Patients known to have had a previous hypersensitivity-type reaction to a drug of this class should not receive any drug in the group as cross sensitivity may occur. They are contraindicated in patients with bone marrow depression or a history of blood dyscrasias or jaundice. (It is desirable that periodic blood counts and liver function tests be performed during prolonged treatment with phenothiazines.)

7. Caution is required in patients with a history of peptic ulcer, glaucoma, or epilepsy. (The dosage of anticonvulsant drugs should be maintained at the usual level while phenothiazines are added gradually to the patient's regimen.)

8. Periodic ocular examinations for the presence of pigmentary deposits are desirable to prevent impairment of the acuity of patient's vision, particularly at night.

9. Remember that these drugs have antiemetic activity and may thus keep patients from vomiting despite overdosage with other drugs. (This action may also mask the presence of signs and symptoms which would help in the diagnosis of brain tumor and intestinal obstruction.)

SUMMARY of Side Effects of Antidepressant Drugs

Tricyclic Type (Amitriptyline, Imipramine, and Others)

Autonomic Side Effects

1. Mouth dryness, blurred vision, constipation, difficulty in voiding the urinary bladder

2. Fall in blood pressure in the standing position (postural hypotension) with resulting feelings of faintness, dizziness, and weakness

3. Localized sweating; male sexual function disturbances (impotence; delayed ejaculation); G.I. disturbances, including nausea and vomiting; headache

Central Side Effects

1. Early feelings of drowsiness and fatigue followed by later signs of mental overstimulation (for example, restlessness, jitteriness, agitation; or hypomania, mania, confusion, hallucinations, and delirium)

2. Motor overstimulation marked by muscle twitching and tremors, hyperreflexia, and possibly convulsive seizures

Peripheral Nerve Effects

Sensory signs of neuritis with possible numbness and tingling (paresthesias) and ringing in the ears (tinnitus)

Hypersensitivity-Type Reactions

Obstructive jaundice; agranulocytosis; skin eruptions, including photosensitivity reactions

Monoamine Oxidase Inhibitors (Phenelzine, Tranylcypromine)—MAOI

Autonomic Side Effects

1. Postural *hypotension* marked by dizziness, weakness, and fainting; occasionally, *hypertension* marked by severe headache, nausea, and vomiting

2. Mouth dryness, blurred vision, constipation, and other G.I. disturbances; male genitourinary disturbances, including difficulty in micturition, delayed ejaculation, or impotence; localized sweating

Central Side Effects

Euphoria leading sometimes to hypomanic and

manic behavior; hyperactivity and hyperreflexia; confusion, agitation, hallucinations, delirium; muscular twitching and tremors, and convulsive seizures

Hypersensitivity, and Other Reactions
Skin reactions, including flushing, photosensitivity, and rashes; edema and weight gain

---

S U M M A R Y of Cautions and Contraindications for Antidepressant Drugs

1. Severely depressed patients with suicidal tendencies are ordinarily not treated with antidepressant drugs alone but may also require electroconvulsive therapy or psychotherapy.

2. Both major types of antidepressant drugs are used with caution, if at all, in patients with a history of glaucoma, difficulty in voiding, hyperthyroidism, epilepsy, and severe cardiovascular disease, including pheochromocytoma. (Patients with angina are cautioned against excessive activity.)

3. Both types of drugs are undesirable for patients who are highly agitated, unless a phenothiazine-type tranquilizer is administered simultaneously.

4. Caution is required in administering MAOI-type drugs to patients with liver function abnormalities. Liver function tests are carried out frequently, and the appearance of changes in these tests may make it necessary to stop the medication.

5. Both types of drugs are *not* ordinarily administered together. A period of at least one week should pass after tricyclic drugs are discontinued before beginning MAOI drug therapy; a two-week drug-free period is recommended when going from MAOI drugs to one of the tricyclic type.

6. Patients taking MAOI-type drugs should be warned against taking any other medication without supervision. This is particularly true of medications containing adrenergic drugs (for example, nose drops and other medications for colds, hay fever, and weight reduction), and caffeine.

7. Drugs prescribed only with caution for patients taking MAOI-type drugs include sedatives (such as barbiturates), analgesics (such as meperidine—Demerol), antiparkinsonism drugs (such as benztropine; levodopa); antihypertensive agents (such as guanethidine), and anesthetics (such as ethyl ether).

8. Patients taking MAOI-type drugs are cautioned against drinking alcoholic beverages, including beer and wine as well as whiskey. Among foods that these patients are warned against are certain cheeses, pickled herring, chicken livers, and canned figs.

S U M M A R Y of Some Points for the Nurse to Remember About the Drug Therapy of Psychiatric Patients

1. Remember that the manner in which psychotherapeutic medications are administered to psychiatric patients is often a factor in their recovery.

(a) When giving medication, foster the patient's self-respect by calling him by name and showing concern for him.

(b) Avoid forcing the patient to take the medication against his will, if this is possible. If he refuses medication, listen to his reasons for doing so and decide what steps are necessary to help the patient deal with the problem. Explain in a positive way that the doctor has ordered the drug in order to help him recover more quickly and explain how he is expected to benefit from taking the medication. (Explain, for example, that the drug is going to make him rest or sleep better.) Avoid implying that the drug is being used to control his behavior and that medication would not be needed if he were not disturbing the ward.

2. Remember to observe how the patient is responding to psychotherapeutic drugs, as these data are useful in planning nursing care and in determining dosage levels. Look for signs of possible adverse effects, report these to the physician, and discuss the problem with him.

(a) Phenothiazines may cause dizziness, weakness, and faintness that can be reduced by the doctor's ordering these drugs in reduced dosage.

(b) Antidepressant drugs may cause an increase in nervousness, agitation, and sleeplessness that can be partly counteracted by administering sedatives and hypnotics.

(c) Patients who show signs of becoming excessively dependent upon drugs can sometimes be taught how to cope with their anxieties by means other than medications.

(d) Stay with the patient until he has taken his medication, as he may try to accumulate enough of the drug to make a suicide attempt.

3. Remember to encourage the psychiatric out-

patient to assume responsibility for taking his prescribed medication after he is released from the hospital.

(a) Suggest to the patient that he take personal responsibility for remembering to take his daily medication, rather than let a member of the family do it for him (if he is able to take this responsibility).

(b) Direct your questions concerning the effects that the medication is having to the patient himself. This is usually preferable to querying other family members who may happen to be present during your interviews with the patient, since it implies that you expect the patient to assume this responsibility.

Discussion Topics: Dealing with Psychotherapeutic Drugs

A. *The Situation*: Six patients who have recently been discharged from a state mental hospital are referred to the psychiatric clinic in which you are a nurse. All of these patients are expected to continue taking the antipsychotic-type drugs that they had been receiving while patients in the institution.

The Problem: Discuss the factors that you would consider to determine whether each of these patients would be capable of profiting from instructions directed to the entire group concerning how best to use the prescribed tranquilizers. (For example: What are some advantages of carrying out group teaching of these patients and what factors might make

this method undesirable for some? Indicate the main material that you would wish to include in your teaching plan.)

B. *The Situation*: You are a public health nurse visiting a schizophrenic patient at his home to see how he is getting along since his release from a mental institution. Every time you ask the patient such questions concerning his medication as the times of day that he takes his drugs and how they make him feel, his mother supplies the answers for him.

The Problem: Discuss what you would do to encourage the patient to answer your questions himself.

DRUG DIGEST

AMITRIPTYLINE HCl U.S.P. (Elavil)
Actions and Indications. An antidepressant drug with a tranquilizing component. It rapidly controls depressive anxiety. Other target symptoms of the various types of depression, including loss of interest and appetite, sleeplessness, headache, and psychomotor retardation, respond more gradually.

Side Effects, Cautions, and Contraindications. Atropinelike side effects include mouth dryness, blurred vision, constipation, urinary retention, and tachycardia. Thus, it is contraindicated in patients with glaucoma or enlarged prostate, and it is used with caution in elderly patients with constipation and in heart disease patients. Patients should be warned against drinking or driving during the early days of drug therapy because of central depressive effects such as drowsiness and impaired alertness. Confusion, jitteriness, tremors, and

occasionally convulsions can occur late in a course of therapy with high doses. Mania and schizophrenic symptoms may be activated.

Dosage and Administration. Most patients are started on 25 mg t.i.d. by mouth, but some require intramuscular administration of 20 to 30 mg q.i.d. for the first week or two. Later most patients may be maintained on oral doses of 25 mg b.i.d. to q.i.d. Some need only 10 mg several times a day, while a few hospitalized patients may require up to 300 mg daily.

CHLORPROMAZINE HCl U.S.P. (Thorazine)
Actions and Indications. This prototype of the phenothiazine antipsychotic agents reduces severe agitation in acute schizophrenic reactions, the manic phase of the manic-depressive psychosis, alcoholism, and brain-damaged senile

patients or mentally retarded children. It also lessens hallucinations, delusions, and other symptoms of psychosis. The drug is also useful in general medicine, surgery, and obstetrics because of its other actions, including potentiation of analgesics, barbiturates, and anesthetics.

Side Effects, Cautions, and Contraindications. Drowsiness, dizziness and faintness are the most common early side effects. Parkinsonism and motor restlessness are more common extrapyramidal reactions than are dystonias, but persistent dyskinesias have also been reported, particularly in brain-damaged elderly women patients. Hypersensitivity reactions including obstructive (cholestatic) jaundice, agranulocytosis, and dermatological disorders develop in rare instances. Caution is suggested in patients with a history of hepatic disease, and a history of hypersensitivity to other phenothiazines is a contraindication.

Dosage and Administration. Dosage ranges from 10 mg t.i.d. by mouth to totals of 1000 mg or more parenterally. Small doses are gradually raised until symptoms of psychosis are controlled. For antiemetic action in vomiting children 25 mg suppositories may be inserted rectally.

FLUPHENAZINE HCl N.F. (Permitil; Prolixin)

Actions and Indications. This is a potent, long-acting phenothiazine-type *major tranquilizer*. It relieves moderately severe anxiety in psychoneurotic patients and reduces the effects of emotional tension in cardiovascular conditions, gastrointestinal disturbances, and other physical disorders. This *antipsychotic* agent controls agitation, and favorably affects behavior in schizophrenia, mania, mental deficiency, and senile psychoses.

Side Effects, Cautions, and Contraindications. Extrapyramidal reactions of various kinds are common. Dystonic-type reactions are particularly alarming but can usually be readily controlled by administration of antiparkinsonism drugs. These and other motor symptoms, including pseudoparkinsonism and akathisia, can usually be minimized by reducing the dose, and they ordinarily disappear when the drug is discontinued. However, involuntary movements sometimes persist. Caution is required in patients with a history of convulsive disorders.

Sedation and hypotensive reactions occur less frequently with this drug than with other types of phenothiazines.

Dosage and Administration. A single oral dose of 1 to 3 mg is adequate for most adult patients. However, some patients may require parenteral doses of 10 mg or more initially. Dosage is reduced to maintenance levels of 0.5 to 1 mg orally once symptoms are controlled. A long-acting ester, fluphenazine enanthate, is administered in a single I.M. or S.C. dose of 25 mg about once in two weeks.

IMIPRAMINE HCl U.S.P. (Tofranil)

Actions and Indications. This prototype of the tricyclic antidepressants is often effective, whether used alone or in combination with psychotherapy or electroconvulsive therapy. It is particularly effective in cases of endogenous depression marked by psychomotor retardation.

Side Effects, Cautions, and Contraindications. Central excitement may be manifested by agitation, confusion, disorientation, and hallucinations requiring dosage reduction and treatment with tranquilizers. Convulsions may occur, particularly in patients with a history of seizures. Atropinelike side effects include dry mouth, constipation, urinary retention, and blurred vision. (Caution in patients with glaucoma or high intraocular pressure.) Cardiac arrhythmias and orthostatic hypotension may occur. Thus, extreme caution is required in patients with cardiovascular disease, and this drug is contraindicated for patients who have had a recent heart attack or who are hyperthyroid or are taking thyroid hormones.

Dosage and Administration. Outpatients are started on daily oral doses of 75 mg which may be raised to as high as 200 mg and reduced during maintenance therapy to as low as 50 mg daily. Hospitalized patients are started on oral or intramuscular doses of 100 mg daily. These doses may be raised gradually over a period of several weeks to 200 mg, 250 mg, or as high as 300 mg daily.

ISOCARBOXAZID N.F. (Marplan)

Actions and Indications. This hydrazide-type inhibitor of the enzyme monoamine oxidase is used for treating selected cases of moderate to severe depression. Used alone or in conjunction with electroshock therapy it is effective for some psychotic patients with depression of the involutional, manic-depressive, and schizophrenic types.

Side Effects, Cautions, and Contraindications. Circulatory side effects are the most common and most dangerous. Postural hypotension may make patients feel weak, faint, dizzy, and result in falls. Patients are warned against taking medications for colds containing sympathomimetic amines, as these may cause a rise in blood pressure. They are also told not to eat certain foods containing tyramine, as this has precipitated hypertensive crisis and fatal intracranial bleeding. Central stimulation may result in various adverse psychological and neurological adverse effects, including mania, muscle tremors, and convulsive seizures.

Dosage and Administration. The drug is usually started at an oral dose level of 30 mg daily. Once the patient shows improvement, dosage is reduced and the patient is maintained on as little as 10 mg daily by mouth.

LITHIUM CARBONATE (Eskalith; Lithane; Lithonate)

Actions and Indications. This drug is used specifically to control acute manic episodes in patients diagnosed as suffering from manic-depressive psychosis. It may also be useful for preventing recurrences. However, the drug is *not* considered effective for control of manic or catatonic excitement in schizophrenia.

Side Effects, Cautions, and Contraindications. Mild nausea, thirst, and fine tremors are common but transient. More serious when they develop during maintenance therapy are vomiting, diarrhea, drowsiness, muscle weakness, and motor incoordination. If such signs and symptoms occur, the patient's plasma lithium levels must be checked and the drug discontinued when this proves to be high. More severe degrees of toxicity may be manifested by: neuromuscular signs, such as tremor, twitching, and sudden spasms; central stimulation, marked by restlessness, confusion, convulsive seizures, stupor, and coma; and/or cardiovascular effects, including cardiac arrhythmias and circulatory collapse.

Dosage and Administration. For control of acute mania, oral doses of 600 mg t.i.d. will usually bring the plasma lithium level into the therapeutic range of 0.5 to 1.5 mEq/liter of blood serum. For long-term maintenance therapy a reduction in dosage to 300 mg t.i.d. is recommended to keep lithium at the desired maintenance level of 0.5 to 1.0 mEq/liter.

THIORIDAZINE HCl U.S.P. (Mellaril)

Actions and Indications. This piperidine-type phenothiazine controls mild to moderate anxiety in psychoneurotic and depressed patients, as well as severe agitation, hallucinations, and delusions in schizophrenics and other psychotics. It is also used in the long-term management of chronic alcoholism, as well as in alcoholic withdrawal syndromes. It is not as effective an antiemetic as other phenothiazines and is thus less likely to mask possible brain tumors, gastrointestinal obstruction, or drug overdosage.

Side Effects, Cautions, and Contraindications. Extrapyramidal reactions are relatively rare except for pseudoparkinsonism and akinesia. Drowsiness and postural hypotensive symptoms occur commonly early in treatment. The drug is contraindicated in patients with severe heart disease and either hypotension or hypertension. Electrocardiographic changes are sometimes seen and may possibly be related to rare cases of sudden death with cardiac arrest. Pigmentation of ocular structures including the retina as well as the conjunctiva, cornea, and lens has developed occasionally.

Dosage and Administration. Total daily dosage ranges from 20 mg in moderately anxious patients up to a maximum of 800 mg in psychosis. The usual initial dosage is 25 mg t.i.d. for neurosis and 50 to 100 mg t.i.d. in psychosis.

TRANYLCYPROMINE N.F. (Parnate)

Actions and Indications. This potent *non*hydrazine monoamine oxidase inhibitor is usually reserved for treating severe depressions that have not responded to other drugs

and in patients for whom electroconvulsive therapy is contraindicated.

Side Effects, Cautions, and Contraindications. The most common effect upon blood pressure is postural hypotension. However, the most important pressure reaction is the occasional development of hypertensive crisis, as this condition can result in fatal intracranial bleeding. Headaches may indicate that this drug should be discontinued. Thus, patients are told to report this symptom promptly. They are also warned against self-medication with

drugs that tend to produce pressure rises (such as remedies for colds and hay fever). Other drugs that are not ordered include narcotic analgesics and antihypertensive agents. Alcoholic beverages and foods of high tyramine content (for example, cheeses, wines, chicken livers) are also contraindicated.

Dosage and Administration. Patients are started on oral doses of 10 mg b.i.d. Later, if necessary, another 10 mg is added to the morning dose. This 30 mg total daily dose may be reduced during maintenance to 20 or 10 mg daily.

References

Ayd, F.J. Jr. A survey of drug-induced extrapyramidal reactions. *JAMA*, 175:102, 1961.

Berger, F.M. The similarities and differences between meprobamate and barbiturates. *Clin. Pharmacol. Ther.*, 4:209, 1963.

Crane, G.E. Tardive dyskinesias, a review of the literature. *Amer. J. Psych.*, 124:8, 1968 (Feb. Suppl.).

Domino, E.F. Human pharmacology of tranquilizing drugs. *Clin. Pharmacol. Ther.*, 3:599, 1962.

Fieve, R.F. et al. The use of lithium in affective disorders. *Amer. J. Psych.*, 125:487, 1968 (Oct. Suppl.).

Hollister, L.E. Adverse reactions to phenothiazines. *JAMA*, 189:311, 1964.

Phinney, R.P. The student of nursing and the schizophrenic patient. *Amer. J. Nurs.* 70:790, 1970.

Rodman, M.J. Drugs for managing mood disorders. *RN*, 33:64, 1970 (Dec.).

———. The major tranquilizers and antidepressants. *RN*, 31:53, 1968 (Aug.).

Travelbee, J. Intervention in Psychiatric Nursing. Philadelphia; F.A. Davis, 1969.

8.

Alcohol and Alcoholism

Drinking and Public Health

Alcoholism is one of this country's most serious public health problems. The more than five million Americans who chronically and compulsively drink to excess are often in need of nursing care. Uncontrolled drinking commonly leads to physical injury and disturbed behavior. Many alcoholics suffer from liver disease and other late medical complications of the prolonged intake of large amounts of alcohol.

The social cost of alcoholism is counted not only in terms of the health of the drinker himself but in the harm done to others. The nurse, both in her professional contacts and in everyday life, sees the results of alcoholism in disrupted families and in the deaths and injuries caused by drunken drivers. More than half of the over 55,000 highway deaths in 1970 involved alcoholics or other problem drinkers.

Problem drinking is now known to exist at every level of society. It has also recently become increasingly clear that there are probably as many women as men who drink to excess. Women with drinking difficulties may keep their secret hidden within the household for longer periods, but the consequences of a mother's alcoholism may be even more devastating to a family's stability than drinking by the father.

In order to aid the alcoholic patient and his family, the nurse needs to know what effects alcohol has on the brain and the body. Her attitudes toward the drinking problem should be based on knowledge of the pharmacological effects of this chemical substance, and not upon myths or old wives' tales. In this chapter, therefore, we shall first discuss the effects of alcohol on the central nervous system and the way in which the body's metabolic processes handle ingested alcohol as an aid to understanding the reasons for the medical measures employed in the management of acute intoxication and the complications of chronic alcoholism.

Pharmacological Actions of Alcohol on the C.N.S.

The central nervous system (C.N.S.) is most sensitive to the depressant effects of ethyl alcohol. This substance is similar to the barbiturates and to general anesthetics such as ethyl ether in the pattern of progressive C.N.S. depression that it is capable of producing. Contrary to common belief, alcohol is *not* a stimulant, and the drinker's excited behavior actually stems from depression of the brain areas which ordinarily exert inhibitory control over psychomotor activity and behavior.

The effects of alcohol on the functioning of the C.N.S. are related to the level of alcohol in the brain. As is true with other drugs, the concentration of alcohol in the C.N.S. at any time after ingestion depends upon the rate of its metabolism. This varies to some extent from person to person, and many heavy drinkers metabolize alcohol more rapidly than most people. However, tolerance of this type is limited, and increasing levels of alcohol in the blood and brain produce degrees of functional impairment that are related to the concentration of alcohol in the C.N.S. (see Table 8-1).

Drinking even a relatively small quantity of alcohol that produces only low levels in the brain results in reduced nervous tension—that is, a sedative or tranquilizing effect. However, even this relaxed feeling and the increase in self-confidence that often accompanies it are an indication of alcohol's ability to affect the highest functions of the cerebral cortex.

Even at alcohol levels of 50 mg per 100 ml of blood—an amount attained by drinking several cocktails or highballs in quick succession (Table 8-2)—a person's thought processes are subtly altered. Thus, he may do or say things in social situations that he would ordinarily not do or say. Presumably, this is because his judgment and inhibitory controls have been affected by the depressant effect of alcohol on nerve pathways that play a part in intellectual function.

When a person drinks alcoholic beverages in somewhat larger amounts, making the blood and brain concentrations rise rapidly to still higher levels, the drinker's judgment is dulled even further. In addition, his ability to make finely coordinated movements and to react to stimuli is reduced. This accounts for the frequency of accidents involving drivers or pedestrians who have been drinking, and for serious injuries and deaths from falls, fires, and industrial accidents.

As blood alcohol levels rise toward 100 mg%, the drinker's weakened ability to evaluate reality and to restrain his impulses, coupled with his increasing clumsiness, may make it dangerous for him to drive a motor vehicle. At an alcohol blood level of 0.1%, most people can be considered mildly intoxicated and unfit to drive. Actually, *much lower levels* of alcohol can cause enough reduction in judgment and skilled motor abilities to make it unsafe for a person to drive. Thus, in view of the disrupting effects of alcohol on these important C.N.S. functions, *no one should attempt to drive while he still feels any effect at all from even moderate drinking.*

Most people with 150 mg% blood alcohol, and just about all people with 200 mg%, may be considered moderately intoxicated, and those with 300 mg% are markedly intoxicated. People who have ingested enough alcohol to have blood levels this high show many signs of rapidly progressive deterioration of higher cortical functions. This appears in the form of increasingly uncontrolled behavior as a result of the release from both emotional and motor inhibitory controls. The person at this stage of an alcoholic episode may become belligerent and pugnacious, or he may have a crying or laughing "jag." At the same time, he tends to have increasing difficulty in locomotion, marked at first by a staggering gait, then by trouble in simply trying to stand and, finally, by his falling and being unable to get up.

People with alcohol blood levels around 300 mg% are often in a stage of acute excitement. The drinker should be kept from harming himself and others. This may require hospitalizing him and administering medications to calm him down (see p. 113). Those with blood levels of 400 mg% are no longer a behavioral problem, as they have usually sunk into a stupor from which they cannot be readily aroused. As the alcoholic's blood level rises above 500 mg%, he lapses into coma, and his breathing becomes shallow and slow. This also

TABLE 8-1 *Alcohol Blood Levels and Effects on C.N.S. Function**

Blood Level	Possible Behavioral Change
20–30 mg%	Slight impairment of psychosensory function.
30–50 mg%	Some impairment of judgment and motor coordination may occur. This level is *not* considered to be legal evidence of "impaired ability" to operate a motor vehicle in the U.S. However, in some European countries, it is illegal to drive with even this level of blood alcohol.
50–150 mg%	Varying degrees of impairment of fine motor coordination and judgment; delayed reaction time. Drivers with blood alcohol between these levels may be required to take tests of gross motor coordination to determine their fitness to drive. The 100 mg% level is now considered to be evidence of "impaired ability" to operate a motor vehicle—a chargeable offense in some states.
150–250 mg%	Moderate intoxication marked by progressive deterioration of higher cortical functions. Levels above 150 mg% are considered to be prima facie evidence of "driving while under the influence of alcohol" in most states of the U.S.
250–400 mg%	Marked intoxication characterized by increasing difficulty in maintaining motor function and by a high degree of uninhibited behavior. The drinker may be boisterous or belligerent and may be involved in violent incidents or accidents.
400–600 mg%	Severe intoxication results in a stuporous state from which arousal is difficult.
600–800 mg% and above	Coma and death from respiratory or cardiovascular failure or complications are likely to occur at these levels of blood alcohol.

* Correlations of blood alcohol levels with changes in functions controlled by the C.N.S. are relatively clear at higher blood levels. However, at the lower blood levels, there may be considerable individual differences in behavior. As with other psychopharmacological agents, the behavioral responses to alcohol may *vary* considerably, depending upon the drinker's "set" and the "setting" in which he does his drinking (Chap. 2).

The amount of alcohol intake required to produce various blood levels also varies, depending upon such factors as the amount of food taken before or during drinking, the interval between drinks, rapidity of absorption of alcohol, and so forth.

requires emergency treatment measures (see p. 113).

Alcohol Metabolism

Before we discuss the management of acutely intoxicated patients and of chronic alcoholism, we shall first review briefly some aspects of how the body handles ingested alcohol. This will help us to understand the basis for some of the treatment measures employed in the emergency management of acute intoxication and in the long-term care of chronic alcoholics.

ABSORPTION

Alcohol is rapidly absorbed from an empty stomach, and its effects on the C.N.S. can often be felt very quickly. Absorption of a drink from the stomach begins immediately and the blood alcohol level may reach a peak within 20 minutes. However, absorption and C.N.S. effects can be considerably delayed when the stomach contains a moderate amount of food. Food tends to dilute the alcohol, interfere with the absorptive processes that begin in the stomach, and—especially with milk and

TABLE 8-2 *Alcohol Content of Beverages**

Beverage and Type or Source	Percent Alcohol by Volume	Proof†
Neutral spirits	90–95	180–190
Vodka (from neutral spirits)	40–55	80–110
Gin (from neutral spirits)	40–45	80–110
Whiskey (from cereal grains)	40–45	80–110
Rum (from molasses)	40–55	80–110
Brandy (from wine)	40–55	80–110
Wine (table, light)	10–12	..
Wine (dessert)	15–22	..
Beer (light)	3–6	..
Ale	6–8	..
Cider (hard)	8–12	..

* The amount of a beverage taken within a brief period of time can be related within limits to the level of alcohol likely to be attained in the blood and brain and to the probable behavior of the individual.
For example, one ounce of a concentrated beverage such as 100 proof whiskey, taken all at once on an empty stomach, might produce an alcohol blood level of 20 mg% (0.02%) within half an hour. Similarly, two to three ounces of whiskey could produce a blood level of 0.05% alcohol; 8 oz (half a pint) 0.15%; 16 oz (one pint) 0.300%, etc.
† *Proof* is the standard of strength for alcoholic liquors. The proof figure in this country is always twice the percentage of alcohol by volume. The term is said to stem from an old test for the alcohol content of whiskey. If gunpowder on which the whiskey was poured ignited, this was "proof" that the whiskey contained at least 50% alcohol.

other fat-containing foods—slow passage of the alcohol into the upper intestine from which most of any drink is usually absorbed.

DISTRIBUTION

Alcohol that enters the bloodstream is carried quickly to the C.N.S., because that system receives such a rich blood supply. It then readily diffuses past the blood-brain barrier and begins to build up to concentrations that depress the functioning of various nerve centers. Later, the alcohol is redistributed to other tissues that have a less abundant blood supply than the brain. Provided that there is no further drinking, the concentration of alcohol in the brain falls and the drinker begins to sober up as the alcohol is redistributed and detoxified.

FINAL FATE

Between 90 and 95 percent of all alcohol that is absorbed is broken down to carbon dioxide and water, with the production of considerable energy. Most of the remaining alcohol leaves the body unchanged in the person's urine and breath. The rate at which body tissues burn up alcohol varies from person to person depending upon the degree of his congenital or acquired tolerance (Chap. 2).

An average person oxidizes about 7 g (10 ml) per hour. This means that it may take the body of an ordinary drinker almost a day to rid itself of the alcohol in a pint of whiskey (see Table 8-2). The fact that alcohol is metabolized at the same slow steady rate, no matter how much is in the body, is of practical importance in the treatment of acute intoxication (see below).

The Management of Acutely Intoxicated Patients

Patients who require treatment may be in any of the following states at the time of admission: (1) stuporous or comatose; (2) excited or combative; (3) suffering the various effects of the withdrawal of alcohol after prolonged drinking. The management of each of these phases of acute alcoholism is, of course, quite different.

ALCOHOLIC STUPOR AND COMA

Most patients who are found in a stuporous state but with normal vital signs need no special treatment. They can usually be left to sleep off the effects of their drinking bout while the body gradually eliminates the alcohol. Occasionally, if the patient's breathing is slow and shallow, respiration may be deepened by having the patient inhale carbon dioxide (5 percent) periodically. The respiratory rate may be increased by parenteral administration of a mild analeptic such as caffeine sodium benzoate.

Comatose patients require more vigorous emergency treatment to prevent respiratory failure and complications such as hypostatic pneumonia. Most important are the general medical and nursing measures for supporting the patient's vital functions that are discussed in Chapter 3. In addition, attempts are sometimes made to lower the level of alcohol in the patient's brain and blood.

Various substances have been recommended for this purpose, including the thyroid hormones and insulin combined with glucose and B-complex vitamins. There is little proof that these measures actually increase the speed of alcohol elimination by the body. Because patients in alcoholic coma often have an extremely low blood sugar level, insulin administration may make them worse. However, starting an immediate I.V. infusion of glucose alone as a 5 percent or even more highly concentrated solution containing B-complex vitamins may have a desirable effect on the comatose patient's condition.

ALCOHOLIC EXCITEMENT

Patients admitted while in the noisy, combative stage of alcoholic intoxication must be calmed and kept from injuring themselves or others by their violent behavior. Although the use of sedatives such as paraldehyde or barbiturates is often effective, these depressant drugs sometimes so intensify the effects of alcohol that the patient may become comatose. Thus, physicians have turned more recently to the minor and major tranquilizers.

Some doctors prefer the parenteral administration of *chlordiazepoxide* (Librium) or *diazepam* (Valium) for this purpose. Others use phenothiazines such as *promazine* (Sparine) and *chlorpromazine* (Thorazine). However, while the phenothiazines also have an antiemetic effect that helps to relieve the patient's nausea, they sometimes set off a severe fall in blood pressure. Thus, patients should be kept lying down following these injections.

Acceptance of the excited alcoholic patient despite his disruptive behavior is an important part of therapy. This is often quite difficult to do, and it is often necessary to set limits on the patient's behavior. However, the nurse who conveys an attitude of calm and firmness can often do much to reduce the patient's agitation and can add to the effectiveness of the sedative drugs that she administers.

ALCOHOL WITHDRAWAL SYNDROMES

People who have been drinking develop mental and physical symptoms when they are deprived of liquor, and the level of alcohol in the blood and brain begins to fall. The severity of this illness, which resembles that seen when barbiturates are withdrawn, depends mainly upon how heavily the alcoholic has been drinking and for how long. Symptoms may range from merely a mild hangover through a state of agitation and tremulousness to potentially fatal delirium tremens (the "D.T.s").

Patients with *"the shakes,"* as they call the tremors of mild to moderate withdrawal, are best treated with general depressant drugs that substitute for the alcohol that is leaving the patient's system. Some doctors still prefer paraldehyde for this purpose; others substitute pentobarbital for alcohol. Injections of *chlordiazepoxide* (Librium) and *diazepam* (Valium) are also used to quiet the agitation and tremulousness of these patients and to assure rest and sleep. These drugs are themselves withdrawn when the patient's symptoms are controlled, to avoid development of dependence.

For the complication that alcoholics call *"the horrors"* and psychiatrists call *"alcoholic hallucinosis,"* phenothiazine-type tranquilizers are often added to the patient's regimen. These drugs help to dampen the patient's fearful response to his auditory and visual hallucinations. Other measures that reduce the patient's tendency to develop hallucinations include considerate nursing care (see p. 114).

Patients with *delirium tremens,* the most serious stage of the alcohol withdrawal syndrome, must be treated by many kinds of vigorous measures, because sudden death from circulatory collapse can occur in this condition. The severely agitated patient must be kept from exhausting himself by treatment with a combination of the substitute-type sedatives such as paraldehyde, chloral hydrate, or barbiturates, together with such sedating phenothiazines as *promazine* (Sparine) and *chlor-promazine* (Thorazine) which potentiate the depressant actions of the stronger hypnotics.

The anticonvulsant drug, *diphenylhydantoin* (Dilantin), may also be administered to control convulsive seizures. If increased intracranial pressure is present as a result of cerebral edema, the patient may also receive infusions of osmotic diuretics such as urea or mannitol. Other measures often used in this dangerous disorder include the administration of intravenous fluids containing vitamins and electrolytes to counteract dehydration resulting from heavy sweating and vomiting and to correct the avitaminosis which is so common in chronic alcoholics.

Sympathetic and understanding nursing care is also most important. The nurse must always explain carefully every procedure that she is about to perform, even when only feeding or bathing the patient or taking his temperature and blood pressure. She avoids restraining the patient physically when feasible, as this may only increase his struggles, while a firm but gentle manner may help to lessen his fear and keep him relatively quiet. The patient's room should be kept well lighted at night, and the patient should not be left unattended. If the nurse cannot remain with the patient, sometimes a member of his family or a friend can stay with him.

The Management of the Chronic Alcoholic Patient

As with other kinds of addiction, getting the alcoholic patient "dried out" is easy compared to the task of rehabilitating him and treating his other illnesses. For one thing, the chronic alcoholic often suffers from physical complications that require care. Even more difficult to manage is the alcoholic's compulsion to return to his pattern of excessive drinking.

PATHOLOGICAL CHANGES

Continued heavy drinking leads almost inevitably to organic damage. Various vital organs, including the liver and brain, suffer from both the direct damaging effect of alcohol or from other, indirect, difficulties mainly caused by malnutrition. This is the result of the alcoholic's failure to eat even a minimally adequate diet while drinking large quantities of distilled spirits.

This failure to eat occurs because of the high caloric value of alcohol when it is being metabolized in the tissues (p. 111). Every gram of alcohol that is oxidized produces seven calories—more energy than is obtained when the body burns an equal amount of carbohydrate or protein, and nearly as much as is derived from fat metabolism. Thus, because the heavy drinker can satisfy a large part of his daily energy requirements by his alcohol intake alone, he fails to eat more nutritious foods containing proteins and vitamins. As a result, he often develops symptoms that stem from a deficiency of B-complex vitamins and other essential food factors.

GASTROINTESTINAL TRACT

High concentrations of alcohol are directly irritating to the mucosal lining of the stomach. Thus, acute and chronic gastritis are quite common in heavy drinkers of concentrated alcoholic beverages such as "straight" whiskey. The nausea and vomiting caused by this inflammatory reaction often keep the drinker from satisfying the requirements of his physical dependence on alcohol, thus precipitating withdrawal symptoms.

Ordinarily, acute gastritis is relieved when the alcoholic stops drinking and begins to eat again. Meanwhile, his symptoms usually respond to treatment with antacids and antispasmodics, and to phenothiazine-type antiemetics. Although alcohol has not been proved to cause peptic ulcer, alcohol does stimulate gastric acid secretion and is thus undesirable in patients who already have ulcers. Gastric bleeding is common in alcoholic patients with ulcers.

EFFECTS OF ALCOHOL ON THE LIVER

Acute and chronic liver disease are commonly seen in people who have been drinking large amounts of alcohol for a long time. Acute alcoholic hepatitis, a condition resembling infectious hepatitis, sometimes develops during a drinking bout. It is characterized by anorexia, nausea, vomiting, abdominal pain, jaundice, and an enlarged liver. The incidence of chronic hepatic disorders such as fatty liver and cirrhosis is much higher in chronic alcoholics than in the general population. However, not all heavy drinkers—and, indeed, only a small proportion of them—develop cirrhosis of the liver.

If the alcoholic can be helped to stop drinking before the degenerative process has gone too far, the liver's remarkable regenerative properties can come into play. Recovery is often rapid when the alcoholic begins to eat again. The nurse encourages the patient to eat the diet prescribed by the doctor, which is high in proteins, lipotropic substances such as choline and methionine, and B-complex vitamins such as folic acid and cyanocobalamin.

NERVOUS SYSTEM DISORDERS

The alcoholic whose drinking has been out of control for many months or years often develops neurologic complications that are the results of a deficiency of vitamin B$_1$ (*thiamine*) and other B-complex vitamins. Such neurologic disorders of nutritional origin include Wernicke's encephalopathy, Korsakoff's psychosis, and alcoholic polyneuropathy.

WERNICKE'S DISEASE. This disorder is marked by the sudden onset of clinical signs of three kinds—ocular muscle paralysis, ataxia, and mental confusion. Once the disease is recognized and treated with massive doses of *thiamine*, the eye signs and muscular incoordination clear up quickly and the patient becomes more alert and responsive.

KORSAKOFF'S PSYCHOSIS. Some patients continue to show mental symptoms even after they have recovered from the acute phase. These alcoholics are suffering from a peculiar kind of intellectual impairment called Korsakoff's psychosis. This is characterized by a disturbance in memory, especially the memory of recent events, as well as an inability to learn new material.

Even when the patient has improved after several months of hospitalization, he still has difficulty in putting past events into their proper sequence. Most victims of this amnesia-type psychosis are unable to function in society and have to be institutionalized. Apparently, in such cases, the severe thiamine deficiency has caused neuropathological lesions in the thalamus that have gone too far to be corrected in the same manner as can the cerebellar lesions of Wernicke's disease.

ALCOHOLIC POLYNEUROPATHY. Many patients show signs of damage to the motor and sensory fibers of peripheral nerves. Most complain of muscle weakness of the legs and arms or numbness and tingling of the skin. A few suffer from burning pain in the feet or hands or deep aching of the legs. Such polyneuropathy is thought to be the result of a multiple vitamin deficiency resulting from a state of semistarvation.

Treatment mainly involves the daily administration of large doses of thiamine, pyridoxine, pantothenic acid, riboflavin, and other vitamins. These may have to be given by injection because of the patient's persistent vomiting or other G.I. complications. Salicylates, and occasionally codeine, may be ordered for relief of the patient's muscle pains during his long weeks of convalescence. He should be encouraged to consume the ordered diet, which is high in calories from protein and which is supplemented by multiple vitamins.

CARDIAC AND RESPIRATORY COMPLICATIONS

Chronic alcoholics sometimes suffer from heart muscle damage. Myocardopathy of this kind may be a manifestation of beriberi, a disease resulting from a deficiency of vitamin B$_1$. As in the latter condition, alcoholic patients may develop congestive heart failure. In addition, prolonged excessive drinking may have a direct toxic effect to the myocardium that makes the heart susceptible to development of cardiac rhythm irregularities during bouts of acute alcoholic intoxication.

Alcoholics suffer frequent acute and chronic bronchopulmonary infections, including tuberculosis. This may occur because the alcoholic's neglect of himself and the unsanitary conditions that often stem from his life style reduce the body's natural defenses against infection. In addition, patients in an alcoholic stupor are prone to develop hypostatic and aspiration pneumonia.

ALCOHOL AND THE KIDNEYS

Despite former claims that alcohol was a cause of nephritis, there seems to be no evidence that alcohol damages the kidneys or even that its use is harmful to patients who have nephritis. Drinking is, however, undesirable for patients with genitourinary tract infections. The increased urinary output induced by drinking alcoholic beverages may cause urgency and frequency in patients with enlargement of the prostate gland.

Rehabilitation Measures

Recovery from alcohol addiction requires long-term treatment. No single form of alcoholism therapy is effective for all patients. However, programs begin with the idea that the problem drinker cannot drink in moderation. Thus, it is absolutely essential that these patients *abstain totally* from alcohol.

No one can make the alcoholic stop drinking by threatening him or by moralizing. However, the nurse can help the patient to recognize that his drinking is out of control and encourage him to seek treatment. Once he himself becomes convinced that he can never take alcohol in any form, various types of treatment measures may prove valuable in the long-term management of alcoholic patients. These include psychotherapy, membership in organizations such as Alcoholics Anonymous (A.A.), and the use of certain drugs that help to deter the patient from drinking.

DETERRENT DRUGS

Patients who are motivated to stop drinking by the help of a physician, nurse, friends, or the former alcoholics that they meet in A.A. often tend to relapse at some point in the course of their recovery. This does not mean that they have failed and should stop trying to control their craving for alcohol. If the patient really wants to stop drinking, his desire can often be reinforced by taking a daily dose of *disulfiram+* (Antabuse) or other deterrent drugs such as *citrated calcium carbimide* (CCC; Temposil) or *metronidazole* (Flagyl; see also Chapter 46).

When a patient who has taken a dose of disulfiram also takes an alcoholic drink a typical reaction soon begins. Within a few minutes, the patient's skin turns bright red and warm as a result of peripheral vasodilation. The vasodilation sets off a pounding vasodilator-type headache, and, as his blood pressure drops, the patient feels faint, weak, and dizzy, and becomes nauseated. Violent vomiting, heart palpitations, chest pains, and dyspnea may develop. Sometimes the cardiovascular complications have proved fatal to patients with myocardial disease or cerebral damage who have begun to drink while under treatment with disulfiram.

The use of deterrent drugs in properly selected patients has proved desirable in various ways. The patient's willingness to take a daily tablet is itself an indication that he really wants to stop drinking. Moreover, those who decide to take the drug each morning are relieved of the need to make countless decisions as to whether or not to take a drink that day. Then, as the days of abstinence lengthen into weeks and months, the patient realizes that he can, after all, get along without drinking. This often serves to reinforce his motivation and increases the likelihood of his profiting from concurrent psychotherapy.

AVERSION THERAPY

Sometimes attempts are made to create a distaste for alcohol in order to help patients resist the temptation to take the first drink that leads, in alcoholics, to many more drinks and to acute intoxication. One way of doing this is for the doctor to inject the emetic drug *apomorphine* soon after the patient has taken a drink of an alcoholic beverage. The nausea and violent vomiting that soon follows is then associated with the drinking in a way that is supposed to create feelings of revulsion at the very thought of alcohol. Although certain clinics claim to have had good results with aversion therapy, this method is not widely used.

PSYCHOTHERAPEUTIC AGENTS

Tranquilizing agents are used during the detoxication period to reduce the patient's nervousness, irritability, insomnia, and tremulousness (p. 113). Daytime doses of *chlordiazepoxide* (Librium) or other antianxiety agents, and bedtime doses of barbiturates, chloral hydrate, or *flurazepam* (Dalmane) are commonly employed for this purpose. However, long-term use of these drugs is not considered desirable during the later rehabilitation period. This is because alcoholics often abuse other depressant drugs also and may become addicted to them.

Patients who suffer periods of anxiety and depression that might make them begin drinking again may receive a major tranquilizer or an antidepressant drug. These agents, including *thioridazine* (Mellaril), *trifluoperazine* (Stelazine), *amitriptyline* (Elavil), and *doxepin* (Sinequan), are claimed less likely to cause dependence than are the other depressant drugs. However, all these agents are less important than psychotherapy and other means of offering the patient human support. Thus, the nurse should know what resources are available in the community that can be mobilized to help the alcoholic patient help himself.

Methyl Alcohol (Methanol; Wood Alcohol)

Methanol has less of a depressant effect on the C.N.S. than ethyl alcohol. However, it is often the cause of serious poisoning when taken internally. This is because it is metabolized in the body to formic acid and formaldehyde, substances that cause the blindness and fatal acidosis of wood alcohol intoxication.

Treatment requires prompt correction of the acidosis by slow I.V. infusion of systemic alkalinizers such as sodium bicarbonate and sodium lactate. The patient's eyes are protected from bright light, and an effort may be made to slow down the rate of methanol's conversion to the toxic metabolites.

One way of doing this, it has been suggested, is to administer repeatedly small amounts of ethyl alcohol (ethanol), which is metabolized by the same enzyme as is methanol. This process then slows oxidation of methanol to formaldehyde, the substance believed to be responsible for retinal damage.

SUMMARY of the Therapeutic Effects of Ethyl Alcohol (Ethanol)

Local Effects

Evaporation from the skin has a cooling effect that is desirable in sponge bathing of feverish patients.

Evaporation from the external ear has a desirable drying effect, helpful for preventing growth of microorganisms in the external ear canal and resulting "swimmer's ear."

Application to the unbroken skin has a disinfecting effect useful in presurgical scrubbing and as an antiseptic for injection sites.

Astringent, cleansing, and skin conditioning effects help to prevent decubitus ulcers.

Rubefacient (skin-reddening) action makes it desirable for use in liniments and skin rubs.

Solvent effect is useful for removing phenol that has been spilled on the skin or for removing toxin-containing oil of the poison ivy plant.

Antifoaming effect when inhaled in the form of fine droplets helps to clear the tracheobronchial tree in acute pulmonary edema.

Local injection close to nerve trunks and ganglia has been employed for pain relief and for producing local vasodilation.

Local effects in throat and stomach may cause reflex respiratory and cardiovascular stimulation in management of faintness.

Systemic Effects

Central effects of small doses,* including sedation, hypnosis, and analgesia, may be desirable for relief of tension and pain and for other purposes in some patients.

(1) In angina pectoris and peripheral vascular diseases, these central effects, rather than vasodilation, are responsible for any benefits of medicinal whiskey.

(2) In cancer, a 5 percent infusion has been used for pain relief and as a source of energy.

(3) In obstetrics, a 5 percent infusion has been used postpartum for relief of pain. (Alcohol infusions have also been employed for preventing premature labor.)

(4) The "digestant" or "stomachic" effects sought when alcoholic drinks are taken before meals are probably brought about by relief of tension and anxiety. (That is, the "appetizer" effect is really due to sedation rather than to an increase in digestive secretions, even though concentrated alcoholic solutions act locally to stimulate gastric secretion in tests of stomach function.)

(5) The diaphoretic (sweat-inducing) action of alcoholic drinks used by laymen for reducing fever (antipyretic) in "head colds" is a central effect.

(6) The hypnotic (sleep-producing) effect may be useful as an occasional "nightcap" but is potentially harmful in people prone to abuse drugs.

---

* Alcohol in large amounts has been used in the past, together with opiates, to produce general anesthesia. However, its prolonged excitement stage and narrow safety margin make it unsuitable for this purpose in modern anesthesia.

S U M M A R Y of Treatment Measures In Acute Alcoholic Coma

The patient's stomach is emptied by gastric lavage if the doctor believes that it still contains large amounts of unabsorbed alcohol. Care is taken, of course, to prevent aspiration of the gastric contents.

Analeptics are occasionally employed parenterally to help the patient's respiration and to reduce the depth of depression. Caffeine sodium benzoate (0.5 g) may be administered parenterally, or the doctor may prefer pentylenetetrazol or one of the other analeptics that are used for barbiturate poisoning.

Attempts may be made to hasten the rate of alcohol metabolism. Among the measures employed for this purpose have been the administration of hormones such as thyroxin and insulin.

The value of such measures is considered doubtful and even dangerous in some circumstances. The removal of alcohol from the body by hemodialysis or by the administration of diuretics to increase urinary flow has recently been recommended.

Artificial respiration with oxygen may be desirable. Maintenance of an open airway by suctioning of secretions or by performing a tracheotomy is important in maintaining respiratory exchange.

Injection of intravenous fluids for combating shock and overcoming the effects of dehydration and malnutrition is desirable. Various vitamins and electrolytes are commonly added to dextrose solutions for intravenous infusion.

S U M M A R Y of Drug Treatment of Alcoholic Excitement and Mild to Moderately Severe Alcohol Withdrawal Syndromes

Acute Alcoholic Excitement

Phenothiazine tranquilizers with sedative and antiemetic components, such as *promazine* (Sparine) and *chlorpromazine* (Thorazine), are administered parenterally to control hyperexcitability, nausea and vomiting. The minor tranquilizers, *chlordiazepoxide* (Librium), *diazepam* (Valium), and *hydroxyzine* (Atarax), are sometimes preferred for this purpose.

Mild to Moderate Alcohol Withdrawal Syndrome

Ethyl alcohol, itself, is *not* ordinarily administered in an attempt to ease the patient's tremulousness and anxiety. Instead, sedative and tranquilizing general depressant drugs may be administered to substitute for the sedative effect of alcohol. *Pentobarbital* (Nembutal), which is commonly employed for treating withdrawal

symptoms due to abuse of other general depressant drugs, may be used here also. Other physicians prefer parenteral *chlordiazepoxide* (Librium) for its prolonged duration of action and relative safety. *Meprobamate* (Miltown; Equanil) also may be employed for this purpose.

Alcoholic Hallucinosis Phase of Withdrawal

Signs of toxic psychosis which sometimes appear on about the second or third day of withdrawal, including auditory hallucinations, confusion, disorientation, and agitation, are best counteracted with increased doses of phenothiazine-type tranquilizers. Some doctors prefer to raise the dosage of promazine and chlorpromazine (see above) to keep patients deeply sedated and to prevent development of delirium. Others employ phenothiazines such as *trifluoperazine* (Stelazine) and other less sedating antipsychotic agents.

S U M M A R Y of Treatment Measures In Delirium Tremens

Sedation of a greater degree than that obtainable with phenothiazines alone may be required for control of extreme agitation. Thus, hypnotic doses of medium- to long-acting barbiturates, such as amobarbital and phenobarbital, or of paraldehyde, may be administered frequently in

addition to full doses of the more sedating phenothiazines, such as promazine and chlorpromazine.

Anticonvulsants, such as I.V. *diphenylhydantoin* (Dilantin) and I.M. phenobarbital, may be administered for the prevention or treatment of withdrawal seizures or "rum fits."

Fluids and electrolytes are administered parenterally to replace the patient's large fluid losses from fever, severe sweating, vomiting, and hyperventilation. A 5 or 10 percent dextrose in saline solution is infused, and potassium or sodium chloride or bicarbonate added as required, in accordance with the result of frequent checks of the patient's serum electrolyte levels. B-complex vitamins may also be administered I.M., or by addition to the infusion fluid, in order to make up for the depletion of these nutrients during the period of drinking.

Osmotic diuretics such as urea or mannitol may be administered by intravenous drip to reduce intracranial pressure, if cerebral edema or "wet brain" develops, or to counteract circulatory overload by parenteral fluids.

Nursing care should be especially sympathetic and understanding. The nurse recognizes the patient's need for care and is aware that his hostile, and even combative, behavior is the result of his illness. Patients should not be restrained, if this can be avoided, and measures for increasing the patient's orientation to his surroundings should be employed. For example, concrete statements telling the patient where he is should be made repeatedly and spoken slowly.

The nurse should always carefully explain what she is about to do before undertaking any procedure, because the patient, reacting in fear to visual, auditory, and tactile hallucinations, may struggle against attempts to feed and bathe him as well as against potentially painful procedures such as blood taking or spinal punctures.

It is desirable to keep the room lighted at night and not to leave the patient unattended. The calm and reassuring presence of the nurse and her firm but gentle manner are most important for keeping the patient relatively quiet. However, if the nurse cannot stay with the patient, it may be permissible to let understanding friends or relatives remain with him to calm him and allay his fears.

SUMMARY of Nursing Points Concerning Alcoholism

The nurse who is caring for an acutely intoxicated patient should both accept the patient and at the same time set limits upon his behavior when it is destructive.

The alcoholic patient's family often needs special consideration and thoughtful explanations concerning the patient's condition and treatment. (Sometimes the family has fostered the patient's drinking without being aware of it. Thus, they, as well as the patient, may benefit from counselling.)

Safety is a paramount consideration when working with a patient who is acutely intoxicated, or with a patient with delirium tremens. Measures that help the patient orient himself to his surroundings and assure him of the presence and concern of those who care for him are essential.

The nurse must be alert to symptoms of the varied complications that can result from alcoholism. For example, nausea and vomiting may indicate gastritis and should be promptly reported to the physician.

The nurse must be prepared to answer questions concerning alcohol and its effects—whether she works in school, hospital, or industry. (For example, many people still believe that alcohol is a stimulant and should be administered for fainting spells.) The public health nurse, particularly, can play an important role in encouraging alcoholics in the community to seek treatment.

Therapeutic measures designed to improve the patient's nutrition and to keep him comfortable should be administered conscientiously. Not only are such measures essential in combating the physical ravages of alcoholism, but they also convey the nurse's personal concern for the patient's welfare and her hopeful attitude toward his eventual recovery.

Care of the alcoholic who is repeatedly readmitted presents a particular challenge, because it is easy for the nurse to lose hope for the patient's recovery. Recognizing and correcting any attitudes of her own toward the alcoholic patient that might adversely affect the quality of the patient's care is necessary.

Clinical Nursing Situation

The Situation: Ms. Mathews has been admitted to the hospital for the fourth time this year. She fell and broke her leg and was admitted by ambulance from her home in a fashionable suburb. Her three other hospital experiences also involved accidental injuries. Ms.

Mathews has a history of chronic alcoholism and she often falls while intoxicated.

Ms. Mathews is extremely nervous and demanding. Her leg is in a cast and she is allowed to move about in a wheel chair. Visitors have come only once since her admission a week ago. A son and daughter-in-law came, stayed very briefly, and the patient seemed upset afterward.

Ms. Mathews is receiving Valium to reduce her restlessness and irritability.

The Problem: Develop a nursing care plan for Ms. Mathews.

DRUG DIGEST

DISULFIRAM (Antabuse)

Actions and Indications. This drug is used as an aid to psychotherapy or other supportive measures in the treatment of chronic alcoholism. It is not a cure for alcoholism but may help selected patients to stay sober. The patient knows that if he takes any alcohol while this drug is still in his system, he will suffer the Antabuse-alcohol reaction. This is marked by such discomfort as a throbbing headache, nausea and vomiting, breathing difficulty, and heart palpitations.

Side Effects, Cautions, and Contraindications. Disulfiram itself causes few ill effects other than skin rashes occasionally, or mild drowsi-ness or headaches that disappear when treatment is continued with smaller doses. However, patients taking alcohol may then suffer severe reactions, including possibly fatal cardiovascular difficulties. The drug is contraindicated in patients with heart disease and in those who are not capable of understanding and following instructions, including psychotic alcoholics. It is never given without the patient's full knowledge or when he has been drinking.

Patients are cautioned not to take alcohol in any form, including cough mixtures or foods containing it, and alcohol should even be avoided in products for external application such as liniments and after-shave lotions. Other drugs to be avoided are paraldehyde and metronidazole. Drug reactions between disulfiram and diphenylhydantoin, isoniazid, and coumarin-type anticoagulants may intensify the toxicity of these drugs. Thus, their dosage may have to be adjusted downward.

Dosage and Administration. Treatment is begun with a single daily dose of 0.5 g, usually taken in the morning. Later, after a week or two, the dose may be reduced to 0.25 or 0.125 g and maintained at this level for months or even years, if necessary.

References

Block, M.A. Medical treatment of alcoholism. *JAMA*, 162:1610, 1956.
———. Preventive treatment of alcoholism. *In* Symposium on the Treatment of Alcoholism. *Mod. Treatm.*, 3:450, 1966 (May).
Campbell, H.E. Traffic deaths go up again. *JAMA*, 201:861, 1967.
Gelperin, A., and Gelperin, E. The inebriate in the emergency room. *Amer. J. Nurs.*, 70:1494, 1970.
Gitlow, S.E. Treatment of the reversible acute complications of alcoholism. *In* Symposium on the Treatment of Alcoholism. *Mod. Treatm.*, 3:472, 1966 (May).
Golder, G.M. The nurse and the alcoholic patient. *Amer. J. Nurs.*, 56:436, 1956.
Himwich, H.E. The physiology of alcohol. *JAMA*, 163:545, 1957.
Kimmel, M.E. Antabuse in a clinic program. *Amer. J. Nurs.* 71:1173, 1971.
Klatskin, G. Effect of alcohol on the liver. *JAMA*, 170:1671, 1959.

McCarthy, R.G. Alcoholism. *Amer. J. Nurs.*, 59:203, 1959.
Morton, E.L. Nursing care in an alcoholic unit. *Nurs. Outlook*, 14:45, 1966 (Oct.).
Quiros, A. Adjusting nursing techniques to the treatment of alcoholic patients. *Nurs. Outlook*, 5:276, 1957.
Rodman, M.J. Alcohol: food, drug, and poison, *RN*, 20:70, 1957 (May).
———. Drugs in alcoholism management. *RN*, 30:51, 1967 (Dec.).
Smith, D.W., and Gips, C.D. Care of the Adult Patient, 3rd ed. Philadelphia: J. B. Lippincott, 1971.
Victor, M. Alcohol and nutritional diseases of the nervous system. *JAMA*, 167:65, 1958.
———. Treatment of the neurologic complications of alcoholism. *In* Symposium on the Treatment of Alcoholism. *Mod. Treatm.*, 3:491, 1966 (May).

9

Psychomotor and Other Central Stimulants

Types of C.N.S. Stimulants
(Table 9-1)

Drugs that increase the excitability of nerve cells in the central nervous system are commonly grouped on the basis of their *primary* sites of action and their clinically significant pharmacological effects as:

1. Cerebral, or psychomotor, stimulants;
2. Brain stem stimulants, or analeptics;
3. Spinal stimulants, or convulsants.

Actually, however, the effects of central stimulants tend to spread to all levels of the C.N.S. when their dosage is increased. Thus, drugs classified as psychomotor or cerebral stimulants (amphetamine and caffeine, for example) may sometimes be used to stimulate the brain stem respiratory control centers, and the effects of analeptics such as pentylenetetrazol may spread from the brain stem to set off spinal convulsions. On the other hand, small doses of a so-called spinal convulsant such as strychnine can, in some circumstances, stimulate respiration *without* causing convulsions.

In addition, some of the drugs that we classify as C.N.S. stimulants can also act at *peripheral* sites. The amphetamines, for instance, act directly at adrenergic neuroeffectors and thus affect the functioning of the heart and blood vessels. Ephedrine+, another adrenergic drug with C.N.S.-stimulating effects, has such potent cardiovascular and other peripheral effects that it is even discussed elsewhere in this text, in Chapter 24.

These secondary effects of stimulation at various central and peripheral sites limit the clinical usefulness of these drugs. Another rea-

T A B L E 9 - 1 *Central Nervous System Stimulants*

Official or Nonproprietary Name	Proprietary Name (or Synonym)	Usual Dosage
Psychomotor (Cerebral) Stimulants		
Amphetamine phosphate N.F.	Raphetamine	5 mg t.i.d.
Amphetamine sulfate N.F.	Benzedrine	10 mg b.i.d.
Dextroamphetamine sulfate U.S.P.	Dexedrine	5 mg q. 4 to 6 hrs.
Dextroamphetamine phosphate N.F.		2.5 to 5 mg t.i.d.
Methamphetamine HCl U.S.P.	Desoxyn; Methedrine, and others	
Methylphenidate HCl U.S.P.	Ritalin	10 mg t.i.d.
Pipradrol HCl	Alertonic	2.5 mg b.i.d.
Caffeine U.S.P.		200 mg
Caffeine and sodium benzoate U.S.P.		500 mg I.M. or S.C.
Citrated caffeine N.F.		60 to 120 mg
Deanol acetamidobenzoate	Deaner	300 mg
Analeptic Agents (Brain Stem Stimulants)		
Doxapram N.F.	Dopram	0.5 to 1.5 mg/kg, I.V.
Nikethamide N.F.	Coramine	1 ml of a 25% sol. I.M. or I.V.
Pentylenetetrazol N.F.	Metrazol	100 mg I.V. or S.C.
Picrotoxin N.F.		3 mg (1 ml) I.V.
Convulsant Poisons and Drugs (Brain Stem and Spinal Stimulants)		
1. POISONS		
Brucine, camphor, cocaine, strychnine, and others		
2. PHARMACOCONVULSANTS		
Flurothyl N.F.	Indoklon	2 to 5 ml by inhalation
Pentylenetetrazol N.F.	Metrazol	500 mg I.V.

son for the declining use of some central stimulants is their abuse potential. For example, the amphetamines, the most widely employed of the C.N.S. stimulants, are now being prescribed much less often than they once were. This is the result of reports indicating that these drugs were being overprescribed for middle-class medical patients and abused by them as well as by members of the drug subculture.

Psychomotor Stimulants (Table 9-1)

CAFFEINE+

Caffeine is the oldest of the drugs that primarily stimulate the mental and motor activities of the cerebral cortex. This alkaloid, found in coffee beans, tea leaves, and kola nuts, produces mild mental stimulation and helps to overcome drowsiness and feelings of fatigue. These alerting and antidepressant actions probably account for the popularity of caffeine-containing beverages, and they play an important part in the few therapeutic applications of caffeine in medical practice.

Caffeine is capable of stimulating all parts of the C.N.S. However, the amounts taken in during ordinary drinking of the beverages containing it affect mainly the mental functions of the cerebral cortex. The effects of drinking coffee and tea have been extensively studied by psychologists. They have shown that small doses of caffeine increase the ability to maintain intellectual effort in the face of weariness.

This is probably the result of the psychic effect of caffeine in counteracting fatigue, boredom, and drowsiness. Although people seem somewhat more alert to sensory stimuli and react more rapidly and with a freer flow of ideas, it is doubtful that caffeine improves learning ability and memory. Caffeine-induced tremors may actually interfere with the efficiency of motor performance requiring coordinated muscular activity.

THE COFFEE HABIT. Coffee is, of course, drunk in enormous quantities in this country. It is hard to think of this dietary beverage as the cause of a "drug habit," and, indeed, for most people the degree of habituation, or psychic dependence, is so mild as to constitute no real problem. On the other hand, the adverse effects of overindulgence may be more common than is generally suspected. People who habitually drink too much coffee may suffer from cardiac irregularities and gastrointestinal upset, as well as restlessness. There is also evidence that they may often be irritable and have headaches when forced to go without their usual amounts of coffee.

THERAPEUTIC USES OF CAFFEINE. This substance has little clinical utility compared to such chemical relatives of the xanthine class as aminophylline. It is often added in small doses to headache remedies that also contain aspirin and phenacetin. (The C in A.P.C. stands for caffeine.) However, it is doubtful that it has a useful effect when taken orally in this way. Injected intravenously, caffeine may help to relieve the throbbing vascular headaches of migraine and high blood pressure, possibly by constricting the painfully pulsating cerebral blood vessels.

Caffeine is also the main ingredient of products that are promoted for preventing drowsiness. Inasmuch as a cup of coffee contains more caffeine than is contained in these proprietary tablets and capsules, it seems to be a waste of money to purchase such products. In addition, the "popping of pills" to change one's mental state should be discouraged.

Sometimes even drinking coffee for its mental effects may be undesirable. For example, people who have been drinking alcoholic beverages are sometimes urged to drink a cup of coffee before attempting to drive. Although the advice to make the "one for the road" coffee instead of alcohol is well intentioned, it is probably unwise. Coffee is unlikely to sober an unfit driver sufficiently to make it safe for him to operate a motor vehicle. He might better be urged not to start out at all until the effects of the alcohol he has imbibed are entirely dissipated.

Caffeine has, however, been used in the treatment of acute alcoholic intoxication to stimulate the patient's depressed respiration and to speed his arousal. Caffeine sodium benzoate is sometimes administered intramuscularly for this purpose. If this parenteral product is unavailable, an infusion of coffee may be prepared which, after cooling to body temperature, may be instilled as a retention enema.

The Amphetamines

Public and professional concern with the abuse of these drugs has resulted in measures that have sharply limited their legitimate medical use. Because of claims that almost half the amphetamines produced by pharmaceutical companies are diverted to illicit channels, the Food and Drug Administration has set quotas limiting the production of these drugs.

Physicians who feel that these drugs were formerly overprescribed recently have voluntarily stopped ordering them. Pharmacists in some areas have agreed among themselves not to dispense these drugs when they are requested for certain indications in which their clinical usefulness is now considered doubtful. Nonetheless, the amphetamines possess pharmacological effects that make them potentially useful for carefully selected cases in several areas of clinical medicine (see *Summary*, p. 128).

PHARMACOLOGICAL EFFECTS

All the amphetamines possess certain central actions that form the basis for their clinical use in the management of many conditions. However, all also act peripherally to varying degrees to bring about side effects which are ordinarily considered undesirable. The doctor tries to use these drugs in small doses that are intended to produce the desired primary effects upon the C.N.S. without adversely affecting cardiovascular function.

Psychopharmacological effects of two types form the basis for the various clinical uses of these drugs and for most of the central side effects that are seen when they are taken in excessive amounts. One of these effects is an increase in alertness and wakefulness. The other action is manifested by a mood-elevating, or euphorigenic, effect. Both effects are dose-related, in the sense that they become progressively more marked as the dosage of these drugs is raised.

The increase in alertness brought about by small doses of these drugs has been used to help counteract feelings of fatigue. A person who is tired and sleepy may take these drugs in order to continue his activities. The trouble with this practice is that the amphetamines only mask feelings of fatigue and are not themselves a source of energy. Thus, people taking these drugs may still have an impaired ability to perform the tasks that they are pushing themselves to complete.

Chronic fatigue is, of course, often of emotional origin. It should not be treated by self-administered amphetamine tablets (or caffeine capsules). The nurse should recognize those patients whose chronic claims of being "dead tired" or "totally exhausted" stem from emotional tension or maladjustment. She may then tactfully guide them to a doctor capable of discovering and dealing with the true cause of their continuous tiredness.

The nurse herself is not immune to physical and mental fatigue that is the result of the nature of her work. She should not attempt to counteract her weariness by the habitual use of amphetamine-type "pep pills," or, for that matter, by an endless round of cups of coffee. Drug-taking of any kind is an unwholesome stopgap remedy for dealing with a condition that requires rest and sleep, rather than the use of chemicals that actually interfere with sleep.

As the dose of these drugs is raised, the person may become aware of an inner tension or irritability which is somewhat discomforting. He may find himself restless, nervous, and "jittery"—a term that he uses to describe his awareness of tremulousness caused by muscular as well as emotional tension.

With still higher doses of these drugs, the patient suffers from insomnia, headache, dizziness, and a variety of side effects (see *Summary*) that are the result of the peripheral actions of these drugs on adrenergic neuroeffectors rather than on extension of their central stimulating action. On the other hand, with continued abuse of amphetamine-type drugs, their adverse effects on brain function are seen, first, in signs of marked agitation and apprehension and, later, in states of panic that may end in a toxic psychosis marked by delirium and visual and auditory hallucinations which elicit paranoid delusions.

The euphorigenic, or mood-elevating, effect is also best brought about by small doses of the amphetamines. Patients with mild mood disturbances caused by distressing events in their life situation sometimes seem to lose interest in their usual activities. Often, they feel fatigued even after a night's sleep, and seem unable or unwilling to meet and to have dealings with other people.

Sometimes small daily doses of an amphetamine bring beneficial changes in the attitudes of patients with mild "reactive" depression. Somehow the patient becomes brighter and more alert and attentive. His depressive apathy gradually disappears, and he regains his desire to take part in normal daily life activities.

Patients with more severe degrees of mental depression are not ordinarily helped by amphetamine therapy and may even be harmed by these drugs. These psychomotor stimulants tend to increase the insomnia and appetite loss of people who are already sleeping and eating poorly. Thus, they are not employed for the more severe neurotic and psychotic depressive symptoms, which require the more potent antidepressant drugs, electroshock therapy, and intensive psychotherapy.

CLINICAL INDICATIONS FOR AMPHETAMINES (SEE SUMMARY)

The alerting and mood-elevating effects of the amphetamines account for the uses to which these drugs have been put in neurology, psychiatry, and general medicine. Among the neurological disorders that sometimes respond to amphetamine treatment are narcolepsy and certain selected cases of epilepsy and postencephalitic parkinsonism. Certain behavioral disorders of childhood believed to be caused by nerve cell malfunction are also sometimes benefited.

Narcolepsy is a neurological condition in which the patient is periodically overcome by uncontrollable drowsiness. Patients may be overwhelmed by a sudden desire to sleep anywhere and at any time. Such "sleep attacks" occur most commonly during an emotional reaction marked by surprise, anger, or laughter. Discovery of the alerting action of amphetamine led to its use in this embarrassing and potentially dangerous condition. Large doses—25 to 50 mg, or more, daily—are required to prevent narcoleptic sleep paroxysms. However, the results seem to make such treatment worthwhile, since most patients are able to remain awake all day—a response to drug therapy that often converts them from social and occupational misfits into useful, productive citizens.

Hyperkinesis, a behavioral disorder of children, is sometimes markedly benefited by treatment with *methylphenidate+* (Ritalin) or *dextroamphetamine+* (Dexedrine). This condition is characterized by hyperactivity and learning difficulties that are thought to be of neurological rather than of psychological origin. This may be the result of slight brain damage sustained at birth or before or after birth. (The condition is also called *minimal brain dysfunction,* or MBD.)

Oddly, in many but not all correctly diagnosed cases of MBD, these psychomotor stimulants exert a paradoxical *quieting* effect. Calmed and relaxed by the action of these drugs, children who have been unable to learn because of their short attention span and easy distractibility become able to profit from school classes and other measures such as psychotherapy. They gain control over their previously unstable emotional state and hostile impulses, and with proper social guidance, they eventually tend to outgrow their difficulties.

Motor disorders caused by hyperactivity of various groups of nerve cells also sometimes respond to treatment with the amphetamines. Some children with petit mal epilepsy have fewer attacks while taking these drugs. In other types of epilepsy, patients who become lethargic from treatment with standard anticonvulsant drugs profit from the alerting effect of amphetamines when these stimulants are added to their drug treatment program.

Postencephalitic lethargy and extrapyramidal motor system symptoms are also often counteracted by treatment with psychomotor stimulants. Amphetamines often reduce parkinsonism tremors, drowsiness, and oculogyric crisis, a distressing complication in which the patient's eyeballs roll far up into the orbits and his head is pulled back by contraction of the neck muscles. Drug-induced dystonias are sometimes relieved by an intravenous injection of caffeine sodium benzoate.

Mild mental depression and withdrawn senile behavior are—as indicated previously— sometimes benefited by small oral doses of amphetamines and methylphenidate. Two other stimulants, *pipradrol* (Alertonic) and *pentylenetetrazol* (Metrazol), have also been advocated for counteracting fatigue, apathy, and lack of energy in such cases. Their usefulness for this purpose seems doubtful as does that of *deanol* (Deaner), a stimulant claimed to aid in treating patients with behavioral and learning problems.

AMPHETAMINES AS APPETITE SUPPRESSANTS. The amphetamines are widely employed in products advocated for use as adjuncts to low-calorie diets in the weight-reducing programs of obese patients and other dieters. These drugs tend, temporarily at least, to lessen the patient's desire to eat. Most authorities feel that the anorectic effect of the amphetamines is related to their mood-elevating action. That is, these drugs are thought to help people stick to a low-calorie diet, despite its discomforts, by making the patient feel better mentally.

The usefulness of this psychopharmacological effect is limited at best. Most patients soon tend to develop tolerance to the psychological lift that the amphetamines offered them at first. If this happens after four to eight weeks, it is not advisable to raise the dose, as this may cause cardiovascular side effects and lead to abuse by addiction-prone patients. Instead, it is best that the medication be discontinued for a few weeks. If drug treatment is then still indicated, it can be begun again following loss of tolerance during the period of abstinence from amphetamine.

The disadvantages and limitations of the amphetamines have led to efforts to find safer, more effective anorectic agents. All that have been introduced so far (Table 9-2) are chemical relatives of the amphetamines that are claimed less likely to cause central stimulation or adrenergic-type cardiovascular effects. In practice, however, all the available appetite suppressants are capable of causing sympathomimetic and central side effects.

Thus, all must be used with caution in patients with cardiovascular disease and the various other disorders in which the amphetamines are often contraindicated (see *Summary,* p. 128). However, certain of the newer appetite suppressants, including *fenfluramine* (Ponderax), do seem somewhat less likely to cause excessive C.N.S. stimulation. In fact, the latter drug has sedative properties which may make it more useful than the amphetamines for patients with the so-called "night eating syndrome" who have insomnia and tend to eat heavily late at night. On the other hand, drowsiness is a more common side effect with this compound, and it has not yet been proved free of drug abuse potential.

Analeptics (Table 9-1)

Analeptics are C.N.S. stimulants that are intended to bring about two main effects:

1. Stimulation of the nerve cells of the respiratory center, when it is depressed by drugs or in disease states.

2. Stimulation of the nerve cell centers that

TABLE 9-2 *Anorexiant Agents*

Official or Generic Name	Proprietary Name	Usual Dose
Amphetamines (see Table 9-1)		
Benzphetamine HCl	Didrex	25 to 50 mg 1 to 3 times daily
Chlorphentermine HCl	Pre-Sate	65 mg daily
Diethylpropion HCl N.F.	Tenuate; Tepanil	25 mg t.i.d.
Fenfluramine	Ponderax	20 mg t.i.d.
Mazindol	Sanorex	1 to 2 mg 1 to 3 times daily
Phendimetrazine tartrate	Plegine	17.5 to 70 mg 2 to 3 times daily
Phenmetrazine HCl N.F.	Preludin	25 mg 2 to 3 times daily
Phentermine resin	Ionamin	15 to 30 mg once daily
Phentermine HCl	Wilpo	8 mg t.i.d.

influence consciousness, when these centers are depressed by drugs.

Unfortunately, when these drugs are administered in the doses needed to produce these clinically desirable effects, they also stimulate other central sites. This can lead to convulsions, vomiting, and cardiovascular or respiratory difficulties. Thus, most authorities are now opposed to the routine use of analeptics for treating the clinical conditions in which these stimulants were once considered indicated. Even those anesthesiologists and others who still employ analeptic therapy do so only in carefully selected patients and with considerable caution.

CLINICAL INDICATIONS FOR ANALEPTICS

These include: (1) the treatment of poisoning by barbiturates and other C.N.S. depressant drugs; (2) shortening the time needed for recovery following anesthesia with barbiturates and other depressants; (3) reducing respiratory complications in the postanesthetic period; and (4) maintaining and restoring acid-base balance in patients with chronic obstructive pulmonary disease. The employment of analeptic therapy in these and other clinical situations is controversial, and these drugs are considered to be of only limited usefulness, at best.

DEPRESSANT DRUG INTOXICATION. Among the analeptics most commonly employed to counteract the effects of overdosage by barbiturates and other C.N.S. depressants are *pentylene-tetrazol+* (Metrazol), a rapid-acting stimulant with a short duration of action, and *picrotoxin*, a stimulant of slow onset but prolonged duration. Both drugs are capable of causing convulsions when administered to patients who are in only a relatively light stupor. They may also bring about recovery of the vomiting reflex mechanism, which may subject the patient to the risk of regurgitating the gastric contents.

Most authorities now maintain that barbiturate poisoning is best managed by measures to help support the patient's respiration and other vital functions. Among the measures employed to avoid atalectasis and pneumonia are: (1) maintaining an open airway with endotracheal and tracheostomy tubes; (2) mechanical assistance to keep the patient well ventilated; (3) turning the patient from side to side frequently and suctioning his respiratory secretions to prevent pulmonary infections; and (4) maintaining fluid and electrolyte balance and administering vasopressor drugs as needed to keep blood pressure at adequate levels.

Those who advocate aggressive supportive measures and superior nursing care are also usually opposed to any use of analeptic drugs. However, others have suggested that analeptics may be useful for determining the depth of a depressed patient's coma. This may be done by administering a single dose of *pentylenetetrazol* I.V. If the patient's reflex activity returns promptly, and he is readily aroused by this so-called "orientation dose," his chances of rapid recovery with supportive care alone are considered good. However, failure to respond to the first dose may mean that the patient's depression is so deep that he may profit from treatment with analeptics in addition to routine supportive care. In addition, overdosage of these drugs is not likely in patients who are very deeply depressed.

POSTANESTHETIC RESPIRATORY DEPRESSION. Patients who have received various central and peripheral depressants before and during surgery sometimes suffer from drug-induced respiratory depression of varying degree postoperatively. Recovery room nurses try to encourage patients to breathe deeply as part of the so-called "stir up" regimen for preventing the development of atalectasis. Some anesthesiologists have recently suggested that respiratory stimulant drugs might be useful to produce deep breathing and physiological sighing and to hasten the return of the protective cough and swallowing reflexes of such patients. *Doxapram* (Dopram), the newest analeptic drug, has reportedly helped to prevent postoperative respiratory complications when infused intravenously for 30-minute periods in such situations.

CHRONIC OBSTRUCTIVE LUNG DISEASES. Patients with chronic respiratory diseases such as pulmonary emphysema may occasionally benefit from very careful infusion of a respiratory stimulant. These drugs cannot, of course, reverse the underlying cause of the patient's hypoventilation. That is, they cannot correct the obstruction caused by the breakdown of the walls of the alveoli, the millions of tiny air sacs that have lost their elasticity and, with it, the ability to expand and contract. Drugs may, however, help to overcome some of the complications that have resulted from the patient's rapid, shallow, labored breathing.

Because of their decreased ability to expel air, patients with pulmonary emphysema tend to retain high levels of carbon dioxide in their blood. This end product of metabolism makes the patient drowsy and may even cause coma. Accumulation of this acid waste product also leads to respiratory acidosis and dyspnea. In such cases, some doctors have reported that administration of the relatively specific respiratory center stimulant *doxapram* (Dopram) has helped to increase the depth of the patient's respiration and improved the ventilation.

Convulsant Drugs and Poisons

Various natural and synthetic substances stimulate motor areas of the C.N.S. so strongly that a person's muscle groups are forced into violent contractions, or convulsive spasms. Alkaloids such as *strychnine* and *cocaine*, and the previously mentioned brain stem stimulants *picrotoxin* and *pentylenetetrazol*, are capable of causing convulsions. *Tetanospasmin*, a substance produced by the pathogenic microorganism, *Clostridium tetani*, is an extremly powerful convulsant toxin.

STRYCHNINE POISONING

Strychnine is a drug that should have no place in modern therapy. It has been used as a respiratory stimulant, digestive tonic, and an ingredient of cathartic combinations. Its usefulness, if any, is far outweighed by the danger of poisoning from accidental ingestion. Similarly, the use of strychnine in so-called mouse "seeds" or rat "poison pellets" and as a bait for field rodents is unjustified in view of the present availability of safer substances.

The incidence of strychnine poisoning has declined as preparations containing it have deservedly lost popularity; however, cases are still reported in which children have died after swallowing a handful of candy-coated "tonic" or cathartic tablets. The quantity of strychnine in a single tablet of aloin, strychnine and belladonna (for example) is harmless—as well as useless—but the total alkaloid contained in several pills may be capable of causing fatal convulsions.

TETANUS TOXIN

Tetanus toxin is set free from anaerobic pathogens multiplying deep in poorly oxygenated dead or dying tissue. Once it spreads to the C.N.S. and becomes bound to motor nerve cells, it exerts a long-lasting stimulating effect. Among the first nerves involved are those that control muscles of the face and jaw. Their contractions keep the patient from opening his mouth completely ("lockjaw"). Later, massive muscle spasms occur suddenly, making the patient's body ramrod stiff or even bending his back until only the head and heels are touching the bed (opisthotonus). Death is caused by prolonged spasm of the muscles of respiration.

CONTROL OF CONVULSIONS

Control of convulsions requires the careful administration of depressant drugs in doses that produce muscle relaxation and light sleep without impairing respiratory center function. Intravenous injection of small doses of an ultrashort-acting barbiturate such as thiopental may be repeated as needed to keep muscular activity under control. This may be followed by intramuscular injection of the long-acting anticonvulsant, phenobarbital. Muscle relaxants such as diazepam and tubocurarine have been found useful in the hands of anesthesiologists called in to aid in controlling the patient's convulsions.

CLINICAL USES OF CONVULSANT DRUGS

The drugs of this class have only limited clinical utility, since convulsions are generally considered a complication to be feared rather than a therapeutically desirable action. However, certain pharmacoconvulsants are occasionally employed in psychiatry and neurology.

Chemoshock is a rarely used alternative to electroshock therapy (EST or ECT) in the treatment of psychotic depressive states and certain schizophrenic reactions. Pentylenetetrazol was the convulsant first employed for this purpose. Injected rapidly by vein, a large dose (5 ml of a 10 percent solution) produces clonic spasms, followed by a massive tonic convulsion. A series of such treatments often improves the patient's mental condition.

Recently, inhalation of the volatile vapors of a drug have been used to produce convulsions in selected psychiatric patients. This convulsant agent, called *flurothyl* (Indoklon), has been employed in the treatment of the same kinds of cases in which pentylenetetrazol was previously thought indicated and for which EST is presently most commonly employed. Like EST, its use is contraindicated in patients with a history of cardiovascular disease and for others who might be endangered by seizure activity.

Epilepsy diagnosis is sometimes aided by the slow intravenous infusion of pentylenetetrazol+, which sets off changes in the patient's electroencephalogram that indicate the presence of neurological abnormalities. Usually this is done by administering the drug alone in subconvulsant doses. Sometimes the I.V. infusion is accompanied by the use of a flickering light to produce an actual clinical convulsion. This can aid the neurologist to determine the patient's exact type of epilepsy and to choose the anticonvulsant drugs best suited for control of seizures.

SUMMARY of Clinical Indications for the Use of Psychomotor Stimulants

Neurological Disorders

Narcolepsy; hyperkinetic behavioral disorders in children with minimal brain dysfunction syndrome; postencephalitic disorders; selected cases of epilepsy.

Psychiatric Disorders

Mental depression of a mild degree and temporary nature secondary to situational stress; senile apathy, withdrawal, and depression (selected cases and brief use only); in psychiatric interviewing.

Obesity

Adjunct to low-calorie diets for brief periods (four to eight weeks), followed by withdrawal when signs of tolerance develop.

Depressant Drug Overdosage

Combined with barbiturates, antihistamine, and anticonvulsant drugs in small oral doses to counteract drowsiness and lethargy; administered parenterally to hasten recovery from anesthetic doses of barbiturates, but *not* for treating poisoning by barbiturates and other depressant drugs when facilities for adequate conservative (supportive) therapy are available.

SUMMARY of Side Effects, Toxicity, Cautions, and Contraindications of Psychomotor Drugs

Central Side Effects and Toxicity

Nervousness, restlessness, jitteriness, irritability, anorexia, insomnia, headache, dizziness; anxiety, tension, difficulty in concentrating; confusion, delirium, hallucinations, toxic psychosis with paranoid delusions.

Peripheral Side Effects and Toxicity

Cardiac palpitations and tachycardia, with possible chest pains and other heartbeat irregularities; elevation of both systolic and diastolic blood pressures; dryness of the mouth, constipation, nausea and vomiting, excessive sweating, dilated pupils.

These drugs are not knowingly ordered for patients who have a history of drug abuse. Only small amounts are made available to patients and prescriptions may be refilled only a limited number of times.

Use of these drugs by patients with a history of cardiovascular disease symptoms is undesirable, and the drugs are contraindicated in patients with advanced coronary or cerebral ar-

teriosclerosis, hyperthyroidism, hypertension, or diabetes.

Use of these drugs for the purpose of counteracting symptoms of fatigue is not desirable. Patients taking these drugs may still have an impaired ability to perform potentially dangerous activities such as driving or operating machinery.

These drugs should not be administered to patients who have been taking guanethidine or drugs of the monoamine oxidase class. Methylphenidate may lead to inhibition of the metabolism of drugs such as coumarin-type anticoagulants and diphenylhydantoin or phenylbutazone. Thus, if signs of drug interaction occur, dosage of these drugs is adjusted downward.

SUMMARY of Nursing Points Related to C.N.S. Stimulants

Teach the obese patient who is taking amphetamines as one aspect of a program of weight reduction to report such symptoms as nervousness, insomnia, or cardiac palpitations.

The nurse, particularly in industrial and school settings, has an opportunity to provide instruction concerning the misuse of caffeine and amphetamines; sometimes she observes individuals misusing these preparations. In the latter instance the individual may be advised to consult his physician so that the reasons for his misuse of these agents can be explored. Sometimes the nurse can provide the necessary information and offer sufficient encouragement so that the patient stops this undesirable and potentially harmful practice.

The depressed patient who is being treated

with amphetamines should be carefully observed for insomnia, loss of appetite, restlessness, and agitation. These symptoms may be related to the patient's illness, but they also can be caused, or be made worse, by the use of amphetamines.

When powerful central nervous system stimulants such as Metrazol and picrotoxin are used, the patient should be observed carefully for symptoms of hypoxia, preconvulsive muscular twitching, and convulsions. Many of the patients who require these stimulants have attempted suicide by taking overdoses of barbiturates or other depressant drugs. As the patient regains consciousness he requires the nurse's careful observation and support in an effort to prevent further suicide attempts.

DRUG DIGEST

CAFFEINE U.S.P.

Actions and Indications. This alkaloid from coffee, tea, and cola is a psychomotor stimulant that increases alertness and wakefulness. It is used by the public in beverages containing it and in solid dosage forms to overcome drowsiness and to counteract the depressant effects of alcohol. The injectable form is sometimes employed medically to hasten recovery from acute alcoholic intoxication. Caffeine is frequently combined with analgesics such as aspirin and phenacetin in proprietary headache remedies and with ergotamine in prescription products for treating migraine and hypertensive headaches.

Side Effects, Cautions, and Contraindications. The adverse effects are mainly those caused by excessive C.N.S. stimulation—for example, insomnia, nervous irritability, and tremors. However, heart palpitations may occur in some sensitive individuals and epigastric distress in others. Many people are both tolerant to and psychologically dependent upon the caffeine in coffee. When deprived of the beverage, they may become irritable and have headaches.

Dosage and Administration. A cup of coffee ordinarily contains 100 to 150 mg of caffeine, but tea and cola beverages contain considerably less. The amount found in

pharmaceutical preparations (50 to 100 mg) is thus less than is available in a cup of coffee. For central stimulation of individuals deeply depressed by alcohol or depressant drugs, caffeine sodium benzoate may be injected intramuscularly or subcutaneously in doses up to 500 mg.

DEXTROAMPHETAMINE SULFATE U.S.P. (Dexedrine)

Actions and Indications. This psychomotor stimulant is now indicated mainly in the management of neurological disorders such as narcolepsy and hyperkinetic behavior in children with the minimal brain dysfunction syndrome. It is also still used as an adjunct to low-calorie diets in the short-term treatment of obesity. It is sometimes added in small doses to prescriptions containing such depressant drugs as antihistamines and anticonvulsants, but it should *not* be used to counteract symptoms of hangover caused by alcohol or barbiturates. It is now rarely used in the treatment of mental depression.

Side Effects, Cautions, and Contraindications. Side effects of central origin include restlessness, irritability, and insomnia; and in overdosage, muscle tremors, increased reflex activity, confusion, and, possibly, panic states. Continued abuse of high doses can cause psychic dependence and possible paranoid reactions. The extreme fatigue and mental depression that follow abrupt withdrawal of this drug may be also an indication of physical dependence. It is contraindicated in patients with a history of having abused other drugs.

Adrenergic stimulation may cause cardiac palpitations and arrhythmias, a rise in blood pressure, and chest pains. The drug is contraindicated in patients with symptoms of cardiovascular disease and hyperthyroidism. It is not administered to patients who have been taking drugs of the monoamine oxidase inhibitor class.

Dosage and Administration. The usual oral dose is 5 mg taken before meals, but daily dosage may range from 2.5 to 30 mg. Sustained-release capsules (Spansules) containing 5, 10, or 15 mg are taken in the morning and, occasionally, about six hours later.

METHYLPHENIDATE U.S.P. (Ritalin)

Actions and Indications. This central stimulant is midway in potency between caffeine and amphetamine.

Small or moderate oral doses may be useful for reducing hyperkinetic behavior in children correctly diagnosed as suffering from minimal brain dysfunction, for maintaining daytime wakefulness in patients with narcolepsy, and possibly in the management of senile patients who are apathetic and withdrawn.

Addition of this drug to the regimen of patients who are made drowsy by depressant drugs such as antihistamines, anticonvulsants, and barbiturates may help to counteract their lethargy. Injections are sometimes used to speed recovery from barbiturate anesthesia. However, in treating acute poisoning by barbiturates, it should be used only if facilities are not available for proper supportive therapy.

Side Effects, Cautions, and Contraindications. Overstimulation of the C.N.S. causes nervousness and insomnia and, in massive overdosage, muscular tremors, twitching, and convulsions. High doses also produce adrenergic effects including cardiac palpitations and acceleration, hypertension, sweating, mydriasis, and mouth dryness. It is contraindicated in agitated patients and in those with glaucoma, and it is administered cautiously to alcoholic patients and others with a history of drug abuse.

Dosage and Administration. Adult oral doses range from 15 to 60 mg daily, with an average of 20 to 30 mg, administered in two or three divided doses before meals. In children, treatment is initiated with 5 mg b.i.d., and dosage is gradually raised, if necessary. Injections of 20 to 30 mg are made I.V., I.M., or S.C.

PENTYLENETETRAZOL N.F. (Metrazol)

Actions and Indications. This brain

stem stimulant has been used mainly as an analeptic for stimulating the respiratory center of patients deeply depressed by overdoses of barbiturates and other central depressant drugs. It is also sometimes used to determine the depth of a patient's depression and his prognosis for recovery when treated with conservative measures for supporting vital functions.

The use of pentylenetetrazol in the chemoshock therapy of depression and schizophrenia has diminished in favor of electroconvulsive therapy. It is sometimes used in subconvulsant I.V. doses as an aid in the diagnosis of epilepsy. Oral doses have been advocated in the treatment of elderly patients who are apathetic or confused and disoriented, but the usefulness of this drug is doubted in such cases of senility.

Side Effects, Cautions, and Contraindications. The utility of this and other analeptic drugs is limited by their lack of specificity for the respiratory center. Thus, the doses that must be employed for effective respiratory stimulation may set off convulsive activity. There is also some danger of stimulating the vomiting center with resulting aspiration of gastric contents, leading to asphyxia or to aspiration pneumonia. Cardiac arrhythmias may also occur.

Dosage and Administration. Intravenous injection of 5 ml of a 10% solution is used to determine the depth of drug-induced coma. Lesser amounts (1 ml or more) may be used to produce convulsive seizures. Oral doses of 200 mg are sometimes taken t.i.d. by elderly patients.

References

Caskey, K., et al. The school nurse and drug abusers. *Nurs. Outlook*, 18:27, 1970.

Clemmesen, C., and Nilson, E. Therapeutic trends in the treatment of barbiturate poisoning. *Clin. Pharmacol. Ther.*, 2:220, 1961.

Connel, P.H. Clinical manifestations and treatment of amphetamine-type dependence. *JAMA*, 196:718, 1966.

Elser, J.R. Acute barbiturate poisoning. *Amer. J. Nurs.*, 60:1096, 1960.

Hadden, J., et al. Acute barbiturate intoxication. *JAMA*, 209:893, 1969.

Kramer, J.C., et al. Amphetamine abuse. *JAMA*, 201:305, 1967.

Modell, W. Status and prospect of drugs for overeating. *JAMA*, 173:1131, 1960.

Rodman, M.J. Use and abuse of the amphetamines. *RN*, 33:55, 1970 (Aug.).

———. The central nervous system stimulants. *RN*, 30:85, 1967 (Sept.).

———. Drugs for dealing with weight problems. *RN*, 26:41, 1963 (May).

Swissiman, N., and Jacoby, J. Strychnine poisoning and its treatment. *Clin. Pharmacol. Ther.*, 5:136, 1964.

Werner, G. Clinical pharmacology of central stimulant and depressant drugs. *Clin. Pharmacol. Ther.*, 3:59, 1962.

SECTION 3

Drugs
Used
in
Neurological
and
Musculoskeletal
Disorders

In the following chapters we shall discuss drugs used in the management of neurological disorders that affect skeletal muscle function. We shall first review briefly some aspects of normal nervous control of movements. This will then help us to understand how drugs act to prevent epileptic seizures, reduce disability in Parkinson's disease, and relieve crippling disability in cerebral palsy and other neurological and musculoskeletal disorders.

Nervous Control of Movements

Every segment of the brain and spinal cord contains nerve cells that exert control over muscle tone and movement. Damage at any level, from the cerebral motor cortex to the spinal cord, can interfere with the flow of nerve impulses that affect muscle function. The result may be motor incoordination, muscle spasm and spasticity and other signs of excessive muscle tone, or sometimes convulsive epileptic seizures.

Spinal reflexes are the simplest circuits for regulating motor responses to sensory stimuli. The simplest reflexes involve only a single sensory neuron connected to one motor neuron. More complex spinal reflexes include a third type of nerve cell, the internuncial neuron. These relay impulses between sensory and motor neurons, sometimes at several spinal segments at once. For example, when a muscle is stretched or tendons and ligaments are torn, streams of sensory impulses pass into the spinal cord. Relayed by interneurons to spinal motor cells, these sensory stimuli set off trains of motor nerve impulses that increase muscle tone and contractions. Sometimes these overactive multineuronal, or polysynaptic, reflexes cause painful muscle spasms.

Supraspinal influences also affect the functioning of spinal motor nerves. For example, fiber tracts from cells originating in the brain stem, basal ganglia, and the cerebral cortex send impulses downstream to the spinal nerve cells. Some of these increase the excitability of the lower motor neurons; others exert inhibitory influences that tend to suppress spinal motor activity. Damage to an inhibitory pathway can result in an imbalance that leads to excessive excitatory-type stimulation of spinal neurons, resulting in muscle spasticity, rigidity, and various other crippling contractures that develop in patients with cerebral palsy, multiple sclerosis, paraplegia, and other neurological disorders.

The *pyramidal tract*, originating in the motor cortex, sends out the signals that set consciously controlled activities into motion. The flow of these impulses is influenced also by feedback messages from the cerebellum and various subcortically located groups of motor neurons. Disease affecting motor neurons in these interacting pathways can set off epileptic seizures.

The *extrapyramidal motor system* makes automatic adjustments in muscle tone and posture. In order for the commands of the motor cortex to be executed with smooth precision, this system must, at the same time, exert its unconscious control of muscles involved in maintaining posture and balance. Injury of the cerebellar portion of this system causes ataxia —unsteady, incoordinated movements; disease in the basal ganglia—the masses of gray matter beneath the cortex—can result in the muscle rigidity and tremors of Parkinson's disease or the violent jerking movements of Huntington's or Sydenham's chorea.

10.

Centrally Acting Skeletal Muscle Relaxants

The Nature of Muscular Spasm and Spasticity

Many disorders of the musculoskeletal and nervous systems cause painful and disabling muscle spasms and spasticity. Spasms are sudden, acute muscle cramps set off by injury or irritation in musculoskeletal areas. In spasticity, the injury or irritation that results in abnormal muscle movements arises within the nervous system. Conditions in which spasm or spasticity occur are treated with drugs that act either centrally or peripherally to reduce excessive reflex activity.

MUSCLE RELAXING DRUGS

Among the drugs that can relax muscle contractions by their effects on the muscles themselves are the neuromuscular blocking agents and the local anesthetics. Centrally acting muscle relaxants include the general anesthetics, barbiturates, and other general depressants. In this chapter we shall discuss a group of drugs that is thought to relieve pain and spasm by a more selective action than other centrally acting drugs.

These centrally acting muscle relaxants, sometimes called neurospasmolytics (Table 10-1), are claimed to be more likely than the general depressants to relax muscle spasm and reduce spasticity without producing excessive sedation or depression of respiration. They are most effective when administered by injection in moderately high doses. The small oral doses in which these drugs are most often prescribed have little antispasmodic activity. Most benefits obtained from low oral doses may be the

T A B L E   1 0 - 1   *Centrally Acting Skeletal Muscle Relaxants*

Nonproprietary Name	Trade Name	Usual Single Dose	Comments
Carisoprodol	Rela; Soma	250–350 mg	Claimed to have analgesic activity
Chlordiazepoxide	Librium	25–50 mg	Antianxiety agent also. See *Drug Digest*
Chlormezanone	Trancopal	100–200 mg	Antianxiety (tranquilizer) also
Chlorphenesin carbamate	Maolate	400–800 mg	Relatively weak central depressant
Chlorzoxazone	Paraflex	250–750 mg	Available in combination with analgesics
Diazepam N.F.	Valium	2–10 mg	Antianxiety also. See *Drug Digest*
Mephenesin	Dioloxol; Tolerol, and others	2000–3000 mg	Weak action; large doses
Mephenesin carbamate	Tolseram	1000–3000 mg	Weak action; large doses
Meprobamate U.S.P.	Equanil; Miltown	400–800 mg	Minor tranquilizer activity also. See *Drug Digest*
Metaxalone	Skelaxin	400–800 mg	Not given for more than 10 consecutive days
Methocarbamol N.F.	Robaxin	500–2000 mg	Analogue of mephenesin carbamate. See *Drug Digest*
Orphenadrine citrate N.F.	Norflex	60–100 mg	Related to the antihistamine, diphenhydramine (Benadryl)
Phenaglycodol	Ultran	200–400 mg	Antianxiety activity also

result of the mild sedative, or antianxiety, effect that most of these drugs exert.

Use in Clinical Disorders

MUSCULOSKELETAL DISORDERS

These conditions (*Summary*, p. 136) are the result of local injury or inflammation in muscles, joints, and related peripheral structures. Local trauma—muscle strains or sprains, for example—sends streams of sensory impulses into the spinal cord. These messages are then relayed to the motor nerves by one or more connecting nerve cells, or internuncial neurons (Fig. 10-1). The spinal motor neurons then send abnormal numbers of nerve impulses to the injured area, thus causing painful muscle spasm. The pain often causes even more muscle spasm in a vicious cycle of spasm-pain-intensified spasm.

Drugs such as *diazepam+* (Valium), *methocarbamol+* (Robaxin), and *carisoprodol* (Rela, Soma), among others of this class, are thought to relieve the reflex spasm set off by muscle or joint injury by reducing the responsiveness of the spinal interneurons to the incoming sensory impulses. This same reduction in polysynaptic reflexes is also claimed to be useful for relief of spasm secondary to local inflammation—in arthritis, bursitis, and fibrositis, for example. However, some authorities suggest that improvement may be the result of the effects on the patient's emotional state of many of these agents, such as *meprobamate+* (Equanil; Miltown), *diazepam*, and others.

Other measures that may give more relief of muscle spasm than oral doses of these drugs include application of heat, massage, traction, and bed rest. These physical and mechanical measures together with parenterally administered diazepam or methocarbamol are particularly useful in acute cases involving pressure on spinal nerve roots. The physician often refers patients with whiplash injuries or other cervical spine or low-back syndromes to a physical therapist for initiating these nondrug aspects of treatment. The nurse then assists the patient with his prescribed exercises during all of her later contacts with him. She also has the responsibility for positioning the patient and assisting or instructing him about aspects of body mechanics and care.

NEUROLOGICAL DISORDERS

The injectable forms of diazepam and methocarbamol are often useful for relief of spas-

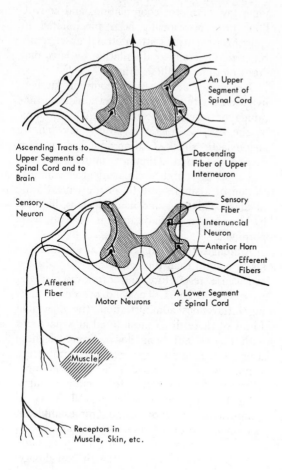

Fig. 10-1. Polysynaptic reflex arc pathways. The neurospasmolytic drugs depress the internuncial neurons in hyperactive reflex pathways (hyperreflexia). This reduces excessive reflex excitability and muscle spasm without affecting normal muscle tone.

In the figure:
- An Upper Segment of Spinal Cord
- Ascending Tracts to Upper Segments of Spinal Cord and to Brain
- Descending Fiber of Upper Interneuron
- Sensory Neuron
- Sensory Fiber
- Internuncial Neuron
- Anterior Horn
- Efferent Fibers
- Afferent Fiber
- Motor Neurons
- A Lower Segment of Spinal Cord
- Muscle
- Receptors in Muscle, Skin, etc.

ticity secondary to such diseases as cerebral palsy and multiple sclerosis, or in cases of hemiplegia (following a stroke, for example) or quadriplegia resulting from cervical spinal cord injury. In all such cases, the patient's excessive muscle tone is the result of the release of lower (spinal) motor neurons from the influence of upper motor neurons that ordinarily tend to exert an inhibitory influence. When these suppressive nerve cells are damaged, certain other areas of the nervous system that send excitatory impulses downstream tend to exert an excessive influence over the lower motor neurons.

These neurospasmolytic drugs are thought to act by depressing the activity of the excitatory interneurons. This helps to restore the balance between inhibitory and excitatory influences upon the spinal motor neurons, with a resulting reduction in muscular spasticity, rigidity, and other movement disorders. The improvement in movement is only temporary and does not ordinarily allow the handicapped patient to function normally. However, the adjunctive use of these drugs often permits nerve-damaged patients to profit from physical therapy.

Some specialists in treating children with cerebral palsy claim, for example, that these central muscle relaxant-tranquilizer drugs can play an important part in the therapeutic program of these patients. Diazepam, administered at first by injection and later by mouth, is said to have helped children handicapped by various movement disorders. The children, it is claimed, became better able to sit up, stand, and walk. They also learned to dress, feed, and bathe themselves. The drug's sedative effects and its ability to reduce involuntary movements helped the children sleep better. By reducing painful cramps, the use of diazepam permitted the performance of previously painful guided exercises, thus preventing crippling contractures from developing.

Injectable methocarbamol, administered by vein to paraplegic patients with multiple sclerosis, has also made it easier to manipulate their spastic limbs during physiotherapeutic procedures. In addition, the oral forms of this drug and of diazepam have been employed during long-term maintenance therapy for improving the patient's muscle strength and mobility. These drugs may also have a desirable calming effect on the emotional state of patients with multiple sclerosis who are subject to periods of anxiety and depression.

The nurse notes the physical and emotional responses of the patients with chronic neurologic disorders to whom she administers these muscle relaxant-tranquilizer drugs. In addition, she helps the patient keep active as long as possible and advises him and his family about measures for maintaining his general health through diet, rest, exercise, and avoiding infection and emotionally upsetting situations.

Injectable diazepam has also been used recently as part of intensive care programs for treating patients with tetanus. This acute nervous system infection is marked by severe convulsive spasms that sometimes go on for weeks, if the patient survives that long. The advantage of using diazepam for control of acute tetanic muscle spasms is that it does not cause the degrees of deep respiratory and circulatory depression sometimes seen when barbiturates are employed. Diazepam also has the advantage of not causing the local adverse effects often reported when other parenterally administered neurospasmolytics such as mephenesin or methocarbamol are employed (see below, *Adverse Effects*). Skilled nursing care of tetanus patients is now recognized as the most crucial factor in pulling them through their ordeal.

ADVERSE EFFECTS
(SUMMARY, p. 137)

The centrally acting skeletal muscle relaxants are relatively safe drugs, particularly when administered in small oral doses. However, severe hypersensitivity reactions have occurred in patients allergic to some of these drugs. The injectable forms of these drugs may sometimes cause local and systemic reactions.

The most common side effect of orally administered muscle relaxants is drowsiness. Although this is less likely to occur than when barbiturates are employed, ambulatory patients should be warned not to drive while taking diazepam, meprobamate, and related drugs, in-

cluding carisoprodol. Larger doses can cause some loss of motor coordination, and convulsions have occasionally been precipitated in epileptic patients. Gastrointestinal upset sometimes results from local irritation by large oral doses of some of these drugs.

Skin rashes are the most common kind of hypersensitivity reaction. Occasionally, histamine-type reactions occur marked by swelling of the lips, asthmatic breathing, and rarely, anaphylactic shock. Carisoprodol has, on rare occasions, caused temporary muscle paralysis and signs of central excitement after administration of a single dose to an idiosyncratic individual. This drug and its relatives is, like the barbiturates, contraindicated in patients with porphyria.

Although these drugs have a much wider safety margin than the barbiturates, overdosage can cause respiratory and cardiovascular depression and coma. To avoid overdosage during intravenous administration, the injectable forms of these drugs are infused at a slow rate with the patient lying down. Some of these drugs—mephenesin, for example—can cause hemolysis of red blood cells and thrombophlebitis when injected into a vein, and intramuscular injections may be painful. Thus, in administering methocarbamol, for example, it is desirable to divide the amount administered into two or more gluteal muscle regions and then to maintain treatment with oral dosage.

S U M M A R Y of Clinical Indications for Centrally Acting Muscle Relaxants

Musculoskeletal Disorders (Peripheral Injury or Inflammation)

Muscle strains as a result of excessive stretching or overuse

Sprains resulting from wrenched joints with stretched or torn ligaments

Whiplash injuries of the cervical spine processes

Cervical root syndromes

Herniated disk syndrome

Low-back syndrome

Dislocations and fractures

Arthritis, myositis, fibrositis, tendosynovitis, bursitis, and neuritis

Neurological Disorders (Hypertonicity Resulting from Central Nervous System Disease and Damage)

Cerebral palsy

Multiple sclerosis

Muscular dystrophy

Poliomyelitis

Amyotrophic lateral sclerosis

Hemiplegia

Quadriplegia

Parkinson's disease

Laminectomy

Spinal tumors

Tetanus

SUMMARY of Side Effects and Toxicity of Centrally Acting Muscle Relaxants

Gastrointestinal (Small Doses)

Epigastric distress, nausea and vomiting, hiccup.

Central Nervous System

Moderate Dosage: Drowsiness, dizziness, vertigo, light-headedness, headache. (Ambulatory patients should not drive or operate dangerous machinery.)

Overdosage: Muscular incoordination (ataxia), loss of flexor reflexes, flaccid paralysis (including muscles of respiration), stupor, coma, respiratory failure.

Cardiovascular Reactions

Facial flushing, bradycardia or tachycardia, hypotension with feelings of faintness and weakness and possible syncope, shock.

Miscellaneous Reactions to Various Agents (Allergic, Idiosyncratic, and others)

Skin rashes, redness, itching, urticaria, angioneurotic edema, asthmatic breathing.

Hemolysis of red blood cells, hematuria (mephenesin).

Thrombophlebitis (methocarbamol).

Dependence—psychological and possibly physical (diazepam, carisoprodol, meprobamate, and others).

Extreme muscle weakness, transient quadriplegia, temporary blindness (carisoprodol idiosyncrasy).

Blurred vision, mouth dryness (orphenadrine).

SUMMARY of Points for the Nurse to Remember About Care of Patients Receiving Muscle Relaxant Drugs for Spasm and Spasticity

1. Patients who require skeletal muscle relaxant drugs often need other measures to relax muscles. The nurse assists the patient with positioning, exercises, rest, and other aspects of total treatment.

2. Patients suffering from spasticity usually need long-term treatment. Drug therapy is only one aspect of total patient care in patients with chronic progressive or improving neurological disorders. Helping patients with cerebral palsy or multiple sclerosis to master tasks of daily living is, for example, as important as monitoring responses to drug therapy.

3. Patients are observed for signs of the hypersensitivity reactions that sometimes occur with various drugs of this class, including carisoprodol and mephenesin (*Summary of Side Effects*, above).

4. Patients receiving drugs of this and other classes in the management of tetanus and other acute central nervous system disorders that cause severe skeletal muscle spasms require special observation and skilled care with which the nurse must be familiar.

Clinical Situation Related to Use of Skeletal Muscle Relaxants

The Situation: Roger is an eight-year-old boy who has cerebral palsy. His life has been centered around hospitals and clinics where he is being helped to perform all the simple motor activities that other youngsters take for granted. He has made especially rapid progress in recent months while taking daily doses of *diazepam* (Valium) and receiving other forms of therapy. Roger is now feeding, washing, and dressing himself. He walks slowly with mechanical aids, talks understandably, and hopes to leave the special class that he is attending for handicapped children in a year or two and join regular classes with other youngsters of his age.

The Problem: You are the nurse at the clinic to which Roger's mother brings him every week for evaluation of his physical, mental, and emotional status, and particularly, his response to treatment with the skeletal muscle relaxant-antianxiety agent that has been prescribed for him. You see him weekly. The physician sees him once a month, unless problems with the medical therapy arise, in which case the physician would see him more frequently.

Describe the observations that you would make of Roger's status, the ways in which you would assess his progress, and the kind of instructions you would give Roger and his mother concerning his drug therapy.

DRUG DIGEST

DIAZEPAM N.F. (Valium)

Actions and Indications. This chemical relative of the minor tranquilizer, chlordiazepoxide, is used for relief of anxiety and tension in many of the same conditions as its prototype. In addition, it is administered parenterally for control of convulsive seizures and skeletal muscle spasticity in such conditions as status epilepticus, tetanus, and cerebral palsy. It is also used for treatment and diagnostic procedures in orthopedics, obstetrics, cardiology, and gastroenterology.

Side Effects, Cautions, and Contraindications. Drowsiness and ataxia are the most common side effects. Patients are warned against drinking alcohol, and the dosage of narcotic drugs is reduced, as these agents and barbiturates have additive effects with diazepam. Coughing, laryngospasm, respiratory depression, and hypotension can occur, and slow I.V. injection is recommended to minimize these and other adverse effects in elderly patients and those with poor pul-

monary function. Paradoxical reactions marked by excitement, insomnia, sleep disturbances, and spasticity occur in rare cases. Acute narrow-angle glaucoma is a condition in which use of this drug is contraindicated.

Dosage and Administration. The usual oral doses range between 2 to 10 mg b.i.d. to q.i.d. Repeated I.M. or I.V. doses of 5 to 10 mg may be needed to control severe convulsions and acute reactions to stress.

METHOCARBAMOL N.F. (Robaxin)

Actions and Indications. This drug depresses spinal interneurons to bring about relaxation of skeletal muscles in spasm or in a spastic state. It is used for such musculoskeletal disorders as strains, sprains, whiplash injuries, herniated disk, and other cervical and lumbar nerve root syndromes. It also relieves spasticity, dystonia, rigidity, and athetosis in patients with cerebral palsy, multiple sclerosis, and other hypertonic muscular states resulting from damage to the central nervous system.

Side Effects, Cautions, and Contraindications. Moderate oral dosage may cause drowsiness, dizziness, light-headedness, and nausea. Too rapid intravenous administration may cause bradycardia and hypotension. Patients receiving the drug by this route should be kept lying down during and for 10 to 15 minutes after the procedure. The parenteral form is contraindicated in patients with kidney disease and in those with a history of skin rashes, fever, and other signs of hypersensitivity to this drug. Thrombophlebitis from I.V. use and painful nodules from I.M. injection may occur with the parenteral product.

Dosage and Administration. Initial oral doses of 6 to 8 g daily are reduced to about 4 g later in treatment. The I.M. dose of 1 g is injected as doses of 500 mg in each gluteal muscle. The I.V. dose of 1 g is injected undiluted at a rate of no more than 300 mg per minute. The total adult I.V. dose does not ordinarily exceed 3 g daily.

References

Clipper, M. Nursing care of patients in a neurological intensive care unit. *Nurs. Clin. N. Amer.*, 4:211, 1969 (June).

Friend, D.G. Pharmacology of muscle relaxants. *Clin. Pharmacol. Ther.*, 9:871, 1964.

Marsh, H.O. Diazepam in incapacitated cerebral palsied children. *JAMA*, 191:797, 1965.

Pothier, P.C. Therapeutic handling of the severely handicapped child. *Amer. J. Nurs.*, 71:321, 1971 (Feb.).

Rodman, M.J. Drugs for neuromuscular pain and spasm. *RN*, 29:62, 1966 (May).

———. Drugs for treating tetanus. *RN*, 34:43, 1971 (Dec.).

Schneider, K. Care of a young patient with paraplegia. *RN*, 32:48, 1969 (Nov.).

11.

Drugs for Treating Parkinsonism

The Nature of Parkinson's Disease

Parkinson's disease is the second most common neurological disorder. An estimated million Americans suffer from this chronic progressively crippling illness. Unlike epilepsy, which afflicts mostly children and young adults, parkinsonism occurs mainly in people past 50 years old. The cause of most cases of parkinsonism is unknown, but some cases are the result of nervous system injury or infection—following viral encephalitis, for example.

Signs of parkinsonism vary considerably depending upon the stage of the disease, which becomes slowly but steadily more disabling. The patient's movements, posture, balance, and speech are often severely affected, but his mind is not ordinarily impaired. In advanced stages, he moves about only very slowly or sluggishly (bradykinesia or akinesia). Some groups of muscles show stiffness or rigidity, while weakness is felt in others. A characteristic tremor of the hands and head while at rest has led to such synonyms for parkinsonism as *paralysis agitans* or "shaking palsy."

Remember that even though the patient's face may seem frozen in an expressionless mask, and his slow slurred speech may be hard to understand, he is not at all defective mentally. However, he may become deeply discouraged and mentally depressed. Thus, it is important to offer the patient support so that he will try to keep active, care for himself, and follow directions for taking antiparkinsonism medications.

The Management of Parkinsonism

Two main kinds of drugs are now available for treating Parkinson's disease. Both kinds are thought to correct a chemical imbalance in the brain. Drugs classed as *anticholinergic and antihistaminic agents* (Table 11-1) may block the effects of an excess of *acetylcholine* in the brain. On the other hand, *levodopa* is thought to act by helping to correct the lack of another neurochemical called *dopamine* (p. 141).

Drugs alone cannot, however, cure a condition that is the result of a loss of nerve cells in the basal ganglia of the brain. Physical therapy is also needed to delay the development of severe disability and invalidism. The nurse can help here by encouraging the patient to do the exercises that the therapist has taught him. However, if no physical therapist is available with whom the nurse can coordinate her own activities, the nurse assumes responsibility for teaching the patient how to perform specialized exercises and for supervising his efforts. She should not help him do simple physical tasks that he can still do by himself, as self-care for as long as possible is an important goal of long-term treatment in parkinsonism. Thus, the patient is encouraged to do all the tasks of daily living that he can still perform.

The nurse cannot, of course, keep the patient from becoming discouraged as his progressive disease begins to limit his activities and eventually leads him to need a wheelchair or results in his being confined to bed. She can be supportive when he is discouraged, and show recognition of his difficulties. She can also discuss with his family the importance of helping the patient avoid stressful, anxiety-provoking situations. Fortunately, recent advances in the drug therapy of parkinsonism now make it possible for the nurse to offer a discouraged patient real hope. For it now seems possible that further discoveries will both help to control the disabling symptoms of this disease and prevent deformity and crippling.

Treatment with Anticholinergic Drugs

The first drugs employed for relief of parkinsonism symptoms were the belladonna plant alkaloids *atropine+* and *scopolamine+*. Although these natural substances are still sometimes used in large doses for younger patients with postencephalitic parkinsonism, their side effects are often so severe that most patients are now maintained on synthetic substitutes that are considered safer.

The synthetic anticholinergic agents such as *trihexyphenidyl+* (Artane, and others), *benztropine+* (Cogentin), and related drugs, often relieve the patient's muscle rigidity. The patient also often feels better mentally, either

TABLE 11-1 *Drugs for Treating Parkinsonism*

Nonproprietary Name	Trade Name or Synonym	Usual Daily Dosage Range	Comments
Synthetic Anticholinergic and Antihistaminic Drugs			
Benztropine mesylate U.S.P.	Cogentin	0.5–6 mg	See *Drug Digest*
Biperiden HCl and lactate	Akineton	2–8 mg	Similar to trihexyphenidyl
Chlorphenoxamine HCl	Phenoxene	50–200 mg	Similar to diphenhydramine
Cycrimine HCl	Pagitane	3.75–15 mg	Similar to trihexyphenidyl
Diphenhydramine HCl U.S.P.	Benadryl	75–150 mg	See *Drug Digest*
Ethopropazine HCl	Parsidol	50–100 mg	Has properties of both trihexyphenidyl and diphenhydramine
Orphenadrine HCl and citrate N.F.	Disipal; Norflex	150–300 mg	Similar to diphenhydramine
Procyclidine HCl	Kemadrin	10–20 mg	Similar to trihexyphenidyl
Trihexyphenidyl HCl U.S.P.	Artane; Pipanol Tremin	6–10 mg	See *Drug Digest*
Other Drugs			
Amantadine HCl	Symmetrel	100–200 mg	Antiviral agent
Levodopa	Dopar; Larodopa; Levopa; L-dopa	4–6 g	Amino acid precursor of dopamine

because of the direct euphoric effects of these drugs, or because of his ability to move about better and to take care of himself more easily. These drugs sometimes also relieve such symptoms of parkinsonism as excessive salivation and drooling, sweating, and skin oiliness.

SIDE EFFECTS (SUMMARY, p. 142)

These drugs are capable of causing atropine-like side effects, including dryness of the mouth and blurring of vision. The nurse can suggest sucking on hard candies or touching the tongue with a slice of lemon as one way of avoiding oral discomfort. She should instruct the patient to report constipation or drug-induced difficulties in voiding urine to his physician. The physician may then prescribe laxatives, fecal softeners, or intestinal and bladder stimulants such as *bethanechol+* and *neostigmine+*. He may also reduce dosage, particularly in elderly patients who tend to become confused or disoriented and even suffer from delirium and toxic psychosis when treated with these drugs.

ADMINISTRATION

To avoid adverse effects, it is desirable to begin treatment with small doses of the safest drugs. The drugs least likely to induce atropinelike side effects are those with primarily antihistaminic activity, including *diphenhydramine+* (Benadryl) and its chemical relatives *chlorphenoxamine* (Phenoxene) and *orphenadrine* (Disipal; Norflex). However, these drugs have only relatively weak antiparkinsonism activity when used alone and are employed mainly in elderly patients and others unable to tolerate the more potent agents.

The latter drugs, including *trihexyphenidyl+* and such chemical relatives as *biperiden* (Akineton) and *procyclidine* (Kemadrin) are preferred for most patients. Treatment is begun with a single dose that is increased only gradually to perhaps four to eight times the initial amount. Ideally, each patient is finally stabilized on an individually adjusted optimal amount at which the patient's movements are maximally improved with minimal side effects. If trihexyphenidyl alone fails to give adequate relief or tolerance to it develops, the more potent antiparkinsonism agent *benztropine+* may be added in small doses to the patient's regimen.

Benztropine+, *biperiden*, and *diphenhydramine+* are available in injectable form, which makes them useful for patients who have difficulty in swallowing or who are suffering from oculogyric crisis, a parkinsonism complication in which eye muscle spasm sends the patient's eyeballs far up or down in the eye socket. These drugs are also employed for treating the acute dystonic reactions that sometimes occur in patients receiving phenothiazine-type antiemetic and antipsychotic agents, or one of the rauwolfia alkaloids or butyrophenones.

Treatment with Levodopa

Levodopa, a drug that differs from those described above, is now considered the drug of choice for treating Parkinson's disease. When it is administered orally, this amino acid is absorbed into the blood stream and carried to the brain. There it is converted into *dopamine*, a neurochemical that is believed to be missing or deficient in the basal ganglia of parkinsonism patients. It can be administered alone or combined with one or more of the acetylcholine-blocking drugs to restore the neurochemical balance of the extrapyramidal motor system (p. 142).

Clinical trials with this compound indicate that about two out of three Parkinson's disease patients benefit to some extent from treatment with levodopa. These patients become better able to move about, stand straight instead of bent over, and can speak more clearly. Maximal improvement occurs about six weeks after treatment is begun with small doses that are gradually raised to optimal levels. Many patients maintain their improvement during long-term treatment with carefully adjusted dosage.

Dosage adjustment is important to avoid the adverse effects of levodopa (*Summary*, p. 143). Early in treatment, many patients suffer gastrointestinal upset. This can be lessened by having the patient take the drug with meals. Later the patient must be watched carefully for signs of cardiac, neuromuscular, and mental side effects. The nurse reports complaints of heart palpitation and feelings of weakness and dizziness to the patient's doctor.

The doctor is also informed of any changes in the patient's behavior, since older patients and those with a history of mental disturbance have reportedly had hallucinations or become mentally depressed while taking levodopa. Some patients show signs of increased sex drive and may make sexual overtures. The nurse who recognizes this as a drug-induced effect can help the patient to understand that these changes are related to his treatment.

In his enthusiasm at his improvement, the patient often has a tendency to become excessively active. This can lead to fatigue and falls. Remind the patient to allow himself time to regain his strength and not to exert himself excessively. Older patients sometimes become dizzy, weak, and faint upon arising—a result of a hypotensive effect of levodopa. The patient must be reminded to get out of bed slowly and helped back to bed whenever signs of drug-induced postural effects on blood pressure appear.

DRUG INTERACTIONS

As previously noted, levodopa may be administered together with trihexyphenidyl and other anticholinergic drugs. However, patients should not receive adrenergic drugs such as ephedrine or antidepressant drugs of the monoamine oxidase inhibitor class, as these substances may set off episodes of high blood pressure. Moderate doses of the B-complex vitamin *pyridoxine* tend to counteract the desired effects of levodopa. Thus, parkinsonism patients who require a multivitamin supplement should take a type that does not contain pyridoxine.

Amantadine

Amantadine (Symmetrel) was introduced originally as a prophylactic to prevent influenza, and was found by accident to benefit some Parkinson's disease patients. Its usefulness for treating parkinsonism has not yet been established. Nurses with patients for whom this experimental drug is prescribed should watch them carefully for signs of potential toxicity including hyperexcitability, restlessness, and insomnia.

Summary

The recent addition of levodopa to the single class of drugs previously available—the synthetic atropinelike agents—has made researchers hopeful that still other effective antiparkinsonism drugs will soon be discovered. It is important to remember that the management of Parkinson's disease involves other factors besides drugs. The nurse can help by offering these patients emotional support and encouraging them to continue their therapy so that they can remain as active as possible.

SUMMARY of Side Effects, Cautions, and Contraindications of Drugs Used in Treating Parkinsonism

Belladonna Alkaloids and Synthetic Drugs with Atropinelike Actions

Mouth Dryness or Xerostomia
May make speaking or swallowing difficult, lead to loss of appetite, and rarely to a mumps-like parotitis.

Blurring of Vision Caused by Cycloplegia and Pupillary Dilation (Mydriasis)
May make reading difficult; possible rise in intraocular pressure in patients with narrow angle glaucoma makes its use in such patients probably contraindicated.

Constipation and, Occasionally, Nausea and Vomiting
Caution in patients with obstipation (tendency toward intestinal obstruction), such as pyloric stenosis.

Urinary Retention or Hesitancy (Dysuria)
Caution in elderly male patients with enlarged prostate and others with genitourinary tract obstruction.

Cardiac Palpitations, Tachycardia, and Hypotension
Caution in patients with cardiovascular instability.

Skin Dryness or Anhidrosis
Lack of sweating may lead to fever with flushed, hot, dry skin and possible heat prostration in hot weather, particularly in chronically ill, elderly, or alcoholic patients.

Central Nervous System Stimulation or Depression
Drowsiness, muscle weakness, and ataxia caused by some of these drugs may make driving and other such activities dangerous. Elderly patients with cerebral arteriosclerosis are particularly prone to reactions marked by mental confusion, memory lapses, disorientation, ex-

citement, or agitation. Visual hallucinations, acute delirium also occur, and even a toxic psychosis is possible, particularly in mental patients.

Miscellaneous

In theory, at least, these drugs may *mask* toxic effects of cholinergic drugs in patients with myasthenia gravis, and of phenothiazine drugs (tardive dyskinesia).

Levodopa

Gastrointestinal Disturbances

Loss of appetite, nausea, vomiting, abdominal pain, and diarrhea or constipation. Caution in patients with a history of peptic ulcer and bleeding.

Cardiovascular Disturbances

Heart palpitation and possible speed-up in rate and rhythm. Flushing; postural hypotension or occasional hypertension. Caution in patients with a history of heart disease (infarction or arrythmias) or stroke (cerebrovascular disease).

Neurological Disturbances

Involuntary movements of the mouth, face, and head. Dyskinetic reactions in large muscle groups, including the neck (torticollis); also possible oculogyric crisis and convulsions. Caution in patients with a history of convulsive disorders.

Psychic Disturbances

Either euphoria and hyperactivity with increased libido or depression with fatigue and drowsiness may develop. Check patients for early signs of mental changes, as suicidal depression or hypomanic behavior with hallucinations and delirium have occurred. Extreme caution in patients with psychoses or severe psychoneuroses.

Visual Disturbances

Blurring of vision, pupillary dilation, double vision. Contraindicated in uncompensated narrow angle glaucoma, caution in controlled, wide angle glaucoma.

Respiratory Disturbances

Postnasal drip, hoarseness, cough; breathing pattern irregularities, and feelings of pressure in the chest. Caution in patients with bronchial asthma or emphysema, as administration of adrenergic bronchodilators is contraindicated in patients taking levodopa.

S U M M A R Y of Points for the Nurse to Remember When Patients Are Taking Antiparkinsonism Drugs

1. Observe the patient carefully for signs of side effects caused by antiparkinsonism drugs and teach the patient to report symptoms promptly to the physician (*Summary*, p. 142).

2. Emphasize to the patient the importance of continued medical care. These patients must return for frequent physical examinations and laboratory tests that are required to evaluate their progress and response to drug therapy.

3. Encourage the patient to help himself as much as he is able in feeding and dressing himself, writing letters, walking, and so on. Sometimes patients who respond favorably to levodopa, in particular, regain feelings of independence and self-esteem along with their greater ability to perform physical tasks.

4. Assist the patient in renewing contacts with other people from whom he may previously have withdrawn because of embarrassment. For example, encourage him to leave his hospital room and go to the ward lounge.

Discussion Topics:
Clinical Situation Involving Patient Taking Antiparkinsonism Drug *

The Situation: Mr. Barnes is a hospitalized 62-year-old patient who is receiving *levodopa* for Parkinson's disease. When first admitted, he always seemed within a hair's breadth of falling as he shuffled forward slowly with small steps, with his body bent over in a stooped position. His hands at rest moved continuously in a marked tremor and his arm movements were stiff and awkward, so that he had difficulty in feeding himself and in swallowing,

* In preparing to discuss nursing situations, students should draw upon information acquired from other sources besides this book.

with the result that his nutritional status was also poor.

During his treatment with levodopa, Mr. Barnes' physical condition has improved considerably. He stands more erect and walks with a more normal gait. His arm movements are more smoothly coordinated, as rigidity has been reduced and tremors have lessened. He speaks more clearly, eats better and looks and acts more lively.

However, shortly after he began taking levodopa in moderate doses (after the initial nausea had subsided and early episodes of weakness and dizziness diminished), Mr. Barnes experienced hallucinations on several occasions, as he later reluctantly admitted to the nurse. Although such psychic phenomena have not occurred since his dosage was adjusted downward, Mr. Barnes is obviously still troubled by the experience, as he asks repeatedly whether he is losing his mind. He is also still shy about receiving physical care by the nurse and still avoids meeting and dealing with other people, as he had during the years when his condition was worsening and embarrassment had led him to lead the life of a recluse.

The Problem: Develop a nursing care plan for Mr. Barnes on the basis of the above information.

DRUG DIGEST

BENZTROPINE MESYLATE U.S.P. (Cogentin)

Actions and Indications. This synthetic antiparkinsonism agent is used mainly to supplement other drugs, or as a substitute for them, when patients with any form of Parkinson's disease are no longer responsive to the drugs that were tried earlier. Its long-lasting skeletal muscle antispasmodic action relieves rigidity and painful cramps, and this together with the drug's sedative effects promotes sleep. The injectable form of this drug is useful for relief of acute, drug-induced dystonic reactions; and oral doses help to reduce extrapyramidal reactions in patients receiving phenothiazines and other antipsychotic neuroleptic agents.

Side Effects, Cautions, and Contraindications. Discomforting atropine-type side effects including dry mouth, blurring of vision, and constipation are common but not serious. However, caution is required in patients with enlarged prostate or intestinal obstruction, and the drug is contraindicated in narrow angle glaucoma. It should be discontinued in hot weather, if the patient's skin becomes flushed

and he develops a fever. Overdosage may lead to mental confusion and excitement, disorientation and delirium; visual hallucinations and delusions may also occur as part of a drug-induced toxic psychosis.

Dosage and Administration. Treatment is started with a small dose of 0.5 to 1 mg at bedtime and raised by 0.5 mg every five or six days. Optimal dosage for most patients is only 1 to 2 mg, but some may require and tolerate 4 to 6 mg daily. For acute dystonic reactions, 2 mg may be administered I.V. or, for less severe reactions, 1 mg may be administered I.M.

TRIHEXYPHENIDYL HCl U.S.P. (Artane; Pipanol; Tremin)

Actions and Indications. This synthetic atropinelike drug is used mainly for relief of Parkinson's disease symptoms. It acts centrally as a skeletal muscle antispasmodic to relieve rigidity. Tremors and slowness in movement (bradykinesia or akinesia) are also counteracted. A mild euphoric effect may lessen mental depression, and peripheral effects may help to reduce excessive salivation and sweating.

This drug also prevents or overcomes some of the symptoms of adverse extrapyramidal reactions that may develop during treatment with antipsychotic drugs such as the phenothiazine and butyrophenone derivatives and reserpine.

Side Effects, Cautions, and Contraindications. Minor side effects are similar to those of atropine and include dryness of the mouth, blurring of vision, constipation, urinary retention, and tachycardia. Caution is required in patients with gastrointestinal and urinary tract obstructions, including elderly males with an enlarged prostate. Older patients are also subject to mental confusion, agitation, and disorientation. Narrow angle glaucoma is a contraindication.

Dosage and Administration. Doses of 1 mg initially are gradually increased to optimal levels, usually 6 to 10 mg daily but sometimes as much as 12 to 15 mg divided into three or four doses administered around mealtimes and at bedtime. One or more sustained-release capsules containing 5 mg may be administered after breakfast and in the early afternoon in similar total daily dosage.

References

Brokken, B., et al. L-dopa: A nursing adventure. *Nurs. Clin. N. Amer.*, 4:733, 1969 (Dec.).

Cotzias, G.C. Metabolic modification of some neurologic disorders. *JAMA*, 210:1255, 1969.

Di Palma, J.R. L-Dopa, a new hope for C.N.S. disease. *RN*, 34:63, 1971 (March).

Haber, M.E. Parkinson's disease: Challenge to the health professions. *Nurs. Clin. N. Amer.*, 4:263, 1969 (June).

Hofmann, W.W., and Hollister, L.E. Pharmacotherapy of Parkinson's disease. *Pharmacol. Physicians*, 4:7, 1970 (July).

Langman, A., and O'Malley, W.E. L-dopa and the patient with Parkinson's disease. *Amer. J. Nurs.*, 69:1455, 1969 (July).

Morgan, J.P., and Bianchine, J.R. The clinical pharmacology of levodopa. *Rational Drug Ther.*, 5:1, 1971 (Jan.).

Rodman, M.J. Advances in treating Parkinsonism. *RN*, 32:73, 1969 (Nov.).

Tyler, E. Management of Parkinson's disease with L-dopa therapy. *Canad. Nurse*, 67:451, 1971 (April).

12.

Drugs for Treating Epilepsy

The Nature of Epilepsy

Epilepsy is a term used to describe a group of nervous system disorders in which patients suffer periodic attacks, or seizures. Epileptic seizures all stem from the sudden discharge of volleys of nerve impulses from abnormally functioning brain cells. However, the signs and symptoms of epileptic seizures of different types are very varied. The nature of the seizure depends upon where in the nervous system the excessive discharges originate and what pathways the nerve impulses take as they spread to other normal neurons from their site of origin in the abnormally functioning nervous tissues.

The most common kinds of epileptic seizures are grouped in one classification scheme as follows:

1. Major motor seizures, such as those of grand mal and focal motor epilepsy
2. Petit mal seizures of the so-called pure, true, or classic type
3. Psychomotor seizures, also sometimes called temporal lobe epilepsy
4. Minor motor seizures, sometimes called petit mal variants, or, more specifically, myoclonic and akinetic attacks

The drugs that have been developed for treating epilepsy differ in the degree to which they are effective for controlling the several different kinds of seizures. Thus, before ordering drugs, the doctor must make an accurate diagnosis of the kind of epilepsy from which the patient is suffering. Then, in starting the patient on drug treatment, and in maintaining the patient on drugs for long periods, the doctor must employ certain important principles (*Summary*, p. 154), in order to gain the goal of therapy in epilepsy—*complete control of seizures without adverse drug reactions.*

The nurse also often plays an important part in the care of the patient. She helps him to stay seizure-free, if possible, and she helps him and his family, friends, and associates deal effectively with actual seizures, if and when they do occur. Thus, in the following discussions of the drugs used in treating the various types of epilepsy, we shall not only take up specific points about the individual antiepileptic drugs, but also indicate some of the general principles of epilepsy therapy that the nurse should know and apply in caring for epileptic patients.

Management of Major Motor Seizures

Seizures that result from discharge of focal lesions may cause only limited sensory and motor changes, during which the patient may not even lose consciousness. On the other hand, focal explosions may spread widely through the brain, resulting in massive convulsions and unconsciousness. Grand mal epilepsy produces generalized seizures following a brief warning, or aura that the patient may perceive as a flash of light, a high-pitched sound, or as other sensations.

The drugs most commonly employed to prevent both grand mal and focal motor seizures are the same—the barbiturates and the hydantoins (Table 12-1). Some doctors start treatment with *phenobarbital+* (Luminal), others prefer *diphenylhydantoin+* (Dilantin). The barbiturate is considered safer for long-term therapy, but diphenylhydantoin is free of the sedative effect of phenobarbital.

Often combinations of carefully adjusted doses of both these drugs are required to bring the patient's seizures under complete control. An amphetamine-type agent may also be added to counteract drug-induced drowsiness. Occasionally, patients who continue to suffer major seizures because they cannot tolerate high doses of phenobarbital may be switched to a third drug, *primidone+* (Mysoline), which is then taken alone or together with diphenylhydantoin.

When administered in accordance with the principles summarized on page 154, these drug combinations are capable of keeping three out of four patients free of major seizures, and some of the rest are moderately improved.

The nurse can help the patient to deal with various kinds of difficulties that may keep him from taking the medications that have been prescribed for him. Sometimes, for example, she may realize that the patient has not really understood the doctor's directions for taking the ordered drugs, or the patient may indicate by his manner, or by something that he says, that he is reluctant to continue taking his medication. If she learns that the patient has problems that might keep him from following his treatment program she can initiate measures to help the patient solve the problem and can share her findings with the doctor and other health workers and tell them what she has done to help the patient.

Other personal problems that may contribute to the patient's failure to take his medication and thus result in his continuing to suffer seizures are poverty and fear of becoming habituated to drugs. Obviously, the epileptic patient who becomes unemployed and unable to find work will not be able to pay for his medication. Or if he becomes worried that his continued need to take drugs will lead to dependence, he may stop the drug despite the doctor's instructions. In both these situations the nurse can help by listening to his views and concerns, so that she, the doctor, the social worker, and others interested in his case can take appropriate action to help him.

DOSAGE ADJUSTMENT AND MAINTENANCE

Successful control of seizures depends upon the patient taking his drugs regularly in the amounts he requires to meet his individual needs. Some patients need high doses because they metabolize the antiepileptic drugs rapidly; others taking ordinary doses of these drugs soon develop signs and symptoms of overdosage because their bodies metabolize the drugs at too slow a rate. Thus, the doctor adjusts the dose in accordance with the patient's clinical response and with the results of laboratory tests that measure the levels of diphenylhydantoin, phenobarbital, and primidone in the patient's blood stream.

Sometimes, other drugs that the patient may be taking at the same time can increase the toxicity of the antiepileptic agents. Patients being treated for tuberculosis as well as epilepsy may, for example, have the level of diphenyl-

TABLE 12-1 *Antiepileptic Drugs*[5]

Nonproprietary Name	Proprietary Name	Usual Daily Dosage Range	Indications by Type of Seizure Benefited			
			Grand mal and Focal	Petit mal	Psycho-motor	Minor motor
First-Line Agents						
Diazepam U.S.P.	Valium	5–30 mg	+[1,2]	+[2]	+[2]	+
Diphenylhydantoin U.S.P.	Dilantin	100–400 mg	+[1]	−	+	+
Ethosuximide U.S.P.	Zarontin	750 mg–1.5 g	−	+	−	+
Paramethadione U.S.P.	Paradione	600 mg–1.8 g	−	+	−	+
Phenobarbital U.S.P.	Luminal	100–400 mg	+[1]	+[2]	+[2]	+[2]
Primidone U.S.P.	Mysoline	250–750 mg	+	−	+	+
Trimethadione U.S.P.	Tridione	900 mg–2.1 g	−	+	−	+
Second-Line Agents						
Acetazolamide U.S.P.	Diamox	250 mg–1 g	+[2]	+[2]	+[2]	+[2]
Bromides (sodium, potassium, calcium, ammonium)		1–3 g	+	−	−	+
Corticotropin U.S.P.	ACTH	40–60 units	−	+	−	+[3]
Dextroamphetamine U.S.P.	Dexedrine	5–15 mg	+[4]	+[2,4]	+[4]	+[4]
Ethotoin	Peganone	1–3 g	+	−	+	−
Mephenytoin	Mesantoin	100–400 mg	+	−	+	−
Mephobarbital N.F.	Mebaral	100–400 mg	+	−	+	+
Methamphetamine	Desoxyn	2.5–5.0 mg	+[4]	+[2,4]	+[4]	+[4]
Metharbital N.F.	Gemonil	100–400 mg	+	−	+	+
Methsuximide N.F.	Celontin	600 mg–1.2 g	−	+	+	+
Methylphenidate U.S.P.	Ritalin	10–60 mg	+[4]	+[4]	+[4]	+[4]
Phensuximide N.F.	Milontin	500 mg–1.2 g	−	+	−	+
Phenacemide	Phenurone	1–2 g	+	−	+	+

[1] Also administered parenterally in status epilepticus.
[2] Used mainly as an adjunct to other drugs in special cases.
[3] Used mainly against infantile spasms (hypsarrhythmia). (Various corticosteroid drugs may also be used for this purpose.)
[4] Used mainly as a psychomotor stimulant to counteract excessive drowsiness.
[5] These are divided into first-line, or primary drugs (safest and most effective), and drugs of secondary importance, some of which may prove effective when some first-line drugs fail. Drugs of lesser importance used occasionally are not listed.

hydantoin in their blood and brain raised to toxic levels. This happens because some of the antituberculosis drugs such as isoniazid, PAS, and cycloserine interfere with the metabolic breakdown of the antiepileptic drug by liver enzyme systems.

Drug interactions of diphenylhydantoin with the alcoholism drug *disulfiram* (Antabuse) and the anticoagulant drugs *dicumarol* and *warfarin* also tend to increase the toxicity of the anticonvulsant. In such cases, doses of the drug that the patient had previously been able to tolerate begin to make him lose his motor coordination (ataxia). He may also become drowsy and confused, complain of double vision (diplopia), and show signs of nystagmus. These central side effects lessen when the dose of diphenylhydantoin is reduced, as it should be whenever any of these drugs are added to the program of a patient who is being maintained on adjusted doses of anticonvulsant drug therapy.

The nurse is often the first person on the health team to learn that a patient is taking other medications. If she sees drug products in the patient's possession on a visit to his home or when he comes to the clinic, she should let the patient know that his taking other drugs may have unexpected effects on the way he will react to the anticonvulsant medication. She advises him to let his physician know that he is taking nonprescription drugs or medications prescribed by another practitioner for some ailment other than epilepsy.

The nurse should make an extra effort to check on whether the patient is taking his medication as directed. She may learn, when she asks how he is getting along, that he is still having seizures and that he has not been taking his drugs regularly. She can help him or his family set up a system of steady medication—for example, by dividing the prescribed tablets or capsules into individual bottles or vials marked to indicate the days of the week. Patients should be told to take any tablets left over at day's end before going to bed. They should also be warned against abruptly stopping drug therapy, as this can set off a severe series of seizures (see discussion of status epilepticus, below).

CHRONIC TOXICITY

The need to take antiepileptic drugs for long periods sometimes leads to the development of drug allergy. Thus, patients taking these drugs must be watched for signs of skin reactons and told to report signs and symptoms of illness, as these may be the first hints of drug-induced blood disorders, liver damage, or other serious drug reactions. Although the first-line drugs used for major seizures are relatively safe in this respect, some types of hypersensitivity reactions do occur that may make a patient want to stop taking his medication.

Diphenylhydantoin, for example, sometimes makes the patient's gum tissue swell and grow over his teeth. This unsightly reaction (gingival hyperplasia) may embarrass a child and keep him from continuing to take his medicine. The patient should be shown how he can help prevent painful gingivitis and bleeding gums by keeping his mouth free of food particles and drug-containing secretions by frequent brushing. If necessary, the excess gum tissue can be removed surgically. Other cosmetic difficulties caused by diphenylhydantoin include skin rashes and growth of hair on the faces of girls. Often these skin reactions are only temporary, but if they persist, or get worse, it may be necessary to discontinue the drug.

STATUS EPILEPTICUS

This condition, in which one major seizure follows another without the patient's regaining consciousness, is most frequently triggered when patients who were previously stabilized on drug therapy suddenly stop taking their medication. Such continuing convulsions—unlike an ordinary grand mal seizure, which is terrifying but not dangerous as long as the patient is kept from being injured—can cause death if they are not brought under control by prompt treatment with anticonvulsant drugs. *Phenobarbital+* is often effective for this purpose when injected parenterally. However, like other general depressant drugs such as paraldehyde and ether, the high doses of phenobarbital required for control of convulsions come close to causing coma and respiratory arrest.

Safer drugs that do not cause excessive depression are now employed for control of status epilepticus. These include the injectable forms of *diphenylhydantoin+* and of *diazepam+* (Valium). Diazepam is more rapid in onset of anticonvulsant action than diphenylhydantoin and does not ordinarily cause cardiac arrhythmias, as the latter drug sometimes does when large doses are injected too rapidly by vein. In this life-threatening emergency, the nurse's duties often include not only obtaining and preparing the anticonvulsant drug injections but also assisting with artificial respiration and monitoring the patient's heart action.

Management of Petit Mal Epilepsy

Petit mal epilepsy of the pure, or classical, type is characterized by brief lapses in consciousness, or so-called "absence" episodes, in which the child stops whatever he is doing and stares blankly for a few seconds. He does not fall down, convulse, or even show any confusion after the attack but simply takes up his activity where he left off when the spell started. Certain so-called petit mal variants, or minor motor seizures, are, on the other hand, marked either by sudden, brief muscular contractions (myoclonic seizures) or by a sudden loss of muscle tone that makes the child fall down (akinetic, or drop, attacks).

Treatment of pure petit mal epilepsy is best begun with *ethosuximide+* (Zarontin), a drug that ordinarily succeeds in bringing three out of four cases under control. Some of those who do not respond may benefit from treatment with *trimethadione+* (Tridione), an equally effective but potentially more toxic drug. Occasionally, a particular patient will do better with one of the chemical relatives of drugs of these two types, such as *methsuximide* (Celontin) and *phensuximide* (Milontin), or *paramethadione* (Paradione).

Patients taking these drugs—and particularly trimethadione and paramethdione—for long periods must be monitored carefully for signs of developing toxicity. Some side effects (Table 12-2, pp. 152-153), such as sedation, nausea and vomiting, and photophobia are not serious, as they either stop as tolerance develops or can be readily controlled. Other types of reactions are very dangerous, as they involve vital organs such as the bone marrow, kidneys, and liver. Thus, the doctor orders laboratory studies at the start of the treatment and periodically during treatment.

If, for example, a patient taking Tridione shows a steady drop in white blood cells or a rise in urinary albumin, the drug may have to be discontinued. Patients are also told to report certain signs and symptoms. Thus, if a nurse learns that a patient has a severe sore throat and fever, or that he has developed bruise marks or bleeding, she tells the doctor. He may then order laboratory blood studies, and if these reveal a reduction in white blood cells and platelets, he may discontinue further therapy because a possible drug-induced blood dyscrasia may be developing.

Children with minor motor seizures do not respond as readily to treatment with these petit mal drugs. However, recent reports indicate that *diazepam* (Valium+) is often effective for control of myoclonic seizures. This drug does not ordinarily cause severe hypersensitivity reactions. Drowsiness produced by the drug may be counteracted by adding a small dose of dextroamphetamine, or by administering it in a lower dose in combination with ethosuximide.

Other drugs sometimes employed for control of resistant cases include *quinacrine* and *chloroquine*, which are sometimes effective for control of akinetic attacks. *Acetazolamide* (Diamox), a diuretic drug that has a dehydrating and acidifying effect, is occasionally a useful adjunct to other antiepileptic treatments. *Corticotropin+* (ACTH), has brought about some improvement in infants subject to attacks of massive myoclonic spasms.

Management of Psychomotor Seizures

Psychomotor seizures are marked by changes in behavior. Because of a victim's strange actions—automatically unbuttoning his clothing and disrobing, for instance—he may be arrested or assumed to be mentally ill. This form of epilepsy sometimes responds to treatment with combinations of the same drugs used against grand mal—*diphenyhydantoin+*, *phenobarbital+*, and *primidone+*. Sometimes, when these drugs, or derivatives such as *ethotoin* or *mephenytoin*, fail to control this form of epilepsy, the doctor may fall back on *phenacemide* (Phenurone). This is an effective but relatively dangerous drug that is administered at first only in patients who are hospitalized so that daily studies of their blood, liver, and kidney function can be carried out. The nurse watches these patients closely for such signs as loss of appetite, sore mouth and throat, jaundice, or fever, which may indicate drug-induced blood dyscrasias or liver damage. Changes in behavior are also noted and reported, as this drug sometimes sets off episodes of depression in patients with psychomotor epilepsy.

OTHER SEIZURES

Not all patients who suffer seizures have epilepsy. An isolated seizure may be a sign of a nervous system disorder as serious as a brain tumor, or it may simply be set off in young children by a high fever. Phenobarbital and aspirin are effective for control of such febrile seizures. Drug abusers who are abruptly withdrawn from barbiturates and other general depressants may also suffer seizures. These are best controlled and prevented by stabilizing the patient on adequate doses of *pentobarbital+* (Nembutal) or phenobarbital. Barbiturates may also be employed for control of seizures in newborn babies. Here, however, the doctor also looks for dietary deficiencies and corrects them —for example, by administration of calcium or the B-complex vitamin, pyridoxine.

TABLE 12-2 *Summary of Side Effects and Toxicity of Antiepileptic Drugs*

Drug Type	Gastrointestinal	Dermatological	Nervous System
Hydantoins Diphenylhydantoin Mephenytoin Ethotoin	Anorexia Epigastric distress Nausea and vomiting	Rashes of measles and scarlet fever and acne-like types Hirsutism or hypertrichosis	Unsteady gait (ataxia) Slurred speech (dysarthria) Double vision (diplopia) Nystagmus; tremors; lethargy
Oxazoladinediones Trimethadione Paramethadione	Epigastric distress Nausea and vomiting Hiccup	Minor rashes also but exfoliative dermatitis, and Stevens-Johnson syndrome (erythema multiforme)	Drowsiness
Succinimides Ethosuximide Methsuximide Phensuximide	Anorexia Nausea and vomiting Hiccup	Minor skin eruptions	Drowsiness, lethargy, fatigue Headache, dizziness Diplopia and ataxia rare
Phenacemide	Anorexia Nausea Vomiting Abdominal discomfort	Minor and major skin reactions	Personality changes Insomnia and restlessness Apathy and withdrawal Toxic psychosis Suicidal depression
Primidone	Nausea and vomiting	Measles-like skin rash	Drowsiness, dizziness Headache, ataxia
Barbiturates Phenobarbital Mephobarbital Metharbital	Nausea and vomiting	Rashes resembling measles or scarlet fever Rarely exfoliative dermatitis or erythema multiforme	Drowsiness, dizziness Headache, lethargy Rarely, restlessness or excitement
Diazepam	Rare G.I. upset	Rare rashes	Drowsiness Ataxia Rarely, paradoxical excitement
Bromides Sodium, Potassium, Calcium, and Ammonium Salts	Anorexia Nausea and vomiting Epigastric distress	Frequent skin eruptions of acnelike, and other types	Drowsiness, dizziness Lethargy, ataxia Personality changes Toxic psychosis

T A B L E   1 2 - 2   *Side Effects and Toxicity of Antiepileptic Drugs (continued)*

Hematological	Hepatic and Renal	Miscellaneous

Megaloblastic anemia
Other blood dyscrasias rare
  (with mephenytoin)
	Rare liver and kidney damage
	  (with mephenytoin)
		Gingival hyperplasia
		  (overgrowth of gum tissue)
		Pseudolymphoma
		Cardiac arrhythmias and arrest

Neutropenia
Thrombocytopenia
Agranulocytosis
Aplastic anemia
	Hepatitis
	Nephrosis
		Photophobia (hemeralopia or
		  blindness) marked by the
		  "Glare phenomenon"
		Pseudolymphoma
		Lupus erythematosus

Rare leukopenia and other blood
  dyscrasias
	Rare nephropathy or hepatitis	Occasional behavior
		  disturbances
		Psychological aberrations, or
		  psychoses

Bone marrow changes resulting
  in agranulocytosis and
  aplastic anemia
	Hepatitis (watch for jaundice
	  and darkening of the urine)
	Nephropathy
		Fever
		General malaise
		Sore throat
		Bruise marks, and other signs of
		  infection or bleeding

Rare megaloblastic anemia or
  leukopenia
	Rare signs of liver or kidney
	  involvement
		General malaise

Rare megaloblastic anemia and
  other blood disorders
	Rare signs of liver or kidney
	  involvement
		Weakness and paralysis in
		  patients with *porphyria*, in
		  whom these drugs are
		  contraindicated

Rare blood disorders	Rare liver or kidney involvement	Rapid I.V. injection can cause cardiac and respiratory failure
Rare blood disorders	Rare liver or kidney involvement	Running nose and eyes resembling common cold Delirium Hallucinations Delusions

S U M M A R Y of General Principles of Antiepileptic Drug Therapy

1. Treatment is started with a single drug selected for its known effectiveness in controlling the kind of seizures to which the patient is subject, and for its relative safety in long-term treatment.

2. *Small doses*—usually about one third of the average daily dose—are administered at first, and dosage is gradually raised at intervals of five to seven days, until the patient's seizures are controlled or significant side effects occur.

3. If the drug is effective but causes minor signs and symptoms of overdosage its dosage is slowly reduced to a level that the patient can tolerate; if seizures are not completely controlled by safe doses of a single drug, a second relatively safe drug is gradually added to the patient's regimen.

4. In adjusting the dosage of a drug or combination of drugs to the needs of each individual patient, the doctor uses various clinical and laboratory aids:

(a) He has the patient or his family keep a record, charting the number of seizures that occur during drug treatment to determine whether attacks are actually occurring less frequently.

(b) He checks the blood levels attained with the doses of certain of the drugs that are being administered and adjusts dosage as necessary to attain optimal plasma levels and clinical control of seizures.

(c) He tries to continue treatment at the highest dose the patient can tolerate and for a long enough trial period (at least two weeks) before deciding to discontinue therapy and switch to another drug.

5. Drugs are discontinued only gradually while another drug is being gradually substituted. Patients are also warned never to discontinue drug therapy abruptly, as this can set off episodes of status epilepticus.

6. Once the patient has been stabilized on optimal dosage, it is essential that he continue to take his medication on a regular schedule. To assure the patient's cooperation, it is important to offer him whatever help he seems to need.

For example, bottles containing medication may be labeled with the names of the seven days of the week and the patient instructed to take leftover tablets at bedtime.

7. Pay attention to the patient's emotional needs and make sure that he understands the nature of his illness and the need to continue drug therapy indefinitely in order to gain the greatest control over his seizures with the least toxicity.

For example, his condition should be explained to him in terms that he can understand, and he should be given an opportunity to ask questions and express himself. If personal, economic, and social problems become apparent that seem likely to keep the patient from cooperating in taking his medication, the doctor, nurse, and social worker must make an effort to help the patient solve them.

8. When it is necessary for the patient to take relatively toxic medications, measures must be taken to detect early signs and symptoms of adverse effects, so that drug therapy may be discontinued if necessary.

For example, the doctor examines the patient periodically for signs of clinical toxicity and orders laboratory studies of blood, liver, and other vital functions. Patients and their families are told to report certain signs and symptoms of illness that might be the result of hypersensitivity reactions to the drugs being taken.

S U M M A R Y of Points for the Nurse to Remember About Treatment with Antiepileptic Drugs

1. A major aspect of the nurse's role in epilepsy management involves helping the patient to control his seizures not only by proper use of medication, but also through measures for reducing nervous tension. The patient can be helped to live more fully and to accept his condition despite still prevalent attitudes that unfortunately tend to stigmatize the epileptic.

2. It is crucial to the success of therapy that the patient continue to take his medication steadily. Thus, it is essential to instruct the patient about the need to take his drugs daily in the dosage prescribed for him.

3. Note whether the patient seems to have any problems that might keep him from following his regimen, and bring such matters to the doctor's attention. Inform the physician also if you learn that the patient is taking other medications, and make the patient aware that he should take no drugs without letting his doctor

know what they are, as drug interactions can cause unexpected responses to anticonvulsant drug therapy.

4. Watch the patient carefully for signs of adverse drug effects both during the early dosage-regulation phase of therapy and during long-term treatment. Teach the patient to note any unusual symptoms and to report them to his doctor.

5. The nurse should take every opportunity to collaborate with the patient's doctor and also with the social worker and other health professionals during long-term treatment.

Discussion Topics:
Dealing With Clinical Situation Involving Anticonvulsant Drugs

The Situation: Joe Marks is a high-school senior who had his first major seizure in school two months ago. During class one day, Joe suddenly slumped to the floor and suffered a grand mal convulsion.

Joe's fellow students were frightened and did not know what to do for him. Fortunately, his teacher had observed such seizures before and was able to protect Joe from injury. She was also able to explain the significance of what they had seen to the students who had observed Joe's seizure. Unfortunately, not all of Joe's teachers understand the situation and some seem reluctant to have him in their classes.

Joe's case was diagnosed as grand mal epilepsy, idiopathic type (that is, of unknown cause). His doctor prescribed *diphenylhydantoin* (Dilantin) and *phenobarbital*. However, his seizures have not yet been entirely controlled, even though he tends to be a bit drowsy during the day at the dose levels of the drug combination that he is taking. Joe has had three more seizures since the first one —one at school and two at home. His parents and teacher realized later in retrospect that just before each seizure occurred, Joe was involved in situations that created considerable nervous tension.

The Problem: Assuming that you were the nurse, in what ways could you help Joe in relation to the following:

(1) Most effective use of the medication that he is taking.

(2) Learning about the nature of his condition and how best to learn to live with it, and gradually bring it under enough control to keep his life from becoming unnecessarily narrowed.

(3) Meeting the needs of Joe's family, so that they recognize his problem and are able to help him cope with it.

(4) Meeting the needs of Joe's teachers and classmates in dealing with seizures that may occur when he is at school.

DRUG DIGEST

DIPHENYLHYDANTOIN U.S.P. (Dilantin)

Actions and Indications. This anticonvulsant is useful for preventing seizures in grand mal, focal, and psychomotor epilepsy. It is not effective in pure petit mal but may help some children with minor motor seizures (myoclonic and akinetic). The injectable form is effective for control of status epilepticus and other recurring seizures. Other conditions in which diphenylhydantoin has been reported useful include trigeminal neuralgia, migraine, personality disorders, and cardiac arrhythmias.

Side Effects, Cautions, and Contraindications. Gastric distress resulting from local irritation may be lessened by administering this drug with meals. Sedation does not occur with ordinary dosage, but overdosage may lead to lethargy. More common nervous system side effects include nystagmus and diplopia (double vision), staggering (ataxia), slurred speech (dysarthria), mental confusion, dizziness, and headache. Too rapid injection by vein can cause cardiac arrest.

Various types of hypersentitivity reactions are seen, of which the most common is gingival hyperplasia, the growth of gum tissue over the teeth. Skin rashes resembling measles may develop. Megaloblastic anemia sometimes results from long-term therapy, but other more serious blood disorders are rare.

Dosage and Administration. Dosage is adjusted individually at between 100 and 600 mg daily by mouth, but oral doses of 100 mg t.i.d. are most common. The parenteral form is injected at a rate of no more than 50 mg per minute I.V. in doses of 150 to 250 mg. It may also be administered I.M. as prophylaxis against seizures prior to neurosurgical procedures.

ETHOSUXIMIDE U.S.P. (Zarontin)

Actions and Indications. This is a desirable drug for first trial in pure petit mal epilepsy because it is both relatively safe and effective. It is also used in minor motor epilepsy of the myoclonic and akinetic types but is less effective for these seizures. It is *not* effective in grand mal epilepsy but may be part of the treatment program of a patient whose major motor seizures are mixed with minor seizures.

Side Effects, Cautions, and Contraindications. Minor side effects include loss of appetite, hiccup, nausea and vomiting, drowsiness, and motor incoordination. Hypersensitivity reactions of the hematologic, hepatic, and dermatological types are relatively rare. However, during long-term therapy, it is desirable that blood studies and liver function tests be carried out periodically and compared with base lines established at the start of treatment.

Dosage and Administration. Children under six years old are started on a daily dose of 250 mg; those over six may begin with 500 mg daily. These doses may be raised by 250 mg a day about once a week until optimal levels are reached. This is usually no more than 1 g in younger children or 1.5 g in older children or adults.

PHENOBARBITAL U.S.P. (Luminal; and others)

Actions and Indications. This long-lasting barbiturate is the preferred anticonvulsant of this group for prevention of seizures in grand mal, focal, and psychomotor epilepsy. The injectable form is effective for control of acute convulsions in status epilepticus and toxemia of pregnancy (eclampsia). Phenobarbital is also used as a sedative and hypnotic.

Side Effects, Cautions, and Contraindications. Long-term use of this drug does *not* cause bone marrow damage or liver and kidney toxicity of the kind sometimes seen with other antiepileptic drugs. Hypersensitive patients may develop a

rash resembling measles or scarlet fever. The drug is contraindicated in patients with porphyria or with nephritis, and it is used with caution in patients in weakened condition or with lung disease.

Side effects are infrequent in ordinary doses, but drowsiness, lethargy, dullness, and headache develop with higher doses. Elderly patients sometimes become confused and excited. Overdosage may result in ataxia and lead to delirium, stupor, and coma.

Dosage and Administration. Dosage in epilepsy ranges between 100 and 200 mg daily for adults and 1 to 6 mg/kg body weight for children. In status epilepticus, parenteral doses of 200 to 300 mg are administered at intervals of several hours.

Daytime sedation is maintained with doses of 16 to 32 mg administered orally b.i.d. or t.i.d. A bedtime dose of 100 mg is used as a hypnotic in insomnia. Doses of 200 to 300 mg are administered for preoperative or postoperative sedation.

PRIMIDONE U.S.P. (Mysoline)

Actions and Indications. This anticonvulsant drug is used to prevent seizures in grand mal, focal, and psychomotor epilepsy. It is administered alone or combined with diphenylhydantoin as a substitute for phenobarbital in cases resistant to other antiepileptic drugs.

Side Effects, Cautions, and Contraindications. Serious toxicity is uncommon, but minor side effects are common at the start of treatment. These include drowsiness, headaches, and ataxia. Occasionally nausea and vomiting, a measles-like rash, and blood changes develop. Routine blood tests are recommended to detect leukopenia and rare development of megaloblastic anemia, for which folic acid may have to be taken in daily doses.

Babies born to mothers taking this drug have sometimes had hemorrhages as a result of low levels of certain clotting factors. This can be avoided by having the

mother take vitamin K for a month before delivery. Nursing mothers may have to discontinue the drug, if their babies become excessively drowsy.

Dosage and Administration. Treatment is begun with a single daily oral dose of 250 mg taken at bedtime for one week. Dosage is then gradually built up to optimal levels —usually from 750 mg to 1.5 g daily. Children are started and eventually stabilized on half the daily adult dosage.

TRIMETHADIONE U.S.P. (Tridione)

Actions and Indications. This is an effective drug for treating petit mal and minor motor seizures, but it is not useful against grand mal and other major motor convulsions. It is often combined with phenobarbital and diphenylhydantoin for patients with mixed seizure patterns.

Side Effects, Cautions, and Contraindications. Minor side effects of early treatment include drowsiness, stomach upset, and a characteristic kind of photophobia called hemeralopia, or day blindness. Patients under long-term therapy should be checked carefully for signs of hypersensitivity reactions involving bone marrow, liver, skin, and kidneys. The drug is discontinued to avoid blood dyscrasias if studies show a steady drop in neutrophils. Regular urinanalyses are performed and the drug is withdrawn if these reveal a continued increase in albuminuria (possible nephrosis). Abnormal liver function tests may also require discontinuing therapy with this drug. Patients and their families are warned to report illnesses with clinical signs and symptoms that may be the result of reactions that require withdrawal of this drug.

Dosage and Administration. The usual adult dosage ranges from 900 to 2100 mg daily. Children receive lower doses, which are adjusted to optimal levels by gradually raising the 150 mg starting dose at intervals to amounts that are effective and still well tolerated.

References

Ausman, J.J. New developments in anticonvulsant therapy. *Postgrad. Med.*, 48:122, 1970.

Geller, M., et al.: Diazepam in the treatment of childhood epilepsy. *JAMA*, 215:2087, 1971.

Griggs, W.L. Epilepsy: Practical medical treatment. *Mod. Treatm.*, 8:258, 1971.

Millichap, J.G. Anticonvulsant drugs in the management of epilepsy. *Mod. Treatm.*, 6:1217, 1969.

Rodman, M.J. Drugs for treating epilepsy. *RN*, 35:63, 1972 (Sept.).

SECTION 4

Drugs

Used

for

Relief

and

Prevention

of

Pain

13.

Potent Analgesics

Pain and Its Relief

Pain is the most common complaint of people seeking medical care. By depriving the patient of rest, sleep, and appetite, pain may undermine his strength and morale. Long-continued severe pain may even set off a cycle of disastrous reactions that can endanger the patient's life. Thus, relieving pain is one of the most important services that doctors and nurses perform for their patients.

Relief of pain can be brought about by several different kinds of drugs. Drugs that relax smooth muscle spasms and those that reduce excessive reflex contractions of skeletal muscles help to relieve pain that originates in these peripheral structures. Local anesthetics lessen the number of pain messages flowing along peripheral nerve fibers toward the central nervous system. General anesthetics suppress the patient's awareness of severe surgical pain, but they usually do so at dose levels that produce unconsciousness.

Analgesic drugs relieve pain primarily by their central actions, and they do so when administered in doses that do not cause loss of consciousness. Such relatively specific pain-relieving agents may be divided into two types: (1) those that relieve only relatively mild degrees of pain; and (2) those that are capable of relieving moderate to severe degrees of pain. Analgesics of the first kind, including aspirin and other salicylates, are taken up in Chapter 16.

In this chapter, we shall discuss the potent, or strong, analgesics. These are also called narcotic analgesics, because they can also cause narcosis, or stupor, when taken in high doses. *Morphine,* an opium alkaloid, is the prototype potent narcotic analgesic. However, drugs from several families of synthetic analgesics are equally effective for relief of severe pain. Since all these natural and synthetic *opioids* possess similar pharmacological effects, we shall discuss the actions of all these drugs and their clinical applications together. The few significant differences in their properties and clinical utility are indicated in the *Drug Digests* of the individual drugs and in Table 13-1.

Pharmacological Effects of the Opioids

CENTRAL EFFECTS

ANALGESIA. Drugs of this kind act in several ways to bring about this therapeutically desirable effect:

(1) They reduce the patient's perception of pain.

(2) They change the patient's reaction to pain.

(3) They can produce sleep despite severe pain.

The most important of these three components of morphine-type analgesia is the change that these drugs often cause in the patient's emotional response to painful stimuli. Somehow the opioids reduce the natural anxiety that pain perception ordinarily provokes. As a result, the patient appears relatively calm and relaxed. Even though he may be aware of painful stimuli, he does not seem to mind them.

This ability of the opioids to change the patient's mental attitude toward pain and to make him unworried and unconcerned about it may also account for the fact that some people tend to become psychologically dependent upon these drugs. People who experience difficulty in coping with their life situation seem most likely to seek the feeling of freedom from worry and concern that these drugs are able to induce, even in patients who would otherwise be in severe physical pain. Those who continue to take *morphine+, heroin, meperidine+* (Demerol), and similar drugs for their euphoric effects also develop *tolerance* and *physical dependence*—the two other components of true addiction. (The nature of addiction to narcotic analgesics and its treatment are taken up in Chapter 4.)

Although morphine analgesia is not neces-

sarily accompanied by drowsiness, the drug does often have a hypnotic action. Such a sleep-producing effect is sometimes desirable for patients whose rest is disturbed by their pain. It is especially important for some pain-tossed patients, such as those who have suffered a coronary occlusion or other condition which requires complete rest and relaxation. On the other hand, excessive drug-induced sedation is undesirable in patients who should remain ambulatory and active in spite of pain.

ANTITUSSIVE. *Cough center depression* by small doses of some analgesic drugs accounts for their use to control coughing. The more potent antitussives, such as *morphine+, methadone+* (Dolophine), and *hydromorphone* (Dilaudid), are usually reserved for certain special clinical situations. They are best suited, for example, to conditions marked by both cough and pain, such as rib fractures, pleurisy, and lung cancer.

Codeine+ and *hydrocodone* are less potent antitussives, but they are much more commonly employed for cough relief. In part, this is because small doses having no adverse effects upon the patient's respiration are adequate for reducing the responsiveness of the cough center. This keeps the streams of sensory impulses that arise in the irritated or inflamed respiratory tract membranes from stimulating the central reflex control area to trigger volleys of unproductive coughs.

Another advantage of codeine is that it does not have as high a capacity for producing dependence as the more potent analgesics-antitussives. However, for treating minor coughs, some physicians prefer to employ medications that are *not* analgesics and that are entirely nonnarcotic (Table 13-2).

Dextromethorphan (Romilar; and others) is the most widely used antitussive of this type. It is claimed less likely to cause such adverse central effects of codeine as drowsiness, dizziness, and headache or such gastrointestinal side effects as constipation. The drug is available in a large number of *non*prescription products for relief of mild coughs due to colds and is considered unlikely to cause dependence.

EMETIC. *Stimulation of the central vomiting mechanism* often occurs following administration of opioids. Nausea, dizziness, and vomiting are most likely to occur in ambulatory patients. Other signs of central stimulation are the restlessness and excitement seen in some patients, instead of the expected sedation. The character-

TABLE 13-1 *Potent (Strong) Analgesics and Related Drugs*

Nonproprietary or Generic Name	Trade Name or Synonym	Usual Dose Range	Remarks
Narcotic Analgesics			
Alphaprodine HCl N.F.	Nisentil	20–60 mg	Short duration
Anileridine HCl N.F. and phosphate	Leritine	25–100 mg	Similar to meperidine but somewhat shorter-acting
Codeine phosphate U.S.P. and sulfate N.F.	Methylmorphine	30–60 mg	Opium alkaloid for mild to moderate pain
Dextromoramide tartrate	Palfium	5–15 mg	Similar to methadone
Dihydrocodeine	Paracodin	10–30 mg	More potent than codeine
Fentanyl citrate	Sublimaze	0.05–0.1 mg	Very potent analgesic and respiratory depressant
Heroin	Diacetylmorphine	2–8 mg	Not used clinically in U.S. (abuse drug)
Hydrocodone bitartrate N.F.	Dicodid; Hycodan; Mercodinone	5–15 mg	More potent than codeine
Hydromorphone HCl and sulfate N.F.	Dilaudid	2–4 mg	More potent than morphine
Levorphanol tartrate N.F.	Levo-Dromoran	2–3 mg	More potent and longer acting than morphine
Meperidine HCl U.S.P.	Demerol; and others	50–100 mg	Less sedating and spasmogenic than morphine
Methadone HCl U.S.P.	Dolophine; and others	2.5–10 mg	Less euphoric than heroin. Now used in management of heroin dependence
Metopon HCl	Methyldihydromorphinone	2–7 mg	Similar to morphine
Morphine sulfate U.S.P.		5–20 mg	Prototype opium alkaloid
Oxycodone HCl and terephthalate	Percodan	5–10 mg	More potent and more dependency-producing than codeine
Oxymorphone HCl N.F.	Numorphan	1.0–1.5 mg	Potent, rapid onset, moderate duration
Pantopium	Pantopon	5–20 mg	Mixture of purified opium alkaloids
Piminodine esylate N.F.	Alvodine	25–50 mg	Similar to meperidine
Potent Nonnarcotic Analgesics			
Methotrimeprazine N.F.	Levoprome	10–30 mg	Does not produce dependence or respiratory depression, but its usefulness is limited by orthostatic hypotension and sedation
Pentazocine HCl and lactate N.F.	Talwin	30–50 mg	Tolerance develops only slowly to therapeutic doses; can produce dependency in abusers
Mild Nonnarcotic Analgesics			
Ethoheptazine citrate N.F.	Zactane	75–100 mg	Related to meperidine, but effective only for mild to moderate pain
Propoxyphene HCl N.F.	Darvon	32–65 mg	About half as potent as codeine but even less likely to produce dependence in normal use. Most effective when combined with aspirin
Propoxyphene napsylate	Darvon-N	50–100 mg	

istic pupillary constriction produced by these drugs is the result of stimulation of the oculomotor center.

Respiratory center depression is the most dangerous central effect of the opioids (see below, p. 166). Most of the newer synthetic analgesics (Table 13-1) were introduced with claims that respiratory depression was less likely

TABLE 13-2 *Centrally Acting Antitussive Agents*

Nonproprietary or Official Name	Proprietary Name or Synonym	Usual Adult Antitussive Dosage
Narcotic Antitussive-Analgesics		
Codeine N.F.	Methylmorphine	15–30 mg
Codeine phosphate U.S.P.	Methylmorphine phosphate	15–30 mg
Codeine sulfate N.F.	Methylmorphine sulfate	15–30 mg
Dihydrocodeine bitartrate	Drocode; Rapacodin; Paracodin	10–20 mg
Hydrocodone bitartrate U.S.P.	Dihydrocodeinone; in Hycodan, and others	5–10 mg
Hydromorphone N.F.	Dihydromorphinone; Dilaudid	2 mg
Methadone HCl U.S.P.	Adanon; Amidon; Dolophine	1.5–2 mg
Morphine sulfate U.S.P.		2–3 mg
Nonnarcotic Antitussives		
Benzonatate N.F.	Tessalon	100 mg
Caramiphen ethanedisulfonate	Toryn	10–20 mg
Carbetapentane citrate N.F.	Toclase	15–30 mg
Chlophedianol HCl	ULO	25 mg
Dextromethorphan HBr N.F.	Romilar; and others	10–20 mg
Dihyprylone	Piperidione; Sedulon	60–120
Dimethoxanate HCl	Cothera	25–50 mg
Levopropoxyphene napsylate	Novrad	50–100 mg
Noscapine HCl N.F.	Narcotine; Nectadon	15–30 mg
Pipazethate HCl	Theratuss	20–40 mg

to occur than when morphine is employed. Actually, however, all the potent analgesics are equally capable of depressing respiration when they are used in doses that produce the same degree of pain relief. Less potent drugs, such as codeine+, do not cause significant respiratory depression in ordinary doses.

PERIPHERAL EFFECTS OF THE OPIOIDS

Morphine and the other opioids produce a variety of peripheral effects, most of which are the cause of discomforting side effects. Sometimes, for example, the patient's skin becomes flushed, sweaty, and itchy, and the mucous membranes of his mouth and nose may be uncomfortably dry. In addition, visceral smooth muscles may be directly contracted by morphine and, to a lesser extent, by meperidine and other synthetic drugs.

Biliary tract pressure may, for example, actually be increased when morphine is administered for relief of pain caused by reflex spasm of the smooth muscle of the bile ducts (biliary colic). Similarly, in renal colic caused by a stone in the ureter, morphine may add to the smooth muscle spasm. Spasm of the sphincter

muscle of the urinary bladder following morphine administration may lead to urinary retention (dysuria) in men with an enlarged prostate gland.

Constipation, a common side effect of the opioids, is in part the result of an increase in the tone of the sphincters and other gastrointestinal smooth muscle. In addition, these drugs decrease the peristaltic movements of the intestine and reduce the secretion of pancreatic fluids and bile. Patients who are immobilized in traction or for other reasons are particularly likely to become constipated when potent analgesics are regularly employed.

This constipating effect of the opium alkaloids is utilized clinically in the management of diarrhea. Paregoric is, for example, a traditional treatment for dysentery. One or two teaspoonsful taken several times daily during acute diarrhea is usually effective for symptomatic relief. Sometimes morphine may be administered parenterally to control diarrhea in colostomy and ileostomy patients to prevent exhaustion and collapse.

The opiates are not used routinely for treating chronic diarrhea because of their potential for causing dependence. Their spasm-producing effect may be undesirable even for control of acute episodes of diarrhea in patients with chronic ulcerative colitis. *Diphenoxylate+* (Lomotil), a synthetic drug related to meperidine, is now often used in place of paregoric for symptomatic relief of diarrhea in various acute and chronic conditions, including the irritable bowel syndrome and gastroenteritis. Although this drug is sometimes abused, it has only a relatively low potential for producing dependence as compared to meperidine and other opioid analgesics.

Clinical Considerations in Opioid Use

The potent analgesics are employed for the relief of acute and chronic pain in a wide variety of clinical conditions (see *Summary*, p. 166). The doctor tries to use these drugs in ways which will reduce the patient's pain most effectively while keeping unwanted side effects to a minimum. The nurse plays an important part in attaining this objective, as the doctor depends upon her reports of the patient's responses to help him evaluate the effectiveness of the analgesic and the need to modify its dosage.

CONTROL OF ACUTE PAIN

Potent analgesics are ordered only after the cause of acute pain has been determined. It would not, for example, be desirable to administer opiates for relief of acute abdominal pain until the possibility of acute appendicitis had been ruled out. These drugs might mask the pain and make diagnosis difficult, with the result that the patient might suffer a ruptured appendix.

Medication ordered for relief of acute pain should be administered promptly. Analgesics are most effective for pain control when given before the pain has fully developed. Once the patient has experienced severe pain, the panic that it can provoke may make it necessary to give much more medication than would have been needed if it had been given earlier.

Postoperative patients may require potent analgesics when the anesthetic wears off. However, narcotics are not given routinely to all surgical patients. The doctor usually decides whether the patient requires medication following surgery after first considering various factors, including the type of general anesthetic that has been employed. For example, patients who have been anesthetized with halothane (Fluothane) or *enflurane* (Euthrane) are more likely to require analgesics after their rapid recovery than those who have been given ether, an anesthetic with long-lasting residual analgesic effects of its own.

The type of surgery is also significant. Following cholecystectomy and other abdominal operations, or chest surgery (thoracotomy), severe pain may lead to reflex splinting of the patient's respiratory muscles. The resulting shallow breathing tends to reduce the exchange of respiratory gases. This can lead to postoperative complications that can be avoided by administering potent analgesic medication to the patient with pain that keeps him from moving, coughing, or even breathing deeply.

Of course, these drugs that depress the respiratory center may themselves cause adverse effects on the patient's breathing. In addition, morphine-type drugs sometimes exert a bronchoconstrictor effect by their ability to cause contraction of smooth muscle (p. 161). This can be particularly hazardous for patients with pulmonary disease, including those with bronchial asthma, emphysema, or cor pulmonale.

Retention of carbon dioxide in such patients may send them into a comatose state. Patients with liver damage may also be precipitated into coma by these drugs that depress the central nervous system and respiratory center. Patients with head injuries may suffer an increase in intracranial pressure as a result of a drug-induced buildup of carbon dioxide that leads to cerebral vasodilation.

The recovery room nurse is often required to judge whether a postoperative patient will need a narcotic and, if so, how much. Later, the nurse on the ward who has been given a p.r.n. order for a narcotic may have to determine whether a dose of the drug should be omitted. This requires experience and good judgment. The skilled nurse recognizes from carefully observing the patient whether he is uncomfortable and in need of the ordered analgesic, or, on the other hand, whether he is excessively sedated and would be better off with the drug withheld.

Preoperative use of opioids for their sedative effects is not as frequent as it once was, as many physicians now prefer to use minor tranquilizers such as parenteral *hydroxyzine* (Vistaril) or *diazepam* (Valium) for this purpose. This is due to such disadvantages of the narcotic analgesics as their previously mentioned tendency to cause nausea, vomiting, and constipation.

In addition, these drugs sometimes cause confusion and even perceptual distortions in some patients who are being prepared for anesthesia and surgery. In fact, many patients suffer dysphoria from opioids, perhaps because they do not like to feel that they are losing control, even temporarily, of their ability to care for themselves. Such patients may find the early phase of their response to these preoperative medications anxiety-provoking, until the drug produces sufficient effect to overcome this apprehension.

Neuroleptanalgesia, a new form of preoperative preparation, does, however, have advantages in some cases. This is a state of reduced awareness of pain produced by administering (1) a neuroleptic agent in combination with (2) a potent analgesic. Under the influence of this drug combination the patient is kept quiet, pain-free, and yet completely cooperative during various diagnostic and neurosurgical procedures that require him to be conscious. If necessary for performing major surgical anesthesia, the patient who has been prepared in this way may then inhale a nitrous oxide-oxygen mixture to induce and to maintain a state of general anesthesia.

Innovar, a clinically available combination of this kind contains (1) *droperidol* (Inapsine), a neuroleptic of the butyrophenone type in combination with (2) a new synthetic analgesic, *fentanyl* (Sublimaze). Fentanyl is about a hundred times more potent than morphine, and its analgesic action is potentiated by the presence of droperidol, a drug that induces a state of detached calmness. Use of this combination is particularly useful for elderly and other poor-risk surgical patients, as it has little adverse effect upon cardiovascular function.

A disadvantage of this neuroleptic combination is its tendency to produce depression of respiration. As is true of all potent analgesics, the pain-relieving potency of fentanyl is matched by an equally powerful depressant effect upon the patient's respiratory center. In addition, this drug often induces skeletal muscle rigidity that may further interfere with the patient's breathing. Sometimes the drug-induced mental detachment may last for a relatively long time after a minor operative procedure has been completed.

Short procedures are best carried out with an-algesic drugs that wear off relatively rapidly, such as *alphaprodine+* (Nisentil). A drug of this kind is particularly useful for managing situations marked by bouts of pain and discomfort that are severe but of short duration. These include the changing of burn dressings, setting of fractures or reduction of dislocations, and passage of a cystoscope in patients with urethral strictures.

In such situations, the sudden disappearance of the pain may leave the patient in a state of deep drug-induced depression when a long-lasting potent analgesic has been employed. For example, when a patient with a renal calculus passes the stone, his pain often vanishes dramatically. This may leave him exposed to the full depressant effect of any previously administered narcotic analgesic.

Women in labor also often receive opioids. These are best administered well before birth of the baby is expected. Given too close to the time of delivery, meperidine+ may, for example, pass to the fetus by way of the placental circulation. This may interfere with onset of spontaneous respiration in the newborn infant. Premedication with *diazepam* (Valium) is said to reduce the need for narcotics during obstetrical procedures, and *alphaprodine+* is said to be safer because of the shorter duration of its depressant effects.

CONTROL OF CHRONIC PAIN

Development of tolerance and dependence is a drawback that limits the usefulness of opioids. Thus, patients with chronic rheumatoid arthritis rarely receive potent analgesics for control of joint pain. In other cases, including cancer, in which the long-term use of pain-relieving medication is necessary, the doctor and nurse must employ various measures to minimize addiction to opioids.

Psychic dependence upon opioids occurs in only a minority of patients. The observant nurse can often detect the addiction-prone patient. Often he has a history of alcoholism or has abused other drugs. The nurse notes whether the patient's complaints of pain or discomfort seem warranted by the nature of the disorder from which he suffers. If she feels that his demands for drugs are greater than those of most patients in similar circumstances, the nurse brings the matter to the doctor's attention.

The doctor may decide that a patient's complaints stem from anxiety rather than actual pain. He may then order a switch to use of a major tranquilizer of the phenothiazine type. Drugs of this kind help to reduce the patient's emotional reaction to physical discomfort. Patients rarely become psychologically dependent upon *chlorpromazine* (Thorazine) and similar tranquilizers.

In such cases, the nurse can also help to reduce the need for pain-relieving medication. She can, for example, offer the patient reassurance and psychological support and be willing to listen as he expresses his concern about his painful condition. Measures that make the patient more physically comfortable also often help to lessen development of dependence upon analgesic drugs. Thus, giving the patient a soothing backrub, changing his position, or even straightening his bedclothes may help to lessen complaints of pain and requests for drugs.

Physical dependence and tolerance to the opioids are inevitable when these drugs are administered regularly. Development of dependence in patients with terminal cancer is sometimes unavoidable. However, tolerance is a more practical problem because these drugs can, in time, lose their effectiveness. To avoid a situation in which even very large doses may not control the patient's pain, the doctor often holds the potent narcotic analgesics in reserve.

He may start the patient on aspirin and phenacetin at first, as these drugs are effective for control of moderate pain. He may also add an antianxiety agent such as *diazepam* (Valium) or *hydroxyzine* (Atarax) to these nonnarcotic analgesics. The addition of *propoxyphene+* (Darvon) to a combination of this type is claimed to offer analgesia superior to that of aspirin alone.

When these *nonnarcotic* drugs fail to control the patient's pain, the physician may begin to employ oral doses of *codeine+* or other opioids that have relatively low dependency-producing effects. If further pain relief is required, the doctor may first administer oral doses, and finally injections, of the potent analgesic *pentazocine+* (Talwin), to which tolerance and dependence develop much less frequently than with the opioids (see below).

If narcotics become necessary, they should be given at irregular intervals rather than on a regular schedule. If the nurse has a choice, she should replace an ordered dose of a potent opioid with a nonnarcotic analgesic or tranquilizer when the patient's pain seems to have subsided. She should not administer narcotics routinely in anticipation of pain or for their sedative effects simply to keep the patient quiet.

Of course, the nurse should not withhold p.r.n. narcotics when the patient is actually experiencing excruciating pain. The purpose of all these delaying tactics is to slow tolerance development so that the opiates will retain their effectiveness when the patient needs them most.

Potent Analgesics Not Subject to Narcotic Controls

Most of the newer synthetic analgesics were prepared with the hope that they would prove less likely to cause dependence and addiction. Yet, all are capable of being abused by people whose personalities predispose them to addiction. All require the precautions previously discussed if addiction is to be prevented during their prolonged use in chronically painful conditions.

Recently, two drugs have become available that appear less likely than the opioids to cause development of tolerance and dependence when administered in doses capable of controlling severe pain. These drugs—*pentazocine+* (Talwin) and *methotrimeprazine* (Levoprome)—have been called "nonnarcotic" and "nonaddicting." However, this does *not* mean that they can be used without taking the same kinds of precautions as are required with the narcotic analgesics. Even though these drugs are not subject to the usual narcotic controls, they are capable of being abused or misused.

Pentazocine is the preferred drug of this type for managing chronic pain in ambulatory patients. Tolerance is said to develop more slowly than when morphine or meperidine are administered in such cases. It is less likely than methotrimeprazine to produce disabling drowsiness and dizziness. However, hallucinations have sometimes occurred, and abuse of the parenteral form of this drug has led to dependence in some cases.

Pentazocine has been claimed less likely to cause the characteristic adverse effects of the opioids (see *Summary*, p. 167), but its use in problem patients requires similar precautions. For example, the same care is needed for patients with bronchial asthma or patients with depressed respiration as when the narcotic opioids are employed. Overdosage is best treated with the new narcotic antagonist, *naloxone* (see below).

Methotrimeprazine (Levoprome), a phenothiazine derivative, is also as effective as the potent narcotic analgesics for relief of moderate to severe pain. Unlike the latter drugs, it does not cause development of dependence or depress respiration and the cough reflex. Unfortunately, it cannot be used continuously in ambulatory patients with chronic pain, because it often causes feelings of weakness, faintness, and dizziness—the result of orthostatic hypotension.

This drug's use is limited largely to control of acute pain in surgical and obstetrical patients. Administered preoperatively, it helps to reduce the patient's apprehension and anxiety. Smaller doses are used for postoperative analgesia, as this drug may potentiate the residual effects of general anesthetics. The solution employed for intramuscular injection is irritating. Thus, it is recommended that injection sites be rotated.

Acute Opioid Toxicity

Opioid overdosage usually produces deep depression of respiration, stupor, and coma. This may occur clinically in patients who are excessively susceptible to the depressant effects of these drugs. Addicts are also frequent victims of fatal heroin overdosage. Here, however, the exact cause of the acute herion reaction syndrome is uncertain, as death occurs with greater suddenness and with different signs than when overdoses of opioid medications have been taken. For example, massive pulmonary edema, rather than respiratory failure, is the most common finding in fatalities from heroin "ODs."

Narcotic Antagonists

Opioid narcosis, coma, and respiratory depression is best treated, *not* with analeptics, but with specific antidotes that act by displacing the narcotic drug molecules from the nerve cell receptors. The most commonly employed of these narcotic antagonists is *nalorphine*+ (Nalline). However, a new drug of this class called *naloxone* (Narcan) has special properties that may make it superior, once more experience in its use has accumulated.

Naloxone, unlike nalorphine and levallorphan, does not cause narcotic-like depression if administered to patients who are not under the influence of an opioid. Thus, it can be used safely for determining whether a patient who is suffering from overdosage of a depressant drug has taken opioids or barbiturates.

If the patient responds to naloxone with increased respiration and lightening of depression, his condition is diagnosed as due to opioid overdosage. If he has taken an overdose of barbiturates, his condition will not be improved by naloxone. However, his depression will not worsen as it would have if one of the other narcotic antagonists had been given.

S U M M A R Y of Main Pharmacologic Actions and Therapeutic Uses of Opiates and Opioids

Analgesic, Sedative, Tranquilizer, Hypnotic

These C.N.S. actions account for the effectiveness of these drugs against even very severe pain, including that caused by acute smooth muscle spasm and chronic bone disease. Among the conditions in which potent analgesics are employed are: acute coronary attacks; biliary and renal colic; trauma caused by fractures or extensive burns; intractable pain of malignancies; control of postoperative pain; preanesthetic sedation; short diagnostic and operative procedures in orthopedics, urology, ophthalmology, rhinology, and laryngology; obstetrical analgesia.

Antiperistaltic, Antisecretory, and Spasmogenic

These peripheral actions on gastrointestinal muscles and glands account for the usefulness of opiate alkaloids in diarrhea, dysentery, and various other gastrointestinal conditions, including peritonitis.

Antitussive

The depressant action of many of these drugs on the medullary cough center mechanism accounts for their usefulness for decreasing the frequency of coughing. Morphine, methadone, and dihydromorphinone are preferred for coughs accompanied by pain, following rib fractures, or in lung cancer, or tuberculosis. Less addicting and less depressant antitussives such as codeine and hydrocodone can control lesser coughs, including those caused by dryness and irritation of the respiratory tract mucosa in the common cold.

S U M M A R Y of Opiate Side Effects, Contraindications, and Toxicity

Central Nervous System Side Effects and Toxicity

Drowsiness, clouding of consciousness, and inability to concentrate; occasionally, especially in women or elderly patients, paradoxical excitement marked by nervousness, restlessness, and even mania may develop. (Excitement is more common with codeine or meperidine overdosage and may progress to convulsions or to disorientation, delirium, or hallucinations.)

Lightheadedness, dizziness, nausea, and vomiting are central in origin and more common when patients are ambulatory. Skin may become warm, flushed, and itchy.

Respiratory depression, especially in elderly and debilitated patients and in those with certain preexisting disorders. Among the conditions in which opiate administration requires caution or in which these depressants may be contraindicated, lest they cause apnea and coma, are:

(a) Head injuries, delirium tremens, increased intracranial pressure

(b) Severe bronchial asthma, emphysema, and other pulmonary diseases

(c) Metabolic disorders, including myxedema, Addison's disease, hepatic cirrhosis, and renal failure.

Circulatory collapse may be the result of severe hypoxia, or direct central and peripheral vasomotor depression. These drugs should be given only very cautiously to patients in shock, and preferably by vein in small fractional doses, because absorption from subcutaneous sites may be poor. Several subcutaneous doses might be absorbed at once if other measures bring blood pressure back to normal.

Peripheral Side Effects

Gastrointestinal tract smooth muscle movements are slowed and muscle tone is increased to the point of spasm. These actions and others, including reduced secretions, lead to constipation, a side effect to which the addict does not develop tolerance.

Biliary and urinary tract muscle is also made spastic, increased choledochal pressure may lead to rupture of *diseased* gallbladder and duct tissues; spasm of the bladder sphincter may act to interfere with urinary flow.

Bronchiolar constriction by morphine is undesirable for asthmatic patients; small doses of meperidine are less likely to cause contraction of bronchial muscles.

S U M M A R Y of Nursing Points Concerning Use of Potent Analgesics

Administer analgesics promptly, as these drugs are more effective when they begin to act before the patient's pain has built up to a high level.

Narcotic analgesics are not a substitute for nursing care measures that also help to make the patient more comfortable. (It is sometimes necessary to help the patient with chronic pain accept the fact that no narcotic drug is going to control his pain completely.)

Generally, however, it is desirable to help the patient feel that the medication you are giving him is going to relieve his pain. The psychological effect of such suggestion often tends to increase the effectiveness of analgesics.

Be alert to the patient's physical and emotional responses to analgesics and report any unusual responses to the doctor, including any indications of dependence or tolerance development.

Be aware that some patients may make excessive demands for analgesic drugs because of their antianxiety and euphoric effects, rather than for pain relief. Other patients are so fearful of becoming addicted that they will refuse even a single dose of analgesic medication. Both kinds of patients require counselling by the physician and the nurse, or in some cases, by a psychiatrist.

Be aware that patients who are not used to narcotic analgesics may suffer dysphoric effects. In addition to such physical discomforts as nausea, vomiting, itching, flushing, and sweating, the patient may be made anxious by the feeling that he is losing control and becoming helpless under the drug's influence.

Patients who receive opioids preoperatively, particularly in combination with potent tranquilizers, sometimes have distortions of visual and auditory perceptions. It is important to stay near the patient in such cases to reassure him. Try to keep him from being exposed to loud noises, bright lights, or sudden jolting of his bed or stretcher.

DRUG DIGEST

ALPHAPRODINE HCl N.F. (Nisentil)
Actions and Indications. This narcotic analgesic has a relatively rapid onset and short duration of action. This makes it useful for preventing pain and discomfort during procedures such as cystoscopy, minor surgery of the eye, nose, and throat, and orthopedic manipulations. When used in obstetrical analgesia, this drug's short duration tends to minimize depression of respiration in the newborn infant.

Side Effects, Cautions, and Contraindications. This drug's depressant effect upon respiration may be intensified in patients who are also receiving barbiturates, phenothiazines, and general anesthetics. Its dose should be reduced in such cases. Excessive depression is best managed with the narcotic antagonist levallorphan, particularly if depression develops during obstetrical analgesia shortly before delivery. After delivery, the same antagonist may be injected into the baby's umbilical vein to counteract any residual respiratory depression caused by administration of this analgesic to the mother. Alphaprodine is not considered desirable in the management of chronically painful disorders. The frequent administration that is required would tend to increase the likelihood of development of dependence.

Dosage and Administration. The usual dose range is 0.4 to 1.2 mg/kg S.C. or 0.4 to 0.6 mg/kg I.V. Early doses are about 60 mg S.C. or 30 mg I.V. The I.M. route is **not** recommended.

CODEINE PHOSPHATE U.S.P. (Methylmorphine)
Actions and Indications. This and other salts of the opium alkaloid have central analgesic and antitussive effects when taken orally in adequate doses. Codeine is most often combined with aspirin for producing additive effects that relieve pain of mild to moderate intensity. It also reduces the frequency of cough volleys by raising the threshold of the cough reflex center to afferent impulses that arise in irritated or inflamed areas of the respiratory tract mucosa. Its sedative effect may also reduce the patient's concern about his coughing.

Side Effects, Cautions, and Contraindications. This drug causes little respiratory depression and fewer of the discomforting side effects that occur with morphine and other more potent opioids. Because of this and its relatively low dependence-producing potential, codeine is preferred for cough control and pain relief in most clinical situations in which it is adequately effective.

The usual oral doses cause few side effects, but some patients may become constipated or complain of nausea, epigastric distress, dizziness, and drowsiness. Large overdoses rarely depress respiration severely, but may cause confusion, agitation, and other signs of central excitement, including delirium and convulsions.

Dosage and Administration. Oral doses of 30 mg are required for relief of pain and are administered every four hours. Oral and subcutaneous administration of up to 60 mg may increase the extent of the drug's analgesic effectiveness. For cough relief, doses of 8 to 15 mg are taken orally several times daily.

DIPHENOXYLATE HCl N.F. (Lomotil)
Actions and Indications. This relative of meperidine (Demerol) is used for its ability to reduce intestinal motility in the treatment of diarrhea. It has been employed: as an adjunct in the management of acute G.I. infections and food poisoning; following gastric surgery, ileostomy, and colostomy; and in the irritable bowel syndrome, malabsorption syndrome, and mild to moderate regional enteritis and ulcerative colitis.

Side Effects, Cautions, and Contraindications. Minor side effects include drowsiness, dizziness, and headache. Overdosage may lead to coma and respiratory depression similar to that which occurs with meperidine and morphine, particularly in children and in patients with hepatic disease. The drug is contraindicated in children less than two years old and in jaundiced patients.

The small subtherapeutic dose of atropine, which is added to diphenoxylate to discourage its abuse, may also produce adverse effects in young children, including flushing and dryness of the skin. This drug does not ordinarily cause dependence. However, caution is required in administering it to patients with a history of heroin dependence or abuse of other drugs. Patients who habitually exceed the recommended dose to gain euphoric effects may become psychologically dependent upon diphenoxylate. If taken together with barbiturates or alcohol, this drug may potentiate the effects of these depressant drugs.

Dosage and Administration. The usual adult dose is 5 to 10 mg t.i.d. or q.i.d. (average dose 20 mg daily). For children, doses range from 2 mg three times daily for those under five years old to 2 mg five times daily for children between eight and twelve years old. The drug is administered orally as 2.5-mg tablets or as a liquid containing 2.5 mg per 5 ml.

MEPERIDINE HCl U.S.P. (Demerol; Mepadin)
Actions and Indications. This synthetic analgesic is similar to morphine in its strong analgesic action. It differs from morphine in having less of a sedative effect and weaker antitussive and spasm-producing actions. When used as an adjunct to

anesthesia or for obstetrical analgesia, it is commonly combined with sedatives such as a barbiturate, diazepam, promethazine, or scopolamine.

Side Effects, Cautions, and Contra-indications. Ambulatory patients are likely to become dizzy and light-headed as a result of postural hypotension. Nausea, vomiting, flushing, and sweating may also occur, as well as feelings of weakness, disorientation, and possibly agitation.

Caution and reduction in dosage are required when other central depressants are also employed, including sedatives, hypnotics, and tranquilizers, as well as tricyclic-type antidepressants. Use of meperidine is contraindicated in patients taking monoamine oxidase (MAO) inhibitor drugs, as severe reactions can occur.

Extreme caution is required in patients with increased intracranial pressure or chronic pulmonary obstruction. The presence of such conditions as supraventricular tachycardias or prostatic hypertrophy requires caution, as this drug has weak atropine-like properties. This drug produces dependence of the morphine type.

Dosage and Administration. Adult dosage ranges between 50 and 150 mg, as needed for relief of pain, by oral and parenteral routes. For preoperative purposes and obstetrical analgesia, only parenteral routes are employed—usually I.M., sometimes subcutaneously, and occasionally I.V.

METHADONE HCl U.S.P. (Dolophine)

Actions and Indications. This strong synthetic analgesic and antitussive drug is as effective as morphine for relief of pain and coughing. It is slower in onset, longer in duration, and less sedating than morphine. It is not ordinarily used for preanesthetic purposes nor in obstetrical analgesia, in which its long-lasting depression of respiration of the fetus is undesirable.

Methadone is used in two ways in the management of addiction: (1) to suppress the abstinence syndrome in patients who are being withdrawn from heroin or other narcotics; and (2) to maintain patients who have been withdrawn from heroin in a state of minimal craving for the illicit narcotic and unresponsive to the euphoric effect of heroin.

Side Effects, Cautions, and Contra-indications. Side effects include drowsiness, dizziness, mouth dryness, nausea, vomiting, and constipation. Overdosage may result in stupor or coma, deep respiratory depression, cardiac slowing or ar-

rest, and hypotension or cardiovascular collapse. Symptoms are of long duration, and repeated injections of the available narcotic antagonists are required to prevent recurrences of respiratory depression and other toxic effects. This drug is capable of causing morphine-type dependence.

Caution is required in patients taking other depressant drugs or the drugs used for treating mental depression, including the monoamine oxidase (MAO) inhibitors, because of potentially dangerous drug interactions. This drug is used with extreme caution, if at all, in patients suffering an acute asthma attack or with head injuries.

Dosage and Administration. The usual adult dosage for relief of pain ranges from 2.5 to 10 mg every three or four hours orally or by injection (I.M. or S.C.). For cough relief the adult dose is 1-2 mg every four to six hours. Dosage for stabilizing addicted patients is variable.

MORPHINE SULFATE U.S.P.

Actions and Indications. This opium alkaloid is the prototype of the potent narcotic analgesics employed for relief of moderate to severe degrees of pain. It also has strong sedative effects that add to its effectiveness in some clinical situations, including preoperatively, and following coronary occlusion. It has antitussive and antiperistaltic effects but is used relatively rarely for relief of cough or diarrhea. Its peripheral vasodilator effect may play a part in its use for relief of acute pulmonary edema following failure of the left ventricle.

Side Effects, Cautions, and Contra-indications. Common side effects include drowsiness, dizziness, light-headedness, sweating and flushing, nausea, and vomiting—particularly in patients who are ambulatory. They should be warned against undertaking potentially hazardous activities that require alertness. Constipation is likely to occur on long-term use, especially in patients confined to bed.

Overdosage causes coma and respiratory depression. Even therapeutic doses can result in stupor and poor ventilation in special risk patients. These include the elderly and others weakened by disease, as well as patients with asthma and other chronic obstructive pulmonary diseases. Morphine may cause a sharp increase in the intracranial pressure of patients in whom cerebrospinal fluid pressure is already high as a result of head injury or other causes. Patients with severe liver disease can readily become comatose following morphine. Others who react ex-

cessively include myxedematous patients and those with Addison's disease.

Dosage and Administration. Subcutaneous administration of about 10 mg per 150 lbs of body weight is commonly employed. Slow I.V. injection of somewhat smaller doses diluted with saline solutions is used for more rapid and more certain action.

NALORPHINE HCl U.S.P. (Nalline)

Actions and Indications. This prototype narcotic antagonist reverses respiratory depression, stupor, and coma caused by overdoses of opioids. It is thought to act by displacing narcotic drug molecules from the receptors of nerve cells. It may be administered to newborn infants who fail to breathe spontaneously because of respiratory center depression caused by narcotic analgesics administered to the mother during labor and delivery. The drug can be used to detect the presence of recently administered narcotics. However, its use for diagnostic testing of narcotism should be limited to physicians familiar with the specialized technique and evaluation procedures.

Side Effects, Cautions, and Contra-indications. Administration of this drug to an individual who is physically dependent upon narcotics can precipitate a severe withdrawal syndrome. Its administration to patients depressed by barbiturates or other sedative hypnotics, rather than by opioids, can cause intensified respiratory depression. Thus, when the cause of drug-induced depression is uncertain, the safer antagonist naloxone should be employed, as it does not cause the depression that nalorphine induces in patients who have not taken narcotics.

Dosage and Administration. Treatment of adults is begun with 5 to 10 mg administered intravenously. This dose may be repeated twice at intervals of 10 to 15 minutes if needed to produce an initial effect. In treating depression by long-acting narcotics such as morphine or methadone, the antagonist is administered in additional doses whenever depression returns. For asphyxia neonatorum, doses of 0.2 to 0.5 mg are injected directly into the baby's umbilical vein.

PENTAZOCINE LACTATE N.F. (and HCl) (Talwin)

Actions and Indications. This strong analgesic for relief of moderate to severe degrees of pain is *non-narcotic* and is actually a weak narcotic antagonist. The injectable lactate salt is also used for preanesthetic medication and as a supplement to surgical anesthesia. The orally administered hydrochloride salt is claimed to be effective against pain in patients with chronic conditions, without leading to development of tolerance or to physical dependence. That is, abrupt discontinuance is *not* followed by withdrawal symptoms.

Side Effects, Cautions, and Contraindications. Patients with a history of drug abuse should be closely supervised to avoid excessive self-administration of the parenteral form of this drug in order to avoid misuse and possible development of psychological and physical dependence. Withdrawal symptoms similar to those that occur in morphine dependence may develop when this drug is abruptly discontinued following long-term use.

Most adverse effects are similar to those seen with narcotic analgesics, including nausea, vomiting, constipation, dizziness, and lightheadedness. In addition, acute mental manifestations such as development of disorientation, confusion, and hallucinations can occur, clear up spontaneously, and

then recur with further administration of the drug.

Overdosage is best treated with the narcotic antagonist *naloxone* (not with nalorphine or levallorphan), or with *methylphenidate* (not with other analeptic agents).

Dosage and Administration. Oral doses of 50 to 100 mg are administered every three or four hours, up to a total dose of 600 mg daily. Single parenteral doses of 30 mg are administered I.M., S.C., or I.V., and repeated every three or four hours. Patients in labor receive only a single I.M. dose of 30 mg but may be given 20 mg I.V. two or three times at two- or three-hour intervals.

PROPOXYPHENE HCl N.F. or NAPSYLATE (Darvon)

Actions and Indications. This chemical relative of methadone is used for relief of mild to moderate pain. It is about half as potent as codeine but can control pain equally well when given in twice the dose of the opiate. Unlike the latter, it is not subject to narcotic law restrictions. The effectiveness of propoxyphene is about equal to that

of aspirin, and a combination of the two drugs is said to produce a better analgesic effect than that of either drug administered alone.

Side Effects. Cautions, and Contraindications. This drug is classified as *non*addicting, but it can produce psychic and physical dependence of the morphine-codeine type when abused. Similarly, massive overdosage causes toxicity similar to that of codeine and other opiates, including convulsions, coma, circulatory collapse, and respiratory failure.

Ordinary doses may cause drowsiness, dizziness, and headache, or, occasionally, excitement and insomnia. Psychomotor impairment may make driving a car hazardous. Epigastric pain, nausea, vomiting, and constipation are also among the minor adverse effects.

Dosage and Administration. The hydrochloride salt is administered orally in doses of 32 or 65 mg; doses of the napsylate salt range from 50 to 100 mg. Both are usually given three or four times daily in combination with aspirin or with aspirin, phenacetin, and caffeine.

References

Council on Drugs. The misuse of pentazocine. *JAMA*, 209:1518, 1969.

Foldes, F.F. The human pharmacology and clinical use of narcotic antagonists. *Med. Clin. N. Amer.*, 48:421, 1964 (March).

Gates, M. Analgesic drugs. *Sci. Amer.*, 215:131, 1966 (Nov.).

Jaffe, J.H. Narcotics in the treatment of pain. *Med. Clin. N. Amer.*, 52:33, 1968.

Kaufman, M.A., and Brown, D.E. Pain wears many faces. *Amer. J. Nurs.*, 61:48, 1961.

Koch, D.M. A personal experience with pain. *Amer. J. Nurs.*, 58:228, 1958.

Morgan, A.J., and Moreno, J.W. Attitudes toward addiction. *Amer. J. Nurs.*, 73:497, 1973.

Murphree, H.B. Clinical pharmacology of potent analgesics. *Clin. Pharmacol. Therap.*, 3:473, 1962.

Rodman, M.J. Drugs for pain problems. *RN*, 34:59, 1971 (April).

Vandam, L.D. The potent analgesics. *New Eng. J. Med.*, 286:249, 1972.

14.

General Anesthetics and Adjuncts to Anesthesia

General anesthetics are central nervous system depressants that are used to bring about loss of pain sensation and consciousness. Their use permits painful surgical procedures to be performed without the patient's being aware of discomfort or even reacting with reflex movements. The modern anesthesiologist administers anesthetics and other drugs in ways that produce minimal changes in the patient's vital functions. Properly employed, these potent drugs are safe for producing the brief loss of consciousness needed for minor procedures or even the deep anesthesia required for performing lengthy major operations.

The general anesthetics are administered mainly by inhalation. Some, such as *nitrous oxide* and *cyclopropane+*, are gases. Others, including *ether+* and *halothane+*, are volatile liquids that give off vapors at room temperature. Still other anesthetics, such as the rapid-acting barbiturates *thiopental+* (Pentothal) and *methohexital* (Brevital), are introduced into the bloodstream by intravenous or rectal administration.

These substances are sometimes classified in terms of their potency and safety under conditions of clinical use. A potent anesthetic produces all the objectives of general anesthesia (see below) with relative safety. *Ether+*, for example, induces full, or complete, surgical anesthesia when inhaled in low concentrations that do not keep the patient from also inhaling adequate amounts of oxygen at the same time. *Nitrous oxide*, on the other hand, is a less potent substance that produces full anesthesia only when the gas is given in such high concentration that the amount of oxygen in the mixture is reduced below safe levels.

The Objectives of General Anesthesia

The potent general anesthetics are capable of producing several clinically useful pharmacological effects. The anesthesiologist tries to use these drugs to achieve these effects safely. Thus, the goals of general anesthesia are the safe attainment of the following effects:

1. *Analgesia,* the loss of pain perception.
2. *Unconsciousness,* a state in which the patient is unaware of what is going on and is later totally unable to recall what took place (amnesia, or loss of memory). (Actually, it is possible to employ ether and certain other general anesthetics in amounts that produce analgesia *without* complete loss of consciousness, but these drugs are rarely used in this way clinically.)
3. *Skeletal muscle relaxation.* Block of the spinal reflexes that maintain muscle tone is often desirable during abdominal surgery. Only the most potent general anesthetics depress these reflexes so completely as to cause abdominal muscle relaxation without, at the same time, dangerously depressing the brain's centers for control of breathing.

Ideally, a potent anesthetic should produce all these effects rapidly without setting off disturbances in cardiac rate and rhythm, sharp drops or rises in blood pressure, or disturbing reflex responses such as involuntary breath holding, laryngospasm, and bronchospasm. In actual practice, there are *no* general anesthetics that meet all the requirements of an *ideal* agent (see *Summary,* p. 179).

BALANCED ANESTHESIA

The lack of any single anesthetic that is ideally suited for use in every patient and in all surgical situations has led to the concept of balanced anesthesia. This involves the use of several different kinds of drugs to counteract the disadvantages of the various potent anesthetics and to make the most of the desirable properties of the less potent agents. (See summary of the advantages and disadvantages of individual anesthetics, pp. 182-184.)

The drugs that are employed for this purpose include such *non*anesthetic central nervous system depressants as: the sedative-

hypnotics and antianxiety agents or minor tranquilizers; the major tranquilizer, or neuroleptic, and antiemetic drugs; and the potent analgesics.

In addition, the general anesthetics and other central depressant drugs are also supplemented by certain peripherally-acting agents. These include *atropine* and other anticholinergic drugs and the neuromuscular blocking agents employed to aid in producing skeletal muscle paralysis (see below).

Before we discuss the use of these drugs in conjunction with the general anesthetics, we shall first indicate briefly what happens when a potent gas or vapor is inhaled and carried by the bloodstream to the patient's brain.

The Pharmacology of the Inhalation Anesthetics

THE ANESTHETIC SYNDROME

These anesthetics produce a progressive depression of the central nervous system. The degree of depression depends upon the concentration of the drug in the C.N.S. This, in turn, depends upon the dynamic balance between the rates at which the gas or vapor is:

(1) Taken up from the alveoli by the blood.
(2) Transported past the blood brain barrier.
(3) Redistributed by the blood and eliminated by the lungs.

As the level of the anesthetic rises, different groups of nerve cells become depressed, and the functions that they normally control are affected. The part of the brain most sensitive to anesthetics is the midbrain reticular activating system (R.A.S.), which functions in keeping a person conscious. Drug-induced depression of this area results in disruption of consciousness during Stage I of anesthesia (see *Summary,* p. 180).

Still higher concentrations knock out more resistant nerve centers. This results in changes in the activity of various reflexes (Fig. 14-1). By noting the state of ocular reflex activity (eye signs) and the nature of respiratory muscle movements, the anesthesiologist can determine how deeply depressed the patient is at any time. The nurse anesthetist also observes these signs during the induction and maintenance of anesthesia and in the recovery room.

Depression of inhibitory neurons may result in signs of excitement even after the patient

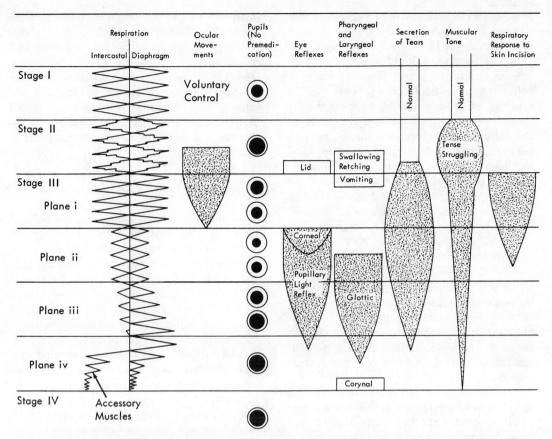

Fig. 14-1. The signs and reflex reactions of the stages of anesthesia. The wedge-shaped areas indicate (1) the variability from individual to individual and (2) the variability of the disappearance of the signs in the several planes of anesthesia. (Gillespie, N. A., *Anesth. Analg.* (Cleveland), 22:275, 1943.)

is unconscious. In Stage II of the anesthetic syndrome (see *Summary*, p. 180) it is important to keep the patient from harming himself. This is why he is secured by straps even before anesthesia is begun. Patients who have been prepared properly with preanesthetic medications and by psychological measures may show only minimal excitement.

It is important to remember that the patient is not responsible for his actions during this excitement stage. He is actually unconscious, even when he may be thrashing about restlessly or laughing, crying, or swearing. The nurse, of course, holds in confidence anything that she may hear the patient say during this delirium stage.

The patient himself should not be told about anything that he may have said or done during induction of anesthesia, as some may be embarrassed to learn later about their behavior. If a patient expresses concern *pre*operatively about how he may act under anes-

thesia, he can be assured that most people who have been adequately sedated only mumble to themselves in a way not understandable to others. The nurse can convey the idea that she is, in any case, accustomed to caring for people who have temporarily lost control and that she understands the cause of their unusual actions.

The nerve cells that are temporarily released from inhibitory control become depressed, and their hyperactivity ceases, as the anesthetic concentration in the brain rises. Depression of the patient's spinal reflex centers results in the relaxation of his skeletal muscles during the middle planes of the third stage of anesthesia (see *Summary*, p. 180).

Loss of these reflexes allows the surgeon to cut through the abdominal wall without setting off powerful contractions. In some surgical situations, it is desirable to supplement this action of the anesthetic with that of a peripherally acting neuromuscular blocking agent (see

p. 177). This makes it easier to carry out abdominal exploration and to perform such procedures as gall bladder and stomach surgery.

In the deepest stage of anesthesia, spontaneous respiration ceases (see *Summary*, p. 180). The anesthesiologist is equipped to maintain pulmonary ventilation mechanically if breathing stops. For some surgical procedures, the patient's respiratory movements are purposely stopped, and assisted or controlled breathing is temporarily employed. Ordinarily, however, the anesthesiologist avoids excessively depressing the patient's respiration, as this can lead to an acid-base imbalance or be followed by collapse of the cardiovascular system.

The anesthesiologist can control the level of anesthesia by balancing the amount of anesthetic that is being inhaled against that which is being eliminated by the lungs. When he wants to lighten anesthesia or terminate it entirely, the anesthetist simply stops the flow of gas or vapor going to the patient's lungs. As the anesthetic level at the various nerve centers falls, the depressed nerve cells regain their activity.

The functions that these neurons control then return at a rate that depends upon how much anesthetic has been administered and upon how long and how deeply the patient has been anesthetized. During recovery from deep anesthesia, the patient's reflexes return in the reverse order from that in which they were lost (Fig. 14-1). The excitement stage during recovery is not dramatic. However, it is important that the patient be properly positioned to avoid aspiration of gastric contents as a result of vomiting before protective gag reflexes have returned.

Clinical Applications of General Anesthetics

The individual anesthetics differ from one another in several of their central depressant properties, including their ability to produce analgesia and skeletal muscle relaxation. They also differ in several of their peripheral effects, including the extent to which they may adversely affect cardiac function. Thus, the anesthesiologist tries to select the anesthetic or combination of drugs best suited to the physical condition of the patient and the surgical operation that is to be performed.

The general anesthetics are used in two main ways: (1) to produce complete anesthesia, in which patients are kept in planes of deep surgical anesthesia for prolonged periods during which major surgery is performed; and (2) to produce basal anesthesia, a state of light anesthesia, in which various minor surgical and diagnostic procedures are carried out. In such states of basal narcosis the patient feels little discomfort and is not aware of what is going on.

USE OF POTENT ANESTHETICS

Only the most potent anesthetics can be used alone for the first purpose—producing full anesthesia safely. (The various advantages and disadvantages of the individual agents are summarized in Table 14-1.) These drugs are rarely used alone. Instead, they are usually supplemented by a combination of less potent, or basal, anesthetics, and by other *non*anesthetic supplementary drugs (see below).

The substances most capable of producing complete anesthesia with safety are the volatile liquids, *ether+* and *halothane+*, and the gas *cyclopropane+*. Various fluorinated hydrocarbons related to halothane, including *methoxyflurane* and *enflurane*, are also effective for achieving full anesthesia. They have the advantage of being nonflammable and nonexplosive.

None of these newer anesthetics is as safe and versatile as ether, the first potent anesthetic employed clinically. Until recently it was the most widely used general anesthetic because of its relatively wide safety margin when inhaled in concentrations that produce excellent analgesia and skeletal muscle relaxation. However, halothane has become more popular because of the rapidity with which it produces unconsciousness and its lack of discomforting postoperative effects. Most of its drawbacks can be counteracted by the use of adjunctive drugs.

USE OF BASAL ANESTHETICS

Even the less potent general anesthetics can all produce complete anesthesia. However, they do so in doses that can also cause various dangerous adverse effects. Thus, *thiopental+*, for example, causes respiratory depression when administered in the amounts needed to relax skeletal muscles and keep the patient from reacting to painful stimuli. For this reason, it is not used by itself to anesthetize patients for major surgery.

One way in which the rapid-acting ultra-short-acting barbiturates such as *thiopental+* and *methohexital* are used is to induce light surgical anesthesia. Injected intravenously, these drugs put the patient to sleep within seconds and carry him to the first plane of Stage III anesthesia. The anesthesiologist may then build upon this state of *basal narcosis* by having the patient inhale a mixture of nitrous oxide-oxygen gases, which adds the analgesic effect that is absent with barbiturates alone.

Combinations of this kind produce anesthesia that is adequate for carrying out various minor surgical and diagnostic procedures. For major surgery, however, more potent inhalation anesthetics must be added to prevent pain and to relax skeletal muscles. The amount of *ether+* or *halothane+* needed for full anesthesia is markedly reduced when the patient has first received an I.V. barbiturate for narcosis and nitrous oxide inhalation for analgesia. Another advantage of the quick unconsciousness induced by the barbiturates is that the patient is spared the stormy induction period experienced when ether alone is administered.

Inhalation of nitrous oxide-oxygen mixtures is used alone for pain relief in brief dental procedures. Other inhalation anesthetics that are too toxic for use in full anesthetic doses may also be used alone for producing a light level of anesthesia that offers adequate analgesia in orthopedic procedures, such as setting a fractured bone, or in urology prior to passage of a cystoscope.

Trichloroethylene, for example, is used in this way and for producing obstetrical analgesia. The small amounts required are safe and free of the potential cardiac toxicity or hepatotoxicity that may sometimes be caused by full doses of trichloroethylene or other halogenated hydrocarbon anesthetics, including ethyl chloride.

Ketamine (Ketalar; Ketaject) is a new nonbarbiturate injectable anesthetic. It is used both for induction prior to administration of more potent anesthetics and alone to prepare patients for minor surgical and diagnostic procedures. It produces profound analgesia and a peculiar mental state in which the patient appears to be awake and yet is unaware of what is taking place. This anesthetic state has been called *dissociative anesthesia*, because the patient seems disconnected from reality rather than asleep.

Injected slowly in the small doses that are adequate for induction and for carrying out painful or discomforting procedures, ketamine does not depress respiration or the cardiovascular system. Some patients become confused or excited and behave irrationally when emerging from anesthesia with this drug. To minimize reactions of this kind, it is best to avoid stimulating the patient in any way during the recovery period.

The Use of Supplementary (Adjunctive) Drugs

As was indicated earlier, the anesthesiologist employs various kinds of centrally and peripherally acting drugs, in addition to inhalation and intravenous anesthetics. Most of these agents are used as preanesthetic medications intended to make the induction of anesthesia go more smoothly. Other drugs are used during or after the operation to counteract various adverse effects of the general anesthetic or to supply a pharmacologic effect that the anesthetic itself lacks.

CENTRAL DEPRESSANT DRUG PREMEDICATION

Various types of depressants are employed to help the patient stay calm and relaxed before being subjected to anesthesia and surgery. Patients who are fearful and apprehensive tend to struggle against going under anesthesia during induction. Those who have been properly premedicated with *sedative-hypnotics*, *antianxiety agents*, or other drugs with a tranquilizing component, tend to slip more smoothly into a state of surgical anesthesia when they then inhale relatively low concentrations of a potent general anesthetic.

Preparing the patient mentally begins the night before the scheduled operation with administration of a hypnotic dose of a short-acting barbiturate such as *pentobarbital+* or *secobarbital+* or a *non*barbiturate sleep-producer such as *chloral hydrate+*. This is intended to give the patient a good night's rest before he undergoes the stress of surgery.

Nursing measures are also helpful in accomplishing this objective, particularly in elderly patients who sometimes tend to become confused and disoriented in the dark. Thus, the nurse may leave a night-light on, and she offers these patients gentle reassurances.

This is particularly true in situations that do not allow for a preoperative visit by the anesthetist the night before surgery. In such cases, the nurse tries to answer the patient's questions and give him some idea of what to expect. If she is unable to tell him what type of anesthesia he will receive or how it will be administered, she should discuss the situation with the patient's doctor, who can then answer his questions.

In the morning, about an hour before anesthesia and surgery, patients receive preanesthetic sedation. The dose should be high enough to prevent fear and apprehension but not so heavy as to depress the patient too deeply, as this could delay his recovery after anesthesia. Some physicians now prefer injectable antianxiety agents for this purpose, rather than barbiturates. For example, *hydroxyzine* (Vistaril) may be administered intramuscularly, and *diazepam* (Valium) is also commonly employed to help patients go under the anesthetic more readily and to emerge from anesthesia with reduced restlessness and confusion.

These drugs are now often administered together with *regional* (for example, *spinal* or *caudal*) anesthesia to reduce discomfort and nervousness during the procedure. They are also useful in obstetrics to smooth the course of labor and delivery. *Diazepam*, for instance, does not depress respiration in the mother or newborn baby as the narcotic analgesics do. Thus, its use reduces the dosage of *meperidine* (Demerol) or *morphine* needed for pain relief.

Narcotic analgesics of this kind have other disadvantages, including production of postoperative vomiting and depression of the cough reflex. They should not be employed routinely but only when the patient is expected to experience postoperative pain. This may occur with *halothane+* and *enflurane* (Ethrane), anesthetics that wear off quickly and leave little residual analgesia. Potent analgesics are often unnecessary when *ether+* or *methoxyflurane* (Penthrane) has been employed because of the prolonged analgesic effects of these anesthetics.

Neuroleptanalgesia is a drug-induced state of preoperative depression produced by administering a combination of a neuroleptic agent and a potent analgesic. A combination of this kind containing the neuroleptic *droperidol* (Inapsine) and the potent narcotic analgesic *fentanyl* is marketed as *Innovar*. Administered parenterally in small doses as preanesthetic medication, the product produces a state of calm detachment and unconcern.

Although various diagnostic and superficial surgical procedures can be performed upon patients put in this state with higher doses, neuroleptanalgesia must still be supplemented with other anesthetics for major surgery. Thus, to convert this state of basal narcosis to one called *neuroleptanesthesia*, the anesthesiologist has the patient inhale a nitrous oxide-oxygen mixture and injects the neuromuscular blocking agent, *succinylcholine+* (see below), to bring about adequate skeletal muscle relaxation.

Phenothiazine-type tranquilizers are also sometimes used preoperatively either alone or to potentiate the analgesic effects of *meperidine* (Demerol) and other opioids. In addition to calming the patient, these drugs exert an antiemetic effect. However, drugs such as *chlorpromazine* (Thorazine), *promazine* (Sparine), and *triflupromazine* (Vesprin) may make the patient's blood pressure drop during anesthesia. Thus, many anesthesiologists now prefer to use these drugs *post*operatively to control actual vomiting, rather than to use them routinely as preoperative prophylaxis.

PERIPHERALLY ACTING ADJUNCTIVE DRUGS

Anticholinergic drugs, such as *atropine* and *scopolamine*, are commonly administered as preanesthetic medications. They are used for two main purposes: (1) to reduce excessive salivation and tracheobronchial secretions of the kind that an anesthetic such as *ether+* tends to stimulate strongly; and (2) to counteract the heart-slowing effects of vagal stimulation of the kind caused by *halothane+* during induction, or as a result of reflexes that are set off by the manipulation of internal organs in some types of surgical procedures.

These drugs are not administered routinely, but only with anesthetics that are known to cause excessive secretions and bradycardia. This is because they not only produce unpleasant mouth dryness and blurring of vision, but can also cause restlessness and mental confusion, particularly in elderly patients or those suffering severe pain. They are also contraindicated for children with fever and in patients with atrial fibrillation or with thyrotoxicosis, because of their heart-stimulating effect.

Antiarrhythmic drugs are sometimes administered to counteract ventricular tachycardia and other rapid irregular rhythms set off by anesthetics. *Procainamide* (Pronestyl) and *lidocaine* (Xylocaine) are most commonly employed for this purpose. Recently, the beta adrenergic blocking agent *propranolol* (Inderal) has proved successful for abolishing rapid cardiac irregularities set off by epinephrine in patients in whom a halogenated hydrocarbon anesthetic had sensitized the heart to this action of the catecholamine.

Neostigmine and other cholinesterase inhibitors may be useful postoperatively for overcoming weakness of certain visceral smooth muscles. These and other cholinergic stimulants are sometimes administered to patients suffering from abdominal distention and urinary retention. By stimulating the smooth muscles of the intestine and the urinary bladder to resume their stalled peristaltic activity, these drugs help to relieve the discomfort caused by retained gases and wastes.

The frequency of these complications can be reduced by various nursing measures administered within the framework of the doctor's orders. For example, helping the patient to turn and walk about can help to relieve such discomforts as distention with flatus. It is also important to provide the patient with privacy and the opportunity to assume a normal position while he is attempting to void or defecate.

If these often overlooked measures fail to relieve the patient's discomfort promptly, the physician should be consulted. He may then suggest the use of physical measures, such as application of heat to the abdomen, or prescribe adjunctive medication, such as neostigmine, in an effort to bring about the return of normal visceral function.

(For fuller discussions of each kind of adjunctive drug described above see the appropriate chapter elsewhere in the text.)

Neuromuscular Blocking Agents

Two types of peripherally acting drugs (see Table 14-2) are used to bring about skeletal muscle relaxation in anesthetized patients. Both kinds of drugs do so by interfering with the transmission of nerve impulses from spinal motor fibers, but the mechanism by which each type of agent does so is different.

One group of drugs, the *competitive blockers*, acts by competing with acetylcholine, the neurohormone that is released from the nerve endings (see Chapter 20 and Fig. 14-2). By occupying the cholinergic receptor site on the motor end plate of skeletal muscle fibers, molecules of tubocurarine, for example, keep the neurohormone from reaching the receptor. This keeps the muscle fibers from contracting, and paralysis results.

The other group of neuromuscular blocking agents—the *depolarizing blockers*—act, at first, like the neurohormone acetylcholine. That is, they first stimulate the muscle fibers to contract. However, after the first increase in contractions, the muscles weaken and quickly become paralyzed. Finally, a flaccid paralysis develops that looks no different from that caused by the competitive blocking agents.

TABLE 14-2 *Neuromuscular Blocking Drugs*

Nonproprietary or Official Name	Proprietary Name or Synonym	Intravenous Dosage Range
Competitive or Nondepolarizing Type		
Dimethyl tubocurarine chloride	Mecostrin	2–3 mg
Dimethyl tubocurarine iodide N.F.	Metubine	1.5–7 mg
Gallamine triethiodide N.F.	Flaxedil	1.0 mg/kg
Pancuronium bromide	Pavulon	2–4 mg
Tubocurarine chloride U.S.P.	Tubarine; Tubadil	6–9 mg
Depolarizing Type		
Succinylcholine chloride U.S.P.	Sucostrin; Anectine; Quelicin	10–40 mg
Decamethonium bromide	Syncurine; C_{10}	0.5–3 mg

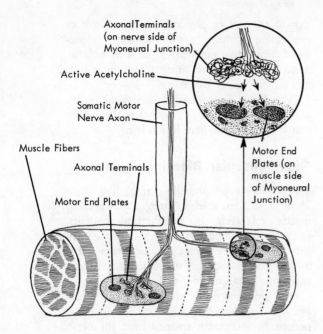

Axonal Terminals
(on nerve side of
Myoneural Junction)

Active Acetylcholine

Somatic Motor
Nerve Axon

Muscle Fibers

Axonal Terminals

Motor End Plates

Motor End
Plates (on
muscle side
of Myoneural
Junction)

Fig. 14-2. Transmission of nerve impulses to skeletal muscle fibers at a myoneural junction. Fiber terminals release acetylcholine.

However, there is one practical difference in case of clinical overdosage by these drugs. The paralysis caused by competitive blockers such as tubocurarine can be counteracted by administering neostigmine as an antidote. This drug does *not* antagonize paralysis produced by overdosage of *succinylcholine+* (Anectine; and others) or other depolarizing-type neuromuscular blockers.

CLINICAL APPLICATIONS

The most common use of these drugs is to bring about skeletal muscle relaxation in patients who are at relatively light levels of anesthesia. Thus, for example, they may be employed after a patient has received *thiopental+* for narcosis and *nitrous oxide* for analgesia. Even when these basal anesthetics have been followed by a potent general anesthetic such as *halothane+*, the administration of succinylcholine may bring about additional relaxation of the abdominal muscle wall.

Succinylcholine+ is preferred to tubocurarine for patients anesthetized by *halothane+*, because tubocurarine is more likely to intensify the fall in blood pressure often produced by this general anesthetic. When *ether* is the anesthetic, the dosage of the neuromuscular blocking agents must be markedly reduced because ether is itself a potent muscle relaxant, and giving full doses of the blocking drug with it can cause prolonged paralysis.

INTUBATION

The administration of muscle relaxants permits the passage of an endotracheal tube down the throat of an anesthetized patient. (Sometimes the anesthesiologist also sprays the patient's throat with an aerosol of a topical anesthetic; see Chapter 15.) Other intubation procedures for which neuromuscular blocking drugs are employed include laryngoscopy, bronchoscopy, esophagoscopy, and sigmoidoscopy.

OTHER USES

Succinylcholine is commonly used today as part of the premedication of psychiatric patients prior to electroshock therapy. Its use helps to dampen the severity of the convulsive spasms set off by passage of the current through the brain. This lessens the likelihood of the massive muscular contractions that might otherwise occur and the consequent vertebral fractures or dislocations. Since the use of this drug together with thiopental increases the likelihood of postseizure apnea, the patient is well oxygenated prior to the procedure and oxygen is kept readily available for administration through an endotracheal tube.

Tubocurarine has also been tried in the treatment of various acute and chronic neuromuscular disorders marked by muscle spasm and rigidity. It has not proved very effective in chronic conditions such as cerebral palsy, because of its relatively short duration of action and the uncertainty of its absorption when it is injected intramuscularly in repository dosage forms. The centrally-acting neurospasmolytics, *diazepam* and *methocarbamol*, are now preferred for treating chronic spastic disorders.

Curarization has, however, become an important measure in treating tetanus. To stop the patient's spasms the patient is completely paralyzed with a curare-type drug such as *tubocurarine* or *gallamine* (Flaxedil) and kept in that condition until the tetanus toxin has been eliminated, often a matter of weeks. The patient's respiration is controlled by pumps that provide intermittent positive pressure for prolonged periods.

Meticulous nursing care is an important part of the curare treatment of tetanus during the weeks in which the patient cannot breathe, move, eat, or communicate in any way. The single most important task is keeping the patient's airway free of secretions. Skillful mouth, throat, and tracheobronchial care helps to safeguard the patient against respiratory infections.

PRECAUTIONS AND TREATMENT OF OVERDOSAGE

The main danger in the use of blocking agents of both types is that paralysis of the diaphragm and chest muscles may cause respiratory difficulty and even apnea. For this reason, these drugs are never used when facilities for controlled respiration are unavailable, nor are they ever to be administered by individuals not completely skilled in their use. The occurrence of apnea following administration of these drugs is no great problem to the experienced anesthesiologist, who merely ventilates the patient artificially until the effects of the drug wear off—usually in a matter of minutes. Indeed, apnea is sometimes deliberately induced in chest and heart surgery without harm, as long as the patient continues to get oxygen by mechanical means.

Although there is no pharmacological antidote for overdosage with a depolarizing-type blocker such as succinylcholine, its effects ordinarily are overcome rather readily by simply supplying the patient with oxygen under pressure—preferably through a previously-inserted airway—until the body's own detoxifying enzymes destroy the excess of the drug. In the relatively rare cases of prolonged apnea following succinylcholine, the administration of whole blood or plasma may be helpful. These fluids contain cholinesterases, the enzymes that account for the ordinarily short action of succinylcholine by their ability to convert it to inactive metabolites. (Prolonged apnea following succinylcholine has been attributed to a lack of circulating cholinesterases.)

It is often important to maintain the patient's blood pressure at adequate levels. In cases of hypotension resulting from curare-induced histamine release and ganglionic blockade the administration of ephedrine or other adrenergic vasopressor drugs may prevent circulatory collapse. Atropine administration also is often desirable to counteract salivation, bronchial mucus secretion, and other muscarinic side effects of curare-drug antidotes such as neostigmine.

SUMMARY of the Characteristics of an Ideal General Inhalation Anesthetic

The vapor or gas should *not* be irritating to the respiratory mucosa or skin, and the patient should *not* be aware of any pungent, unpleasant odor in the few moments before he loses consconsciousness.

Induction of the surgical stage of anesthesia should occur rapidly and easily. The excitement stage should be brief and free of excessive psychomotor activity, salivation, or bronchial secretions of the kind that cause pharyngeal and laryngeal hyperreflexia, marked by coughing, gagging, laryngospasm, or bronchospasm.

The anesthetic should be potent enough to produce full anesthesia (unconsciousness, analgesia, and skeletal muscle relaxation) when inhaled in a low concentration that allows inhalation of oxygen in adequate amounts at the same time.

Recovery of consciousness should be rapid after the anesthetic is discontinued. The patient should *not* be confused, excited, disoriented, or subject to hallucinations. His thought processes should be lucid, and he should be free of discomforting feelings such as dizziness, heaviness, headache, grogginess, or pain. Nausea and vomiting should not occur, and his appetite should return promptly.

The anesthetic should not adversely affect vital functions during induction or prolonged maintenance of deep surgical planes:

1. It should *not* cause cardiac depression or arrhythmias, even when catecholamines such as epinephrine are administered; but both heart rate and blood pressure should remain stable.

2. The rate and depth of respiration should *not* become excessively depressed but, if this does occur, it should be easy for the anesthetist to take over the respiration with mechanical ventilation measures.

3. It should not adversely affect brain metabolism or set off electroencephalic abnormalities and seizure activity.

The anesthetic should have no adverse postanesthesia effects on such vital organs as the liver and kidneys. (That is, it should not be hepatotoxic, nephrotoxic, or adversely affect other parenchymatous organs, or metabolic processes and laboratory tests.)

The anesthetic should possess physical properties that make it nonflammable and nonexplosive:

1. It should not react chemically with the alkali used for absorbing carbon dioxide in closed anesthesia systems.

2. It should not have a corrosive effect on metallic equipment or damage rubber or plastic materials.

3. It should be chemically stable when stored indefinitely in clear glass containers without the need to add any stabilizers.

S U M M A R Y of the Stages and Planes of Anesthesia*
(The Anesthetic Syndrome)

Stage I: Early Induction

Consciousness becomes progressively clouded.

The patient's awareness of sensory stimuli is disrupted:

Sight, hearing and other perceptions are distorted

Feelings of floating and numbness

Analgesia (loss of pain sensation) may be profound with some anesthetics (for example, ether; methoxyflurane†).

Complete loss of consciousness marks the end of this stage.

Stage II: Delirium or Excitement

Patient is unconscious but may show signs of psychomotor excitement which are the result of drug-induced depression of inhibitory areas of the C.N.S.

Respiratory and cardiovascular reflexes may be hyperactive.

No surgical procedures are carried out. Efforts are made to minimize excitement and to protect the patient from injury.

Stage III: Surgical Anesthesia

Begins with a change from irregular to regular breathing and a loss of eyelid reflexes.

Artificially divided into four planes to indicate an increasing depth of anesthesia:

Plane 1: Eyeball movements; regular breathing.

Plane 2: Eyeballs fixed; breathing less deep or full; skeletal muscle tone reduced.

Plane 3: Chest breathing shallow; abdominal respiration deeper; no wink response when the cornea is touched.

Plane 4: Chest breathing stops; abdominal breathing becomes increasingly shallow.

Stage IV: Medullary Paralysis

Respiration ceases; cardiovascular collapse may occur if respiratory arrest is not corrected by resuscitative measures.

* This classic (Guedel) pattern applies mainly to ether anesthesia. It varies somewhat when other anesthetics are employed. (For instance, the first two stages are scarcely seen when anesthesia is induced with a rapid-acting barbiturate.)

† Guidelines developed for this drug include five levels of deepening anesthesia. Analgesia and loss of consciousness occur at Level 3, which is similar to Stage III. However, analgesia also is evident earlier, while the patient is still conscious. (That is, at Level 2, which corresponds to Stage I of the classic pattern.)

S U M M A R Y of Clinical Uses and Adverse Reactions of the
Neuromuscular Blocking Agents

Clinical Uses

Adjuvant in anesthesia.

Adjuvant in electroconvulsive shock therapy.

Intubation procedures (bronchoscopy, esophagoscopy, laryngoscopy, sigmoidoscopy).

Orthopedic procedures (reduction of dislocations and fractures).

Neuromuscular spastic disorders (cerebral palsy, hemiplegia, paraplegia, poliomyelitis, athetosis, dystonia, hyperkinesis).

Acute convulsive states (status epilepticus, tetanus, arachnidism).

Adverse Reactions

Respiratory: Hypoxia and apnea, following respiratory embarrassment and paralysis or bronchial constriction.

Use with caution in patients with asthma or myasthenia gravis; succinylcholine chloride contraindicated in patients with liver disease, malnutrition, anemia, or plasma cholinesterase deficiency.

Circulatory: Hypotension and possible circulatory collapse from partial ganglionic blockade, histamine release (for example, tubocurarine); cardiac arrhythmias from hypoxia or vagal blocking actions (for example, gallamine).

S U M M A R Y of Points for the Nurse to Remember About Administration of Anesthetics and Adjunctive Medications

In the Preanesthesia Period

1. Encourage your patient to ask questions and express his concern about the forthcoming anesthesia and surgery. Let him know that you will take the time to listen and that you want to help him learn what to expect.

2. Show your concern for your patient's welfare by paying attention to his physical comfort, as well as by talking to him. A soothing backrub, for instance, can promote relaxation.

3. Encourage your patient to be as self-reliant as possible before the operation. Thus, if he is able to bathe himself, allow him to do so. Allowing him to stay active and help himself can help reduce his anxiety about undergoing surgery. Diversions such as reading, watching television, and listening to the radio are desirable for the same reason.

4. Administer all preoperative medications at the times specified by the doctor and observe your patient's reactions to drugs.

5. If the patient is unable to sleep the night before surgery, try nursing measures before asking the physician to order more sedation. Spend some time with the patient to give him an opportunity to talk about the experience. This and such measures as straightening the bed and rubbing his back may help him fall asleep.

6. Make certain that you have completed all the details of preoperative care before administering the preoperative sedative, so that the patient can rest undisturbed. Explain that he should not get out of bed without assistance, or smoke while unattended, once he has been given the preanesthetic medication.

7. Observe the patient frequently after preoperative medication has been given to note his response to it. Avoid exposing the patient to loud noise, physical jolts, and glaring lights, as he is especially sensitive to such undesirable stimuli at this time.

In the Postanesthesia Period

1. Follow the physician's orders as to positioning the patient. If no specific orders have been left, the patient is usually positioned on his side with the head of the bed flat and with no pillow provided. This position helps prevent aspiration of respiratory secretions and vomitus. Suction the patient as necessary.

2. Observe the patient's vital signs as ordered. If no specific orders have been given, the blood pressure, pulse, and respiration are usually recorded every fifteen minutes until stabilized.

3. Observe the patient for any evidence of hemorrhage or signs of inadequate pulmonary ventilation.

4. Speak to the patient calmly and quietly as he regains consciousness, thus helping him to orient himself to his surroundings.

S U M M A R Y of Nursing Points Concerning Neuromuscular Blocking Drugs Used as Anesthesia Adjuncts and in Tetanus Treatment

Make certain that equipment and antidotal drugs (for example, neostigmine; edrophonium) that may be required for resuscitation are readily available.

Observe the patient for signs of respiratory embarrassment or apnea and be prepared to assist with such measures as artificial respiration and oxygen administration to sustain the patient until normal breathing resumes. Note also any signs of asthmatic breathing as a result of tubocurarine-induced release of tissue histamine.

Watch the patient's pulse and blood pressure carefully; circulatory collapse is a possible effect of tubocurarine administration.

With tetanus patients on long-term curarization treatment, employ measures for keeping the airway free of secretions in attending to the patient's tracheostomy toilet.

Remember that although the tetanus patient paralyzed with curare cannot move, he is conscious and aware of what is going on and of what is being said. Thus, be discreet in what you say in his presence and take every opportunity to reassure him and allay his alarm by providing simple explanations of each procedure.

Move the curare-paralyzed patient periodically to help prevent hypostatic pneumonia and to relieve limb discomfort. Supply a footboard and opportunities for passive exercise to prevent contractures.

Protect the curare-paralyzed patient's open eyes by shielding them and by instilling eyedrops periodically. Also provide skin care at pressure points.

SUMMARY of Characteristics of Individual Anesthetics

Nonproprietary or Generic Name	Trade Name, Synonym, or Chemical Name	Chemical or Physical Characteristics	Remarks Concerning Clinical Status	
			ADVANTAGES	**DISADVANTAGES**
Inhalation Anesthetics				
Chloroform N.F.	Trichloromethane	Volatile liquid; chlorinated hydrocarbon	Potent analgesic; good muscle relaxant; nonflammable and nonexplosive	Toxic to the liver and to the heart; rarely used today
Cyclopropane U.S.P.	Trimethylene	Cyclic hydrocarbon gas	Rapid, pleasant induction and recovery; potent analgesic; good muscle relaxant; relatively wide safety margin	Cardiac irregularities occur when epinephrine is employed; post-operative nausea, vomiting, headache, and delirium; flammable and explosive
Enflurane	Ethrane	Volatile liquid; fluorinated hydrocarbon	Rapid induction and recovery; pleasant odor; good muscle relaxation; nonflammable and nonexplosive	Analgesia not great; cardiac arrhythmias possible; respiratory depression may develop rapidly together with EEG abnormalities
Ether U.S.P.	Ethyl ether; diethyl ether	Volatile liquid ether	*See Drug Digest*	
Ethyl chloride N.F.		Volatile liquid, chlorinated hydrocarbon	Rapid induction and recovery; vapors not irritating	Toxic to the liver and the heart; not a good muscle relaxant in safe doses; flammable
Ethylene N.F.		Gas with an unpleasant odor	Rapid induction and recovery; good analgesia; not toxic to heart, lungs, liver, or kidneys	Highly explosive; not potent enough for full anesthesia; must be supplemented by potent analgesics and other depressant drugs

Drug	Physical form	Advantages	Disadvantages
Fluroxene N.F. (Fluoromar; trifluoroethyl vinyl ether)	Volatile liquid; fluorinated ether	Rapid induction and recovery with little nausea or excitement, and little effect upon blood pressure or cardiac rhythm; excellent analgesia	Not a good muscle relaxant; requires supplementation for full anesthesia; potentially toxic to liver; flammable
Halothane U.S.P. (Fluothane)	Volatile liquid; halogenated hydrocarbon	*See Drug Digest*	
Methoxyflurane N.F. (Penthrane)	Volatile liquid; halogenated ethylmethyl ether	Very potent anesthetic with prolonged analgesic effect; nonflammable and nonexplosive	Prolonged recovery from anesthesia; deep respiratory depression and hypotension at levels required for muscle relaxation; fatal liver and kidney damage have occurred
Nitrous oxide U.S.P. (Nitrogen monoxide)	Gas with little odor or taste; nonflammable	Produces good analgesia promptly and quick recovery; has no adverse effects on vital organs and does not cause nausea, vomiting, salivation, or respiratory tract irritation	Not a potent anesthetic or skeletal muscle relaxant; hypoxia occurs with high concentrations; low safe concentrations require supplementation by various other anesthetics, hypnotics, and relaxants
Trichloroethylene U.S.P. (Trilene; Trimar)	Volatile liquid with characteristic odor; halogenated hydrocarbon	Potent analgesic at safe levels of anesthesia; useful in obstetrics	Slow induction and recovery; not a good muscle relaxant; causes cardiac arrhythmias and rapid shallow breathing; potentially toxic to liver
Vinyl ether N.F. (Vinethene; divinyl oxide)	Volatile liquid chemically related to ether and ethylene	Rapid, smooth induction and recovery; potent analgesic for short operations and in obstetrics	Not a good skeletal muscle relaxant at safe levels; respiratory depression can develop rapidly; prolonged use may lead to liver damage

S U M M A R Y of Characteristics of Individual Anesthetics *(continued)*

Nonproprietary or Generic Name	Trade Name, Synonym, or Chemical Name	Chemical or Physical Characteristics	Remarks Concerning Clinical Status	
			ADVANTAGES	**DISADVANTAGES**
Intravenously and/or Rectally Administered Anesthetics (Basal Anesthetics)				
Hydroxydione sodium succinate	Viadril	Steroid solution (1%) for I.V. injection	Produces unconsciousness without depressing respiration or causing laryngospasm	Relatively slow onset and recovery compared to barbiturates; requires supplementation with potent analgesics, and skeletal muscle relaxants
Ketamine HCl	Ketalar; Ketaject	Phencyclidine (*non-barbiturate*) solution for I.V. and I.M. administration	Produces a dissociative state in which patient seems to be conscious but is unaware of pain in minor surgical and diagnostic procedures	May cause delirium or hallucinations during recovery; requires supplementation with muscle relaxants, nitrous oxide, and others, for major surgery
Methohexital sodium N.F.	Brevital sodium	Barbituate solution (1%) for I.V. use	Rapid onset of hypnosis with recovery of consciousness more rapid than with thiopental	Can cause respiratory depression and apnea; can cause laryngospasm, particularly in asthmatic patients; *not* a good analgesic or skeletal muscle relaxant
Thiamylal sodium N.F.	Surital sodium	Barbiturate solution (2.5%) for I.V. use	Similar to thiopental in its rapid onset and ultrashort recovery time	Similar to thiopental in its adverse effects upon respiratory system and lack of analgesic or skeletal muscle relaxant properties

		See *Drug Digest*
Thiopental sodium U.S.P.	Pentothal sodium	Barbiturate solution (2.5%) for I.V. use and 10% for rectal administration	Produces gradual basal narcosis without excitement; one of the first preanesthetic medications of this kind
Tribromoethanol solution N.F.	Avertin fluid	Brominated ethanol in amylene hydrate solution for rectal administration	Potentially toxic to heart and liver; rarely used today

Clinical Nursing Situation Concerning Preparation of the Patient for General Anesthesia

The Situation: You are caring for a patient who is to have a cholecystectomy. After the patient has received the preoperative medication she seems troubled and restless. Seeing you approach the patient, a colleague says, "Leave her alone so the medication can work."

The Problem: 1. Would you follow your colleague's advice? What would you do in this situation? Explain the rationale for your approach.

2. A few moments later the operating room calls for the patient. Would you: (1) ask the aide who is helping you to take the patient to the operating room (assisted by another aide, who works in the operating room) while you make the patient's bed, or (2) ask the aide to make the patient's bed while you accompany the patient and the O.R. aide to the operating room?

Explain the reason for your decision.

DRUG DIGEST

CYCLOPROPANE U.S.P. (Trimethylene)

Actions and Indications. This potent gas is capable of promptly producing complete anesthesia. Recovery is also rather rapid. It has a relatively wide safety margin when inhaled in amounts that give good analgesia and adequate muscle relaxation. It can be used prior to every kind of surgical operation and is said to be particularly useful for patients in shock because of the stability of the blood pressure. (The pressure may even rise slightly because of sympathetic nervous system stimulation.)

Side Effects, Cautions, and Contraindications. Postoperative headache is common, as is nausea and vomiting. Delirium may also develop during recovery, but it can be prevented by pretreatment with a potent analgesic. Respiratory acidosis sometimes occurs, and this, in turn, may lead to vasodilation, a fall in blood pressure, and reflex tachycardia.

Cardiac irregularities may be precipitated by the administration of epinephrine or other catecholamines and adrenergic vasopressor drugs, particularly if patients are not adequately oxygenated, or if carbon dioxide levels have been allowed to rise. This gas is flammable and explosive.

Dosage and Administration. The gas is administered by means of a closed or semiclosed system provided with carbon dioxide-absorbing chemicals. Induction of anesthesia may require 15 to 30 volumes-percent of gas, which may then be reduced to lower levels for maintaining adequate analgesia. The gas may have to be supplemented with a neuromuscular blocking agent when a lower volume-percent is employed. Atropine premedication is desirable.

ETHER U.S.P. (Ethyl ether; diethyl ether)

Actions and Indications. This potent general anesthetic produces excellent analgesia and skeletal muscle relaxation. It is a relatively safe agent because it rarely causes cardiac irregularities and does not damage the liver. Reflex stimulation of the respiratory and cardiovascular system is an added safety factor.

Side Effects, Cautions, and Contraindications. Ether irritates the respiratory mucosa and stimulates the flow of bronchial and salivary secretions. The induction of anesthesia is relatively slow, as is recovery. Postoperative nausea and vomiting is common, and gastrointestinal tone and motility are decreased. Ether is flammable and explosive.

Caution is required in administering adjunctive neuromuscular blocking agents in order to avoid excessive and prolonged skeletal muscle paralysis. Patients who have been receiving high doses of certain antibiotics such as kanamycin, polymyxin, and colistimethate, which also possess neuromuscular blocking properties, must also be carefully observed to avoid muscle paralysis.

Dosage and Administration. The amount of ether required varies depending upon the condition of the patient and the depth of anesthesia desired. The initially relatively high vapor concentrations required during induction are reduced for maintenance of surgical anesthesia.

Patients are commonly premedicated with atropine and sedative drugs to reduce induction stage difficulties, or they may first receive basal anesthetics such as thiopental or a nitrous oxide-oxygen mixture.

HALOTHANE U.S.P. (Fluothane)

Actions and Indications. The vapors of this nonflammable liquid produce rapid induction of anesthesia with little excitement, respiratory tract irritation, salivation, nausea, or vomiting. It tends to produce bronchodilation rather than bronchospasm. It may be used to lower blood pressure deliberately in order to produce a bloodless surgical field. Its relaxant effect on the uterine musculature may be useful in some obstetrical situations.

Side Effects, Cautions, and Contraindications. Halothane often produces hypotension and bradycardia, and occasionally causes cardiac arrhythmias, particularly in the presence of epinephrine and other catecholamines. Neuromuscular blocking agents of the tubocurarine type may intensify the fall in blood pressure, while use of succinylcholine may add to the drug's heart-slowing tendency.

Liver damage may occur, particularly if this anesthetic is employed repeatedly over a short period of time. Patients who develop fever and vomiting after exposure to halothane should not be anesthetized with it again, as fatal hepatic necrosis has occurred in such cases. Relaxation of the uterine musculature may inhibit normal labor.

Dosage and Administration. A special vaporizer is employed to control the concentration of vapors delivered to the lungs. Surgical levels of anesthesia are induced by administering a 2 to 2.5 percent concentration of the vapors in a stream of nitrous oxide-oxygen mixture. This is then reduced to a level of 0.5 to 1.5 percent for maintenance of anesthesia. Atropine premedication is desirable to prevent bradycardia. Intravenous barbiturates administered for basal narcosis reduce the concentration of halothane required for induction.

SODIUM THIOPENTAL U.S.P. (Pentothal sodium)

Actions and Indications. This rapid-acting drug causes unconsciousness within 30 to 60 seconds after intravenous administration of a hypnotic dose. It is used mainly for inducing light surgical anesthesia. However, it lacks good analgesic or skeletal muscle relaxing properties. Thus, it is rarely used alone, except in certain brief procedures lasting only about 15 minutes.

Thiopental is most commonly followed by administration of a more potent general anesthetic. The basal narcosis that it produces is also used to supplement nitrous oxide analgesia and regional anesthesia. It is also used to control drug-induced convulsions and in psychiatry for facilitating narcoanalysis procedures.

Side Effects, Cautions, and Contraindications. Overdosage can cause severe respiratory and myocardial depression and cardiac irregularities. Resuscitative equipment, including an endotracheal tube and oxygen, must always be available. The drug is employed with caution in patients with bronchial asthma, as they are most prone to develop laryngospasm, bronchospasm, and cough. Other conditions requiring caution are liver disease, myxedema, and increased intracranial pressure.

Dosage and Administration. For induction of anesthesia, 2 or 3 ml of a 2.5 percent solution (50-75 mg) may be administered intermittently at intervals of 30 to 60 seconds as needed. It may also be administered by the rectal route for preanesthetic hypnosis and basal narcosis in doses of about 1 g per 50 to 75 lbs. The total dose for children should not exceed 1 g, and for even large adults no more than 3 or 4 g should be given by this route.

SUCCINYLCHOLINE CHLORIDE U.S.P. (Anectine; Quelicin; Sucostrin)

Actions and Indications. This is the prototype neuromuscular blocking agent of the depolarizing or *non*-competitive type. After a brief period of muscular twitching or fasciculation, it produces flaccid paralysis. This is ordinarily of only short duration, but the drug-induced paralysis may be maintained by infusing the drug continuously at a slow rate.

It is best employed for producing skeletal muscle relaxation during short surgical procedures carried out at the light levels of anesthesia produced by nitrous oxide-oxygen inhalation and thiopental agents that do not give good muscle relaxation.

It is also employed clinically for facilitating endotracheal intubation by relaxing the muscles of the jaw and other structures, in orthopedic manipulations and ophthalmological surgery, and as part of the premedication of psychiatric patients prior to electroconvulsive therapy.

Side Effects, Cautions, and Contraindications. Patients may complain of muscle soreness caused by the initial contractions that often occur prior to the onset of paralysis. Cardiac slowing sometimes occurs as a result of stimulation of vagal neuroeffectors.

Respiratory paralysis *cannot* be treated with cholinergic drugs such as neostigmine. Thus, facilities must be available for intubation and for administration of oxygen by assisted or controlled respiration. Prolonged apnea sometimes occurs in patients who lack the enzyme that detoxifies this drug. The drug is contraindicated in patients with this hereditary enzyme defect and also in those weakened by malnutrition, anemia, or severe liver disease.

Dosage and Administration. Slow I.V. injection of a 0.1 percent solution in amounts of 10 to 40 mg produces prompt muscle relaxation. This lasts only about two to five minutes, but paralysis may be maintained by prolonged infusion at a carefully adjusted rate.

TUBOCURARINE CHLORIDE U.S.P. (Tubarine; Tubadil)

Actions and Indications. This curare alkaloid salt is the prototype neuromuscular blocking agent of the competitive or *non*depolarizing type. It produces muscular relaxation and flaccid paralysis by preventing the motor end plates of skeletal muscle fibers from reacting to acetylcholine. (This neurohormone normally transmits motor nerve impulses when it is released from somatic motor nerve endings and makes contact with the motor end plates.)

Tubocurarine is used mainly as an adjunct to general anesthetics. Its supplementary use in combination with anesthetics that are not good skeletal muscle relaxants produces abdominal muscle paralysis of a degree that permits performance of major surgical procedures at relatively light levels of anesthesia. It has also been employed recently in the management of patients with tetanus to control convulsive spasms by producing continuous paralysis.

Side Effects, Cautions, and Contraindications. This drug is administered only by anesthesiologists and others especially trained to use equipment for maintaining the patient's pulmonary ventilation mechanically during periods of drug-induced respiratory muscle paralysis.

Tubocurarine sometimes causes cardiovascular collapse, not only secondary to apnea and hypoxia, but also because it may interfere with sympathetic ganglion transmission of vasomotor impulses. It may also cause release of histamine in the tissues and thus cause further vasodilation as well as bronchoconstriction (particularly in patients with bronchial asthma).

Dosage and Administration. Dosage varies in each individual situation. Most commonly a dose of 6 to 9 mg is slowly injected by vein over a period of 30 to 90 seconds. Supplementary doses of 3 to 5 mg may be added as needed.

References

GENERAL ANESTHESIA

Adriani, J. Some newer anesthetic agents. *Amer. J. Nurs.*, 61:60, 1961.

Adriani, J., and Zepernick, R. Anesthesia for infants and children. *Amer. J. Nurs.*, 64: 107, 1964.

Rapper, E.M. The pharmacologic basis of anesthesiology. *Clin. Pharmacol. Ther.*, 2: 141, 1961.

Rodman, M.J. Drugs used in anesthesia. *RN*, 33:53, 1970 (July).

Weaver, D.C. Preventing aspiration deaths during anesthesia. *JAMA*, 188:971, 1964.

Woolbridge, P.D. The components of general anesthesia. *JAMA*, 186:641, 1963.

NEUROMUSCULAR BLOCKING AGENTS

Foldes, F.F. The pharmacology of neuromuscular blocking agents in man. *Clin. Pharmacol. Ther.*, 1:345, 1960.

Friend, D.G. Pharmacology of muscle relaxants. *Clin. Pharmacol. Ther.*, 5:871, 1964.

Levine, I.M. Muscle relaxants in neurospastic diseases. *Med. Clin. N. Amer.*, 45:1017, 1961.

McIntyre, A.R. Some physiological effects of curare and their application to clinical medicine. *Physiol. Rev.*, 27:464, 1947.

Rodman, M.J. Drugs for treating tetanus. *RN*, 34:43, 1971 (Dec.).

15.

Local Anesthetics

General Considerations

Local anesthetics are drugs that prevent the patient from feeling pain when they are applied to parts of the peripheral nervous system. Depending on which portion of this system's nerve roots and fibers is affected, the loss of sensation may be limited to a small part of the body or involve quite a large area. However, unlike the general anesthetics, these drugs are *not* used clinically to cause unconsciousness.

The effects of local anesthetics are not necessarily limited to the sensory fibers alone. When these drugs are brought into direct contact with other parts of mixed spinal nerves, they can also affect the functioning of somatic motor and sympathetic efferent nerve fibers. This can then interfere with the tone of the skeletal and smooth muscles innervated by these nerves.

In addition, local anesthetics that are systemically absorbed from the site of their application may be carried by the bloodstream to the brain, heart, liver, and other organs. The effects of these drugs on the central nervous system and the circulatory system can then cause serious toxic reactions (see *Summary*, p. 197).

Thus, the anesthesiologist employs special techniques of administration. These are intended to: (1) place the local anesthetic solution at some precise local point along the course of the peripheral nerves; and (2) to keep the drug's systemic absorption at a rate so slow that it does not build up to toxic levels.

Techniques of Administration

Three general procedures are employed to bring local anesthetics into contact with nerve endings, nerve roots, or along the nerve fibers, or trunks, that run between the nerve's root and its ending. These are:

(1) *Topical application* to nerve endings in mucous membranes or broken skin.

(2) *Infiltration* along the line of a surgical incision or deep into the structures within the wound. (This affects local nerve endings but not nerve trunks.)

(3) *Regional or conduction anesthesia* is carried out, *not* in the surgical field itself, but by injections made into or around the nerve or group of nerves that supply the area in which the operation is to be performed.

Nerve blocks of this kind differ depending upon the anatomic point at which the solution of the local anesthetic is injected. Some are called peripheral nerve blocks, because specific nerves such as the sciatic-femoral, ulnar, or intercostal nerves, or the brachial plexus are blocked. Others are called central nerve blocks, because injections are made close to the spinal cord portion of the cerebrospinal axis—the central nervous system. Spinal anesthesia (see below, p. 194) is one form of central nerve block; caudal anesthesia is another example of this kind of conduction anesthesia.

Types of Local Anesthetics

Hundreds of chemicals have the ability to interfere with the conduction of impulses in nervous tissue. However, only relatively few of these compounds have proved clinically useful. Those that are available differ in several of their pharmacological properties and in their suitability for use in different clinical situations. Thus, the doctor tries to select the local anesthetic that seems most suitable for each surgical procedure or medical disorder.

Before discussing the clinical applications of this class of drugs, we shall briefly mention some significant differences in the properties of individual drugs (see Table 15-1).

TABLE 15-1 *Drugs Used for Local Anesthesia*

Nonproprietary or Generic Name	Trade Name	Main Use* and Maximal Dose†	Remarks
Benoxinate HCl	Dorsacaine	Topical	Used for opthalmic anesthesia
Benzocaine N.F.	Ethyl aminobenzoate; Anesthesin; and others	Topical	Used on broken skin and on mucous membranes
Butacaine sulfate	Butyn sulfate	Topical	Rapid and long action in eye, nose, and throat
Bupivacaine	Marcaine	Infiltration and conduction; 15–25 mg	Produces long-lasting nerve blocks in obstetrical and surgical procedures
Butethamine HCl N.F.	Monocaine	Infiltration and conduction; 100–150 mg	Used as a spinal anesthetic more active than procaine
Butyl aminobenzoate N.F.	Butesin	Topical	Used on burns and broken skin
Chloroprocaine HCl N.F.	Nesacaine	Infiltration and conduction; 750–1000 mg	More potent and less toxic than procaine
Cocaine N.F. and Cocaine HCl U.S.P.	. . . . . .	Topical; 150 mg	See *Drug Digest*
Cyclomethycaine sulfate	Surfacaine	Topical; 750 mg	Used on urethral, rectal, and vaginal mucosa, as well as on broken skin
Dibucaine HCl U.S.P.	Nupercaine HCl	Topically, and by infiltration and conduction; 7.5–100 mg	Most potent, toxic, and long-lasting spinal and surface anesthetic action

T A B L E   1 5 - 1   *(Continued)*

Nonproprietary or Generic Name	Trade Name	Main Use* and Maximal Dose†	Remarks
Dimethisoquin HCl N.F.	Quotane	Topical	Used as anogenital antipruritic, and for skin lesion pain relief
Diperodon	Diothane	Topical	Claimed as potent as cocaine and longer-lasting for surface anesthesia
Dyclonine HCl	Dyclone	Topical	Used to deaden mucous membranes prior to endoscopy
Ethyl chloride U.S.P.	Monochlorethane; Kelene	Topical	Sprayed on skin prior to making incisions
Hexylcaine HCl N.F.	Cyclaine	Infiltration and conduction; 250–500 mg	Used topically prior to intubations and for spinal anesthesia more prolonged than with procaine
Lidocaine HCl U.S.P.	Xylocaine	Infiltration and conduction; 200–500 mg	See *Drug Digest*
Mepivacaine HCl N.F.	Carbocaine	Infiltration and conduction; 100–400 mg	Claimed more rapid and longer-acting than lidocaine
Oxethazaine	Oxaine	Topical	Claimed to relieve gastritis and peptic ulcer pain when swallowed
Phenacaine HCl N.F.	Holocaine	Topical	Used mainly in the eye
Piperocaine HCl	Metycaine	Topical and infiltration; 50–300 mg	More potent than procaine but also more toxic
Pramoxine HCl N.F.	Tronothane	Topical	Used on broken skin and on anogenital membranes but not in the eye or nose
Prilocaine HCl	Citanest	Infiltration and conduction; 200–600 mg	Claimed as effective as lidocaine for nerve block procedures
Procaine HCl U.S.P.	Novocaine	Infiltration and conduction; 150–1,000 mg	See *Drug Digest*
Proparacaine HCl U.S.P.	Ophthaine	Topical	Rapid but short ocular anesthesia
Propoxycaine HCl N.F.	Blockaine	Infiltration and conduction; 20–200 mg	More intensive and prolonged action than procaine
Pyrrocaine HCl	Dynacaine	Infiltration and conduction; 20–200 mg	Rapid onset and long duration of action in dental and other peripheral nerve blocks
Tetracaine HCl U.S.P.	Pontocaine	Infiltration and conduction; 4–100 mg	See *Drug Digest*

* Agents for topical use may, in some cases, be applied only to the eye or only to the skin; in other cases, these agents are also administered by injection.

† Lower doses apply usually to concentrated solutions for conduction anesthesia or to application to respiratory and urethral mucosa; higher doses apply to infiltration of tissues with much more dilute solutions.

Cocaine+, an alkaloid extracted from the leaves of the South American coca shrub, was the first important local anesthetic. It was first found useful for relief of pain when applied to the conjunctiva prior to eye surgery. However, its high toxicity and addictive properties upon injection limited its usefulness. This led to efforts to synthesize safer local anesthetics.

Procaine+ (Novocaine), one of the first synthetic compounds, is an anesthetic of relatively low toxicity. Unlike cocaine, it is not very effective when applied to the mucosa of the eye. When injected, it is rather rapidly destroyed. Thus, compounds of the same chemical series were sought which would have a more prolonged duration of action.

Tetracaine+ (Pontocaine), a chemical relative of procaine, exerts an anesthetic effect that is more than twice as long as the prototype drug. It is commonly employed for producing spinal anesthesia.

Dibucaine (Nupercaine), mepivacaine (Carbocaine), bupivacaine (Marcaine), and prilocaine (Citanest) are other drugs with a prolonged duration of action when injected to produce peripheral and central nerve blocks.

Lidocaine+ (Xylocaine) is one of the most versatile of the potent long-lasting local anesthetics. It is available in many pharmaceutical forms for use in every kind of injection procedure and for topical application to the skin and to the mucous membranes of the eye, nose, throat, and even of the gastrointestinal tract.

Proparacaine (Ophthaine) and benoxinate (Dorsacaine) are particularly useful for application to the surface of the eye. Unlike cocaine and other topically effective agents, these newer compounds cause relatively little ocular irritation.

Dimethisoquin (Quotane) is considered too irritating for use in the eye. However, it is safe and effective enough when applied to other less sensitive mucosal surfaces or to the skin. Pramoxine (Tronothane) is another effective surface anesthetic used in similar clinical situations. Cyclomethycaine (Surfacaine) is, like procaine, poorly absorbed when applied to the mucosa of the eye, mouth, or nose, but it can penetrate the rectal and urethral mucosa to reach and anesthetize nerve endings.

Benzocaine (Anesthesin; and others) and butyl aminobenzoate (Butesin) exert a relatively long-lasting local anesthetic action when applied to broken skin. This is because they are only slightly soluble and thus are not swept away by the blood and other body fluids.

Clinical Applications of Local Anesthetics

TOPICAL BLOCKS (SURFACE ANESTHESIA)

The skin, when damaged or diseased, permits penetration of topically applied local anesthetics. The drugs' action on nerve endings then deadens pain and itch sensations. Thus, drugs such as dimethisoquin, pramoxine, and benzocaine (see above) offer effective relief in many dermatological disorders that are marked by minor but annoying symptoms.

Among the skin conditions in which topical anesthetics of this kind are employed are: dermatoses marked by pruritis, including poison ivy; burns, including sunburn; fissured nipples in the postpartum period; ulcerations, abrasions, and lacerations from minor injuries; and painful surgical incisions, such as following an episiotomy.

Pain and itching of the anogenital area may also be relieved by application of local anesthetic creams, ointments, jellies, or suppositories. Thus, these products are employed for pruritus ani or vulvae, and following hemorrhoidectomy or repair of fissure in ano, or in other proctologic procedures involving the skin and perianal mucosa.

Adverse reactions of the systemic toxicity type (see p. 196) are rare with these poorly absorbable agents. However, allergic reactions can occur in patients who have become sensitized to topically applied local anesthetics. Thus, the long-term use of these drugs in chronic dermatoses is not advisable, particularly in patients with atopic dermatitis.

If signs such as redness, swelling, oozing, and pain develop during use of a topical anesthetic, treatment is discontinued. (Sometimes, a local anesthetic of a different chemical class can be substituted, but patients whose skin is predisposed to react to chemicals can become sensitized to any of these agents.)

The ocular mucosa can be deadened readily by eye drops containing topical anesthetics. Surface anesthesia produced by proparacaine or benoxinate (see above) or by butacaine or dibucaine permits removal of foreign bodies from the cornea. Drops are also applied to the conjunctiva prior to performance of such ophthalmological diagnostic procedures as tonometry and gonioscopy, or diagnostic conjunctival scraping.

Simple surgical procedures such as the opening of a small sty, or eyelid tumor (chalazion), can be carried out after topical application of a soluble anesthetic. More complicated ocular surgery such as cataract removal or iridectomy requires retrobulbar injection of local anesthetics. Such injections are made only after the conjunctiva and cornea are first desensitized by surface anesthesia.

Local irritation limits the usefulness of some agents for these purposes. Cocaine, for example, can cause dryness and other damage to the epithelium of the cornea. The newer ophthalmic anesthetics cause little early stinging or burning, and their use is rarely followed by the clouding, pitting, or ulceration of the cornea sometimes seen with cocaine.

Other mucous membranes, including those of the tracheobronchial, gastrointestinal, and genitourinary tracts are also often anesthetized with local anesthetic solutions that penetrate to the free nerve endings just below the mucosal surface. The resulting reduction in sensation is useful for facilitating passage of instruments and for relief of pain.

The mouth, throat, and upper gastrointestinal tract may be anesthetized by swishing and then swallowing a viscous solution of *lidocaine* or by gargling with a solution of *dyclonine* or other surface anesthetic. This helps to reduce irritation in inflamed oral mucous membranes or to relieve the pain following dental procedures or tonsillectomy. Local anesthesia is also attained by spraying or swabbing the throat prior to passage of a tube down the esophagus for endoscopy.

Endotracheal intubation of patients who require support of respiration is also made easier by reducing the reflex activity that results in gagging and bucking. This is done by spraying the larynx and trachea with a fine aerosol of a local anesthetic solution. This procedure is also used prior to broncoscopy to prevent laryngeal spasm, coughing, and the dangerous heart-slowing reflexes that are sometimes set off when a tube is introduced into the throat.

Absorption of the local anesthetic from these membrane surfaces or those of the genitourinary tract (following instillation into the urethra or bladder before cystoscopy) may be dangerously rapid. A sudden rise in the blood levels of certain local anesthetics can cause systemic toxicity similar to that seen with accidental intravenous administration (see p. 196).

This hazard may be reduced by use of the smallest amount of the lowest concentration of local anesthetic needed to deaden mucosal nerve endings. The anesthesiologist may also have the nurse keep a record of the actual amount of anesthetic (in milligrams) that has been administered in the fine spray or instilled as a solution. She also often has this responsibility when local anesthetics are being administered by the infiltration method.

LOCAL INFILTRATION AND FIELD BLOCKS*

The injection of local anesthetics can also result in pharmacological effects that are not limited to local sites. Solutions injected into or under the skin and into muscles to anesthetize the nerve fibers in these tissues are, before long, absorbed into the systemic circulation. If the plasma level rises too rapidly, the anesthetic can adversely affect the functioning of the heart, brain, and other tissues.

Local infiltration of a highly vascular area such as the scalp or face with a too concentrated solution of a local anesthetic can lead to absorption of toxic doses of the drug. Similarly, during the performance of extensive *field blocks* in preparation for major surgery, large amounts of solution may have to be injected. Thus, care is required to avoid the absorption of high doses of these drugs at a rate so rapid that adverse systemic reactions develop.

Precautions employed to prevent rapid systemic absorption from the skin, subcutaneous tissues, fascia, and muscles, or accidental I.V. injection, include the following:

1. Injecting only the least amount of the most dilute solution that is effective for anesthesia.

2. Aspiration is performed in several injection planes to be sure that the needle has not entered a blood vessel, or the needle and syringe are kept moving back and forth constantly during field block or local infiltration

---

* Field block is a form of peripheral nerve block in which the nerve pathways from an operative field are blocked off by a wall of injected local anesthetic solution. It differs from local infiltration, in which the solution is injected directly into the operative area, and it differs also from ordinary nerve blocks because it is *not* aimed at any specific individual nerve but at all the nerves that lie within the circular ring of local anesthetic injections made around the surgical site.

to ensure against the needle's staying in any vein that it may accidentally enter.

3. Injections are not made haphazardly, but solutions are instead placed systematically in intradermal, then subcutaneous, and finally intrafascial and intramuscular sites.

4. A record is kept of the total amount of solution that has been injected, and the actual number of milligrams that have been administered is calculated. Thus, the total dose is kept constantly within safe limits for the particular anesthetic that is being employed.

5. Enough time is allowed to elapse for the drug's local action to take effect and for any systemically absorbed drug to be largely eliminated before further injections are made.

6. Observations are made of the patient's behavior, and his pulse, blood pressure, and rate of respiration are carefully watched.

7. Vasoconstrictor drugs such as epinephrine are added in low concentrations to local anesthetic solutions in order to: (1) reduce the rate of systemic absorption and toxicity; and (2) to prolong the local block of nerve conduction.

Solutions that contain epinephrine in a 1:100,000 concentration are used in areas rich in blood vessels such as the scalp and face; for less vascular areas such as the skin of the back or the extremities, more dilute solutions (for example, 1:200,000) are adequate.

Higher concentrations of epinephrine are no more effective for these purposes and can cause adrenergic side effects such as a rise in blood pressure, tachycardia, tremors, and nervousness. Vasoconstrictors are *not* added to local anesthetic solutions that are to be used for infiltrating areas of relatively restricted circulation such as the fingers, toes, tip of the nose, ears, or penis. Excessive local ischemia and vasospasm in such areas could result in gangrene.

CENTRAL NERVE BLOCKS

Regional anesthesia of extensive areas can be obtained by injecting local anesthetic solutions at points close to where the spinal nerves emerge from the cord. *Conduction anesthesia* of this kind includes spinal, saddle, epidural, and caudal blocks—terms that refer mainly to the anatomical sites at which the injections are made.

SPINAL ANESTHESIA. Spinal anesthesia is induced by introducing the needle between two lumbar vertebrae, puncturing the dural and subarachnoid membranes, and injecting the local anesthetic solution into the spinal fluid in the subarachnoid space (Fig. 15-1). The drug blocks conduction quickly in spinal nerve roots but has little effect on the spinal cord itself.

All three types of fibers—autonomic, sensory, and motor—can be blocked. As the drug's effects come on, the patient first loses the ability to perceive pain. A little later the skeletal muscles become relaxed and paralyzed. This and autonomic blockade may bring about blood pressure changes (see below). Muscle tone and sensation return in reverse order as the drug's effects wear off.

Spinal anesthesia is most useful for surgery of the lower extremities and the lower abdomen. It is preferred to inhalation anesthesia for patients with asthma, emphysema, and other pulmonary diseases which might be made worse by the irritating action of some volatile agents. Elderly patients with cardiac or renal disease, and also diabetics, may do better with spinal rather than general anesthesia. For emergency surgery in patients who have eaten recently and have a full stomach, spinal anesthesia is indicated.

COMPLICATIONS. Spinal anesthesia requires strict adherence to a careful routine in order to avoid complications during and after the procedure. For example, the patient must be carefully positioned so that the injected local anesthetic solution does not diffuse upward to block the medullary respiratory center or the roots of the phrenic and intercostal nerves, which control the movements of the diaphragm and other respiratory muscles.

In addition to possible respiratory complications, spinal anesthesia is often accompanied by sharp drops in blood pressure. Hypotension is, in part, the result of blockade of sympathetic vasomotor nerve fibers in the spinal nerves. Reduction in the flow of vasoconstrictor impulses to the arterioles leads to dilatation of these blood vessels and a steady fall in pressure. Other factors, including muscular relaxation and cardiac slowing, contribute to this hypotensive reaction to spinal anesthesia. Blood pressure falls may be prevented or counteracted by the prior administration of long-acting vasopressor amines such as ephedrine, phenylephrine, and methoxamine.

It is usually necessary to give the patient sedative premedication to prevent the natural

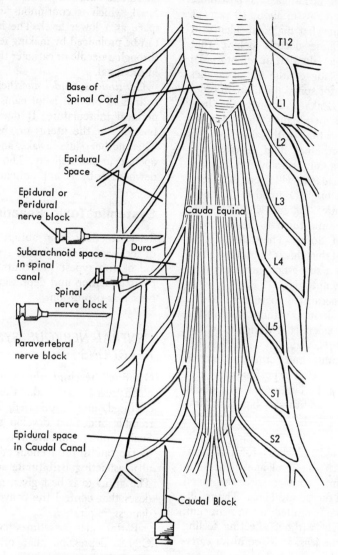

Fig. 15-1. Sites of injection for spinal anesthesia, showing position of needle for spinal and epidural types. Letters indicate vertebral level of injection.

anxiety he may feel when fully awake during procedures carried out under regional anesthesia. Of course, patients who would be extremely apprehensive should be given general anesthesia; or, if the potent inhalation anesthetics are contraindicated, basal anesthesia with a barbiturate may be employed prior to spinal anesthesia. If the patient is only lightly sedated, all operating room personnel should be careful not to say anything that might upset him.

POSTSPINAL AFTEREFFECTS. Neurological complications occur only rarely today and then mostly in people for whom spinal anesthesia was undesirable because of some preexisting vertebral or spinal nerve abnormality. However, patients often fear that they have suffered a spinal injury when they find themselves unable to move their legs after spinal anesthesia. Therefore, it is important to explain in advance that this will occur and will last only a short while. Similarly, patients should also be told to expect feelings of numbness and "pins and needles" as sensation returns and that this will shortly disappear. Sometimes nerve palsies and paresthesias of longer duration occur, but even these are usually minor and transient.

A more common occurrence is postspinal headache, which develops in about 10 percent of cases, with a somewhat higher incidence in women patients. Some doctors believe that these are caused by a reduction in cerebrospinal fluid pressure. They suggest the use of needles of narrow diameter for spinal puncture in order to minimize fluid leakage through the hole made in the dural membrane. They also advise hydrating the patient with saline solution to keep his cerebrospinal fluid pressure up.

A measure commonly employed to reduce the chances that headache will occur is to keep the patient flat on his back for 6 to 12 hours after spinal procedures. Patients should be told that their doctor wants them to lie flat for a specific number of hours. They should not, however, be warned that this is to prevent headache, because such a suggestion may only help to bring on this symptom.

The patient is permitted to turn from side to side, if he so desires, without raising his head. The use of siderails is desirable in the care of these patients, who may be drowsy because of barbiturates and other adjunctive medications; yet this detail of postoperative care may be overlooked because the patient under conduction anesthesia has not lost consciousness.

SADDLE BLOCK. Saddle block is a form of spinal anesthesia in which the local anesthetic solution is brought into contact with the sacral nerves that run to the perineal area. The resulting loss of sensation is limited to the perineum, buttocks, and thighs without affecting feeling or movement in the legs. It is useful for carrying out obstetrical procedures during the second stage of labor and delivery, and for gynecological, urological, and rectal surgery.

EPIDURAL (PERIDURAL) ANESTHESIA. Epidural, or peridural, anesthesia is induced by inserting the needle in the same way as in spinal anesthesia, but without breaking through the spinal dural membrane. The space between the dura and the spinal canal's periosteal lining (the epidural space) is then flooded with local anesthetic solution. This results in block of conduction in the spinal nerves without some of the complications that can occur when the dura is penetrated in spinal (subdural) block.

CAUDAL ANESTHESIA. Caudal anesthesia is a form of epidural block in which the local anesthetic solution is deposited in the sacral canal, which is continuous with the epidural space at a lower level. The block that results can be prolonged by making repeated injections through a needle or catheter that is left in place in the canal.

Continuous caudal anesthesia is used in obstetrics to prevent labor pains and to relax the perineal musculature. It does not affect contractions of the uterus or abdominal muscles. The mother stays awake and is able to cooperate in the delivery. The breathing of the newborn baby is not ordinarily depressed.

Systemic Toxic Reactions

Toxic reactions from abrupt rises in the level of local anesthetics in the systemic circulation are of two types: (1) central nervous system overstimulation and depression; and (2) cardiovascular depression.

CENTRAL NERVOUS SYSTEM REACTIONS

Overdoses reaching the brain by way of the bloodstream may make the patient nervous, confused, and disoriented; he may begin to tremble and then develop convulsive spasms. Such motor stimulation is best counteracted by the careful intravenous administration of an ultrafast-acting barbiturate such as thiopental. The antidote is best given repeatedly in small doses that control the convulsions but do not depress respiration.

Barbiturates sometimes tend to intensify the C.N.S. depression that often follows initial nervous system stimulation by local anesthetics. Such a double depressant action could result in coma and respiratory failure. Consequently, facilities and equipment for administering oxygen should always be available when local anesthetics are employed in infiltration, conduction, and respiratory tract spraying procedures.

CARDIOVASCULAR REACTIONS

Administration of oxygen and manual massage of the heart may revive the rare patient who suffers cardiac arrest from rapid delivery to the myocardium of a large dose of an absorbed anesthetic. In such cases, cardiac standstill may occur with dramatic suddenness and require the use of immediate heroic measures.

Other circulatory collapse, caused more by

vasodilatation than by myocardial depression, is slower in onset and easier to correct when the warning signs are noted in time. The patient, in these cases, may turn pale and get drowsy or dizzy; his heart may race, but the beats become progressively fainter until finally the pulse cannot be felt, and he becomes comatose. This vascular reaction—the result of direct depression of arteriolar smooth muscle—is best treated in the same way as the hypotensive reactions of spinal anesthesia; that is by parenteral administration of sympathomimetic vasopressor substances, such as ephedrine, phenylephrine, or methoxamine.

S U M M A R Y of Toxic Reactions to Local Anesthetic Drugs

Central Nervous System Reactions

Stimulation. Excitement marked by nervousness, apprehension, disorientation, confusion, and, possibly, dizziness, vertigo, nausea, and vomiting. This may be followed by tremors and tonic-clonic convulsions.

Depression. Convulsions may be quickly followed by loss of reflexes, coma, and respiratory depression and failure.

Cardiovascular Reactions

Hypotensive Reaction. Blood pressure falls gradually or abruptly. Patient shows pallor and may complain of feeling faint and dizzy; cardiac palpitations occur when the heart reflexly speeds up. Patient may become drowsy and pass into comatose state as blood pressure falls to shock levels.

Cardiac Reaction. Heart rate may slow down markedly; pulse pressure is reduced. Cardiac standstill or ventricular fibrillation may develop suddenly.

Miscellaneous Reactions

Allergic Reactions. Skin rashes, urticaria, bronchospasm, and laryngeal edema may develop in sensitized individuals.

Local Tissue Damage. Application of cocaine and other topical anesthetics may cause itching, burning, redness, and possible corneal ulcerations.

Postspinal Sequelae. Headaches and, occasionally, paresthesias (numbness and tingling), palsies, and paraplegia.

S U M M A R Y of Cautions and Contraindications in the Administration of Local Anesthetics

Local anesthetics should be used in the lowest concentration and amount of solution that will produce the desired degree of blockade.

The total amount of the local anesthetic agent (in mg) should be recorded each time a solution is injected or applied, and the maximum safe dose for each agent should not be exceeded.

Local anesthetic solutions should not be injected into areas of infection or applied to traumatized mucous membranes.

Injections of local anesthetics should always be made slowly and cautiously and the syringe plunger should be pulled back periodically. If blood is aspirated, the needle should be withdrawn and the injection made in another area.

Epinephrine or a similar sympathomimetic vasoconstrictor drug should be added to delay systemic absorption of the local anesthetic, except when patients are known to react adversely to epinephrine-type agents (for example, severe cardiovascular disease), or in areas with relatively restricted circulation.

Patients should be placed in proper position for injection of spinal anesthetics to avoid upward diffusion of the anesthetic in the spinal fluid.

Patients should be kept lying flat or with head down (Trendelenburg position) after spinal anesthesia. (This and the use of a narrow gauge needle may minimize postspinal headache.)

Oxygen, rapid-acting barbiturates, and vasopressor drugs, together with apparatus for their proper administration, should be readily available whenever any procedure utilizing local anesthetics is to be carried out.

S U M M A R Y of Points for the Nurse to Remember Concerning Local Anesthetics

Be particularly careful during procedures conducted under local anesthesia to assure that nothing is said that may be upsetting to the patient.

Use suitable nursing intervention measures to make it easier for the patient to tolerate the procedure for which employment of a local anesthetic is necessary. This may help to lessen the amount of local anesthetic that has to be used, and this in turn may reduce systemic side effects.

Remember to explain to the patient who has had spinal anesthesia that his legs will feel numb until the effects of the anesthetic have worn off. This may help to allay unnecessary concern during the hour or more it often takes for full feeling to return after the operation.

Instruct patients to seek medical assistance instead of relying on local anesthetic preparations to allay skin irritation or chronic anal or vaginal pruritus, as extended use of such products for palliative purposes over long periods may result in allergic reactions.

Clinical Nursing Situations Concerning Local Anesthesia

1. *The Situation:* Twelve-year-old Johnny severely cut his hand while building a tree house. His mother, accompanied by a neighbor, rushed him to the emergency room of the hospital, with his hand bleeding severely.

The Problem: Describe the actions you would take when admitting Johnny to the emergency room, and while assisting the physician with administration of a local anesthetic and with care of the wound.

2. *The Situation:* Mr. Robertson has had an appendectomy performed under spinal anesthesia. Approximately two hours after the operation, Mr. Robertson asks "May I have the head of my bed rolled up?" and "Why do my legs feel numb?"

The Problem: How would you answer each of his questions?

D R U G   D I G E S T

COCAINE HCl U.S.P. AND COCAINE N.F.

Actions and Indications. This alkaloid obtained from the coca shrub was the first clinically important local anesthetic. It is also a potent psychomotor stimulant and possesses sympathomimetic properties upon injection.

Cocaine is used mainly for producing topical anesthesia when applied to mucous membranes. It may be sprayed into the throat and tracheobronchial tree prior to passage of an endotracheal tube. Dropped into the eye, it produces prompt surface anesthesia, vasoconstriction, and mydriasis.

Side Effects, Cautions, and Contraindications. Pupillary dilatation may be a drawback, particularly in patients with narrow-angle glaucoma. Dryness and damage to the cornea (clouding, stippled pitting, and ulcerations) may occur following topical application. The patient's eye should be kept well irrigated with saline solution during the time that the protective wink reflex is inactive.

This drug is not administered by injection as its systemic absorption can result in a marked rise in blood pressure, tachycardia, tremors, and possible convulsive seizures and respiratory failure. This drug can cause psychological, and possibly physical, dependence. Thus, it is handled in accordance with regulations for control of dangerous drugs.

Dosage and Administration. For topical application to the nasal and pharyngeal mucosa 5 to 10 percent solutions are employed. Lower concentrations (1 to 2 percent) are used for surface anesthesia of the urethra, and solutions as dilute as 0.25 to 0.5 percent are effective for anesthetizing the cornea, although higher concentrations are often used.

LIDOCAINE HCl U.S.P. (Xylocaine)

Actions and Indications. This versatile local anesthetic is used for local infiltration, peripheral nerve blocks, and central (epidural, caudal, spinal) nerve blocks. It is also effective when applied topically to the mucous membranes of the mouth and throat, anorectal area, urethra, and skin for relief of pain and itching, and for facilitating instrumentations in endoscopy. A form for intravenous administration is employed in the management of cardiac arrhythmias.

Side Effects, Cautions, and Contraindications. Injections are made slowly with frequent aspirations to minimize inadvertent intravascular administration and possible systemic reactions. These include signs of stimulation *or* depression of the central nervous system such as drowsiness, dizziness, tremors, convulsions, unconsciousness, and respiratory arrest. Cardiovascular toxicity includes hypotension, bradycardia, or cardiac arrest.

This drug is contraindicated in patients hypersensitive to local anesthetics of the amide type. Allergic reactions involve mainly the skin, but may also be of the systemic anaphylactoid type.

Dosage and Administration. Injections are made with 1 to 5 percent solutions in amounts that vary widely depending upon the procedure. Total doses of solutions administered without epinephrine should not exceed 300 mg; with epinephrine, the maximum recommended dose is 500 mg, or no more than 7 mg/kg of body weight.

This anesthetic is applied topically to the skin and mucous membranes in the form of ointments (2 percent or 5 percent); as a jelly (20 mg/ml); in suppositories (100 mg); and as a viscous solution (2 percent).

PROCAINE HCl U.S.P. (Novocaine)

Actions and Indications. This prototype local anesthetic is rapidly effective when injected, but it is not effective as a topical anesthetic. Its duration of action is relatively short, but it can be lengthened considerably by the addition of a low concentration of epinephrine. It is used for peripheral and central nerve blocks prior to surgery, and in various diagnostic and therapeutic procedures.

Side Effects, Cautions, and Contraindications. Procaine possesses relatively low local and systemic toxicity. Injections are not irritating to soft tissues or nerves. The absorbed drug is rapidly destroyed by circulating enzymes before high blood levels are reached.

However, inadvertent intravenous administration, and injection of single doses above 1,000 mg, can cause central and cardiovascular toxicity. Central stimulation may be manifested by mental effects such as nervousness, or motor system toxicity, including tremors, muscle twitching, or convulsive spasms. Cardiovascular toxicity includes hypotension, bradycardia, and possible cardiac arrest.

Dosage and Administration. Local infiltration and field block is carried out with solutions of 0.5 to 1 percent in amounts up to 1,000 mg, or 300 ml. Solutions of 1 to 2 percent are employed for central nerve block procedures. The total dose for spinal anesthesia is 50 to 200 mg injected intrathecally. For intravenous anesthesia, a 0.1 percent or 0.2 percent solution is infused slowly at a rate of 10 to 15 ml per minute for several hours.

TETRACAINE HCl U.S.P. (Pontocaine)

Actions and Indications. This is a potent, long-acting spinal anesthetic that is particularly useful for prolonged (two- to three-hour) surgical operations. Because analgesia may last as long as five or six hours, its use reduces the need for potent narcotic analgesics postoperatively. The onset of anesthesia is relatively slow (15 to 45 minutes). This local anesthetic may also be used for infiltration and for peripheral nerve blocks, as well as for epidural, including caudal, anesthesia and as a surface anesthetic in the eye, nose, and throat or on the skin.

Side Effects, Cautions, and Contraindications. This anesthetic is about ten times as toxic as procaine but, because it is effective at about one tenth the dose of procaine, it can be used in solutions of low concentration that are safe when precautions for preventing too rapid systemic absorption are employed.

The chief adverse effect is spinal anesthesia is hypotension as a result of depression of conduction in vasomotor fibers. A marked decrease in blood pressure may be manifested by pallor, sweating, restlessness, and vomiting. It should be treated by administration of vasopressor drugs. Oxygen and equipment for artificial respiration should be available for counteracting the effects of respiratory motor nerve or center paralysis from upward diffusion of the anesthetic.

Dosage and Administration. Dilute solutions (0.1 to 0.25 percent) are employed for local infiltration in amounts that should not ordinarily exceed 100 mg. For spinal anesthesia, doses of no more than 15 mg are employed. Topical application of 0.1 ml of a 0.5 percent solution is sufficient for surface anesthesia. A 2 percent solution may be applied to the nose and throat in an amount of 1 ml. Ointments of 0.5 to 1 percent are available for application to the skin.

References

Adriani, J. Local anesthetics. *Amer. J. Nurs.,* 59:86, 1959.
———. Clinical effectiveness of drugs used for topical anesthesia. *JAMA,* 188:711, 1964.
——— et al. The comparative potency and effectiveness of topical anesthetics in man. *Clin. Pharmacol. Therap.,* 5:49, 1964.
Covino, B.G. Comparative clinical pharmacology of local anesthetic agents. *Anesthesiology,* 35:158, 1971.

———. Local anesthesia. *New Eng. J. Med.,* 286:975, 1035, 1972.
Lowenthal, W. Factors affecting drug absorption. *Amer. J. Nurs.,* 71:1391, 1973.
Moore, D.C., and Bridenburgh, L.D. Oxygen: The antidote for systemic toxic reactions from local anesthetic drugs. *JAMA,* 174:842, 1960.
Rodman, M.J. Local anesthesia. *RN,* 24:47, 1961 (Jan.).
———. Pain-relieving drugs in labor and delivery. *RN,* 27:95, 1964.

SECTION 5

Drugs

for

Inflammation,

Allergy,

and

Related

Disorders

Inflammation and *immunity* are natural processes by which the body protects itself against injury by foreign invaders or damage by a wide variety of adverse environmental factors. Both of these biochemically complex defense mechanisms have some steps in common in the sequence of events triggered by exposure to various types of stress, and both make use of some of the same chemicals. Both the inflammatory process and the immune response can also be the cause of discomforting and even life-threatening symptoms when something goes wrong with one or more steps in what was supposed to be a protective process.

Many of the chemical substances that are produced and released by the body to protect it against tissue injury are also capable of causing trauma to the tissues. Substances such as histamine, for instance, help to bring about changes in function that aid body defenses. Yet these same substances can also damage various organs and interfere with their function. This can result in chronic tissue destruction or even in severely acute and fatal reactions.

Many different kinds of drugs may be useful for preventing or limiting the adverse effects of an excess of the chemicals released in inflammatory and allergic reactions. These drugs often differ very greatly in their pharmacological effects; yet, when properly employed, some are effective for relief of such symptoms as pain, redness, and swelling, and others can help to counteract possibly fatal respiratory and cardiovascular reactions. Thus, the drugs discussed in this section can be useful in the management of many disabling disorders such as arthritis, gout, migraine, and many allergic conditions. They can even be lifesaving—in anaphylaxis, for example, and other hypersensitivity reactions.

16.

Analgesic-Antipyretics, Antiinflammatory Agents, and Other Drugs for Rheumatic Disorders and Headaches

Drugs Used for Pain of Mild to Moderate Severity

In this chapter we shall take up several types of analgesic drugs that do not have the degree of pain-relieving potency of the narcotic analgesics previously discussed. These drugs, which are effective mainly in mild to moderate, rather than very severe, *pain* are sometimes called "non-narcotic," or "nonaddicting," or "mild" and "weak" analgesics. It may be better to describe them—in terms of their most important pharmacological effects—as *analgesic-antipyretic* and *antiinflammatory agents*.

Drugs of this kind differ from the potent narcoatic analgesics in some ways that are advantageous for patients with certain chronically painful conditions. They may, for example, be taken in daily oral doses for long periods *without* producing *tolerance* or *physical dependence*. They are also relatively free of serious side effects when taken in doses that are adequate for relief of acute pain of moderate severity that arises in such structures as the joints, muscles, and the head.

Thus, in addition to discussing the pharmacology of the salicylates and other analgesic-antipyretic agents listed in Table 16-1, we shall also take up in this chapter their uses alone, or in combination with the drugs listed in Table 16-4, in the management of various rheumatic disorders and headaches.

TABLE 16-1 *Nonnarcotic Analgesics and Antipyretics*

Official or Generic Name	Synonym or Trade Name	Dose
Salicylates and related drugs		
Aluminum aspirin N.F.	Aluminum acetylsalicylate	670 mg
Aspirin U.S.P.	Acetylsalicylic acid	300–1000 mg
Calcium acetylsalicylate carbimide	Calurin	300–600 mg
Choline salicylate	Arthropan liquid	870 mg
Methyl salicylate U.S.P.	Oil of wintergreen	Topical
Salicylamide N.F.	o-Hydroxybenzamide	300 mg
Salicylsalicylic acid	Salysal (ingredient of Persistin)	300 mg
Salicylic acid U.S.P.	o-Hydroxybenzoic acid	Topical
Sodium salicylate U.S.P.	. . . . . .	300–1000 mg
Para-aminophenol, coal tar, or aniline derivatives		
Acetanilid	Antifebrin	200–300 mg
Acetaminophen N.F.	N-acetyl-p-aminophenol (in Tylenol and others)	650 mg
Phenacetin U.S.P.	Acetophenetidin	300–600 mg
Pyrazolon derivatives		
Aminopyrine	Pyramidon	300–600 mg
Antipyrine N.F.	Phenazone	300–600 mg
Dipyrone	Methampyrone	300–600 mg
Oxyphenbutazone N.F.	Tandearil	300–400 mg per day
Phenylbutazone U.S.P.	Butazolidin	300–600 mg per day
*Newer nonaddicting agents of codeine-like action**		
Ethoheptazine citrate N.F.	Zactane (also in Zactirin)	75–150 mg
Propoxyphene HCl U.S.P.	Darvon	32–65 mg
Propoxyphene napsylate	Darvon N	300–400 mg per day

* See Chapter 13.

Of course, these are not the only kinds of painful conditions for which the salicylates and similar drugs are used. They may even be ordered for managing pain in patients with cancer, in order to delay the need to employ narcotic drugs. Thus, although these drugs are called "mild" analgesics, the nurse should not think that the patient is not suffering just because the doctor ordered "only aspirin." She should always administer these pain-relievers with the same care and concern for the patient's comfort as when the potent narcotic analgesics of the opioid type are ordered.

The Salicylates (Table 16-1)

The most important chemical class of analgesic-antipyretics are derivatives of *salicylic acid*, called salicylates. These include: the simple salts, such as sodium salicylate; esters such as *methyl salicylate*; and, most important of all, the salicylate ester of acetic acid, *acetylsalicylic acid*, or *aspirin+*. (Over 35 million pounds of this drug are produced annually in

the United States for use mostly in *non*prescription products for relief of pain and fever.

PHARMACOLOGICAL EFFECTS OF ASPIRIN (Table 16-2)

The effects of aspirin and related salicylates are related to the dose that is taken. Small doses (300 to 600 mg—the amounts in one or two ordinary 5-grain tablets) are usually effective in producing analgesia and an antipyretic effect in feverish patients. Larger doses—about 4 to 6 grams—are required for maintaining the drug's desirable antiinflammatory effect in rheumatic disorders such as chronic arthritis. At higher doses, aspirin produces many other pharmacologic effects, but these are of no practical therapeutic significance because of the toxicity that occurs at such high dose levels.

ANTIPYRETIC EFFECT

Historically, the natural salicylates found in willow bark were first used by the ancient

TABLE 16-2 *Pharmacological Actions and Therapeutic Uses of the Salicylates*

Pharmacological Action	Clinical Uses
Analgesic Especially useful against pain originating in the joints, muscles, teeth, head, skin, and connective tissues	Headache, toothache, arthritis and related musculoskeletal conditions, general malaise, dysmenorrhea, and other similar conditions
Antipyretic To reduce fever	Respiratory viral illnesses, such as influenza and the common cold
Antiinflammatory or antirheumatic	Acute rheumatic fever, acute and chronic rheumatoid and osteoarthritis, and related rheumatic disorders
Uricosuric Increased excretion of uric acid	Chronic gout management

Greeks for treating fevers. Later, during the last century, a search for quinine substitutes to be used in the management of malarial fevers led to the discovery of such synthetic salicylates as sodium salicylate and aspirin. Today doctors feel that it is better to treat the cause of the fever with antibiotics and other antiinfective agents rather than merely to relieve the symptom. However, salicylates are still considered desirable for reducing a fever in order to make some febrile patients more comfortable. Symptomatic relief with salicylates is especially useful for reducing the restlessness of young children who may sometimes convulse if their very high temperatures are not brought down rapidly.

The salicylates lower body temperature in feverish patients by their action on the heat-regulating centers located in the hypothalamus. By somehow resetting this central thermostat, aspirin and similar drugs increase the body's ability to rid itself of excessive heat. The patient loses heat from his skin surfaces as a result of the evaporation of sweat and the conduction of internal heat from dilated cutaneous blood vessels to the cooler external environment.

The nurse checks the patient's temperature after administering salicylates and records the response to the drug. As the patient's feverish temperature falls to lower levels, he may perspire profusely; so, to prevent his becoming chilled, the nurse may have to change the patient's gown and even his bedding. She may also apply cool, wet cloths or use alcohol sponge baths as adjunctive measures for removing excess body heat. Tact and gentleness

are often needed to get feverish, irritable children to accept the aspirin that they need.

ANALGESIC ACTION

Aspirin and related drugs are believed to relieve pain by a combination of central and peripheral actions. The effects on the central nervous system are said to be exerted at subcortical sites such as the thalamus rather than on the cerebral cortex. Thus, these drugs do not affect psychological functioning or alter the patient's mental or emotional state. Although these analgesics dull the patient's perception of pain, they do so without causing the drowsiness or the kind of euphoric feelings that are a factor in producing addiction to the opioid-type analgesics.

Recent evidence suggests that the salicylates and other nonnarcotic analgesics also act at the point of origin of the pain impulses. These drugs may act, according to one theory, by blocking the action of an injury-released polypeptide called *bradykinin* upon pain receptors located in the traumatized tissues. Other peripheral pain-relieving mechanisms of aspirin's action have also been suggested.

Aspirin and related drugs are particularly effective for the relief of aching-type pain arising in the outer areas of the body. Pain of this moderate degree occurs much more commonly than does the severe pain that requires opiates for relief. (The salicylates are relatively ineffective against pain arising in visceral organs or against sudden, sharp pain.) Thus, in many conditions marked by mild to moderate pain and discomfort, the public employs aspirin and its relatives in huge amounts for self-medication. Among the common conditions for which people take aspirin without prescription are headaches, toothaches, neuralgia, arthritis, dysmenorrhea, and the general malaise that accompanies "colds" and "the flu."

SELF-MEDICATION WITH ANALGESICS

Despite the widespread use of nonprescription analgesics and the extent to which these products are advertised to the public, many people are not very well informed about them. The nurse should be prepared to offer people information as to how salicylate-based analgesics can be used with greatest effectiveness and safety. She should also be able to answer questions that arise from the conflicting claims of greater effectiveness for one or another type of product advertised for relief of minor pain.

One kind of common claim, for example, is that particular salicylate products are specially formulated to foster more rapid, intense and prolonged analgesic activity. Despite many conflicting scientific reports about the effect on absorption of incorporating alkali or buffering agents with aspirin, there is still no proof that the addition of such substances actually increases the analgesic effectiveness of these products. Thus, most patients may be well-advised to purchase the less expensive plain aspirin products. Patients with stomach problems may profit from products specially formulated to minimize gastric irritation by aspirin (see *Adverse Effects*).

ANTIINFLAMMATORY ACTION

One of the most valuable properties of the salicylates is their ability to suppress inflammatory reactions in connective tissues. The mechanism of this antirheumatic effect is not known. One theory is that the salicylates stimulate increased production of adrenal cortex hormones, which have potent antiinflammatory activity. A more recent view is that the salicylates act directly upon rheumatic joints to counteract one or more of the components in the complex tissue-damaging reaction of the joints to the still unknown causative factor that triggers rheumatic disorders.

Salicylates are the mainstay of the conservative management of rheumatoid arthritis. Administered in large daily doses, aspirin is said to delay the joint damage that is the cause of crippling in this condition. Patients are encouraged to keep taking salicylates regularly in the largest doses that they can tolerate, as these drugs not only relieve pain but also reduce inflammation and, possibly, slow degenerative processes in the affected joints.

The nurse should take every opportunity to assure impatient arthritis sufferers that simple aspirin is the safest and most effective antirheumatic drug in most cases. She should try to keep people from wasting their money on the more expensive and less effective arthritis remedies that are often promoted as "miracle cures." The nurse teaches patients to follow faithfully the regimen of salicylates, rest, and special exercises that are the cornerstones of therapy in most cases of arthritis.

In rheumatic fever, the administration of aspirin or sodium salicylate in very high doses usually brings about rapid symptomatic relief. The patient's hot, red, painfully swollen joints often return to almost normal appearance in 24 to 48 hours. However, salicylate administration is continued even after all symptoms are gone. The nurse's observations of the patient's response to therapy help the doctor to adjust the dosage of salicylates to a safe level that the patient can tolerate (see *Adverse Effects* below).

ADVERSE EFFECTS

The salicylates are relatively safe drugs when taken occasionally for relief of minor pain. The much larger doses needed to control rheumatoid inflammation often cause gastrointestinal upset and other discomforting symptoms. The chronic abuse of analgesics containing salicylates, or the accidental ingestion of massive overdoses, can cause severe and sometimes fatal salicylate intoxication (*Summary*, p. 216).

Small doses of aspirin are well tolerated by most people. However, people who have a history of allergic hypersensitivity may react adversely after taking a single tablet. The nurse should pay attention to the patient who tells her that he has suffered skin eruptions or breathing difficulties from aspirin. If the doctor is told of this, he can often safely substitute one of the *non*salicylate-type analgesics. On the other hand, the nurse should not give in to a patient's demands for aspirin or any other medication that the doctor has not ordered.

Some patients complain that even small doses of aspirin cause stomach irritation. Recent reports indicate that slight gastric bleeding often follows ingestion of only one or two tablets. Occasional occult bleeding of this kind is not ordinarily dangerous. However, serious overt hemorrhages have occurred in people with previously undetected gastric lesions such as peptic ulcer. Nonsalicylate-type analgesics, such as acetaminophen, are preferred for patients with a history of chronic gastritis or esophagitis, as well as peptic ulcer.

Although it has not been proved that aspirin products containing alkaline buffers cause less distress than plain aspirin, aspirin that is presented in an alkaline solution is probably preferable to tablets of the drug. Enteric-coated tablets may be preferred for arthritic patients who are taking large daily doses of salicylates. The nurse can help minimize gastric distress in such patients by administering the drug with meals or with a small snack of milk and crackers, and the doctor may order a teaspoonful of sodium bicarbonate with each dose of aspirin.

Salicylism, or early salicylate toxicity, is seen in patients with acute rheumatic fever who are receiving large daily doses of aspirin. One danger sign is development of *tinnitus*—a ringing, roaring, buzzing, or blowing sound in the patient's ears. The nurse reports such complaints to the doctor, who then orders a slight reduction in dosage so that salicylate blood levels will drop to a point that is safer but still effective for maintaining antirheumatic activity.

ACUTE POISONING

The accidental ingestion of aspirin or of methyl salicylate can cause severe toxicity in young children (*Summary,* p. 216). Often salicylate intoxication results from overtreatment of a feverish, already dehydrated infant. Sometimes youngsters eat the contents of a bottle of tablets or drink an external-use liniment containing methyl salicylate. Treatment of the sometimes severe metabolic imbalances that follow such ingestion is much more difficult than preventing salicylate poisoning in the first place. Thus, the nurse should instruct parents in how to use aspirin properly and in the need to store salicylates safely.

Nonsalicylate Analgesic-Antipyretics (Table 16-1)

Several other classes of chemicals are as effective as the salicylates for relief of pain and reduction of fever. They are not as widely used as the salicylates, however, mainly for the following reasons: (1) Some, such as the aniline *derivatives,* (see below) lack adequate anti-inflammatory activity. (2) Others, such as the *pyrazolon derivatives* (see below) are considered potentially too toxic for routine use. Many nonprescription products contain one or more nonsalicylate analgesics in combination with aspirin or with one another.

ANILINE OR para-AMINOPHENOL DERIVATIVES
(Table 16-1)

The currently most commonly employed drug of this class is *acetaminopen+*. It has, to some extent, displaced its chemical relative *phenacetin+* although the latter is still frequently found combined with aspirin in proprietary remedies of the A.P.C. type (Table 16-3). *Acetanilid,* the third analgesic of this class, is now no longer used to any extent in this country. The present status of these three related analgesics is primarily the result of currently held opinions concerning their relative safety.

ADVERSE EFFECTS. The toxic effects most commonly reported when drugs of this class are taken in excessive amounts or by sensitive patients involve the circulating blood and the kidneys. Phenacetin, for example, has caused hemolytic anemia and kidney damage; acetanilid often has produced methemoglobinemia; acetaminophen has little tendency to cause the latter condition, nor has it been involved in production of other blood disorders or of nephrotoxicity.

Other safety advantages claimed for acetaminophen are: (1) that it does not cause stomach upset of the kind common with aspirin; and (2) that it can be given to patients sensitive to aspirin without causing an allergic reaction. It is claimed less likely than the salicylates to cause undesirable interactions with anticoagulant drugs, but this has not been established.

T A B L E 16-3 *Contents of Some Analgesic Combination Products**

Product	Analgesics	Other Drugs
Alka-Seltzer	Aspirin 325 mg	Sodium bicarbonate Citric acid Calcium phosphate
Anacin	Aspirin 400 mg	Caffeine
A.P.C. Tablets	Aspirin 225 mg Phenacetin 160 mg	Caffeine
A.S.A. Compound	Aspirin 225 mg Phenacetin 160 mg	Caffeine
Bromo-Seltzer	Acetaminophen 195 mg Phenacetin 130 mg	Caffeine
Bufferin	Aspirin 324 mg	Aluminum dihydroxyaminoacetate Magnesium carbonate
Empirin Compound	Aspirin 233 mg Phenacetin 166 mg	Caffeine
Excedrin	Aspirin 190 mg Salicylamide 130 mg Acetaminophen 90 mg	Caffeine
Medache	Acetaminophen 150 mg Salicylamide 150 mg	Caffeine
PAC	Aspirin 228 mg Phenacetin 163 mg	Caffeine
Vanquish	Aspirin 227 mg Acetaminophen 194 mg	Caffeine

* The formulations of proprietary analgesic products are often changed without direct notice to the public.

COMBINATIONS OF ANILINE ANALGESICS AND ASPIRIN

Headache remedies (p. 213) often contain aspirin combined with phenacetin or acetaminophen and other nonanalgesic drugs, including caffeine (Table 16-3). In theory, administering combinations of these drugs in fractional doses rather than full doses of each should reduce their adverse effects. In practice, however, there is no proof of lessened toxicity, and, in fact, a person sensitive to one of the drugs in such fixed-dose combinations could suffer an allergic reaction which would not have occurred had he taken a full dose of only the one analgesic to which he was not sensitive.

Similarly, such combinations are not any more effective than full doses of aspirin, phenacetin, or acetaminophen taken alone. There is also no reason to think that the small dose of caffeine traditionally added to such analgesic combinations actually makes them more effective for pain relief. On the other hand, the addition of a *weak* narcotic analgesic such as *codeine* or *oxycodone* to mixtures of aspirin with acetaminophen or phenacetin *does* often add to the pain relieving effectiveness of the *non*narcotic analgesic-antipyretic agents. The reason for this is that the two different types of analgesics act at different places in the pain pathway and thus produce additive effects.

PYRAZOLONE DERIVATIVES
(Table 16-1)

The analgesic-antipyretic drugs of this chemical subclass also possess potent antiinflammatory activity. However, these drugs are used relatively rarely today in this country because of their potential toxicity. *Aminopyrine*, for example, is capable of causing fatal agranulocytosis in certain sensitive patients. Thus, the risk of using it or the related drugs *antipyrine* and *dipyrone* for routine pain relief is not warranted, and they should be reserved mainly for reducing high fever in the rare cases that do not respond to other safer antipyretic drugs and simple measures such as sponge baths.

On the other hand, the chemically related compound, *phenylbutazone+* (Butazolidin) which shares the toxic properties of this drug class *does* have wider therapeutic applications. Its excellent antiinflammatory activity makes it particularly valuable for treating certain acute and chronic rheumatoid disorders. However, as indicated in the following section, its use requires considerable caution to avoid the adverse effects that this drug may produce in a considerable proportion of arthritic patients taking it for prolonged periods.

Mefenamic acid (Ponstel) is a new analgesic that differs chemically from the other three classes of analgesic-antipyretic-antiinflammatory agents. It does not appear to have any advantages over the older drugs, and it may, in fact, cause a higher incidence of adverse effects. For this reason, its use for longer than one week is not recommended, and this, of course, means that it cannot serve as a substitute for salicylates in the management of patients with chronic rheumatoid disorders. The drug commonly causes gastrointestinal upset and is contraindicated in patients with gastritis or peptic ulcer. If diarrhea develops and persists, mefenamic acid must be discontinued.

Drugs Used for Rheumatic Disorders

Arthritis and related rheumatic disorders are chronic, potentially crippling diseases of the musculoskeletal system. In most of these conditions, the underlying cause is not known. Thus, the drugs used for treating rheumatoid arthritis, spondylitis, and osteoarthritis, for example, relieve joint pain and reduce inflammation without really stopping the disease process. In gout, on the other hand, other drugs besides analgesics and antiinflammatory agents are employed to counteract the better understood metabolic abnormality of this disorder. Thus, we shall discuss drugs used in this special form of arthritis separately (see pp. 212-213).

Salicylates, as we have already indicated, are the most important drugs for relief of pain and inflammation in the long-term treatment of rheumatic disorders. Taken regularly as part of the patient's total program, aspirin and similar salicylates play an important role in relief of the discomforting symptoms of the various kinds of arthritis. This may help the patient to profit from the physical therapy that is often needed for maintaining joint mobility and preventing crippling contractures.

Sometimes, however, salicylates alone may not be enough to control the rapidly progressive stages of certain rheumatic diseases. In such cases, the patient's doctor may add other antiinflammatory agents to his basic regimen of rest, exercise, and physical therapy. In the remainder of this section, we shall discuss the status of several kinds of other analgesic and antiinflammatory drugs that are now available for treating the various types of rheumatic disorders.

Nonsalicylate-Nonsteroid Drugs

Phenylbutazone+ (Butazolidin) is a useful antiinflammatory agent with analgesic-antipyretic and uricosuric actions. However, because of its many potential adverse effects, it is not used for simple pain relief, merely reducing fever, or for only increasing the excretion of uric acid. It is reserved instead for treating selected patients with rheumatoid arthritis who have not responded adequately to salicylates.

It is also particularly useful for reducing joint inflammation during acute gout attacks in patients who can not tolerate *colchicine+*, the preferred drug for aborting acute attacks. Similarly, patients with ankylosing spondylitis who do not respond to the safer drug *indomethacin* may profit from phenylbutazone treatment.

Phenylbutazone often acts quickly to relieve such symptoms of acute inflammatory disorders as pain and tenderness, heat and redness, and swelling that interferes with mobility. When patients with acute gout or thrombophlebitis, for example, take this drug for the few days of peak inflammation, adverse effects do not commonly develop. However, the long-term use of this drug may be hazardous for many patients. Thus, the doctor carefully selects patients for treatment with phenylbutazone or the related compound *oxyphenbutazone* (Tandearil). He avoids ordering these drugs for elderly patients or for those with a history of various kinds of ailments that make them particularly susceptible to the potential adverse secondary effects of these drugs.

Because this drug is capable of causing bone marrow depression, gastrointestinal irritation,

T A B L E   1 6 - 4   *Drugs Used in the Management of Arthritis, Gout, and Migraine Headache**

Nonproprietary or Official Name	Proprietary Name or Synonym	Dosage
ANTIRHEUMATICS		
Antimalarial-type		
Chloroquine phosphate U.S.P.	Aralen, and others	250 mg daily
Hydroxychloroquine sulfate U.S.P.	Plaquenil	200–600 mg daily
Quinacrine HCl U.S.P.	Atabrine	200–800 mg daily
Gold Salts		
Aurothioglucose U.S.P.	Solganal; gold thioglucose	10 to 50 mg weekly I.M. up to a total dose of 1.5 g per course of treatment
Aurothioglycanide	Lauron	25 mg I.M. initially; gradually increased by increments of no more than 25 mg at weekly intervals for 22 weeks to a maximum single dose of 150 mg
Gold sodium thiomalate U.S.P.	Myochrysine	10 mg I.M. initially, increasing to 50 mg per week to a total dose of 750 to 1,500 mg
Gold sodium thiosulfate N.F.	Sanochrysine	5 to 75 mg weekly dosage range, to a total dose of 500 to 1,000 mg per course
Miscellaneous Antiinflammatory Agents		
Indomethacin N.F.	Indocin	50–150 mg
Oxyphenbutazone N.F.	Tandearil	300–600 mg daily
Phenylbutazone U.S.P.	Butazolidin	300–600 mg daily
GOUT TREATMENT		
Allopurinol U.S.P.	Zyloprim	200–600 mg daily
Colchicine U.S.P.		1 mg q. 2 hours for 6–8 doses as suppressant: 0.5 mg maintenance.
Probenecid U.S.P.	Benemid	500 mg–2 g daily
Sulfinpyrazone U.S.P.	Anturan	200–800 mg daily
MIGRAINE TREATMENT		
Ergotamine tartrate U.S.P.	Ergomar Gynergen	Oral 1–2 mg immediately, repeated if necessary at 30-minute intervals up to a total dose of 6 mg in 24 hours and no more than 12 mg in one week Parenteral: 0.25–0.5 mg immediately, repeated if necessary every hour up to a total 1 mg in 24 hours and no more than 2 mg per week (also administered by buccal and sublingual routes and by inhalation)
Ergonovine maleate U.S.P.	Ergotrate	0.2–0.4 mg immediately by oral, sublingual, or intramuscular routes. Repeat every 2 hours if necessary up to a total of 1.6 mg daily
Methylergonovine maleate U.S.P.	Methergine	0.2–0.4 mg immediately by oral, sublingual, or intramuscular routes. Repeat every 2 hours if necessary up to a total of 1.6 mg daily
Methysergide maleate N.F.	Sansert	Total oral daily doses of 4 to 8 mg, divided into four doses taken with food

* The analgesics listed in Table 16-1 and the corticosteroid drugs and corticotropin are also employed in treating these disorders.

and fluid retention, it is not ordinarily administered to patients with a history of blood dyscrasias, peptic ulcer, or cardiac and renal disorders. Patients are instructed to return for frequent blood checks during the period of continued treatment with doses that have been adjusted down to the smallest effective level. They must be told to report such signs and symptoms as sore mouth or throat, fever, weight gain, stomach pain or black, tarry stools —all signs of potentially severe toxicity.

Indomethacin (Indocin) has pharmacological effects like those of phenylbutazone and the salicylates. It causes more side effects than aspirin and thus is reserved for rheumatoid arthritis patients who do not respond to salicylates or are sensitive to these drugs. On the other hand, it is safer than phenylbutazone, and some physicians prefer it for treating cases of ankylosing spondylitis. It is also used for treating osteoarthritis and some cases of acute gout.

Adverse effects of indomethacin are mainly central in origin, but—as with other antiarthritic drugs—it often causes epigastric distress and is used with caution in patients with a past history of gastritis and dyspepsia, and is contraindicated in those with active peptic ulcer or ulcerative colitis. Headache is the most common of the central side effects of indomethacin. Patients occasionally show signs also of mental confusion, light-headedness, and vertigo. Patients taking this drug for long periods should have eye examinations performed to detect possible adverse ocular changes. About 10 to 15 percent of patients are forced to discontinue the drug because of persistent gastrointestinal or nervous system side effects.

Chrysotherapy, or treatment with gold salts, seems effective for suppressing cases of rheumatoid arthritis that are still showing active inflammation despite salicylate treatment. It is used in early cases before cartilage has been destroyed and joints have degenerated. Most people respond well to small doses that cause little toxicity, particularly when the patients are also benefiting from general conservative management measures.

Gold salts are given in courses lasting many weeks or months, during which time dosage is increased only gradually. Patients are watched closely for signs of toxicity, including various kinds of skin reactions. Dermatitis may make it necessary to discontinue treatment. Less common but more serious complications include kidney and bone marrow damage. Thus urinanalyses and blood tests are performed before each injection in the series, and patients are questioned closely about whether they have had such symptoms as itchy skin rashes, sore mouth, and other early indications of adverse reactions.

The antimalarial drugs *chloroquine* and *hydroxychloroquine* benefit some rheumatoid arthritis patients. However, improvement appears only slowly when these drugs are administered in small safe doses. Larger doses have caused damage to the retina, resulting in permanent blindness. To avoid retinopathy during long-term maintenance therapy, patients must be examined by an ophthalmologist at the start of treatment and at frequent intervals afterwards. The drug is discontinued at the first sign of any ocular change such as retinal edema. Hydroxychloroquine is less likely than chloroquine to cause such other side effects as gastrointestinal discomfort, headache, and skin rash.

Immunosuppressive drugs, including *azathioprine* (Imuran) and certain anticancer agents, sometimes suppress inflammation in active cases of rheumatoid arthritis that have not responded to other antiarthritic drugs. However, these drugs are highly toxic, so they are still reserved mostly for patients whose disease is very severe or even life-threatening.

Corticosteroid Therapy of Rheumatic Disorders

As we shall see (Chapter 17), the corticosteroid drugs are extremely effective for suppressing inflammatory processes in the joints and elsewhere. These drugs are very valuable, for example, for control of acute rheumatic fever symptoms, particularly when the patient shows signs of systemic toxicity including heart muscle inflammation. Administered in massive doses for only a few days, these drugs usually bring the patient's symptoms under control without causing significant toxicity.

On the other hand, even relatively low doses of corticosteroids inevitably cause metabolic toxicity, when these drugs are administered for long periods. Thus, the steroids are employed in chronic rheumatic disorders only after the salicylates, gold salts, and other safer antiarthritic drugs have first been tried and found ineffective. The doctor turns to long-term steroid therapy when the rapid progress of uncontrolled rheumatoid arthritis threatens to disable the patient and keep him from his customary and necessary activities.

In such cases, corticosteroid drugs are added to the patient's basic program in low daily doses that are then raised only very slowly to the lowest level that will keep inflammation under control. The doctor does *not* try to relieve *all* the patient's symptoms, as the doses needed to do so may produce toxic symptoms too rapidly. Another reason for not trying to eliminate all of the patient's arthritic complaints is that he may become so dependent upon steroids that he will not be willing to give them up. He may, in fact, even refuse to reduce his daily dosage when the doctor decides that it is desirable to do so in order to prevent adverse drug reactions.

The physician always tries to keep corticosteroid dosage at a low level and to reduce or even to eliminate these drugs whenever the patient's arthritis passes into an inactive phase. Often the patient resists attempts to employ alternate day therapy or other efforts to cut back corticosteroid dosage because he has come to depend on these drugs for relief of rheumatic discomfort.

The nurse can often help the patient understand how important it is for him to follow the doctor's orders, even though reducing dosage seems to make his symptoms worse. The nurse explains why this is necessary in order to avoid the toxic effects of these drugs. She provides emotional support and encourages the drug-dependent patient to get along without steroids whenever his disease is in one of its periods of spontaneous remission.

One way of avoiding systemic toxicity is to administer corticosteroids by direct injection into inflamed joints. This may prove satisfactory when only a few joints are involved, and sometimes just one injection of a long-lasting acetate ester may give relief lasting several weeks. However, patients should be warned not to become too active, because they may then tend to overwork the damaged joint. This can then actually increase the rate of progressive joint destruction, as corticosteroid drugs do not counteract the underlying disease process of rheumatoid arthritis. Despite their ability to suppress such signs and symptoms of inflammation as pain, swelling, heat, and redness, the corticosteroids—like all other antiinflam-matory drugs—are no cure for arthritis nor do they prevent structural joint damage.

Drug Treatment of Gout

Gout is a metabolic disorder marked by high levels of uric acid in the blood. Patients with hyperuricemia (7 mg or more of uric acid per 100 ml of plasma) are subject to acute attacks of gouty arthritis. The extreme pain is the result of an inflammatory reaction caused by uric acid microcrystals that settle out of solution in the affected joints.

Acute and chronic gout can be treated today more successfully than any other form of arthritis. Three types of drugs are employed: (1) drugs for controlling the acute inflammation of an attack; (2) drugs for increasing the excretion of uric acid by the kidneys—uricosuric agents; and (3) drugs for reducing the production of uric acid by the body. The regular use of the two types of drugs that affect uric acid metabolism is intended to prevent recurrences of gout attacks. Early administration of certain specific antiinflammatory agents at the first warning sign often terminates an acute attack that develops despite prophylactic treatment.

TREATMENT OF AN ACUTE ATTACK

Gout tends to flare up in a sudden, almost unbearably painful, attack. Sometimes only a single joint such as that of the big toe or the knee becomes red hot, swollen, and extremely tender; sometimes several small joints of the feet and hands are involved simultaneously. Prompt administration of *colchicine+*, a drug that most chronic gout patients should carry with them, will very often abort the acute attack before it becomes incapacitating.

Oral colchicine must be taken in a special way to gain its benefits with least toxicity. The patient takes one or two tablets immediately and continues to take a tablet every hour until his pain is relieved or he begins to suffer gastrointestinal distress, including diarrhea. Usually, relief begins in a few hours and before the gastrointestinal symptoms develop. However, some patients may have to take paregoric or an antiemetic for control of diarrhea, nausea, or vomiting.

Attacks that are not promptly treated with colchicine may then not respond to oral doses that the patient can tolerate. The drug may then be injected by vein to lessen gastrointestinal irritation. The total dose must be limited in such cases to avoid kidney and bone marrow damage. Some specialists now prefer to use other antiinflammatory agents that they consider safer than colchicine and that are almost as effective as the traditional gout remedy.

Phenylbutazone+ (Butazolidin) is often effective when taken in high doses for a brief period. The patient is told to take 400 mg at once and an equal amount divided into four doses taken at 4-hour intervals. This regimen may be repeated on the following day if full relief is not obtained. The patient may also be given an intramuscular injection of *corticotropin* (ACTH) in gel form, and if a large joint such as the knee is involved, a corticosteroid ester may be injected directly into the joint after excess fluid has been drawn off. *Indomethacin* (Indocin) is somewhat safer than any of these drugs, but it is not as specific for the type of inflammatory reaction that is characteristic of gout.

The nurse should see that the patient understands and follows the doctor's instructions for taking these drugs and that he carries out other measures also. Bed rest is desirable during the attack, for example. However, once the pain is completely relieved and the affected joint can bear the patient's weight, he should be encouraged to walk about. Exercise of pain-free joints is necessary to avoid muscle weakness and atrophy.

PROPHYLACTIC TREATMENT OF CHRONIC GOUT

Acute attacks can be prevented today by proper use of drugs that keep blood and tissue levels of uric acid below 7 mg%. The drugs most commonly employed for this purpose are the uricosuric agents *probenecid+* (Benemid) and *sulfinpyrazone* (Anturane). These drugs act in kidney tubules where they keep uric acid that has entered the tubules by glomerular filtration from being reabsorbed back into the blood. This results in the removal of greater amounts of uric acid in the urine and a drop in the plasma urate level.

Certain precautions are required when treatment with uricosuric drugs is being initiated. The patient should, for example, force fluids before receiving his first relatively small doses of the drug. The reason for this is that uric acid may form urate stones in the urinary tract

when the drug's action causes more of this metabolite to be excreted than can stay in solution in the urine. Drinking fluids produces a large volume of urine and thus keeps the uric acid in a dissolved state. Sometimes it is also desirable to make the uric acid even more soluble by alkalinizing the dilute urine. This is done by having the patient take a teaspoonful of sodium bicarbonate or a dose of potassium citrate several times a day.

Allopurinol+ (Zyloprim), a drug that reduces the production of uric acid instead of increasing its excretion, is also useful for long-term treatment that is intended to increase the intervals between attacks. The resulting decrease in the amount of uric acid that needs to be excreted in the urine makes this drug especially useful for treating gout patients whose kidneys are damaged. Such patients do not respond well to probenecid and other uricosuric drugs. They are also the ones most likely to form urate stones in the urinary tract when treated with uricosuric drugs.

DRUG COMBINATIONS. Allopurinol and probenecid or sulfinpyrazone may be administered together in a combined attack intended to keep uric acid at low plasma levels. Small daily doses of colchicine may be added to prevent flareups of inflammation at the start of such prophylactic therapy.

Pain relievers such as *meperidine* (Demerol) may have to be employed at the height of an acute attack, and an analgesic-antipyretic may be needed for less severe joint pains. However, aspirin should not be used by patients who are taking probenecid, as salicylates antagonize the uricosuric effect of this drug. A more dangerous drug interaction may occur if allopurinol is taken together with full doses of the antineoplastic agent, mercaptopurine. Patients with leukemia who are treated with both drugs should receive only one third or one quarter the usual dose of mercaptopurine.

In summary, gout is the rheumatic disorder most readily controllable by drug therapy, provided that patients follow directions for their proper use.

Drugs for Headache Relief

Headache is one of the most common complaints for which people seek relief. In most headaches that all people have occasionally the pain is minor and is readily relieved by aspirin or one of the other mild analgesics. However, people whose headaches recur frequently should be advised to see a doctor. The physician studies such patients to rule out the presence of organic disorders such as sinusitis, glaucoma, or even brain tumor.

Actually, few headaches turn out to be symptoms of serious structural changes within the patient's cranium. The most common kinds of chronic headaches stem from bodily reactions to situations that people find stressful. The two most important types are: (1) tension, or muscular contraction headaches; and (2) vascular headaches, including classic migraine.

TENSION HEADACHES

Recurring headaches of this type often result from a person's unconscious reaction to stress. This causes the muscles of the neck and scalp to go into a sustained state of contraction. Sometimes, the same kind of muscle tension occurs in people who keep the head in a set position as they work. Headaches of this kind are best managed by eliminating the cause rather than by the repeated use of drugs.

Helping the patient change his work routine often relieves recurrent tension headaches. Getting a person to change his life style and his emotional responses to stress is, of course, much more difficult even when his physician employs psychotherapeutic measures. Often the nurse can suggest certain safe *nondrug* measures for dealing with headache pain. Certainly, setting aside some time for a quiet rest period, a warm, relaxing bath, or a gentle massage of the back of the neck is better than becoming dependent upon the repeated use of potentially toxic drugs.

Of course, a medically supervised program of adjunctive drug therapy may be a helpful part of a total program for tension headache control. The safest and simplest drugs for occasional adjunctive use in such cases are the mild analgesics discussed earlier in this chapter. As indicated previously, the best procedure is to have the patient take a full dose of a single analgesic—preferably *plain aspirin* if, as is true for most people, the patient tolerates this salicylate. Patients sensitive to salicylates should receive a full dose of *phenacetin* or *acetaminophen* alone rather than a complex mixture of drugs.

For occasional tension headaches of more than ordinary severity, the patient may profit from the addition of a weak narcotic analgesic such as *codeine* or *oxycodone* to the single salicylate or other mild analgesics. The many other kinds of drugs that are so often combined with analgesics are not now considered to make the resulting product any more effective for tension headache relief. The doctor can occasionally prescribe an additional drug of a different class when it seems desirable for a particular patient. Such drugs include: (1) sedative-hypnotics and antianxiety agents; (2) skeletal muscle relaxants; and even occasionally (3) antidepressant drugs.

VASCULAR HEADACHES

Dilation of blood vessels in the tissues surrounding the brain results in throbbing headaches that are particularly painful. The cause of cranial vasodilation in some kinds of vascular headaches is well understood and relatively easy to correct through treatment of the underlying disorder—high blood pressure or infection, for example. *Migraine* headaches, on the other hand, have complex psychological and biochemical causes that are not easy to counteract. Nevertheless, drugs are available that can be quite effective for relief of an acute attack of migraine, and at least one drug has proven useful for prevention of migraine attacks in some patients.

TREATMENT OF AN ACUTE ATTACK. The ergot alkaloid *ergotamine tartrate*+ (Gynergen and others) is relatively specific for control of migraine attacks. Taken at the first sign of an oncoming episode, this drug is capable of aborting over 90 percent of attacks. The patient is taught to take the entire amount of ergotamine that he has learned from experience will stop the progress of his migraine episodes. He should also cease his activities and lie down in a darkened room to rest during the time that the drug is acting.

Patients should limit their ergotamine intake to avoid toxicity. Some side effects, such as nausea and vomiting, are not serious. However, misuse of this drug might cause severe vasoconstriction and result in damage to peripheral blood vessels that could lead to gangrene. Safe doses taken occasionally contract the smooth muscles of the dilated cerebral vessels and thus relieve the pain, but frequent administration of overdoses can cause constriction of vessels in the fingers and toes or even in the coronary arterioles of the heart. Thus, numbness and tingling in the legs and arms, muscle cramps in the extremities, and anginal-type chest pains indicate that the patient has been taking too much ergotamine. (See also Chapter 47 for a further discussion of ergot toxicity.)

PREVENTION OF MIGRAINE ATTACKS. Ergotamine is not effective for reducing the number of migraine episodes a person suffers, and its long-term use for preventive purposes might, in any case, cause chronic toxicity. However, a chemically related drug called *methysergide* (Sansert) has proved useful for prophylaxis. It is reserved for use in patients who suffer frequent migraine attacks of a kind not readily controllable by safe doses of ergotamine.

Methysergide is itself a potentially toxic drug that must be used only when the patient can be kept under close medical supervision. Some side effects, such as gastrointestinal upset, are not serious and can be minimized by having the patient start with small doses that are taken with meals. Other effects are similar to those of ergotamine and are equally serious. Thus, patients are warned to report signs of vasospasm such as cold or numbness in the hands, cramping leg pains while walking, or pains in the chest and abdomen.

In addition to such vascular complications methysergide has caused serious chronic effects by bringing about fibrous tissue changes in the pelvic region, lungs, and elsewhere. The doctor is particularly watchful for signs of retroperitoneal fibrosis, a condition that can cause urinary tract obstruction. This requires immediate discontinuance of further treatment with this drug. In any case, the drug is gradually discontinued toward the end of every six-month period to give the patient a drug-free period of three or four weeks.

SUMMARY of Points for the Nurse to Remember About Salicylates and Other Analgesic and Arthritis Drugs

Be prepared to answer questions that people may ask you about the conflicting claims for pain relief and arthritis products that are advertised directly to the public.

Instruct parents of young children in the safe use and storage of aspirin, which is the most common cause of accidental poisoning in youngsters.

Be tactful and helpful in persuading feverish, irritable children to accept salicylates and to drink plenty of fluids. Change gown and bedding when patients perspire profusely. Note and record temperature changes.

Help to lessen gastric irritation from aspirin by giving the drug with fluid after the patient has taken some food. Notify the physician if stomach pains persist in patients taking salicylates or other antirheumatic drugs.

Carefully observe patients receiving salicylates in high doses for such symptoms as ringing or buzzing in the ears, which may signal the onset of early toxicity.

Pay attention to patients who volunteer the information that they "can't take aspirin." Such possibly sensitive patients should not receive salicylates until the doctor has decided that there is little risk of a severe allergic reaction.

Remember that patients for whom aspirin and other mild analgesics are prescribed may have serious illnesses and severe discomfort and that these drugs should be administered promptly and with as much care and concern as when potent narcotic analgesics are prescribed.

Note the time required for a patient to feel relief of pain following the administration of analgesic-antirheumatic drugs and the extent of such relief. Record this information on the patient's chart.

Remember that these nonnarcotic drugs can be misused and abused. Advise patients who seem to be taking these nonprescription products too often that they should consult their physician about the symptoms that they are trying to treat by excessive self-medication.

Help arthritic patients to understand why they must accept a reduction in corticosteroid dosage when acute exacerbations seems to be subsiding. Look for symptoms of steroid toxicity in patients who require long-term use of these drugs.

Make sure that patients with arthritic disorders, and gout in particular, understand how to use the various drugs to get their greatest benefits with fewest side effects.

Help arthritic patients maintain their general health and avoid fatigue, emotional stress, infection, and other conditions that may set off acute episodes.

S U M M A R Y of the Side Effects and Toxicity of Salicylates and Other Nonnarcotic Analgesics

Salicylates

Allergic hypersensitivity. Skin, gastrointestinal, and respiratory effects of varying severity may develop suddenly.

Early salicylism. Gastrointestinal upset including nausea, vomiting, pain, and gastric bleeding; tinnitus, partial deafness, diplopia, dizziness, drowsiness, lethargy, mental confusion.

Salicylate poisoning. Central stimulation may lead to convulsions, followed by respiratory and cardiovascular failure. Stimulation of respiratory center causes hyperpnea, which in turn leads to respiratory alkalosis. Metabolic acidosis and disturbances such as *hyper-* or *hypo*glycemia and hypokalemia may also occur. Bleeding disorders caused by hypoprothrombinemia or thrombocytopenia may develop.

Acetanilid, Phenacetin, and Related Drugs

Hematological effects include methemoglobinemia marked by cyanosis, headache, chest pain, and dyspnea; also hemolytic anemia, which may lead to hematuria, anuria, and acute kidney failure.

Nephritis with papillary necrosis may develop in patients who abuse these drugs.

Aminopyrine and Related Drugs

Agranulocytosis manifested by very low leukocyte counts, severe sore throat, and fulminating infection.

Propoxyphene (Darvon)

Gastrointestinal upset—nausea, vomiting, gastric pain.

Central nervous system depression (drowsiness and dizziness) and, with massive dosage, stimulation that may lead to convulsions.

Clinical Nursing Situation

The Situation: Mrs. O'Connor has had rheumatoid arthritis for six years and has been admitted to the hospital three times in the past year when severe pain and swelling of her knee joints and those of her hands and feet had become particularly disabling. She seldom complains and typically responds to the nurse's questions by saying that she is sure there are others worse off than she. Each time that she has returned home Mrs. O'Connor has worked too hard taking care of her two children, aged eight and nine, and maintaining her home in accordance with her high standards of meticulous housekeeping. She is now rather thin and listless.

Mrs. O'Connor currently takes 0.6 g of aspirin at least four times a day, and she has a prescription for Valium that she takes to help her rest and to relieve anxiety. However, she would like to be taking the corticosteroid Decadron, which her doctor sometimes prescribes in small doses when she suffers acute flare-ups of her chronic arthritis. She says this is the only drug that really gave her dramatic relief.

The Problem: Develop a nursing plan for Mrs. O'Connor. How would you reply to her wistful comments about wanting to take corticosteroids along with her regular aspirin? What suggestions might you make to help reduce gastric irritation when Mrs. O'Connor has to raise her aspirin dosage to six times a day or more?

DRUG DIGEST

ACETAMINOPHEN N.F. (APAP, Tempra; Tylenol; and others)

Actions and Indications. This relative of phenacetin is an effective analgesic and antipyretic, but it has little or no antiinflammatory activity. It may be substituted for aspirin to relieve mild to moderate pain (but not in the management of rheumatic disorders) for patients who are hypersensitive to salicylates or who have low tolerance for the irritating effects of aspirin on the gastrointestinal mucosa.

It is also preferred to aspirin for relief of pain in gout patients who are taking probenecid or other uricosuric drugs that might be antagonized by salicylates. This drug does not seem to have the platelet-aggregating or prothrombin-prolonging effects of aspirin, and thus it may be preferable for pain relief in patients with hemorrhagic disorders or those who are receiving anticoagulant therapy.

Side Effects, Cautions, and Contra-indications. Ordinary doses cause few side effects. This drug has rarely been reported to cause the kinds of renal damage, hemolytic anemia, and methemoglobinemia that have been recorded for the related drugs phenacetin and acetanilid. However, such adverse effects should be watched for; further administration of the drug would be contraindicated in those who showed symptoms of these disorders. Similarly, the drug is discontinued if such signs of hypersensitivity as skin redness, itching, or urticaria occur.

Accidental or deliberate massive overdosage has caused severe illness and death from acute hepatic necrosis and other complications, such as hypoglycemia and metabolic acidosis.

Dosage and Administration. The usual adult dose is 300 to 600 mg repeated in four hours; for children 6 to 12 years old, half this dose is employed, and youngsters 1 to 6 years old receive only 60 to 120 mg at four- to six-hour intervals if necessary.

ALLOPURINOL U.S.P. (Zyloprim)

Actions and Indications. This drug reduces the production of uric acid, which lowers the level of uric acid in both the blood and urine of patients with primary gout. Those who tend to form kidney stones or whose kidneys are damaged are most likely to benefit from the fact that this drug does not increase the concentration of uric acid in the urine.

The drug is also employed when high blood and urine levels of uric acid are the result of neoplastic diseases. The drug prevents gouty arthritis and nephropathy from developing secondary to treatment of leukemias, lymphomas, and other malignancies with antineoplastic drugs or radiation, because of its ability to reduce formation of excess uric acid from the destroyed proliferating cells.

Side Effects, Cautions, and Contra-indications. Skin rashes, mostly of the measles-like type, are the most common adverse effect. Other

signs of hypersensitivity include chills and fever, nausea, vomiting, epigastric distress, and diarrhea, and more serious skin lesions, including purpura and exfoliative dermatitis. Further use of the drug is contraindicated in patients who have had such severe idiosyncratic reactions. Its use in patients with a history of liver disease requires caution, and periodic liver function tests are done early in treatment of all cases because of occasional hepatotoxicity.

Dosage and Administration. Low doses—100 to 200 mg—are employed daily, at first. This is increased gradually to 200 or 300 mg for mild cases or 400 to 600 mg for more severe gout, administered in several divided doses after meals and with high daily fluid intake.

ASPIRIN U.S.P. (Acetylsalicylic acid)

Actions and Indications. Aspirin in ordinary doses possesses analgesic, antipyretic, and antiinflammatory properties. It is used mainly for relief of headache and relatively minor muscle and joint discomfort but is also effective for relief of mild to moderate postpartum and postoperative pain. Somewhat higher doses are employed in the management of chronic rheumatoid arthritis, and dosage may be pushed to the limit of tolerance in treating acute rheumatic fever.

Side Effects, Cautions, and Contra-indications. Ordinary doses produce few side effects, except for gastrointestinal discomfort, nausea, and occult bleeding in some individuals. A few hypersensitive people may suffer allergic reactions, including the severe anaphylactoid type. Caution is required in patients with a general history of allergy, and the drug is contraindicated in those who are known to be sensitive to aspirin specifically.

Moderately high therapeutic doses may produce salicylism, mild toxicity marked by ringing in the ears (tinnitus), visual disturbances, dizziness, restlessness, and confusion. Massive overdosage leads to serious acid-base imbalances in young children that can result in coma, convulsions, cardiovascular collapse, and fatal respiratory failure.

Dosage and Administration. The usual dose is 600 mg which may be repeated in two to four hours. In rheumatic disorders, total daily doses of 3.6 g to as much as 10 g may be employed to maintain therapeutic blood levels. Each dose is taken with large amounts of water, milk, and food, and dosage is re-

duced if tinnitus or other signs of salicylism appear.

COLCHICINE U.S.P.

Actions and Indications. This is a specific drug for aborting acute attacks of gout. It also helps to prevent recurrences when taken in smaller daily doses together with a uricosuric agent such as probenecid. Colchicine itself does not affect uric acid metabolism, and although it is not an analgesic nor a general antiinflammatory agent, it relieves pain and suppresses the inflammatory response to uric acid in the joints of patients with gouty arthritis.

Side Effects, Cautions, and Contra-indications. Diarrhea, nausea, and vomiting may develop with high oral doses, but such symptoms are less likely to occur when the drug is administered by the intravenous route. Overdosage may cause kidney damage, and shock may occur as a result of damage to blood vessels and bleeding from gastroenteritis. Prolonged administration may cause bone marrow damage and peripheral neuritis. Caution is required in elderly or weakened patients and those with gastrointestinal or cardiovascular disease.

Dosage and Administration. At the first warning sign of an attack, 1 or 2 tablets containing 0.5 or 0.6 mg may be administered by mouth, or 1 or 2 mg may be injected intravenously with care to avoid leakage into the subcutaneous tissues. These initial doses may be followed by one tablet every one or two hours until pain is relieved or diarrhea develops; or 0.5 mg may be administered I.V. every three to six hours up to a maximum of 4 mg in 24 hours.

For prophylaxis, 0.5 or 0.6 mg may be administered several times a week or taken once or twice daily.

ERGOTAMINE TARTRATE U.S.P. (Gynergen)

Actions and Indications. This is a specific drug for control of acute attacks of migraine. It acts to abort vascular headaches by constricting dilated cerebral arterioles. Its use for prophylactic purposes is not desirable, and it should not be taken daily for longer than one week.

Side Effects, Cautions, and Contra-indications. Nausea, vomiting, epigastric distress, and diarrhea may occur with large doses. Potentially more serious are signs indicating peripheral vasoconstriction, including numbness and tingling of fingers and toes, muscle cramps and pain in the legs, and chest pain. Overdosage can cause gangrene.

The drug is contraindicated in patients with peripheral vascular disease. It should not be taken during pregnancy or by individuals known to be hypersensitive to it—for example, those who react with severe itching and local edema.

Dosage and Administration. This drug is administered by many routes, but is most effective when injected intramuscularly or subcutaneously at the start of an attack. Dosage by this route is 0.25 to 0.5 mg. This may be repeated in one hour, but no more than 1 mg may be given in one 24-hour period, or 2 mg per week.

Oral administration of 1 or 2 mg at the start of an attack may be followed by additional doses every half hour up to a maximum of 6 mg in 24 hours.

The drug is also available as an aerosol for inhalation and as sublingual or buccal tablets, and it may be administered also by the rectal route.

PHENACETIN U.S.P.
(Acetophenetidin)

Actions and Indications. This drug has analgesic-antipyretic properties similar to those of aspirin, with which it is commonly combined in products for relief of headache and mild to moderate muscle, joint, and other pain. However, phenacetin has *little* of the antiinflammatory activity of aspirin and can*not* be substituted for it in the management of rheumatic disorders. It may be used in place of aspirin in individuals sensitive to salicylates or in gout patients who are being treated with a uricosuric agent, the effects of which might be antagonized by aspirin.

Side Effects, Cautions and Contraindications. Ordinary doses normally produce few side effects. However, some individuals with a congenital deficiency of the enzyme glucose-6-phosphate dehydrogenase (G-6PD) may suffer hemolytic anemia from only small doses. (This disorder may also develop in others as a result of a hypersensitivity-type reaction, usually after a high intake of the drug.)

Prolonged intake of high doses has also reportedly resulted in kidney damage (nephritis with papillary necrosis). However, it is uncertain whether this substance, or other drugs in the combination products that the patient has been abusing, is the actual cause of this manifestation of chronic toxicity. Large doses may lead to production of methemoglobinemia, but this is much less likely than with the related drug, acetanilid.

Dosage and Administration. The dose when used alone is 300 to 600 mg up to a total of no more than 2.4 g daily. However, this drug is more commonly administered in fractions of the full dose combined with fractional doses of aspirin plus a small amount of caffeine in the common APC products.

PHENYLBUTAZONE U.S.P.
(Butazolidin)

Actions and Indications. The antiinflammatory effects of this drug makes it valuable in selected cases of rheumatoid arthritis and other kinds of inflammatory disorders that are not controlled by other safer analgesic-antipyretic, antiinflammatory agents. It is useful, for example, in rheumatoid arthritis not relieved by salicylates, ankylosing spondylitis not responsive to indomethacin, and acute gout attacks not controlled by colchicine. The drug is also useful for suppressing inflammatory symptoms of acute thrombophlebitis.

Side Effects, Cautions, and Contraindications. Patients must be carefully selected and observed frequently to avoid the various kinds of dangerous reactions to this drug. Frequent blood tests are required to detect early signs of possible blood dyscrasias. The drug is contraindicated in patients with a history of hematological disorders, peptic ulcer, and cardiovascular, kidney, or liver diseases.

Dosage and Administration. Dosage varies depending upon the age of the patient, his physical condition, and the nature of the disorder being treated. Adults with most rheumatoid disorders receive between 300 and 600 mg daily. This is divided into three or four doses, each of which is taken immediately before or after meals or with a glass of milk to minimize epigastric distress. (A form containing this drug combined with antacids may also be employed.) Acute gouty arthritis requires higher doses for shorter periods—400 mg initially followed by 100 mg every four hours until joint inflammation subsides. Acute thrombophlebitis is treated with daily doses of 600 mg for the first few days, followed by 300 mg daily for the final few days.

PROBENECID U.S.P. (Benemid)

Actions and Indications. This drug's most common use is in the treatment of gout. It acts to increase the amount of uric acid excreted by the kidneys. This uricosuric effect results in the reduction of plasma and tissue levels of uric acid and thus tends to prevent gout attacks.

Probenecid is also administered together with the penicillins in order to raise the level of these antibiotics in infected tissues, and prolong their bactericidal activity against relatively resistant strains of susceptible pathogens that are the cause of severe infections.

Side Effects, Cautions, and Contraindications. This drug is well tolerated but may cause reactions in hypersensitive patients. Those with a history of itchy rashes and other signs of sensitivity to probenecid should be treated with another type of uricosuric agent to avoid more severe actions, including anaphylaxis.

Early treatment sometimes sets off an acute attack of gout, but this may be prevented or treated by the administration of colchicine at the same time. Acetaminophen is the preferred analgesic for relief of mild pain in patients taking this drug, as aspirin and other salicylates tend to antagonize this drug's uricosuric action.

Dosage and Administration. Initial doses of 0.25 g twice daily are raised to 0.5 g after one week or to higher levels (up to 2 g) in patients with impaired kidney function. It is important to force fluids to avoid formation of urate stones. Total daily dosage as an adjunct to penicillin therapy is 2 g for most adult patients.

References

ANALGESIC-ANTIPYRETICS

Boyd, E.M. The safety and toxicity of aspirin. *Amer. J. Nurs.*, 71:964, 1971 (May).

De Kornfeld, T.S. Aspirin. *Amer. J. Nurs.*, 64:60, 1964.

Gross, M. The salicylates. *Amer. J. Nurs.*, 55: 1372, 1955.

Rodman, M.J. Drugs for pain problems. *RN*, 34:59, 1971 (April).

RHEUMATIC DISORDERS

Bayles, T.B. Salicylate therapy of rheumatoid arthritis. *Med. Clin. N. Amer.*, 52:703, 1968 (May).

Magginniss, O. Rheumatoid arthritis—my tutor. *Amer. J. Nurs.*, 68:1699, 1968 (Aug.).

Rodman, M.J. Drugs for rheumatic disorders. *RN*, 31:55, 1968 (Sept.).

Weaver, A.L. Management of rheumatoid arthritis. *Bedside Nurse*, 4:14, 1971 (May).

GOUT

Ball, G.V., and Freeman, D. Management of chronic and recurrent gout. *Mod. Treatm.*, 8:829, 1971 (Nov.).

Bartels, E.C. Acute gout—definitely a medical emergency. *Med. Clin. N. Amer.*, 53:455, 1969 (March).

Johnson, S.B. Understanding hyperuricemia. *Nurs. Clin. N. Amer.*, 7:399, 1972 (June).

Talbott, J.H. Gout. *Med. Clin. N. Amer.*, 54:431, 1970 (March).

———, and Ricketts, A. Gout and gouty arthritis. *Amer. J. Nurs.*, 59:1405, 1959.

Rodman, M.J. Drug treatment of gouty arthritis. *RN*, 23:33, 1960 (Dec.).

HEADACHE

Friedman, A.P. Treatment of migraine. Symposium on the treatment of headache. *Mod. Treatm.*, 6:1363, 1964 (Nov.).

Graham, J.R., et al. Fibrotic disorders associated with methysergide therapy for headache. *New Eng. J. Med.*, 274:359, 1966.

Rodman, M.J. Drugs for recurring headache. *RN*, 29:65, 1966 (June).

17.

Adrenocorticosteroid Drugs and Corticotropin

Adrenal-Pituitary Physiology

The adrenocorticosteroid drugs are among the most important substances employed in modern medicine. The antiinflammatory and other pharmacological actions of these agents have proved useful in the treatment of countless clinical disorders. However, these drugs are not a cure for any of the scores of conditions in which they are administered but only suppress the signs and symptoms of disease. In addition, their long-continued administration in high doses can be quite harmful. Thus, in order to understand the principles that the physician employs in making the best use of these drugs, we should first review briefly the physiological effects of the adrenal cortex hormones and their relationship to the pituitary hormone, corticotropin.

PITUITARY-ADRENAL GLAND RELATIONSHIPS

The anterior pituitary gland controls the production of the hormones secreted by the outer shell, or cortex, of the adrenal glands. Certain pituitary cells secrete a substance, the *adrenocorticotropic hormone (corticotropin—ACTH)*. Carried by the bloodstream to the two adrenal glands just above each kidney, this substance stimulates the adrenal cortex tissues to make and release certain steroid hormones including cortisol, or hydrocortisone, and cortisone (Fig. 17-1).

REGULATION OF HORMONE SECRETION. The secretion of these hormones does not occur at a steady rate but varies at different times during

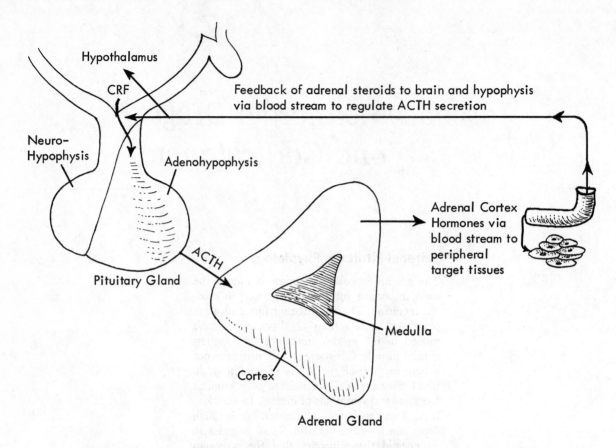

Fig. 17-1. Interrelationships between corticotropin secretion and adrenal cortical function.

the day. Corticotropin, for example, is manufactured by the pituitary during the night and is released in largest amounts in the early morning hours. This, in turn, causes the adrenocorticosteroid hormones to be secreted at their highest level of the day at that time. The level of natural steroid hormone secretion then drops during the day and reaches its lowest levels late at night.

This fall in circulating steroids serves as a stmulus to the pituitary gland, which then steps up its production of corticotropin, the adrenal cortex stimulating hormone. The administration of high doses of adrenocorticosteroids does the opposite; that is, an excess of substances with adrenal hormone activity suppresses this pituitary-adrenal secretory mechanism (see p. 223).

Physical and emotional stress may cause a tenfold increase in the production of both these types of hormones. Thus, for example, people who are injured and suffer severe blood loss may secrete 250 mg of cortisol in 24 hours instead of the usual 25 mg daily. However, this lifesaving response to stress, including anesthesia and surgery, or severe infection and fever, may fail to occur in patients whose pituitary-adrenal function has been suppressed by prior treatment with high doses of adrenocorticosteroid drugs.

Natural steroids of three kinds are secreted by the adrenal cortex. These substances, which differ in their physiological functions are:

1. The *glucocorticoids*—substances such as *cortisol* (hydrocortisone) and *cortisone*, which mainly affect carbohydrate metabolism, but also affect protein and fat metabolism.

2. The *mineralocorticoids, aldosterone,* and *desoxycorticosterone*, which influence salt and water metabolism, help the kidneys hold sodium in exchange for potassium ions.

3. Certain *male* and *female sex hormones.* These are of only minor importance in normal metabolism compared to similar substances secreted by the testes and the ovaries. However, their presence in excess sometimes causes pathologic symptoms.

The glucocorticoids and mineralocorticoids

play an important part in helping the body adjust to changes in environment. Through their metabolic effects these adrenal hormones influence the functioning of most organs and systems. Their importance for human survival becomes obvious in the imbalances that result from a lack of these hormones (*hypocorticism*) or from their presence in excess amounts (*hypercorticism*).

Adrenal Insufficiency and its Treatment

Hypocorticism occurs mainly as a result of adrenal gland damage, atrophy, or surgical removal. Addison's disease is an example of a disorder that results in adrenal lesions that lead to insufficient hormone production. Adrenal insufficiency also often follows adrenalectomy, an operation sometimes performed in patients with certain kinds of cancers.

Pituitary failure can, of course, also lead to a secondary lack of adrenal secretions caused by the absence of the adrenocorticotropic hormone of the anterior pituitary gland (see p. 221). As also mentioned above, the long-term administration of high doses of corticosteroid drugs may also act to suppress pituitary function and thus indirectly bring about adrenal insufficiency. Surgical excision of the pituitary gland—an operation called *hypophysectomy* that is sometimes performed for treating severe diabetes—also leads to loss of the adrenal stimulating hormone. The result in all such situations is partial or complete atrophy of the adrenal glands.

REPLACEMENT THERAPY

Patients with chronic adrenal insufficiency can usually be kept in good health today. They regularly take small amounts of substances which have the activity of the missing hormones. The natural glucocorticoid *hydrocortisone+* (which also has some mineralocorticoid activity) keeps many patients in metabolic balance when taken in replacement doses of 15 to 30 mg daily. However, most patients require the addition of a more potent, pure mineralocorticoid such as *desoxycorticosterone acetate+* or the potent synthetic adrenal hormone substitute *fludrocortisone acetate* (Florinef) to prevent dangerous dehydration and drops in blood pressure.

When these patients catch a heavy cold or suffer some other concurrent illness, the doses of these substitutes are doubled. Patients who show sudden signs of acute adrenal insufficiency require prompt treatment with massive doses of steroids. The soluble salts and esters of hydrocortisone are commonly infused by vein along with a large volume of fluid in the form of isotonic sodium chloride and glucose solution. The nurse in the intensive care unit must often monitor the patient's central venous pressure to avoid fluid overload while checking the effect of this treatment upon his arterial blood pressure. The underlying stressful cause of adrenal cortex insufficiency—severe injury, overwhelming infection, or heavy bleeding for example—must also be treated at the same time, while the steroids are helping to tide the patient over the life-threatening crisis.

Patients who would once not have survived acute and chronic adrenal insufficiency can now usually be saved and then kept alive indefinitely. The physician determines the daily doses of adrenal hormones needed to substitute for those that are lacking. The nurse often checks the patient's blood pressure, muscle strength, and general health to be sure that the missing hormones and salt are being properly replaced.

The Therapeutic Uses of Natural and Synthetic Glucocorticoids

PHARMACOLOGICAL EFFECTS

The corticosteroids are used clinically in many disorders besides adrenal insufficiency. Administered in doses larger than the small amounts employed in replacement therapy, the natural and synthetic glucocorticoids produce various pharmacological effects. Among the biological effects that are brought about by doses greater than the amounts produced physiologically by the adrenal glands, the most widely useful is the ability to suppress inflammatory and allergic tissue responses.

These related *antiinflammatory* and *antiallergy actions* account for the effectiveness of corticosteroids in treating many clinical conditions. These include rheumatoid arthritis and other diseases that affect connective tissue protein of the collagen type. Other so-called collagen diseases in which the pathologic process can be temporarily suppressed by corticosteroid drugs include systemic lupus erythematosus and pemphigus (see also *Summary*, p. 230, for other classes of responsive clinical conditions).

High doses of glucocorticoids also seem to increase the body's capacity to withstand stress. That is, these substances somehow act to help the body mobilize its defenses to resist all kinds of severe challenges. Part of this *antistress action* of the corticosteroids may have to do with their ability to aid circulating vasopressor substances in keeping the patient's blood pressure up. In the case of the natural glucocorticoids such as hydrocortisone, a sodium- and water-retaining component also helps to counteract shock by raising the blood volume. Yet, the newer synthetic steroids that have little or no mineralocorticoid activity are also often useful for maintaining cardiovascular function during life-threatening illnesses.

ADVERSE EFFECTS

The relative freedom of the synthetic steroids from mineralocorticoid activity makes these drugs safer for use in some patients. A drug such as *dexamethasone+*, for example, produces its desired antiinflammatory action without causing salty fluids to accumulate or loss of potassium. This makes it particularly useful for patients with heart disease and high blood pressure, in whom the drug-induced edema caused by hydrocortisone or cortisone could prove dangerous.

In all other respects, however, the natural and synthetic corticosteroids produce the same kinds of chronic toxicity (see p. 227, and *Summary*, p. 231). This occurs because the doses needed to produce the therapeutically desirable antiinflammatory and antiallergy effects also eventually bring about metabolic toxicity, pituitary gland suppression, and changes in central nervous system function that can be disabling and dangerous. This is as true of the potent synthetic steroids such as dexamethasone+ and betamethasone, which produce an antiinflammatory effect in doses of less than 1 mg, as it is of the natural steroids that require doses as much as thirty times higher (Tables 17-1 and 17-2).

DOSAGE ADJUSTMENT

The fact that the long-continued use of *any* corticosteroid will inevitably produce adverse effects makes these drugs a two-edged sword. Thus, the doctor first has to decide whether the risks of starting a patient on long-term steroid therapy of a chronic disorder are worth taking. If he does decide that the benefits outweigh the risks, the doctor adjusts the dose of these drugs to the minimal amount needed to relieve each patient's symptoms. He keeps the patient under close observation and tries to reduce dosage periodically or even discontinues these drugs entirely if possible. The nurse also observes the patient for side effects and encourages him to get along on lower doses whenever the doctor orders dosage reduction. (Local administration of steroids, whenever possible, also helps to lessen the likelihood of systemic toxic reactions.)

CLINICAL USES

The dosage of adrenocorticosteroids needed to produce clinically desirable effects while keeping adverse effects at a minimum varies very widely. How much will be required to suppress a patient's signs and symptoms depends upon many factors that the doctor must consider, including particularly whether the condition is a chronic one that will need prolonged drug treatment. Here are some examples of the problems that arise in different kinds of cases that respond to treatment with corticosteroid drugs (see also the *Summary of Dosage and Administration Principles*, pp. 231-232).

Chronic conditions such as rheumatoid arthritis and bronchial asthma are often benefited by treatment with steroids. Yet the cautious physician turns to these agents only after other measures have failed to keep these conditions under adequate control. This is because the corticosteroids do not cure these chronic disorders and their continued use will inevitably cause some adverse effects. In addition, once patients have experienced the symptomatic relief that these drugs can produce, they often resist attempts to reduce their dosage or to discontinue corticosteroid therapy.

As indicated in the more detailed discussions of the use of corticosteroids in asthma (Chap. 19) and arthritis (Chap. 16), patients with these chronic disorders are kept on the lowest doses capable of providing symptomatic relief and preventing crippling disability. Whenever the patient's symptoms seem to be subsiding spontaneously, the steroid dosage is slowly reduced. The nurse teaches the patient why it is important for him to get along on the lower doses of these drugs, even though he may feel less comfortable than when taking larger amounts. She provides the encouragement and emotional support that these patients usually

TABLE 17-1 *Adrenocorticosteroid Drugs**

Nonproprietary or Official Name	Synonym or Proprietary Name	Usual Doses† and Dosage Ranges
Betamethasone N.F.	Celestone	600 mcg to 4.8 mg daily, oral
Cortisone acetate U.S.P.	Cortogen; Cortone	Oral 25 mg q.i.d.; I.M. 100 mg daily
Dexamethasone U.S.P.	Decadron; Deronil; Decameth; Gammacorten; Hexadrol	500 mcg to 6 mg daily; 750 mcg 2 to 4 times daily
Dexamethasone sodium phosphate U.S.P.	Decadron phosphate	0.4 to 6 mg per local injection
Hydrocortisone U.S.P.	Cortisol; Cortef; Cortifan; Cortril; Hydrocortone	10 to 300 mg daily; oral 10 mg up to 4 times a day
Hydrocortisone acetate U.S.P.	Cortef acetate	10 to 50 mg intraarticular
Hydrocortisone cypionate	Cortef fluid	Initially 20 to 500 mg; maintenance 10 to 260 mg
Hydrocortisone sodium succinate U.S.P.	Solucortef	50 to 300 mg daily I.V. or I.M.
Methylprednisolone sodium succinate N.F.	Solu-medrol	10 to 40 mg daily I.V. or I.M.
Methylprednisolone N.F.	Medrol	Oral 4 mg q.i.d. or 2 to 60 mg daily
Paramethasone acetate N.F.	Haldrone	Oral 6 to 12 mg initially; 1 to 8 mg maintenance
Prednisolone U.S.P.	Delta Cortef; Hydeltra; Meticortelone; Metiderm; Paracortol; Sterane; Sterolone	Oral 5 mg 1 to 4 times daily for 2 to 7 days; then 5 mg one or more times a day. Range: 5 to 80 mg daily
Prednisolone acetate U.S.P.	Sterane	5 to 50 mg intraarticular; 5 to 80 mg daily I.M.
Prednisolone sodium phosphate U.S.P.	Hydeltrasol	10 to 100 mg I.M. or I.V.
Prednisone U.S.P.	Deltasone; Deltra; Meticorten; Paracort	Initially 5 mg 2 to 4 times a day for 2 to 7 days; maintenance, up to 5 mg one or more times a day. Range: 5 to 80 mg daily
Triamcinolone U.S.P.	Aristocort; Kenacort	Initially 8 to 30 mg daily orally for adults; 4 to 16 mg daily for children; reduce for maintenance

* These drugs are administered orally or parenterally for systemic or intraarticular actions of an antiinflammatory or antistress type. Other steroids and dosage forms are available for topical application and for mineralocorticoid activity.

† Doses vary very widely, depending on the nature and severity of the condition that is being treated. Equivalent milligram dosages of the glucocorticoids are given in Table 17-2.

need in order to profit from the total therapeutic plan for treating these chronic disorders.

Acute flare-ups of these chronic conditions are handled differently. Instead of starting with the small doses of steroids that are used when the patient's symptoms worsen only slowly, the doctor orders quite large doses. This, together with other emergency measures, is intended: to bring about prompt relief of bronchial obstruction in a condition such as status asthmaticus; to counteract widespread, severe joint inflammation in an exacerbation of rheu-

matoid arthritis; or to stop signs of the systemic toxicity of an acute rheumatic fever attack, particularly when myocarditis (heart muscle inflammation) is present. High steroid dosage does *not* cause much metabolic toxicity when administered for only a few days and then slowly reduced to low maintenance dose levels.

Acute crises in the course of potentially fatal infections and other serious illnesses are also sometimes treated with massive doses of corticosteroids. For example, patients in shock from septicemia caused by gram-negative bac-

TABLE 17-2 *Comparison of Common Corticosteroid Drugs*

Name of Glucocorticoid	Relative Antiinflammatory Potency*	Relative Mineralocorticoid Activity†	Relative Duration of Activity‡
Hydrocortisone	1 (20 mg)	Strong (2+)	Short (1½ days)
Cortisone	0.8 (25 mg)	Strong (2+)	Short (1½ days)
Prednisone	3.5 (5 mg)	Moderate (1+)	Short (1½ days)
Prednisolone	4 (5 mg)	Moderate (1+)	Short (1½ days)
Methylprednisolone	5 (4 mg)	Little (0+)	Short (1½ days)
Triamcinolone	5 (4 mg)	Little (0+)	Intermediate (2+ days)
Paramethasone	10 (2 mg)	Little (0+)	Intermediate (2+ days)
Dexamethasone	25 (0.75 mg)	Little (0+)	Long (more than 2½ days)
Betamethasone	30 (0.60 mg)	Little (0+)	Long (more than 2½ days)

* Compared to hydrocortisone, which here has the arbitrary value of 1 and the actual dosage of 20 mg. (The weaker compound cortisone, only 0.8 times as potent as hydrocortisone, requires a higher dose (25mg). The synthetic steroids are arranged in accordance with their increasing potency and consequently lower dosage for equivalent antiinflamatory activity.)

† Compared to the purely mineralcorticoid compound fludrocortisone with activity of 5+. (Only hydrocortisone and cortisone cause enough sodium retention to make them useful for treating some cases of acute and chronic adrenal insufficiency.)

‡ Compared in terms of duration of hypothalamo-pituitary-adrenal suppression rather than in terms of the biological (plasma) half-life of the compounds.

teria have reportedly been helped by the timely infusion of a soluble steroid such as hydrocortisone sodium succinate+ in large doses, together with antiinfective agents and other drugs and measures for treating shock. Once the patient has weathered the crisis and is recovering, corticosteroid therapy can then be quickly reduced and discontinued.

Massive doses of steroids may also be employed during the acute crises that develop periodically in certain potentially fatal chronic disorders such as systemic lupus erythematosus and pemphigus. Here, however, the patient is usually continued on high steroid dosage even after the immediate danger has passed. This is because the complications that often occur in these dangerous disorders are considered to be worse than the inevitably toxic effects of large daily doses of steroids. Of course, every effort is made to minimize the adverse effects of drug-induced hypercorticism (p. 227).

Corticosteroids are most effective for use in conditions that are acutely disabling for a brief period but are not of a chronic nature. Hay fever and poison ivy are examples of such acute, self-limiting ailments. One way of producing rapid symptomatic relief in such cases is by administering steroids orally in a so-called "step-down," or "cut-down," dosage schedule.

In this regimen the patient takes high doses for the first two or three days; then, as his symptoms begin to subside, each day's dosage is reduced for the next few days. Finally, after one week to ten days, steroids are discontinued entirely without having caused any significant side effects. Patients with pollinosis may continue to have symptomatic relief for the remaining several weeks of the hay fever season.

Topical administration of steroids is another means of minimizing systemic toxicity while attaining their beneficial effects locally. Steroids, applied topically to the skin in the form of creams, lotions, ointments and aerosols have been particularly effective for symptomatic relief of various acute and chronic dermatologic disorders, including atopic (eczematous) dermatitis, contact dermatitis, and psoriasis.

In psoriasis, wrapping an occlusive dressing around the parts to which the steroid has been applied permits it to penetrate deeply through the superficial scales and exert its antiinflammatory effect on underlying areas. Some cases of psoriasis and other dermatologic disorders such as lichen planus and neurodermatitis are also treated by infiltrating the lesion with a local injection of a poorly absorbable steroid ester such as *triamcinolone acetonide*+.

Such intralesional injections sometimes produce long-lasting remissions of these chronic skin disorders. As is the case also with occlusive dressings, systemic (metabolic or endocrine) toxicity does not ordinarily occur. Thus, this method may be preferable to oral steroid dosage in these chronic skin disorders. Sometimes, however, the high local concentration of the steroid in the injected area may cause the underlying tissues to become atrophied. Usually such shrinkage or dimpling of the skin, though somewhat disfiguring, is only temporary.

Acute ocular inflammation in outer eye tissues may also be suppressed by topically applied steroids that attain high local concentrations in the anterior chamber. Unlike the oral and injectable steroids that must be administered for more deep-seated ocular inflammation involving structures *behind* the iris, steroid eye drops do not cause systemic toxicity. However, repeated application of corticosteroids has reportedly caused a rise in intraocular pressure (and possibly glaucoma) in some patients and development of cataracts (clouding of the lens) in others. Thus, patients who require long-term topical ocular steroids must be observed for signs of these adverse local effects or of thinning of the cornea.

The principle of delivering high corticosteroid concentrations to local sites for greater effectiveness with little risk of systemic toxicity is also employed in some cases of arthritis and of respiratory allergy. In osteoarthritis, for example, and in rheumatoid arthritis when only a few joints are involved, long-acting steroid suspensions may be injected directly into the patient's joints. Such intra-articular injections often produce long-lasting relief without causing systemic steroid toxicity. However, strict sterile technique is needed to avoid joint infection, and patients must be cautioned to avoid excessive activity that may cause further joint damage.

The Adverse Effects of Corticosteroid Therapy

The administration of corticosteroids in amounts capable of producing clinically desirable pharmacological effects can lead to many complications. These are most likely to occur in patients with chronic conditions that require long-term therapy. Complications are most likely to have serious consequences in patients with underlying disorders that make them particularly susceptible to the adverse pharma-

cological effects of steroid therapy. (*Summary of Contraindications and Precautions*, p. 231.)

The adverse effects can be classified in general as follows:

1. *Metabolic effects.* These are the result of excessive glucocorticoid and mineralocorticoid activity, which lead to very many signs and symptoms of toxicity and make patients susceptible to many complications.

2. *Central nervous system effects.* These are manifested mainly by various kinds of mental changes brought about by high doses of corticosteroids in susceptible individuals.

3. *Endocrine effects.* These result from the effects of the prolonged action of steroids upon anterior pituitary gland function which, in turn, leads to secondary effects upon the adrenal glands and on body tissues in general.

One type of metabolic effect—the mineralocorticoid activity that can lead to sodium retention, edema, and potassium loss—is minimal with the newer synthetic glucocorticoids. These steroids are therefore preferred to the natural adrenal hormones in patients with heart disease and high blood pressure. However, because some patients gain weight when on corticosteroid therapy, it is important that a careful record of weight be kept.

Metabolic toxicity of the glucocorticoid type is very much more common, because scientists have not yet been able to make any synthetic steroids in which these side effects can be separated from the desired antiinflammatory and antiallergy effects. The signs and symptoms of excessive glucocorticoid activity (hypercorticism) resemble those seen in Cushing's syndrome, a disorder caused by certain types of pituitary or adrenal gland tumors. Such Cushingoid signs include a characteristic fullness or rounding of the face and an abnormal distribution of body fat (*Summary of Side Effects*, p. 231).

The drug-induced changes in metabolism of carbohydrates, protein, and fat make some patients particularly prone to certain kinds of complications. Diabetes mellitus symptoms, may, for example, show up in patients who have no previous history of high blood glucose or sugar in the urine. Similarly, some patients may develop peptic ulcer, and others may be found to be suffering from osteoporosis, a condition that can result in compression fractures of the vertebrae.

None of these conditions necessarily contraindicates the use of corticosteroids in patients who require these drugs. Patients with diabetes may be maintained on oral hypoglycemic agents or adjusted doses of insulin. Patients with osteoporosis may be helped by eating a high protein diet, taking calcium salt supplements, and by the administration of anabolic agents while they are being maintained on corticosteroid therapy. Nursing care of these patients includes measures to prevent injury that may result in fracture. Patients with a history of peptic ulcer receive antacids routinely and also antispasmodic drugs occasionally. Gastrointestinal tract x-rays are taken periodically during treatment, and the patient's stools are checked for the presence of occult blood. (Corticosteroids may mask the pain of a peptic ulcer that could be approaching the perforation stage.)

Infection may also be masked, even while it is spreading, because the patient's defenses against invading microorganisms are lowered by the metabolic effects of corticosteroids. This resistance-reducing effect of the steroids does not mean that these drugs cannot be used in the presence of infection. However, heavy doses of effective antiinfective agents must be administered at the same time. The nurse needs to make careful observations to detect even slight signs of infection. Thus, even though corticosteroids may reactivate healed lesions in tuberculosis patients, use of these drugs may be justified provided that the doctor also orders antituberculosis medication such as isoniazid to prevent a flare-up of active infection.

The danger of steroid-spread infection is most serious when viruses and fungi are involved because of the lack of effective antiviral agents and the difficulty of treating widespread systemic fungal infections. Thus, steroids are used with caution, if at all, in patients with herpes simplex virus infections of the eye or in children with chicken pox, for example. Caution is also required in chronic diseases in children because of the tendency of steroids to suppress growth.

CENTRAL NERVOUS SYSTEM TOXICITY

Corticosteroid therapy often affects the patient's mental state. Most commonly, the patient becomes happy and talkative. This sometimes happens so soon after treatment with steroids is started that it was thought to be the patient's natural response to the drug-induced relief of pain or other discomforting physical symptoms. Actually, this euphoric effect is now known to result from an action of corticosteroids on the CNS. Some patients so enjoy this feeling of well-being that they become, in effect, psychologically dependent upon steroids. This is one reason why they resist attempts to reduce dosage or to withdraw these drugs.

The continued use of corticosteroids sometimes leads to excessive excitement, restlessness, and sleeplessness. The patient's mood may become manic and then swing back to a stage of agitated depression. The nurse should watch for such mood swings and behavioral changes and report them to the patient's physician. He will then try to reduce dosage to avoid possible psychotic complications, including suicide attempts. Such mood swings require nursing intervention: for example, reducing stimuli and thus helping the manic patient to become calmer, and supporting the patient who is depressed and thus helping him combat this distressing symptom.

Serious reactions of this kind are relatively rare. More often, the main difficulty caused by drug-induced mental changes is a decrease in the patient's ability to cope with his chronic illness constructively. The nurse must make a special effort to help the patient meet his problems realistically and maintain his relationship with other people, despite the adverse effects of steroid medication on his mood and emotional state.

The cause of manic-depressive, schizophrenic, and other psychotic reactions to corticosteroids is uncertain. Unlike other types of steroid toxicity, the adverse central effects are not closely related to the length of time patients have been taking high supraphysiologic (pharmacologic) doses. A more important factor in determining which patients will react abnormally is the patient's personality before treatment is begun. People with a history of emotional and psychological difficulties develop these kinds of complications more often than other patients. Thus, the doctor tries to avoid steroid use in such cases, particularly in patients who are already psychotic.

ENDOCRINE TOXICITY

As mentioned earlier, long-term steroid treatment tends to suppress certain anterior pituitary gland functions. This may partially account for the failure of children to grow during prolonged administration of corticosteroids for nephrosis, severe bronchial asthma, and other conditions in which these drugs offer symptomatic relief. More common is the occurrence of suppression of production of the pituitary's adrencorticotropic hormone. This in turn leads to reduction in the size of the patient's adrenal glands and in their ability to produce adrenal cortex hormones.

The danger in such cases of partial adrenal atrophy is that even though the patient may normally show no signs of adrenal insufficiency, he may not be able to withstand any unusual stress. Thus, a patient who suffers a severe injury or illness or who requires surgery—even many months after steroids have been withdrawn—may develop acute adrenal insufficiency. This requires immediate treatment with massive doses of corticosteroids to avoid severe, possibly fatal collapse. This situation underscores the necessity that the nurse listen intently to the patient's account of previous illnesses and their therapy, when she is carrying out her assessment of the patient.

STEROID WITHDRAWAL

Doctors have tried to avoid steroid-induced adrenal insufficiency by reducing steroid dosage only very slowly. This is thought to help the patient's pituitary gland to regain its normal function. Some authorities have suggested that also administering injections of the adrenal-stimulating pituitary hormone corticotropin increases the rate at which the adrenal glands recover their function. Other authorities deny that the administration of this pituitary hormone helps to hasten a return to normal pituitary-adrenal function, and they even claim that corticotropin dosage may actually delay the process. All do agree that patients who become seriously ill during the year after they have been withdrawn from prolonged steroid therapy should be put back on supplemental doses of these drugs during the course of the acute illness.

INTERMITTENT DOSAGE SCHEDULES

In order to minimize the inevitably toxic effects of prolonged treatment with pharmacologic doses of steroids, doctors have been trying to devise new dosage schedules. Instead of ordering the drugs to be taken in the traditional way—in three or four divided daily doses, for example—they now often suggest that the patient take the total daily dose all at once on several days of the week and no drug at all on other days.

The best time of day to take the total steroid dose is in the morning between 7:00 and 8:00 a.m. This time is believed to cause the least interference with the patient's pituitary gland production of corticotropin. This, in turn, lessens the drug-induced depression of the patient's adrenal gland activity. Other types of toxicity, including reduced growth in children, may also be minimized when this dosage schedule is employed.

Alternate day therapy is possible in many patients. Here, the patient takes the total dose that would ordinarily be spread over 48 hours every other morning. This schedule seems especially useful for reducing metabolic and endocrine toxicity in children who require lengthy steroid treatment for control of nephrosis or severe bronchial asthma. However, even though side effects may also be reduced in other patients, some of them complain of discomfort late on the second—or "no-medication" day—when the level of steroids in their inflamed tissues falls below the point of effectiveness.

Therefore, in order to profit from alternate day therapy and other intermittent dosage schedules, many patients require emotional support. The nurse teaches the patient the reasons for continuing to take steroid drugs in this way. He should understand that even though this method does not give him complete relief of all his symptoms, it helps to prevent toxicity that might otherwise make it necessary to discontinue corticosteroids completely. In any case, the patient who receives personal assurance of the nurse's concern for his health and well-being is more likely to profit from long-term treatment of his chronic disorder.

Corticotropin (ACTH) [+]

The adrenocorticotropic pituitary hormone has been employed in the past for treating most of the same disorders that are relieved by corticosteroid therapy. This is understandable, as injections of this hormone stimulate normal adrenal glands to secrete increased amounts of all three types of adrenocorticosteroid hormones.

However, doctors now prefer to employ corticosteroid drugs rather than this adrenal cortex stimulating hormone.

DISADVANTAGES

One reason for the superiority of steroids in most conditions is that the foreign protein in the ACTH preparation may cause allergic reactions in sensitive patients. Skin tests are sometimes done before beginning treatment, and patients should be observed for a few minutes following injections to detect and to counteract anaphylaxis. In addition, oral doses of corticosteroid drugs are more convenient to administer and less expensive than corticotropin injections. The synthetic steroids produce a more predictable antiinflammatory effect, and they are free of the usually undesirable mineralocorticoid and sex hormone effects that corticotropin produces by its actions on the patient's own adrenal glands.

DIAGNOSIS AND TREATMENT OF ADRENAL INSUFFICIENCY

Corticotropin is not, of course, useful for treating adrenal insufficiency in patients who have had their adrenal glands removed. It is also ineffective in patients with Addison's disease or other disorders in which the patient's damaged adrenal glands do not respond to his own pituitary adrenocorticotropic hormone. Although corticotropin has, in the past, been advocated for stimulating the partially atrophied adrenal glands of patients who have been on long-term steroid therapy, it is rarely recommended today for reactivating adrenal function. (Some authorities suggest that once spontaneous recovery of adrenal secretion begins, corticotropin injections may help to shorten the lengthy recovery period.)

Corticotropin can, however, be useful in laboratory procedures for testing a patient's adrenal function. Patients with normal adrenal glands respond to an intravenous infusion of corticotropin with a marked increase in measurable levels of adrenal steroid hormones in the blood and urine. Patients with Addison's disease and other forms of adrenal insufficiency do not show the expected increase in steroid levels. This test can also be done periodically to determine the extent to which a patient's adrenal glands are regaining their function after corticosteroid therapy has been discontinued.

S U M M A R Y of Some Clinical Conditions Responsive to Corticosteroid Therapy

Collagen Diseases and Nonarticular Musculoskeletal Disorders

Rheumatoid arthritis (and related disorders, such as rheumatoid spondylitis, Still's disease, psoriatic arthritis, acute and chronic gout, and gouty arthritis)
Acute rheumatic fever
Bursitis, fibrositis, synovitis, myositis, tendinitis
Disseminated lupus erythematosus
Pemphigus
Scleroderma
Periarteritis nodosa
Dermatomyositis

Allergic, Infectious, and Other Inflammatory Disorders of the Skin and Ocular and Respiratory Mucous Membranes

Bronchial asthma, including status asthmaticus
Pulmonary fibrosis and emphysema
Pollinosis (hay fever)
Rhinitis (perennial vasomotor; allergic)
Skin disorders such as atopic dermatitis (eczema), contact dermatitis, poison ivy dermatitis, neurodermatitis, exfoliative dermatitis, angioneurotic edema, urticaria, seborrheic dermatitis, pruritus vulvi or ani, dermatitis herpetiformis
Eye disorders such as allergic conjunctivitis, iritis, iridocyclitis, choroiditis, chorioretinitis, keratitis, uveitis, corneal ulcers, secondary glaucoma
Severe allergic reaction including anaphylactic shock, transfusion reactions, Stevens-Johnson syndrome

Hematological and Neoplastic Conditions

Acute leukemia; chronic lymphocytic leukemia
Autoimmune hemolytic anemia
Acquired hemolytic anemia
Idiopathic thrombocytic purpura
Blood dyscrasias such as agranulocytosis and aplastic anemia
Breast cancer (advanced metastatic mammary carcinoma)

Hodgkin's disease and other lymphomatous neoplasms
Pulmonary granulomatosis

Miscellaneous

Nephrotic syndrome
Adrenogenital syndrome
Ulcerative colitis
Thyroiditis

Sarcoidosis
Hepatitis and cirrhosis
Parotitis (mumps)
Neuritis
Bell's palsy
Myocarditis and other cardiac conditions, including heart block and congestive heart failure
Shock—hemorrhagic, endotoxic, bacteremic, postoperative, and related types
Adrenocortical insufficiency

S U M M A R Y of Side Effects and Toxicity of Adrenocorticosteroid Drugs

Cushingoid signs such as:
Rounding of the face (moon face), with flushing, sweating, acne, and hirsutism; thinning of hair on the scalp, supraclavicular fat pads, buffalo hump, abdominal distention, and striae; weight gain
Thrombophlebitis, thromboembolism, petechiae, purpura, necrotizing angiitis
Peptic ulcer, gastrointestinal hemorrhage, ulcerative esophagitis, acute pancreatitis
Headache, vertigo, increased intracranial pressure, increased intraocular pressure, posterior subcapsular cataracts requiring extraction

Psychic disturbances, marked mainly by euphoria but sometimes by depression; insomnia, fatigue; convulsions
Protein depletion, with osteoporosis and spontaneous fractures; myopathy, with weakness of muscles, thighs, pelvis, and lower back; aseptic necrosis of the hip and humerus
Suppression of growth in children
Aggravation of infection
Aggravation of diabetes mellitus
Increase in blood pressure
Amenorrhea and other menstrual irregularities

S U M M A R Y of Contraindications and Precautions with Corticosteroid Drugs

Contraindications (Absolute and Relative)

Infections, including active, questionably healed, or latent tuberculosis; herpes simplex keratitis; and sometimes fungal or exanthematous diseases, such as chickenpox
Osteoporosis; myasthenia gravis
Peptic ulcer, diverticulitis, fresh intestinal anastomoses; thrombophlebitis
Diabetes mellitus; hyperthyroidism
Psychic or marked emotional disturbances
Hypertension; acute coronary disease, acute glomerular nephritis, and renal insufficiency
Pregnancy, especially in first trimester

Precautions

Patients with a history of peptic ulcer are placed on an antiulcer regimen, including antacid and anticholinergic drugs, diet, and rest. If they complain of abdominal pain, they are x-rayed (steroids may mask symptoms of perforation).
Patients with a history of tuberculosis should receive prophylactic doses of antituberculosis drugs. If infection develops in these or other patients, high dosage of appropriate antiinfective drugs is required. Steroids should *not* be withdrawn abruptly in acute infections (or other severe stress, such as surgery or trauma); dosage may actually be increased.
Patients with a history of well controlled diabetes are closely watched and their insulin dosage increased if glycosuria or hyperglycemia develops.
Patients should be closely watched for signs of possible adrenocortical insufficiency, periarteritis nodosa, and ocular changes. Children on prolonged steroid therapy are observed for signs of growth retardation.

S U M M A R Y of Principles of Corticosteroid Dosage and Administration

Chronic Nonfatal Disorders (for example, rheumatoid arthritis; asthma)

Steroids are reserved for use in cases not controlled by safer, more conservative measures.

Steroids are added to the patient's regular regimen in small doses that are then raised slowly.

Administration is continued at the lowest daily

dose levels needed for symptomatic relief and for the shortest possible time.

Acute exacerbations of these chronic conditions can be treated with large doses for short periods with relatively little danger, but dosage must be slowly reduced once the acute stage is brought under control.

During periods of disease remission, drug dosage is gradually reduced and, if possible, an attempt is made to discontinue steroid therapy.

If possible, steroids are administered locally rather than systemically (for example, intra-articular injections; topical application).

If the patient's condition can be kept under control by intermittent rather than daily drug administration, such a method of administration should be tried (such as alternate day therapy).

Acute Stages of Chronic, Possibly Fatal Diseases (for example, lupus erythematosus; pemphigus)

Massive doses of steroids are administered during the life-threatening episodes and then reduced to somewhat lower levels. (To avoid the dangerous complications of these chronic conditions, the development of hypercorticism from large daily doses is considered acceptable.)

Acute Crises Caused by Severe Infection or Other Forms of Stress (for example, gram-negative bacterial endotoxic shock; surgical shock; anaphylactic shock)

Massive doses of a soluble steroid are administered by vein several times daily during the critical period, whether or not there is acute adrenal insufficiency. (Steroids are adjuncts to other drugs such as vasopressors, vasodilators, antibiotics, and replacement fluids and electrolytes.)

Acute, Self-Limiting Episodes of Allergic and other Disorders (for example, in conditions not of a dangerous nature, such as hay fever or poison ivy)

Large oral doses are administered at once, and dosage is then "stepped down" every day or two until discontinued entirely after a week to ten days.

Topical corticosteroid therapy is employed promptly whenever the symptoms can be controlled in this alone.

SUMMARY of Nursing Points to Remember in Corticosteroid Therapy

Observe the patient carefully for signs of metabolic toxicity such as Cushingoid effects, report these to the physician, and consider nursing measures relevant to these toxic effects, should they occur.

Observe the patient for changes in mood, as patients who have periods of euphoria and depression find it more difficult to cope with their chronic conditions.

Be aware of the potential adverse effects of steroids to which patients with certain secondary conditions are particularly prone. This may help to prevent such complications as a perforated peptic ulcer.

Remember that the steroids can also mask the spread of an infection or such symptoms of acute appendicitis as abdominal pain and fever. Thus, be particularly alert to even slight signs and symptoms that may point to the presence of a serious secondary disorder that requires treatment.

Remember that patients who have been withdrawn from long-term steroid treatment may respond poorly to stress and that they may require prompt administration of high doses of steroids if they suffer an infection, are injured, or require anesthesia and surgery.

Encourage the patient on long-term corticosteroid therapy to keep his appointments with his doctor or the clinic for the necessary clinical observations and laboratory tests that help to detect improvement in his condition or the development of adverse drug effects.

Help the chronically ill patient to understand from the start of steroid therapy that he may not be able to take these drugs indefinitely despite the symptomatic relief that they may offer.

Reinforce explanations to the patient of why it is necessary to reduce dosage of steroids at times or to employ dosage schedules that keep the patient from getting complete relief of all his discomforting symptoms.

Offer the patient emotional support and reassurance when it becomes necessary to reduce steroid dosage or even to withdraw these drugs entirely because of toxicity.

Clinical Nursing Situation

The Situation: Miss Washington suffers from severe rheumatoid arthritis. Her pain is no longer relieved by salicylates, and the physician has ordered 5 mg of prednisone t.i.d. Miss Washington's symptoms were markedly relieved, and the physician advised decreasing the dose gradually to 5 mg b.i.d., and finally to 5 mg q.d. Miss Washington confided to the clinic nurse that because she had recurrence of symptoms when the amount of medication was decreased, she has continued taking three tablets daily, despite the physician's recommendation.

The Problem: How would you, as the clinic nurse, deal with this problem in your interaction with Miss Washington and her physician?

DRUG DIGEST

CORTICOTROPIN INJECTION U.S.P. (ACTH; Acthar, and others)

Actions and Indications. This pituitary hormone stimulates the patient's adrenal glands to secrete several kinds of steroid hormones. It has been used clinically to treat the same disorders that respond to the antiinflammatory effects of the natural and synthetic adrenocorticosteroid drugs, including gout and other rheumatic disorders. However, oral steroids are generally preferred for producing a more predictable therapeutic response more conveniently, safely, and cheaply. The main use of corticotropin today is in the diagnosis of primary adrenal insufficiency.

Side Effects, Cautions, and Contraindications. Corticotropin can cause all the types of toxicity caused by corticosteroid therapy. Thus, the same precautions are required in patients who are particularly susceptible to steroid toxicity. In addition, the foreign protein in this animal-derived pituitary preparation may produce allergic reactions in sensitive patients. Skin tests are sometimes employed to detect reactors prior to treatment, and all patients should be observed for a few minutes following an injection so that treatment may be begun promptly if signs of a reaction are seen.

Dosage and Administration. Dosage is individualized, but ranges between 10 to 80 units daily depending upon the patient's response. The usual dose is 40 units daily by the intramuscular or subcutaneous route. Doses of 10 to 25 units dissolved in 500 ml of a 5 percent solution of dextrose in water may be infused intravenously over a period of eight hours.

DEXAMETHASONE U.S.P. (Decadron; Deronil; Dexameth; and others)

Actions and Indications. The potent antiinflammatory effect of this synthetic steroid accounts for its usefulness in rheumatic disorders, collagen diseases, and dermatological conditions. This steroid also controls signs and symptoms of respiratory and skin allergies and of blood disorders and leukemias. The highly soluble and absorbable sodium phosphate salt is used as an adjunct in acute life-threatening emergencies whether or not adrenal insufficiency exists.

Side Effects, Cautions and Contraindications. This steroid is relatively free of the kind of mineralocorticoid activity that leads to edema. However, it causes all the side effects typical of glucocorticoids when administered for more than a brief period. These include: Cushing's syndrome and other signs of metabolic toxicity; suppression of growth in children and of pituitary-adrenal gland function (endocrine toxicity); and psychological disturbances, which contraindicate its use in psychotic patients. It is also contraindicated in systemic fungal infections and viral infections, including ocular herpes simplex, chicken pox, and vaccinia, as well as in most cases of tuberculosis.

Dosage and Administration. Dosage ranges from 0.5 to 3 mg daily in mild cases, or to 10 mg orally in more severe disorders. The sodium phosphate salt is injected I.V. or I.M. in doses as high as 20 mg, which may be repeated if necessary in acute emergencies. It is also injected directly into joints in doses of about 2 to 4 mg, and it may be administered by inhalation for local effects on respiratory membranes or applied topically to the skin and eyes.

DESOXYCORTICOSTERONE ACETATE U.S.P. (Cortate; Doca; Percorten)

Actions and Indications. This steroid possesses almost pure mineralocorticoid activity and produces prompt retention of sodium and water. Administered as replacement therapy to patients with primary and secondary adrenal insufficiency including Addison's disease, Simmond's disease, or the Waterhouse-Fridrichsen syndrome, this hormone helps to overcome the characteristic hypotension, salt loss, and potassium retention (hyperkalemia) of these disorders.

Side Effects, Cautions, and Contraindications. Overdosage of this drug together with an excessive salt intake may lead to the development of edema, high blood pressure, and cardiac enlargement, particularly in patients with essential hypertension or heart disease. Treatment is stopped if a significant gain in weight or rise in blood pressure is detected. Local irritation and symptoms of hypersensitivity may develop occasionally.

Dosage and Administration. An oily suspension is administered in initial doses of 2 mg daily by intramuscular injection into the upper outer quadrant of the buttocks. Dosage for maintenance is then adjusted between 1 and 5 mg daily. Initial dosage for the first few days of treatment of patients with the salt-losing adrenogenital syndrome may be somewhat higher but should never exceed 10 mg.

Pellets for implantation in subcutaneous sites have long-lasting effects. The amount implanted for a six- to eight-month period is based more or less upon the daily maintenance dose of the oily suspension. Buccal tablets are also available for maintenance dosage of 1 to 5 mg daily.

HYDROCORTISONE U.S.P. AND ITS ESTERS AND SALTS (Cortisol; Cortef; Cortril; and others)

Actions and Indications. This natural adrenal cortex hormone has high glucocorticoid and moderate mineralocorticoid activity which makes it useful in cases of chronic and acute adrenal insufficiency as replacement therapy, and for meeting stressful emergency situations.

Hydrocortisone exerts the antiinflammatory and antiallergy actions that account for the effectiveness of corticosteroid therapy in controlling signs and symptoms of many conditions including rheumatoid arthritis, bronchial asthma, and various collagen diseases. It is also effective for bringing about temporary remissions in certain hematologic and neoplastic disorders.

Side Effects, Cautions, and Contraindications. The mineralocorticoid activity of this compound causes sodium and fluid retention and potassium loss. Thus, the synthetic glucocorticoids are preferred for patients with cardiovascular disorders. Prolonged use may also lead to metabolic, endocrine, and central nervous system toxicity. Cushingoid signs and symptoms, pituitary gland suppression with secondary adrenal atrophy, and euphoria or depression may result.

Dosage and Administration. Dosage is individually adjusted. Replacement therapy usually requires only 15 to 30 mg daily, while 40 to 80 mg a day are needed to maintain an antiinflammatory effect. In acute emergencies, 100 to 250 mg of the sodium succinate ester or sodium phosphate salt may be administered by vein or intramuscularly and repeated if needed. The acetate ester may be injected into joints in amounts of 10 to 50 mg or applied topically to the skin and membranes.

PREDNISONE U.S.P. (Deltasone; Deltra, Meticorten, and others)

Actions and Indications. This synthetic derivative of cortisone has greater glucocorticoid activity and much less mineralocorticoid activity than the natural steroid. It is used for its antiinflammatory and antiallergic effects in the treatment of rheumatic and collagen diseases, and in dermatologic and ophthalmic disorders marked by acute or chronic inflammatory and allergic processes. It is also used in hematologic disorders and neoplastic diseases and numerous other conditions in which it offers symptomatic relief.

Side Effects, Cautions, and Contraindications. It is not as likely to cause sodium retention as the natural hormones, but is more likely to do so at higher dosage levels than the newer steroids that have relatively greater antiinflammatory activity. It causes the typical metabolic, endocrine, central, and other adverse effects of all corticosteroids. Susceptible patients may develop peptic ulcer with perforation and bleeding, hypertension and congestive heart failure, signs of diabetes mellitus, muscle weakness and wastage and osteoporosis.

Dosage and Administration. Dosage varies depending upon the severity of the disease and the patient's response. Thus, depending upon the disease, treatment may be begun with doses ranging from 5 to 60 mg daily. Later, the first dosage is gradually adjusted downward to the least amount required for maintaining adequate symptomatic relief with minimal toxicity. When treatment is to be discontinued, the drug is withdrawn very gradually.

TRIAMCINOLONE U.S.P. AND ITS DERIVATIVES* (Aristocort; Kenacort; and others)

Actions and Indications. This synthetic corticosteroid produces potent antiinflammatory effects when administered for systemic or only local responses in the many disorders responsive to steroid therapy. The diacetate and hexacetonide forms are injected directly into joints in rheumatoid arthritis and osteoarthritis.

The diacetate may also be injected directly into skin lesions in psoriasis and various dermatoses. The acetonide is applied topically for symptomatic relief of skin disorders, including contact dermatitis, atopic and seborrheic dermatitis, neurodermatitis, and eczema.

Side Effects, Cautions, and Contraindications. This steroid can cause the various metabolic, endocrine, and central side effects seen during chronic use and systemic absorption of all corticosteroids. It tends to cause mood depression more often than euphoria, and it reduces rather than stimulates the patient's appetite. Thus, weight gain from overeating (as well as from fluid retention) is less likely to occur than with other steroids. However, muscle wastage may occur more commonly. Myopathy is marked by weakness of the muscles of the thighs, lower back, and pelvis.

Dosage and Administration. Dosage varies depending upon the nature and severity of the disorder, but it usually ranges between 4 and 16 mg daily. Intralesional skin injections range from 5 to 50 mg, and intraarticular dosage ranges from 2 to 20 mg, depending upon size of the lesions or joints.

* Triamcinolone acetonide, diacetate, and hexacetonide.

References

Frawley, T.F. Treatment of adrenal insufficiency states, including Addison's disease. *Mod. Treatm.*, 3:1328, 1966 (Nov.).

Frohman, I.P. The steroids. *Amer J. Nurs.*, 59:518, 1959.

Harter, J.G. Reddy, W.J., and Thorn, G.W. Studies on an intermittent corticosteroid dosage regimen. *New Eng. J. Med.*, 269:591, 1963.

Liddle, G.W. Clinical pharmacology of the anti-inflammatory steroids. *Clin. Pharmacol. Ther.*, 2:615, 1961.

Rodman, M.J. The corticosteroids. *RN*, 32:69, 1969 (Sept.).

Soyka, L.F., and Saxena, K.M. Alternate day steroid therapy for nephrotic children. *JAMA*, 192:125, 1965.

Thorn, G.W. Clinical considerations in the use of corticosteroids. *New Eng. J. Med.*, 274:775, 1966.

Treadwell, B.L.J., et al. Pituitary-adrenal function during corticosteroid therapy. *New Eng. J. Med.*, 272:522, 1965.

Weaver, A. L. Management of rheumatoid arthritis. *Bedside Nurse*, 4:14, 1971 (May).

18

The Antihistamine Drugs

The Nature of Allergy

Allergic disorders affect only a minority of people. Most of these individuals are *atopic*—that is, they have a hereditary or familial tendency to develop sudden allergic reactions involving mainly the skin, mucous membranes of the nose, and bronchial smooth muscles. The reasons for their tendency to react in this way upon contact with foreign substances (*antigens*) that are harmless to most people are still not certain, but are now beginning to be understood better.

IMMUNOLOGIC BASIS

Exposure to antigens stimulates production of specific antibodies. Some of these protect the body against bacteria and viruses by making the person immune to the infections that these microorganisms can cause. Other types of antibodies produced when the body is exposed to the foreign proteins in foods, plant pollens, and other substances are thought to be the cause of allergic reactions. These antibodies, called *reagins*, are now known to belong to the immunoglobulin E (IgE) family of body proteins.

When a previously exposed, or *sensitized*, person with large amounts of IgE in his body comes in contact with the same specific antigen again, an *antigen-antibody reaction* occurs that is damaging to the tissues in which it takes place. As a result of this reaction in the target tissues, or shock organs, certain pharmacologically active chemicals, or *autacoids*, are released, including: (1) *histamine*; (2) *brady-*

kinin; and (3) SRS-A (slow-reacting substance A).

All three of these substances can cause bronchial muscles to contract. Histamine and bradykinin also make blood vessels dilate and increase the permeability of capillaries so that fluid leaks out. These effects account for the signs and symptoms of sudden severe anaphylactic reactions and other allergic disorders.

Histamine

In this chapter, we shall limit our discussion mainly to certain allergic conditions in which the clinical signs and symptoms are believed to stem from the liberation of histamine. Other kinds of allergic disorders are taken up in Chapters 3, 17, and 19.

Histamine is a substance present in bound form in most body tissues. Its function in normal physiology is uncertain at present, except that it is thought to play a part in setting off protective inflammatory reactions to injury in skin and other tissues. However, it now seems certain that the sudden release of histamine has effects on the sensitized individual's blood vessels, bronchial muscles, and exocrine glands that account for many (but not all) of the pathological effects of various allergic disorders, including allergic rhinitis and urticaria.

Arterioles respond to released histamine by dilating as a result of the chemical's relaxing effect on their smooth muscle walls. At the same time, the tiny arterial and venous capillaries become more permeable, with the result that plasma fluid leaks out into the surrounding tissues. These actions account for the reddened swellings, or wheals, seen in the patient's skin, and for the congestion in the mucous membranes of his nose and lungs.

Bronchial smooth muscle is contracted by histamine and *bronchial gland secretions* are stimulated. The chemical also increases nasal, lacrimal, and gastric gland secretions. This accounts for the running nose and eyes noted in certain allergic illnesses and for some of the epigastric distress that occurs in others. (Histamine is sometimes injected deliberately to stimulate the *gastric glands* in certain diagnostic studies of the secretory capacity of the patient's stomach.)

Histamine-Antagonizing Drugs and Procedures

Allergists employ various measures and drugs to prevent the release of histamine or to counteract the effects of this potent chemical on body tissues. *Sympathomimetic (adrenergic) drugs* are used, for example, to produce effects that directly oppose those of histamine (and the other autacoids) upon arterioles and bronchioles. (See Chapter 19 for a discussion of the uses of these drugs in treating bronchial asthma, anaphylactic shock, and nasal congestion.) *Corticosteroid drugs* reduce the responsiveness of the sensitized patient's tissues to the actions of the autacoids released in antigen-antibody reactions.

Hyposensitization is a procedure employed to make allergic patients less reactive when exposed to the antigens to which they have become sensitive. The patient receives periodic injections of gradually increasing doses of dilute extracts of substances to which previous tests have shown him to be allergic—plant pollens, house dust, or mold spores, for example.

Such controlled exposure is believed to stimulate the body to produce so-called "blocking" antibodies, mainly of a class called immunoglobulin G (IgG). The gradual build-up of IgG-type antibodies, that do *not* cause tissue damage when they later combine with the allergen to which the person is sensitive, serves to protect the patient. That is, by competing with the IgE antibodies (reagins) that are thought to be responsible for histamine-releasing reactions, the IgG, or blocking, antibodies which were built up by the long series of allergy "shots" keep the patient from suffering allergy symptoms.

The nurse asks patients to remain in the clinic or doctor's office for at least twenty minutes following each desensitization injection. During this time she unobtrusively observes him for signs of an excessive reaction of a kind that might require emergency treatment. She also tells the patient to call the doctor if any symptoms develop when he gets home. He is also advised to take an antihistamine drug to counteract such symptoms.

Antihistamine Drugs

MANNER OF ACTION

The drugs classified as antihistaminic agents (Table 18-1) differ from adrenergic and corticosteroid drugs in their manner of antiallergy action. That is, the antihistaminics do not produce pharmacological effects that oppose those of histamine on the patient's tissues.

T A B L E 1 8 - 1 *Official Antihistamine Drugs**

Nonproprietary or Official Name	Synonym or Proprietary Name	Usual Single Oral Dose
Antazoline phosphate N.F.	Antistine	100 mg
Bromdiphenhydramine HCl N.F.	Ambodryl	25 mg
Brompheniramine maleate N.F.	Dimetane	4 mg
Carbinoxamine maleate N.F.	Clistin	4 mg
Chlorcyclizine HCl N.F.	Di-Paralene; Perazil	50 mg
Chlorothen citrate N.F.	Tagathen	25 mg
Chlorpheniramine maleate U.S.P.	Chlor-Trimeton, and others	4 mg
Cyproheptadine HCl N.F.	Periactin	4 mg
Dexbrompheniramine maleate N.F.	Disomer	2 mg
Dexchlorpheniramine maleate N.F.	Polaramine	2 mg
Dimethindene maleate N.F.	Forhistal	1 to 2 mg
Diphenhydramine HCl U.S.P.	Benadryl	25 mg
Methapyrilene HCl N.F.	Histadyl, and others	50 mg
Methdilazine HCl N.F.	Tacaryl	8 mg
Phenindamine tartrate N.F.	Thephorin	25 mg
Promethazine HCl U.S.P.	Phenergan	25 mg
Pyrilamine maleate N.F.	Antihist; Neo-Antergan	25 mg
Pyrrobutamine phosphate N.F.	Pyronil	15 mg
Trimeprazine tartrate N.F.	Temaril	2.5 mg
Tripelennamine citrate U.S.P.	Pyribenzamine citrate	50 mg
Tripelennamine HCl U.S.P.	Pyribenzamine HCl	50 mg
Tripolidine HCl N.F.	Actidil	2.5 mg

*Other antihistamines that are used mainly as motion sickness remedies and antiemetics are listed in Table 45-0.

Nor do these drugs keep free histamine from being released. Instead, they act by competing with the allergy-liberated histamine for receptor sites in the patient's arterioles, capillaries, and glands.

When antihistamine drug molecules have occupied such cellular receptors, the histamine which is being released in the antigen-antibody reaction cannot attach itself to these histamine-reactive sites. As a result, the histamine molecules fail to set off the pharmacological effects that are the source of the main signs and symptoms of certain allergic disorders.

OTHER ACTIONS

Although the primary effect of these drugs is the antagonism of histamine in the manner just described, these agents are also capable of exerting effects of their own. Some of these secondary effects are clinically useful in the treatment of allergy and other disorders.* Other

* Certain antihistamine drugs are used in the management of anxiety, nausea and vomiting, motion sickness, extrapyramidal motor system disorders, and parkinsonism (see Chaps. 6, 7, 11, and 45).

actions of these drugs can lead to side effects that sometimes limit the usefulness of these agents for treating allergic patients (p. 239).

Clinical Indications in Allergy Treatment (Summary, p. 240)

The antihistamine drugs are not equally effective for treating all types of allergic disorders. They have *not*, for example, proved very useful in bronchial asthma. This may be because the persistent bronchospasm of this condition is caused mainly, not by histamine, but by such other autacoids as SRS-A and bradykinin (p. 239). However, in allergic conditions with symptoms that stem mainly from free histamine, these drugs are much more effective when properly employed. These disorders include upper respiratory tract and dermatological allergies of various kinds.

ALLERGIC RHINITIS

The mucous membrane lining the nose is often the target tissue for allergic reactions. People allergic to plant pollens or molds may suffer from nasal allergy at certain seasons of the year. Such seasonal allergy is known as *pollinosis*, or hay fever. In other individuals, the nasal mucosa stays sensitive without regard to the season, and, in fact, the patient's symptoms need not be set off by inhaled allergens. Thus for example, in this condition, called *perennial rhinitis*, recurrent attacks can be precipitated by eating certain foods or by the exposure to bacteria, chilling, and other factors.

Both seasonal and perennial rhinitis are marked in their early stages by repeated sneezing, running nose (*rhinorrhea*) and nasal obstruction. In hay fever, the patient's eyes (as well as his nose) are reddened, running (*lacrimation*), and itchy. Patients with perennial rhinitis tend, in time, to develop pathologic changes of the nasal membrane that are the result of chronic inflammation and frequent secondary infections.

Antihistamine drug therapy is most effective in pollinosis, particularly when the drugs are taken regularly in the early edematous stage. By blocking the action of the histamine that is released when the allergenic pollen grains react with IgE antibodies on the mucosal surface of the nose and eyes, these drugs often effectively prevent the typical nasal symptoms from developing.

When protected by the presence of antihistamine molecules, the arterioles that run through the nasal mucosa do not dilate, nor does fluid leak out of the capillaries. Thus, the nasal mucosa does not become swollen and congested, and the nasal air passages are kept open. The patient's nasal and lacrimal glands do not secrete excessively, and itchiness of the nose and eyes is minimal.

Later in the hay fever season, particularly when pollen counts are heavy, antihistamine drug blockade becomes less effective. Similarly, in perennial rhinitis, administration of antihistamine drugs alone is rarely capable of controlling the condition or preventing nasal obstruction and pathologic changes in the patient's nasal mucosa.

In such cases, the antihistamines are commonly supplemented by topical therapy with *nasal decongestants*—that is, with adrenergic drugs that shrink the swollen membrane by their vasoconstrictor effect on the arterioles. Occasionally, difficult cases of perennial rhinitis also require treatment with systemic or topically applied corticosteroid drugs.

ALLERGIC SKIN DISORDERS

The antihistamine drugs are most effective in control of skin symptoms that stem directly from the effects of histamine; other allergic dermatoses do not respond as well. *Acute urticaria* (hives, nettle rash) is most readily responsive to antihistamine drug therapy. The crops of intensely itching skin wheals that characterize this condition are caused by the effects of histamine upon blood vessels in the patient's skin. Drug-induced blockade of histamine prevents the edema and itching, or pruritus. Chronic urticaria symptoms are less easily relieved by these drugs. However, certain antihistaminic drugs that also have sedative or tranquilizing effects often suppress pruritus even when the skin swellings persist.

Among the more sedating antihistamines that may be useful here and for relief of itching in atopic dermatitis and contact dermatitis is *diphenhydramine+* (Benadryl). Also useful as *antipruritics* are the antihistaminic-minor tranquilizer *hydroxyzine* (Atarax; Vistaril) and the antihistaminic-phenothiazine tranquilizers *trimeprazine* (Temaril), *methdilazine* (Tacaryl), and *cyproheptadine* (Periactin). All are thought to act mainly in the central nervous system rather than in the skin.

Some antihistaminic agents possess a *local anesthetic* effect when applied topically to itching skin. *Tripelennamine+* (Pyribenzamine), applied in ointment or cream form, may relieve the itching that makes patients with atopic dermatitis tear at their irritated skin, even though histamine does not play an important part in producing the symptoms of this allergic skin condition.

Unfortunately, the already excessively sensitized skin of such a patient may be further sensitized by continued topical application of these chemicals. This can cause contact dermatitis, a skin condition that does not respond very well to treatment with even orally administered antihistamine drugs. (See Chapters 17 and 46 for discussions of the use of the much more effective topical corticosteroids and other antipruritic agents in the management of dermatitis of the atopic and contact types.)

Acute Anaphylactic Reactions (See Chap. 23)

Antihistamine drugs do *not* have great value in the emergency management of acute anaphylactic reactions. This may be because some of the most severe immediate effects of an antigen-antibody reaction are the result of the release of other substances besides histamine. Parenterally administered histamine-antagonizing drugs may be helpful for control of cutaneous reactions such as urticaria and pruritus that are caused by the release of histamine. However, these drugs do not antagonize such other autacoids as SRS-A and bradykinin—the substances believed to be most responsible for the severe, sustained bronchospasm and the sudden circulatory collapse that are the usual cause of death.

The emergency kit for use in anaphylactic reactions should of course include an injectable form of an antihistamine drug such as *diphenhydramine+* (Benadryl). However, it should be employed only after other more immediately effective measures have first been employed. These include keeping the patient's airway open and maintaining his heartbeat and blood pressure by mechanical and pharmacological means. (See Chapter 23 for a discussion of the use of *epinephrine+*, the most valuable drug for counteracting both respiratory and circulatory failure.)

Once the patient's breathing and blood pressure have been stabilized by administration of adrenergic drugs, including vasopressors such as *levarterenol+* and *metaraminol+*, the doctor may make use of the antihistamine injection and other slower-acting adjunctive drugs, including an infusion of a water-soluble corticosteroid such as *hydrocortisone sodium succinate+* (Solu-Cortef). The emergency materials should also include oxygen, the *non*-adrenergic bronchodilator *aminophylline+*, and such equipment as an oral airway, endotracheal tube, tourniquets, and a tracheotomy set.

Prevention of anaphylactic reactions is more desirable than attempting to treat a patient suffering such a sudden life-threatening situation. Although products are available that contain an antihistamine drug combined with such common allergy-provoking substances as penicillin, these are not considered desirable for preventing penicillin reactions. Presence of the antihistamine in such an injection may, in fact, mask such early warning signs as itching, flushing, and skin wheals without helping to overcome the much more serious respiratory

and cardiovascular effects of anaphylaxis. Thus, knowing the patient's history and keeping him under close observation after he has been exposed to a substance to which he may be sensitive are more important preventive measures.

THE COMMON COLD

The common cold is commonly treated with antihistamine drugs. Contrary to what was once claimed, these drugs do *not* abort or cure a cold. They may, however, offer some symptomatic relief in the early stages of a cold. Drugs such as *diphenhydramine+* that possess an atropine-like drying effect may be particularly useful for relief of a running nose. However, this drying action may make such antihistamine drugs undesirable for patients with bronchial asthma, because it tends to aid formation of obstructive mucous plugs in the bronchi.

Side Effects and Toxicity (Summary, p. 241)

Drowsiness is the main drawback of some antihistaminic agents. Thus, the nurse instructs the patient who is taking one of these drugs for the first time to observe how it affects him. If he finds that he gets sleepy, he should not drive a car or engage in other activities that require mental alertness and motor coordination. The nurse also warns against drinking, as antihistamines and alcohol may have additive depressant effects on the nervous system.

Encourage the allergic patient to tell the doctor, if a prescribed antihistamine continues to make him drowsy. The physician may then order a different drug of this class that may not have so strong a sedative effect. Two of the least sedating antihistamines are *phenindamine* (Thephorin) and *dimethindene* (Forhistal). However, patients differ in their responses and the best antihistamine for regular daytime use may have to be determined by trial and error in each individual.

Sometimes the physician may deliberately order one of the more hypnotic antihistamines for bedtime use by patients whose allergic symptoms interfere with sleep. *Promethazine*

(Phenergan), for example, may be used in this way. Sometimes, a small dose of a psychomotor stimulant such as caffeine, an amphetamine, or *methylphenidate* (Ritalin) may be added to a moderately sedating antihistamine such as *tripelennamine* (Pyribenzamine) or *chlorpheniramine maleate* (Chlor-Trimeton).

TOXICITY

Patients taking antihistamines for chronic allergic disorders often ask whether long-term use of these drugs is dangerous. Actually, these are relatively safe drugs when taken in ordinary doses for even long periods. The nurse should refer such questioners to the physician who will probably reassure the patient that such use of antihistamines—unlike long use of corticosteroids—is generally harmless.

However, patients should be warned that the antihistamines may be dangerous when taken in overdoses. Children are particularly likely to suffer severe ill effects when they accidentally ingest an excess amount. Convulsive seizures, coma, cardiovascular collapse, and respiratory failure may occur. The nurse should teach parents that products for treating colds, cough, and allergies should be safely stored where youngsters cannot readily reach these medications.

Summary

The antihistamine drugs are often useful for control of symptoms in patients with various kinds of allergies. They must, however, be properly employed to avoid side effects involving the central nervous system. Precautions must be taken to prevent accidents that might result from the effects that these drugs sometimes have on the patient's mental and motor functions.

The patient should understand that these drugs are *not* a cure and will not eliminate his allergy. He should be taught to protect himself from exposure to the substance to which he is sensitive. He should also be advised to avoid becoming fatigued or emotionally upset, as allergic symptoms are sometimes set off or become worse in such circumstances.

Hyposensitization, or desensitization, treatment often helps to prevent the release of histamine and thus makes antihistaminic and other drug treatments unnecessary. However, hyposensitization is itself not without danger. The dosage of the dilute antigen must be very carefully and accurately measured in the finely calibrated syringe used in this procedure. Drugs for treating severe reactions, such as epinephrine and corticosteroids, as well as antihistamines, must be kept ready together with tourniquets, needles and syringes, and tracheotomy and intubation equipment.

S U M M A R Y of the Clinical Indications for Antihistamine Drugs

Histamine Antagonism and Antipruritic

Seasonal allergic rhinitis (hay fever; pollinosis)
Perennial and vasomotor rhinitis
Allergic conjunctivitis
Urticaria (hives), acute and chronic
Contact dermatitis, including poison ivy
Dermographism (skin writing wheals)
Physical allergy (such as a cold)
Insect sting allergic reactions, mild and local
Reactions to blood, plasma, serum, and drugs (for relief of pruritus and mild angioedema)
Acute anaphylactic reactions—as an adjunct following epinephrine and other more immediately effective measures

Selective Central Nervous System Depression

Insomnia—for sedative-hypnotic effects
Anxiety and psychomotor excitement—especially in *some* hyperactive, emotionally disturbed children
Preoperative and postoperative sedation
Postoperative and postanesthetic nausea and vomiting—for antiemetic effects
Motion sickness prevention and treatment
Parkinson's disease—mild cases in elderly patients
Parkinsonism, drug-induced—extrapyramidal motor reactions to phenothiazines and other antipsychotic drugs.

S U M M A R Y of Adverse Effects of Antihistamine Drugs and of Cautions and Contraindications*

Central Nervous System Depression

Drowsiness, dizziness, disturbed motor co-ordination and difficulty in concentrating may occur during the first few days of treatment. Caution patients against driving or engaging in other potentially hazardous activities; also against drinking or taking other sedatives, hypnotics, or tranquilizers.

Central Nervous System Stimulation†

Restlessness, nervousness, confusion, and, occasionally, insomnia.

Convulsions, following tremors, have occurred in children taking large overdoses. Death has sometimes resulted.

Atropinelike Peripheral Effects

Dryness of the mouth, nose, and throat. Thickening of mucous secretions may lead to tightness in the chest, wheezing, and dyspnea in asthmatic patients.

Vision may be blurred. Contraindicated in patients with narrow-angle glaucoma.

Urination may be difficult. Contraindicated in patients with enlarged prostate or obstructions of the neck of the bladder.

Constipation or diarrhea, also nausea, epigastric distress, heartburn, and vomiting. Contraindicated in patients with G.I. obstructions or stenosis.

Hypersensitivity Reactions

Sensitized patients may develop skin eruptions and other signs and symptoms of allergic reactions, including even anaphylactic shock.

Cardiovascular Effects of Parenteral Administration

Hypotension, heart palpitations, and irregularities with faintness, weakness, sweating, and pallor.

* The several different chemical classes of drugs that act to antagonize histamine may differ in their other pharmacological effects. Thus, the drugs may not *all* produce the same side effects.
† CNS stimulation is most likely to occur in drugs with a strong anticholinergic (atropinelike) component.

S U M M A R Y of Points for the Nurse to Remember Concerning Allergy Treatment

1. Teach your patient to take the necessary precautions to prevent accidents that might result from the central effects of antihistamine drugs.

(a) He should know that these drugs sometimes cause drowsiness, dizziness, light-headedness and unsteadiness, particularly if taken with alcoholic drinks.

(b) If he has such reactions, the patient should not drive or use potentially hazardous tools (for example, a home power saw).

2. Suggest that your patient discuss with his doctor any reactions that he may be having to the antihistaminic medication that has been prescribed for him. The doctor may then try a different antihistamine that may not make him as drowsy.

3. Help the patient to understand his allergic condition and how he can best help himself.

(a) He should take the medication that has been prescribed for him but with the realization that he may continue to suffer some symptoms.

(Some patients expect drugs to rid them of their allergy; they should understand that antihistamines are *not* a cure but are given only for temporary relief.)

(b) He should know the types of substances to which he is sensitive and try to protect himself from exposure to them by various common sense measures.

(c) If possible, the patient who is allergic to pollen should air-condition his home, or at least one room in it, and spend a good deal of his time in the protected environment during the allergy season.

(d) The patient should try to avoid situations that are physically or emotionally stressful, as fatigue and tension may make some allergy symptoms worse, while rest and relaxation may tend to lessen discomforting symptoms.

4. Instruct the patient who is receiving desensitization treatment to remain in the clinic or the doctor's office for at least twenty minutes after he has had an injection of an allergen.

(a) Watch the patient without making him aware that he is being observed for respiratory, skin, and other signs of an allergic reaction.

(b) Have available the necessary drugs and supplies for treating a severe allergic reaction.

(c) Call the doctor's attention immediately to any reaction that occurs and be prepared to assist him with emergency measures if necessary.

Clinical Nursing Situation: I

The Situation: Mr. Jameson has been coming to the clinic to receive a series of "shots" containing diluted ragweed pollen preparations. On this occasion, he is sitting in the clinic waiting room not far from the nurse who can observe him periodically. About 10 minutes after he has had his injection, the nurse notes that Mr. Jameson becomes restless, suddenly starts scratching at the injection site, and begins to sneeze repeatedly.

The Problem: Describe what you would do, if you were the nurse in this situation. Indicate also how you would react if the patient began to experience respiratory difficulties (wheezing, dyspnea, cough); his skin became pale and sweaty, then cyanotic; and he collapsed on the floor of the clinic.

Clinical Nursing Situation: II

The Situation: Janet, a 15-year-old high school student, began to sneeze during the late summer. By early fall, when she saw the school nurse about her "cold," she felt nearly incapacitated by the constant watery discharge from her nose and eyes. She was also concerned about her appearance, as her eyes were red, swollen, and "teary," and her face was puffy. The nurse persuaded her to visit an allergist.

The physician found from skin tests that Janet was highly sensitive to ragweed pollen. He advised her to have a course of injections and to take an antihistamine tablet that he prescribed for use several times daily. He quickly gave her various oral instructions together with a printed list to take home.

Janet agreed to undertake the treatment after talking it over with her parents. However, she was impatient about "having to hang around the waiting room" after her desensitization injections, and she was puzzled about some of the written instructions and had forgotten most of what the doctor had told her. So she took the list to the school nurse and asked some questions.

The Problem: Assume that you are the nurse. Describe how you would explain to Janet what allergy is and the reasons for the various instructions that she has to follow. How would you explain why it is important for her to stay at the doctor's office for 20 to 25 minutes after each injection? What would you teach Janet about taking an antihistamine medication such as Benadryl, Pyribenzamine, or Chlor-Trimeton?

DRUG DIGEST

DIPHENHYDRAMINE U.S.P. (Benadryl)

Actions and Indications. This prototype histamine antagonist is often effective for symptomatic relief of various allergic disorders. It is a particularly effective palliative in seasonal allergic rhinitis (pollinosis) for reducing sneezing, running nose, and eyes, and itching of the nasal and conjunctical membranes. Its secondary anticholinergic (atropinelike) drying action may add a drying effect that is desirable in upper respiratory allergy and infections but undesirable in most asthmatic patients. Administered parenterally, diphenhydramine may be useful in the management of minor signs and symptoms (urticaria, angioneurotic edema) of anaphylactic reactions, but epinephrine is the preferred treatment for more severe allergic responses.

Side Effects, Cautions, and Contraindications. This antihistamine agent often causes drowsiness, which may make driving or operating machinery hazardous. Its atropinelike activity may make the drug undesirable for patients with asthma, and its use is contraindicated in patients with narrow angle glaucoma, enlarged prostate, and other obstructive disorders of the genitourinary and gastrointestinal tracts. Parenteral administration may cause tachycardia of a degree that could be dangerous to patients with heart disease.

Dosage and Administration. The usual oral dose for adults is 50 mg t.i.d. or q.i.d. and for children 12.5 to 25 mg. The drug is also administered intravenously or by deep intramuscular injection in doses of 10 to 50 mg for adults and 10 to 30 mg for children. Daily dosage should not ordinarily exceed 300 mg.

TRIPELENNAMINE HCl U.S.P.
(Pyribenzamine)

Actions and Indications. This prototype antihistamine drug is used for symptomatic relief of upper respiratory allergies such as hay fever and for dermatological allergic reactions of the urticarial and contact dermatitis types. It is used occasionally for control of cough in asthmatic children with excessive respiratory tract secretions, but it is generally not considered desirable for patients with bronchial asthma. It is sometimes administered by injection as part of the emergency treatment of severe allergic (anaphylactic) reactions, but epinephrine is the most important agent for immediate use in such situations.

Side Effects, Cautions, and Contraindications. Drowsiness is a common side effect, and dizziness, confusion, and excitement sometimes occur. Such central symptoms may be most severe in patients also taking sedatives or hypnotic drugs, or drinking alcoholic beverages. Patients who react in this way are cautioned against driving or engaging in other activities that require alertness. Epigastric distress, nausea, mouth dryness, and difficulty in urination may occur but are rarely severe enough to require discontinuing the drug.

Dosage and Administration. The usual oral adult dose is 50 mg taken once or twice daily, but dosage may range between 25 mg and 600 mg or more daily, depending upon individual need and tolerance. The drug may be administered intramuscularly or by slow intravenous injection of 25 mg for rapid control of severe drug and transfusion reactions.

References

Hildreth, E.A. Some common allergic emergencies. *Med. Clin. N. Amer.*, 50:1313, 1966 (Sept.).

Falleroni, A.E. Treatment of allergic emergencies. *Mod. Treatm.*, 5:782, 1968(Sept.).

Norman, P.S. Treatment of allergic rhinitis. *Mod. Treatm.*, 3:881, 1966 (July).

Rodman, M.J. Drugs for allergic disorders: part 1, anaphylaxis and asthma. *RN*, 34: 63, 1971 (June).

————. Drugs for allergic disorders: part 2, pollinosis, perrenial rhinitis, dermatitis. *RN*, 34:53, 1971 (July).

Valentine, M.D., and Sheffer, A.L. The anaphylactic syndromes. *Med. Clin. N. Amer.*, 53:249, 1969 (March).

19.

Drugs Used for Respiratory Tract Obstruction

Chronic disorders of the respiratory tract are an increasingly common cause of disability. These pulmonary diseases are marked by pathologic changes of a kind that tend to block the air passages. Airway obstruction of this kind accounts for the distressing symptoms of *emphysema, chronic bronchitis,* and *bronchial asthma.* In this chapter, we shall emphasize mainly certain classes of drugs that are used in the management of patients with chronic asthma and the acute attacks that often occur in the course of this disease.

Bronchial asthma is a chronic condition in which the patient periodically suffers acute attacks. As his bronchial passages become narrowed and congested, the patient has difficulty in breathing (dyspnea). His expired breath makes a characteristic wheezing sound, and he coughs frequently in an effort to clear his tracheobronchial tree of accumulating mucous secretions.

Most cases of asthma occur in allergic patients—that is, in *atopic* people who have become sensitized to antigenic substances in their external environment. (This type is often called *extrinsic* asthma.) Other patients with no history of allergy up to about the age of 35 or 40 begin to suffer asthmatic attacks in their later years. Their bouts of breathing difficulty, unproductive cough, and wheezing seem to be set off mainly by microorganisms that live in their lungs and other parts of the respiratory tract and cause chronic infections. (This form of asthma is now often called *intrinsic.*)

Drugs Used in the Management of Bronchial Asthma

Patients with the allergic (extrinsic) type of asthma may stay free of attacks for long periods by protecting themselves against exposure to the allergens against which their respiratory tract tissues react. Often the use of measures that eliminate specific allergens from the patient's environment, together with a course of *hyposensitization* treatments, will keep his condition under control. However, these procedures do *not* help patients with intrinsic asthma who cannot be shown to be reacting to any specific substance with which they are coming into contact. Patients with this type of asthma sometimes suffer fewer attacks while on long-term antibiotic drug prophylactic therapy.

Actual attacks of asthma—no matter what the underlying cause—are treated with drugs that are intended to relieve their symptoms. These include *bronchodilator drugs* for relaxing spasm of the smooth muscles of the bronchial passages, and *expectorant* and *mucolytic agents* for clearing mucus from these tubes. In more severe forms of asthma, the doctor may attempt to suppress bronchial tissue reactions with *corticosteroid drugs*. We shall discuss the use of these kinds of drugs in the control of chronic asthma symptoms and in overcoming life-threatening *acute* attacks of status asthmaticus.

BRONCHODILATOR DRUGS

Two types of drugs are used to relax bronchial muscle spasm and thus relieve symptoms that stem from respiratory tract obstruction. These are: (1) *adrenergic drugs* such as *ephedrine*+, *epinephrine*+ (Adrenalin), and *isoproterenol* (Isuprel; Norisodrine); and (2) *theophylline-type* agents such as *aminophylline*+. Because the use of adrenergic antiasthmatic drugs is discussed in Chapter 23 and its *Drug Digest*, we shall discuss here only bronchodilators that are derivatives of theophylline.

TABLE 19-1   *Some Drugs Used in Respiratory Tract Obstruction*

Nonproprietary Name	Proprietary Name or Synonym	Usual Adult Dosage	Remarks
Bronchodilator Drugs			
ADRENERGIC TYPE (see also Table 23-1)			
Ephedrine sulfate U.S.P.		25–50 mg oral	Best for treating and preventing mild attacks of bronchospasm
Epinephrine U.S.P.	Adrenalin	0.2 to 0.5 mg s.c. or I.M. as 0.2–0.5 ml of 1:1000 sol.; 1:100 sol. for inhalation	Best for treating acute asthmatic attacks
Isoproterenol HCl U.S.P.	Isuprel	Inhalation of 1:100 or 1:200 sol.; sublingual 10 to 15 mg	Effective for mild to moderately severe asthmatic attacks
Metaproterenol	Alupent	2 or 3 inhalations 60.65 mg/ inhalation	Less likely than isoproterenol to cause cardiac stimulation
THEOPHYLLINE TYPE			
Aminophylline U.S.P.	Theophylline ethylenediamine	250 mg oral; 250–500 mg rectal; 250–500 mg by slow I.V.	I.V. for acute bronchospasm and status asthmaticus; oral and rectal for milder attacks & prevention
Diphylline	Dilor; Lufyllin; Neothylline	100–300 mg oral; 250–500 mg I.M.	Less irritating and better absorbed than theophylline
Oxtriphylline N.F.	Choledyl	100–400 mg oral	Less irritating and better absorbed than theophylline

TABLE 19-1 *(Continued)*

Nonproprietary Name	Proprietary Name or Synonym	Usual Adult Dosage	Remarks
Theophylline U.S.P.	Elixophylline; Optiphyllin, and others	100–200 mg oral	
Theophylline meglumine	Glucophylline	500 mg rectal	Effective alone or combined with ephedrine for relief and prevention of mild to moderate bronchospasm
Theophylline monoethanolamine	Monotheamin, and others	250–500 mg rectal	
Theophylline sodium acetate N.F.		100–200 mg oral	
Theophylline sodium glycinate N.F.	Glynazan; Synophyllate	330–780 mg oral and rectal; also I.V. 200–400 mg	
Expectorants			
Ammonium chloride U.S.P.		300 mg orally	Most of these drugs act mainly by stimulating the flow of respiratory tract fluids reflexly by irritating the gastric mucosa
Glyceryl guaiacolate N.F.	Robitussin	100–200 mg orally	
Iodinated glycerin	Organidin	30–60 mg	
Ipecac Syrup U.S.P.		0.5–2 ml orally	
Potassium guaiacolsulfonate N.F.		500 mg orally	
Potassium iodide U.S.P.		300 mg orally	see *Drug Digest*
Sodium iodide U.S.P.		300 mg orally or I.V.	
Terpin hydrate N.F.		5 ml orally	May act directly on bronchial secretory cells
Mucolytic Agents			
Acetylcysteine	Mucomyst	1–10 ml of 10% sol by nebulizer; 1–2 ml by instillation	
Tyloxapol	Alevaire	Continuous inhalation of mist delivered through a nebulizer	
Adrenocorticosteroids (see also Chapter 17)			
Dexamethasone phosphate aerosol N.F.	Decadron Respihaler	18 mg per spray by inhalation	
Hydrocortisone sodium phosphate U.S.P.	Cortiphate; Hydrocortone	100–250 mg I.V. or I.M.	
Hydrocortisone sodium succinate U.S.P.	Solu-Cortef	100–250 mg I.V. or I.M.	
Methylprednisolone sodium succinate N.F.	Solu-Medrol	100–250 mg I.V.; 40–120 mg I.M.	
Prednisolone sodium phosphate U.S.P.	Hydeltrasol	50–150 mg I.V.	
Prednisolone sodium succinate N.F.	Meticortilene Soluble	50–150 mg I.V.	
Miscellaneous Drugs			
Cromolyn sodium	Aarane Intal	Inhale contents of 1 capsule 4 times daily	Used to prevent attacks, not to treat them

Theophylline and its derivatives (Table 19-1) are administered orally or rectally as part of treatment programs aimed at preventing attacks of wheezing. Although often effective for control of symptoms during long-term therapy of asthma, these bronchodilators have drawbacks that limit their usefulness. They are usually administered in oral doses that are too low to be fully effective for relaxing spasm in bronchial smooth muscle. Higher oral doses tend to cause gastrointestinal irritation that results in epigastric distress, nausea, and vomiting.

Certain derivatives are said to be more soluble and more readily absorbable from the intestine. *Oxtriphylline* (Choledyl), for example, is a theophylline salt that is claimed to cause less gastrointestinal upset when administered in doses that are readily absorbed to reach effective levels in the lungs. *Aminophylline+*, another solubilized theophylline, is readily but irregularly absorbed through the mucosa of the lower intestine when taken in suppository form or by retention enema. However, when used repeatedly in this way it can cause anorectal irritation. The nurse should look for signs of such irritation in this area and listen for complaints of rectal pain or discomfort. Report this to the doctor who may then order another derivative or another route. *Dyphilline*, for example, is a neutral salt said to be less irritating when taken orally and less painful when injected intramuscularly.

Theophylline derivatives are often combined with ephedrine or other orally effective adrenergic drugs. Taken together, the two types of bronchodilator drugs seem to produce greater effects than either drug alone, and the presence of theophylline tends to delay development of tolerance to ephedrine during long-term treatment. A possible disadvantage of such combinations is the added likelihood of overstimulating the nervous system, since both drugs are central stimulants. A barbiturate is commonly added to theophylline-ephedrine products to counteract any tendency toward insomnia in patients taking such combinations to prevent nighttime asthmatic attacks.

Aminophylline+, administered by slow intravenous injection, is often effective for rapid relief of bronchospasm in patients who no longer respond to aerosol therapy with adrenergic drugs such as epinephrine and isoproterenol. This occurs in *status asthmaticus*, a severe form of the disease that can cause fatal respiratory center depression. Aminophylline helps here both by its direct relaxing effect on bronchial smooth muscle and by stimulating the patient's depressed breathing center.

One reason for carefully regulating the flow of aminophylline solution is that too rapid administration may cause cardiac irregularities in severely ill asthmatic patients. Yet, the heart-stimulating effect of aminophylline is sometimes useful for cardiac patients who develop pulmonary edema as a result of failure of the left ventricle. In such patients, a slow infusion of aminophylline strengthens the heart beat and increases the cardiac output more rapidly than do most digitalis derivatives. (Perhaps the low oxygen and high carbon dioxide levels in severe asthma makes *these* patients more prone to develop drug-induced arrhythmias.)

Drugs and Other Measures for Removing Secretions

Patients with asthma and chronic bronchitis tend to produce excessive amounts of sticky secretions. This adds to air flow obstruction in bronchial passages already narrowed by smooth muscle spasm and by congestion of the mucous membranes of the respiratory tract. Sometimes this retained sputum hardens into masses that may completely block many of the bronchial tubes. This, of course, keeps aerosol sprays of isoproterenol or epinephrine from reaching their sites of action in the smooth muscles of the respiratory tract—a possible factor in setting off status asthmaticus attacks.

Keeping airways free of mucous masses is an important consideration in managing chronic asthmatics, and removing solid plugs becomes a lifesaving emergency measure in patients with status asthmaticus. The best way to prevent respiratory tract obstruction by sticky sputum is to make it less viscid. Measures that increase the water content of the bronchial secretions are employed to accomplish this. The simplest way to reduce sputum viscosity is to keep the patient himself well hydrated.

Asthmatic patients, even when not seriously ill, should drink large quantities of water. The nurse who is caring for such a patient encourages him to drink the dozen or so glasses of water he needs daily, when fluids are being forced. Patients severely ill with status asthmaticus are usually dehydrated when hospitalized. They often have to be rehydrated by receiving intravenous fluids before bronchodilators can become effective again. Often, after hydration has helped to thin the patient's tenacious bronchial secretions, he responds to treatment with an adrenergic bronchodilator drug such as isoproterenol or epinephrine.

EXPECTORANT DRUGS (TABLE 19-1)

Certain substances that have traditionally been taken in the form of cough syrups are also used to make bronchial gland secretions more watery. These expectorants—the term means "out of the chest"—help to liquefy mucus and thus make it easier for the patient to clear his bronchial tree by coughing more productively. These substances do this by stimulating the secretion of a natural lubricating fluid, called *respiratory tract fluid* (RTF).

Potassium iodide+, ammonium chloride, and *syrup of ipecac* are among the most commonly employed expectorants in chronic bronchitis and bronchial asthma. These substances do not, of course, enter the respiratory tract when they are swallowed. Instead, upon reaching the stomach, they irritate the gastric lining. This sets off a reflex that results in an increased flow of RTF.

The same reflex also accounts for the nausea, retching, and vomiting that may occur when patients take too much of these expectorants. Larger doses of syrup of ipecac—as indicated in Chapter 3—are used to induce vomiting in the emergency treatment of patients who have ingested poisons. The much more potent fluidextract of ipecac should *never* be employed either as an emetic or in *sub*emetic doses, as an expectorant, when the syrup of ipecac is ordered.

Cough medication products containing centrally acting *antitussive agents* such as codeine or antihistamines are *not* ordinarily considered desirable in treating asthmatic patients. Occasionally, however, codeine may be ordered to suppress an irritating, unproductive cough in chronic bronchitis. Similarly, an antihistamine such as *diphenhydramine+* (Benadryl) or *tripelennamine+* (Pyribenzamine) may sometimes be combined with codeine, ephedrine, and expectorants for control of certain types of allergic (and other) coughs.

MUCUS-DISSOLVING DRUGS (SEE MUCOLYTIC AGENTS, TABLE 19-1)

Substances that act locally to liquefy mucus masses are also sometimes employed to open blocked passages. These include detergents and other wetting agents that are intended to draw water into the thickened mucus in order to thin down these secretions. Other chemicals break down the mucus chemically or by enzymatic action. Unfortunately, the irritating and sensitizing properties of these substances limit their usefulness for routine use in asthmatic patients.

Even when used in *non*asthmatic patients with obstructive pulmonary diseases such as emphysema and chronic bronchitis, administration of these substances is not always effective. Bulb atomizers and ordinary nebulizers may not deliver enough of the vaporized solution into the bronchioles. However, hospitalized patients are sometimes helped when an oxygen stream is used to pick up a mucolytic mist that is then pumped deep into the lungs by an intermittent positive pressure apparatus.

Patients close to asphyxia because of bronchus-blocking plugs may benefit from having the drug solutions instilled directly into the tracheobronchial tree. In such cases, sterile solutions are instilled through an endotracheal tube, tracheostomy, or bronchoscope. After about 20 minutes of direct contact with the mucus plugs, the solution and the dissolved material are removed by mechanical suction or postural drainage.

Sometimes, after the accumulated sputum is successfully cleared out in this way, the patient's constricted bronchi can respond to and be relaxed by aerosolized adrenergic bronchodilators. Epinephrine and isoproterenol can now reach the previously blocked off parts of the bronchi in the form of oxygen-nebulized droplets delivered by an air compressor apparatus. Later, following recovery from the acute attack for which he was hospitalized, the patient can administer his own inhalant medications at home.

The nurse instructs the patient in how best to use his nebulizer, mask, or mouthpiece in order not to lose any of the mist. She also teaches the asthmatic patient and his family how to make the epinephrine injections that may be needed to terminate sudden severe attacks of bronchospasm. Elderly, disease-weakened patients with chronic bronchitis or emphysema are helped to sit up and encouraged to cough productively. The nurse then examines the contents of the patient's sputum cup and reports its appearance to the physician.

CORTICOSTEROID DRUGS

Corticosteroids are often useful for treating severe asthma in both its acute and chronic stages. Their use in patients suffering severe, life-threatening status asthmaticus is considered particularly useful and relatively safe. Long-term treatment of chronic asthma with steroid drugs involves hazards that make their use desirable only in carefully selected cases.

In *status asthmaticus* marked by severe, continuous bronchial spasm that does not readily respond to treatment with bronchodilator drugs, the addition of steroid therapy to other supportive measures often produces dramatically beneficial effects. Water-soluble steroid esters such as *hydrocortisone sodium succinate+* (Solu-Cortef) are infused intravenously in very large doses. Within a few hours the patient's labored breathing becomes easier, and his general condition also seems much better. Apparently, the steroid drugs both relieve bronchial obstruction by their antiinflammatory effects and somehow strengthen the patient's defenses against the extreme stress of such severe acute attacks.

The administration of massive amounts of water-soluble steroids in this way for only a day or two to tide the asthmatic patient over the emergency does *not* lead to the typical metabolic toxicity seen during long-term steroid therapy (*Summary of Cushingoid Signs and Symptoms*, p. 230). However, patients with a history of hypertension, peptic ulcer, or emotional disturbances should be observed carefully for signs of flare-ups of these disorders during even short-term emergency treatment of severe asthma with high steroid dosage. In any case, steroid dosage is reduced rapidly to maintenance levels or discontinued entirely after a few days.

Severe chronic asthma is also often improved when steroid drugs are added to the patient's regular regimen. However, because of the hazards of long-term steroid therapy, the doctor usually decides to use these drugs only after very careful evaluation of the patient's condition. He bases his decision mainly on signs that the patient's condition is no longer under control by conventional antiasthma measures. The development of rib cage deformities or emphysema and other signs of rapidly progressive disability justify the use of steroids despite the danger of their continuous use.

The doctor begins by adding low doses of steroids and raising dosage only gradually. He does *not* try to relieve *all* of the patient's discomforting symptoms. Instead, he makes an effort to establish the least dose needed to halt

progress of the disabling effects of the disease. Whenever the patient's asthma improves, the doctor gradually reduces steroid dosage and even tries to discontinue these drugs entirely.

Patients often resist attempts to wean them away from steroids. The nurse helps here by explaining why it is so important to follow the doctor's orders for reducing the dosage of these drugs. She encourages the patient and offers him emotional support when his asthmatic symptoms seem to get worse as the daily steroid dosage is reduced. Pointing out the improvement in his appearance that results from lower steroid dosage (and subsequent lessening of cushingoid type toxicity signs) as well as the lessening of other side effects often helps the patient to hold out during this difficult dosage adjustment period.

The doctor often tries to lessen systemic steroid toxicity in chronic asthma by the use of other measures for keeping the amount of medication at the minimal level needed for preventing disability. One way of doing so is by inhalation of the steroid in aerosol form. This is thought to deliver a high local concentration of the drug to respiratory tract tissues. Steroids can, of course, be absorbed from the lungs. Thus, the number of daily inhalations of a drug such as *dexamethasone sodium phosphate* (Decadron Respihaler) must be carefully controlled to keep the total daily dose at a level low enough to avoid systemic toxicity. Patients who make excessive use of steroid aerosols may suffer typical metabolic toxicity and suppression of adrenal function.

To lessen the likelihood of such adverse steroid effects, dosage schedules have been devised that are aimed at minimizing the suppressant effect of steroids on the patient's pituitary and adrenal glands. The most commonly employed of these intermittent dosage plans is *alternate day therapy*, a method in which the total steroid dosage for two days is administered early in the morning every other day (see Chapter 17, p. 229, for details). Although such schedules seem safer for many asthmatic patients, some become quite uncomfortable in the last part of the 48-hour period between doses of the drugs such as prednisone that are used for this purpose. This is particularly likely to occur when the patient is being switched from divided steroid dosage to the alternate day therapy plan. Here too, the nurse encourages the patient to accept the return of some of his asthma symptoms during the dosage adjustment period. She helps him understand the benefits of taking fewer doses of steroid drugs.

Other Drugs in Pulmonary Disease Management

Antibiotic drug therapy for preventing and treating respiratory tract infections is often employed in the management of patients with chronic bronchitis and asthma. *Tetracycline+* and *ampicillin+* are considered to be the most effective antibiotics for routine long-term prophylaxis against the kinds of infections that set off acute attacks. These broad spectrum antibiotics are also employed as soon as a patient develops a respiratory infection even before the specific pathogen has been determined. Of course, once laboratory reports have identified any unusual organism and showed it to be especially sensitive to a particular antiinfective agent—such as *cephalothin+*, for example—the patient seriously ill with a respiratory infection is switched to that drug for further treatment.

Sedative drugs in small doses are sometimes useful for relief of anxiety in asthmatic patients. Emotional upset often plays a part in triggering attacks of wheezing in chronic asthmatic patients, and, of course, severe dyspnea frightens the patient and adds to his agitation during a severe attack. Unfortunately, the continued use of barbiturates and other antianxiety agents could lead to *dependence* (Chapter 6) in chronic cases. In acute cases, the administration of depressant drugs may further reduce the rate and depth of the patient's already inadequate breathing.

The nurse can help to minimize the patient's need for sedative drugs by helping him to deal with the anxiety typically associated with these attacks. Simply staying with the seriously ill asthmatic and listening as he expresses his concerns helps to lessen his nervousness. If she cannot stay with him, she should provide him with a way to signal when he feels that he needs help. She looks in on him frequently and makes him feel by her words and actions that he is in the hands of competent staff who understand his illness and know how to help him.

Cromolyn sodium (Aarrane; Intal) is a drug that is neither a bronchodilator nor a bronchial mucus liquefier nor an antiinflammatory agent.

This drug is used to *prevent* attacks rather than to treat them. It is thought to do so by interfering with the release of tissue autocoids during an antigen-antibody reaction. That is, the lung tissue of a patient who is exposed to a substance to which he is sensitive does not release such substances as histamine and SRS-A, when he has been pretreated with cromolyn.

RESPIRATORY FAILURE IN PULMONARY DISEASE PATIENTS

Patients with advanced asthma or chronic bronchitis and emphysema sometimes suffer physiologic stress so severe that they may die of respiratory failure. When hospitalized, the patient may be in great distress as he struggles to breathe. He is often severely dehydrated, fearful, and hypoxic. (His pale or cyanotic face often shows his fright and the poor oxygenation of his tissues.) The patient obviously requires prompt, effective medical treatment and intelligent skillful nursing care.

Emergency treatment of this kind is best carried out in an intensive respiratory care unit (I.R.C.U.) by a team of nurses and doctors knowledgeable in respiratory physiology and skilled in the use of vigorous measures for reversing the effects of acute pulmonary obstruction. In addition to measures already described for hydrating the patient, relieving his bronchoconstriction, allaying his apprehension, and fighting infection, the I.R.C.U. team must also often administer carefully controlled oxygen therapy.

Oxygen administration to counteract tissue hypoxia is usually part of patient management in acute pulmonary obstructive episodes. The equipment for delivering oxygen to the patient's lungs—face mask, mouthpiece, nasal catheter, or tent—may make him nervous. Thus, the nurse should try to reduce his apprehension by such measures as calmly stating that breathing through the mask or another device will lessen his distress. She then stays with the patient until he gets used to the procedure and sees that it does indeed aid his breathing.

Patients must be closely observed during oxygen inhalation therapy. Oxygenation may lead indirectly to a rise in serum levels of carbon dioxide and to the development of acidosis. The patient's respiration may then require mechanical assistance to remove the excess carbon dioxide. *Systemic alkalinizers* such as sodium bicarbonate, sodium lactate, or tromethamine (Tham-E) may be administered to counteract metabolic acidosis.

Occasionally, a patient's breathing has to be completely controlled. That is, an intermittent positive pressure breathing machine may be employed to do the exhausted patient's breathing for him. In such cases, an anesthesiologist on the I.R.C.U. team may deliberately depress the patient's respiratory reflex activity with ether or halothane. The patient may also receive a skeletal muscle relaxant such as succinylcholine or tubocurarine to aid the passage of an endotracheal tube. Then, various substances such as sterile saline solution or a mucolytic agent may be instilled for bronchial lavage, or bronchoscopy may be employed to dislodge and remove the resistant bronchial plugs that may be contributing to the patient's asphyxia.

Summary

Patients with chronic obstructive diseases of the respiratory tract often require treatment with several different types of drugs. The nurse can help to teach them how best to treat themselves with the bronchodilator drugs and others that are to be taken by various routes—as aerosol inhalants, retention enemas and suppositories, orally, and by injection.

Patients hospitalized with acute attacks of severe asthma need particularly skilled nursing care not only to administer oxygen and drugs that help the patient to breathe more easily, but also to allay his fears and thus increase the effectiveness of the drugs with which he is being treated. Nurses also play an important part in the work of the emergency teams that treat critically ill patients who require intensive respiratory care.

S U M M A R Y of Points for the Nurse to Remember Concerning Drug Therapy of Respiratory Tract Obstructive Disorders

Try to detect factors involved in causing acute attacks in patients with chronic obstructive conditions and help the patient to avoid exposing himself to such situations.

Advise the patient and his family to remove substances to which the patient is allergic from his home environment.

Keep chronic bronchitis patients from becoming chilled or exposed to infection.

Help patients avoid situations that may upset them emotionally.

Encourage patients to stop smoking.

Observe how patients respond to drug treatment to see whether they get prompt relief from their medication or are becoming resistant to bronchodilator aerosols and other types of medication.

Observe patients for adverse effects such as signs of central nervous system stimulation (nervousness, trembling) from einephrine, or heart palpitations from isoproterenol. Check the patient's anorectal region for signs of irritation from aminophylline suppositories.

Teach patients and their families how to prepare and administer medications such as subcutaneous epinephrine injections, theophylline retention enemas, and aerosol inhalations of isoproterenol or mucolytic agents.

Use adjunctive nursing measures to help patients who are receiving expectorants to cough more productively. For example, encourage the patient to maintain a high intake of fluids. Help him to sit up when he has to cough.

Encourage asthmatic patients to withstand the discomfort of reduced dosage of corticosteroids when the doctor tries to wean the patient away from these drugs periodically. Help the patient to understand the desirability of trying to get along without these drugs whenever possible.

Use nursing measures to relieve the alarm of patients hospitalized with severe asthmatic attacks. Convey a feeling of calmness and of confidence that the drugs and other measures that are being employed will soon prove effective for relieving his breathing difficulty. Stay with the patient as long as possible and provide a call bell to summon you promptly when you have to be away from him.

Clinical Nursing Situation

The Situation: Mrs. Logan began having asthmatic attacks soon after her daughter brought home a kitten. Because they had become fond of it, they decided not to give it up. Instead, Mrs. Logan began to get a series of injections to densensitize her to the animal's dander.

This course of hyposensitization therapy did

not prove very successful, and Mrs. Logan continued to have asthmatic attacks, though at somewhat less frequent intervals. The physician finally concluded, from things that Mrs. Logan told him during her visits, that the kitten was probably no more than a trigger and that emotional stress may have been a more important factor underlying her allergic response. Mrs. Logan agreed that financial difficulties and the need to care for her aged mother who had had a stroke might have made her more susceptible to asthmatic attacks.

The doctor, who worked with a nurse in the long-term care of patients such as Mrs. Logan, realized that medication alone would not be enough, but that gradual re-education and an effort to change some of the stress-producing factors in the patient's life situation would be necessary. Thus, he conferred with the nurse about these matters as well as about the prescribed regimen which included: an ephedrine-phenobarbital combination and chlorpheniramine for regular daily use along with a liberal fluid intake; aminophylline suppositories for use when wheezing developed; and Librium which was to be taken when the patient felt herself tense and upset.

The Problem: Place yourself in the role of the nurse who was to visit Mrs. Logan at home each week to provide assistance with some of her practical problems. What observations would you make of the physical environment and of the interpersonal relationships within the household, which included Mrs. Logan's partially paralyzed mother, her daughter, her husband, and a pet kitten? What factors would you plan to assess in relation to Mrs. Logan's care of her mother and her feelings about the situation? What observations would you make to evaluate Mrs. Logan's response to each of the drugs that she is taking and the adequacy of her fluid intake?

DRUG DIGEST

AMINOPHYLLINE U.S.P.
(Theophylline ethylenediamine)
Actions and Indications. This theophylline-type bronchodilator drug is used alone or combined with adrenergic drugs such as ephedrine for preventing attacks of bronchial asthma. It is also often effective for rapid relief of bronchospasm in patients with status asthmaticus whose severe acute attacks do not respond to treatment with epinephrine. Aminophylline is also sometimes useful for relief of dyspnea in pulmonary edema following left ventricular heart failure.

Side Effects, Cautions, and Contraindications. Gastrointestinal irritation may cause epigastric distress, nausea, and vomiting. Caution is required in patients with healed peptic ulcer. Children receiving overdoses have sometimes suffered persistent severe and bloody ("coffee grounds") vomitus, also nervous system stimulation leading to delirium, convulsions, and shock. Too rapid intravenous injection may cause a rapid drop in blood pressure and cardiovascular collapse.

Dosage and Administration. Aminophylline is effective when administered orally, rectally, or parenterally. Oral adult dosage is about 130 to 250 mg t.i.d. or q.i.d. Administered rectally by suppository or retention enema, the drug's dosage is about 300 mg for adults and 50 to 100 mg for children up to three times a day. The intravenous dose of 250 to 500 mg is injected slowly over a period of about 10 to 20 minutes up to three times daily.

POTASSIUM IODIDE U.S.P.
Actions and Indications. This expectorant is used to reduce the viscosity of thick bronchial secretions in asthma and chronic bronchitis. Administered with moderate amounts of fluid, it may stimulate the flow of respiratory tract fluid, a natural watery liquid that loosens mucous plugs. This may result in a cough that helps to remove sputum previously retained in the respiratory tract.

Side Effects, Cautions, and Contraindications. Gastrointestinal upset caused by irritation of the gastric mucosa is the most common side effect. It may cause nausea, vomiting, and diarrhea.

Patients sensitive to iodides may develop painful swelling of the parotid glands and acnelike skin eruptions. Drug fever and anaphylactic reactions have also been reported. Use of this drug is undesirable in patients with tuberculosis or thyroid disease. It may interfere with the interpretation of tests of thyroid function.

Chronic intake may cause iodism, a condition that may be confused with a heavy head cold, as it often begins with a sore throat and is followed by a running nose and nasal and chest congestion.

Dosage and Administration. This drug is administered q.i.d. in oral doses of 300 mg. Each dose should be taken with a glass of water or milk to reduce gastric irritation and to keep the patient well hydrated.

References

Bocles, J.S. Status asthmaticus. *Med. Clin. N. Amer.*, 54:493, 1970 (March).
Dines, D.E. Medications in pulmonary insufficiency. *Mod. Treatm.*, 6:346, 1969 (March).
Ebert, R.V., and Pierce, J.A. Therapy in

chronic bronchitis and pulmonary emphysema. *JAMA*, 184:490, 1963.

Foss, G. Postural drainage. *Amer. J. Nurs.*, 73:666, 1973.

Rodman, M.J. Drugs for allergic disorders, part 1, anaphylaxis and asthma. *RN*, 34:63, 1971 (June).

———— Drugs for respiratory tract disorders. *RN*, 37:57, 1974 (Feb.).

Segal, M.S., and Weiss, E.B. Current concepts in the management of the patient with status asthmaticus. *Med. Clin. N. Amer.*, 51:373, 1967 (March).

Shapiro, A.G., and Walker, C.G. Respiratory intensive care. *Med. Clin. N. Amer.*, 55:1217, 1971 (Sept.).

Sheffer, A.L., and Valentine, M.D. The treatment of bronchial asthma. *Med. Clin. N. Amer.*, 53:239, 1969 (March).

Weiss, E.B., et al. Current concepts in pathophysiology and management of status asthmaticus. *Mod. Treatm.*, 6:278, 1969 (March).

SECTION **6**

Drugs

Acting

on

Autonomic

Neuroeffectors

20.

The Autonomic Nervous System

Introduction

In the several chapters of this section, we shall discuss the so-called *autonomic* drugs—agents that affect the functioning of organs that receive nerve impulses from the *autonomic nervous system (the A.N.S.).* These drugs produce their effects mainly by acting upon the smooth muscle, cardiac muscle, and gland cells in which the autonomic nerve fibers end. These autonomically innervated muscle and gland structures are called *effectors,* or *neuro-effectors,* because they respond to nerve impulses by *doing* something. Thus, as we shall see in detail, the several classes of autonomic drugs that we shall be studying produce changes in smooth muscle tone and motility, in the rate and strength of heart muscle contractions, and in the secretions of glandular tissues.

In this chapter, we shall review the anatomy and physiology of the autonomic nervous system. Once the student understands how this system functions normally, she can often predict what effects the different kinds of drugs are likely to have on the activity of the various organs that receive autonomic nerve fibers.

Students often find the study of this class of drugs difficult. However, this need not be so if the student first takes time to understand how this system normally functions and then learns the "lingo," the special terms for describing the different kinds of drug actions.

We shall also discuss some aspects of the ways in which nerve impulses are transmitted by the release of certain chemicals from nerve endings. Drugs that affect the chemical transmission of nerve impulses affect the functioning not only of autonomically innervated organs but also of skeletal muscle and of the central nervous system (Sections Two, Three, and Four).

General Functions of the Autonomic Nervous System

The autonomic nervous system regulates the functioning of the viscera, or internal organs, and other structures that function in ways which we cannot control by an act of the will; it is also called the *visceral* or *involuntary nervous system*. Although we can not consciously influence its activity, the A.N.S. *is* influenced by areas of the cerebral cortex and by other central nervous system (C.N.S.) nerve centers. Similarly, although we tend to think of the A.N.S. mainly in terms of the nerve fibers that carry motor and secretory messages *from* the C.N.S., these efferent impulses are actually set off by streams of afferent impulses that travel to the C.N.S. from the viscera and other autonomically innervated structures.

The main nerve centers for these autonomic reflex arcs are located in the hypothalamus, medulla oblongata, and spinal cord. Nerve impulses that arise in peripheral structures are carried to these centers by afferent fibers. The integrating centers at various levels of the C.N.S. then respond by sending out efferent impulses via A.N.S. pathways. These then adjust the functioning of the various visceral organs in ways that keep the body's internal environment constant (homeostasis). The A.N.S. regulates blood pressure, breathing, body temperature, water balance, and urinary bladder and digestive functions, among others. This moment-to-moment control is exerted by a never-ending interplay between two opposing subdivisions of the peripheral part of the A.N.S.: (1) *the sympathetic* and (2) *the parasympathetic systems*.

The Divisions of the Autonomic Nervous System

In each of the two divisions of the autonomic nervous system, nerve impulses are carried from the central nervous system (C.N.S.) to outlying organs and structures by way of a two-neuron chain. Nerve cell bodies located at various levels of the cerebrospinal axis send their fibers out toward the periphery. However, these fibers do *not* pass directly to the organs that they innervate.

Instead, the fibers from the first, or central, neuron end in *ganglia*, groups of nerve cell bodies packed together in various locations outside the C.N.S. These second neurons then receive impulses from the *preganglionic* fibers and relay the messages down the *postganglionic* fibers. When these nerve impulses finally reach the ends of the second fibers, they release chemicals that transmit impulses to the neuroeffector cells located in the innervated smooth and cardiac muscle and exocrine gland cells.

This differs from the way in which the one-celled pathway that nervous messages take from the C.N.S. travels to skeletal muscle fibers. That is, the somatic fibers of mixed spinal nerves go directly to the skeletal fibers from the C.N.S. without any intervening nerve cells to relay the messages that make the voluntary muscles move.

The two-neuron pathways of both subdivisions of the A.N.S. differ from each other in several ways: (1) the location within the central nervous system of the first nerve cell body of the two neuron chain; (2) the location of the ganglia containing the second cells in the link; and (3) the relative lengths of the preganglionic and postganglionic nerve fibers that connect these subdivisions of the A.N.S. with the visceral organs which they innervate (Table 20-1 and Fig. 20-1).

ANATOMY OF THE SYMPATHETIC SYSTEM

This system is also called the *thoracolumbar* system, because the first nerve cell bodies are located in the part of the spinal cord that runs through the chest, or thorax, down into the lumbar region of the back. These centrally located cells send out relatively short *preganglionic* fibers that synapse with nerve cells in ganglia located mostly in chains that run like a paired string of beads just outside the spinal cord (Fig. 20-1). Relatively long *post*ganglionic fibers then make their way to the autonomically innervated visceral organs.

ANATOMY OF THE PARASYMPATHETIC SYSTEM

This system is also called the *craniosacral* system, because its cells of origin lie centrally at the two extreme ends of the cerebrospinal axis. Some are located at subcortical levels of the brain (that is, within the cranium), while

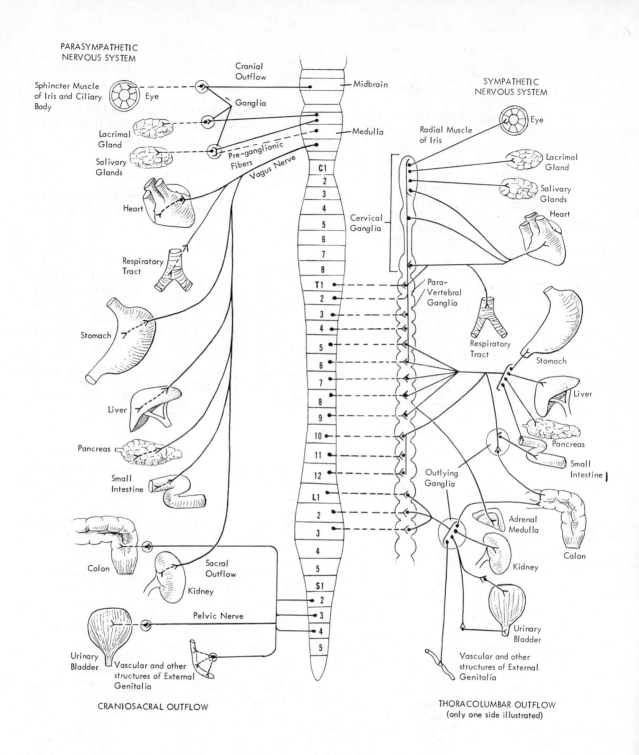

Fig. 20-1. The autonomic nervous system. Solid lines from cranial and sacral portions of the cerebrospinal axis indicate *pre*ganglionic fibers of the parasympathetic nervous system. Short broken lines within or just outside organs indicate *post*ganglionic fibers.

Short broken lines from thoracolumbar portions of the spinal cord to chain of paravertebral ganglia indicate *pre*ganglionic fibers of the sympathetic nervous system. Long solid lines indicate *post*ganglionic fibers.

TABLE 20-1 *Anatomical and Physiological Characteristics of Sympathetic, Parasympathetic, and Somatic Nerves*

Characteristics	Sympathetic Nervous System (Involuntary)	Parasympathetic Nervous System (Involuntary)	Somatic Motor Neurons (Voluntary)
Structures innervated	Heart, smooth muscles of blood vessels, viscera, ocular structures, glands	Heart, smooth muscles of blood vessels, viscera, ocular structures, glands	Skeletal muscles
Origin of centrally located neuron	Thoracolumbar portion of spinal cord (that is, lateral horn cells in T_1–T_{12}; L_1 and L_2)	Cranial and sacral portion of the cerebrospinal axis (such as cells in midbrain, medulla, and S_2, S_3, and S_4 of spinal cord)	Anterior horn of spinal cord at all levels.
Axonal pathway from C.N.S. nerve cell body	Short, myelinated preganglionic fibers (for example, white rami communicantes to vertebral ganglia), and other relatively short fibers	Relatively very long myelinated preganglionic fibers travel in cranial (for example, facial; vagus) and spinal (for instance, pelvic) nerves	Myelinated motoneuron axons lead directly to skeletal muscles, where they divide into many branches
Final distribution of terminations of central neuron	Terminals in contact with many neurons in a single ganglion (preganglionic fiber may pass through many ganglia before synapsing with as many as 20 or more ganglionic neurons which also receive ends of other preganglionic fibers)	Terminals synapse with only one *or* two neurons of terminal ganglia lying near, or even in, the visceral or other organs usually (for instance, make contact with nerve cells in ganglia of abdominal, pelvic, and thoracic organs)	Each axon makes contact with 100 or more muscle fibers (that is, a motor unit is formed). Axon ending becomes *non*myelinated to form nerve end plate, which comes in contact with muscle sole plate in invagination of muscle membrane, thus forming the motor end plate. Acetylcholine released by axon ending depolarizes the motor end plate (nicotinic type of cholinergic transmission). Impulses can be blocked by certain anticholinergic agents (for example, curare)
Impulse transmission (nicotinic type of cholinergic transmission in *both* types of autonomic ganglia and at the myoneural junction of the skeletal muscle fibers)	Acetylcholine released at preganglionic nerve terminals stimulates neurons in ganglia located relatively close to C.N.S. Impulses can be blocked by certain anticholinergic agents (for example, C_6)	Acetylcholine released at preganglionic nerve terminals stimulates neurons in ganglia located relatively far from C.N.S. Impulses can be blocked by certain anticholinergic agents (such as C_6)	
Postganglionic fiber distribution	Gray rami communicantes from ganglia join spinal nerves and travel to junctions in smooth muscle and gland cells	Very short fibers from ganglia terminate in smooth muscle and gland cells (that is, in neuroeffectors)	
Impulse transmission at postganglionic neuroeffectors (that is, junction between terminations of nerve fibers and receptors of cardiac and smooth muscle and gland cells)	Norepinephrine released and stimulates neuroeffectors except in sweat glands and some blood vessels. Impulses can be blocked by alpha or beta blocking agents (for example, alpha by phenoxybenzamine; beta by propranolol)	Acetylcholine released to stimulate smooth muscle, cardiac and gland cells (for instance, muscarinic type of cholinergic transmission). Impulses can be blocked by certain anticholinergic agents (for example, atropine)	

other nerve cell bodies are located in the sacral portion of the spinal cord. Thus, some parasympathetic fibers run in cranial nerves such as the facial and vagus nerves. Other axons, originating at lower levels of the spinal cord, form the pelvic nerves, which send branches to organs such as the urinary bladder and lower large intestine.

COMPARISON OF PHYSIOLOGICAL FUNCTIONS

The *sympathetic system*, working together with the adrenal medulla, which it innervates, tends to regulate the expenditure of energy, especially in times of stress. The *parasympathetic system*, on the other hand, mainly influences functions that help the body to store up and save energy.

The opposing functions of the two divisions of the A.N.S. may be grasped by a thoughtful study of Table 20-2. A typically *sympathetic response* is the "fight or flight" reaction that occurs when the organism feels threatened and reacts with rage and fear: the heartbeat speeds up, blood pressure rises, blood leaves the constricted vessels of the skin and viscera and is shunted to the dilated arterioles in the hardworking heart and skeletal muscles; at the same time, the extra amounts of oxygen and glucose that these muscles require are supplied by liver glycogen breakdown and by rapid deep breathing to take in air through widely dilated lung bronchi.

The *parasympathetic system*, on the other hand, slows the heart, constricts the dilated pupils of the eyes to protect the retinas from excessive light, and restarts the temporarily stalled gastrointestinal movements and secretions so that digestion and assimilation of foodstuffs can once more proceed. It helps also to rid the urinary bladder and the rectum of body wastes.

We must not think of these systems only as emergency mechanisms, however; their work goes on continuously, making possible the delicate adjustments needed to keep up with the ever changing environment. It is perhaps better to think of the two systems as functioning like the handlebars of a bicycle, which help the rider keep to a straight course when he automatically puts pressure on one handle or the other to correct any tendency of the bike to veer too far to either the right or left.

Actually, this picture is somewhat simplified.

Both divisions of the A.N.S. do not exert equal control over all organs. For example, the parasympathetic system has greater influence on gastrointestinal tract function than does the sympathetic, whereas the latter regulates blood vessel tone and blood pressure to a much greater extent than does the parasympathetic system.

Nonetheless, the general concept of two opposing systems in a state of tonic, or continuous, activity designed to achieve an unstable, shifting functional balance is a useful one for helping us understand the actions of the various autonomic drugs. For, by acting at the same synapses and neuroeffectors as do the A.N.S. nerve impulses, these drugs tend to upset the temporary balance in one direction or another. Thus, some drugs may imitate, or *mimic*, the effects either of sympathetic or of parasympathetic stimulation in slowing down or speeding up a particular function. On the other hand, some drugs may keep nerve impulses from reaching the muscle or gland cells through one or the other division of the A.N.S. In that case, the still active division tends to exert a disproportionate influence upon the functioning of most of the organs, structures, and systems that have had part of their tonic nervous control blocked out.

Chemical Transmission of Nerve Impulses

It is now known that when nerve impulses reach the endings of nerve cell fibers they trigger the release of chemical substances from the nerve endings. These chemicals then transmit the nerve impulse across the microscopic gap between the end of the nerve and the structure which it innervates. This may be another nerve cell, a smooth or skeletal muscle cell, or a gland cell. These second cells in the series then respond to the chemical messages from the nerve fiber in their characteristic ways. That is, nerve cells—in the ganglia, for example—are stimulated to fire impulses, muscle cells contract or relax, and glandular cells secrete.

Several kinds of chemical substances are synthesized by nerve cells and stored in the nerve endings. The two neurohormones released by peripheral autonomic nerves are *acetylcholine* (ACh) and *norepinephrine* (NE). Most peripheral nerve fibers release ACh, and all the nerves that do so are called *cholinergic*. NE is

TABLE 20-2   *Results of Autonomic Nervous Stimulation (Comparison of Responses to Sympathetic and Parasympathetic Nerve Impulses)*

Organs and Structures	Sympathetic (Adrenergic) Nerve Impulses	Type of Adrenergic Receptor	Parasympathetic and Other Cholinergic Nerve Impulses
Heart	Increase in rate, contractility, and conduction speed	Beta 1	Decrease in rate, contractility, and A-V conduction
Blood Vessels			
1. Skin and mucous membrane	Constriction	Alpha	Dilatation
2. Skeletal muscle	Dilatation (usually)	Beta 2	Dilatation*
3. Coronary	Dilatation (may be due to indirect, metabolic effects)	(?)	Dilatation
Bronchial Muscle	Relaxation (lumen dilated)	Beta 2	Contraction (lumen constricted)
Gastrointestinal			
1. Muscle motility and tone	Decrease	Beta 2	Increase
2. Sphincters	Contraction (ordinarily)	Alpha	Relaxation (ordinarily)
3. Exocrine glands	Secretion reduced (?)	(?)	Secretion increased
4. Gallbladder	Relaxation	(?)	Contraction
Urinary Bladder			
1. Detrusor	Relaxation	Beta 2	Contraction
2. Trigone and sphincter	Contraction	Alpha	Relaxation
Ocular Structures			
1. Iris radial muscle	Contraction (pupil dilates)	Alpha	. . . .
2. Iris sphincter muscle	. . . .	. . .	Contraction (pupil constricts)
3. Ciliary muscle	Relaxation (but with relatively little effect on lens movement)	Beta 2	Contraction (lens adjusted for near vision)
Skin Structures			
1. Sweat glands	Increased palmar and other localized sweating	Alpha	Generalized increase* in sweating
2. Pilomotor muscles	Contracted (gooseflesh)	Alpha	. . . .
Miscellaneous			
1. Salivary glands	Thick, viscid secretion	Alpha	Copious, watery secretion
2. Lacrimal and nasopharyngeal glands	. . . .	. . .	Increased secretion
3. Liver	Glycogenolysis	. . .	. . . .
4. Male sex organs	Ejaculation	. . .	Erection (vascular dilatation)

* Cholinergic transmission, but nerve cell chain originates in thoracolumbar portion of spinal cord and is, therefore, sympathetic.

released by postganglionic sympathetic nerve endings, except for those that innervate the sweat glands and some blood vessels. These fibers are referred to as *adrenergic*.

CHOLINERGIC TRANSMISSION

Several different kinds of peripheral nerves transmit nerve impulses by releasing acetylcholine as the chemical mediator between the neuron and the second cell in the series. *The three major classes of cholinergic nerves are:*

1. *Postganglionic cholinergic fibers.* These include all the parasympathetic postganglionic fibers and a few exceptional sympathetic postganglionic fibers—those to the sweat glands and to some blood vessels (as mentioned above).

2. *Preganglionic cholinergic fibers.* These include *all* of the preganglionic fibers of *both* the sympathetic and parasympathetic divisions of the A.N.S. (The cells of the adrenal medulla—a structure that is similar to autonomic ganglia except that it is made up of gland cells instead of nerve cells—are also innervated by cholinergic nerves that originate in the spinal cord.)

3. *Somatic motor nerve fibers.* These fibers, although they are *not* part of the A.N.S., also release acetylcholine from their endings in skeletal (voluntary) muscle. (Cholinergic transmission is not limited to nerves of the A.N.S. nor even to peripheral nerves alone. ACh is also the chemical mediator at certain synapses in nerve pathways that run entirely within the central nervous system.)

All these cholinergic nerves contain acetylcholine molecules stored in a bound, or inactive, form in the nerve endings. Nerve impulses that reach these storage sites release ACh in a free form from the tiny blisterlike storage sacs. The freed ACh molecules then flow out of the nerve ending and cross the tiny junctional space. The ACh molecules that bridge this gap then make contact with a chemically specialized spot on the membrane of the second cell—a *cholinergic receptor*, or *cholinoceptive site*.

The combination between the ACh molecule and the specially designed cholinergic receptor of the postjunctional cell sets in motion changes in the activity of the second nerve cell (in autonomic ganglia), the gland cells, or the smooth and skeletal muscle fibers. As indicated above, the second nerve cell then sends an impulse down the postganglionic fibers, exocrine gland cells then secrete fluids, and muscle cells contract or, in some cases, relax.

Once the neurohormone has transmitted its message and the neuroeffector cell has responded, any remaining ACh molecules are immediately destroyed. This destruction of excess ACh is carried out by an enzyme called *acetylcholinesterase* (AChE). This enzyme, which is packed into synaptic and neuromuscular junctions, catalyzes the conversion of active ACh molecules to acetic acid and choline. These metabolites are not active as neurotransmitters. The membrane of the postjunctional nerve, muscle, or gland cell recovers excitability and is now ready to respond to the next volley of cholinergic nerve impulses.

ADRENERGIC TRANSMISSION

Adrenergic nerves contain molecules of *norepinephrine (NE)* that are stored in granules close to the endings of postganglionic sympathetic fibers. Sympathetic nerve impulses release molecules of NE, and the freed neurohormone then flows out of the nerve endings and makes contact with a specialized site on the membrane of the muscle cell that receives the nerve fiber—the *adrenergic receptor* or *adrenoceptive site*. This sets in motion biochemical changes that result in the contraction of some smooth muscle cells and in the relaxation of others.

The responses of the various organs and structures to sympathetic nerve impulses depend upon which of two kinds of adrenergic receptors they mainly contain. Smooth muscle cells that for the most part contain receptors of the *alpha* type respond by contracting. This is seen, for example, in the blood vessels of the skin and mucous membranes, in which sympathetic impulses cause contraction of the muscular walls and narrowing of the vascular space (vasoconstriction, Table 20-2).

Smooth muscle cells that contain mainly receptors of the *beta* 2 type—those of the bronchial tubes, for example—respond by relaxing. In the case of the heart, however, sympathetic nerve stimulation releases NE molecules that react with cardiac muscle cell beta 1 type adrenergic receptors in a way that makes the heart muscle cells contract more forcefully and rapidly (Table 20-2).

Once the adrenergic neurohormone has transmitted its message to smooth and cardiac muscle cells, any excess molecules must be removed from the alpha and beta receptor sites. Most of the free NE molecules are taken up by the adrenergic nerve endings that had released them. Some of those recaptured NE molecules are stored in the granules, from which they will later be released again by another volley of sympathetic nerve impulses. Free NE that does not get back into the nerve cells diffuses away from the nerve-muscle junction. Molecules of NE that are carried to the liver and other tissues are destroyed in a series of enzymatically catalyzed steps. The enzymes involved in the destruction of norepinephrine and of other endogenous catecholamines, such as the adrenal medulla hormone epinephrine and the C.N.S. neurotransmitter dopamine, are (1) *monoamine oxidase (MAO)* and catechol-O-methyl transferase (COMT).

Pharmacological Actions

The various organs and structures that respond to autonomic nerve impulses are also responsive to the actions of the various kinds of autonomic drugs. Drugs producing effects that *imitate* stimulation by nerve impulses from the two divisions of the A.N.S. are called *sympathomimetic (adrenergic)* and *parasympathomimetic (cholinergic)*. Drugs that interfere with transmission of nerve impulses by acetylcholine are called *cholinergic blockers*; those that interfere with transmission by norepinephrine are called *adrenergic blockers*.

Drugs that *imitate* cholinergic transmission include not only the parasympathomimetic drugs which act upon postganglionic neuroeffectors but also agents that act upon autonomic ganglia, skeletal muscle, and even cells of the C.N.S. (See *classes of cholinergic drugs*, p. 267). Drugs that imitate the effects of acetylcholine—cholinomimetic drugs—are sometimes said to have "*muscarinic*" and "*nicotinic*" effects.

The term "*muscarinic*" refers to drug actions that take place at postganglionic cholinergic neuroeffectors—that is, at cholinoceptive sites in the same cells that react to the acetylcholine released by *parasympathetic* nerve impulses.

The term "*nicotinic*" refers to drug actions that resemble those of the acetylcholine released in autonomic ganglia and in skeletal muscle. Since some drugs have *both* muscarinic (parasympathomimetic) and nicotinic effects, they are best called cholinergic, or cholinomimetic agents (Tables 20-3 and 21-1). One of the characteristics of drug action at nicotinic

sites (ganglia and skeletal muscles) is that overdoses first cause a stimulation of function, followed by later depression and failure.

Cholinergic blocking drugs are agents that keep cells from responding to the acetylcholine released by the various kinds of cholinergic nerves. *Atropine*, for example, blocks cholinergic nerve impulses to smooth muscle, cardiac muscle, and exocrine gland cells that receive parasympathetic and other postganglionic cholinergic nerves. Thus, it is classified as an *antimuscarinic-type* cholinergic blocker (Table 20-3). Curare, on the other hand, blocks cholinergic transmission at nicotinic sites—particularly skeletal muscle, and only to a lesser extent the autonomic ganglia (see Table 20-3). Still other drugs block cholinergic transmission, primarily at autonomic ganglia (see *ganglionic blocking agents*, Tables 20-3, 26-1, and 32-1).

Drugs that *imitate adrenergic* transmission (Table 20-3) do so in various ways. Some, such as epinephrine, set off effects similar to those of the neurohormone norepinephrine (NE) when they come in contact with alpha or beta adrenergic receptors. Other sympathomimetic drugs—ephedrine, for example—act by increasing the release of NE from adrenergic nerve endings. Still other indirect-acting adrenergic drugs such as cocaine are thought to act by keeping adrenergic nerve endings from taking up previously released free NE. (See *adrenergic transmission*, p. 263.)

Adrenergic blocking drugs, agents that prevent sympathetically innervated cells from responding to the norepinephrine released by nerve impulses, fall into two classes. Some interfere with transmission to the alpha-type adrenergic receptors; others decrease the responsiveness of beta adrenergic receptors. Clinically effective *alpha adrenergic blockers* are used mainly to alter the responses of blood vessel smooth muscle to norepinephrine and to circulating epinephrine from the adrenal medulla. The *beta adrenergic blockers* are used clinically for their effects upon cardiac function (see *propranolol*, Chapters 24, 29, and 30).

Adrenergic neuron blocking drugs also interfere with sympathetic nervous system impulse transmission. These drugs do so by reducing the rate of release of norepinephrine from sympathetic postganglionic nerve endings rather than by blocking the action of released norepinephrine upon adrenergic receptors. Drugs of this kind are employed mainly in the management of hypertension (Chapter 26).

TABLE 20-3 *Autonomic Drugs Classified by Site and Type of Action*

Site of Action	Stimulants	Blocking Agents
Cholinergic autonomic neuroeffectors (such as smooth and cardiac muscle; exocrine glands)	*Parasympathomimetics* (muscarinic type cholinergic agents)* Acetylcholine and the synthetic choline esters (for example, methacholine) Cholinomimetic alkaloids (such as muscarine; pilocarpine) Anticholinesterase agents (for example, neostigmine)	*Antimuscarinic type cholinergic blockers* Natural solanaceous alkaloids† (for example, atropine) Synthetic anticholinergic agents‡ (for example, methantheline bromide)
Autonomic ganglia (both sympathetic and parasympathetic)	*Nicotinic type cholinergic agents (in low doses)* Acetylcholine and certain synthetic choline esters* (for example, carbachol) Anticholinesterase agents* (for example, neostigmine) Nicotine Dimethylphenylpiperazinium (DMPP)	*Ganglion cell transmission blockers* Large doses of most of the nicotinic type stimulants listed at the left will interfere with impulse transmission Ganglionic blocking agents§ (for example, mecamylamine)
Somatic neuromuscular junctions‖ (motor end plates of skeletal muscle fibers)	*Nicotinic type cholinergic agents (in low doses)* Acetylcholine* Anticholinesterase agents, low doses* (for example, edrophonium) Phenyltrimethylammonium (PTMA)	*Neuromuscular blocking agents*** Competitive type (for example, curare) Depolarizing type (for example, succinylcholine) Large doses of most of the nicotinic type stimulants listed at the left will interfere with impulse transmission.
Adrenergic neuroeffectors (for example, in cardiac tissues, smooth muscle of blood vessels, bronchioles)	*Sympathomimetics†† (Adrenergic receptor stimulants)* Catecholamines (for example, epinephrine) Alipatic amines (for example, phenylephrine)	*Adrenergic blocking agents* Alpha type blockers‡‡ (for example, tolazoline) Beta type blockers (for example, propranolol)
Adrenergic nerve endings	*Sympathomimetics (acting at nerve ending, rather than at postjunctional receptor)* Tyramine, ephedrine, cocaine	*Adrenergic nerve transmission blockers* Reserpine, guanethidine, methyldopa

* See Table 21-1 for detailed listing.
† See Table 22-1 for detailed listing.
‡ See Table 22-2 for detailed listing.
§ See Table 26-1 for detailed listing.
‖ These are *not* autonomic sites but drugs acting at these sites are included here because some also act simultaneously (especially in large doses) at autonomic sites.
** See Table 14-2 for detailed listing.
†† See Table 23-1 for detailed listing.
‡‡ See Chapter 24.

Summary

In this chapter, we have reviewed the anatomy and physiology of the autonomic nervous system and introduced the terms that are employed in discussing autonomic nerve impulse transmission and the drugs that imitate the natural transmitters or that block their effects.

We have also seen that it is often possible to *predict* the effects that an autonomic blocking drug of any particular class is likely to produce. Thus, for example, if we know that the sympathetic nervous system tends to speed up the heart, we can *predict* that a sympathomimetic drug should do the same, and that a beta adrenergic blocker such as propranolol should slow the heart. Similarly, if we know that parasympathetic nervous system activity tends to cause gastrointestinal smooth muscle to contract, we can *predict* that a parasympathomimetic drug may cause cramps and that an antimuscarinic-type cholinergic blocker such as atropine should relieve gastrointestinal spasms.

The nurse who administers these drugs should know as much as possible about all of their varied pharmacological effects. Autonomic drugs exert many powerful effects that can help patients or harm them. The better the nurse understands what these drugs actually do, the more effective is the care she can offer to patients receiving these potent agents. The nurse who knows the effects that these drugs can have on her patient's condition can help him to gain their maximum therapeutic benefits while avoiding the many possible adverse effects of autonomic drugs.

21.

Cholinergic
(Parasympathomimetic)
Drugs in the Management of
Myasthenia Gravis, Glaucoma,
and Other Disorders

Classes of Cholinergic Drugs
(Table 21-1)

The cholinergic drugs are chemicals that act at the same sites as the neurohormone, *acetylcholine*. Their actions upon the structures that receive cholinergic nerves are similar to those of stimulation of the same organs by the several kinds of nerves that transmit impulses by the release of acetylcholine. Thus, these drugs can also be called *cholinomimetic*.

Parasympathomimetic-type cholinergic drugs have effects that are largely limited to the cells that receive postganglionic fibers from the parasympathetic division of the A.N.S. Cholinergic drugs of this kind act directly upon postganglionic neuroeffectors of the *muscarinic* type. That is, these chemicals combine with the *cholinoceptive sites*, or *cholinergic receptors*, in such structures as smooth muscle, cardiac muscle, and exocrine gland cells. This then produces effects similar to those brought about by stimulation of the parasympathetic nerves that innervate these structures (Table 20-2).

The parasympathomimetic drugs are divided into two subgroups: (1) the *synthetic choline esters*—drugs chemically similar to the neurohormone acetylcholine but with a much longer duration of action; and (2) the *cholinomimetic*

267

alkaloids—plant products that differ from acetylcholine chemically but which produce the same kinds of effects when their molecules occupy cholinergic receptors in postganglionic neuroeffectors. Muscarine, the mushroom derivative from which the term "muscarinic" is derived, is one such alkaloid, and pilocarpine is another.

Anticholinesterase-type cholinergic drugs act *indirectly* to produce acetylcholinelike effects not only at muscarinic, but also at "nicotinic" sites. That is, they are capable of affecting the functioning of skeletal muscle and ganglion cells as well as smooth muscle, cardiac muscle, and glandular tissues. (Some even affect transmission at cholinergic nerve pathways in the central nervous system.) These drugs have relatively little direct effect upon cholinergic receptors. They act, instead, by *inhibiting acetylcholinesterase*, the enzyme that is responsible for the immediate destruction of free acetylcholine (ACh) molecules.

As a result of this interference with enzyme function, the acetylcholine that is being constantly freed from cholinergic nerves tends to accumulate at all kinds of postjunctional cells. At muscarinic sites, the resulting rise in the local levels of free undestroyed ACh leads to intensified parasympathomimetic activity of smooth and cardiac muscle and gland cells. The drug-induced inhibition of the enzyme also leads to the accumulation of undestroyed ACh at nicotinic sites. This, in turn, causes stimulation of skeletal muscle and autonomic ganglion cells *at first*. Later, however, the excessive accumulation of ACh that occurs indirectly as a result of the enzyme-inactivating action of anticholinesterase-type cholinergic drugs leads to depression of skeletal muscle tone and ganglion nerve cell impulse transmission.

There are two types of anticholinesterase drugs and chemicals: (1) those with a relatively short duration of inhibitory effect upon the enzyme, that are thus often referred to as "*reversible*" inhibitors of acetylcholinesterase; and (2) those with a prolonged inhibitory effect —called "*irreversible*" inhibitors.

Drugs of the first group include *neostigmine*+ and other chemicals of the quaternary ammonium class (Table 21-1). Their effects are readily controlled by careful dosage adjustment. Thus, these drugs are used in the treatment of various kinds of clinical disorders (see *Summary of Therapeutic Uses*, p. 276).

Chemicals of the second kind are rarely used clinically as they are considered too toxic to be administered *systemically* in most circumstances. (Some are applied *topically* to the eye in glaucoma treatment, p. 271.) These acetylcholinesterase inhibitors are organophosphorus compounds that are used, instead, mainly as insecticides (see *Insecticide Poisoning*, p. 275). They have also been extensively studied as "nerve gases" for use in chemical warfare.

Clinical Pharmacology

The cholinergic drugs have many potential therapeutic uses. However, their clinical usefulness is limited by the many discomforting side effects that often occur. To minimize these adverse reactions, the doctor tries to adjust cholinergic drug dosage very carefully. Even so, the doses required for producing therapeutically desirable actions also often cause unwanted effects.

The nurse must sometimes warn the patient to expect certain discomforting side effects. She should, at the same time, point out any signs of improvement that may appear as a result of cholinergic drug treatment. The patient often tends to tolerate annoying drug effects if he knows in advance what to expect and if he sees evidence of the benefits of drug therapy. The nurse watches the patient closely for early signs of adverse drug effects. Dosage of the cholinergic drug can then be reduced and other medications can be administered to relieve some of the almost inevitable side effects.

In the following discussion, we shall indicate the pharmacological effects that cholinergic drugs exert upon various visceral organs and other structures. Then we shall point out, in each case, the clinical applications of these actions in the treatment of various disorders. The adverse effects of these drugs on each organ will then be discussed together with the reasons for the precautions required in administering these drugs.

GASTROINTESTINAL TRACT

The cholinergic drugs increase the tone and motility of G.I. tract smooth muscles. Thus, some of these drugs are used to treat patients with poor peristaltic activity. Among clinical conditions of this kind are *postoperative abdominal atony and distention. Bethanechol*+ is often preferred for stimulating G.I. motility

TABLE 21-1 *Cholinergic Drugs*

Nonproprietary or Official Name	Trade Name or Synonym	Dosage	Remarks
Parasympathomimetic Drugs			
Bethanechol chloride U.S.P.	Urecholine	Oral 5 to 30 mg; s.c. 2.5 to 5 mg	See *Drug Digest*
Carbachol U.S.P.	Carcholin; Doryl	. . . .	See Table 21-2
Methacholine bromide and chloride N.F.	Mecholyl	Oral 200 mg; s.c. 20 mg	Used mainly for its effects on heart and blood vessels
Pilocarpine HCl and nitrate U.S.P.	. . . .	. . . .	See Table 21-2
Anticholinesterase Agents			
QUATERNARY AMMONIUM COMPOUNDS			
Ambenonium chloride N.F.	Mytelase	5 to 25 mg	Antimyasthenic agent
Benzpyrinium bromide	Stigmonene	2 mg I.M.	Smooth muscle stimulant
Demecarium bromide U.S.P.	Humorsol	Topical ophthalmic	See Table 21-2
Edrophonium chloride U.S.P.	Tensilon	5 to 20 mg	See *Drug Digest*
Neostigmine bromide U.S.P.	Prostigmin Br	10 to 30 mg, oral	See *Drug Digest*
Neostigmine methylsulfate U.S.P.	Prostigmin Methylsulfate	0.25 to 1 mg I.M. or s.c.	See *Drug Digest*
Physostigmine and its salicylate and sulfate salts U.S.P.	. . . .	Topical ophthalmic	See Table 21-2
Pyridostigmine bromide U.S.P.	Mestinon	180 to 600 mg daily	See *Drug Digest*
ORGANOPHOSPHATE COMPOUNDS			
Echothiophate iodide U.S.P.	Phospholine	Topical ophthalmic	See Table 21-2
Isoflurophate U.S.P.	Floropryl; DFP	Topical ophthalmic	See Table 21-2
Malathion	. . . .	. . . .	Insecticide
OMPA	. . . .	. . . .	Insecticide, for example
Parathion	. . . .	. . . .	Insecticide
Sarin	. . . .	. . . .	Nerve gas
Soman	. . . .	. . . .	Nerve gas
Tabun	. . . .	. . . .	Nerve gas

in such cases, as the effects of ordinary doses are limited largely to smooth muscle. *Neostigmine+* is also sometimes used for this purpose, but its tendency to affect various nicotinic as well as muscarinic sites tends to produce more circulatory (and other) side effects. (Physical and mechanical measures such as the use of a rectal tube, applying heat to the abdomen, and the use of daily enemas and laxatives are often tried for several days before resorting to cholinergic drugs.)

The predictable G.I. side effects of cholinergic drugs include intestinal cramps and diarrhea. Increased secretion of gastric acid may also cause heartburn and belching. If taken too soon after eating, these drugs may cause nausea and vomiting. However, giving them with a little milk helps to prevent epigastric distress. It is also desirable to have a syringe available containing a solution of the anticholinergic drug *atropine+* to counteract excessive G.I. tract stimulation in patients receiving injections of cholinergic drugs for other conditions—for example, when *methacholine* is employed in treating patients with peripheral vascular or other circulatory disorders (see below). In such situations, it is advisable to place the patient on a bedpan.

GENITOURINARY TRACT

Cholinergic drugs cause the detrusor muscle of the urinary bladder to contract. This action is often useful for treating *bladder atony* and for bringing about micturition (evacuation of urine). Thus, subcutaneous injection of *bethanechol+* or of *neostigmine+* is sometimes employed for relief of *postoperative* or *postpartum urinary retention*. Pharmacological "catheterization" of this kind may help to prevent the urinary tract infections that sometimes follow mechanical catheterization of these patients, or of those with spinal cord injuries that cause neurogenic atony of the urinary bladder.

The nurse makes sure that patients receiving cholinergic drugs have a urinal or bedpan close at hand. She answers their calls quickly, as these drugs often produce a feeling of urgency to void. Patients with mechanical obstructions of the neck of the urinary bladder (or within the G.I. tract) must not be treated with cholinergic drugs.

CARDIOVASCULAR SYSTEM

Cholinergic drugs tend to slow the heart rate, dilate the blood vessels, and bring about a fall in blood pressure. However, these effects are not entirely predictable, as compensatory reflex responses may counteract the expected circulatory effects in some patients. The synthetic choline ester, *methacholine*, is the cholinergic drug most commonly employed in the treatment of circulatory disorders. However, its tendency to cause numerous discomforting side effects limits the usefulness of methacholine.

In treating attacks of *paroxysmal atrial tachycardia*, for example, many other drugs and measures are now preferred to methacholine administration. Similarly, in the management of *peripheral vascular diseases* (Chapter 32), other vasodilator drugs are considered less toxic than this cholinergic drug and more effective for producing a sustained increase of blood flow to the skin of patients with Raynaud's disease, acrocyanosis, and so forth. In treating essential hypertension, many more dependable drugs of other classes are used clinically for maintaining blood pressure at lower levels, and cholinergic drugs are not now employed for this purpose.

Adverse cardiovascular effects are not common when cholinergic drugs are administered in ordinary therapeutic doses. However, overdosage or poisoning may cause not only excessive slowing of the heart (bradycardia), but also such arrhythmias as atrial fibrillation and even cardiac arrest. Patients with hyperthyroidism have suffered episodes of heart block when methacholine was employed to control their tachycardia. A too steep fall in blood pressure has followed administration of this drug to patients with high blood pressure. In mushroom poisoning, the actions of the alkaloid muscarine have caused cardiovascular collapse and convulsions secondary to a reduction in blood flow to the brain.

OCULAR EFFECTS

Cholinergic drugs have effects on smooth muscle structures within the eye. They cause a contraction of the sphincter of the iris that results in constriction of the pupil, or *miosis*. Contraction of the ciliary bodies, structures that control the movements of the lens, causes a spasm of accommodation, the process by which the eye is adjusted to see at various distances. These and other actions tend to cause a reduction in the abnormally high intraocular pressure of glaucoma.

Glaucoma is a common cause of blindness. Most of the estimated one million people with this disease do not know that they have it, as it causes few symptoms at first. However, unusually high fluid pressure within the eye can cause optic nerve and retinal damage resulting in visual loss. Thus, public health nurses and others should suggest that people—particularly those over 40 years old—have their eyes examined periodically. (Ophthalmologists and optometrists can detect high intraocular pressure by a simple test with a tonometer.)

The most common kind of primary glaucoma is the chronic simple kind, also called the *open-angle* or *wide-angle* type, which can be readily treated by cholinergic miotics and other drugs that reduce intraocular pressure. This angle is the space between the base of the iris and the place where the cornea comes in contact with the sclera, or outer layer of the eye (Fig. 21-1); it contains the channels through which fluid normally flows out of the eye. In glaucoma, the flow of fluid is interfered with by a block within the channels (open-angle type), or by an obstruction within the angle (*narrow-angle* or *angle-closure type*). The more serious but much less common narrow-angle, or angle-closure, kind of glaucoma is best treated by iridectomy, a procedure for draining off excess intraocular fluid. Drugs are, in most of these cases, used only preoperatively in preparing these patients for the ocular surgery.

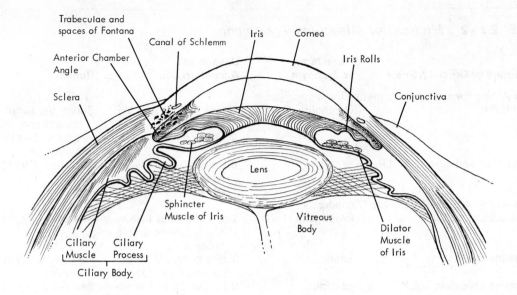

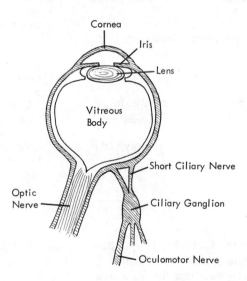

Fig. 21-1. (*Top*) The angle of the eye. An attack of glaucoma can occur when the folds of the iris and the ciliary processes crowd into the angle and block the outflow of fluid from the eye. (*Bottom*) Innervation of the eye.

MIOTIC THERAPY. The cholinergic drugs most commonly used in the preoperative emergency management of acute angle-closure glaucoma are the short-acting agents *pilocarpine*+ and *physostigmine*+. Solutions of these relatively safe drugs are dropped into the affected eye repeatedly until the angle opens. The more potent long-acting anticholinesterase-type miotics (Table 21-2) are contraindicated in such cases of acute congestive narrow-angle glaucoma, as they may actually cause a rise in intraocular pressure.

Patients with the chronic simple (noncongestive) open-angle type of glaucoma are most commonly treated at first with *pilocarpine*+, the least toxic miotic. However, tolerance tends to develop to its desired action, and it often becomes necessary to instill more highly concentrated solutions of pilocarpine more frequently than at first. This may cause local irritation and allergic conjunctivitis. Therefore, patients who seem to be developing resistance to pilocarpine are sometimes switched to another parasympathomimetic miotic, *carbachol*

TABLE 21-2   *Miotics for Glaucoma Treatment*

Nonproprietary or Official Name	Trade Name or Synonym	Dosage and Administration	Remarks
Short-Acting Parasympathomimetic Drugs			
Carbachol U.S.P.	Carcholin; Doryl	0.1 ml of 0.75 to 3.0% solution; 1 to 4 times daily	Substitute for pilocarpine in open-angle glaucoma
Pilocarpine HCl and nitrate U.S.P.		0.1 ml of 0.5 to 4% solution; 1 to 6 times daily	See *Drug Digest*
Short-Acting Anticholinesterase Compounds			
Neostigmine bromide U.S.P.	Prostigmin	1 or 2 drops of 0.25 to 5% solution; 2 to 6 times daily	See *Drug Digest*
Physostigmine U.S.P.	Eserine	0.25% ointment for application as needed	For use mainly at bedtime
Physostigmine salicylate U.S.P.	Eserine salicylate	0.1 ml of 0.2 to 1% solution several times daily	See *Drug Digest*
Physostigmine sulfate U.S.P.	Eserine sulfate	0.1 ml of 0.25 to 1% solution up to 4 times daily	See *Drug Digest*
Long-Acting Anticholinesterase Compounds			
Demecarium bromide U.S.P.	Humorsol	1 or 2 drops of 0.25% solution once or twice daily or less often	See *Drug Digest*
Echothiophate iodide U.S.P.	Phospholine iodide	1 drop of 0.06 to 0.25% solution once or twice daily	See *Drug Digest*
Isoflurophate U.S.P.	Floropryl; DFP	1 drop of 0.1% solution every 12 to 72 hours	For cases resistant to short-acting miotics

or to *physostigmine+*. Carbachol is less effective than pilocarpine, and physostigmine is more irritating. However, their use for a time as substitutes for pilocarpine may allow the patient's eyes to become responsive once again to the safer, standard drug.

Patients with chronic simple wide-angle glaucoma that can no longer be controlled with these safer, short-acting miotics may be managed with the long-acting anticholinesterase-type miotics, *demecarium+*, *echothiophate+*, and *isoflurophate*. A single instillation of these agents produces a decrease in intraocular pressure that lasts from 12 hours to several days. Thus, they need not be given very frequently. However, their use is often accompanied by numerous local side effects and occasionally by systemic toxicity similar to that seen in poison-

ing by organophosphate insecticides (see below).

❪ *Adverse effects*. Patients often resist further treatment with miotics when they feel discomfort from miotic eye drops during early treatment. The nurse should reassure such patients that such local effects as browaches and headaches, some pain and redness in the eyes, and blurring or dimming of vision will disappear within a week or ten days. She stresses that the temporary side effects of the eye drops are harmless, especially when compared to the possible consequence of neglecting to treat glaucoma—blindness.

Patients are watched closely for signs of systemic absorption such as gastrointestinal spasm or diarrhea, bronchospasm and wheezing, or salivation and sweating. The drug is discontinued at least temporarily in such cases. During long-term treatment children are observed for signs of cysts developing along the pupillary margin of the iris, and older patients are watched for development of lens opacities from prolonged use of high concentrations of the long-lasting anticholinesterase-type miotic agents.

❨ *Ophthalmic administration.* The systemic absorption of potent miotic solutions can be avoided by teaching the patient the proper technique for instilling eye drops. This involves application of finger pressure at the inner canthus for a minute or two following instillation. This area near the nose contains the lacrimal ducts, through which the solution may otherwise rapidly run into the upper respiratory tract and be absorbed into the bloodstream. Keeping the patient's lids apart for several seconds while applying such pressure tends to retain the drug solution on the surface of the eye and to prolong the action on eye structures. (Some eye drops contain adjunctive thickening agents such as methylcellulose and its derivatives, which also tend to delay absorption and enhance local activity of topically applied ophthalmic solutions.)

To avoid loss of the medication and lessen the likelihood of local irritation, the patient should be taught how to instill eye drops and apply ophthalmic ointments. One or two drops are placed carefully in a sac made by gently everting the lower lid, instead of dropping the drug directly on the sensitive cornea. The patient then closes his eyelids gently instead of squeezing them tightly together. Ointments are squeezed in a thin ribbon onto the inner surface of the lower lid which is then gently massaged.

All equipment for administering ophthalmic medications, including droppers, tubes, or plastic containers, must be sterile. The tip of the tube or dropper is not permitted to touch the eye, for the container may then become a vehicle for the spread of infection. To prevent the container from being thrust into his eye if the patient moves, it is good practice to support your hand by placing a finger on his forehead.

In administering ophthalmic products, it is important to read the label carefully and comply with all instructions for storage. Physostigmine solutions, for example, should be stored in a cool place and protected from light to reduce the rate of deterioration. Solutions should be checked before they are used, for physical changes may make them ineffective or irritating. Cloudy or discolored solutions may have to be discarded. (For example, physostigmine tends to turn pink or red.)

OTHER MUSCARINIC EFFECTS

Cholinergic drugs stimulate increased secretion by various exocrine glands, including those of the skin, mouth, stomach, and respiratory tract. *Pilocarpine+* is particularly likely to cause profuse sweating and salivation when taken by mouth or injected. These effects have few uses in modern treatment, and this parasympathomimetic drug is administered mainly by topical application in the eye (see above).

More serious than excessive salivation, sweating, and flushing are the effects of overdoses of cholinergic drugs upon the mucus-secreting glands of the respiratory tract. The outpouring of such secretions, together with drug-induced contractions of the bronchial smooth muscles, causes some patients to cough, choke, or wheeze when these drugs are administered. Such cholinergic side effects are particularly likely to occur in patients with a history of bronchial asthma. Thus, the use of drugs such as bethanechol+, methacholine, and neostigmine+ is avoided in such patients.

SKELETAL MUSCLE EFFECTS AND MYASTHENIA GRAVIS

Certain cholinergic drugs of the anticholinesterase type have effects upon the functioning of skeletal muscle which have therapeutic applications. Small doses increase the strength of muscular contractions in patients with myasthenia gravis, a disease marked by muscle weakness. Larger doses of these drugs can cause a block of neuromuscular transmission, resulting in a decrease in muscle strength, or even in skeletal muscle paralysis.

Myasthenia gravis is a chronic disease caused by a defect in neuromuscular transmission. This leads to rapid development of weakness and fatigue when the person performs simple movements repeatedly. In some patients, the disease is mild and may be marked only by drooping of one eyelid (ptosis). Other untreated patients may be totally incapacitated, and some die of respiratory complications.

The exact pathologic defect in myasthenia

gravis is still uncertain. Recent evidence indicates that: (1) the somatic motor nerve fibers release inadequate amounts of acetylcholine; and (2) the motor end plates on the patient's skeletal muscle fibers are relatively unresponsive to the acetylcholine that is released by his nerve endings. In any case, the patient's muscle strength is improved by the administration of the anticholinesterase drugs, which act indirectly to raise the amount of acetylcholine in the neuromuscular junction.

DIAGNOSIS. *Edrophonium*+ (Tensilon), an anticholinesterase agent with a rapid onset and short duration of action, is used in the differential diagnosis of myasthenia gravis from other disorders in which muscle weakness occurs. Administered by vein in a small dose that has little effect on the muscle weakness of patients who have no defect in neuromuscular junctional transmission, edrophonium brings about a short but dramatic increase in the muscle strength of myasthenic patients.

Neostigmine+ (Prostigmin), a longer-acting anticholinesterase, is preferred to edrophonium in the long-term management of myasthenic patients. However, it must also be administered fairly frequently, and because myasthenic patients often tend to become resistant to its action, the dose must be raised to high levels to maintain the muscle-strengthening effects. In such cases, the drug's action at autonomic neuroeffectors also increases. This causes a variety of muscarinic side effects, including abdominal cramps, diarrhea, nausea and vomiting, and increased secretion of sweat, saliva, tears, and bronchial mucus.

Other drugs for treating myasthenia have been introduced, with claims that they have certain advantages over neostigmine. Pyridostigmine+ has a somewhat longer duration of action, which is further increased by presenting it in a slow-release form. The main advantage is that patients taking the drug at bedtime need not be wakened during the night to take more medication. In addition, patients who used to waken too weak to swallow their morning dose of neostigmine, and thus had to receive their medication by injection, do not suffer from morning dysphagia when taking the sustained-action oral form of the longer-acting drug.

A further advantage claimed for this and another, newer, antimyasthenic drug, *ambenonium*+, is that they cause fewer muscarinic effects. Pyridostigmine, for example, is said to cause much less gastrointestinal stimulation than neostigmine, a fact that might make it more desirable for myasthenics unable to take effective doses of the latter drug without suffering from severe cramps. Similarly, ambenonium may be better for myasthenics who are being maintained in a respirator, because this agent causes less bronchial secretions than the other anticholinesterase drugs.

Some authorities suggest that a reduction in muscarinic side effects, such as may be achieved with these newer drugs or by the simultaneous administration of atropine, is not always desirable. They argue that drug-induced gastrointestinal upset and glandular secretions of increasing severity serve as a useful warning against development of the much more dangerous nicotinic effects of overdosage, which may come on insidiously and can result in increasing skeletal muscle weakness and, finally, paralysis.

Because of the tendency of myasthenics to suffer from the effects of underdosage or overdosage of medication, they must be taught the importance of adjusting dosage to their individual needs and then maintaining their muscle strength at optimal levels by regular administration of the drug. Their families also should learn how to help the patient, in case he is left helpless either by waiting too long between doses or by taking too much medication. In either case, he may waken in the morning unable to move, swallow, or call for help. Thus, he has to arrange his living accommodations so that he can get assistance from another person when he requires it. Someone in the family, for example, should be able to administer a parenteral form of an antimyasthenic agent if the patient becomes unable to swallow his tablets.

Because the course of the disease is unpredictable, the patient's response to drug treatment must be observed often and with care. Any change in his condition must be reported to the doctor, who may then order a change in drug dosage. This is true not only for the patient who suffers a flare-up in intensity of the disease, requiring an upward adjustment of dosage. The patient in remission must reduce his dosage, lest maintenance of the same amount of medication result in overdosage and an insidious return of muscle weakness which is actually drug-induced. Raising the dosage in such circumstances can cause cholinergic crisis.

CHOLINERGIC CRISIS. Administration of over-doses of anticholinesterase-type medications to myasthenic patients sometimes sets off a serious cholinergic crisis. This is marked not only by muscarinic side effects that can be counter-acted by atropine but also by skeletal muscle weakness and respiratory difficulties, which do not readily respond to treatment with this anti-muscarinic antidote. This drug-induced muscle weakness stems from the accumulation of ex-cessive amounts of acetylcholine at the motor end plates, with a resulting reduction in im-pulse transmission.

It is often difficult to differentiate choliner-gic crisis from *myasthenic crisis*, a situation in which, for poorly understood reasons, the pa-tient suffers a sudden flare-up of his underlying disease. This, like cholinergic crisis, is mani-fested by respiratory muscle weakness. How-ever, whereas cholinergic crisis calls for *with-drawal* of anticholinesterase drug therapy, patients in myasthenic crisis require *more* anti-myasthenic medication.

It is, of course, essential for the nurse to recognize that, regardless of whether the crisis is cholinergic or myasthenic, this is an acute emergency requiring medical intervention and she should promptly call the physician to see his patient. The doctor, who then is faced with what has been called "a desperate dilemma" in deciding how to handle his rapidly weakening patient, now has available a useful drug to help determine the myasthenic patient's true status.

Edrophonium+ (Tensilon) is used to deter-mine whether patients are suffering from cho-linergic crisis or myasthenic crisis. A small dose is injected into the vein of a myasthemic patient suffering from severe respiratory dif-ficulties. If the patient's condition *improves* dramatically—even if for only a couple of min-utes—he is probably suffering from *myasthenic* crisis and requires treatment with larger doses of one of the longer-acting anticholinesterase compounds. If, on the other hand, the edro-phonium injection makes the myasthenic pa-tient even *weaker*, this is an indication that all medication except atropine must be withdrawn and that he should be managed by mechanical and surgical measures such as endotracheal in-tubation, suction, tracheotomy, and artificial respiration. Atropine is useful no matter what

the diagnosis, and the nurse should always have it available both in oral and parenteral form when she is caring for any myasthenic patient. Small oral doses counteract the com-mon G.I. discomforts; large parenteral doses of atropine aid the breathing of patients in cholinergic crisis, although mechanical meas-ures are also often required.

Insecticide Poisoning

Certain chemicals employed in agriculture as insecticides exert potent cholinergic activity. *Parathion* and other organophosphorus-type chemicals have been a frequent cause of poison-ing in workers and others exposed to them. These poisons that inhibit cholinesterase cause acetylcholine (ACh) to build up in the body. The accumulation of excess ACh at *all* sites of cholinergic transmission produces very many signs and symptoms of poisoning. (See *Sum-mary of Side Effects of the Muscarinic, Nico-tinic, and Central Types*, pp. 276-277.)

Public health nurses can help prevent poison-ing by parathion and related chemicals by calling attention to the danger of using these insecticides without proper protection. This includes measures to prevent contact of these chemicals with the skin and to keep their vapors from being inhaled. These precautions apply not only to workers who are occupation-ally exposed to parathion; home gardeners and others using the less toxic compound *malathion* should also be warned to read the label of the products containing it and to avoid careless handling. If an accident does occur, people who call should be asked to bring the container or a sample of the material to the hospital emergency room or doctor's office.

TREATMENT

Atropine, administered repeatedly in large doses, is a specific antidote against cholinergic poisoning of this kind. It often gives dramatic relief of muscarinic-type symptoms and also helps to prevent C.N.S. toxicity, including res-piratory center depression and failure. How-ever, atropine does *not* prevent paralysis of the muscles of respiration. Thus, artificial respira-tion with oxygen inhalation may be required until these muscles resume their function.

Pralidoxime (Protopam) is an antidote of a different type. It helps to reactivate molecules of the enzyme acetylcholinesterase that have been poisoned by organophosphorus chemicals. The enzyme molecules are then able to destroy the excess acetylcholine that has accumulated in the body. Administered intravenously together with atropine, pralidoxime has proved lifesaving in some severe cases of poisoning by cholinesterase inhibitor-type chemicals.

S U M M A R Y of the Pharmacological Actions and Therapeutic Uses of Cholinergic Drugs

Pharmacological Actions

Gastrointestinal
Increased tone and motility of musculature, leading to defecation; increased secretion of gastric and other glands

Genitourinary
Increased tone of detrusor muscle of bladder and relaxation of trigone and sphincter results in stimulation of micturition

Cardiac
Decrease in heart rate (bradycardia); decrease in atrial contractility, impulse formation and conductivity

Vascular
Vasodilation resulting in rise in skin temperature and local flushing

Ocular
Contraction of sphincter muscle of iris causes miosis; contraction of ciliary body causes spasm of accommodation

Respiratory
Bronchial constriction and increased mucus secretion

Skeletal muscle
Stimulation of muscle fibers improves strength of abnormally weak motor units but causes fasciculation and weakness of normal muscles

Glandular effects
(1) Diaphoresis—profuse sweating with some drugs
(2) Sialagogue—profuse salivary secretion with some drugs

Therapeutic Uses

Gastrointestinal
Relief or prevention of postoperative abdominal distention and of gastric atony following vagotomy; management of megacolon and of constipation induced by ganglionic blocking agents

Genitourinary
Relief or prevention of postoperative and postpartum urinary retention; management of patients with neurogenic bladder

Cardiac
Arrest of attacks of atrial tachycardia, especially when combined with ocular pressure and carotid sinus massage

Vascular
Relief of local pain, coldness, and cyanosis in selected cases of peripheral vascular disease

Ocular
Reduction of intraocular pressure in chronic simple wide-angle glaucoma. Alternated with mydriatics to break up adhesions between the iris and the lens

Respiratory
Not a therapeutically useful action

Skeletal muscle
Long-term relief of myasthenia gravis; emergency treatment of myasthenic crisis; differential diagnosis of myasthenia gravis and of myasthenic from cholinergic crisis; curare antidote

Glandular effects
(1) Diagnosis of peripheral nerve injuries and, rarely, for removal of waste materials in acute renal failure
(2) Used to counteract xerostomia (mouth dryness) in some situations

---

S U M M A R Y of the Side Effects, Cautions, and Contraindications of Cholinergic Drugs

Side Effects

Muscarinic-Type
Gastrointestinal: Heartburn, belching, epigastric distress, abdominal cramps, tenesmus (painful anal spasms), diarrhea, nausea, and vomiting.

Genitourinary: Involuntary micturition; increased tone and motility of ureters.
Cardiovascular: Bradycardia and hypotension usually, but with reflex cardioacceleration and hypertension in some individuals exposed to overdoses of some agents.

Ocular: Blurring of vision and miosis; aching of brow and eyes; photophobia, myopia, and others.

Respiratory: Bronchoconstriction and increased bronchial mucus secretion may cause wheezing cough, feelings of tightness, and pain in chest.

Glandular: Profuse sweating, salivation, lacrimation.

Nicotinic-Type

Initial skeletal muscular fasciculations, twitching, and cramps followed by fatigue, weakness, and paralysis of all striated muscles including the diaphragm and intercostals, leading to respiratory distress and failure.

Central

The organic phosphate (*non*quaternary amine) compounds may cause anxiety, confusion, restlessness, disorientation, difficulty in concentrating, slurring of speech, apathy, and drowsiness. Also ataxia, dizziness, headache, weakness, tremor, and convulsions. Finally, depression of respiration with Cheyne-Stokes breathing, cyanosis, coma, cardiovascular collapse, arreflexia, respiratory failure, and death.

Contraindications

Muscarinic-Type

Gastrointestinal: In patients with peptic ulcer or spastic or obstructive gastrointestinal disturbances.

Genitourinary: In patients with vesical neck obstruction.

Cardiovascular: In patients with vasomotor instability, recent myocardial infarction, or hyperthyroidism. Use with caution in patients being treated with ganglionic blocking agents.

Ocular: In narrow-angle glaucoma.

Respiratory: In patients with bronchial asthma and with pulmonary edema.

Glandular: Possible loss of fluids and electrolytes undesirable in patients with acute renal failure.

Nicotinic-Types

In patients in cholinergic crisis. Possible sympathetic ganglionic and adrenal medullary stimulation may cause occasional cardioacceleration and elevation until counteracted by parasympathetic stimulation and late ganglionic depressant effects.

SUMMARY of Adverse Effects of Topically Applied Cholinergic Miotics

Local Early Effects

Browache, headache, ocular pain, and congestion

Blurring and dimness of vision, particularly in poor light

Twitching of the eyelids

Late Local Effects

Allergic conjunctivitis and dermatitis

Cyst development at pupillary margins of the iris in children

Lens opacity and cataracts, particularly in elderly patients

Systemic Absorption Signs

Gastrointestinal spasm; nausea, vomiting, and diarrhea

Salivation, sweating, and lacrimation

Bronchoconstriction, with wheezing and chest tightness

Bradycardia, hypotension, possible respiratory muscle weakness, and paralysis

---

SUMMARY of Points for the Nurse to Remember Concerning Cholinergic Drugs

Cholinergic drugs have a wide range of effects. Note carefully the patient's response to therapy, both those that are desired and those that are unwanted.

Emphasize the progress that the patient is making as a result of cholinergic drug therapy even though he may be experiencing some discomfort as a result of the medication. Make certain that distressing symptoms are brought to the attention of the physician so that the patient

can benefit from any measures to minimize discomfort that may be available.

Be alert for any comment by the patient concerning previous illnesses, such as asthma or peptic ulcer, that he may have neglected to mention to the physician. Report such information to the doctor, because it may mean that the patient should not receive a cholinergic drug.

Remember that atropine is an antidote for cholinergic drugs, and make certain that a supply, along with equipment for parenteral injection, is available at all times.

For patients with myasthenia gravis, stress the importance of regular timing of the medication, careful observation of symptomatic response, and the necessity of providing for assistance from others when the patient's symptoms result in sudden helplessness.

Insecticides such as parathion can cause serious toxic effects. Be alert to the hazards of injudicious use of such chemicals and explain these to others in an effort to avert accidental poisoning. When instilling eye drops containing potent cholinergic miotics, apply finger pressure to the inner canthus for a minute or two following instillation to lessen the systemic absorption of these drugs.

If the ophthalmic medication is likely to cause early local discomfort, let the patient know this and assure him that the initial irritation will subside shortly. (It is important that the patient not discontinue miotic therapy for any reason, so he should be encouraged to bear with transient discomfort.)

Keep ophthalmic solutions and their containers sterile and do not touch the patient's eye with the dropper or plastic container. Place drops gently into the sac made by everting the lower lid, and apply ophthalmic ointments in a thin ribbon on the inner surface of the lower lid. Then have the patient close his eyes without squeezing the lids together tightly and massage the area gently to spread the medication around.

Clinical Nursing Situation

The Situation: Mr. Johnson, who is 64 years old, has chronic glaucoma, a condition that first appeared after his son was killed in an automobile accident. Mr. Johnson's symptoms are controlled by instillation of pilocarpine 2 percent q.i.d. and Diamox 125 mg t.i.d. Mr. Johnson's ophthalmologist has explained to him that surgery may become necessary in the future, if these measures fail to relieve his symptoms.

Mr. Johnson has several other conditions, too. He has mild diabetes, which is controlled by diet; he tests his urine twice daily. He also has chronic congestive heart failure, for which he takes digitoxin 0.1 mg once daily, and he is on a low sodium diet.

The Problem: Assume you are the nurse at the neighborhood clinic where Mr. Johnson receives treatment. You see Mr. Johnson every week to assess his condition and his response to therapy. Mr. Johnson sees the ophthalmologist and the internist once a month, unless you or the patient thinks he should make more frequent visits.

Describe how you would assess Mr. Johnson's status in relation to his chronic glaucoma, diabetes, and congestive heart failure, his response to the therapy prescribed for each of these conditions, and how you would identify his nursing requirements.

DRUG DIGEST

BETHANECHOL CHLORIDE U.S.P.
(Myocholine; Urecholine)

Actions and Indications. This choline ester exerts parasympathomimetic effects upon the smooth muscle of the G.I. tract, urinary bladder, and other structures innervated by postganglionic cholinergic nerves. Its muscarinic effects upon the G.I. tract are used to increase muscle tone and peristaltic motility in such disorders as: postoperative abdominal distention; paralytic, or adynamic, ileus in patients suffering from severe injury or infections; and gastric atony following bilateral vagotomy or stomach surgery.

The drug's stimulating effect upon the urinary bladder is often effective in postoperative and post-partum urinary retention or in similar situations resulting from neurogenic atony or from overdosage of cholinergic blocking drugs, including ganglionic blocking agents. Its use for treating dysphagia in patients with scleroderma has also been suggested.

Side Effects, Cautions, and Contraindications. This drug is best administered on an empty stomach to avoid nausea and vomiting. Atropine should be available to counteract cramps, diarrhea, and other undesirable effects that may follow injection. The drug is contraindicated in obstructive G.I. and G.U. disorders. Although ordinary doses have few cardiovascular and respiratory effects in most individuals, this drug is contraindicated in patients with an unstable circulatory system, a history of a recent myocardial infarction, or a history of asthma.

Dosage and Administration. Bethanechol may be administered orally in doses of 5 to 30 mg t.i.d. or q.i.d. before meals. It is also administered subcutaneously—*never* I.M. or I.V.—in doses of 2.5 to 5 mg repeated t.i.d. or q.i.d. If trial with these doses does not produce the desired response, a single dose of 10 mg may be given subcutaneously.

DEMECARIUM BROMIDE U.S.P.
(Humorsol)

Actions and Indications. This anticholinesterase-type cholinergic drug exerts a long-lasting miotic action when applied topically to the eye. Its use reduces intraocular pressure for 12 hours to several days in the eyes of patients with primary open-angle glaucoma which has not responded adequately to treatment with shorter-acting miotics. The drug is also sometimes employed in secondary glaucoma that occurs following removal of the lens (aphakia) but never in glaucoma secondary to iritis or other ocular inflammatory disorders. It is sometimes used for treating the inturning squint of children with accommodative convergent strabismus or osotropia.

Side Effects, Cautions, and Contraindications. Demecarium is contraindicated in acute narrow-angle glaucoma as it can cause a further *rise* in intraocular pressure as a result of actions that add to local congestion and interfere with the free flow of fluid within the eye (pupillary block). Other local effects besides redness include blurring and dimness of vision and difficulty in accommodating for distant vision. Spasm of the ciliary muscles may cause browache, eye pain, and headache, and some eyelid twitching may develop. Chronic use may lead to cyst formation along the inner margin of the iris.

Dosage and Administration. Treatment is started with the lowest effective concentration and maintained at the longest possible intervals. One drop of a 0.125 percent or 0.25 percent solution may be instilled only once or twice a week or as often as every 12 hours. Measures for minimizing systemic absorption should be employed in order to avoid abdominal cramps, bronchoconstriction, and other adverse cholinergic effects.

ECHOTHIOPHATE IODIDE U.S.P. (Phospholine Iodide)
Actions and Indications. This cholinergic drug exerts a prolonged miotic effect when instilled into the eyes of patients with primary glaucoma of the chronic simple type. It is reserved for use in those cases in which high intraocular pressure cannot be kept adequately reduced by the short-acting miotic agents, including pilocarpine. In such cases, the relatively long duration of this drug's effect permits around-the-clock control of the patient's intraocular pressure with relatively infrequent instillation of a single drop of the ophthalmic solution.

Side Effects, Cautions, and Contraindications. This miotic is contraindicated in acute congestive cases of angle-closure glaucoma, even though it is occasionally employed in *noncongestive* chronic cases of the narrow-angle type following surgery, or in patients in whom surgery may be unsafe. Similarly, it is contraindicated in secondary glaucoma caused by acute inflammation, although it is employed in glaucoma secondary to aphakia (absence of the lens).

Early local side effects include dimness and blurring of vision, eye redness, browache, and headache. Late effects include cysts of the iris and clouding of the lens. Systemic absorption may cause G.I. discomfort, bronchospasm, salivation, and sweating.

Dosage and Administration. A single drop instilled at bedtime and in the morning usually produces reduction in intraocular pressure for a full 24-hour period. Solutions are available in various strengths (0.03, 0.06, 0.125 and 0.25 percent), and the lowest effective concentration is employed.

EDROPHONIUM CHLORIDE U.S.P. (Tensilon)
Actions and Indications. This rapid-acting cholinergic drug of short duration is used mainly in the differential diagnosis of myasthenia gravis and for differentiating myasthenic crisis from cholinergic crisis. However, its muscle-strengthening action is too short to be useful in the maintenance therapy of myasthenia gravis.

Side Effetcs, Cautions, and Contraindications. Overdosage may cause muscarinic side effects such as abdominal cramps and diarrhea, bronchoconstriction and increased bronchial secretion, and bradycardia and hypotension. These can be corrected by administration of atropine, which should always be available in a syringe for injection. Respiratory failure may also result from skeletal muscle paralysis and respiratory center depression.

Dosage and Administration. In the test for differentiating between myasthenia gravis and other disorders marked by muscle weakness, 0.2 ml (0.2 mg) is injected by vein and followed by 0.8 ml (0.8 mg) more, if no muscarinic reactions occur after 45 seconds. The test may also be performed with 1 ml (10 mg) injected I.M. These doses increase muscle strength in myasthenic patients but produce muscle weakness in others.

In differentiating between myasthenic and cholinergic crisis, 0.1 ml (0.1 mg) is injected I.V., and the patient is observed for improvement of muscle strength (myasthenic crisis) or for further weakness (cholinergic crisis). If no change in the patient's respiration occurs, an additional 0.1 ml may be injected and observation continued.

NEOSTIGMINE BROMIDE AND METHYLSULFATE U.S.P. (Prostigmin)
Actions and Indications. This prototype anticholinesterase agent increases transmission from cholinergic nerves to smooth and skeletal muscles. It may be used postoperatively to prevent and treat gastrointestinal and genitourinary atony. Its action reduces abdominal distention and helps to evacuate the urinary bladder.

The drug is useful in the diagnosis and treatment of myasthenia gravis, as it increases the strength of the patient's disease-weakened muscular contractions. Applied topically, a solution of this drug can reduce the high intraocular pressure of patients with primary, chronic simple (wide-angle) glaucoma.

Side Effects, Cautions, and Contraindications. Overdosage may cause abdominal cramps and diarrhea which can be counteracted by atropine. The drug is contraindicated in patients with asthma, as it can cause bronchoconstriction and increased bronchial gland secretions. Overdosage can cause cholinergic crisis, a condition marked by respiratory muscle weakness and possible paralysis. Once this condition is diagnosed, this drug is immediately discontinued.

Dosage and Administration. Oral doses of the bromide salt are administered in very variable doses depending upon the needs of the individual myasthenic patient (for example, 15 mg to 375 mg daily). The methylsulfate salt is injected s.c. or I.M. in doses of 0.25 to 0.5 mg for prevention and treatment of postoperative abdominal distention or urinary retention.

PHYSOSTIGMINE SALICYLATE (AND SULFATE) U.S.P. (Eserine)
Actions and Indications. The salts of this alkaloid produce miosis, spasm of accommodation, and a reduction in intraocular pressure when applied topically to the eye. These effects make the drug useful in the management of primary open-angle glaucoma. It is also instilled alternately with pilocarpine in the emergency treatment of acute attacks of narrow-angle glaucoma. This helps to reduce angle closure and intraocular pressure prior to definitive surgical intervention (iridectomy). Physostigmine is occasionally applied topically to counteract mydriasis induced by anticholinergic drugs, and it may be administered parenterally

to counteract symptoms of central toxicity produced by atropine, scopolamine, and similar anticholinergic agents.

Side Effects, Cautions, and Contraindications. Local side effects include conjunctivitis and contact dermatitis as a result of irritation and allergic sensitivity. This is most likely to occur if partially decomposed salt solutions are employed. Thus, darkened solutions should be discarded.

Some blurring and dimming of vision may occur early in treatment, and long-term use may lead to development of follicular cysts of the conjunctival space. Eyelid twitching and headache may also occur.

Dosage and Administration. One or two drops of solutions ranging from 0.1 to 1 percent are instilled in each eye several times daily in primary, open-angle glaucoma. In acute angle-closure attacks, one or two drops of a 0.25 percent solution may be applied alone or alternately with pilocarpine very frequently until the angle opens. Physostigmine base is available as a 0.25 percent ointment for application at bedtime to produce an intense, prolonged effect.

PILOCARPINE HCl (AND NITRITE) U.S.P. (Almocarpine; Pilocar, and others)

Actions and Indications. The salts of this alkaloid are the most commonly employed miotics used in the early management of primary open-angle glaucoma. Solutions penetrate the cornea rapidly and produce their maximal reduction in intraocular pressure in about 30 to 60 minutes. Its effects are of relatively short duration (about four to eight hours) and tend to lessen as tolerance develops. Thus, this drug is administered in higher concentrations and at more frequent intervals during long-term maintenance therapy. Pilocarpine is also instilled repeatedly in order to open the angle prior to surgery for acute closed-angle glaucoma or for congenital glaucoma. It is sometimes employed to shorten atropine-induced mydriasis and cycloplegia, and is used alternately with atropine to prevent adhesions from forming between the iris and the lens.

Side Effects, Cautions, and Contraindications. Pilocarpine produces fewer side effects than most miotics. However, too frequent instillation of high concentrations (above 4 percent) can cause conjunctival irritation and allergic sensitization. Systemic absorption may lead to salivation, sweating, epigastric distress, and cramps.

Dosage and Administration. Treatment may be initiated with relatively weak solutions (0.5 to 2 percent) and raised as required to concentrations of 4 percent or more. (Solutions of up to 10 percent strength are available but are rarely more effective than the 4 percent dilution.) In open-angle glaucoma, one or two drops are instilled every six to eight hours at first and as often as every two hours later. For treating acute narrow-angle glaucoma, one or two drops are instilled in the affected eye every few minutes in attempts to open the angle.

PYRIDOSTIGMINE BROMIDE U.S.P. (Mestinon)

Actions and Indications. This cholinergic antimyasthenia drug counteracts the muscle weakness of myasthenia gravis by increasing the rate at which nerve impulses pass the neuromuscular junction to skeletal muscle. It is claimed to cause fewer muscarinic effects upon the G.I. tract than does neostigmine, and its duration of action is said to be longer.

Side Effects, Cautions, and Contraindications. Overdosage can cause muscarinic as well as nicotinic type side effects. Muscarinic effects include increased peristaltic activity; the drug is contraindicated in patients with organic obstructions of the G.I. and g.u. tracts. Increased bronchial secretions and bronchoconstriction can occur. Therefore, the drug is contraindicated in patients with bronchial asthma. It may also cause breathing difficulties that result in weakness or paralysis of the skeletal muscles of respiration when overdosage causes nicotinic interference with transmission. In such cases, the drug must be discontinued, atropine administered, and measures taken to control ventilation—for example, by tracheostomy and assisted ventilation.

Dosage and Administration. Daily dosage is adjusted to the needs of each patient individually. Thus, the needs of different patients may vary from 1 to 25 tablets of 60 mg each (average dose 10 tablets). A syrup is now available for easier dosage adjustment when fractions of 60 mg are required. Also available are sustained-action tablets containing 180 mg each, which have a duration of action between two and three times that of ordinary tablets. A dose of one to three of these at intervals of at least six hours is usually effective.

References

Abrams, J. D. The nature of glaucoma. *Nursing Times*, 68:767, 1972.

Clagett, O.T. Myasthenia gravis. *Amer. J. Nurs.*, 51:654, 1951.

Grob, D. Myasthenia gravis. *Arch. Intern. Med.*, 108:615, 1961.

Hayes, W.J. Parathion poisoning and its treatment. *JAMA*, 192:49, 1965.

Leopold, I.H., and Keates, E. Drugs used in the treatment of glaucoma. *Clin. Pharmacol. Ther.*, 6:130, 262, 1965.

Osserman, K.E., and Shapiro, E.K. Nursing care in myasthenia gravis. *Nurs. World*, 130:12, 1956.

Periera, P. Screening for glaucoma. *Nursing Times*, 68:771, 1972.

Rodman, M.J. Muscle relaxants and stimulants. *RN*, 2:54, 1958 (Feb.).

———. Drugs used in eye disorders. *RN*, 30:63, 1967 (Feb.).

Spaeth, G.L. General medications, glaucoma, and disturbances of intraocular pressure. *Med. Clin. N. Amer.*, 53:1109, 1969 (Sept.).

Schwab, R.S. The pharmacological basis of the treatment of myasthenia gravis. *Clin. Pharmacol. Ther.*, 1:319, 1960.

22.

Cholinergic Blocking Drugs

General Considerations

We have seen that various drugs can interfere with the transmission of nerve impulses from cholinergic nerves to the organs and structures that they influence. In this chapter we shall discuss one of these kinds of cholinergic blocking drugs—*anticholinergic drugs* of the *antimuscarinic class*.

These are drugs—*atropine* is the prototype—that keep postganglionic parasympathetic nerves from exerting their full control over the functioning of the smooth muscle, cardiac muscle, and exocrine glands cells that they innervate. Since these postganglionic neuroeffectors respond to the neurohormone acetylcholine released by these nerves in much the same way as they do to the mushroom alkaloid muscarine, drugs that block transmission at these sites may also be called *antimuscarinic*.

Drugs of this class are not very selective in the organs that they affect. Thus, for example, when the physician orders atropine for its therapeutically desirable effects in reducing stomach acid secretions, he knows that the patient will often complain of side effects caused by atropine's concurrent actions on his salivary glands and eyes. Because of this, chemists have synthesized other chemicals that are claimed to have a greater affinity for specific sites, such as the gastrointestinal tract, than do the natural belladonna family alkaloids (Table 22-1).

TABLE 22-1

*Natural Alkaloids, Preparations, and Quaternary Ammonium Derivatives**

Nonproprietary, Official, or Generic Name	Synonym or Trade Name	Usual Range of Single Oral Doses	Remarks
Atropine	dl-Hyoscyamine	0.4–0.5 mg	Free alkaloid of belladonna, stramonium, and other solanaceous plants
Atropine methylnitrate	Eumydrin	0.5–1.5 mg	Quaternary ammonium derivative of atropine
Atropine sulfate U.S.P.	. . . .	0.3–1.2 mg	See *Drug Digest*
Belladonna extract N.F.	. . . .	10–40 mg	Contains about 0.2 mg of atropine
Belladonna (leaf) fluidextract N.F.	. . . .	0.06–0.1 ml	Very potent (1 ml contains 3 mg of alkaloids)
Belladonna (leaf) tincture U.S.P.	. . . .	0.3–2.4 ml	Only 1/100 as potent as the fluid extract
Homatropine methylbromide N.F.	. . . .	2.5–7.5 mg	Less potent antimuscarinic activity than atropine
Hyoscyamine HBr and sulfate N.F.	. . . .	0.25–1.0 mg	Salts of alkaloid of hyoscyamus
Methscopolamine bromide N.F.	Scopolamine methylbromide; Pamine; and others	2.5–5 mg	Less potent than atropine orally but equally potent by I.M. or s.c. injection
Methscopolamine nitrate	Scopolamine methylnitrate	2–4 mg	Similar to the above quaternary ammonium derivative of scopolamine
Scopolamine HBr U.S.P.	Hyoscine HBr	0.3–0.8 mg	See *Drug Digest* and Table 22-4

* See also Table 22-4.

The search for synthetic anticholinergic drugs led to the development of drugs quite different from the alkaloids in chemical structure. Some of these, such as *dicyclomine* (Bentyl; Table 22-2), are so different that they produce fewer of the desirable actions of atropine, as well as less of the side effects typical of that alkaloid. Others are synthetic compounds that are claimed to have more potent gastrointestinal actions than the natural products. However, the advantages claimed for the prototype of this group, *methantheline bromide* (Banthine) and its successors (Table 22-3) are said by some authorities to be unimportant (see discussion below).

In the following discussion of the pharmacological effects of atropinelike drugs on the various organs, structures, and systems, we shall proceed as follows: After indicating what atropine and its relatives do to alter the functioning of the particular tissue, we shall point out the clinically significant aspects of each particular action. Thus we shall take up, together, both the therapeutic use of each action and also its undesirable aspects, particularly those that make atropine and similar drugs unsafe for patients with various pathological states that increase susceptibility to such adverse actions. All the therapeutic uses, side effects, cautions, and contraindications will be found summarized on pp. 290-292.

Pharmacological Actions and Applications

Atropine+ and *scopolamine+* have many and varied actions, not only peripherally at neuroeffector cells innervated by postganglionic autonomic nerve fibers, but also centrally through blocking effects upon cholinergic nerve pathways within the central nervous system (C.N.S.).

T A B L E 2 2 - 2 *Synthetic Antispasmodic Drugs**

Nonproprietary Name	Trade Name	Dosage
Adiphenine HCl	Trasentine	75 to 150 mg
Alverine citrate N.F.	Spacolin	120 mg
Amprotropine phosphate	Syntropan	50 to 100 mg
Anisotropine methylbromide	Valpin	10 mg
Carbofluorene HCl	Pavatrine	125 mg
Dicyclomine HCl N.F.	Bentyl	10 to 20 mg
Flavoxate	Urispas	100 to 200 mg
Methixene HCl	Trest	1 mg
Triphenamil HCl	Trocinate	100 to 400 mg

* These drugs are claimed to act mainly by a *direct* action on the contractile mechanism of smooth muscle and only slightly by producing blockade of parasympathetic motor impulses. This is the basis for claims that they are likely to cause few atropinelike side effects. Nevertheless, caution is reuired in administering these drugs to patients for whom belladonna alkaloids and synthetic anticholinergic drugs would be contraindicated.

T A B L E 2 2 - 3 *Synthetic Anticholinergic Agents Used In Treating Peptic Ulcer**

Nonproprietary Name	Trade Name	Dosage
Clidinium Br	Quarzan (in Librax)	2.5 to 5 mg
Dibutoline sulfate	Dibuline	25 mg
Diphemanil methylsulfate N.F.	Prantal	100 mg, oral; 25 mg, parenteral
Glycopyrrolate	Robinul	1 mg
Hexocyclium methylsulfate	Tral	25 mg
Isopropamide iodide	Darbid	5 mg
Mepenzolate bromide	Cantil	25 mg
Mepiperphenidol bromide	Darstine	50 to 100 mg
Methantheline bromide N.F.	Banthine	50 mg
Oxyphencyclimine HCl	Daricon	10 mg
Oxyphenonium bromide	Antrenyl	10 mg, oral; 1 to 2 mg, parenteral
Pentapiperidine methylsulfate	Quilene	10 to 30 mg
Penthienate bromide N.F.	Monodral	5 mg
Pipenzolate bromide	Piptal	5 to 10 mg
Piperidolate HCl	Dactil	50 mg
Poldine methylsulfate	Nacton	5 to 10 mg
Propantheline U.S.P.	Pro-Banthine	15 mg
Thihexinol methylbromide N.F.	In Sorboquel	15 to 30 mg
Tricyclamol chloride	Elorine; Tricoloid	50 mg
Tridihexethyl chloride N.F.	Pathilon	25 to 50 mg
Valethamate bromide	Mureal	10 to 20 mg

CENTRAL NERVOUS SYSTEM

The two belladonna alkaloids differ in their central effects when administered in small therapeutic doses. Atropine is a weak C.N.S. stimulant, while scopolamine produces mainly depressant effects upon the C.N.S. This depressant effect of scopolamine accounts for its use clinically for several therapeutic purposes.

For example, it is a component of sleep-producing and antianxiety products promoted for use by the public, and it is advocated for the prevention of motion sickness. Both alkaloids are still employed in the management of parkinsonism, although certain synthetic anticholinergic drugs are now preferred for most patients.

Atropine is sometimes administered in large

doses to counteract the central effects of poisoning by insecticides of the organophosphate type. In such cases of cholinergic poisoning even massive doses of atropine produce few side effects. However, high doses of both atropine and scopolamine have been responsible for such symptoms of central toxicity as restlessness, dizziness, disorientation, and delirium (see the discussion of atropine poisoning, below). Elderly patients are particularly prone to suffer the toxic central effects of anticholinergic drugs, but young drug abusers are also often affected.

Peripheral Effects

Atropine and related drugs that block cholinergic nerve impulses to various visceral organs, exocrine glands, and the heart often produce effects on several organs and structures at once. This means that the anticholinergic drugs often cause undesired side effects when they are administered orally or by injection in doses needed for producing any particular therapeutic effect. Thus, before we discuss the use of belladonna, its derivatives, and related drugs in the management of gastrointestinal disorders —their most common clinical indication—we shall first review the effects of these drugs that account for their most common undesired effects.

GLANDULAR SECRETIONS

Anticholinergic drugs reduce the rate of secretion of the gastric glands when administered in doses that also slow fluid secretion by the salivary, bronchial, and sweat glands. Thus, for example, when these drugs are employed in the management of acid-peptic diseases (see p. 287), patients often complain of mouth dryness, and other of the *anhidrotic*, or secretion-drying, effects of these drugs may cause discomfort in some cases.

SALIVARY GLAND SECRETION. Atropine, scopolamine, and synthetic substitutes such as *methantheline* (Banthine) and *propantheline+* (Pro-Banthine) act in relatively small doses to block transmission of parasympathetic nerve impulses to the salivary glands. The patient's mouth becomes uncomfortably dry (*xerostomia*), and he has difficulty in swallowing and talking.

The patient who receives atropine preoperatively is especially likely to have a very dry mouth after surgery. Thus the nurse should see that he gets thorough mouth care, including frequent rinsings and cold drinks if oral fluids are permitted. Similar measures may be suggested to patients taking belladonna derivatives, for gastrointestinal disorders or other conditions, and the patient should be told that sucking hard candies or chewing a stick of gum may stimulate some salivation when xerostomia is especially discomforting. It may help, too, to let him know that tablets containing these products are to be swallowed and not chewed.

Respiratory tract gland secretion is also suppressed. The inhibition of nasal secretion is the basis for the use of belladonna alkaloids in various products sold to the public for treating symptoms of the common cold (Contac, for example). One of the main reasons for administering atropine or scopolamine preoperatively is to reduce the likelihood that an inhalation anesthetic such as ether will stimulate an excessive flow of bronchial, nasal, and salivary gland secretion, which might interfere with the patient's breathing. These drugs also tend to reduce the reflex laryngospasm which is sometimes set off by such secretions.

The reduction of bronchial gland secretions is occasionally useful in the treatment of an allergy-induced cough. More often, such drug-induced dryness is considered undesirable for patients with chronic respiratory difficulties for, when respiratory tract fluids are reduced, they may thicken, harden and plug up narrow passages. Because asthmatic patients often already have difficulty in coughing up thick secretions, anticholinergic drugs are used with caution, if at all, in such cases.

Sweat gland secretions are reduced by the blocking action of atropinelike drugs upon transmission of sympathetic postganglionic nerve impulses to these structures. This action is rarely used for relief of excessive sweating (*hyperhidrosis*) because of side effects brought about by the doses that reduce perspiration. The sweat-stopping effect of drugs with anticholinergic activity can sometimes cause fever (*hyperpyrexia*).

This is especially likely in warm weather when the body rids itself of excess heat mainly by evaporation of fluid (perspiration) from the skin. By causing cessation of sweating, atropine-type drugs may sometimes precipitate a dangerous hyperpyrexic reaction. The nurse should be alert to the possibility that a feverish patient with a hot, dry, flushed skin or even a scarlatinoform rash may be suffering from atropine poisoning (see p. 289).

CARDIAC EFFECTS

Moderate doses of atropine tend to speed the rate of the heart. Anticholinergic drugs do this by blocking the braking action of vagus nerve impulses upon the heart. By reducing the inhibiting influence of the vagus nerves on the sino-auricular (S-A) node pacemaker and upon the atrioventricular (A-V) node, atropinelike drugs permit sympathetic cardioaccelerator impulses to predominate.

Atropine-induced tachycardia is not in itself clinically useful. In fact, it is usually considered a side effect that is especially undesirable for patients with a history of heart disease. Thus, the nurse should always be alert to changes in pulse rate after atropine has been administered. Atropine and related drugs must be used cautiously, if at all, in patients with angina pectoris, because they may set off an episode of coronary insufficiency. Too rapid heart action may also cause cardiac decompensation in patients with heart failure, by interfering with diastolic filling of the heart's chambers and thus reducing cardiac output.

Atropine is, however, useful for treating conditions in which the patient's heart is slowed down by excessive numbers of vagus nerve impulses. *Bradycardia* and *partial heart block* of this kind occurs, for example, in some patients who have suffered a coronary attack. This can often be counteracted by intravenous administration of atropine.

Atropine premedication is also used to prevent excessive reflex bradycardia during induction of anesthesia with halothane and other general anesthetics. Oral doses also help to prevent sudden blackouts in patients with the *carotid sinus syndrome,* a condition in which even slight pressure in the neck sets off a reflex stream of heart-slowing vagus nerve impulses.

OCULAR EFFECTS

Atropine and similar drugs produce two types of effects in the eye: (1) *mydriasis,* or dilation of the pupils; and (2) *cycloplegia,* or paralysis of accommodation, which keeps the patient from making the adjustments of the lens that are needed for near vision (see Table 22-4).

The ophthalmologist makes clinical use of these actions in the diagnosis and treatment of various ocular disorders. By inducing mydriasis and the loss of the light reflex that also occurs, drops of an anticholinergic drug allow the ophthalmologist to examine the inner structures at the back of the eye more easily. Production of cycloplegia permits the doctor to

TABLE 22-4 *Mydriatics and Cycloplegics*

Nonproprietary or Official Name	Trade Name or Synonym	Topical Application	Remarks
Atropine sulfate U.S.P.	. . . .	1 or 2 drops of 1% solution	Prolonged duration of action
Cyclopentolate HCl U.S.P.	Cyclogyl	2 drops of 0.5% solution or 1 drop of 1.0% solution	Relatively brief action
Eucatropine HCl U.S.P.	Euphthalmine	1 or 2 drops of 2–5% solution	Mainly mydriatic with little cycloplegia
Homatropine HBr U.S.P.	Homatrocel	1 or 2 drops of 1–2% solution	Relatively brief action
Scopolamine HBr U.S.P.	Hyoscine	1 or 2 drops of 1% solution	Moderate duration of action
Tropicamide U.S.P.	Mydriacyl	1 or 2 drops of 0.5% solution for mydriasis; 1 or 2 drops of 1% solution repeatedly for cycloplegia	Rapid onset and brief duration of action

examine the eye for refractive errors without interference by the patient's involuntary adjustment of the position of the lens.

The long-lasting cycloplegic effect of atropine may make it difficult for the patient to read for some time after a refractive examination. Thus, such other short-acting cycloplegic agents as *cyclopentolate+* (Cyclogyl) and *homatropine hydrobromide+* are often preferred, as their vision-blurring effects tend to wear off more rapidly. When *only* mydriasis is desired, the physician may employ a solution of *tropicamide* (Mydriacil), or *eucatropine+* (Euphthalmine), anticholinergic drugs which in low concentrations produce mainly mydriasis alone, or he may use an adrenergic drug such as *phenylephrine* or *hydroxyamphetamine*, which have *only* mydriatic effects.

Atropine is preferred when the doctor wishes deliberately to induce prolonged rest, relaxation, and even paralysis of the sphincter muscles of the iris and the ciliary body. This is often desirable in treating inflammatory disorders of the inner eye, for it helps to relieve painful reflex spasm of these smooth muscle structures. It also tends to prevent contact and subsequent formation of adhesions between these and other ocular structures such as the lens and cornea. (Sometimes combinations of shorter-acting mydriatic-cycloplegic drugs are alternated with miotics in an effort to break up adhesions that have begun to form.)

Adverse ocular effects of atropinelike drugs may be brought on when they are taken orally or injected for treatment of other conditions. The thoughtful nurse lets the patient know that his vision will be blurred for a while. This both helps to keep him from becoming alarmed and helps him plan his work when it requires reading or other tasks for which near vision is needed. Operating a car or other types of machinery can cause a problem whenever the patient has blurred vision due to atropinelike drugs. When blurred vision is to be expected, stress to the patient the importance of allowing time for the drug's effects to wear off before he resumes such activity.

All drugs with an anticholinergic action are contraindicated in patients with narrow-angle glaucoma, as their ocular effects can set off an acute attack of angle closure. Caution is also required in patients over 40 years old, as people in this age group are most prone to have glaucoma without being aware of it.

The nurse who administers eye drops never administers mydriatic-cycloplegics routinely. She checks carefully to avoid errors that might result in an acute angle closure attack and possible blindness. She also advises patients about the use of these drugs in order to prevent other kinds of accidents and discomforts. Elderly patients, who may already have visual difficulties and who may be unsteady on their feet should, for example, be warned to take special care in walking down stairs after receiving a drug that blurs their vision. Other patients may be advised to wear dark glasses when they go outdoors after treatment with these drugs, which may interfere with the reflex constriction of the pupils that usually occurs in sunlight.

SMOOTH MUSCLE EFFECTS

Smooth muscles of various visceral organs are relaxed by the *antispasmodic action* of atropine and related natural and synthetic drugs. This is especially desirable in conditions marked by painful hypertonicity and hypermotility of the gastrointestinal and genitourinary system smooth musculature.

The *urinary bladder and the ureters* are affected by the ability of atropinelike drugs to block parasympathetic nerve impulses to visceral smooth muscle. Patients with cystitis, for example, often have an urgent need to void because of reflex spasms that are set off by bladder inflammation. Belladonna derivatives reduce such bladder irritability by blocking the excessive motor impulses.

This quieting action of atropine also often helps to increase the urine-holding capacity of the bladder. Thus, this drug and *methantheline* (Banthine), as well as other drugs with an anticholinergic component, are sometimes prescribed for children with a bed-wetting problem (*nocturnal enuresis*) or for paraplegic patients who suffer from *urinary incontinence*.

The loss of bladder tone produced by atropine may make micturition difficult in some cases. This is especially true in elderly men with an enlarged prostate gland which already partially obstructs urine flow. Thus, the drug is contraindicated in patients with prostatic hypertrophy, because its use may result in *dysuria* and urinary retention. If the nurse notes that a man of upper middle age who is receiving atropine for peptic ulcer tends to get up and go to the bathroom every two hours or so, she should report this to the doctor, who may not know that the patient has a voiding problem. Often the patient fails to tell the physician because he is embarrassed or does not understand the significance of this troubling symptom.

GASTROINTESTINAL EFFECTS

The gastrointestinal actions of the anticholinergic drugs are the ones of greatest clinical importance. Atropinelike drugs are used mainly to reduce gastrointestinal spasm and secretions in conditions marked by hypersecretion of gastric acid. Among the disorders in which these drugs are employed are *peptic ulcer, gastritis, cardiospasm, pylorospasm, ileitis, diverticulitis, ulcerative colitis* and other functional and organic inflammatory and infectious diseases of the upper and lower gastrointestinal tract.

ACID-PEPTIC DISEASES. These disorders are marked by distress caused by the action of acid digestive juices on the mucous membranes of the upper gastrointestinal tract. These symptoms that people call "heartburn," "indigestion," or "dyspepsia" are often relieved by measures for neutralizing or reducing the production of stomach acid. In peptic ulcer, the most serious of the acid-related disorders, management with anticholinergic and antacid drugs is employed both for relief of pain and for helping to heal the ulcerated area.

The main objective of treatment in peptic ulcer is to protect the irritated or eroded gastrointestinal mucosa from acid gastric juices. This has two purposes: (1) it reduces the reflex smooth muscle spasm that is the source of the boring, burning pain; and (2) it reduces the digestive action of pepsin, the acid-activated enzyme that breaks down mucosal tissue.

[*Antisecretory agents*. In theory, the anticholinergic drugs should be effective for reducing gastric acid production, which is in large part under the influence of parasympathetic (vagal) nerve impulses. Thus, block of the released acetylcholine should halt the secretion of acid. In practice, it is difficult to stop acid secretion completely with safe doses of belladonna alkaloids or the newer synthetic substitutes. In part, this is because many patients are unwilling to tolerate the mouth dryness, blurred vision, and other discomforting side effects that accompany significant reduction in acid production by these drugs.

Nevertheless, the use of anticholinergic drugs in combination with antacid drugs does seem desirable for bringing about pain relief in peptic ulcer. In part, this is because the antispasmodic effect of the cholinergic blocking drugs relieves the painful reflex spasm set off by gastric acid stimulation of the sensory nerve endings in the ulcer crater. In addition, by prolonging the emptying time of the stomach, the anticholinergic drugs tend to keep the acid-neutralizing antacid agents at the place in the gastrointestinal tract where they act most effectively.

[*Antacid therapy*. Drugs that neutralize gastric acid *after* its secretion are considered the most effective means of relieving peptic ulcer pain. Whether their use alone or combined with anticholinergic drugs also speeds healing of the ulcer is controversial. In any case, they should be administered at the appropriate times for producing maximal pain relief (see Table 22-5).

[*Administration*. The frequency with which antacids are given depends primarily upon the severity of the patient's pain. Ordinarily, such substances as *aluminum hydroxide gel+, magnesium hydroxide+,* and *calcium carbonate* are administered about an hour after each meal and at bedtime. Their acid-neutralizing effect is more prolonged when the patient has also taken an anticholinergic drug about half an hour *before* the meals and at bedtime for reducing acid production during the night. However, patients suffering from the severe pain of an acute ulcer need to take antacids much more often and in much larger amounts.

The patient with an acute bleeding ulcer may require almost continuous medication. Sometimes an antacid suspension is dripped steadily into his stomach through an intragastric tube. This medication may be alternated with milk and cream mixtures to which a hemostatic powder has been added to counteract local bleeding. Even after bleeding is controlled, the patient may still need hourly feedings, followed every half hour by an antacid mixture. Later, however, when his illness is less severe and he does not require as much care, observation, and emotional support, the patient can be taught to take over a good deal of his own treatment.

As part of his preparation for leaving the hospital, the patient should be helped to set up a schedule of medication and taught that he must adhere to this schedule rigorously. He

TABLE 22-5 *Gastric Antacids*

Official, Chemical, or Nonproprietary Name	Synonym or Trade Name	Dosage	Remarks
Aluminum Compounds			
Aluminum hydroxide gel U.S.P.	Amphojel	5–40 ml	See *Drug Digest*
Aluminum hydroxide gel dried U.S.P.	Amphojel	300–600 mg	See *Drug Digest*
Aluminum carbonate, basic	Basalgel	8–30 ml	Used to treat nephrolithiasis
Aluminum phosphate gel N.F.	Phosphalgel	15–45 ml	Does not cause phosphate deficiency
Dihydroxyaluminum amino-acetate N.F.	Alglyn; Robalate; and others	500 mg–2 gm	Available as tablets and as a magma, or liquid suspension
Dihydroxyaluminum sodium carbonate N.F.	Rolaids	600–1320 mg	Relatively rapid action; in part, systemically absorbable
Calcium Compounds			
Calcium carbonate, precipitated U.S.P. (and tablets, N.F.)	Precipitated chalk; in Titralac, Ducon, and others	1–2 gm	See *Drug Digest*
Calcium phosphate, dibasic and tribasic N.F.	. . . .	1–4 gm	Relatively low, and short, neutralizing activity
Magnesium Compounds			
Magnesium carbonate N.F.	. . . .	500 mg–2 g	Liberates some carbon dioxide during slow neutralization of acid
Magnesium hydroxide N.F.	. . . .	300–600 mg	See *Drug Digest*
Magnesium oxide U.S.P.	. . . .	250–1500 mg	Same properties as the hydroxide
Magnesium phosphate N.F.	. . . .	1–2 g	Less neutralizing power
Magnesium trisilicate U.S.P.	. . . .	1–4 g	Lowest in neutralizing capacity of the magnesium compounds
Milk of magnesia U.S.P.	. . . .	5–30 ml	Suspension, or magma, of magnesium hydroxide
Mixtures of Aluminum and Magnesium Compounds *			
Alumina and magnesia oral suspension U.S.P.	Creamalin; and others	5–30 ml	. . . .
Aluminum hydroxide and magnesium hydroxide tablets U.S.P.	Aludrox; and others	300–600 mg	. . . .
Aluminum hydroxide and magnesium trisilicate oral suspension U.S.P.	Tricreamalate; and others	5–30 ml	. . . .
Aluminum hydroxide and magnesium trisilicate tablets U.S.P.	Gelusil; Trisogel; and others	300–600 mg	. . . .
Magaldrate N.F.	Riopan	400–800 mg	A complex hydroxy-magnesium aluminate compound
Magnesia and alumina oral Suspension U.S.P.	Maalox	5–30 ml	. . . .
Sodium Compounds			
Sodium bicarbonate U.S.P.	Baking soda	1–4 g	See *Drug Digest*
Sodium biphosphate N.F.	. . . .	1–2 g	Systemic absorption possible
Sodium phosphate N.F.	. . . .	1–2 g	

* Similar products made up of mixtures of these substances, alone or combined with calcium carbonate simethicone, and others, include: Bidrox, Camalox, Delcid, Ducon, Malcogel, Mylanta, Tri-Droxal, and Win Gel.

should be made to understand that, to be truly effective, antacids must be kept in the stomach continuously, because this both prevents pain and helps the ulcer to heal. Thus, it is not only permissible but actually desirable that the patient take his own medicine during his convalescence.

To help the convalescent patient assume this responsibility, he should be furnished with a bedside supply of antacid tablets or suspension and told how to take it. Some tablets need to be chewed or sucked slowly; others can be swallowed whole. If a suspension is employed, the patient should be instructed to shake the bottle each time before pouring his dose of the sticky stuff and washing it down the esophagus and into his stomach with a little water. He should be supplied with paper cups and a wastebacket to avoid the discouraging prospect of being surrounded by a growing mound of dirty glasses. If the disposable cups are not calibrated, a clearly marked measuring cup should be furnished to ensure ease in pouring an accurate dose even when the patient's eyesight is poor.

The nurse can reinforce the doctor's instruction to the patient and his family. She should stress the importance of timing his daily medication precisely, help him to understand why he must continue his ulcer treatment on his own for several months, and warn against giving in to any temptation to switch to some other type of antacid without consulting his doctor. Patients may sometimes read in a newspaper or magazine article about some new "wonder drug" or fad diet for curing ulcers quickly and effortlessly. These ulcer "cures" usually injure only his pocketbook, but their real danger is that the patient may be persuaded to drop the more burdensome but incomparably more effective antacid-diet regimen prescribed by his doctor.

INTESTINAL SPASM. The *antiperistaltic-antispasmodic* effects of the belladonna alkaloids and of the synthetic anticholinergic compounds are useful in the management of gastrointestinal conditions that are marked by diarrhea and painful smooth muscle spasm. These drugs seem most effective in the *irritable colon syndrome*, a functional disturbance of the gastrointestinal tract marked by excessive activity of parasympathetic nerves. This may be because these cholinergic blocking drugs keep the acetylcholine released by these nerves from increasing the motility of the patient's colon.

This helps to reduce the diarrhea and spasm of spastic, or mucous, colitis.

Drugs of this class are not very effective against diarrhea and intestinal spasm that are caused by chronic inflammatory disorders such as ulcerative colitis or by acute bacterial, viral, or amebic infections. In such cases *paregoric* is preferred for control of excessive intestinal motility, corticosteroids for reducing local inflammation, and antibiotics or sulfonamides for fighting the pathogenic microorganisms.

For those patients with functional disorders marked by gastrointestinal hypermotility and spasm who are sensitive to the side effects of anticholinergic drugs, certain synthetic antispasmodics (Table 22-2) are sometimes preferred. *Dicyclomine+* (Bentyl), for example, produces fewer atropine-type side effects such as mouth dryness and blurring of vision. It may be used for relief of spasm with greater safety in patients with narrow-angle glaucoma, for example, as it is less likely than atropine+ and propantheline+ to cause angle closure.

POISONING

Poisoning by belladonna alkaloids and other drugs with an anticholinergic component causes a wide variety of dramatic signs and symptoms. The peripheral and central effects previously described have led to patients poisoned by atropine being described as: "Hot as a hare, blind as a bat, dry as a bone, and mad as a hatter."

Fatal reactions to overdosage with atropine medication are rare despite the patient's great discomfort and the many alarming signs and symptoms. However, fatalities have occurred in infants given overdoses of belladonna preparations for colic. Recently, reports of atropine-scopolamine type toxicity have increased due to deliberate abuse of products containing these alkaloids by those seeking the *hallucinogenic* effect of overdoses of these drugs. The anticholinesterase-type cholinergic drug *physostigmine* (eserine) has reportedly proved effective as an antidote to anticholinergic drug intoxication. It is said to reverse very promptly the patient's confusion, agitation, delirium, stupor, and other signs and symptoms of central toxicity, as well as the peripheral effects of atropine poisoning.

The nurse should take special care in administering atropine to see that the patient is receiving the right dose. The small doses of this drug are sometimes ordered in the apothecary system and at other times in the metric system, which could lead to confusion and result in a patient's getting a dangerous overdose. In these situations the nurse should work toward patient safety by advocating use of the metric system for all drug measurements. The nurse should be especially cautious when an atropine solution is to be mixed in the same syringe with a narcotic analgesic for preoperative administration.

SUMMARY of the Pharmacological Actions and Therapeutic Uses of Atropine-type Drugs

Pharmacological Actions

Gastrointestinal
Smooth muscle: Antispasmodic and antiperistaltic actions reduced the tone and motility of the stomach and intestines.
Gastric glands: Large doses reduce secretion of acid and of digestive enzymes.

Other Smooth Muscle
Urinary tract: Reduces tone and motility of ureters, fundus of the bladder, and possibly the uterus; increases tone of the bladder sphincter.
Biliary tract: Weak antispasmodic action on gallbladder and bile ducts accounts for its use combined with morphine.
Bronchial muscle is only slightly relaxed to cause relatively weak bronchodilation.

Cardiovascular System
Cardiac actions: Small doses of atropine slow the heart rate slightly and larger doses accelerate it markedly. The decrease in rate is more marked with scopolamine.
Vascular: Local vasodilation often causes flushing of the face. Blood pressure is not much affected, except that the hypotension caused by cholinergic drugs can be prevented and counteracted.

Ocular Effects
Produce dilation of the pupil (mydriasis) and paralysis of accommodation (cycloplegia) by blocking tonic impulses to the sphincter muscle of the iris and to the ciliary muscles. This may raise the intraocular pressure in the eyes of patients with narrow-angle glaucoma.

Glandular Secretions
Small doses markedly reduce sweating, salivation, and the secretions of the nose, throat, and bronchial glands.

Central Nervous System
Atropine, in therapeutic doses, has a slight excitatory action, whereas scopolamine in equivalent amounts causes depressant effects including drowsiness, sleep, and amnesia. Both alkaloids depress motor mechanisms responsible for abnormal skeletal muscle tone. Toxic doses of atropine cause excitement, restlessness, disorientation, and delirium.

Therapeutic Uses

Gastrointestinal
Used to reduce hypermotility and hypersecretory activity in such conditions as peptic ulcer, gastritis, cardiospasm, pylorospasm, regional enteritis (that is, ileitis, ulcerative colitis, diverticulitis), diarrhea in mild dysentery, and constipation of the hypertonic or spastic type.

Other Smooth Muscle
Used to increase bladder capacity in children with nocturnal enuresis and in spastic paraplegics and others with urinary incontinence; in cystitis and other irritative conditions to relieve urinary urgency and frequency; as an antispasmodic in renal colic to relax ureters or to counteract added spasm caused by morphine; for relief of pain in dysmenorrhea.
For relief of biliary colic.
Although it is not very useful in bronchial asthma, this action is useful for counteracting bronchoconstriction caused by cholinergic drugs, including methacholine and the anticholinesterase insecticides and nerve gases.

Cardiovascular System
Used to prevent or counteract reflex bradycardia caused by excessive vagal tone: in anesthesia (for example, with halothane); during certain surgical procedures; in the carotid sinus syndrome; and in certain kinds of heart block.

Ocular Effects
Used in ophthalmologic examinations of the retina and optic disk and for measuring refractive errors. Mydriasis alone or alternated with miosis is used to keep the lens from adhering to the iris in iritis. Also used to relax ocular muscles and reduce irritation in inflammatory conditions such as iridocyclitis and choroiditis.

Glandular Secretions
Used prior to inhalation anesthesia to reduce respiratory tract secretions.

Used to reduce nasal secretions in acute rhinitis of the common cold and hay fever.

Used to reduce excessive sweating in hyperhidrosis and in the night sweats of tuberculosis.

Central Nervous System

Used to reduce tremor and rigidity in Parkinsonism.

Used as prophylaxis against motion sickness.

Scopolamine is an ingredient of sleep-producing products advertised to the public for self-medication of insomnia.

Scopolamine was once widely used for its sedative and amnesic effects, when combined with opiates as a preoperative adjunct to general anesthesia. It has been largely replaced by phenothiazine-type tranquilizers for this purpose and for quieting manic patients and alcoholics with delirium tremens.

S U M M A R Y of the Side Effects, Cautions, and Contraindications of Atropine-type Drugs

Mouth

Mouth dryness, due to reduced salivation: may make swallowing difficult; dryness of respiratory tract and hardening of reduced bronchial secretions may be bad for patients with asthma and other chronic lung diseases.

Skin

Skin dry, hot, red, due to abolition of sweating, and vasodilation. The interference with heat loss may lead to fever, especially in infants and young children; patients may suffer hyperpyrexia in warm weather or hot climates.

Eyes

Possible photophobia results from widely dilated pupils; vision blurred, due to paralysis of accommodation. Crowding of iris and ciliary muscle into angle of eye chamber may raise intraocular pressure by interfering with drainage of aqueous humor. Thus, these drugs are contraindicated in patients with narrow-angle glaucoma, and caution is required in all patients over 40 years old because of their increased susceptibility to attacks of acute glaucoma.

Urinary Tract

Urinary retention may occur, owing to loss of bladder tone, especially in elderly males with an enlarged prostate gland. Thus, these drugs are contraindicated in patients with prostatic hypertrophy. Synthetic atropinelike drugs with ganglionic blocking component may produce impotence in young men.

Cardiac

Heart palpitations and tachycardia may occur, owing to loss of vagal control. This may cause coronary insufficiency, chest pain, and cardiac decompensation in patients with a history of heart disease. Thus, caution is required in patients with angina, for example.

Gastrointestinal

Constipation and possible obstipation, due to reduced tone and motility of gastrointestinal musculature. Thus, caution is required in patients with partial pyloric stenosis, because of the danger that the narrowed passageway may become completely obstructed.

S U M M A R Y of Adverse Effects of Gastric Antacids

Gastrointestinal Side Effects

Nausea and vomiting, occasionally (aluminum salts).

Constipation (calcium and aluminum compounds).

Diarrhea (magnesium salts).

Flatulence from release of CO_2 gas (bicarbonate and carbonates).

Systemic Toxicity

Metabolic alkalosis (in patients with kidney disease who take sodium bicarbonate in large amounts).

Edema (due to sodium retention in patients with kidney disease who take sodium bicarbonate in large amounts).

Osteomalacia—softening of the bones due to phosphate depletion by fecal elimination (aluminum hydroxide).

S U M M A R Y of Points for the Nurse to Remember about Atropine and Related Drugs

Take special care in checking dosages as they are often unusually small (for example, 0.4 mg of atropine), and an error resulting from a misplaced decimal point is both possible and dangerous.

Be alert for signs and symptoms of atropine overdosage, and inform the physician of any marked changes in pulse rate, visual acuity, bladder function, or behavior.

Tell the patient that certain side effects such as mouth dryness and blurring of vision are likely to occur, as this can spare him needless concern. (Parents should be told that children often look flushed and feel warm after taking atropine, so that they will not think that the children are feverish from an infection.)

Advise the patient that he can relieve mouth dryness discomfort by sucking on hard candies and that he can minimize photophobia by wearing dark glasses.

Caution elderly and other ambulatory patients to take special care during physical activity (for example, walking down stairs) when they have drug-induced blurring of vision. Driving a car and operating machinery may be particularly hazardous when vision is blurred.

Mydriatic-Cycloplegic Eye Drops

Let patients who have had eye drops know when the visual effects will wear off so that they can plan their activities accordingly.

Be aware of the potential seriousness of accidentally administering a mydriatic instead of a miotic to a patient with narrow-angle glaucoma. (It may precipitate an acute attack which could lead to blindness.)

Never administer mydriatics routinely when eye examinations are being performed. Always ask the physician which patients are to receive mydriatics prior to the examination.

Clinical Nursing Situation

The Situation: Mr. West's physician is treating him at home for peptic ulcer. In addition to rest and a bland diet, the doctor has ordered Amphogel 8 cc every hour, Prantal 50 mg t.i.d., a.c., and h.s., and Librium 10 mg t.i.d.

Mr. West appears very nervous. Although he has been staying at home until his symptoms improve, he is surrounded by papers and ledgers.

The Problem:
What directions should the public health

nurse give Mr. West about taking his Amphogel?

Mr. West mentions that his mouth is very dry. What suggestions could the nurse make to him for relieving the dryness?

During your visit, Mr. West receives several urgent business telephone calls. Describe what you consider to be a useful approach toward helping him lessen tension and achieve the rest that is essential.

DRUG DIGEST

ALUMINUM HYDROXIDE GEL U.S.P. (Amphogel; and others)
Actions and Indications. This nonabsorbable antacid reacts slowly with hydrochloric acid to form aluminum chloride and other compounds, including aluminum phosphate, which are then eliminated in the feces. The neutralizing action of the dried gel is relatively low compared to that of the liquid suspension. This chemical also has adsorbent, astringent, and demulcent properties, but their value in ulcer treatment is uncertain.

In addition to its use alone or combined with magnesium compounds for relief of peptic pain, aluminum hydroxide is also sometimes used in the management of patients who tend to form phosphate-type kidney stones (nephrolithiasis).

Side Effects, Cautions, and Contraindications. This compound does not cause metabolic alkalosis, and its potential for systemic toxicity is relatively low. However, high daily doses taken for long periods by a person eating a phosphate-poor diet might mobilize phosphate from the bones and result in osteomalacia, a softening or bending of the bones.

Gastrointestinal side effects—possibly from its astringent action—include occasional nausea and vomiting, and frequent constipation. Administration with magnesium hydroxide tends to counteract constipation.

Dosage and Administration. Dose of the solid gel is 300 to 600 mg several times daily before meals in tablets that are chewed before being swallowed. Dose of the liquid suspension ranges from 5 to 40 ml. The latter dose, diluted with water, may be administered by intragastric drip in severe cases. It should not be taken at the same time as tetracycline-type antibiotics or anticholinergic drugs, as its adsorbent action interferes with their absorption.

ATROPINE SULFATE U.S.P.

Actions and Indications. This belladonna alkaloid is the prototype of cholinergic blocking drugs. It is used mainly for its antispasmodic and antisecretory effects in the management of peptic ulcer, gastritis, spastic colitis, and other gastrointestinal disorders marked by hypertonicity and hypermotility of smooth muscle and by excessive gastric acid production.

Atropine is also used to prevent or counteract excessive cardiac slowing caused by vagus nerve stimulation. In the eye, it produces mydriasis and cycloplegia, effects useful for ocular examination and measurement of refractive errors. It is also used in treating parkinsonism.

Side Effects, Cautions, and Contraindications. Common side effects of therapeutic doses include dryness of the mouth and blurring of vision. Toxic doses may cause flushing of the skin, fever, and such signs of C.N.S. stimulation as confusion, restlessness, hallucinations, and delirium. This drug is contraindicated in patients with narrow-angle glaucoma and is used

only with caution in open-angle glaucoma. Caution is also required in patients with coronary insufficiency and other cardiac disorders. The drug is contraindicated in the presence of organic obstructions of the gastrointestinal tract (pyloric stenosis, for example) and of the genitourinary tract (enlarged prostate gland, for example).

Dosage and Administration. Oral and subcutaneous doses of 0.3 to 1.2 mg (average 0.5 mg) may be administered every four hours. One or two drops may be applied topically to the eye and repeated two or three times daily.

CALCIUM CARBONATE, PRECIPITATED U.S.P. (Precipitated Chalk)

Actions and Indications. This is the least expensive antacid and one that has high neutralizing activity, which is relatively rapid and prolonged. It is best administered in combination with magnesium compounds or alternated with them. Relatively frequent administration of high doses is required for full effects in reducing peptic activity in ulcer patients.

Side Effects, Cautions, and Contraindications. Local gastrointestinal side effects include constipation most commonly, flatulence and belching sometimes, and nausea rarely. Constipation is counteracted by administration of magnesium hydroxide, as is the occasional formation of fecal concretions.

Systemic absorption of some calcium occurs. However, hypercalcemia is not significant, except possibly in patients with kidney dysfunction. It is contraindicated in such patients, as metabolic alkalosis is possible, particularly when large amounts of milk or cream are also being taken. It is also contraindicated in patients with a history of kidney stones, as it can cause hypercalciuria and calcium calculi.

Dosage and Administration. The usual oral dose is 1 to 2 g taken with water several times daily before meals. However, amounts as high as 2 to 4 g every hour may be needed in severe cases to keep gastric acidity below the level at which the enzyme pepsin stays active.

CYCLOPENTOLATE HCl U.S.P. (Cyclogyl)

Actions and Indications. This anticholinergic agent is applied topically to the eye to bring about rapid mydriasis and cycloplegia of relatively short duration. This offers an advantage over atropine in diagnostic ophthalmology, since the patient recovers normal vision

within one day compared to the relatively prolonged blurring of near vision produced by atropine. This drug has also been used therapeutically to produce reflex paralysis of ocular muscle structures in the management of iritis, iridocyclitis, choroiditis, and keratitis.

Side Effects, Cautions, and Contraindications. Caution is required to avoid accidental application of eye drops containing this or other anticholinergic drugs to the eyes of individuals with a narrow ocular angle, as mydriatics may precipitate an acute glaucoma attack in such people. The solutions should be used with caution, in any case, in those—particularly elderly patients—whose intraocular pressure has not been measured by tonometry.

Care should be taken to minimize systemic absorption, especially when drops of a more concentrated solution are applied to the eyes of young children. This has resulted in signs and symptoms of central and peripheral atropinelike toxicity, for which treatment with physostigmine may be required.

Dosage and Administration. Ophthalmic solutions of several strengths are available. Two drops of a 0.5 percent solution or one drop of a 1 percent solution are usually effective for cycloplegia. For darkly pigmented irises and in other relatively resistant eyes, a 2 percent solution is used.

DICYCLOMINE HCl N.F. (Bentyl)

Actions and Indications. This antispasmodic drug produces its main effects by directly relaxing gastrointestinal smooth muscle. It is used for relief of spasm in organic gastrointestinal disease, including gastritis and peptic ulcer, but it does not reduce gastric acid secretion.

Side Effects, Cautions, and Contraindications. This drug does not ordinarily cause atropinelike side effects. However, in high doses or in susceptible patients, mouth dryness and blurring of vision may occur. Thus, caution is required in patients with narrow-angle glaucoma, as well as in those with a tendency toward urinary retention, or with obstructive gastrointestinal disease such as pyloric stenosis.

Central effects such as drowsiness, euphoria, or feelings of fatigue and headache, have sometimes occurred. Nausea, vomiting, and, rarely, skin rashes have also been reported.

Dosage and Administration. Oral doses of 10 to 20 mg may be taken three or four times daily in tablet, capsule, or syrup form, alone or combined with phenobarbital. I.M. injections of 20 mg may be made every four to six hours.

EUCATROPINE HCl U.S.P. (Euphthalmine)

Actions and Indications. This anticholinergic agent produces mydriasis rapidly when applied to the eye in concentrations too low to cause significant cycloplegia. Thus, it does not cause blurring of vision by interfering with accommodation for near vision when it is employed to aid ophthalmoscopic examination of the retina, optic disk, and other structures in the fundus of the eye. The effectiveness of this relatively weak mydriatic is increased when it is administered together with an adrenergic-class mydriatic such as phenylephrine or ephedrine.

Side Effects, Cautions, and Contraindications. Like other anticholinergic-type mydriatics, this drug is contraindicated in patients whose intraocular pressure is not known to be in the normal range and in people with a shallow anterior chamber and narrow ocular angle. It is used with caution in elderly patients, and systemic absorption should be particularly avoided in children by gentle pressure on the inner canthus following topical application.

Dosage and Administration. One or two drops of 2 to 5 percent solutions are applied topically to the conjunctiva of each eye for rapid mydriatic action within one half to one hour.

HOMATROPINE HBr U.S.P. (Homatrocel; and others)

Actions and Indications. This anticholinergic agent brings about both mydriasis and cycloplegia. It has the advantage of wearing off more rapidly than atropine when employed as a diagnostic agent in ophthalmology. However, for therapeutic purposes, the more prolonged and complete cycloplegia produced by atropine is preferred —for example, in the treatment of keratitis and uveitis.

The mydriatic action of this agent is useful for examining ocular structures in the fundus and elsewhere. The cycloplegic effect is employed in measuring errors in refraction, as the partial paralysis of accommodation prevents involuntary reflex responses that interfere with measurement.

Side Effects, Cautions, and Contraindications. This drug is contraindicated in patients with narrow-angle glaucoma, in whom its use

may precipitate angle closure and an acute attack. It is used with caution in patients over 40 years old, who may be more subject to unexpected rises in intraocular pressure produced by mydriatics.

Dosage and Administration. One or two drops of a 1 percent solution is employed to produce mydriasis. For cycloplegia, a 2 to 5 percent solution is preferred. Topical administration of the 2 percent solution several times at 10-minute intervals may be necessary for maintaining cycloplegia.

MAGNESIUM HYDROXIDE N.F.

Actions and Indications. This compound, particularly in the form of the magma or suspension called milk of magnesia, is a popular antacid and laxative. It reacts rapidly with gastric acid to neutralize large amounts. A remaining residue produces a more prolonged antacid effect. For long-term treatment of peptic ulcer, it is best administered in combination with aluminum and calcium compounds.

Side Effects, Cautions, and Contraindications. The doses required for continuous acid neutralization are high enough to cause catharsis. Thus, diarrhea occurs commonly, unless magnesium hydroxide is administered together with astringent or constipating aluminum hydroxide and calcium carbonate, or given alternately with them.

The small amount of magnesium absorbed does not cause significant metabolic alkalosis or systemic toxicity. However, its use is contraindicated in patients with severe renal impairment, as systemic accumulation of magnesium may cause C.N.S. depression marked by drowsiness, stupor, coma, and possible respiratory paralysis or circulatory collapse.

Dosage and Administration. The powder or tablet form is taken with water in doses of 300 to 600 mg several times daily before meals and at bedtime. Milk of magnesia is given in doses of as little as 5 ml or as much as 30 ml four or many more times daily, depending upon the degree of severity of the condition that is being treated.

PROPANTHELINE BROMIDE U.S.P. (Probanthine)

Actions and Indications. This synthetic anticholinergic drug produces peripheral effects similar to those of the chemically related prototype, methantheline, and of the natural cholinergic blocking alkaloids, atropine and scopolamine. It is used mainly as an antispasmodic-antisecretory agent for

symptomatic relief in patients with peptic ulcer, pancreatitis, and gastritis. It reduces gastrointestinal hypermotility in functional gastrointestinal disorders, including the irritable bowel syndrome and in diverticulitis, ulcerative colitis, and others. It also relieves spasms of the ureters and urinary bladder.

Side Effects, Cautions, and Contraindications. The side effects are similar to those of atropine— mouth dryness, blurring of vision, tachycardia, and possible urinary hesitation and retention. Thus, it is used with caution in patients with coronary insufficiency and in elderly male patients with prostatic enlargement, and it is contraindicated in cases of narrow-angle glaucoma.

Central toxicity from overdosage is not as likely as with the natural anticholinergic alkaloids. However, the ganglionic blocking effects of this drug can cause episodes of postural hypotension and impotence. Massive overdosage may cause a curarelike neuromuscular blockade, leading to muscle weakness and paralysis.

Dosage and Administration. Orally, 15 mg is administered with each meal and 30 mg at bedtime. Parenterally, 30 mg is injected I.M. or diluted with 10 cc of saline solution I.V. Up to 60 mg may be injected for prompt action in acute pancreatitis or spasm.

SCOPOLAMINE HBr U.S.P. (Hyoscine HBr)

Actions and Indications. This alkaloid of solonaceous plants produces peripheral effects similar to those of atropine. Thus, it is used for its cholinergic blocking effects at several of the same neuroeffector sites. Its anticholinergic effects at ocular structures are, for example, used to produce mydriasis and cycloplegia for ophthalmological purposes.

Scopolamine differs from atropine in its effects on the C.N.S., where it causes depression in therapeutic doses. It has been employed as a motion sickness preventive, a sedative-hypnotic, and in parkinsonism treatment. It is also used for its amnesic effect in obstetrics, and preoperatively for increasing the pain-relieving potency of narcotic analgesics without a proportionate increase in respiratory depression.

Side Effects, Cautions, and Contraindications. Scopolamine causes peripheral side effects similar to those of atropine, including mouth dryness, blurring of vision, constipation, and tachycardia. It is used with caution in patients with prostatic hypertrophy, partial gastrointestinal tract obstructions, and angina pectoris, and its use is contraindicated in narrow-angle glaucoma. Overdosage and drug abuse have resulted in signs and symptoms of central toxicity, including excitement, confusion, delirium, and hallucinations.

Dosage and Administration. Oral or subcutaneous dosage ranges between 0.3 and 0.8 mg (usual dose 0.6 mg). It is also applied topically to the eyes as a 1 percent solution (1 or 2 drops).

SODIUM BICARBONATE U.S.P. (Baking Soda)

Actions and Indications. This soluble, absorbable alkalizer is widely used by the public for the rapid relief of hyperacidity symptoms. It is an ingredient of the once widely used Sippy powders, but it is not now often prescribed by physicians for peptic ulcer treatment because of its too brief action and possible adverse effects.

Side Effects, Cautions, and Contraindications. The release of carbon dioxide in the immediate reaction with hydrochloric acid causes belching and stomach distention. This may be dangerous for patients with a peptic ulcer that is close to the point of perforation. This compound, when taken in excess, is systemically absorbed and then excreted by the kidneys. It is contraindicated in patients with renal insufficiency because of possible development of metabolic alkalosis and of edema.

Dosage and Administration. Oral doses of 1 to 4 g are taken for relief of gastric hyperacidity at frequent intervals.

References

Di Palma, J.R. Drugs in the management of peptic ulcer. *RN*, 26:71, 1963 (April).

Friend, D. Gastrointestinal anticholinergic drugs. *Clin. Pharmacol. Ther.*, 4:559, 1963.

Kirsner, J.B. Facts and fallacies of current medical therapy for uncomplicated duodenal ulcer. *JAMA*, 187:423, 1964.

Librach, I. M. Peptic ulcer: facts and figures. *Nursing Mirror*, 134:23, 1972.

Rodman, M.J. Drugs for peptic pain. *RN*, 21:64, 1958.

————. Drugs in the management of peptic ulcer. *RN*, 26:71, 1963 (April).

Schiff, E.R. Treatment of uncomplicated peptic ulcer disease. *Med. Clin. N. Amer.*, 55:305, 1971 (March).

Sodeman, W.A., Jr., et al. Physiology and pharmacology of belladonna therapy in acid-peptic disease. *Med. Clin. N. Amer.*, 53:1379, 1969 (Nov.).

Woldman, E.E. Peptic ulcer: current medical treatment. *Amer. J. Nurs.*, 59:222, 1959.

23.

Sympathomimetic (Adrenergic) Drugs

General Considerations

ADRENERGIC TRANSMISSION

The sympathetic nervous system transmits impulses to the heart and the smooth muscles of blood vessels, bronchi, and other structures by releasing the neurotransmitter, norepinephrine. The medulla releases a similar hormone, epinephrine, which acts at the same receptors that respond to the neurohormone norepinephrine. Because epinephrine (also known as adrenaline) was the first such substance studied, the passage of nerve impulses from sympathetic nerve endings to the innervated organs and structures is called *adrenergic transmission.*

Adrenergic Drugs

Certain synthetic substances that imitate many of the effects of the natural sympathetic nervous system neurohormone and of the adrenal medulla hormone are used for treating various clinical conditions. These adrenergic, or sympathomimetic, drugs do not all produce exactly the same effects. Some, for example, are more likely than others to cause cardiac stimulation. Some sympathomimetic drugs exert their main effects on blood vessels of the kind that respond to sympathetic stimulation by constricting; other adrenergic drugs act mainly on the vessels which tend to dilate when they are stimulated by impulses from the sympathetic nervous system (see Table 20-2). Other adrenergic drugs act mainly on bronchial or on ocular smooth muscle.

Thus, in treating various clinical conditions

with adrenergic drugs, the doctor tries to select the specific sympathomimetic agent that he knows is most likely to act on the organ at which he is aiming. But because all these drugs act to some extent on other structures, side effects occur fairly frequently during adrenergic drug therapy.

Pharmacology and Clinical Applications of Adrenergic Drugs

CARDIAC EFFECTS OF ADRENERGIC DRUGS

The two adrenergic drugs with the most powerful direct actions on the heart are *epinephrine+* (Adrenalin) and *isoproterenol+* (Isuprel). (See Chapter 25, *The Heart and Blood Vessels in Health and Disease*, for a refresher on some principles of cardiac function.) This is because they have the greatest affinity for adrenergic receptors of the beta (β_1) type, the predominant type of adrenergic receptors in cardiac tissue. The main useful effects that these (and other sympathomimetic amine-type drugs) have on the heart are the following:

1. They strengthen the heart beat.
2. They speed up the heart rate.
3. They increase the rate of impulse conduction from atria to ventricles.

These combined actions of adrenergic drugs usually result in an increase in cardiac output, which—together with the vasoconstrictor effect upon blood vessels (discussed below)—leads to a rise in arterial blood pressure. Sometimes, if the blood pressure rises rapidly and steeply, it sets off reflex activity that acts indirectly to produce yet another potentially useful cardiac effect—a *slowing* down of the heart rate.

Ordinarily, the heart muscle itself is the first organ to benefit from the increase in cardiac output brought about by the effects of adrenergic drugs. The coronary arterioles, which branch off from the aorta into the myocardium, carry a better flow of blood to this muscle when adrenergic drugs are increasing the speed and strength with which the left ventricle contracts. Sometimes, however, if the myocardium is made to work too hard, the patient's coronary arteries may not be able to carry enough blood to keep up with the heart muscle's greatly increased demands for oxygen. When the heart muscle becomes hypoxic, it is particularly sensitive to yet another cardiac

action of adrenergic drugs—a tendency to *increase cardiac irritability*. This can sometimes cause dangerous cardiac arrhythmias, including fatal ventricular fibrillation.

CLINICAL APPLICATIONS OF CARDIAC EFFECTS

The administration of certain adrenergic drugs is indicated for treating those cardiac conditions that are marked by an excessively slow heart beat or even sudden stoppage of rhythmic contractions. These conditions include the Stokes-Adams syndrome, the carotid sinus syndrome, A-V block and bradycardia in digitalis intoxication, and cardiac arrest.

CARDIAC ARREST. The adrenergic drugs most commonly employed in this acute emergency are *isoproterenol+* and *epinephrine+*. Isoproterenol is preferred for intracardiac administration because it is as useful as epinephrine for restarting a heart that is in standstill (asystole), and even more effective than epinephrine when the heart's failure to pump blood into the arteries is the result of ventricular fibrillation. Both of these sympathomimetic amines are more effective when administered following infusion of sodium bicarbonate solution, a systemic alkalinizer that counteracts the metabolic acidosis caused by the building up of lactic acid in the heart and in other tissues during periods of hypoxia.

NURSE'S ROLE IN CARDIAC ARREST. In this emergency, other measures for maintaining cardiopulmonary function are actually more important than drug therapy. Until medical help arrives, the nurse who has to cope with a patient in cardiac arrest is more concerned with establishing an airway through which oxygen can be delivered by mouth-to-mouth breathing or by way of a mechanical ventilating device. She may also perform closed cardiac massage or administer electrical defibrillating shock, if this is one of her recognized duties as a member of a hospital's cardiac arrest team. When the doctor orders adrenergic (and other) drugs, it is often the nurse's responsibility to prepare the injections and to monitor the patient's responses to drug therapy.

PAROXYSMAL SUPRAVENTRICULAR TACHYCARDIA. The rapid heart beat that suddenly develops in this condition is best controlled by physical measures and drugs (such as digitalis), that increase vagal control of the heart rate.

Two adrenergic drugs, *phenylephrine+* (Neosynephrine) and *methoxamine+* (Vasoxyl) are used for this purpose. These drugs, which act mainly at the alpha-type adrenergic receptors in blood vessels, have no *direct* effect on the heart itself, which contains mainly beta receptors. However, when injected intravenously at a slow rate during an attack, these sympathomimetic agents sometimes restore normal sinus rhythm within one minute. They do so by their ability to constrict blood vessels in the systemic circulation, thus raising the peripheral resistance and blood pressure (see below). This in turn produces a reflex bradycardia, because the rise in blood pressure stimulates the brain's cardioinhibitory center to send more heart-slowing impulses down the vagus nerve to the heart.

STOKES-ADAMS SYNDROME. Intravenously infused *isoproterenol* solution is also the most effective adrenergic drug for treating the attacks of asystole that occur periodically in this condition, particularly when the heart of a patient with partial heart block goes suddenly into complete A-V block. Administered during such a seizure, isoproterenol acts to overcome the patient's cerebral symptoms by stimulating the heart to pump more blood to the brain.

It does so by bringing about the three main effects of sympathomimetic amines listed above, but because overdosage can cause a dangerous increase in cardiac irritability, the I.V. drip of this potent drug must be carefully regulated. To avoid producing too rapid cardiac arrhythmias, the infusion rate is slowed down when the patient's pulse has returned to about 60 beats per minute; if the pulse rises to much higher levels, or if premature ventricular contractions appear on the electrocardiogram, isoproterenol must be discontinued.

A sublingual dosage form of isoproterenol is available for routine use several times daily for preventing Stokes-Adams seizures. This rapidly disintegrating tablet may also be placed under the patient's tongue for rapid action, if he complains of feeling faint or lightheaded. (The patient is told not to swallow his saliva until the drug is absorbed.) This can help prevent the falls and physical injuries that often occur when patients with this cardiac condition "black out" as the result of a syncopal attack. Other adrenergic drugs occasionally ordered for oral administration in this condition include *ephedrine+* and *hydroxyamphetamine* (Paredrine). Because these drugs have central

actions that can cause nervousness and insomnia, they are often combined with a barbiturate or other sedative hypnotic. Many patients with this condition are now maintained in stable rhythm by means of electrical pacemakers—a method considered more certainly effective than daily adrenergic drug therapy.

ADVERSE CARDIAC EFFECTS OF ADRENERGIC DRUGS

As was previously indicated, the most dangerous effect of adrenergic drugs is their tendency to cause rapid cardiac arrhythmias in some circumstances (see *Summary of Side Effects*, p. 305). This is particularly true when the drugs have caused myocardial hypoxia by driving the heart beyond the capacity of its coronary arterioles to deliver oxygen. Ventricular premature beats, tachycardia, and fibrillation can also develop when adrenergic drugs are administered to patients under anesthesia with halothane or cyclopropane.

Sympathommietic drugs should also be used with caution, if at all, in patients with angina pectoris or hyperthyroidism. Patients with these conditions are particularly likely to complain of cardiac palpitations and pounding, and chest pains, if they take adrenergic drugs: for treating a cold; as a weight-reducing measure; or for management of asthma or other disorders unrelated to their heart ailment.

VASCULAR EFFECTS OF ADRENERGIC DRUGS

Most adrenergic drugs act to constrict arterioles and venules, but some sympathomimetic amines produce local vasodilation. The vasoconstrictor effects of adrenergic drugs on blood vessels of the skin and mucous membranes have clinical applications in stopping bleeding and bringing about nasal and ocular decongestion. These and other uses of local vasoconstriction are discussed on p. 302. The clinical applications of those adrenergic drugs that dilate the blood vessels of skeletal muscles are discussed in Chapter 32, *Drugs for Peripheral Vascular Disease.*

Doses of adrenergic drugs large enough to constrict the vessels of vascular beds all through the body, and particularly the splanchnic arterioles of the abdominal viscera, produce a rise in arterial blood pressure. Various *vasopressors*—as the adrenergic drugs that cause such generalized vasoconstriction are called—are employed in the management of acute hypotension and circulatory shock (Table 23-1).

VASOPRESSORS FOR TREATING SHOCK

Circulatory failure can result from many causes. Loss of blood volume as a result of uncontrolled bleeding is a common cause of shock. Such hemorrhagic shock is best treated by stemming the flow of blood and by replacement of the loss by transfusions of whole blood, plasma, or plasma substitutes. In other kinds of shock, including that caused by drug overdosage, acute coronary attacks, severe infections, injuries, and burns, no actual loss of blood occurs. Yet the amount of blood pumped by the heart into the arterial circulation is markedly reduced. The poor flow of blood to vital organs such as the brain, kidneys, and the heart muscle itself can lead to cellular damage, and—if shock is not counteracted—to death.

In such shock states, the administration of adrenergic vasopressors often helps to keep blood flowing to the brain, heart, and other organs in adequate amounts to ward off the development of so-called *"irreversible" shock.* Doctors often differ in the adrenergic drugs that they prefer to employ. The choice, in many cases, depends upon whether the patient's state of shock stems mainly from impaired peripheral vessel function, cardiac failure, or both. We shall discuss the treatment of several types of shock with adrenergic drugs that differ somewhat in their effects. These differences may· make one kind or another

TABLE 23-1   *Adrenergic Drugs Used In Treating Shock*

Nonproprietary or Official Name	Trade Name or Synonym	Dosage
Ephedrine sulfate* U.S.P.		25 to 50 mg I.V. or I.M.
Epinephrine injection* U.S.P.	Adrenalin	0.1 to 0.5 ml of 1:1,000 solution s.c., I.M., or I.V., diluted in 10 ml of saline solution for slow I.V. infusion
Isoproterenol HCl† U.S.P.	Isuprel	5 ml of 1:5,000 solution diluted with 500 ml of 5% dextrose for slow I.V. infusion
Levarterenol bitartrate‡ U.S.P.	Levophed	4 ml of a 0.2% solution diluted in 1,000 ml of a 5% dextrose solution for slow I.V. infusion
Mephentermine sulfate* U.S.P.	Wyamine	500 mg to 1g diluted in 1,000 ml of 5% dextrose solution for slow I.V. infusion
Metaraminol bitartrate‡ U.S.P.	Aramine	2 to 10 mg I.M.; 15 to 100 mg diluted in 500 ml of 5% dextrose or saline solution for slow I.V. infusion
Methamphetamine HCl* U.S.P.	Drinalfa, and others	10 to 30 mg I.M.; 5 to 10 mg by slow I.V.
Methoxamine HCl§ U.S.P.	Vasoxyl	10 to 15 mg I.M.; 3 to 5 mg by slow I.V.
Phenylephrine HCl§ U.S.P.	Neo-Synephrine	2 to 5 mg I.M. or s.c.; 1 ml of a 1% solution diluted in 500 ml of dextrose or saline solution for slow infusion

The reference marks refer to the manner in which each drug is thought to bring about its clinically desirable hemodynamic effects in shock states.

* Produces pressor effects mainly by stimulating the heart, thus increasing cardiac output; some types of blood vessels are constricted while others are dilated. (Epinephrine is used mainly in anaphylactic shock.)

† Produces improved tissue perfusion by stimulating the heart while dilating peripheral vessels; to assure increased cardiac output, blood volume must be maintained by administration of fluids.

‡ Produces pressure effects mainly by constricting blood vessels and thus raising peripheral resistance; cardiac output is increased by an increase in contractile strength, but heart rate need not be accelerated.

§ Produces pressure effects mainly by constricting arterioles and thus raising peripheral resistance; heart is *not* stimulated and its rate may even be slowed.

adrenergic drug preferred for treating each type of shock (Table 23-1).

NEUROGENIC HYPOTENSION AND SHOCK. Drugs that reduce the normal flow of nerve impulses to the blood vessels produce dilation of the arteries and pooling of blood in the veins. This can lead to acute hypotension and shock of a kind that is best treated or prevented with drugs that cause vasoconstriction. Among adrenergic drugs that do this—and thus increase the venous return of blood to the heart—are *phenylephrine+*, *methoxamine+*, and *ephedrine+*. A nonadrenergic drug that also raises peripheral arterial resistance is *angiotensin amide* (Hypertensin). Even though only ephedrine stimulates the heart directly, all of these drugs increase the cardiac output and produce a better flow of blood to the vital organs.

Among the kinds of drugs that can cause a fall in blood pressure to shock levels by cutting off nerve impulses to blood vessel walls are the spinal and general anesthetics and toxic doses of barbiturates. Overdoses of drugs that are used in treating high blood pressure, including guanethidine, reserpine, and ganglionic and adrenergic blocking agents, can also cause shock of this kind. In all of these situations, intramuscular administration of the adrenergic drugs listed above produces a long-lasting rise in blood pressure that keeps the vital tissues well supplied with blood. In acute emergencies, I.V. infusion of *levarterenol+* (Levophed) may be preferred for its immediate vasopressor effect.

CARDIOGENIC SHOCK. The heart muscle of a patient who has suffered an acute coronary attack may fail to pump enough blood to meet its own need for oxygen. In about 10 to 15 percent of cases this leads to cardiac shock, a condition with a very high mortality rate. Certain adrenergic drugs that promote better blood flow through the coronary arteries may help to reduce the high death rate in this cardiac disorder. However, these drugs must be very carefully administered to avoid doing further damage to the ischemic myocardium.

The drugs most commonly recommended are *levarterenol+*, which is usually administered by intravenous infusion in a hospital setting, and *metaraminol+* (Aramine) which can be administered intramuscularly in the patient's home or in the ambulance as well as intravenously in the hospital. Both drugs act mainly on alpha adrenergic receptors in the blood vessels. The resulting rise in peripheral arterial resistance and constriction of the veins leads to an increase in cardiac output, aortic pressure, and coronary artery blood flow. These drugs also make the myocardium contract more forcefully without accelerating the heart excessively.

《 *Administration of levarterenol.* To avoid drug-induced hypertension and cardiac arrhythmias, levarterenol must be administered very carefully. The nurse never leaves the patient unattended. She checks his blood pressure every two minutes at first and every five minutes later, after blood pressure has risen to the desired level—usually 90 to 100 mm of Hg systolic. Headache is a symptom and projectile vomiting a sign that blood pressure is building up to a level that adversely affects brain function.

Care is also taken to avoid local leakage of the levarterenol solution with resulting ischemia, necrosis, and sloughing of tissue, or even gangrene. The nurse checks the infusion site frequently to be sure that the solution is flowing freely. The injection is best made into a large antecubital or femoral vein rather than one on the back of the hand or in the ankle. If signs are seen that indicate excessive local vasoconstriction, the infusion must be stopped immediately. When the physician has been notified, he may order that the infusion be restarted in another area. If the first site stays blanched, the doctor may infiltrate the area with *phentolamine+* (Regitine), an alpha adrenergic blocking agent that antagonizes the local vasoconstrictor effect of levarterenol. Promptly administered in this way, phentolamine may prevent tissue damage and necrosis.

BACTEREMIC (SEPTIC) SHOCK. Patients with serious infections often suffer circulatory collapse when bacteria spread to the bloodstream. Gram-negative pathogens produce and release an endotoxin that is believed to play a part in causing shock in such cases. Because endotoxic shock is marked by severe constriction of blood vessels in visceral and other organs, some authorities advocate the use of *vasodilator* drugs rather than vasoconstrictors. Alpha adrenergic blocking agents are being tried experimentally for treating endotoxic shock. Two adrenergic vasodilator drugs that also stimulate the heart —*isoproterenol+* and *mephentermine* (Wyamine)—have also been employed in endotoxic and other kinds of shock.

The use of isoproterenol for this purpose requires constant monitoring of the patient's heart rate, blood pressure, and central venous pressure to avoid overdosage. The rate of infusion flow is reduced whenever the patient's heart begins to beat at a rate above 110 per minute, or discontinued, if blood pressure begins to fall. To prevent a drop in pressure due to vasodilation, it is important to correct hypovolemia before administering isoproterenol. The nurse takes frequent readings of central venous pressure before and during administration of isoproterenol, blood, plasma, and plasma expanders to avoid either excessive vasodilation or overloading the circulation with fluid.

In addition to preparing and administering adrenergic and other drugs for treating shock, the nurse watches the patient's responses to treatment. She also offers the patient emotional support by her words and actions, as it is important for the shock patient to be kept calm and quiet. Often, just watching the skilled nurse go about her many tasks in caring for him competently serves as a source of reassurance to the shock patient. The patient's alarmed family may also require special consideration and counseling, particularly in explaining that the patient needs to be kept quiet, making limitations on visiting necessary.

LOCAL VASOCONSTRICTION

Adrenergic drugs are often applied topically or injected subcutaneously to produce constriction of blood vessels at several local sites. Sometimes, for example, *epinephrine+*, *phenylephrine+*, or other sympathomimetic amines are added to solutions of local anesthetics to reduce the rate at which these nerve-numbing drugs are swept into the systemic circulation. Vasoconstriction serves two purposes here: (1) it prolongs the local pain-preventing effect of the anesthetic; and (2) it keeps the anesthetic from being absorbed too rapidly with possible toxic effects on the heart and brain.

Epinephrine solution 1:1,000 is often applied topically to stop nosebleed or to stem bleeding after a tonsillectomy. The same solution, injected subcutaneously in acute allergic emergencies (see p. 303), owes some of its effectiveness to its ability to constrict vessels in the skin and mucous membranes. This helps to halt development of urticarial wheals and angioneurotic edema.

Epinephrine is also often applied to the surface of the eye in treating open-angle glaucoma. The resulting constriction of ocular blood vessels helps to reduce the flow of fluid into the eye and thus lowers intraocular pressure. Patients should be warned in advance that these eye drops may sting and be reassured that the discomfort will not last long. Such stinging ordinarily stops with continued treatment. However, some patients become sensitive to this drug and it may have to be discontinued if persistent redness, itching, and burning develop.

NASAL DECONGESTION

Certain adrenergic drugs (see Table 23-2) are used mainly for relief of symptoms in the common cold and in seasonal and perennial allergic rhinitis. They are usually applied topically as nose drops or sprays. This constricts the dilated arterioles of the mucous membranes of the nose and sinuses, thus shrinking the swollen membranes and opening clogged nasal passages.

Overuse of nasal decongestants can cause an undesirable secondary, or rebound congestion. Systemic absorption can cause nervousness, heart palpitations, and other side effects of sympathomimetic drugs. To avoid letting the drops trickle down the throat, the patient should be instructed to keep his head down below the side of the bed when applying adrenergic vasoconstrictor-decongestant drug nose drops.

BRONCHIAL EFFECTS OF ADRENERGIC DRUGS

Certain sympathomimetic amines (see Table 23-3) stimulate beta (β_2, inhibitory)-type adrenergic receptors in bronchial smooth muscle. This action relaxes bronchospasm and relieves such symptoms of bronchial asthma as wheezing and dyspnea. The bronchospasmolytic and vasoconstrictive effects brought about by these drugs is also useful for symptomatic relief of other acute and chronic conditions in which the pulmonary tract becomes obstructed.

CLINICAL APPLICATIONS OF BRONCHIAL EFFECTS. Bronchial asthma is a chronic disorder marked by frequent attacks that are triggered by exposure to pollens and other specific allergens, or by respiratory tract infections and

TABLE 23-2 *Adrenergic Nasal Decongestant Drugs**

Nonproprietary or Official Name	Trade Name or Synonym	Dosage
Cyclopentamine HCl N.F.	Clopane	0.5–1% topically
Ephedrine (and its salts) U.S.P. and N.F.		0.5–3% topically
Mephentermine sulfate U.S.P.	Wyamine	0.5% topically
Naphazoline HCl N.F.	Privine	0.5% topically
Oxymetazoline HCl N.F.	Afrin	0.5% topically
Phenylephrine HCl U.S.P.	Neo-Synephrine	0.125–0.5% topically
Phenylpropanolamine HCl N.F.	Propadrine	25–50 mg orally
Propylhexedrine HCl N.F.	Benzedrex	Topically by inhaler
Tetrahydrozyline HCl N.F.	Tyzine	0.05–0.1%
Tuaminoheptane sulfate N.F.	Tuamine	1–2%
Xylometazoline HCl N.F.	Otrivin	0.05–0.1%

* These sympathomimetic amines are usually instilled in dilute solution as drops and occasionally as nasal packs or tampons. Some are inhaled as vapors; others, including ephedrine, phenylephrine, and phenylpropanolamine, are effective when taken by mouth.

TABLE 23-3 *Adrenergic Bronchodilator Drugs*

Nonproprietary or Official Name	Trade Name or Synonym	Dosage
Epinephrine bitartrate U.S.P. in Medihaler-Epi		0.3 mg per inhalation
Epinephrine U.S.P.	Adrenalin	0.2–0.5 mg I.M., s.c., or by inhalation
Ephedrine sulfate U.S.P.		25 to 50 mg orally
Isoproterenol HCl U.S.P.	Isuprel	10 to 15 mg sublingually
Isoproterenol sulfate U.S.P.	Norisodrine	3 mg orally or 0.125 mg per inhalation
Metaproterenol	Alupent	0.65 mg per inhalation (2 to 3 inhalations)
Methoxyphenamine HCl	Orthoxine	50–100 mg orally
Protokylol HCl	Caytine	2 to 4 mg orally; 0.1 to 0.5 mg I.M. or s.c.
Pseudoephedrine HCl N.F.	Sudafed	30–60 mg orally

emotional upset. Several classes of drugs are employed for symptomatic relief, including not only adrenergic drugs, but also corticosteroids, expectorants, and other mucus-liquefying and bronchodilator drugs.

Patients who suffer recurrent but relatively mild attacks often get rapid relief by inhaling aerosol mists containing *epinephrine*+ (Adrenalin) or *isoproterenol*+ (Isuprel; Norisodrine). The nurse often teaches the patient how to use the nebulizer. He should be told to press his lips tightly around the plastic mouthpiece before releasing the medicated mist. This allows the entire dose to reach the bronchi without any loss.

Epinephrine solution is also injected subcutaneously for treating more severe attacks. Here too, the nurse can help teach the patient and members of his family how to make such injections. They should be given opportunities to practice, using a sterile saline solution, so that they can perform the injection properly in an actual acute attack, despite nervousness and dyspnea.

Ephedrine+ is an orally effective adrenergic drug with a more prolonged bronchodilator and decongestive action. Taken regularly, it reduces the frequency of mild asthmatic attacks, but— like other drugs of this class—it tends to become less effective when used steadily. Thus, it is often alternated with or combined with a *non*adrenergic theophylline-type bronchodilator. It is also often combined with a barbiturate or other sedative to counteract the nervousness and insomnia sometimes caused by the stimulating effect of ephedrine on the central nervous system.

ACUTE ANAPHYLACTIC REACTIONS
(See also Chapter 18.)

Epinephrine 1:1,000 solution is the best drug for treating anaphylactic shock. It must be administered immediately, as death can occur very quickly in this acute medical emergency. A dose of 0.3 to 0.5 ml is administered intramuscularly or by deep subcutaneous injection, and the area is massaged to speed its absorption. However, if circulatory collapse has occurred, the dose is diluted with 10 ml of saline solution and injected slowly into a vein. The nurse may have the responsibility of preparing solutions of epinephrine and other drugs for injection in this emergency. She also keeps the allergy emergency kit stocked with drugs and equipment for performing a tracheotomy or endotracheal intubation.

OCULAR EFFECTS OF ADRENERGIC DRUGS

Sympathomimetic drugs have two types of effects on the eye:

1. They cause the radial muscle of the iris to contract in a direction that leads to dilation of the pupil (*mydriasis*).

2. Applied topically, they cause ocular blood vessels to constrict, thus reducing redness that is the result of congestion. This vasoconstricting effect also tends to reduce the pressure of fluids within the eye.

These ocular actions account both for the usefulness of these drugs in the diagnosis and treatment of certain eye disorders and for their potentially harmful effects in some patients.

CLINICAL APPLICATIONS OF OCULAR EFFECTS. Topical application of *epinephrine+* and *phenylephrine+* solutions, for example, is employed in the management of *open-angle glaucoma*. The vasoconstricting effect of these drugs tends to reduce the production and inflow of fluid into the eye. Thus, when applied together with a miotic such as pilocarpine, these and other adrenergic drugs help to produce an additive drop in intraocular pressure. However, their use is contraindicated in narrow (closed)-angle glaucoma, because the mydriatic effect of adrenergic drugs may make the iris muscle crowd back into the angle, thus blocking fluid outflow. The resulting rise in intraocular pressure could set off an attack of acute glaucoma in such patients.

The mydriatic action is desirable for diagnostic purposes when the ophthalmologist wants to examine internal structures within the patient's eyes. Applications of a strong (10 percent) solution of phenylephrine, for example, widens the pupil in a way that lets the doctor see the entire eye more easily. Adrenergic drugs do *not* ordinarily cause *cycloplegia* (paralysis of accommodation). Therefore, these drugs are not used alone for refraction, although they are occasionally combined with cycloplegic drugs of the anticholinergic class such as atropine and homatropine for this diagnostic purpose (Chapter 22).

Adrenergic and anticholinergic drugs are also sometimes applied together for preventing adhesions from forming as a result of inner eye inflammation—in uveitis, for example. However, adrenergic vasoconstriction is sometimes followed by a rebound congestion and redness. If allergic sensitivity occurs, it may be necessary to discontinue further application of phenylephrine or epinephrine. Because both these drugs can cause a stinging sensation, it is desirable to warn the patient to expect this and to assure him that it won't last long. The doctor may, of course, order prior application of a topical anesthetic solution to prevent pain caused by concentrations of adrenergic drugs that tend to cause irritation.

Even when applied topically, enough epinephrine may be absorbed to produce systemic side effects (see *Summary*, p. 305). Thus, the nurse should employ the same measures for minimizing absorption of adrenergic drug solutions as were recommended for cholinergic (miotic) agents (Chapter 21).

ADRENERGIC DRUG EFFECTS ON OTHER ORGANS

Although adrenergic drugs may affect the functioning of uterine and gastrointestinal smooth muscles, they are rarely used clinically for this purpose because of adverse effects produced elsewhere by the high doses needed to influence these organs. *Epinephrine* is sometimes used to relax uterine spasms during labor. *Isometheptene* (Octin) has been employed as an intestinal antispasmodic, but anticholinergic drugs are usually preferred. This drug is also sometimes used in treating migraine headaches in patients unable to tolerate ergotamine (see Chapter 16).

SUMMARY of Chief Pharmacological Actions and Clinical Uses of Adrenergic Drugs

Cardiac Actions and Uses

Increase in rate and strength of heartbeat:
Useful in treating cardiac slowing and heart block in Stokes-Adams disease and the carotid sinus syndrome; may help to resuscitate heart in cardiac standstill, or asystole, but not in ventricular fibrillation.

Decrease in heart rate as a result of reflex vagal stimulation:
May be useful for terminating paroxysmal atrial (supraventricular) tachycardia.

Strengthening and slowing of heart and coronary vasodilation:
These actions may be desirable in adrenergic drugs used in cardiogenic shock.

Vascular Actions and Uses

Local vasodilation by some adrenergic drugs is useful for treating certain peripheral vascular diseases.

Local vasoconstriction is useful in many circumstances:

1. Nasal decongestant in acute and chronic inflammatory and allergic disorders, including the common cold, hay fever, vasomotor rhinitis, and others
2. Ocular decongestant in conjunctivitis and in some forms of glaucoma
3. Hemostatic in epistaxis (nosebleed) and after tonsillectomy and other throat surgery
4. Additive to local anesthetic solutions for reducing systemic absorption of these drugs
5. Antiallergic *action* in urticaria, angioneurotic edema, and anaphylactoid reaction

Systemic vasoconstriction to raise blood pressure, in:

1. Acute hypotension caused by drug-induced reduction of sympathetic vasomotor tone (for example, spinal and inhalation anesthetics, ganglionic and adrenergic blocking agents, and others)
2. Cardiogenic shock following myocardial infarction
3. Circulatory collapse from other causes, including that resulting from severe hemorrhage (here, replacement of blood or restoration of blood volume with plasma or other fluids is the most important measure and the use of adrenergic vasopressors is only adjunctive)

Bronchial Muscle Actions and Uses

Stimulation of beta, β_2, type (inhibitory) receptors in smooth muscle of bronchi relaxes spasm and dilates bronchial tubes in the following conditions:

1. Acute and chronic asthmatic states
2. Pulmonary emphysema and fibrosis
3. Chronic bronchitis and bronchiectasis

Miscellaneous Actions and Uses

Stimulation of alpha type (motor) receptors in radial muscle of the iris results in mydriasis, which is useful for facilitating ophthalmological examinations

Gastrointestinal, genitourinary, and biliary tract musculature may occasionally be relaxed to relieve spasm of these viscera in ureteral and biliary colic and in dysmenorrhea and labor

Skeletal muscle is sometimes strengthened by ephedrine in myasthenia gravis

Dilated cerebral vessels are sometimes constricted by isometheptene in migraine headaches

Increased tone of trigone and sphincter of urinary bladder brought about by ephedrine may be helpful in nocturnal enuresis (bedwetting)

Central stimulation by amphetamines and ephedrine may be useful in narcolepsy, and in other clinical situations

SUMMARY of Side Effects, Toxicity, and Contraindications of Adrenergic Drugs

Side Effects

Cardiovascular:
Cardiac palpitations, possible precordial pain, pallor, headache, hypertension.

Nervous:
Anxiety, nervousness, vertigo tremor, insomnia.
Other:
Dilated pupils, nausea, vomiting, glycosuria.

Severe Toxicity

Cardiac arrhythmias ranging from tachycardia to bradycardia and various other irregularities, including possible fatal ventricular fibrillation. Severe hypertension may result in cerebral hemorrhage, especially in patients with cerebral atherosclerosis. Cardiac dilatation and pulmonary edema may also develop as a result of a sharp, sustained rise in blood pressure.

Cautions and Contraindications

Give with extreme caution, if at all, to patients with coronary artery and other organic heart disease, hypertension, hyperthyroidism, and diabetes. These drugs are also undesirable for elderly patients and should not be employed during inhalation anesthesia with halogenated hydrocarbons (for instance, chloroform; trichlorethylene) and cyclopropane.

Patients receiving intravenous infusions of potent vasopressors should not be left unattended; blood pressure should be taken frequently; the site of infusion should be frequently inspected for signs of extravasation and tissue infiltration.

S U M M A R Y of Some Points for Nurses to Remember in Administering Vasopressors and Vasodilators for Shock

1. Apply all the nursing measures that are part of the nurse's responsibility in any emergency. These include not only concern for the patient's welfare during the emergency, but also relating to the patient and his family in a beneficial manner after the emergency is over.

2. During the intravenous administration of adrenergic vasopressors such as *levarterenol,* observe the patient constantly for signs of toxicity (for instance, take the patient's blood pressure every two to five minutes or at other intervals specified by the physician).

3. During the intravenous administration of adrenergic vasodilator-heart stimulant drugs such as *isoproterenol,* constant monitoring of the patient's blood pressure, heart rate, and central venous pressure is necessary to avoid overdosage.

4. When administering vasopressor infusions, take extra care in moving the patient to keep the needle from being dislodged. Check the injection site frequently for signs of leakage and tissue infiltration, which require that the flow of solution be stopped. Notify the physician so that the infusion can be restarted as soon as possible.

5. Remember that these are very powerful drugs and that errors in dosage are especially serious. Take special note of the strength of the solution (is it 1:100 or 1:1,000?), the dosage (0.10 ml or 1.0 ml), and the route of administration (spray for inhalation, subcutaneous injection).

6. Adrenergic drugs are usually kept on emergency trays. Be sure that the solutions are in good condition (for instance, have not turned brown) and in ample supply. Check the tray frequently and replace used materials as soon as the emergency is over.

Clinical Nursing Situation: I

The Situation: Mr. Strauss, age 48, received an intramuscular injection of penicillin in a hospital outpatient department for treatment of a carbuncle. As Mr. Strauss was walking out of the door of the treatment room he suddenly slumped to the floor. A nurse and a physician rushed over to him. The patient was unconscious, pale, his pulse was thready and barely perceptible.

The physician asked the nurse to prepare and administer s.c. 0.30 cc of epinephrine immediately. He stated that he believed Mr. Strauss to be in anaphylactic shock as a result of the penicillin. After Mr. Strauss had received the injection of epinephrine, he began to respond, his pulse became stronger, and his blood pressure reading was 75. At this time, Mr. Strauss was placed in a bed and the physician ordered an infusion started with 1,000 cc of 5 percent dextrose in distilled water. The doctor stated that, depending on the patient's response, it might be necessary for Levophed to be given intravenously. Oxygen was administered by face mask at the rate of 5 liters per minute.

The Problem: Assume that you are the nurse in this situation.

(1) Describe the observations you would make and record concerning Mr. Strauss's condition.

(2) Discuss the legal implications of the physician's verbal order for epinephrine in this situation.

(3) Describe the observations you would make if Mr. Strauss were to be given Levophed.

Clinical Nursing Situation: II

The Situation: Ms. Watton was unconscious and had extremely profuse vaginal bleeding when brought by ambulance to the emergency room. Her pulse was barely perceptible and a blood pressure reading could not be obtained. Her circulatory collapse even made it hard to get an I.V. infusion started while waiting for blood units of her type to arrive.

After the blood transfusion was begun, Ms. Watton was transferred to the intensive care unit with a provisional diagnosis of hemorrhagic shock resulting from abortion. Despite the transfusion, her blood pressure remained low and her pulse was very weak and rapid. After 15 minutes, the house physician decided to order an infusion containing Levophed.

The nurse stayed with the patient recording pulse rate, central venous pressure, and blood pressure. These and other vital signs soon started to show improvement, the vaginal bleeding began to abate somewhat, and Ms. Watton regained consciousness. Finally, when her rapid pulse slowed to about 88, the CVP read 15 cm H_2O and blood pressure stabilized at 110/80, the vasopressor drug was stopped and a saline infusion only was continued at a rate of 40 drops per minute.

Unfortunately, another patient in the intensive care unit with a tracheostomy began to suffer difficulty in breathing, and the nurse had to suction her until respiration became easier. Upon her return to Ms. Watton's bedside after a period of about 20 minutes, during which vital signs had not been checked, the nurse noted that *she* was now having breathing difficulty, as indicated by rapid respiration and moist sounds. She also saw that the infusion was running at a more rapid rate than that at which she and the doctor had initially regulated it.

The Problem: Assume that you are the nurse caring for Ms. Watton. Describe what steps you would take and the order in which you would take them. State your rationale for each of these actions, and for the earlier steps in treatment of this patient.

DRUG DIGEST

EPHEDRINE AND ITS HYDROCHLORIDE AND SULFATE SALTS U.S.P. AND N.F.

Actions and Indications. This adrenergic drug is an effective bronchodilator employed in asthma to prevent and treat mild attacks when taken orally. Applied topically to the nasal mucosa, it opens blocked nasal and sinus passages but tends to cause rebound congestion if used excessively in acute and chronic rhinitis. It produces a prolonged vasopressor effect that helps to prevent falls in blood pressure during spinal and general anesthesia. It has been used for treating nocturnal enuresis (bed wetting), as an adjunct to cholinergic drugs in myasthenia gravis, and for its central stimulating effect in narcolepsy.

Side Effects, Cautions, and Contraindications. Caution is required in patients with hyperthyroidism, diabetes, coronary insufficiency, and hypertension. Its use by patients taking tricyclic-type and mono-amine oxidase inhibitor-type antidepressants may set off a sharp rise in blood pressure. Caution is also required in elderly men with enlarged prostate glands to avoid urinary retention. Insomnia, nervousness, and restlessness may result from this drug's stimulating effect on the central nervous system.

Dosage and Administration. Administered orally or parenterally in adult doses of 25 to 50 mg and doses of 12.5 to 25 mg. three to six times daily for children. Nose drops or sprays contain 0.5 to 1 percent concentrations. An ophthalmic solution of 3 percent is employed as a mydriatic by topical applications to the eye.

EPINEPHRINE AND ITS BITARTRATE AND HYDROCHLORIDE SALTS U.S.P. (Adrenalin)

Actions and Indications. This prototype sympathomimetic amine has many potent actions. It is most useful as a bronchodilator for treating acute asthma attacks. This effect and its vasoconstrictor and cardiac stimulating action can be lifesaving in anaphylactic shock, cardiac arrest, and other acute emergencies.

Topical application stops bleeding from the skin and mucous membranes of the nose and throat. Applied to the eye, alone or together with miotics, it produces a drop in intraocular pressure in wide-angle glaucoma, but because of its mydriatic action, its use is contraindicated in closed-angle glaucoma. Epinephrine is often added in low concentrations to injectable solutions of local anesthetics to delay their systemic absorption.

Side Effects, Cautions, and Contra-indications. Overdosage can cause dangerous cardiovascular reactions, including hypertensive headache and crisis, and rapid cardiac irregularities including fibrillation. More commonly, overdosage is marked by pallor, heart palpitations, and feelings of anxiety and nervousness. Caution is required in patients with angina pectoris to avoid causing coronary insufficiency and chest pains; care is also required in patients with diabetes, hyperthyroidism, and hypertension.

Dosage and Administration. Doses of 0.2 to 0.5 ml of a 1:1,000 solution are injected s.c. or I.M. in acute asthma attacks, or I.V. after dilution in dextrose or saline solution, in extreme emergencies. Aqueous and oily solutions—1:400

and 1:500 I.M.—give more prolonged bronchodilator effects. Other solutions (0.1 to 1 percent) are inhaled as a mist. Topical nasal and ocular solutions (0.5 to 2 percent) are instilled in drop dosage.

ISOPROTERENOL HCl U.S.P. (Isuprel; and others)

Actions and Indications. This adrenergic drug produces cardiac stimulation, peripheral vasodilation, and relaxation of bronchial spasm. The heart stimulating effect is often useful for counteracting cardiac slowing in Stokes-Adams disease and the carotid sinus syndrome and in treating cardiac standstill. Drug-induced vasodilation and increase in cardiac output may be beneficial in some forms of circulatory shock. Symptomatic relief of bronchial spasm is desirable in asthma, bronchitis, bronchiectasis, and pulmonary emphysema and fibrosis.

Side Effects, Cautions, and Contra-indications. Tachycardia with heart palpitations felt as pounding in the chest is a side effect that accounts for this drug's being contraindicated in patients with rapid cardiac rhythm irregularities. It is used with caution in patients with angina pectoris and other forms of coronary insufficiency, hyperthyriodism, and diabetes. It should not be administered together with epinephrine, which also stimulates the heart. When infused by the I.V. route for treating shock, the solution's rate of flow is slowed or discontinued if the patient's heart rate goes above 110 beats per minute.

Dosage and Administration. Solutions are available for forming mists that are inhaled in doses adjusted to the needs of each patient for control of acute asthma attacks. The drug is also administered sublingually in doses of 10 to 15 mg several times a day up to a maximum of 60 mg daily. A 1:5,000 sol is diluted for I.V. infusion in shock, or 1 ml may be injected undiluted by the I.M., subcutaneous, or intracardiac routes.

LEVARTERENOL BITARTRATE U.S.P. (Levophed)

Actions and Indications. Shock from all causes including acute coronary attacks, severe infection, injury, bleeding, and surgery is treated with this potent vasoconstrictor. The drug's ability to constrict arterioles without excessively increasing the heart rate makes it useful for counteracting loss of vasomotor tone during spinal anesthesia or after drug-induced or surgical sympathectomy

and following removal of pheochromocytoma tumors.

Side Effects, Cautions, and Contra-indications. Patients are watched constantly during I.V. infusion, and the rate of flow is carefully controlled to avoid development of hypertension, cardiac arrhythmias, and local tissue damage. The drug is contraindicated in patients anesthetized with halothane, cyclopropane, and other agents that tend to sensitize the heart to the arrhythmia-producing effect of this drug. It is also contraindicated in patients with blood clots in mesenteric vessels, and the infusion is administered cautiously to elderly patients and those with peripheral vascular diseases to avoid obstructions to flow that could lead to local leakage of the solution with possible development of necrosis and sloughing or gangrene.

Dosage and Administration. Four ml of a 0.2 percent solution is diluted in 1,000 ml of a 5 percent dextrose solution and administered by I.V. infusion in individually adjusted dosage. Blood pressure is taken every two minutes until it rises to the desired low normal level; then it is checked every five minutes. The number of drops administered per minute is estimated by use of a drip bulb.

METARAMINOL BITARTRATE U.S.P. (Aramine)

Actions and Indications. This adrenergic vasopressor drug raises low blood pressure in acute hypotensive states and shock. It constricts the patient's arterioles and increases the strength of his heartbeat. Because this drug does not ordinarily speed up the heart rate or cause cardiac irregularities, it is safer than most other sympathomimetic amines for treating cardiogenic shock. It is also used to prevent sharp drops in blood pressure during spinal anesthesia and as an adjunct to other measures in the management of various other kinds of shock.

Side Effects, Cautions, and Contra-indications. To avoid causing cardiac arrhythmias, this substance should *not* be injected when patients have been anesthetized with halothane or cyclopropane. Too rapid a rise in blood pressure can also set off heart rhythm irregularities as well as hypertensive reactions. Caution is needed in patients with a history of hypertension, hyperthyroidism, diabetes, or heart disease.

Dosage and Administration. Intramuscular injection of 2 to 10 mg produces a relatively prompt and prolonged rise in blood pressure. Intravenous injection of 0.5 to 5 mg, which is reserved for extreme emergencies, acts within one or two minutes. Slow intravenous infusion of a dilute solution of the drug in 5 percent dextrose or isotonic saline is more commonly used, because it is considered safer when the rate of flow is properly adjusted in accordance with the patient's response.

METHOXAMINE HCl U.S.P. (Vasoxyl)

Actions and Indications. This sympathomimetic amine raises low blood pressure by constricting the arterioles. Unlike most other adrenergic drugs, it does not cause cardiac irregularities in patients anesthetized with halothane or cyclopropane. Thus, it is particularly useful for overcoming hypotensive reactions that develop during surgery conducted under these general anesthetics. This vasopressor is also employed to prevent or counteract drops in blood pressure following administration of spinal anesthetics. It can be used to end episodes of paroxysmal supraventricular tachycardias in less than a minute.

Side Effects, Cautions, and Contraindications. Overdosage that produces too high blood pressure can cause severe headache with projectile vomiting and excessive slowing of the heart rate. Particular care is required in administering this drug to patients with higher grades of hypertension and those with hyperthyroidism.

Dosage and Administration. Intramuscular dosage of 10 to 15 mg is usually enough to prevent or correct hypotension. In emergencies, 3 to 5 mg may be administered by slow intravenous injection. In treating prolonged shock and for hypertension following an acute coronary attack, 35 to 40 mg may be diluted in 250 ml of 5 percent dextrose solution and administered by slow I.V. infusion. The usual dose for restoring normal rhythm in paroxysmal tachycardia is 10 mg given by slow I.V. injection.

PHENYLEPHRINE HCl U.S.P. (Neo-Synephrine)

Actions and Indications. This adrenergic vasoconstrictor is applied topically to nasal or ocular mucous membranes to produce decongestive effects or administered parenterally for cardiovascular effects.

It is used for symptomatic relief of the common cold, in hay fever, sinusitis, and perennial rhinitis. Intraocular pressure is reduced in wide-angle glaucoma and congestion lessened in intraocular inflammation.

Injected solutions prevent hypotension in spinal anesthesia and are useful for raising blood pressure in drug-induced shock. The drug may also bring about sinus rhythm in patients with paroxysmal tachycardia.

Side Effects, Cautions, and Contraindications. Overdosage may cause hypertensive headache and cardiac arrhythmias. The drug should be used with caution, if at all, in patients with hypertension, hyperthyroidism, diabetes, or coronary disease. It is contraindicated in patients receiving monoamine oxidase inhibitor agents or oxytocic drugs. Ophthalmic administration is contraindicated in narrow-angle glaucoma.

Dosage and Administration. For intranasal administration, it is available as drops, spray, or jelly in concentrations of 0.125 to 1 percent. Ophthalmic solutions of 2.5 percent and 10 percent are instilled in drop dosage. Parenteral solutions are injected s.c., I.M., or I.V. in doses usually ranging from 0.5 to 5 mg.

References

TREATMENT OF SHOCK

Alexander, S., and Fonad, G.A. Treatment of cardiogenic shock. *Med. Clin. N. Amer.*, 53:309, 1969 (March).

Chandler, J.G. The physiology and treatment of shock. *RN*, 34:42, 1971 (June).

Dietzman, R.H., et al. Drugs in the treatment of shock. *Pharmacol. Physicians*, 4:1, 1970 (Aug.).

Lambert, K., et al. Pathophysiology and management of bacteremic shock. *AORN J.*, 10:67, 1969 (Nov.).

Morris, D.G. The patient in cardiogenic shock. *Cardiovasc. Nurs.*, 5:15, 1969 (July-Aug.).

O'Donohue, W.J., Jr. Current concepts in the pharmacologic approach to shock. *Southern Med J.*, 62:1402, 1969 (Nov.).

Rodman, M.J. Vasopressors vs. vasodilators in treating shock. *RN*, 31:59, 1968 (Dec.).

Shoemaker, W.C., et al. The dilemma of vasopressors and vasodilators in the therapy of shock. *Surg. Gynec. Obstet.*, 132:51, 1971 (Jan.).

TREATMENT OF ANAPHYLACTIC SHOCK

Craven, R. F. Anaphylactic shock. *Amer. J. Nurs.*, 72:718, 1972 (April).

Hildreth, E.A. Some common allergic emergencies. *Med Clin. N. Amer.*, 50:1313, 1966 (Sept.).

Falleroni, A.E. Treatment of allergic emergencies. *Mod. Treatm.*, 5:782, 1968 (Sept.).

Lister, J. Nursing intervention in anaphylactic shock. *Amer. J. Nurs.*, 72:720, 1972 (April).

Rodman, M.J. Drugs for allergic disorders. Part 1. Anaphylaxis and asthma. *RN*, 34: 63, 1971 (June).

24.

Adrenergic Blocking Drugs

A few drugs are available that occupy adrenergic receptors in various organs *without* setting off the responses produced by norepinephrine, epinephrine, and the sympathomimetic drugs that were discussed in the preceding chapter. In fact, by attaching themselves to alpha- or beta-type adrenergic receptors, these drugs often interfere with the transmission of nerve impulses from the sympathetic nervous system to the blood vessels and other organs. These *adrenergic blocking agents*, as they are called, can also keep epinephrine from exerting its effects.

Alpha Adrenergic Blocking Agents

Drugs that block the alpha adrenergic receptors in the smooth muscle walls of blood vessels cause these muscles to relax. This results in dilatation of the vessels and an increased flow of blood to the skin and other structures that receive their blood supply from the dilated arterioles. This local effect on blood flow is sometimes useful clinically for treating patients suffering from *peripheral vascular diseases*. The use of such alpha adrenergic blocking agents as *azeptine* (Ilidar), *phenoxybenzamine+* (Dibenzyline), and *tolazoline+* (Priscoline) for this purpose is discussed in Chapter 32, *Drugs for Peripheral Vascular Disease*.

Doses of these drugs large enough to cut off sympathetic nerve impulses to the splanchnic arterioles and other vessels involved in maintaining systemic blood pressure produce a pressure drop that could, in theory, be useful in treating essential hypertension. In practice, however, the alpha adrenergic blocking agents have not proved clinically effective for this purpose compared to the ganglionic blocking agents and the new drugs that affect the function of adrenergic nerves (see below).

In one type of hypertension, however, certain adrenergic blockers are sometimes useful for diagnosis and treatment. *Phentolamine+* (Regitine), for example, is used to help determine whether a patient's high blood pressure is caused by *pheochromocytoma*, a tumor of the adrenal medulla that produces large amounts of epinephrine. Phentolamine blocks the blood pressure elevating effect of epinephrine when this adrenergic blocker is administered in doses that do *not* lower high blood pressure in other kinds of hypertension. Thus, a sharp fall in blood pressure following the administration of phentolamine is a positive test for pheochromocytoma; if, on the other hand the patient's high blood pressure stays steady, the patient probably has essential hypertension.

One alpha adrenergic blocking agent, *phenoxybenzamine+* (Dibenzyline) is being tested in the treatment of certain types of shock including, particularly, bacteremic shock (p. 311). Its use in such cases is said to cut off some of the sympathetic impulses that have caused excessive vasoconstriction. The resulting vasodilation is claimed to produce the following desirable effects on the flow of blood in the patient's body:

1. Blood pooled in the veins is freed to return to the right side of the heart.

2. The cardiac output is increased, and

3. The flow of blood to the brain, the heart muscle, and the viscera by way of dilated arterioles is increased.

Despite these advantages, there is a danger in administering a drug that expands the circulatory space. Sudden drug-induced vasodilation can reduce the venous return to the heart rather than increase it. To prevent this, it is very important to keep the patient's blood volume at normal levels. This is done by infusing plasma, plasma expanders, or other fluids in the required quantities. As indicated previously (Chapter 23), the nurse often has the responsibility of monitoring the shock patient's central venous pressure to check for hypovolemia and to avoid overloading the heart with excessive amounts of fluid.

Beta-Type Adrenergic Blocking Agents

Drugs that block transmission of sympathetic nerve impulses to the beta (β_2) receptors of the heart can be expected to slow its rate. The one drug of this kind currently available in this country is *propranolol+* (Inderal). Its use in the treatment of various kinds of cardiac rhythm irregularities is discussed in Chapter 29, *Antiarrhythmic Drugs*.

ADRENERGIC NEURON BLOCKING DRUGS

Certain other drugs reduce transmission of sympathetic nerve impulses to the cardiovascular system. They do so by their effects on the *endings* of the *adrenergic nerves* rather than on adrenergic receptors in the heart and blood vessels. Drugs of this kind including *reserpine+*, *guanethidine+*, and *methyldopa+* are discussed in Chapter 26, *Drugs Used in Treating Hypertension*.

DRUG DIGEST

PHENTOLAMINE MESYLATE U.S.P. (Regitine)

Actions and Indications. This alpha adrenergic blocking agent is used mainly for the diagnosis of pheochromocytoma. A positive test for this tumor is suggested by a prompt and persistent fall in blood pressure by more than 35 mm of Hg systolic and 25 mm diastolic.

This drug is also injected intravenously during surgery for pheochromocytoma, if manipulation of the tumor leads to sudden release of large amounts of epinephrine with a resulting rapid rise in blood pressure to dangerous level (hypertensive crisis).

Side Effects, Cautions, and Contraindications. The drug-induced fall in blood pressure may set off reflex tachycardia. Thus, this drug is contraindicated in patients with coronary artery disease, including angina pectoris. Overdosage may also cause a severe, sustained fall in blood pressure. This is best treated by infusion of fluids to fill the dilated vascular tree, followed by administration of levarterenol to counteract adrenergic blockade of the blood vessels.

Dosage and Administration. For diagnosis, a single dose of 5 mg is injected intravenously or intramuscularly under standard conditions. For treatment of hypertensive crisis, this dose may be administered repeatedly or the drug solution may be infused continuously.

To prevent sloughing from leakage of levarterenol infusion solutions, infiltration of the affected area with 10 to 15 ml of phentolamine solution (5 to 10 mg) is recommended.

An oral dosage form, phentolamine HCl N.F., is available for use in doses of 50 mg four to six times daily for use in the period prior to surgery.

SECTION 7

Drugs

Acting

on

the

Heart

and

Circulation

25.

The Heart and Blood Vessels in Health and Disease

Cardiovascular disease causes more disability and death than any other kind of illness. Very many of the patients for whom the nurse cares suffer from diseases of the heart and blood vessels. She often administers cardiovascular drugs both in emergency situations and to patients in the chronic stages of these diseases. The following chapters of this section deal with the various classes of drugs that are used to counteract the complications caused by diseases of the circulatory system.

In order to understand how drugs are best used to bring about their therapeutic effects, we have to know how the circulatory system functions in health and disease. You have already studied the anatomy and physiology of the cardiovascular system and, in each of the following chapters, brief explanations will be offered concerning various disorders that are treated with the drugs that are to be discussed. Here, we shall review briefly some of the concepts of cardiac function and blood flow that are most pertinent to the topics that are taken up in this section of the textbook.

The Heart

The heart is a muscular organ with four hollow chambers (Fig. 25-1). Actually, there are two hearts—a right one and a left. Each is divided into two parts, an upper *atrium* and a lower *ventricle*. Blood that returns to the heart by way of the venous system first pours into the right side of the heart. The right ventricle contracts to drive the oxygen-spent blood into the lungs, where it is reoxygenated and carried to the left side of the heart by way of the

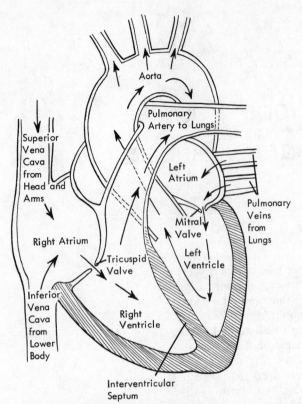

Fig. 25-1. Blood flow, into and out of the heart.

pulmonary blood vessels. Contractions of the thick muscular wall of the left ventricle then drive the blood out into the aorta, the body's largest blood vessel, and then through the rest of the circulatory system.

THE NORMAL HEART BEAT

The cardiac contractions that drive blood into the pulmonary and systemic circulation are set off by electrical impulses. These impulses arise spontaneously in specialized cells and then spread swiftly through the rest of the heart muscle. The heart cells that discharge in this way more rapidly than any others are located in a knot of tissue on the rear wall of the right atrium called the *sino-atrial*, or S-A, node.

The impulses that originate in this pacemaker are conducted across both atria, exciting the cardiac muscle cells of these chambers to contract. The wave of impulses also reaches other automatic cells located at the junction of the atria and the ventricles. This *atrioventricular*, or A-V, node is discharged by the arriving impulses and, in turn, transmits the signals to a mass of specialized conducting tissue called the A-V *bundle*, or *bundle of His*,

located in the wall (septum) between the two ventricles. This bundle divides into smaller branches that break up into a network of fine fibers within the walls of both ventricles (*Purkinje fibers*). These carry the command to contract to both ventricles.

The heart's ability to act as a forcefully contracting muscular pump depends on the precise operation of these electrical processes— *automaticity, excitability,* and *conductivity.* Normally, impulses are generated and transmitted in a manner that produces coordinated contractions of the atria and ventricles following a period in which the hollow chambers have filled with blood. If—as sometimes happens in heart disease—groups of cardiac fibers are stimulated to contract irregularly, the patient's cardiac output may be sharply reduced.

IRREGULAR HEART BEATS

Poorly coordinated cardiac contractions may have many causes. Sometimes impulses arise in automatic cells other than the S-A node more rapidly than they do in that normal pacemaker. Impulses from such so-called *ectopic* sites may then set off *premature contractions,* or *extrasystoles.* On the other hand, impulses may take abnormal pathways, or they may run into cardiac tissue that cannot conduct them properly. If the ventricles then receive too many or too few signals, they will respond with contractions at a too rapid and irregular rate, or with beats that occur too slowly. In both cases, the ventricles may fail to pump adequate quantities of blood to body tissues, including the myocardium, or heart muscle, itself.

THE ELECTROCARDIOGRAM

Abnormal formation and transmission of cardiac impulses can be readily detected by monitoring the patient's electrocardiogram (EKG). Nurses in coronary care units have learned to detect the appearance of EKG abnormalities that indicate potentially dangerous changes in cardiac function. Often, for example, the nurse is the first to see the so-called *premature ventricular complexes,* the abnormal electrical tracings that indicate the development of dangerous extrasystoles. She may then administer drugs that reduce the rate at which impulses are arising at ectopic sites, and she notes the effect that these drugs have in returning the EKG picture to normal.

On the other hand, the drugs that a heart patient is receiving may be the cause of EKG changes that are signals of potentially dangerous overdosage. For example, digitalis and various cardiac depressant drugs such as quinidine may interfere with impulse conduction through the cardiac tissues. A lengthening of the *P-R interval*—the part of the EKG picture that reflects the passage of electrical activity from the atria through the A-V conducting tissues—may indicate the onset of drug-induced *heart block*. Similarly, a gradual widening of the *QRS complex*, the wave caused by passage of the electrical impulse through the ventricles, may signal an adverse effect of these drugs on impulse conduction through these cardiac tissues. Correct interpretation of these and other EKG abnormalities, such as an inversion of the T wave that indicates recovery of cardiac excitability, for example, is essential for regulating the response of the patient's heart to these potent drugs.

THE CORONARY CIRCULATION

The heart muscle needs a constant supply of blood containing oxygen and nutrients. Deprived of part of its blood supply, the hypoxic heart can no longer continue to contract efficiently. Heart muscle ischemia of this kind causes the severe chest pains of angina pectoris and coronary occlusion. The most common cause of poor blood flow through the heart muscle is a narrowing of the coronary arteries by atherosclerosis.

The coronary vessels branch off from the aorta at the point where that vessel leaves the left ventricle. The right and left coronary arteries then subdivide into smaller and smaller vessels that move down from the surface of the myocardium to form a meshwork that feeds blood to every portion of the cardiac tissues. The coronary vessels normally widen in response to acid metabolites formed when the heart is being forced to work harder during physical exertion.

Diseased coronary vessels that are unable to dilate cannot carry enough blood to meet the increased demands of the hard-working myocardium for oxygen. Pain then forces the person with this condition to stop his activity and rest in order to bring his oxygen needs back into balance with the amount of oxygen that his coronary arteries can supply. However, when a major branch of a coronary vessel is blocked by a blood clot, rest alone will not relieve the severe ischemic pain. (See Chapter 30 for a fuller discussion of myocardial infarction following a coronary occlusion.)

NERVOUS CONTROL OF CARDIAC ACTION

Normally—as we have indicated—the heart beats at a rate set by the S-A nodal pacemaker, which operates automatically. However, the rate of this spontaneous firing, or electrical depolarization, can be altered by influences from outside the heart itself. The heart receives impulses by way of nerves from both divisions of the autonomic nervous system. The sympathetic branch sends nerve fibers to the heart that carry cardioacceleratory impulses; the parasympathetic sends impulses by way of the vagus nerves that slow the cardiac rate.

These adjustments are the result of reflex actions that are set off by stimulation of sensory receptors located in the aorta, the carotid arteries (the vessels that carry blood to the brain), and elsewhere in the body. As a result, the heart can beat harder and more rapidly when the tissues require greater amounts of oxygenated blood—during physical exercise, for example—and it can be slowed down to conserve its energy when the emergency is over. In heart failure, however, these compensatory mechanisms may fail to function efficiently, and the heart may then beat too rapidly and use up too much oxygen. The action of cardiotonic drugs of the digitalis type may then be required to reduce cardioacceleratory nerve activity, to restore vagal control, and to slow and strengthen the heart beat in other ways also (Chapter 28).

The Blood Vessels

Blood flow through the heart-lung (*pulmonary*) and myocardial (*coronary*) circulations has been discussed above. Now we shall review some of the principles of blood flow through the rest of the body by way of the so-called *systemic circulation*. The arteries and veins of this system transport oxygen and nutrients to the body tissues and carry away carbon dioxide and other waste products. The heart supplies the head of pressure that forces the blood through the entire circulatory tree and back to the right atrium. However, other factors also influence the amount of blood flowing through the blood vessels of the various body tissues at any moment.

The *peripheral arterioles* offer resistance to the blood flowing through them. This peripheral resistance changes in response to sympathetic nervous system impulses that affect the extent of contraction of arteriolar smooth muscle. An increase in vasoconstrictor impulses narrows the arterioles. This reduces blood flow in local vascular beds but tends to raise the systemic arterial blood pressure.

Drugs that block transmission of vasoconstrictor impulses tend to relax arterial smooth muscle walls. The resulting reduction in resistance to blood flow in various local regions brings more blood to those areas—an effect sometimes useful in the treatment of certain peripheral arterial diseases. The generalized reduction in peripheral resistance often helps to produce a fall in high blood pressure in patients with hypertension.

The *peripheral venules* are also constricted by sympathetic nerve impulses and dilated when sympathetic vasomotor tone is reduced. This also affects the blood pressure, particularly when a person is standing or sitting upright. The thin-walled venules can distend to hold large amounts of blood. Thus, when certain of these so-called *capacitance vessels* become distended, they tend to trap large amounts of blood. This blood that is pooled in the dilated venules does not readily return to the right atrium of the heart. The resulting reduction in venous return leads to a drop in cardiac output and, in some circumstances, to a fall in systemic blood pressure.

Drugs that constrict the venules and increase the return of blood to the right atrium are often effective for treating shock. The pressure in the right atrium, the *central venous pressure*, may also be raised by infusing fluids that bring depleted blood volume back to normal. Nurses in intensive care units often monitor the patient's central venous pressure. They do this to prevent the right heart from being overloaded with infused fluid, or to guard against an excessive reduction in the venous return of blood to the heart following administration of drugs that dilate the vessels and thus cause blood to pool peripherally.

An abnormal rise in venous pressure and in pressure in the right and left atria often occurs in patients with heart failure. The patient's weakened myocardium cannot pump all of the venous return out into the arterial circulation. As a result of this decrease in cardiac output or of an increase in atrial pressure, complex compensatory mechanisms come into play in an effort to keep the circulation functioning normally.

Unfortunately, if the heart muscle weakness continues, these reflex and hormonal mechanisms may cause the kidney to retain salty fluids. Fluid retention leads, in turn, to a rise in pressure within the venous capillaries and leakage of the fluid into the tissue spaces (edema). To overcome the edema of congestive heart failure, the doctor orders drugs that strengthen cardiac contractions and drugs that aid sodium and fluid removal by the kidneys.

In summary, we have briefly reviewed some aspects of normal circulatory system function. We have also emphasized some of the abnormalities that occur in various clinical disorders, including cardiac arrhythmias, congestive heart failure, angina pectoris, peripheral vascular diseases, and hypertension. In each case we have indicated that drugs are available for counteracting many of the complications of circulatory ailments. In the ten chapters that follow, we shall discuss in detail the many kinds of drugs that are used in the treatment of cardiovascular diseases.

26.

Drugs Used in Treating Hypertension

The Nature of Hypertension

Hypertension is a condition in which a person's blood pressure *stays* at levels higher than normal. A patient whose blood pressure reads consistently above 90 mm of Hg diastolic, measured on several different occasions during physical examinations, is usually considered to have hypertension, even when there are little or no other signs or symptoms. The higher an individual's diastolic pressure, the greater is the grade or degree of severity of the disease and the more likely he is to develop signs of organ damage that may lead to dangerous complications.

CAUSES

In most cases of chronic hypertension, the cause is unknown; in some, the patient's high pressure can be linked to a specific cause. Examples of such *secondary* hypertension include cases resulting from *pheochromocytoma* (chromaffin cell tumors); the blockage of a kidney artery, or other kinds of *renal* disease. In these conditions surgical removal of the tumor or repair of the kidney artery defect can often cure the secondary hypertension. However, there is at present no cure for high blood pressure of the first and most common kind, *primary* or *essential* hypertension, in which the causes are uncertain.

Fortunately, remarkable advances in drug therapy during the past two decades now make it possible to bring the blood pressure of most patients down to normal levels. Even though antihypertensive drugs do not counteract the unknown underlying causes of essential hypertension, drug therapy has proved capable of preventing the complications of this condition. These result from damage to vital organs so often seen in patients with severe degrees of the disease. Properly employed, drugs for treating hypertension can keep the pressure elevation from going higher and doing further damage.

COMPLICATIONS

Long-sustained elevation of systolic and diastolic blood pressure leads to damage to the walls of blood vessels in the brain, heart, kidneys, and elsewhere. The doctor can often detect the results of such pressure-induced damage by a battery of clinical and laboratory tests. In advanced cases, the patient's eyes may show abnormally constricted arterioles in the retina, with signs of swelling and bleeding near the optic nerve. The patient's heart may be enlarged, or his electrocardiogram may be abnormal. Protein may appear in the urine, and tests of the patient's blood may show abnormally high levels of blood urea nitrogen (BUN) and of serum creatinine. All this may indicate that the patient's chances of having a heart attack, stroke, aortic aneurysm, or other catastrophic cardiovascular or kidney complications are above average.

Indications for Drug Treatment

The goal of treatment in chronic essential hypertension is to lower the patient's blood pressure to normal levels and to keep it there indefinitely. The patient has to adhere quite steadily to his treatment regimen of rest, modified diet, and drug therapy. The nurse can often help the patient accept the need for drug treatment over a prolonged period.

The drugs that are so effective for helping to prevent damage to the patient's vital organs sometimes cause unpleasant side effects. Patients who have few disease-induced symptoms may want to stop taking their medication when they experience drug-induced discomfort. The nurse can play an important part in getting the patient to accept the need for treatment. He must be helped to find a middle ground between the extremes of becoming excessively preoccupied with the state of his blood pressure or of not being at all concerned about it even when he is warned that it has risen too high.

The physician has to select the drugs best suited for each individual's condition and administer them in carefully regulated dosage. The doctor's choice of drugs for a particular patient is based on the severity of his hypertension and on his ability to withstand adverse drug effects. This, in turn, depends not only upon how high his pressure is, but also on how badly damaged his vital organs already are and on how well they are functioning. The physician also considers such factors as the patient's age, sex, and even race in deciding whether what the patient is likely to gain from treatment with certain drugs is worth the risks.

MILD HYPERTENSION

Often, patients with *mild* hypertension need no drug treatment at all, or at most only a sedative. Thus, a patient whose pressure rises in response to emotional stress (*labile* hypertension) may maintain normal pressure with only an antianxiety agent such as *chlordiazepoxide+* (Librium), *meprobamate+* (Equanil; Miltown) or related minor tranquilizers. Other patients with only early essential hypertension of mild degree—for example, with diastolic pressure below 105 mm of Hg and no signs of organ damage—may be managed by a program of weight reduction, lower salt intake, and a recommendation that they get more rest and sleep.

Patients whose diastolic pressure has risen above 105 mm of Hg but stays below 115 mm are best treated with one of the *diuretic drugs* discussed below. Most cases can be controlled by small daily doses of a diuretic alone or combined with a rauwolfia alkaloid such as *reserpine+* (Serpasil, and others). Such combinations are also employed in the management of *moderate* hypertension—for example, patients with diastolic pressure above 115 mm of Hg but below 130 mm and not much evidence of organ damage. Often, the doctor adds a third drug, such as *hydralazine* (Apresoline) to the rauwolfia-diuretic regimen, if the first two together fail to keep the patient's pressure at the desired level.

SEVERE HYPERTENSION

Patients with more *severe* hypertension—for example, with diastolic pressure persistently above 130 mm of Hg and with obvious evidence of organ damage—may receive *methyl-*

dopa+ (Aldomet) as a substitute for reserpine or hydralazine. The diuretic drug is continued, as it markedly increases the hypotensive effect of methyldopa and other antihypertensive agents, including *guanethidine*+ (Ismelin). The latter is particularly useful for patients whose severe hypertension shows signs of entering the malignant, or accelerated, phase which, if not quickly checked, will cause rapid renal and other organ damage and failure of various vital functions.

In *hypertensive crisis*, an acute medical emergency marked by signs of neurological deficit, parenterally administered reserpine and methyldopa are often employed, along with high oral doses of guanethidine. In addition, some otherwise rarely used antihypertensive agents are sometimes infused slowly into a vein to bring down the extremely elevated diastolic pressure before it does irreversible brain damage or leads to death from heart failure, uremia,

or hemorrhage. Among these are the ganglionic blocking agent, *trimethaphan* (Arfonad), and *sodium nitroprusside* (p. 325; Table 26-1).

In the following discussions of the various kinds of drugs that the doctor may order for treating patients with hypertension of different degrees of severity, we shall show how each drug should best be used to make the most of its desirable properties. We shall also indicate the limitations of each drug and suggest ways to recognize its adverse effects in order to take precautions against dangerous drug-induced complications.

Types of Antihypertensive Drugs

All the drugs currently available for treating hypertension affect the circulation in two main ways: (1) by *reducing peripheral resistance*; or (2) *decreasing the cardiac output*. Some drugs do both. That is, they lower the

TABLE 26-1 *Antihypertensive Agents**

Nonproprietary Name	Trade Name	Usual Daily Dosage Range	Remarks
Alkavervir	Veriloid	9–15 mg	Mixture of *Veratrum* alkaloids
Alseroxylon	Rauwiloid	2–4 mg	*Rauwolfia* serpentina root extract (see reserpine)
Deserpidine	Harmonyl	0.25–0.5 mg	*Rauwolfia serpentina* alkaloid
Guanethidine sulfate U.S.P.	Ismelin	25–75 mg	See *Drug Digest*
Hydralazine HCl N.F.	Apresoline	40–200 mg	Blood flow to the kidneys is not reduced
Mecamylamine HCl U.S.P.	Inversine	10–25 mg	Ganglionic blocking agent
Methyldopa U.S.P.	Aldomet	750–200 mg	See *Drug Digest*
Methyldopate HCl U.S.P.	Aldomet ester	2–4 grams	See *Drug Digest*
Pargyline N.F.	Eutonyl	25–50 mg	Monoamine oxidase inhibitor
Pentolinium tartrate	Ansolysen	60–600 mg	Ganglionic blocking agent
Rauwolfia serpentina N.F.	Raudixin	50–300 mg	The whole dried root of the plant
Rescinnamine N.F.	Moderil	0.25–0.5 mg	*Rauwolfia serpentina* alkaloid
Reserpine U.S.P.	Serpasil, and others	0.25–0.5 mg	See *Drug Digest*
Sodium nitroprusside			Pharmacy prepares a fresh solution containing 60 mg per liter of dextrose for closely monitored infusion at a rate of 1 or 2 ml per minute in hypertensive crises.
Syrosingopine N.F.	Singoserp	1–3 mg	Synthetic derivative of reserpine
Trimethaphan camsylate U.S.P.	Arfonad	I.V. at a rate of 1–4 mg per minute	Rapid-acting ganglionic blocking agent

* The sulfonamide-type diuretics that are used in hypertension are listed in Chapter 27, *Diuretic Drugs*; the adrenergic blocking agents are discussed in Chapter 24.

elevated pressure within the patient's circulatory system both: (1) by dilating the arterioles so that the vessels offer less resistance to blood flowing through them; and (2) by making the heart pump less blood out into this increased circulatory space.

SYMPATHOLYTIC AGENTS

Several classes of antihypertensive agents reduce the peripheral resistance and cardiac output by interfering with nerve impulses passing over the sympathetic nervous system to the heart and blood vessels. The drugs do this by blocking the pathway at any of several points between the brain's vasomotor and cardiac control centers and the circulatory end organs.

(1) The *ganglionic blocking agents,* for example, stop the stream of impulses at the sympathetic ganglia, the relay stations between the nerves originating centrally and the outlying nerves that carry commands to the heart and blood vessels.

(2) The *adrenergic neuron blocking agents,* including such important pressure-reducing drugs as the *rauwolfia alkaloids, methyldopa+,* and *guanethidine+,* keep the terminals of sympathetic (adrenergic) nerves from transmitting impulses by reducing the amount of the neurotransmitter in the nerve ending.

(3) The *adrenergic blocking agents* keep receptors in the heart and vessels from responding to the released neurohormone when it reaches them.

Other drugs, including hydralazine (p. 324) and the diuretics, also reduce pressure but do so in other ways.

THE DIURETICS (SEE TABLE 27-1)

The thiazide-type diuretics such as *hydrochlorothiazide+* (Esidrix; Hydrodiuril, and others) are the drugs most commonly employed in treating hypertension. Used alone in small doses, these drugs produce adequate blood pressure reduction in about two out of three patients with a *mild* degree of hypertension. They do so without ordinarily producing salt and water imbalances or other kinds of side effects that occur more commonly when larger doses of diuretics are employed in treating patients with edema. Patients can take these drugs for long periods without much loss of blood pressure-lowering effectiveness.

Diuretics are also capable of increasing the effectiveness of other antihypertensive drugs when administered *in combination.* Patients with moderately severe hypertension get a much greater decrease in pressure, for example, when *methyldopa+* (Aldomet) is administered together with a diuretic than when the adrenergic nerve blocker is given alone. *Guanethidine+* (Ismelin) is also more effective for treating severe degrees of hypertension when it is combined with a diuretic. Another advantage of combining these drugs with diuretics is a reduction in certain side effects of the nerve blocking drug.

For treating patients with *malignant hypertension* or in *hypertensive crisis,* some doctors now order one of the more powerful and rapid-acting diuretics. Injected I.V. in an emergency, together with parenterally administered antihypertensive agents, *ethacrynate sodium+* (Edecrin) and *furosemide+* (Lasix) are particularly useful in acute hypertensive patients with pulmonary edema caused by left ventricle failure. After the acute crisis has been controlled, the safer oral diuretic drugs are substituted for the potent parenteral agents.

SYMPATHETIC BLOCKING DRUGS (SEE TABLE 26-1)

The manner of action by which most drugs of the several subtypes reduce blood pressure in hypertensive patients is essentially the same. That is, although drugs of different subclasses may differ in the details of their precise neurochemical mechanisms, they all act to reduce the outflow of sympathetic nerve impulses to the cardiovascular system. This, in turn, affects blood flow through the vessels to and from the heart in ways that lead to a lowering of elevated blood pressure.

All of these drugs reduce the tone of the smooth muscle in blood vessel walls. Relaxation of these vascular muscles dilates both the arterioles and venules. Arterial vasodilation results in reduced peripheral resistance and pressure; dilation of the veins leads to pooling of blood and a reduction in the amount of blood that is being returned to the heart. This reduced venous return results, in turn, in the heart's having to pump smaller amounts of blood into the arteries. Most of the sympathetic blocking drugs also reduce cardiac output directly by tending to slow the heart and to weaken the force of its contractions.

OVERDOSAGE. The shift of blood from the arterial to the venous system by the actions of these antihypertensive drugs helps to lower elevated pressure to normal. However, even slight overdosage of the potent drugs of this class can cause blood pressure to fall too far. This is most likely to occur when a patient who has been lying down stands up too suddenly. The brain is then deprived of blood, because these drugs tend to block the reflex responses that ordinarily compensate for the fall in pressure that occurs upon standing.

Postural hypotension of this kind makes the patient feel dizzy, weak, and faint. Thus, when a patient who is hospitalized during dosage adjustment of potent hypotensive drugs wants to get out of bed, the nurse assists and supports him. She also suggests that he sit on the edge of the bed for a couple of minutes before getting up and moving about. He is also told how to protect himself from falls when he will be taking the drug at home. He should sit down promptly with his head between his knees or even lie horizontally on the floor whenever he feels himself getting faint and weak while standing or walking about.

Sudden drops in blood pressure are particularly bad for elderly patients and others with poor circulation, especially if they have already had a recent stroke or heart attack. A drug-induced reduction in blood flow through cerebral and coronary vessels that are narrowed by disease may set the stage for clot formation, or otherwise deprive brain or heart muscle of needed oxygen and nutrients. Similarly, poor perfusion of kidney tissue as a result of too great a reduction in the patient's blood pressure can lead to both kidney failure and congestive heart failure.

Other side effects common to all these drugs are the result of reduced transmission of sympathetic nerve impulses to other organs and structures besides the heart and blood vessels. Block of sympathetic impulses to the gastrointestinal tract, for example, can cause increased muscle contractions, leading to cramps and diarrhea. Patients with peptic ulcer or colitis may suffer especially from such a drug-induced increase in G.I. motility and secretion. Similarly, block of sympathetic outflow to the male genitalia by these drugs may have adverse effects on sexual function.

THE RAUWOLFIA ALKALOIDS (TABLE 26-1).
Reserpine+ (Serpasil) is the most widely used of the various available natural and semisynthetic derivatives of the *Rauwolfia*, or snakeroot, plant, which has been used for centuries in India for treating many ailments. Because it acts in the brain as well as on the circulation, this nerve blocker was once widely used in this country as a tranquilizer but has now been largely replaced by the phenothiazines and other more effective antipsychotic agents. However, reserpine still has an important place in the management of hypertension.

A single daily dose of this drug is enough to maintain the blood pressure at normal levels in mild cases that respond to the drug's gradual pressure-reducing effect. It is most often administered in combination with a thiazide diuretic, particularly in cases of moderate hypertension not controlled by either type of agent alone. The drug's heart-slowing action may add to the effectiveness of digitalis in patients with hypertensive heart disease, and this drug-induced bradycardia tends to counteract the tachycardia of hydralazine when these two agents are combined in treating resistant cases of moderately severe hypertension.

Reserpine is often injected I.M. or I.V. in treating hypertensive emergencies. It is slower than certain other drugs used in such crises, and it sometimes makes the patient excessively sleepy. However, despite these drawbacks, reserpine is relatively safe, as overdosage rarely leads to too rapid a fall in pressure to hypotensive levels. Other side effects of reserpine and the precautions needed for its safe use are discussed further in the *Drug Digest*.

Methyldopa+ (Aldomet) is an antihypertensive drug that acts by reducing adrenergic nerve stimulation of the cardiovascular system. It seems less likely, however, than other drugs of this type to reduce cardiac output and blood flow through the kidneys. Thus, postural hypotension appears to be less of a problem than with the more potent drugs. Because kidney perfusion is not reduced, this drug is considered most desirable for patients with poor kidney function that might be made worse by pressure-reducing drugs which reduce renal blood flow excessively.

For best results in patients with moderate hypertension that has not responded to treatment with reserpine and a diuretic, this drug is substituted for the reserpine while continuing with the diuretic. In hypertensive emergencies, the injectable form of methyldopa is employed. It is also most likely to prove effective when administered together with a diuretic. Like reserpine, this drug enters the central nervous system and can cause drowsiness and mental depression.

Although methyldopa is considered one of the safest of the sympatholytic drugs, its use has on rare occasions resulted in hypersensitivity-type reactions affecting liver function. Hemolytic anemia has also occurred. Thus, tests of liver function are made during treatment, and the drug is not administered to patients who already have liver disease or blood dyscrasias. Dosage may have to be reduced in elderly patients who are excessively susceptible to the drug's pressure-reducing effects and in patients in whom ordinary doses have cumulative effects because of poor renal excretion.

Guanethidine (Ismelin) is one of the most dependable drugs available for bringing down highly elevated pressure and reversing deterioration of kidney function in patients with severe, and even malignant, hypertension. It is *not*, however, used to reduce high blood pressure caused by pheochromocytoma, because it may stimulate the tumor tissue to release large amounts of epinephrine. Similarly, it is *not* given by injection to patients in hypertensive crisis, as large parenteral doses can release norepinephrine from sympathetic nerve endings. In both such cases, the result would be a *rise* rather than the expected fall in blood pressure.

Ordinarily, however, administration of just one daily oral dose of this potent and long-acting drug gradually reduces the amount of neurohormonal transmitter substance in the sympathetic nerves. This accounts for the drug's vasodilating and heart-slowing actions, leading in turn to the desired reduction in high blood pressure. Combining guanethidine with a diuretic permits the use of smaller doses. This then helps to lessen certain dose-related side effects of this drug, such as epigastric distress, diarrhea, and a tendency to cause fluid retention.

Other common side effects such as feelings of faintness, dizziness, and weakness are best avoided by careful dosage adjustment to prevent postural hypotension. It is important that the nurse teach patients or members of their families to take their own blood pressure readings at home before taking each morning's dose of the drug. However, because not all patients wish to assume responsibility for taking their own blood pressure, it is important for the doctor and nurse to discuss the desirability of the patient's carrying out this aspect of his own care. In some cases, they may decide that it would be better for a family member to check the patient's blood pressure to avoid administering a dose that he does not need and that could cause discomforting and possibly dangerous drops in his pressure.

Pargyline (Eutonyl) is one of the class of drugs called *monoamine oxidase inhibitors* that are used mainly as antidepressants in the management of mentally depressed patients. It is capable of causing all of the varied adverse effects and drug interactions that have limited the usefulness of this drug class in patients with affective disorders (see Chapter 6 and the *Summary of Side Effects of Antidepressant Drugs*, p. 104).

For the same reasons, the use of this drug as an antihypertensive agent is reserved for the relatively few patients with moderately severe hypertension who have not responded to treatment with such other antihypertensive agents as reserpine, methyldopa, and guanethidine. It is not used in treating either mild or malignant hypertension or patients whose pressure is elevated because of the presence of pheochromocytoma. As is true with depressed patients taking drugs of this type, the nurse warns the patient on pargyline not to treat himself with nonprescription cold remedies or to eat certain cheeses and other foods that may cause dangerous drug or food interactions with this agent.

OTHER ANTIHYPERTENSIVE AGENTS

Various other drugs effective for reducing high blood pressure also have drawbacks that limit their usefulness to special situations. At present, drugs of the ganglionic and adrenergic blocking classes, and sodium nitroprusside, are for example, used mainly in emergency situations. *Hydralazine* is also used in hypertensive crisis, but unlike the others it is often administered orally in combination with other drugs in the management of less serious stages of hypertensive disease.

Hydralazine acts mainly by relaxing the smooth muscle walls of the arterioles. The resulting vasodilation and reduction in peripheral resistance accounts for its pressure-reducing effect, particularly when it is combined with reserpine and a diuretic such as hydrochlorothiazide. The direct dilating effect of this drug on the arterioles of the kidney is claimed to make it useful for patients with poor kidney function. Thus, it is often effective when administered parenterally to patients in hypertensive crisis with acute glomerulonephritis or toxemia of pregnancy.

Side effects that limit the routine use of hydralazine in less serious cases include headache, dizziness, and heart palpitations. The drug's tendency to speed the heart may be counteracted by combining it with reserpine or other heart-slowing drugs. However, patients with angina pectoris are told to report any increase in chest pains, and the drug is not considered suited for routine use in patients with hypertensive heart disease. Unusual reactions marked by joint pains and fever are sometimes reported.

GANGLIONIC BLOCKING AGENTS. These drugs have been largely replaced by guanethidine and other adrenergic nerve blocking drugs. The newer drugs have the advantage of not blocking transmission in parasympathetic nerve pathways. Thus, they are free of the constipating and the bladder-paralyzing effects that sometimes result from blockade of parasympathetic ganglia. However, the depressant action of some of these drugs on transmission through sympathetic ganglia is still often employed in the management of patients in hypertensive crisis who require a prompt drop in blood pressure.

Trimethaphan (Arfonad) is a ganglionic blocker with a very rapid onset of action. Administered by intravenous drip, this drug usu-ally produces an immediate drop in pressure in most patients with acute hypertension. Often, the doctor also orders that the head of the patient's bed be raised to increase the drug's pressure-reducing effectiveness. The patient must be closely monitored to prevent too rapid infusion with a resulting fall in pressure to shock levels.

Sodium nitroprusside is similar to the ganglionic blocker in the speed of its pressure-lowering effect, and is sometimes used to follow trimethaphan when that drug proves ineffective in an acute hypertensive emergency. Patients receiving infusions of this potent antihypertensive agent must also be closely observed to avoid overdosage.

The adrenergic blocking drugs *phentolamine+* (Regitine) and *phenoxybenzamine+* (Dibenzyline) are reserved for patients whose high blood pressure results from the actions of circulating catecholamines released by the tumor tissue of a pheochromocytoma. These drugs block the effects of epinephrine on the patient's arterioles but not on his heart. To counteract the cardiac stimulation, the beta adrenergic blocker, *propranolol* (Inderal), is employed. This drug is at present also being tested in the treatment of other types of hypertension.

The alkaloids of the *Veratrum* plant, including alkavervir, cryptenamine, and proto-veratrine, are rarely employed today for treating hypertension. Although they are effective for reducing blood pressure, the doses that do so very often cause nausea, salivation, and vomiting.

S U M M A R Y of Points for the Nurse to Remember about Drugs Used in Treating Hypertension

1. Help the patient to understand the need for prolonged treatment. The discomforts of drug therapy are relatively mild compared to the possible complications to which a person with hypertension is particularly susceptible, including strokes and heart attacks.

2. Follow the physician's instructions for regulating drug dosage very carefully. Because the state of the patient's blood pressure is one basis for determining the dosage of antihypertensive agents, it is essential to take pressures accurately under specified conditions (for example, sitting or standing) and at the times requested by the physician.

3. Observe the patient carefully for any side effects and early signs and symptoms of drug toxicity (see *Summaries*) and report these promptly to the physician.

4. Instruct the patient who is troubled by symptoms of postural hypotension as to how these can be alleviated or minimized. (For example, he should avoid standing up suddenly, but instead sit on the edge of the bed for a couple of minutes before arising; he should lie down whenever he feels faint and weak to avoid falling and possibly injuring himself).

Clinical Nursing Situation

The Situation: Mrs. Black, age 52, has essential hypertension, which had its onset after her husband's sudden death in an automobile accident about ten years ago. Her condition has been quite well stabilized by treatment with a combination of reserpine 25 mg and hydrochlorothiazide 25 mg.

Mrs. Black has been referred for continuing care and observation to a nurse at the neighborhood health clinic. The nurse, Mrs. O'Neil, sees her patient once weekly to assess the state of her illness and her response to antihypertensive drug therapy.

The Problem: If you had Mrs. O'Neil's responsibility, what factors do you think it would be important to consider in evaluating Mrs. Black's response to long-term therapy with reserpine and hydrochlorothiazide? What kinds of symptoms might indicate that you should consider referring Mrs. Black to her physician?

DRUG DIGEST

GUANETHIDINE SULFATE U.S.P. (Ismelin)

Actions and Indications. This adrenergic nerve blocking drug has largely replaced the ganglionic blocking agents in the management of moderate to severe hypertension. It is slow in onset but then exerts a prolonged antihypertensive effect that permits once daily administration in chronic cases. It is most effective when combined with a diuretic; this also permits lower dosage and thus results in a reduction in certain side effects.

Side Effects, Cautions, and Contraindications. Postural hypotension resulting in feelings of dizziness, weakness, and faintness often occurs, particularly upon arising in the morning. The drug's dose-responses must be closely monitored, especially in elderly patients and others with a history of cardiovascular-renal disorders. Too great a fall in blood pressure can cause episodes of renal, cerebral, or coronary insufficiency in such patients or precipitate congestive heart failure. The drug can cause epigastric distress, diarrhea, and disturbances in male sex function.

Dosage and Administration. A single daily dose of 10 mg is administered orally at first. This is gradually raised in increments of 10 mg in accordance with the patient's blood pressure response. Optimal daily dosage usually varies between 25 and 75 mg. Diuretics are often combined with lower doses of this drug.

METHYLDOPA AND METHYLDOPATE HCl (Aldomet)

Actions and Indications. This drug reduces elevated blood pressure in patients with moderate hypertension without reducing blood flow through the kidneys. This makes it a desirable drug for treating hypertension in patients whose kidney function is impaired. The parenterally administered form is effective for producing gradual reduction of the dangerously high pressure in hypertensive emergencies. Administration with a diuretic increases the effectiveness of this drug.

Side Effects, Cautions, and Contraindications. This drug produces less postural hypotension than other more potent adrenergic neuron blocking drugs. However, some older patients may become dizzy, weak, or light-headed. They and patients with kidney disease require reduced dosage to avoid excessive hypotensive effects.

Drowsiness is the most common side effect. Headache, mouth dryness, nasal stuffiness, and diarrhea are also reported. Mild hepatitis has sometimes occurred; thus, caution is required in patients with a past history of liver disease, and use of the drug in patients with active liver disease is contraindicated. Liver function and blood tests are recommended.

Dosage and Administration. Oral doses of 250 mg are administered t.i.d. at the start of treatment. Later, dose levels of 1 or 2 g may be reached if needed. A dose of 500 mg may be administered by vein, and, if necessary for adequate effect, an additional dose of 1 g may be administered several hours later.

RESERPINE U.S.P. (Serpasil; and others)

Actions and Indications. Small oral doses of this rauwolfia alkaloid are useful for bringing about a gradual reduction of blood pressure in patients with mild degrees of hypertension. It is often combined with a diuretic and sometimes also with hydralazine for treating moderately severe hypertension. The injectable form of this drug is used in treating hypertensive emergencies, such as malignant hypertension and acute crisis.

Side Effects, Cautions, and Contraindications. The central effects of this drug tend to cause drowsiness and feelings of fatigue and weakness. Patients with a history of suicidal tendencies should not receive reserpine, and other patients should be watched carefully for possible signs of mental depression induced by this drug.

Increased gastrointestinal motility and secretion may cause epigastric distress, cramps, and diarrhea. The drug is contraindicated in patients with active cases of peptic ulcer or colitis.

Generalized vasodilation leading to postural hypotension is rare with oral dosage, but local vasodilation in the nasal mucosa commonly causes congestion and stuffiness.

Dosage and Administration. Treatment is usually begun with oral doses of about 0.5 mg daily, which may later be lowered to 0.25 mg daily or less. Intramuscular or intravenous doses of about 1 or 2 mg may be used at first and followed by similar or somewhat higher doses at intervals of 4 to 24 hours.

References

Aagaard, G.M. Treatment of hypertension. *Amer. J. Nurs.*, 73:620, 1973 (April).

Bourne, H.R., and Melmon, K.L. Guides to the pharmacologic management of hypertension. *Rational Drug Ther.*, 5:4, 1971 (April).

Gilmore, H.R. The treatment of chronic hypertension. *Med. Clin. N. Amer.*, 55:315, 1971 (March).

Hamilton, M. Management of hypertension. *Nurs. Mirror*, 132:33, 1971 (Jan.).

Foley, M.L. Variations in blood pressure in the lateral recumbent position. *Nursing Res.*, 20:64, 1971 (Jan.-Feb.).

Fries, E.D. Hypertensive crisis. *JAMA*, 208:338, 1969.

————. Medical treatment of chronic hypertension. *Mod. Conc. Cardiovasc. Dis.*, 40:17, 1971 (April).

Rodman, M.J. Drugs used in treating hypertension. *RN*, 36:41, 1973 (April).

————. Managing high blood pressure. *RN*, 32:73, 1969 (May).

Vaamonde, C.A., et al: Hypertensive emergencies. *Med. Clin. N. Amer.*, 55:325, 1971 (March).

Veterans Administration Cooperative Study Group on Antihypertensive Agents. Effects of treatment on morbidity in hypertension. *JAMA*, 213:1143, 1970.

27.

Diuretic Drugs

The Kidneys in Health and Disease

Diuretics are drugs that increase the amount of urine produced by the kidneys. The most important clinical use of these drugs is in the management of *edema*—an abnormal increase in the amount of fluid outside the body's cells. Diuretic therapy aids in eliminating this extra fluid by increasing the excretion of sodium by the kidneys. Sodium that is transferred from the tissues to the urine carries with it the water that was retained in the tissues. Before we discuss the actions and uses of the several classes of diuretic drugs, it is desirable that we review briefly how the kidneys handle sodium and other substances in health and disease.

KIDNEY FUNCTIONS IN HEALTH

All the body's cells need a constant internal environment in which to function efficiently. The kidneys play a very important part in adjusting the amount of fluid and essential chemicals inside body cells and in the extracellular fluids that surround these cells. In the course of their constant activity to *keep the volume and composition of the body fluids within normal limits*, the kidneys work in various ways to retain substances vital to the body and to discard chemicals that are present in excess.

As a result of these renal activities, the body: (1) rids itself of the nitrogenous waste products of protein metabolism; (2) stays in acid-base balance; and (3) keeps such substances as sodium, potassium, chloride, and bicarbonate ions in correct balance within the body's several separate fluid compartments. (Body water

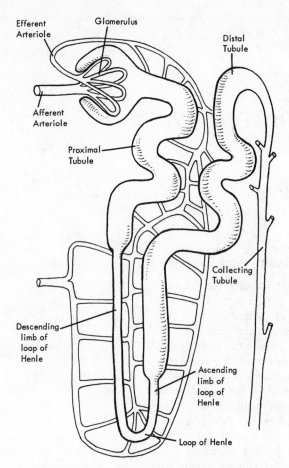

Fig. 27-1. The nephron—the functional unit of the kidney. Secretion and absorption of water, electrolytes and other solutes in the proximal and the distal tubule can be influenced by drugs of many types.

is distributed as follows: (1) *intra*cellular and (2) *extra*cellular, which is in turn subdivided into (a) the blood plasma, and (b) the interstitial fluid that makes its way out of the blood vessels to surround and bathe the body cells.)

The three processes by which the kidneys accomplish all this are: (1) glomerular filtration; (2) tubular reabsorption; and (3) tubular secretion.

GLOMERULAR FILTRATION. This is a process in which certain substances in solution in the blood plasma make their way out of the systemic circulation and into the *nephrons*, the tiny functional units of the kidneys (Fig. 27-1). Each of the two million or so nephrons consists of a *glomerulus* and a *tubule*. The glomerulus is made up of a ball of tiny blood vessels enclosed in a membranous capsule. Fluid is forced through the capillary membranes into

the tubular portion of each nephron. It contains most of the plasma constituents except for proteins and lipids.

TUBULAR REABSORPTION. About 99 out of every 100 ml of the glomerular filtrate is returned to the blood during its passage down the tubules. The cells that line the tubules have the ability to reabsorb substances in the filtrate that the body needs, including glucose, vitamins, and dissolved electrolytes, such as sodium and chloride ions. A small amount of sodium (about 1 percent) normally is not reabsorbed and ends up in the urine along with other filtered waste materials and the water in which they are dissolved. This reabsorptive process is very important for keeping the extracellular fluids at just the right volume and composition for serving the needs of the tissue cells that they surround.

TUBULAR SECRETION. The cells that line the kidney tubules can also secrete substances *from* the blood *into* the tubular fluid. Secretion of hydrogen ions helps to keep body fluids from becoming acidic. Excess potassium ions may also be secreted into the tubular fluid to be passed out of the body in the urine. Uric acid is another substance that may be either reabsorbed from the renal tubules or secreted into them.

KIDNEY FUNCTION IN DISEASE

In certain diseases, including heart failure and liver disorders, the kidneys lose some of their capacity to keep sodium in proper balance. In health, any reduction in the amount of fluid filtered by the glomeruli leads to a proportional reduction in the amount of sodium that the tubules reabsorb. In heart failure, however, when the failing heart pumps less blood through the kidneys and glomerular filtration falls, the amount of sodium that is reabsorbed by the tubules often rises. This extra sodium then leaks into the extracellular spaces to trap fluids in the form of edema.

Edema is both discomforting and, in some cases, dangerous. Fluid that accumulates within the abdomen (that is, *ascites*) or in the patient's legs and ankles (*anascara*) may make it difficult for him to move. Pulmonary edema filling up lung space can make breathing so difficult that the patient may die if the excess fluid is not promptly removed. Various measures are used to overcome edema.

Management of edema is best aimed at correcting its cause. In heart failure, for example, edema stems primarily from the reduced ability of the weakened heart muscle to handle the load of blood that it must pump to the kidneys and other tissues. Edema may be reduced by bed rest to reduce the work of the heart. Similarly, restricting the salt and water intake of patients with cirrhotic ascites or nephrotic edema and employing other measures for improving hepatic, renal, and cardiac function can lessen edema.

DIURETIC THERAPY

Even in ordering drugs, the doctor may first use those that come closer than diuretics to affecting the primary pathogenetic cause. He may administer a *non*diuretic drug of the digitalis type which often relieves edema by strengthening the contractions of the weakened cardiac muscle of heart failure patients. Or, he may order corticosteroid drugs in an attempt to stop the loss of plasma proteins through the leaky glomerular membranes that is the cause of nephrotic edema.

In almost every case of edema, however, the doctor does have to employ the diuretic drugs that act directly on the kidney to alter the abnormal way in which the tubules reabsorb sodium in pathologic states. Potent diuretics are now available for rapidly removing edema from the lungs in an emergency or for more slowly removing ascitic fluid that has accumulated in the abdomen of a patient with cirrhosis of the liver. Once the patient has attained his "dry weight," milder diuretics may be employed daily or on alternate days to keep fluid from again accumulating.

The nurse's role is important to the success of diuretic therapy. She usually has the responsibility for keeping an accurate record of the patient's daily intake of fluid, his output of urine, and changes in his body weight during the first several days of diuretic administration. Weighing the patient should be done at the same time each day.

Even after the patient has reached his "dry weight," continued checks are desirable, as body weight is the best index of whether the patient is beginning to retain fluid again. If the nurse notes that a patient's weight is going up (even though his food intake and activity remain the same) she reports this to the doctor. He may then raise the dose of the diuretic or try giving it in combination with another diuretic of a different class (see below).

The nurse also shows concern for the patient's physical comfort and emotional state when he is receiving diuretics. In making intramuscular injections of organic mercurials and other parenterally administered diuretics, she avoids edematous areas and subcutaneous fat pads and massages the muscle site vigorously to reduce local irritation and pain. She keeps the patient from becoming alarmed by the urgency of his need to void by explaining in advance that these drugs are expected to cause a copious flow of urine.

The time of administration of a diuretic drug is another factor that affects the patient's comfort. Although this consideration must be put aside in emergency situations that require immediate administration of the drug for removing edema fluid from the lungs and elsewhere, the nurse should consider the patient's comfort in this regard when she has a choice in the matter of diuretic timing. The organic mercurial *meralluride* (Mercuhydrin), for example, should be given in the morning rather than the evening. This diuretic can be expected to produce a strong diuretic effect several hours after its administration and it is desirable that the patient's sleep not be disturbed by his need to void frequently.

Finally, the nurse sees to it that a urinal or bedpan is readily available. This is particularly important for weak or elderly patients. Sometimes, the urgent need to void leads such patients to make a sudden unaccompanied trip to the bathroom, even though this may be beyond their strength. If walking to a toilet facility is permitted at all, these people should be helped and given physical support. If not, the side rails of the bed should be kept up to remind the elderly or confused patient that he must not get out of bed. In that case, place the call bell within easy reach of the patient and instruct him to call when he feels the urge to void. Such calls should be answered promptly.

The patient's response to diuretic therapy is often quite dramatic. This can be very encouraging to the patient and satisfying to those who care for him. Improvement is often detected first by a change in the patient's appearance, as edema fluid leaves his face and his features lose their flabby, bloated look. Loss of ascitic fluid from the abdomen makes it easier for the patient to move about—which he often wants to do, as his earlier feelings of fatigue and lethargy are replaced by feelings of energy and renewed strength, and his appetite for food returns. Most dramatic of all is the obvious well-being of the patient with pulmonary edema that had caused dyspnea accompanied by rales and frothy, pink-tinged sputum, as his breathing becomes easier, his dull, dusky (cyanotic) skin color turns to a brighter, healthier tone, and his coughing stops.

The nurse should try to capitalize on such marked symptomatic improvement to help the patient renew his hopefulness. Often, the patient with chronic cardiac, liver, or kidney disease has become discouraged by his own fruitless physical efforts to cope with edema-induced symptoms. Pointing out how readily such symptoms can often be kept under control by a careful diuretic treatment regimen may help to motivate the patient in making an effort to follow instructions about diet, medication and other matters.

DIURETIC EFFECTS ON SODIUM AND OTHER IONS

All the diuretics that are most useful for treating edema act in one main way: *they interfere with the tubular reabsorption of sodium.* That is, these drugs keep the cells that line the tubules from reabsorbing an excessive proportion of the sodium ions from the glomerular filtrate. As a result, sodium and other ions such as chloride enter the urine along with the water in which they are dissolved, instead of being returned to the blood and then leaking into interstitial spaces and body cavities.

The several different types of diuretics act in different ways to prevent sodium from being carried back into the blood plasma and the interstitial spaces. Depending upon which of several different renal tubular transport systems they affect, these drugs also remove other ions such as potassium, hydrogen, chloride, and bicarbonate. Excessive diuretic actions can cause complications that are the result of electrolyte and acid-base imbalances. This can lead to the development of many discomforting and dangerous signs and symptoms.

Among the imbalances resulting from the excessive activity of most diuretics are hypokalemia, hypochloremia, and metabolic alkalosis or acidosis. The most common of these conditions is *hypokalemia*—a *low* level of plasma *potassium*. It is also the most dangerous

because it can lead to heartbeat irregularities in patients who are taking digitalis as well as diuretics. Loss of potassium may also cause patients with cirrhosis of the liver to lapse into hepatic coma. Hypokalemia also often leads to muscle weakness and pain, drowsiness, dizziness, confusion, and other nervous system and neuromuscular signs and symptoms. *Hyperkalemia*—a *high* serum level of *potassium*—is a condition that can occur during treatment with certain other diuretics. If not detected and corrected, hyperkalemia can cause cardiac arrest.

Alkalosis is an acid-base imbalance that develops when diuretics remove not only sodium but also excessive amounts of other ions such as potassium, hydrogen, and chloride (*hypochloremia*). In these circumstances, bicarbonate ions tend to accumulate in the extracellular fluid, and the patient may become nauseated, drowsy, and complain of muscle weakness and pain.

Acidosis, on the other hand, is an acid-base imbalance caused by overtreatment with diuretics that remove too much bicarbonate from the body with an accompanying accumulation of chloride ions in the extracellular fluids (*hyperchloremia*). This condition is sometimes seen in patients who are being treated with the class of diuretics called carbonic anhydrase inhibitor-type diuretics or with ammonium chloride and other acidifying salts (Table 27-1).

In addition to resulting in adverse effects, diuretic-induced electrolyte and acid-base imbalances can interfere with the further effectiveness of diuretic therapy. That is, when alkalosis or acidosis develops, the patient's edema may no longer respond to drug treatment. Therefore, the doctor sometimes alternates one type of diuretic drug with another to prevent or correct imbalances that interfere with diuretic therapy. In order to understand the reasons for changes in the doctor's orders for diuretic therapy, we should know the properties of the several different classes of diuretic drugs.

Classes of Diuretic Drugs

Diuretics are divided into several classes on the basis of their chemical structures and the ways in which they bring about their effects. Although they may differ chemically and in the details of their pharmacological effects, certain classes of diuretics act in essentially the

TABLE 27-1 *Diuretic Drugs*

Nonproprietary Name	Trade Name	Daily Dosage Range	Remarks
Oral Sulfonamide-Type Diuretics			
Bendroflumethiazide N.F.	Naturetin	2.5 to 20 mg	Potent, long acting
Benzthiazide N.F.	Aquatag; Exna	25 to 200 mg	Moderate duration and potency
Chlorothiazide N.F.	Diuril	500 to 1000 mg	Prototype thiazide
Chlorthalidone U.S.P.	Hygroton	50 to 200 mg; 3 times weekly	Very long-acting nonthiazide
Cyclothiazide N.F.	Anhydron	1–2 mg	High potency; long duration
Hydrochlorothiazide U.S.P.	Esidrix; Hydro Diuril; Oretic	25–200 mg	See *Drug Digest*
Hydroflumethiazide N.F.	Saluron	25–200 mg	Moderate duration and potency.
Methyclothiazide N.F.	Enduron	2.5–10 mg	High potency; long duration
Polythiazide N.F.	Renese	1–4 mg	High potency; long duration
Quinethazone U.S.P.	Hydromox	50–200 mg	Nonthiazide of moderate potency and duration
Trichlormethiazide N.F.	Metahydrin; Naqua	2–4 mg	High potency; long duration
Newer High Potency Diuretics			
Ethacrynic acid U.S.P.	Edecrin	25–200 mg orally	See *Drug Digest*
Ethachynate sodium U.S.P.	Edecrin sodium	0.5 to 1 mg per kg of body weight I.V.	See *Drug Digest*
Furosemide U.S.P.	Lasix	40–80 mg orally; 20–40 mg I.V.	Potent short-acting nonthiazide sulfonamide
Organic Mercurial Diuretics			
Chloromerodrin N.F.	Neohydrin	55–110 mg	Relatively weak mercurial but often effective by oral administration
Meralluride sodium U.S.P.	Mercuhydrin	1–2 ml I.M. or s.c.	See *Drug Digest*
Mercaptomerin sodium U.S.P.	Thiomerin	0.2–2 ml I.M. or s.c.	Relatively low tissue irritancy
Mercurophylline	Mercuzanthine	1 ml I.M.	Rarely used now
Merethoxylline procaine	Dicurin; Procaine	0.5–2 ml I.M. or s.c.	Not in common use
Mersalyl sodium and theophylline	Salyrgan; Theophylline	0.5–2 ml I.M. or I.V.	Not in common use
Carbonic Anhydrase Inhibitors			
Acetazolamide U.S.P.	Diamox	250–375 mg orally once daily	See *Drug Digest*
Acetazolamide sodium U.S.P.	Diamox Parenteral	250–500 mg I.V.	See *Drug Digest*
Dichlorphenamide U.S.P.	Daranide; Oratrol	50–200 mg orally q. 6–8 hours	Used to reduce intraocular tension in glaucoma
Ethoxzolamide U.S.P.	Cardrase; Ethamide	62.5 to 200 mg orally q. 4–8 hours	Used in glaucoma and epilepsy
Methazolamide U.S.P.	Neptazane	50–100 mg q. 8 hours orally	Lowers intraocular pressure in glaucoma
Osmotic Diuretics			
Mannitol U.S.P.	Osmitrol	50 to 100 g I.V. in 15–20% solution	Infused slowly in oliguria or certain types of edema

TABLE 27-1 *Diuretic Drugs (continued)*

Nonproprietary Name	Trade Name	Daily Dosage Range	Remarks
Urea, sterile U.S.P.	Ureaphil; Urevert	40–120 g I.V. in 4% or 30% solution	See *Drug Digest*
Potassium-Sparing Diuretics			
Spironolactone U.S.P.	Aldactone	25 mg orally 2–4 times daily	See *Drug Digest*
Triamterene U.S.P.	Dyrenium	100–200 mg orally	Used with thiazides to counteract potassium loss
Acid-Forming Salts			
Ammonium chloride U.S.P.	. . . .	1 g 4 times daily by mouth	Potentiates organic mercurials
Lysine monohydrochloride	. . . .	10 g 4 times daily by mouth	Used for patients who do not tolerate ammonium chloride
Xanthine Compounds			
Aminophylline U.S.P.	Theophylline ethylenediamine, and others	100–200 mg orally	See *Drug Digest*
Oxtriphylline N.F.	Choledyl	200–600 mg orally	Bronchodilator
Theophylline N.F.	Theocin	200–800 mg orally	Bronchodilator
Theobromine calcium salicylate	Theocalcin	500–1500 mg orally	Used in cardiac conditions

same way. For example, the sulfonamides and the organic mercurials both bring about a loss of sodium and chloride ions in close to equal amounts, as do the new, more potent diuretics, *furosemide* and *ethacrynic acid*.

The diuretics classified as carbonic acid inhibitors, on the other hand, cause a loss of sodium accompanied by bicarbonate ions rather than chloride. A third group, called the potassium-sparing diuretics, including *spironolactone* and *triamterene*, differ from other diuretics in being able to remove sodium without causing any loss of potassium. These differences help to explain why some drugs often cause one type of electrolyte imbalance, while other diuretics cause excessive loss of different ions. The doctor often orders one or another type of diuretic in order to prevent or correct complications of imbalances that stem from their different effects on the electrolytes of the extracellular fluids.

SALIURETICS

The diuretics that cause the kidneys to produce an increased volume of urine that is high in both sodium and chloride—the elements in common salt—are sometimes called salt removers, or saliuretic drugs. The most important saliuretics are the sulfonamides, the organic mercurials, ethacrynic acid, and furosemide. Administered in overdosage, all of these drugs can cause a condition called the *low-salt syndrome*. To varying degrees, these classes of diuretics also have in common a tendency to cause hypochloremia, hypokalemia, and alkalosis.

THE SULFONAMIDE DIURETICS (SEE TABLE 27-1).

❨ *Status*. The most commonly used diuretics are drugs related chemically to the antibacterial sulfonamide drugs. The first to be introduced, *chlorothiazide* (Diuril), is still widely used despite the introduction of many much more potent relatives. Although these drugs are not as effective against severe edema as the older mercurial diuretics or the newer drugs, ethacrynic acid and furosemide (all of which are discussed below), the thiazides, and related sulfonamides have several important advantages. The orally effective thiazides are, for example, convenient to administer and relatively safe compared to the mercurials, which must usually be injected in doses that sometimes cause direct tissue toxicity. The thiazides are also less likely to cause excessive diuresis and severe electrolyte imbalances than are the more potent but often less readily controllable compounds furosemide and ethacrynic acid.

For these reasons, many doctors today prefer to begin treatment of most edematous patients with a moderately potent diuretic such as *hydrochlorothiazide+* (Esidrix; Hydro-Diuril; and others). If this fails to remove the edema from the patient's tissue spaces, the physician may then employ one of the more potent agents. Once the edema fluid has been mobilized by the action of a mercurial diuretic or ethacrynic acid, the doctor may switch the patient back to a sulfonamide diuretic to keep him at his "dry weight" during long-term maintenance therapy in heart failure, cirrhosis, and similar serious disorders. In minor degrees of edema such as that which develops in premenstrual edema or in fluid retention from treatment with corticosteroid drugs, the thiazide diuretics may be administered for brief periods as needed. The thiazides are also used in the treatment of high blood pressure, even in patients without any edema (Chapter 26).

◖ *Adverse effects.* The sulfonamide diuretics do not differ significantly from one another in their effectiveness or safety. Even though some compounds are effective for producing diuresis when taken in much smaller doses than other drugs, this is not a practical advantage. Some, including the *non*thiazide sulfonamide diuretic, *chlorthalidone* (Hygroton), have a longer-lasting action than others. Although these diuretics of long duration have the advantage of not needing to be taken daily, any toxicity that they may cause is also prolonged.

The sulfonamides do not ordinarily cause direct tissue toxicity of the kinds sometimes seen with organic mercurial diuretics or ethacrynic acid. Rarely, individuals allergic to the sulfonamide type chemical structure may develop dermatologic reactions or blood dyscrasias. Much more common, however, in patients who have been overtreated with these dieuretics, are such electrolyte and acid-base imbalances as hypokalemia, hypochloremia, and alkalosis.

All the thiazide diuretics tend to cause hypokalemia to about the same extent. That is, all of these drugs remove sodium and potassium in the same ratio. Even though some compounds are much more potent than others, milligram for milligram, in their ability to remove sodium, all drugs of this class tend to cause the loss of potassium in proportional amounts. Thus, to prevent hypokalemia when any of these diuretics is being used, the doctor often suggests that the patient eat foods containing natural potassium, including bananas and citrus fruits.

In addition, the doctor may order the routine administration of potassium salt supplements to make up for the loss of this ion, along with sodium. There are now various products available containing potassium, preferably as the chloride salt, in flavored solutions or in the form of powders or tablets that are dissolved in water and taken orally. Another method used to prevent potassium loss is to administer a thiazide diuretic in combination with one of the so-called potassium-sparing diuretics such as spironolactone or triamterene.

Other metabolic effects occasionally seen in patients taking thiazide diuretics include a rise in blood levels of uric acid and glucose. This can cause an attack of gout or set off symptoms of diabetes mellitus. The use of these diuretics is not contraindicated in patients with gout or diabetes. However, the doctor keeps such patients under close observation, and, if necessary, prescribes higher doses of the patient's antigout drugs or raises his insulin dosage. Caution is also required in patients with severe liver or kidney disease to avoid diuretic-induced hepatic coma or kidney failure. However such complications of excessive diuretic activity are less likely to occur with the thiazides than with the more potent agents.

POTENT NEW DIURETICS. Two of the most potent diuretics now available are *ethacrynic acid+* (Edecrin) and *furosemide* (Lasix). These drugs are often effective in patients who have failed to respond to thiazides and other diuretics. Their rapid onset of diuretic action when injected intravenously makes these drugs useful for treating patients with acute pulmonary edema. These drugs are even sometimes effective in patients with advanced kidney disease and in patients with electrolyte and acid-base imbalances which would interfere with the diuretic action of organic mercurials and the thiazides.

Because of their potency, the use of these

drugs requires considerable care to avoid too rapid a loss of too much body fluid. This is particularly true in older patients with blood vessels narrowed by disease, as too sudden and massive a diuresis can cause cardiovascular collapse or blood clot formation resulting in a heart attack or stroke. These drugs are even more likely than the thiazides to cause electrolyte and acid-base imbalances such as hypokalemia and alkalosis.

To avoid overtreatment, particularly in patients with liver damage or those taking digitalis, the doctor has the hospital laboratory keep a close check on the patient's serum electrolyte levels. The nurse watches these patients closely for signs and symptoms known to stem from excessive loss of fluid or of sodium and potassium, or as a result of alkalosis (see *Summary of Side Effects*, p. 338). She also measures fluid intake and output carefully and weighs the patient once daily. On the basis of the nurse's notes, as well as laboratory reports and his own observation of the patient's response to treatment with ethacrynic acid or furosemide, the doctor adjusts the dosage of these potent drugs to the patient's precise needs. This usually means administering doses that remove relatively small amounts of edema daily (except in emergencies), as this procedure is safer than using these drugs at their full strength.

THE ORGANIC MERCURIAL DIURETICS (TABLE 27-1).

¶ *Status.* These are the oldest of the potent diuretics. They are used less frequently today than they once were, as the thiazides are generally preferred for patients with moderate edema, and ethacrynic acid or furosemide are preferred for severe edema. The drawbacks of the mercurials include the need to administer them by injection for full effectiveness and their tendency to cause direct tissue toxicity. An advantage may be that they are somewhat less likely to cause hypokalemia than are the other classes of potent diuretics.

Despite their drawbacks, the mercurials are still considered to be dependable drugs for producing a rapid diuretic action in emergencies such as congestive heart failure with acute pulmonary edema. Drugs such as *meralluride sodium+* (Mercuhydrin) and *mercaptomerin* (Thiomerin) are still commonly employed for starting treatment to eliminate edema. They are administered in daily injections until the patient has reached his "dry weight." The doctor may then order daily or alternate day doses of an *oral* diuretic such as a thiazide alone or in combination with spironolactone. However, if the patient's body weight builds up only slowly, the physician may continue with injections of mercurials administered at intervals of several days.

Patients may become unresponsive to mercurials if the drugs are administered too frequently, resulting in loss of excessive amounts of chloride ions. To counteract the resulting hypochloremic alkalosis and restore responsiveness to mercurial injections, the doctor may order oral administration of ammonium chloride or other acidifying salts. However, care is required in patients with cirrhosis of the liver and renal insufficiency, as metabolic acidosis and hepatic coma may result from such pretreatment.

THE POTASSIUM-SPARING DIURETICS (TABLE 27-1)

Certain diuretics, including *spironolactone+* (Aldactone), *triamterene* (Dyrenium), and *amiloride* (Colectril), have the ability to remove sodium-containing edema fluid without causing a loss of potassium. They are especially effective when combined with thiazide or organic mercurial diuretics. Such combinations not only cause an increased excretion of sodium, but also counteract the tendency of the other diuretics to cause hypokalemic alkalosis. However, if patients have been taking a potassium salt supplement together with a thiazide diuretic, the potassium is discontinued when one of these drugs is added to the patient's treatment regimen. This is because the potassium-retaining effects of these diuretics could lead to hyperkalemia, particularly in patients with poor kidney function.

Spironolactone is most effective in disorders in which the adrenal cortex secretes high levels of the mineralocorticoid hormone *aldosterone*. The level of this hormone is often high in patients with cirrhosis of the liver and the nephrotic syndrome, and causes the kidney to retain sodium and to lose potassium. Spironolactone, a steroid drug, blocks the effects of this adrenal steroid on kidney tubule reabsorption of sodium. The other two drugs of this class do not act by blocking the effects of aldosterone. However, triamterene and amiloride do reduce the reabsorption of sodium by the renal tubule, and they do so while retaining potassium. Thus, these drugs are also best administered in combination with thiazide diuretics during long-term maintenance therapy in order to keep the patient at "dry weight" without causing such electrolyte imbalances as either hypokalemic alkalosis or hyperkalemic acidosis.

THE CARBONIC ANHYDRASE INHIBITORS (TABLE 27-1)

STATUS. Drugs of this class are relatively weak but safe diuretics. They are effective in mild causes of edema, including premenstrual and pregnancy edema, and fluid retention during treatment of patients with corticosteroid drugs. They are not ordinarily used alone for removing accumulations of edema in cases of congestive heart failure. However, they may be employed as part of a long-term program for maintaining a patient at "dry weight."

CLINICAL USE. They are best used alternately with drugs of other classes such as the thiazides, ethacrynic acid, or furosemide, and organic mercurials. Drugs of this class, such as *acetazolamide+* (Diamox), tend to cause a metabolic acidosis by excreting sodium with bicarbonate while retaining chloride and hydrogen ions. This leads to a loss of further diuretic activity after a couple of days. However, when administered alternately with drugs such as the organic mercurials, which tend to become less active because of the alkalosis they cause, the two types of drugs each overcome the acid-base imbalance caused by the other, and this reinforces the diuretic activity of both.

Because both these classes of diuretics tend to cause a loss of potassium, patients must be monitored for hypokalemia, and administration of potassium supplements is desirable, particularly in heart failure patients taking digitalis and in patients with cirrhosis of the liver or severely impaired kidney function. Small doses employed with rest periods of a day or two are often more effective than large doses administered more frequently. However, relatively large doses of various carbonic anhydrase inhibitors are employed for reducing intraocular pressure in glaucoma and as adjuncts to other anticonvulsants in epilepsy.

THE OSMOTIC DIURETICS

Certain substances, including *urea+* (Ureaphil) and *mannitol* (Osmitrol), that cause an increase in the amount of urine produced by the kidneys, are used clinically for various purposes in addition to the management of edema. They are, in fact, used only rarely for ridding the body of sodium and retained fluids. Instead, the most important uses of these drugs depend upon their ability to keep the kidneys producing urine in circumstances that could cause the kidneys to shut down.

Thus, in clinical situations in which blood flow through the kidney and the rate of glomerular filtration is severely reduced, these diuretics help to prevent renal failure. In certain severely injured and burned patients, and in others following heart surgery and other operations, a marked reduction in urine production occurs that can in itself lead to kidney damage. These osmotic substances can, by their ability to hold water within the renal tubules, keep production of urine going, and in this way overcome oliguria and prevent tubular damage.

The osmotic action of molecules of these substances in the bloodstream also tends to draw fluid from the extravascular spaces into the plasma. This action is useful for reducing abnormally elevated intracranial and intraocular pressure. The reduction of cerebral edema and of pressure upon the brain is often useful during neurosurgery and in patients who have suffered head injuries. Reduction of pressure within the eye with these drugs is sometimes employed prior to surgery for acute closed-angle glaucoma or for a detached retina. Use of these drugs is undesirable in patients with severely impaired kidney, liver, or cardiac function.

MISCELLANEOUS DIURETICS

Certain substances which are only weak diuretics are sometimes employed as adjuncts to more potent drugs in the management of edema. *Acidifying salts*, such as ammonium chloride, are (as indicated above), sometimes useful when administered orally prior to injection of organic mercurial compounds. Patients with cirrhotic ascites and others who do not tolerate this drug very well sometimes receive arginine monohydrochloride or lysine monohydrochloride for the same purpose: counteracting hypochloremic alkalosis and thus restoring responsiveness to the mercurials.

Xanthines are a class of weak diuretics that includes caffeine, theobromine, and theophylline. The most useful of these drugs in the management of certain cases of pulmonary edema following left-sided heart failure is *aminophylline+*. This drug's beneficial effects in such cases result more from its actions on cardiac and bronchial muscles than from its weak direct action on kidney tubule transport mechanisms for handling sodium.

SUMMARY of Side Effects, Toxicity, Cautions, and Contraindications of Certain Diuretic Drug Classes

Organic Mercurial Compounds

Hypersensitivity reactions: Dermatitis, fever, dizziness, stomatitis, nausea, and vomiting; intravenous injections have caused fatal ventricular arrhythmias.

Local irritation: Pain at sites of injection; epigastric distress from tablets; proctitis from suppositories.

Electrolyte depletion: Excessive salt loss may cause muscle weakness or cramps, lethargy, circulatory collapse, oliguria, and azotemia.

Contraindications: Acute nephritis; repeated injections should not be given to patients who fail to respond. (Hypertonic chloride injections may be required to correct low-salt syndrome, or ammonium chloride to correct hypochloremic alkalosis.)

Sulfonamide-Type Compounds (Benzothiazides, and others)

Electrolyte imbalances: Muscle weakness or cramps, thirst, dizziness, paresthesias, nausea, vomiting, diarrhea; (if severe and unrecognized) oliguria, hypotension, convulsions, coma. (Administer sodium chloride for hyponatremia and hypochloremia, potassium salts for hypokalemia and alkalosis.)

Hypersensitivity reactions: Skin eruptions of maculopapular type, photosensitivity, leukopenia, agranulocytosis, thrombocytic purpura.

Cautions and contraindications: Patients with poor kidney functions may retain blood urea nitrogen (BUN), nonprotein nitrogen (NPN), and creatinine; gout patients may get acute attacks from higher uric acid levels; diabetes patients may need more insulin; heart irregularities may occur in digitalized heart patients.

New Potent Diuretics (Furosemide and Ethacrynic Acid)

Electrolyte imbalances: Too vigorous diuresis may lead to dehydration and excessive loss of sodium, chloride, and potassium ions. Signs of hyponatremia, hypokalemia, and hypochloremic alkalosis include muscle cramps, weakness, thirst, and paresthesias. (Weigh the patient daily during the period of dosage adjustment to avoid excessive diuresis. Administer supplemental potassium chloride to prevent hypokalemia.)

Other adverse effects: Gastrointestinal complaints include anorexia, nausea, and vomiting. Mild diarrhea may occur with both compounds, but the occasional profuse watery diarrhea caused by ethacrynic acid requires discontinuation of drug treatment. Readministration of this diuretic in such cases is contraindicated.

Other cautions and contraindications: These drugs are contraindicated in the presence of anuria and should be withdrawn if increasing oliguria or azotemia is noted during treatment. Particular caution is required with the following patients:

1. Those with advanced liver cirrhosis: diuretic drug-induced electrolyte imbalances may lead to encephalopathy, hepatic coma and death

2. Patients receiving digitalis for cardiac decompensation: diuretic drug-induced hypokalemia can cause fatal arrhythmias

3. Patients taking antihypertensive drugs, who are subject to episodes of postural hypotension

4. Diabetic patients, in whom hyperglycemia may develop

5. Gout patients in whom an acute gout attack may be precipitated by a rise in plasma levels of uric acid

6. Patients who have previously exhibited sensitivity to these drugs resulting in leukopenia or thrombocytopenia

Carbonic Anhydrase Inhibitors

Electrolyte imbalances: Potassium depletion and sodium bicarbonate loss cause hypokalemia and mild metabolic acidosis, leading to gastrointestinal upset (anorexia, nausea, vomiting, mouth dryness), nervous system signs and symptoms (drowsiness, dizziness, headache, tinnitus, tremor, paresthesias—numbness and tingling of face and extremities, especially lips, fingers, and toes).

Hypersensitivity reactions: Skin rashes, fever, bone marrow depression, crystalluria, and renal calculi.

Cautions and contraindications: Patients with renal failure; Addison's disease and adrenocortical insufficiency; respiratory disorders with reduced pulmonary ventilation leading to hyperchloremic acidosis.

Potassium Sparing Diuretics

Electrolyte imbalances: Caution is required in

patients with impaired renal function because of the danger of potassium retention, leading to serious hyperkalemia. Patients with severe liver disease may lose excessive sodium and suffer the effects of hyponatremia and subsequent stupor or transient hepatic coma.

S U M M A R Y of Points for the Nurse to Remember During Diuretic Therapy

1. The nurse has the responsibility of assessing and recording the patient's response to diuretic therapy. She keeps an accurate daily record of the patient's fluid intake, urinary output, and body weight changes, whether or not such observations have been specifically ordered by the physician.

2. Look for signs of symptomatic improvement in the patient's appearance such as: reduction in the protrusion of his abdomen, in pitting when fingers are pressed into the flesh of the extremities; healthier skin tone and color; easier breathing, freedom from cough, and so on. Capitalize on this improvement to encourage the patient to follow the physician's instruction concerning all aspects of his treatment regimen (for example, low sodium diet)

3. Know the signs and symptoms of the various syndromes that may result from excessive loss of electrolytes and water. For example, patients taking potent diuretics should be carefully observed for signs of dehydration, the low-salt syndrome, acid-base imbalance, and hypokalemia (potassium depletion). Listen for complaints such as muscle cramps or weakness, listlessness, and fatigue, and loss of appetite (anorexia). Also, know the signs and symptoms of the hypersensitivity reactions and direct tissue toxicity caused by organic mercurials, sulfonamides, and other diuretics.

4. Be sure that patients who are taking diuretics regularly for long periods have been advised to eat foods that are rich in potassium (such as bananas, citrus fruits, tomatoes) to replace potassium lost as a result of diuretic action. Alert the doctor to the patient's need for supplementary potassium (and other electrolytes), if the patient shows signs of depletion, including, for example, reduced responses to diuretic medication after repeated drug administration.

5. Avoid injecting diuretics (or other drugs) into edematous areas because of their poor absorption from such sites. Make injections of mercurials (and other diuretics) deep into the muscles. Massage the area vigorously to increase the rate of absorption and to reduce local pain and irritation. (When mercurial suppositories are employed, examine the patient's rectum for signs of irritation.)

6. Explain to the patient that the diuretic may produce a copious flow of urine within a few hours, so that he won't be alarmed by the frequency and urgency of his need to void. Administer once-a-day diuretics in the morning so that the patient's sleep will not be disturbed. See to it that the patient has a urinal or bedpan handy, or, if he is ambulatory, put the call bell within his easy reach and instruct him to call for assistance when he wants to make a trip to the bathroom. This is especially important for elderly, weak, or confused patients who could suffer injury in trying to get out of bed to go to the bathroom by themselves (side rails may be necessary).

Clinical Nursing Situation*

The Situation: Mrs. Cohen, age 68, lives alone in a two-room apartment. Her nearest relative is a son now living abroad. She has suffered from congestive heart failure for the past five years, for which she has been taking digoxin 0.25 mg once daily. This and a low sodium diet have been successful in keeping her edema-free.

During the past two weeks, Mrs. Cohen has

noted the development of increasingly severe swelling of her ankles during the day, a feeling of fatigue and general malaise, bloating, and considerable shortness of breath. She comes to a neighborhood health clinic a few blocks from her apartment for treatment by a doctor-nurse team.

The physician recommends the addition of *hydrochlorothiazide* (Hydro Diuril and others)

* Other sources of information besides this textbook should be consulted, if needed, for full discussion of various aspects of this problem.

to her treatment regimen in a daily dose of 25 mg. The plan is that Mrs. Cohen will see the nurse twice weekly and the doctor every other week until her symptoms are brought under better control. She has also been instructed to call the clinic at any time if her symptoms should become more severe.

The Problem: Assume that you are the nurse who will see Mrs. Cohen twice weekly. What factors would you consider in evaluating her response to diuretic therapy? What health topics may it be necessary to teach this patient?

Give examples of some signs and symptoms that you might observe which would lead you to recommend that Mrs. Cohen see the doctor *before* her next scheduled appointment with him.

DRUG DIGEST

ACETAZOLAMIDE U.S.P. (Diamox)

Actions and Indications. This carbonic anhydrase inhibitor-type diuretic is used mainly in mild edema, including that of pregnancy, premenstrual tension, and drug-induced edema. Although it is not used for removing edema already accumulated in cases of congestive heart failure, acetazolamide is often effective for maintaining a patient at "dry weight," particularly when alternated with a thiazide or mercurial diuretic. This drug is also used in the management of epilepsy and glaucoma (chronic open-angle and acute closed-angle).

Side Effects, Cautions, and Contraindications. Drowsiness and feelings of numbness and tingling are the most common side effects. Hypersensitivity-type reactions including skin rashes, fever, and, rarely, blood dyscrasias have been reported. The drug causes the excretion of sodium bicarbonate and potassium. This and the retention of chloride ions may result in hyperchloremic acidosis as well as hypokalemia. Thus, the drug is contraindicated in patients with severe kidney and liver disease, in whom these acid-base and electrolyte imbalances are dangerous. Acetazolamide should not be administered over the long term to patients with chronic closed-angle glaucoma, although it may be used in acute congestive ocular emergencies.

Dosage and Administration. A morning dose of 250 to 375 mg is administered for one or two days, alternating with a rest day. In chronic open-angle glaucoma 250 to 1000 mg is administered orally; in acute closed-angle glaucoma 250 mg may be given orally or I.V. every four hours. Daily dosages in epilepsy ranges between 375 mg and 1 gram.

ETHACRYNIC ACID U.S.P. (Edecrin)

Actions and Indications. This potent diuretic is often effective for treating edema in patients who do not respond to therapy with thiazides and other drugs. Its action, coming on within a few minutes after I.V. administration, may be lifesaving in patients with acute pulmonary edema. This drug is often effective in patients with poor kidney function, including children with nephrotic edema. Its activity may continue even in patients with electrolyte and acid-base imbalances.

Side Effects, Cautions, and Contraindications. Care is required to avoid too sudden loss of large amounts of fluid to prevent complications from dehydration and depletion of sodium, potassium, and other electrolytes, particularly in patients with severe heart, liver, or kidney disease.

Signs of excessive electrolyte loss include loss of appetite, lethargy, muscle cramps, and weakness. The drug's direct effects may lead to abdominal discomfort and pain; occasionally, the drug may have to be discontinued because of development of severe, watery diarrhea or gastrointestinal bleeding. Patients with poor kidney function have sometimes suffered vertigo and temporary deafness while taking this drug.

Dosage and Administration. Treatment is begun with a single small (50 mg) dose administered by mouth after a meal. Dosage is then raised just enough to cause a weight loss of only one or two pounds daily. Once dry weight is reached, this drug is best given only two or three times a week, except in cases of resistant edema. In emergencies, the sodium salt is administered in a single I.V. dose of 50 to 100 mg.

FUROSEMIDE U.S.P. (Lasix)

Actions and Indications. This potent sulfonamide diuretic is often useful for treating edematous patients who have not responded well to treatment with thiazides and other diuretics. It is employed in the management of edema in congestive heart failure, hepatic cirrhosis, and the nephrotic syndrome.

Side Effects, Cautions, and Contraindications. Drug-induced electrolyte imbalances can result from excessive diuretic activity. Loss of sodium and chloride in excess may cause muscle cramps. Potassium loss may be particularly dangerous for patients taking digitalis. Hypokalemic alkalosis may also occur, as can other metabolic imbalances, including rises in blood glucose and uric acid levels. Elderly patients may suffer circulatory collapse or blood clots as a result of dehydration and a drop in blood volume following a too-strong response to this drug.

Dosage and Administration. This drug may be administered orally in doses of 40 to 80 mg and followed by a second dose 6 to 8 hours later, if necessary. Individually determined higher doses may be administered twice daily up to a maximum daily dose of 600 mg. For rapid onset of action in acute pulmonary edema or other emergencies, a single dose of 20 to 40 mg is administered I.M. or I.V.

HYDROCHLOROTHIAZIDE U.S.P. (Esidrix; Hydro Diuril; and others)

Actions and Indications. This thiazide diuretic is useful in the management of edema and in hypertension. Used alone, it reduces mildly elevated blood pressure. For treating moderate to severe degrees of hypertension, this drug is commonly combined with other antihypertensive agents, such as reserpine and guanethidine. Among the edematous states that respond to treatment with this diuretic are congestive heart failure, hepatic ascites, the nephrotic syndrome, and less serious disorders such as premenstrual tension and edema.

Side Effects, Cautions, and Contraindications. Side effects of this drug mainly result from excessive loss of fluid and electrolytes such as sodium, chloride, and potassium. Patients are watched for such warning signs of the low-salt syndrome, hypochloremic alkalosis, and hypokalemia as: mouth dryness and thirst, feelings of fatigue, weakness and drowsiness, muscle cramps and pain, and nausea, vomiting, and diarrhea.

Special care is required in patients with cirrhosis of the liver, in whom drug-induced hypokalemia and alkalosis can set off hepatic coma. The drug is contraindicated in patients with renal shutdown and in those with a history of hypersensitivity to thiazides and other sulfonamide drugs.

Dosage and Administration. The usual oral doses for maintaining patients at dry weight in edema are 25 to 100 mg daily or intermittently. At least twice these doses is needed for initiating treatment of edema. The dosage range in hypertension is from 25 to 150 mg daily.

MERALLURIDE SODIUM U.S.P. (Mercuhydrin)

Actions and Indications. This organic mercurial produces rapid diuretic action when administered by injection to patients with congestive heart failure, cirrhosis of the liver with ascites, and the nephrotic syndrome. Patients who lose the ability to respond to this diuretic may have their responsiveness restored by the prior administration of ammonium chloride or other acidifying salts.

Side Effects, Cautions, and Contraindications. Direct tissue toxicity can cause stomatitis (mouth lesions), colitis, and renal tubular damage. Elderly patients with reduced renal function should be given only small doses cautiously to avoid accumulation of the drug

in kidney tissues. Its use is contraindicated in patients with acute nephritis. Hypersensitivity reactions resulting in skin rashes, fever, and, rarely, cardiac arrhythmias, may occur. Electrolyte imbalances and dehydration may result from excessive elimination of fluid containing sodium, chloride, and potassium ions. Patients may complain of muscle cramps or weakness, and gastrointestinal upset. Hypotension and clot formation leading to cardiac, kidney, or other vital organ damage may also result.

Dosage and Administration. The usual dose for initiating treatment of severe edema is 1 or 2 ml of the injection solution administered intramuscularly or subcutaneously. This may be continued once daily or every other day until "dry weight" is attained. Then the drug may be administered intermittently whenever the patient's body weight begins to rise.

SPIRONOLACTONE U.S.P. (Aldactone)

Actions and Indications. This diuretic removes sodium and chloride ions with water in various edematous states without causing any loss of potassium. It is particularly indicated in disorders in which the adrenal hormone aldosterone is secreted in large amounts, including cirrhosis of the liver, the nephrotic syndrome, and in congestive heart failure. Spironolactone is commonly combined with thiazide diuretics in treating edema and for reducing high blood pressure in patients with essential hypertension.

Side Effects, Cautions, and Contraindications. This drug may cause potassium retention, particularly in patients with poor kidney function. Such patients should have their plasma potassium levels checked to detect any tendency toward development of hyperkalemia, a condition that can cause cardiac arrest. Other imbalances include occasional mild acidosis and hyponatremia (low serum sodium), which may be marked by thirst, dry mouth, and drowsiness.

This steroid drug sometimes produces sex hormone-type side effects, including growth of hair

and deepening of the voice in women and painful swelling of the breasts in men.

Dosage and Administration. For treating edema, a daily dose of 100 mg is administered orally in four doses of 25 mg. This may be combined with a thiazide or mercurial diuretic for further effects. Higher doses may be needed in cases of resistant edema, but lower doses may be adequate in the management of essential hypertension.

UREA, STERILE U.S.P. (Ureaphil; Urevert)

Actions and Indications. This osmotic diuretic is used clinically for several purposes other than control of edema. These are based upon the drug's ability to keep water within the kidney tubules and thus bring about an increase in urine production. This helps to prevent oliguria and kidney damage in patients severely injured or burned, or following surgery, including prostatectomy. The drug is also useful for reducing intracranial and intraocular pressure during neurological surgery and in acute glaucoma attacks.

Side Effects, Cautions, and Contraindications. Care is needed in patients with kidney diseases, and the drug is contraindicated when kidney function is severely impaired. This diuretic should not be administered to severely dehydrated patients or during active intracranial bleeding. Infusions should not be made into leg veins of elderly patients because of possible thrombophlebitis and blood clot formation. Avoid letting the solution leak into tissues around the injected vein, as this may cause local irritation, leading occasionally to tissue necrosis.

Dosage and Administration. Solutions of sterile urea are prepared by adding fluid in amounts needed to make 4 percent or 30 percent solutions. These solutions are infused intravenously in amounts from 1 to 1.5 g per kg body weight per day in adults or 1 g per kg body weight per day in children. The rate of injection should be no greater than 3 to 4 ml per minute.

References

Cannon, P.J. Use of diuretics in liver disease with ascites. *Mod. Treatm.*, 7:420, 1970 (March).

Di Palma, J. The diuretic drugs. RN, 30:59, 1967 (April).

Heinemann, H.O. Use of diuretics in congestive heart failure, pulmonary edema, and cor pulmonale. *Mod. Treatm.*, 7:380, 1970 (March).

Perez-Stable, E.C., and Materson, B.J. Diuretic drug therapy of edema. *Med. Clin. N. Amer.*, 55:359, 1971 (March).

Rodman, M.J. Roundup of the diuretics. *RN*, 26:77, 1963 (Nov.).

———. Drugs for congestive heart failure and cardiac arrhythmias. *RN*, 30:51, 1967 (Nov.).

Special feature. Drugs used in the care of the cardiac patient. *Nurs. Clin. N. Amer.*, 4:645, 1969 (Dec.).

Spencer, R. Problems of drug therapy in congestive heart failure. *RN*, 35:46, 1972 (Aug.).

28.

Digitalis and Related Heart Drugs

The Plant and Its Principles (Table 28-1)

Digitalis is a drug of great value in the treatment of congestive heart failure and various cardiac disorders marked by irregular rhythms. No synthetic drug has yet been discovered that is able to strengthen the beat of the failing heart as well as the glycosides that are the active constituents of this plant. In this country, two species of foxglove—*Digitalis purpurea* and *Digitalis lanata*—are the source of the most commonly employed plant principles, *digoxin* and *digitoxin*. Other glycosides, including some obtained from other families of plants, also have the same kind of *cardiotonic*, or heart-strengthening, activity. For example, *ouabain*, a rapid-acting emergency heart drug, comes from the plant *Strophanthus gratus*.*

PREPARATIONS

Many different types of products are available. Doctors sometimes order pills or capsules containing dried, powdered digitalis leaves. Occa-

---

* Plants of other families that contain principles with digitalis-like cardiac actions include the lily of the valley (*Convallaria*), the sea onion (Squill), the oleander shrub (Thevetia), and the Christmas Rose (*Helleborus*). These plants and their principles are rarely used for medicinal purposes in this country, but cases of accidental poisoning from eating parts of ornamental shrubs or flowers may occasionally be of concern to the nurse. Other glycosides of *Digitalis lanata* include acetyldigitoxin, deslanoside, lanatoside C, and a mixture of lanatosides A, B, and C. A mixture of amorphous (*non*-crystalline) glycosides of *Digitalis purpurea*, called gitalin, is also available.

TABLE 28-1 *Cardiotonic Drugs and Dosage Schedules**

Nonproprietary Name	Proprietary Name or Synonym	Range of Total (Full) Digitalizing Doses	Daily Maintenance Dose
Acetyldigitoxin N.F.	Acylanid	1.0–2.0 mg oral	0.1–0.2 mg
Deslanoside U.S.P. and Deslanoside injection U.S.P.	Cedilanid D	1.2–1.6 mg I.V.	0.4 mg I.V.
Digitalis, powdered (dried leaf) U.S.P.	Digifortis; Digitora; Pil-Digis	1.0–2 g oral	100–200 mg
Digitalis, tincture		10–15 ml oral	0.75–1.5 ml
Digitoxin U.S.P. and Digitoxin injection N.F.	Crystodigin; Digisidin; Digitaline Nativelle; Myodigin; Purodigin	1.0–1.5 mg oral or I.V.	0.05–0.2 mg
Digoxin U.S.P. and Digoxin injection U.S.P.	Lanoxin; Davoxin	2.0–3.0 mg oral; 1 mg I.V.	0.25–0.75 mg
Gitalin (amorphous) N.F.	Gitaligin	4.0–8.0 mg oral	0.25–1.0 mg
Lanatoside C, N.F.	Cedilanid	5.0–10.0 mg oral; 1.2–1.6 mg I.V.	0.5–2.0 mg
Lanatoside A, B, C, mixed	Digilanid	3.0–6.0 mg oral; 0.8–0.16 mg I.V.	0.33–0.66 mg
Ouabain injection U.S.P.	G-Strophanthin	0.5–1 mg I.V.	

* These doses should be considered as approximations and used as a guide in checking dosage, which is, of course, highly individualized. Full digitalization may be achieved by a series of fractional doses or by a single larger dose (p. 349).

sionally, the drug may be administered in liquid form, as a tincture. More commonly, today, the purified, highly potent glycosides (Table 28-1) are prescribed because of the relative dependability with which a given amount will produce the desired effect. In spite of differences in milligram for milligram potency and in their speed of onset and duration of action, all the available products have almost exactly the same kinds of effects on the heart and other organs.

Cardiac and Circulatory Effects of Digitalis

Digitalis has two main types of actions on the heart:

1. It increases the strength of the heartbeat (positive inotropic action).

2. It alters the electrophysiological properties of the heart and thus affects its rate and rhythm.

The ability of digitalis to make the myocardium contract more forcefully when this muscular pump is weakened by disease is the main action that accounts for this drug's usefulness in treating congestive heart failure. Administered to patients with hypodynamic heart ac-

tion, digitalis glycosides help the heart muscle to drive more blood out of its chambers with each beat. This increase in stroke volume and cardiac output improves the patient's pulmonary and systemic circulations and relieves the signs and symptoms that stem from edema fluid that has accumulated in his tissues.

The effects of digitalis upon the electrical properties of the heart muscle fibers and on the specialized conducting tissue play an important part in bringing about changes in the rate and rhythm of the patient's heartbeats. Depending upon the dose of the drug and the state of the patient's heart, these effects of digitalis can either be therapeutically useful or a cause of cardiac toxicity.

Among clinical conditions in which digitalis is often beneficial to the patient are some in which the ventricles are being driven to beat too rapidly because of overstimulation by impulses that originate in the atria. In such supraventricular tachyarrhythmias as atrial and nodal tachycardia, atrial flutter, and atrial fibrillation, digitalis helps to slow and to stabilize the rapid, irregular ventricular rhythms.

On the other hand, digitalis is also capable of *causing* every kind of cardiac irregularity. Overdoses of digitalis can *slow* the heartbeat to the point of causing cardiac standstill (*asystole*). On the other hand, an excess of digitalis can also make the heart beat in a rapid, irregular rhythm. This too, can lead to cardiac arrest —in this case, as a result of ventricular fibrillation. The nurse's observations are often very important for preventing digitalis intoxication (see p. 347).

Therapeutic Applications

CONGESTIVE HEART FAILURE

The term "failure" refers to the fact that the patient's heart is failing to pump enough blood to meet the body's needs for oxygen and nutrients. The term "congestive" refers to the fluid that accumulates in tissue spaces and cavities as a result of this primary pump failure. As indicated in Chapters 26 and 27, most of the discomforting and often dangerous complications of heart failure stem from this fluid, which leaks into the tissues from the overfilled venous capillaries.

The signs and symptoms of congestive failure (Table 28-2) vary greatly, depending upon whether the right or left ventricle is failing or if both sides of the heart are involved. The clinical picture is also affected by whether the condition is chronic or acute and by the nature

T A B L E 2 8 - 2 *Cardiac Decompensation and Response to Digitalis*

Signs and Symptoms*	During Decompensation	After Full Digitalization†
Heart rate, rhythm, and size	Heart hypertrophied and dilated; rate often rapid, rhythm irregular (for example, gallop rhythm, pulse alternation). Patient may complain of awareness of palpitations.	Resting rate slowed to between 70 and 80 beats per minute. Heart size (dilation) reduced, but hypertrophy may still exist.
Lungs	Dyspnea ("breathlessness," or "shortness of breath") on slight effort or when lying flat in bed (orthopnea). Sudden attacks of breath shortness (paroxysmal nocturnal dyspnea or cardiac asthma), and periodic (Cheyne-Stokes) breathing. Pulmonary edema, rales at base of lungs, cough, expectoration, and hemoptysis (bloody sputum).	Breathing improved, but other drugs (such as aminophylline and mercurial diuretics) may also be required for relief of bronchospasm and edema, and morphine may be desirable for allaying restlessness, struggling, and excitement.
Peripheral congestion	Pitting edema of dependent parts (feet, legs, lower abdomen); enlarged liver; accumulation of fluid in abdominal cavity (ascites); veins distended with rise in venous pressure; prolongation of circulation time; cyanosis—dusky blue color of lips, nail beds, and elsewhere on the skin surfaces; oliguria and nocturia (increased urine volume at night).	Increased cardiac output and relief of renal anoxia leads to diuresis. Loss of large quantity of salty fluids in urine results in relief of all congestion symptoms and better skin color.
Other	Weakness, fatigue, insomnia; anorexia, nausea, vomiting, abdominal pain.	Strength and appetite return.

* Because the clinical picture in heart failure varies with stage and degree of severity, the signs and symptoms may vary considerably in different patients.

† Digitalis will not overcome similar symptoms when they are caused by conditions other than heart failure. Overdosage may actually cause symptoms similar to those of heart failure (for example, anorexia, nausea, and vomiting; cardiac arrhythmias; peripheral congestion).

of the underlying disease that has led to heart failure. For example, a patient with chronic hypertensive or mitral valvular heart disease may have an enlarged rapidly beating heart and show signs and symptoms (such as fluid in the lungs) that stem from gradual left-sided heart failure. A patient who has suffered an acute pulmonary embolus may have mainly right-sided heart failure and his symptoms may be mainly the result of systemic circulatory difficulties. In all such cases, the administration of digitalis can often increase cardiac output and counteract signs and symptoms of cardiac failure.

DIGITALIS EFFECTS. As digitalis accumulates in the myocardium it produces effects on cardiac function that set into motion a train of events resulting in remarkable improvement in the condition of the heart failure patient. The ventricles, contracting more powerfully, empty themselves of their contents more completely. This improved ability to handle the load of blood brought to it by the veins helps the heart itself to function more efficiently. If, for example, the heart has been excessively dilated and rapid as a result of its efforts to compensate, it often tends to become smaller and slower under the influence of digitalis. Such cardiac changes help the heart to pump more blood out into the arteries without wasting its energy and its own oxygen supply.

The improved circulation of the blood in both the systemic and pulmonary vessels results in reduced edema in such areas as the abdominal cavity, the lungs, and the legs. In part, this stems from a lessening of hydrostatic pressure within the venous capillaries, when the digitalis-strengthened heart muscle becomes better able to transfer more blood from the venous to the arterial side of the circulatory tree. In addition, the fuller flow of blood through the arterioles of the kidneys reverses certain compensatory mechanisms that had resulted in excessive reabsorption of filtered sodium by the renal tubules.

The kidneys become better able to handle the load of salty fluids that then leaves the interstitial spaces and body cavities and enters the bloodstream. As a result, much of the edema that had accumulated in the lungs, abdomen, legs, and elsewhere leaves the body in a heavy flow of urine. This diuresis and the resulting relief of signs and symptoms of heart failure such as breathlessness, abdominal fluid accumulation (ascites), pitting edema (ana-

sarca), and others listed in Table 28-2 stems from the primary action of digitalis—the drug's ability to strengthen the contractions of a weakened (hypodynamic) heart which has lost its ability to compensate for the inefficiency of its cells in converting chemical (metabolic) energy into mechanical (pumping) power.

The nurse observes the patient for signs of improvement brought about by digitalis. She notes gross changes, such as reduction in the size of the patient's fluid-swollen abdomen and the absence of pitting when she presses the thumb against the patient's ankles. She records the amount of urine produced in response to digitalis therapy and weighs the patient daily, because these data are important in determining the best dose of digitalis and whether to add a diuretic to the patient's treatment regimen, as well as in planning nursing care.

The nurse also keeps particularly close check on how the patient's cardiac and respiratory functions respond to digitalization. For example, if the patient had shown signs of pulmonary edema, the nurse looks for signs of improvement such as a lessening of lung sounds (rales) and sputum-laden coughing, easier breathing, and better skin color. The rate and rhythm of the patient's heart action are noted, as digitalis often causes a rapid, irregularly beating heart to become slower and steadier.

CARDIAC ARRHYTHMIAS. The first slowing of the heart that often develops in patients with failure who are digitalized is the result of the drug-induced circulatory improvement. That is, if the patient's failing heart has speeded up because of autonomic nervous reflexes set off to compensate for low cardiac output, the heart slows down again after digitalis has increased the cardiac output and thus removed the stimuli that caused the cardioacceleratory reflex activity. However, digitalis also helps to slow the ventricular rate by directly affecting the rate at which the impulses arise in the atria and travel through conducting tissues.

In therapeutic doses, digitalis increases the sensitivity of S-A and A-V nodal tissues to the braking action of the vagus nerves. In addition, digitalis depresses the rate at which impulses are conducted from the atria to the ventricles by way of the A-V transmission system. This combination of vagal and extravagal effects of digitalis protects the ventricles from overstimulation of excessive numbers of impulses arising rapidly in atrial tissues other than the S-A nodal pacemaker.

In *paroxysmal atrial tachycardia* (PAT), for example, digitalis not only keeps the rapidly generated atrial impulses from reaching the ventricles but also often converts this arrhythmia to a normal sinus rhythm. Intravenous administration of a relatively rapid-acting digitalis glycoside such as *digoxin*+ (Davoxin; Lanoxin) for example, is more effective than cholinergic and adrenergic drugs for stopping this type of tachyarrhythmia attack. Once the condition is brought under control, daily oral administration of digoxin may be even more effective for preventing recurrences than taking other antiarrhythmic drugs such as quinidine and procainamide.

Digitalis is not often as effective for converting the atria to a normal sinus rhythm in other supraventricular arrhythmias such as atrial fibrillation and atrial flutter. This drug does, however, block bombardment of the ventricles by the hundreds of impulses that arise at ectopic sites in the atria. Ordinarily, in these arrhythmias, even though the conducting tissues are refractory to most of the impulses crowding into them from the atria, enough stimuli get through to make the heart beat rapidly and irregularly. This can reduce the heart's pumping power, and the resulting reduction in cardiac output and mechanical efficiency can then lead to congestive heart failure.

In *atrial fibrillation,* for example, impulses arising in the atria at a rate of 400 to 600 per minute may drive the ventricles at rates between 100 and 200 beats per minute. These rapid systolic contractions leave little time for filling of the ventricles during diastole. Thus, some rapid, irregular beats by the ventricle drive little or no blood out into the systemic circulation. The nurse can often detect this as *a pulse deficit*—a difference between the patient's apical pulse and the pulse taken at the wrist. When she takes the patient's pulse following full digitalization, the beats are slower and more regular, and there is usually no longer any pulse deficit.

The nurse also watches for any signs of excessive actions of digitalis on the patient's heart rate and rhythm. Digitalis can cause various degrees of heart block by prolonging the refractory period of the conducting tissues and slowing the rate at which atrial impulses reach the ventricles to too great an extent. The nurse notes any tendency of the apical rate to fall below 60 per minute, as this is a sign that the next dose of digitalis should be withheld until the doctor has been consulted. Continuing the administration of the drug without a careful evaluation of the patient's cardiac status can result in dangerous digitalis intoxication.

The Toxic Effects of Digitalis Overdosage

Digitalis intoxication is one of the most common kinds of drug poisoning. It accounts for about one out of every five drug reactions in hospitalized patients. About one out of three digitalis-poisoned patients dies. Thus, the nurse must be able to recognize the early signs of toxicity in patients who are receiving digitalis. The doctor who is alerted by the nurse's observations can then discontinue digitalis and order tests for determining the exact state of the patient's cardiac function.

Prevention of toxicity is, of course, primarily the doctor's problem. He has the often difficult task of determining the best digitalizing and maintenance doses (see pp. 349-350) for each individual patient. However, the nurse can help the physician to regulate digitalis dosage in order to get the desired effects and avoid adverse effects. This involves not only noting changes in the rate and rhythm of the patient's pulse, but also other signs that often serve as early warnings of digitalis toxicity.

EXTRACARDIAC SIGNS AND SYMPTOMS

Often, patients who are approaching cardiac toxicity first show other adverse effects. Most commonly, the patient may refuse food when his tray is brought to him. The nurse should report such instances of anorexia, as this is often an early sign of toxicity. The patient's loss of appetite may be accompanied by nausea and is often followed by vomiting.

Of course, if a patient vomits shortly after he has received his very first dose of digitalis, he is probably *not* suffering from overdosage. Some products, such as powdered digitalis or tincture of digitalis, tend to cause early gastrointestinal tract irritation. Also, patients with congestive heart failure are often nauseated to begin with. In such cases the nurse gives the digitalis preparation before meals to reduce the local irritation that may cause vomiting. However, the development of these gastrointestinal complaints after several days of digitalis treatment is a more significant sign that the patient may be approaching cardiac toxicity too.

Other ill effects that should alert the nurse are complaints of headache, drowsiness, and fatigue. Question the patient about his eyesight. He may then mention that he is seeing double, or that his vision seems blurred. Reports of flickering lights or colored dots and flashes also often indicate that digitalis toxicity is close. Elderly patients who become confused and disoriented during digitalis administration may also be suffering from the drug's central effects.

CARDIAC TOXICITY

Digitalis can cause almost every known kind of cardiac rate and rhythm irregularity. In general, digitalis-induced arrhythmias are of two types:

(1) *Bradycardias*—conditions in which the ventricular rate becomes excessively slow.

(2) *Tachystolic arrhythmias*—marked by rapid, irregular rhythms.

Both kinds of irregularities can be dangerous because the heart may then be unable to keep pumping an adequate flow of blood to the tissues. An excessive reduction of cardiac output can, of course, lead to a return of the signs and symptoms of congestive heart failure. Thus, the doctor may then not be sure whether the patient needs more digitalis or whether he has already had too much.

DIGITALIS-INDUCED BRADYCARDIA. This sometimes results from the same action of the drug that is useful for protecting the ventricles from the effects of atrial arrhythmias. That is, toxic doses of digitalis may depress the conducting tissues excessively. If too few impulses from the sinus node pacemaker reach the ventricles, they may beat at too slow a rate. This may make the patient dizzy, weak, and faint, or he may complain of chest pains—symptoms that stem from poor blood flow to the patient's brain or through the coronary vessels that supply the heart muscle with blood.

The nurse can help prevent this type of cardiac toxicity by her observations while taking the patient's apical pulse with a stethoscope. A drop in the patient's heart rate to levels below 60 beats per minute may mean that digitalis is producing toxic effects at the S-A or A-V nodes or on ventricular tissues.

When the nurse reports this to the doctor, he may order digitalis to be discontinued. If the slow rhythm persists, the physician may call for the administration of such autonomic drugs as *atropine* or *isoproterenol*. Occasionally, a pacemaker may have to be employed to convert the patient's rhythm to a safer rate.

DIGITALIS-INDUCED TACHYARRHYTHMIAS. Sometimes, a patient whose heart has been slowed by digitalis therapy to a desirable rate of about 70 to 80 beats per minute may begin to develop a rapid, irregular heartbeat. This can be confusing to the doctor who then has to decide whether the patient is *over*digitalized or *under*digitalized. The nurse's recorded observations can often be of great help here, if they show that she had detected occasional ectopic beats even while the patient's heart rate was otherwise normal.

Ectopic beats, or extrasystoles, are the most common early signs of digitalis cardiotoxicity. They are most likely to occur when a patient has lost much plasma potassium as a result of diuretic therapy, because such hypokalemia sensitizes the heart to the toxic effects of digitalis upon the cardiac property called *automaticity*. This may then make certain latent pacemaker cells discharge spontaneously, often at a rate more rapid than the regular pacemaker.

The most characteristic pattern of extra heartbeats, or premature ventricular contractions, caused by digitalis overdosage is *bigeminy*, or "coupling"—a weak beat alternating with a strong one. These sounds can be heard clearly when the stethoscope is placed above the apex of the patient's heart. Sometimes, when the patient's radial pulse is taken at the same time as the weak apical beat is heard, no corresponding pulsation is felt at the patient's wrist (*pulse deficit*).

Promptly detecting and reporting such irregularities as bigeminy, trigeminy, and pulse deficit can help the doctor prevent development of further dangerous toxicity. When the nurse quickly reports such warning signals, the doctor will usually withhold the patient's medication and perhaps order an electrocardiogram and various laboratory tests to confirm the diagnosis of digitalis overdosage. He may then also order several different drugs to counteract toxicity.

Treatment of tachyarrhythmias may require no more than discontinuing digitalis and diuretic therapy. If extrasystoles continue, the doctor may order the administration of potassium salts by mouth, or—in cases with severe ventricular tachycardia—by intravenous infusion. To prevent potassium overdosage, the doctor makes sure that the patient's kidney function is normal and monitors his heart action by electrocardiograms during the potassium salt infusion. The reason for this is that although potassium salts suppress the digitalis-induced automaticity of the ventricles, they may also increase the A-V conduction defect. This could cause complete heart block followed by cardiac standstill (asystolic cardiac arrest).

The antiarrhythmic drugs, such as *quinidine* and *procainamide*, have also been used to control digitalis tachyarrhythmias. Like potassium salts, these agents can also cause cardiac arrest. The newer antiarrhythmic agents, *lidocaine*, *propranolol*, and particularly *diphenylhydantoin+* (Dilantin), are claimed to be safer and more effective for treating digitalis toxicity. Diphenylhydantoin is said to suppress ventricular irregularities when administered in low doses that do *not* depress the A-V conducting tissues or stop ventricular contractions. Nevertheless, the effects of this drug on the patient's heart must be carefully followed on the electrocardiogram, so that the drug may be discontinued if signs of A-V block and myocardial depression do appear.

Prevention of digitalis toxicity is obviously better than having to treat toxicity after it has developed. The nurse can begin to instruct patients who are likely to require maintenance therapy while they are still hospitalized, as well as when she meets them as outpatients. She teaches them to follow directions concerning proper dosage and regular timing of administration of this useful but potentially dangerous medication.

Dosage and Administration of Digitalis Products

DIGITALIS PREPARATIONS

All the different types of digitalis products have the same kinds of actions and do not differ much in their effectiveness and safety. However, they do differ in how they are handled by the body. Some are rapidly absorbed and excreted; others reach effective concentrations in the heart relatively slowly and are only eliminated slowly by the body. Thus, the physician often prefers some digitalis glycosides for rapid action in emergencies and others for long-term treatment of chronic cardiac disorders.

Rapid-acting glycosides such as *ouabain* and *deslanoside+* (Cedilanid-D) are administered parenterally for emergency management of acute pulmonary edema and rapid supraventricular arrhythmias. The long-lasting glycoside, *digitoxin+* (Crystodigin; and others) (or the powdered crude leaf and tincture of which it is the active constituent) is often preferred for prolonged administration. Actually, the intermediate-acting glycoside *digoxin+* (Lanoxin; Davoxin; and others) is probably the most commonly employed preparation of all today. It is fast-acting enough (particularly when administered parenterally) to establish quick control, and its action after oral administration is long enough to maintain day-to-day control for long periods.

DIGITALIZATION

Digitalization is the process of bringing the patient's decompensated or irregularly beating heart under control. Often this is done by administering relatively large doses of digitalis preparations within a few hours. This type of intensive administration of "loading" doses can cause toxic reactions, as these potent drugs have only a moderate safety margin. Thus, the administration of initial doses at a slower rate is often desirable. The doctor can order slower digitalization to lessen toxicity, particularly when he is uncertain of how much of the drug may still be in the patient's system from prior administration, or when the patient's case is a mild one in which a very rapid return to normal is not essential.

The nurse observes patients carefully during the administration of these relatively large initial doses. As already indicated, she looks both for signs of improvement and signs of cardiac and extracardiac toxicity (see Table 28-2 and *Summaries*, pp. 351-352) before administering each successive ordered dose in a series. She takes particular care in checking that she has read the dosage on the order and the label correctly, and measured it very accurately, as errors of only fractions of a milligram of the potent pure glycosides can cause cardiac toxicity.

MAINTENANCE DOSAGE

Once the patient's condition has responded to digitalization, he may have to continue taking a digitalis product indefinitely. The doctor tries to determine what daily dosage is needed to keep the patient's heart action at its optimal level. Doses are ordered that are just enough to replace the amount of digitalis eliminated since administration of the previous dose. Even though these daily maintenance doses are much lower than the original digitalizing doses, the risk of toxicity remains.

The amount of digitalis needed for maintenance varies not only in different patients but even in the same patient from time to time. Even though all authorities agree, in theory, that patients should be seen often and observed carefully to be sure that they are taking the dose that will keep optimal control over their cardiac action, this is often not carried out in practice. As a result, some patients gradually accumulate excessive amounts of digitalis and develop signs and symptoms of toxicity. Others may be taking daily doses that are lower than the amounts their bodies eliminate each day, with the result that they gradually slide back into heart failure. Patients whose cardiac function changes for the worse may suffer adverse effects from a maintenance dose that they have been taking for years without any difficulty. Similarly, a patient who eats foods containing too much sodium may suffer an episode of failure because his maintenance digitalis dosage is not enough to meet the added load the extra sodium may put on his barely compensated heart.

The nurse takes time to teach the patient and his family that it is important to make regular visits to the doctor and to follow the physician's directions during long-term maintenance therapy. She is particularly concerned with instructing elderly patients because they are the ones most likely to become confused by a rapid-fire barrage of directions, as well as being the group most susceptible to digitalis toxicity from overdosage.

The nurse's role as a teacher of patients and their families during long-term digitalis treatment of cardiac failure has recently assumed increasing importance. Nurses now often work, for example, with elderly patients in housing projects and other neighborhood communities. Helping these people to understand the nature of their drug therapy and the need to follow directions when they take *any* prescribed drug is an important part of the nurse's functions in such situations.

Thus, the nurse often sits down with the patient and writes down a simple summary of his instructions for him. She gives the patient an opportunity to ask questions and explains in simple language how taking the drug will help his heart so that he will be better able to carry on his daily activities. In ways that won't alarm the patient, she points out that, though the drug is safe and not "habit-forming" in the ordinary sense, it is important for him not to skip any prescribed doses and to watch for certain signs and symptoms of underdosage or overdosage. (See *Summaries of Cardiac Actions of Digitalis* and *Points to Remember about its Administration*, pp. 351–352.)

It is also often helpful to teach the patient how to make up a daily and weekly medication check-off card in order to avoid missing a day's digitalis therapy or taking the drug twice on the same day due to forgetfulness. Each time the nurse sees the patient, she should ask him direct questions, such as: "How many pills do you take? How often do you take them?" This is better than just repeating advice that the patient may really not be hearing even though he nods his head as though he understands.

Communicating details is, of course, part of conscientious care of a patient with any condition, and it reflects the nurse's personal concern for his well-being. However, it is particularly important in the long-term care of patients taking potent digitalis products for a chronic cardiac illness, as attention to such details can make the difference between sudden fatal heart failure and several years of independence and productivity.

S U M M A R Y of Pharmacological and Toxicological Effects of Digitalis Glycosides

Cardiac Effects (Therapeutically Desirable)

Increased contractility (positive inotropic).

Strengthening of the beats of the hypodynamic heart increases the stroke volume and cardiac output. This sets in motion a series of circulatory changes that relieve congestion.

Slowing of the heart (negative chronotropic).

(1) Heart slows as circulation improves, and the stimuli that had caused reflex cardioacceleration are removed, thus increasing vagal tone.

(2) Heart slows as a result of sensitization of the vagal mechanism which leads to increased vagal (braking) control over the heart.

(3) Heart slows because of direct (as well as vagal) depression of the A-V node and other conducting tissues. (The effective refractory period of the atrioventricular transmission system is increased.)

Cardiac Effects (Toxic)

Partial or complete heart block.

Slowing of the ventricular rate (apical pulse) well below 60 beats per minute may lead to poor cerebral and coronary circulation manifested by dizziness, weakness, fainting spells, and even signs and symptoms of congestive heart failure.

Increased automaticity.

Leads to patterns of premature beats, including bigeminy or coupling, trigeminy, pulse deficit, and ventricular tachycardia. Together with depressed ventricular conduction, this action can result in fatal ventricular fibrillation.

Extracardiac Effects (Signs and Symptoms of Toxicity)

Gastrointestinal.

Anorexia, nausea and vomiting are early signs of overdigitalization; epigastric pain and diarrhea occur less frequently.

Nervous system.

Drowsiness, fatigue, and headache are common; facial pain as a result of neuralgia is relatively rare as are convulsions.

Elderly patients may show such mental symptoms as confusion, disorientation, and even delirium.

Visual effects.

Vision may be blurred and diplopia (double vision) may also develop; flashes and flickering lights, halos, white or colored dots; yellow or green vision is common, brown, blue, and red less frequent.

Miscellaneous.

Gynecomastia (painful breast swellings) occurs sometimes in male patients treated with these glycosides, which are chemically related to sex hormones such as the estrogens; dermatological reactions include urticarial (hives) eruptions and scarlatiniform rashes.

S U M M A R Y of Clinical Indications for Digitalis Therapy

Congestive heart failure

Both right- and left-sided failure, especially in hypertensive heart disease or failure secondary to valvular or atherosclerotic disease.

Cardiac arrhythmias

Paroxysmal tachycardia. Both atrial (PAT) and A-V nodal types may be converted to a normal sinus rhythm.

Atrial fibrillation. Digitalis does not ordinarily convert to a normal sinus rhythm, but it protects the ventricles from overstimulation, thus reducing their rapid rate and restoring myocardial efficiency.

Atrial flutter. Digitalis acts indirectly to restore sinus rhythm in some cases, but even if the flutter is not converted, the ventricles are kept from being driven at an excessively rapid rate.

S U M M A R Y of Points that the Nurse Should Remember During Digitalis Administration

Before administering an ordered dose of a digitalis product:

(1) Take special care to check the label to be sure that you have picked out the digitalis preparation that was ordered. Names of the various glycosides are sometimes similar and may be easily confused—for example, *digoxin* and *digitoxin*. This could lead to errors in dosage and frequency of administration.

(2) Take particular care to check the accuracy

of measurements of these medications. These extremely potent drugs must be administered in precisely correct amounts to assure the success of treatment of the patient's cardiac condition, as well as his safety.

Observe the patient for signs of clinical improvement, including the following:

(1) Gradual slowing of the pulse to between 70 and 80 beats per minute, with reduction in pulse deficit (the difference between the patient's apical pulse and that taken at the wrist). In counting the pulse, for at least a full minute, observe its rhythm as well as its rate.

(2) Reduction in signs and symptoms of pulmonary congestion such as dyspnea, orthopnea, cyanosis, cough, hemoptysis, and anxiety, restlessness, or other emotional reactions.

(3) Reduction of generalized edema, as indicated by reduced abdominal size and lessened discomfort or pain upon pressure; absence of pitting when the surfaces of the extremities are pressed; an increase in the patient's daily urinary output and a decrease in his daily weight, both of which should be recorded.

Before giving each dose of the drug, observe the patient for signs of digitalis overdosage, including:

(1) An excessive slowing of the heart or the appearance of rhythmic changes such as bigeminy. If the apical pulse rate falls below 60 per minute, the next dose is usually withheld until the doctor has been consulted. (Do not withhold digitalis on the basis of the radial pulse, which may well be below 60, while the apical rate is, for example, 84.)

(2) Loss of interest in food by a patient who has usually had a good appetite. Ask him whether he feels nauseated and, if so, report this to the doctor to avoid the discomforting vomiting which will probably follow further dosage, and, of course, to prevent cardiac toxicity.

(3) Listen for complaints of headache, neuralgic facial pain, and unusual visual disturbances.

Teach the patient who is going to continue on long-term digitalis therapy:

(1) What the doctor's purpose is in prescribing this potent drug for treating his cardiac condition.

(2) Why it is important for him to take the medication regularly each day without missing a dose or taking any extra tablets. (Emphasize the importance of his administering this medication exactly as directed.)

(3) How to keep an accurate record of the medication taken and the medication remaining over a period of time.

(4) Which symptoms to report to the doctor, because they may indicate a need for upward or downward adjustment of dosage. The patient should, for example, recognize that fatigue and difficulty in breathing may be caused by fluid beginning to build up in his lungs and that these are not merely symptoms of a chest cold coming on, or that nausea and loss of appetite may not just be the result of something that he ate. (Of course, this instruction should be given in a way that warns the patient without alarming him.)

Be aware that elderly patients taking digitalis may have special problems, if they are short of funds, have no family or friends, and their eyesight or memory is failing.

Clinical Nursing Situation

The Situation: Ms. Whitaker is a 52-year-old patient with rheumatic heart disease. Until recently, she managed to carry out her daily activities without discomfort by avoiding excessive fatigue, and limiting intake of sodium. A few months ago Mr. Whitaker lost his job and Ms. Whitaker returned to work as a secretary. She had not worked for many years and found the adjustment very stressful. She began having dyspnea upon exertion and noted ankle edema late in the day. She developed a persistent fatigue which left her irritable, and with barely enough energy to complete her daily tasks.

The doctor decided that it was desirable to hospitalize Ms. Whitaker for a brief period in order to give her a rest, and to begin therapy with digitalis and a diuretic. He ordered the following:

1. Bed rest with bathroom privileges.
2. Diet low in sodium.
3. Furosemide (Lasix) 40 mg daily.
4. Chlordiazepoxide (Librium) 5 mg t.i.d.
5. Chloral hydrate 250 mg at bedtime.
6. Digoxin (Lanoxin) 1.5 mg, followed at six-hour intervals by 0.25 mg until fully digitalized, with maintenance dosage of 0.25 mg daily.

The Problem: Assume that you are the nurse caring for Ms. Whitaker. Describe the observations you would make and the care that you would provide particularly in relation to her drug therapy.

Ms. Whitaker was discharged from the hospital after five days, and is to return to her physician once a month. It is anticipated that she can return to work after a two-week rest at home. You plan to make a home visit during this two-week interval to assess Ms. Whitaker's progress and to evaluate how well she has learned to follow her therapy.

Develop a written observational guide which would help you in carrying out this assessment.

DRUG DIGEST

**DESLANOSIDE U.S.P.
(Cedilanid D)**

Actions and Indications. This soluble glycoside is administered by injection when rapid action is required for control of acute left heart failure with pulmonary edema or for conversion of paroxysmal atrial tachycardia. The relative rapidity with which full digitalization can be obtained—one or two hours in some cases—also makes it useful for protecting the ventricles from the effects of atrial fibrillation or flutter and in other types of congestive heart failure.

Side Effects, Cautions, and Contraindications. The relatively rapid rate of elimination of this glycoside is a safety factor in the event of overdosage. Extracardiac effects such as anorexia, nausea, and vomiting, headache, listlessness, and confusion, and visual blurring, flickering, and color disturbances often come on at about the same time as electrocardiographic evidence of toxicity. As with other digitalis preparations, cardiac toxicity may take the form of A-V conduction block, ventricular premature beats, or tachycardia or both. Caution is required in patients with hypokalemia.

Dosage and Administration. A single I.V. or I.M. injection of 1.6 mg (8 ml) may be administered for rapid loading, or the total dose may be divided into two injections of 0.8 mg (4 ml) and administered at half-hour intervals. The solution is said to be less irritating than other digitalis injections but, because some pain is likely, the I.M. injections may be made at different sites.

DIGITOXIN U.S.P. (Crystodigin; Myodigin Purodigin; and others)
Actions and Indications. This pure, potent digitalis glycoside has a relatively slow onset (6 to 12 hours for maximum effects) and a prolonged duration of action. Thus, it is preferred for maintenance therapy rather than for use when rapid digitalization is required in emergencies. Like other digitalis preparations, it is indicated for increasing the cardiac output and for removing edema in patients with congestive heart failure and for protecting the ventricles from the effects of supraventricular arrhythmias such as atrial fibrillation and atrial flutter.

Side Effects, Cautions, and Contraindications. Overdosage with this glycoside may be particularly dangerous because of its slow elimination from the body. Patients may require prolonged observation and treatment for either slow rhythms resulting from conduction defects or rapid rhythms caused by an increase in automaticity.

Cardiac toxicity is most likely in elderly or weakened patients with advanced disease of the heart, liver, and kidneys. Early extracardiac signs of toxicity include: anorexia, nausea, and vomiting; visual disturbances, such as blurred and flickering colored vision; and headache, depression, confusion, or disorientation.

Dosage and Administration. Rapid digitalization is often accomplished by administering an initial oral dose of 0.6 mg followed by a dose of 0.4 mg and one of 0.2 mg at intervals of four and six hours (total dose of 1.2 mg). Maintenance dosage is about 0.15 mg but may range between 0.05 and 0.3 mg daily.

DIGOXIN U.S.P. (Lanoxin; Davoxin; and others)

Actions and Indications. This is a pure, potent glycoside with a relatively rapid onset of action and an intermediate duration of effects. Thus, it is often used for both rapid initial digitalization (full effects developing in about 2 to 6 hours) and for maintenance therapy in chronic cardiac cases.

Like other digitalis preparations, it is useful for control of congestive heart failure and in the management of various kinds of cardiac arrhythmias, including atrial tachycardia, atrial fibrillation, and atrial flutter. In such cases it both protects the ventricles and sometimes brings about conversion to a sinus rhythm.

Side Effects, Cautions, and Contraindications. Periods of toxicity from overdosage with this drug do not last long because it is eliminated from the body rather rapidly (as compared to digitoxin). However, the drug can accumulate to toxic levels in patients with poor kidney function. Caution is also required in elderly patients with advanced heart disease and in patients with acute carditis. Cardiac toxicity can cause almost every kind of slow or rapid arrhythmia. Extracardiac warning signs include anorexia, nausea and vomiting, and visual and mental disturbances.

Dosage and Administration. Rapid digitalization may be accomplished by both the oral and I.V. routes by administering divided doses—for example, an initial oral dose of 1.5 mg followed at six-hour intervals by 0.25 to 0.5 mg. Maintenance doses range between 0.25 to 0.75 mg daily for adults, by both oral and parenteral routes.

References

Friend, D.W. Current concepts of therapy with cardiac glycosides. *New Eng. J. Med.*, 266:88, 187, 300, 400, 1962.

Hecht, A. B. Self medication inaccuracy and what can be done.

Modell, W. The clinical pharmacology of digitalis materials. *Clin. Pharmacol. Ther.*, 2:177, 1961.

Rodman, M.J. Drugs for heart failure and arrhythmias. *RN*, 30:51, 1967 (Nov.).

———. Drugs used in managing cardiac emergencies. *RN*, 36:55, 1973 (May).

Spann, J.F., Jr., et al. Recent advances in the understanding of congestive heart failure. *Mod. Conc. Cardiovasc. Dis.*, 39:73, 1970 (Jan.); 39:79, 1970 (Feb.).

Spencer, R. Problems of drug therapy in congestive heart failure. *RN*, 35:46, 1972 (Aug.). *Nurs. Outlook*, 18:30 1972 (April).

Wilson, W.S. Newer concepts regarding digitalis therapy. *Med. Clin. N. Amer.*, 53: 1279, 1969 (Nov.).

29

Antiarrhythmic Drugs

The Nature of Cardiac Arrhythmias

We have seen that the heart's ability to pump blood with power depends upon the coordinated contraction of the atria and the ventricles. The muscular walls of these cardiac chambers are activated to contract by impulses that arise regularly at the sinoatrial (S-A) pacemaker. These impulses, spreading swiftly through the atria, the A-V node, and the specialized conducting tissues in the ventricles, trigger the powerful beats that propel blood into the pulmonary and systemic circulations.

Cardiac arrhythmias—conditions in which the atria and ventricles contract at an abnormal rate or rhythm—are the result of two main types of impairment of the triggering mechanisms that activate cardiac contractions:

1. Impulses that arise in areas of cardiac tissue outside of the normal sinoatrial pacemaker (that is, at ectopic sites).

2. Impulses that spread through the heart by way of abnormal pathways (for instance, "circus" movements).

These kinds of disorders—disturbances of impulse formation and of impulse conduction—can make the heart beat both too slowly or too rapidly. The irregular, poorly coordinated contractions may then be unable to supply the needs of the body's tissues for blood.

In this chapter we shall discuss only those drugs that are used clinically to treat *rapid* atrial or ventricular arrhythmias. The treatment of cardiac disorders marked by development of excessively slow rhythms and of cardiac arrest is discussed in the section dealing with autonomic drugs—for example, *atropine* and *isoproterenol* and *epinephrine* (Chapters 22 and 23).

The Pharmacologic Effects of Antiarrhythmic Drugs

The drugs used in the management of rapid cardiac arrhythmias belong to several different chemical classes. However, they are all similar in their *main* effects upon the electrical activity of cardiac muscle cells. In this section, we shall summarize the cardiac effects of the older drugs, *quinidine+* and *procainamide+*. Then, in our later discussion of the therapeutic uses of the antiarrhythmic drugs, we shall point out certain significant differences in the effects of several newer drugs that have come into use in recent years, including *lidocaine+* (Xylocaine), *diphenylhydantoin+* (Dilantin), and *propranolol+* (Inderal). (The uses of *digitalis* as an antiarrhythmic agent are discussed in Chapter 28.

CARDIAC EFFECTS OF QUINIDINE AND PROCAINAMIDE

These two drugs exert the same kinds of effects on cardiac function, even though quinidine is a natural alkaloid derived from the cinchona plant and procainamide is a synthetic chemical related to the local anesthetic *procaine* (Novocain). We shall first summarize here the effects of these drugs that are therapeutically useful for treating cardiac arrhythmias and then discuss those effects on cardiac rate and rhythm that may prove toxic.

Therapeutic doses of both drugs produce the following effects:

1. Both drugs *suppress ectopic automaticity.* That is, they reduce the rate at which impulses arise spontaneously in cardiac tissues outside the normal pacemaker cells. This helps to halt some abnormally rapid arrhythmias and to restore a normal sinus rhythm in such disorders as atrial or ventricular premature beats or tachycardias, atrial fibrillation, and atrial flutter.

2. Both drugs *prolong the effective refractory period* of all parts of the heart, including the specialized conducting tissues. This lengthening of the period of time during which the excitability of cardiac tissues is reduced also tends to abolish arrhythmias. The drug-induced decreased excitability in certain areas of atrial and ventricular muscle often helps to halt trains of impulses that are traveling in abnormal pathways (for example, the so-called "circus" movements that are a factor in fibrillations).

In toxic doses, other effects of quinidine and procainamide on cardiac function can seriously interfere with the patient's circulation. These are among their most dangerous effects:

1. *Excessive slowing of conduction.* Some slowing of the rate at which abnormal impulses that arise in the atria are conducted to the ventricles is, of course, desirable, as it helps to keep the ventricles from being driven at too rapid a rate. However, doses that depress conduction through the A-V node too much can lead to dangerous arrhythmias that may end in cardiac arrest.

2. *Depression of myocardial contractions.* These drugs sometimes so weaken the heartbeat that heart failure may develop. When combined with the tendency of these drugs to dilate the arterioles, this cardiac effect can lead to severe hypotension and possibly to circulatory collapse.

The nurse may observe such early signs of heart failure as ankle edema, fatigue, and dyspnea in patients taking oral doses of quinidine at home. She should report these signs of toxicity to the patient's doctor and advise the patient to space his activities and to rest at intervals in order to avoid fatigue. (The responsibilities of the intensive coronary care unit (I.C.C.U.) nurse in avoiding toxicity are discussed below and in Chapter 30.)

SUMMARY

We have emphasized here how the two traditional antiarrhythmic drugs, quinidine and procainamide, can produce cardiac effects that are both desirable and potentially dangerous.

In the following two sections on therapeutic uses and toxicity we shall discuss the clinical applications of these pharmacologic effects in the treatment of patients with cardiac arrhythmias. We shall also show how the newer antiarrhythmic drugs—lidocaine, diphenylhydantoin, and propranolol—are similar in most of their cardiac effects but different in others. It is the differences in the cardiac effects of these newer drugs that account for the special effectiveness of one or another of them against various arrhythmias.

Therapeutic Uses of Antiarrhythmic Drugs

Drug treatment of cardiac irregularities is not always necessary. Some people with normal hearts may occasionally develop abnormal beats that need no specific drug treatment. The doctor simply assures the patient that the condition is temporary and harmless. He may prescribe a minor tranquilizer such as *chlordiazepoxide+* (Librium), if the patient's condition seems to stem from anxiety and tension. However, the doctor avoids ordering any of the potentially dangerous drugs discussed below if he finds no evidence of organic heart disease, and if he feels that the patient's irregular heartbeat will not in any way adversely affect his cardiac function or the flow of blood to vital organs.

The various arrhythmic drugs are reserved for use in the following kinds of clinical situations:

1. When the ventricles beat so rapidly and irregularly that the cardiac output is reduced. This, in turn, results in signs of impaired cerebral and coronary circulation.

2. When a relatively minor arrhythmia, such as premature ventricular contractions (extrasystoles), seems likely to develop into a more dangerous one, such as ventricular tachycardia.

3. When a dangerous irregularity has already developed and may prove rapidly fatal if not brought promptly to a halt. For example, when ventricular tachycardia seems likely to result in cardiac arrest.

In all of the above circumstances involving atrial and ventricular arrhythmias, the antiarrhythmic drugs are administered for two main purposes:

1. To abolish the abnormal rhythm and restore normal sinus rhythm.

2. To prevent further recurrences of the arrhythmias by means of maintenance therapy.

ATRIAL TACHYARRHYTHMIAS

Rhythm disorders originating in the atria include atrial extrasystoles, paroxysmal atrial tachycardia, atrial flutter, and atrial fibrillation. Often, abnormal atrial impulses reach the ventricles and cause them to contract so rapidly and irregularly that the systemic circulation becomes impaired. Antiarrhythmic drugs are used for two purposes in treating such so-called *supraventricular* arrhythmias: (1) to protect the ventricles from being driven at an excessive rate by the atrial impulses; and (2) to terminate the atrial arrhythmia (see *Summary*, p. 360).

In *atrial fibrillation*, for example, quinidine and procainamide can often abolish the abnormal rhythm. They do so by their ability to increase the length of the refractory period of the atrial muscle tissue, as well as by depressing excessive automaticity in ectopic pacemaker tissue. In this respect these drugs differ from digitalis, a drug that protects the ventricles from the effects of atrial fibrillation without converting the atria to a normal sinus rhythm.

Digitalis is, however, administered before trying to treat this disorder (and atrial flutter) with antiarrhythmic drugs. The reason for doing so is that quinidine and procainamide sometimes decrease the effect of vagus nerve control over atrioventricular conduction. This can cause a greater number of impulses from the fibrillating or fluttering atria to reach the ventricles, and thus make them speed up suddenly. Prior digitalization helps to prevent this paradoxical increase in the ventricular rate by reinforcing vagal control over A-V conduction.

On the other hand, the use of these drugs to abolish atrial tachycardia caused by digitalis intoxication can be dangerous. This is because quinidine and procainamide may intensify a digitalis-induced conduction block. The combined use of both digitalis and quinidine or procainamide could cause even more serious cardiac arrhythmias and even lead to cardiac arrest (see discussion of the *Toxic Effects* of these drugs, p. 359).

Diphenylhydantoin (Dilantin) is now the preferred antiarrhythmic drug for treating atrial (and ventricular) irregularities that are the result of digitalis toxicity. The main reason for this is that this drug, unlike the older antiarrhythmic agents, does *not* depress A-V conduction when administered in ordinary therapeutic doses. Thus, it often halts digitalis-induced atrial tachycardia without intensifying the heart block that is also often caused by digitalis overdosage. (See Chapter 28 for a further discussion of digitalis toxicity and p. 360 for precautions in using diphenylhydantoin).

Today, many atrial arrhythmias are brought under control, not by drugs, but by the application of direct current electrical shock. However, when the underlying cardiac disorder cannot be corrected, the irregularity often tends to occur again and again. Thus, even when the doctor decides to employ electrocardioversion, he may still administer quinidine orally both before and after this procedure. The prior presence of adequate blood levels of

TABLE 29-1 *Drugs for Rapid Arrhythmias**

Nonproprietary Name	Trade Name	Usual Dosage	Remarks
Digitalis glycosides			See Chapter 28, Table 28-1
Diphenylhydantoin sodium U.S.P.	Dilantin	5 to 10 mg/kg of body weight I.V. slowly; also I.M. 125–250 mg or orally 100–200 mg	Particularly useful in digitalis toxicity, as it does not ordinarily increase A-V block
Lidocaine HCl U.S.P.	Xylocaine	Single I.V. dose of 50–100 mg, followed by a continuous infusion of 1–4 mg per minute I.V.	See *Drug Digest*
Procainamide HCl U.S.P.	Pronestyl	0.5–1 orally or I.M.; 0.2–1 I.V.	See *Drug Digest*
Propranolol HCl	Inderal	10–40 mg orally; 0.5–1 mg I.V. repeated up to 0.1 mg/kg	Particularly effective in pheochromocytoma and when sympathetic stimulation is excessive
Quinidine salts, such as:			
Quinidine sulfate U.S.P.	Quinora; Quinidex	200–600 mg orally	See *Drug Digest*
Quinidine gluconate U.S.P.	Quinaglute	300–600 mg orally; I.M. 200 mg	
Quinidine polygalacturonate	Cardioquin	275–825 mg orally	
Quinidine HCl		200 mg diluted by slow I.V.; also I.M.	

* Drugs for *slow* arrhythmias, include *atropine* (Chapter 22) and *isoproterenol* (Chapter 23).

quinidine helps to keep the converted rhythm stable. Then, the continued use of prophylactic long-term treatment with oral quinidine or procainamide often helps to prevent recurrences of attacks of atrial (and ventricular) tachyarrhythmias.

VENTRICULAR TACHYARRHYTHMIAS

Rapid, irregular rhythms originating in the ventricles include premature ventricular contractions (PVCs), ventricular tachycardia, and ventricular fibrillation. Quinidine and procainamide are still used for treating the first of these conditions but are now rarely employed for reverting the more serious ventricular arrhythmias. Administered by mouth to a patient without serious heart disease, these drugs will often abolish ventricular as well as atrial PVCs. Once such ventricular extrasystoles have been halted, continued oral doses of these drugs will prevent return of the arrhythmia for long periods.

CORONARY ATTACKS. Premature ventricular contractions that develop in a patient who has suffered a heart attack are today not ordinarily treated with oral quinidine or procainamide. Now the appearance of such extrasystoles in a patient hospitalized after an acute myocardial infarction is taken as a warning sign that dangerous ventricular tachycardia may soon develop. This rapid, irregular heartbeat can lead to further cardiac damage and fatal ventricular fibrillation. The prompt parenteral administration of a rapid-acting antiarrhythmic drug is required to suppress the ectopic focus and eliminate the PVCs.

Lidocaine+ (Xylocaine) is the antiarrhythmic drug that is now preferred for this purpose. It is considered safer and more effective than quinidine and procainamide for intravenous administration to patients who have suffered an acute myocardial infarction. This drug differs from the older drugs mainly in its greater safety margin. Administered by vein to patients who develop premature ventricular contractions following a heart attack, this drug usually succeeds in controlling these arrhythmias without depressing cardiac conduction or reducing the heart muscle's contractile strength.

The short duration of lidocaine's action is also a safety factor when overdosage occurs. However, rapid elimination of single doses often makes it necessary to continue its administration by slow intravenous infusion for several days in order to keep the ventricular arrhythmias from recurring. The nurse must monitor the rate of infusion very carefully in such cases to be sure that the patient is receiving enough of the drug to keep his rhythm normal while also avoiding overdosage. The patient's electrocardiogram is also monitored for signs of delayed conduction (lengthening of the P-R interval) or of myocardial depression (widening of the QRS complex).

Lidocaine is a drug that can affect the central nervous system as well as the heart. Like other local anesthetics, it can cause combined stimulating and depressant effects.* Patients are watched for signs of central excitement, followed by drowsiness and disorientation. Dosage of lidocaine is decreased at the first sign of central toxicity and stopped completely if the patient has difficulty in breathing or goes into convulsions or coma. (See Chapter 30 for a further discussion of the use of lidocaine in treating patients in the intensive coronary care unit following an acute myocardial infarction.)

Arrhythmias in anesthesia and surgery may also be prevented or corrected by the administration of antiarrhythmic drugs. For example, lidocaine has proved useful for control of cardiac irregularities that develop during open heart surgery. Procainamide is sometimes employed during chest surgery procedures to check arrhythmias. It is also often administered orally or intramuscularly just before patients with heart disorders go to the anesthesia room and again during the induction of anes-

---

* Never store lidocaine for intravenous use together with the local anesthetic preparation that also contains *epinephrine*. Accidental I.V. use of the latter product in place of lidocaine could cause fatal cardiac arrhythmias in a heart attack patient with PVCs.

thesia. *Propranolol+* (Inderal), a beta adrenergic blocking agent, is also used to prevent arrhythmias during general anesthesia with halothane, cyclopropane, and other drugs that sensitize the heart to circulating catecholamines and thus tend to set off arrhythmias during the induction of anesthesia.

Propranolol is also particularly useful for control of other cardiac rhythm disorders that are set off by excessive sympathetic nervous system activity or adrenal medulla hormones. In treating pheochromocytoma patients, for example, this drug is now administered together with an *alpha* adrenergic blocker such as *phentolamine+* (Regitine) to protect the patient's cardiovascular system from the effects of epinephrine released from the tumor tissue.

Other cardiac conditions in which propranolol helps to slow a rapid, irregular heartbeart include thyrotoxicosis, hypertrophic subaortic stenosis, and digitalis intoxication. Propranolol protects the heart against digitalis-induced ventricular tachycardia, and digitalis, in turn, helps to counteract the tendency of this drug to depress the heart muscle's pumping power.

Toxic Effects of Antiarrhythmic Agents (See Summary, p. 361)

CARDIOVASCULAR TOXICITY

Overdosage of any drugs of this class can cause dangerous arrhythmias. As indicated in our earlier discussion of the pharmacological effects of quinidine and procainamide, toxic doses of all these drugs are capable of slowing cardiac impulse conduction excessively. They may also depress the heart muscle's contractile strength. These toxic effects can lead to heart failure or even to cardiac arrest.

The nurse in intensive coronary care units helps to avoid overdosage with these drugs by her monitoring of the patient's electrocardiogram and his vital signs. She notifies the physician, for example, when she observes a widening of the P-R interval and other indications of an increasing atrioventricular block. Similarly, she takes action when the electrocardiogram reveals a widening of the QRS complex and shows other indications of slowed ventricular conduction and myocardial contractions.

The doctor may then administer molar sodium lactate or sodium bicarbonate and isoproterenol to counteract the cardiotoxic effects of such drugs as quinidine, procainamide, and propranolol, as well as of the safer but still potentially toxic agents lidocaine and diphenylhydantoin. The nurse makes sure that all the drugs and equipment needed for cardiopulmonary resuscitation and support of the patient's circulation are available for emergency use. She also makes such measurements as taking the patient's blood pressure every two minutes during the intravenous administration of procainamide, a drug that sometimes tends to produce a steep drop in blood pressure, particularly when it is infused too rapidly.

EXTRACARDIAC TOXICITY

The antiarrhythmic drugs cause a variety of ill effects besides those that affect cardiac function. Some of these adverse effects may make it necessary to discontinue one drug and possibly to substitute another. Patients who develop *cinchonism* and other signs of sensitivity to quinidine (see *Summary*, p. 361) for example, may be successfully switched to procainamide, if the nurse detects these characteristic side effects and brings them to the physician's attention. Similarly, patient's taking procainamide must be watched for signs of the peculiar idiosyncratic reactions that this drug causes occasionally (see *Summary*, p. 361).

Propranolol, because of its beta adrenergic blocking effects, tends to produce *non*cardiac side effects that can be particularly dangerous for some patients. For example, by cutting off sympathetic nerve impulses to the bronchial smooth muscles of asthmatic patients, propranolol may cause bronchoconstriction and thus set off an acute attack. Drugs such as isoproterenol in aerosol form and aminophylline should be readily available to counteract bronchospasm. Similarly, the nurse should watch diabetic patients with particular care, because propranolol tends to mask the signs of insulin overdosage. (The beta adrenergic blocking drugs keep epinephrine from exerting some of its characteristic effects when the body releases that hormone in an effort to counteract the insulin-induced hypoglycemic reaction.)

Diphenylhydantoin can interact with such anticoagulant drugs as dicumarol and warfarin in ways which may endanger the patient who is being treated with both types of drugs. Because of possible potentiation of the action of the anticoagulants, patients should be observed especially carefully for bleeding tendencies when diphenylhydantoin is added to their therapeutic regimen for control of cardiac arrhythmias. (This drug sometimes colors the patient's urine reddish brown. This should not be confused with bleeding, and the patient can be reassured if he detects the color change.)

Lidocaine's effects on the central nervous system have already been discussed above.

SUMMARY

The antiarrhythmic agents can be lifesaving in acute cardiac emergencies. Yet these drugs themselves have potentially toxic effects that can make their use hazardous for heart patients. The nurse's careful observations of the effects of these drugs on cardiovascular function, and of the extracardiac effects of these drugs, can help bring the patient the maximum benefits of treatment of heart rhythm irregularities with minimum danger of suffering severe adverse effects. Dosage can be adjusted to optimal levels only on the basis of continuous careful observation of the patient.

SUMMARY of Clinical Indications and Objectives of Antiarrhythmia Drug Treatment

Clinical Indications	Objectives
Atrial tachyarrhythmias Atrial premature beats Atrial flutter Atrial fibrillation Atrial tachycardia (paroxysmal and *non*paroxysmal)	Drugs are used mainly to protect the ventricles from excessive supraventricular impulses. Drugs may also prevent recurrences of atrial arrhythmias when administered as maintenance therapy, following electrical cardioversion to restore normal sinus rhythm.

Ventricular tachyarrhythmias

Premature ventricular contractions
(Ventricular extrasystoles; PVCs)
Ventricular tachycardia
Ventricular fibrillation

Drugs are used to restore normal rhythm by abolishing PVCs and thus preventing their extension to more serious arrhythmias in various clinical situations.*

---

* Among the clinical situations of varied etiology in which various antiarrhythmic drugs are employed are:
1. Patients who have suffered an acute myocardial infarction (AMI).
2. Patients who have received overdoses of digitalis.
3. Patients with arrhythmias set off by anesthetics such as cyclopropane and halothane.
4. Patients undergoing cardiac (open-heart) surgery and other kinds of thoracic surgery.
5. Patients with conditions marked by excessive sympathetic nervous system stimulation or excessive circulating catecholamines (such as pheochromocytoma).

S U M M A R Y of the Cardiac Effects of Antiarrhythmic Agents that Account for their Therapeutic Effects and Cardiotoxicity

Suppress automaticity.

Therapeutic doses depress spontaneous depolarizations in ectopic automatic cells; toxic doses can also depress atrial, nodal, and ventricular pacemakers.

Prolong the effective refractory period.

Therapeutic doses reduce the responsiveness of cardiac tissues to abnormally generated impulses and impulses travelling in abnormal pathways. This often helps to abolish arrhythmias and restore normal sinus rhythm.

Depress conduction in all types of cardiac tissues.

Therapeutic doses slow the rate at which impulses are transmitted through the automatic conduction system. This helps to control the ventricular rate in supraventricular tachyarrhythmias.

Toxic doses of these drugs can cause various degrees of heart block (as indicated by lengthening of the P-R interval on the electrocardiogram) and depression of conduction in the ventricles (as indicated by widening of the QRS complex). Thus, these drugs are contraindicated in patients who already have heart block, and they are used with caution in patients in whom A-V conduction may be depressed as, for example, in digitalis intoxication. (Diphenylhydantoin, which is less likely to depress conduction than procainamide, is preferred for treating digitalis overdosage.)

S U M M A R Y of Signs and Symptoms of Extracardiac Toxicity of Antiarrhythmic Drugs

Diphenylhydantoin (See *Summary,* Chapter 28)

Dizziness, weakness, fatigue, muscular incoordination, and ataxia, nystagmus.
Nausea and vomiting.
Skin rash, itching.

Lidocaine

Drowsiness, dizziness, nervousness, confusion.
Paresthesias (generalized numbness and tingling).
Muscular tremors, twitching, convulsions.

Procainamide

Nausea, vomiting, bitter taste, loss of appetite.
Macropapular skin rash, urticaria, angioneurotic edema, fever.
Dizziness, weakness, mental depression.
Rare idiosyncracies include agranulocytosis and collagen disease syndrome resembling lupus erythematosus.

Propranolol

Nausea, vomiting, lightheadedness.
Weakness, fatigue, possible mental depression.
Rarely, respiratory distress, wheezing, laryngospasm. (Contraindicated in patients with bronchial asthma and allergic rhinitis.)
Rarely, a red rash and paresthesias.

Quinidine

Cinchonism—tinnitus, visual disturbances, dizziness, headache, confusion.
Gastrointestinal—nausea, vomiting, abdominal cramps, and diarrhea.
Hypersensitivity—fever, skin rashes, angioneurotic edema, asthma, respiratory depression, cyanosis, thrombocytic purpura.

SUMMARY of Points for the Nurse to Remember about Antiarrhythmic Drugs

1. Observe patients for signs of cardiac and extracardiac toxicity and report these promptly to the doctor, if they should occur. (See *Summary of Toxic Effects.*)

2. Carefully note the rate and character of both the apical and radial pulse rates of patients receiving these drugs. Make repeated counts of at least one full minute and look for any detectable disturbances in rhythm.

3. In observing the electrocardiogram of patients under intensive care, look particularly for lengthening of the P-R interval and for a widening of the QRS complex of more than 25 percent. Report these signs of impending toxicity promptly to the patient's doctor and discuss their significance with him.

4. Place ward patients where they can be observed frequently—preferably, for example, in a room directly across from the nurse's station rather than in a room at the far end of the corridor.

5. Check the availability of drugs for treating cardiac toxicity caused by these drugs and the working order of emergency equipment such as pacemakers, and defibrillators.

6. When visiting patients who take these drugs at home, look for such early signs of drug-induced congestive heart failure as ankle edema, fatigue, and dyspnea.

7. Even though these patients may show no signs of congestive heart failure at home or on their visits to the clinic, these myocardial depressant drugs may interfere with their cardiac reserve.

Thus, it is advisable to ask the patient about any symptoms that he may be experiencing, such as early fatigue during periods of activity. Explain why he should space his activities and rest at intervals to make up for his drug-induced decreased ability to tolerate physical activity.

Clinical Nursing Situation

The Situation: Mr. Weatherby is a 67-year-old retired factory foreman. He has lived alone (following his wife's death a year ago) in a small bungalow in a suburban town. Two months ago he suffered an acute myocardial infarction complicated by episodes of ventricular tachycardia. This acute arrhythmia was brought under control in the I.C.C.U. with repeated infusions of lidocaine, but bouts have tended to recur during the past month since his return home from the hospital.

Mr. Weatherby's physician has put him on a maintenance dose of quinidine sulfate 0.2 g orally, q.i.d. He has also suggested a regimen of rest, gradually increasing activity, and weight reduction. He is to see the nurse at the recently established health clinic for older citizens each week and will be seen by the doctor at least once a month or oftener (depending upon the nurse's assessment of his condition).

The Problem: Assume that you are the clinic nurse. Describe the observations that you would make when you see Mr. Weatherby every week, particularly as regards the following: (1) his therapy with quinidine; (2) his dietary regimen of 1,800 calories daily; (3) your asssesment of his ability to tolerate activity; (4) Mr. Weatherby's total life situation and such aspects of it as his adaptation to the loss of his wife, his retirement, and his recent life-threatening illness.

DRUG DIGEST

LIDOCAINE HCl U.S.P. (Xylocaine)
Actions and Indications. This local anesthetic drug is used not only for relief of pain but also for treating cardiac arrhythmias. It controls premature ventricular contractions and tachycardia in patients with an acute myocardial infarction. It also stops rapid cardiac irregularities caused by digitalis overdosage or manipulation of the heart during surgery or cardiac catherization.

Side Effects, Cautions, and Contraindications. Overdosage can cause hypotension, bradycardia, and even cardiac arrest. Thus, the electrocardiogram must be monitored for signs of depressed conduction (prolongation of P-R interval and widening of QRS complex) and blood pressure must be taken frequently.

Drowsiness, lightheadedness, and dizziness are early central signs of overdosage. Higher doses may also cause muscular twitching, tremors, and convulsions, or even coma and respiratory failure.

Dosage and Administration. Various dosage forms and concentrations are available for infiltration, regional, and topical anesthesia (see other sources for details).

The 2 percent solution is administered intravenously for control of cardiac arrhythmias in two ways: (1) a single injection of 50 to 100 mg at a rate of 25 to 50 mg per minute, followed by a second dose within five minutes if needed. A total of no more than 200 to 300 mg may be administered within one hour; (2) a continuous infusion of 1 to 4 mg per minute may be made in the form of a 0.1 to 0.2 percent solution until the patient's rhythm is stabilized.

PROCAINAMIDE HCl U.S.P. (Pronestyl)

Actions and Indications. This derivative of the local anesthetic procaine is used clinically for control of cardiac arrhythmias. It is particularly effective for terminating rapid ventricular irregularities. It is employed: for counteracting or preventing ventricular and supraventricular tachycardia that may develop following an acute myocardial infarction; in digitalis intoxication; or during anesthesia and chest surgery.

Side Effects, Cautions, and Contraindications. The drug is infused by vein very slowly and with electrocardiographic monitoring and frequent measurements of blood pressure, when it is being employed for emergency conversion of arrhythmias. It is discontinued if blood pressure falls rapidly or signs of A-V conduction disturbances appear. Complete heart

block is a contraindication, and caution is required in digitalis intoxication and other conditions in which partial heart block may develop. Extracardiac adverse effects that may appear during prolonged oral administration include loss of appetite, nausea, and vomiting, and occasional reduction of white blood cell counts.

Dosage and Administration. In emergencies, procainamide is injected slowly at rates between 25 and 50 mg per minute in total amounts that do not exceed 1 g. It is also administered intramuscularly in doses between 250 and 750 mg, when patients cannot take the usual oral doses of 1.0 to 1.25 g initially, followed by doses of 500 to 1000 mg every four to six hours.

PROPRANOLOL (Inderal)

Actions and Indications. This prototype beta adrenergic blocking agent is used mainly in the management of cardiac arrhythmias of the supraventricular type, including paroxysmal atrial tachycardia (PAT) and atrial fibrillation, flutter, or premature beats. Among the disorders in which it has been employed are digitalis intoxication, pheochromocytoma, hypertrophic subaortic stenosis, and, experimentally, in angina pectoris and essential hypertension.

Side Effects, Cautions, and Contraindications. This drug can cause excessive cardiac slowing and myocardial weakness. Patients should be carefully observed for signs of drug-induced congestive heart failure. The drug is not ordinarily administered to patients who are already in failure or who have a high degree of heart block or bradycardia. It is contraindicated in bronchial asthma and in allergic rhinitis patients during the pollen season.

Dosage and Administration. The usual oral dose ranges from 10 to 40 mg three or four times daily and at bedtime. It may also be admin-

istered by slow I.V. (1 mg per minute) in doses of 1 to 3 mg in the management of emergencies requiring quick control of rapid cardiac irregularities.

QUINIDINE SULFATE U.S.P. (Quinidex; Quinora)

Actions and Indications. This cinchona alkaloid is a prototype agent for prevention and treatment of atrial and ventricular arrhythmias. However, it is now used only occasionally to terminate attacks of atrial tachycardia, fibrillation, and flutter or to abolish atrial tachycardia, as electrical conversion is more commonly employed. Similarly, other somewhat safer drugs are now preferred for converting ventricular irregularities to normal. Nonetheless, quinidine is still commonly employed for long-term maintenance therapy, once a normal sinus rhythm has been attained by such other measures.

Side Effects, Cautions, and Contraindications. Overdosage tends to impair cardiac impulse conduction. This can *cause* arrhythmias and even cardiac arrest. Thus, the drug is contraindicated in patients with heart block. The patient's electrocardiogram must be monitored during emergency parenteral use of quinidine for conversion.

Cinchonism, a syndrome marked by gastrointestinal disturbances, tinnitus (ringing in the ears), blurring of vision, lightheadedness, dizziness, and tremors, is the main type of *extra*cardiac toxicity. Patients should receive a test dose to detect signs of drug allergy or quinidine idiosyncracy.

Dosage and Administration. The usual oral doses are 0.2 to 0.6 g every two to four hours (up to five doses) for several days, until effective concentrations are reached. The patient may then be maintained on daily oral doses of 0.2 g administered up to six times a day or by 0.6 g administered b.i.d. in the form of extended action tablets.

References

Alexander, S. Treatment of arrhythmias associated with acute myocardial infarction. *Med. Clin. N. Amer.*, 53:315, 1969 (March).

Bernstein, H. Drug treatment of cardiac arrhythmias. *Amer. J. Nurs.*, 64:118, 1964 (July).

Bigger, J.T., and Heissenbuttel, T.H. The use

of procainamide and lidocaine in the treatment of cardiac arrhythmias. *Progr. Cardiovasc. Dis.*, 11:515, 1969.

Damato, A.N. Diphenylhydantoin: Pharmacological and clinical use. *Progr. Cardiovasc. Dis.*, 12:1, 1969.

Fowler, N.O. Modern treatment of cardiac arrhythmias: A perspective. *Mod. Treatm.*, 7:13, 1970 (Jan.).

Lemberg, L., et al. The treatment of arrhythmias following acute myocardial infarc-

tion. *Med. Clin. N. Amer.*, 55:273, 1971 (March).

Rodman, M.J. Drugs for the irregular heart. *RN*, 25:53, 1962 (Aug.).

———. Drugs for congestive heart failure and arrhythmias. *RN*, 30:51, 1967 (Nov.).

———. Drugs used in managing cardiac emergencies. *RN*, 36:55, 1973 (May).

Thielen, E.O., and Wilson, W.R.: Beta-adrenergic receptor blocking drugs in the treatment of cardiac arrhythmias. *Med. Clin. N. Amer.*, 52:1017, 1968 (Sept.).

30.

Drugs Used in Coronary Artery Disease

Coronary Heart Disease

Disease of the heart muscle's arteries is the most common cause of death in the United States. Coronary artery disease is the cause of one out of every three deaths in people 35 to 64 years old. The underlying cause of this kind of heart disease is coronary atherosclerosis, a narrowing of the arterial channels by the formation of fatty deposits within the inner lining of the heart's blood vessels.

In this chapter, we shall discuss the following aspects of coronary heart disease:

1. *Angina pectoris* and the drugs used to treat and prevent painful anginal attacks.

2. *Acute myocardial infarction* (A.M.I.) and the use of various drugs in the management of the complications of such heart attacks.

Drugs used in attempts to prevent and treat coronary atherosclerosis are taken up in the next chapter, *Drugs for Reducing Elevated Plasma Lipids*.

Angina Pectoris

Attacks of this type are usually marked by the sudden onset of chest pains that radiate up into the throat, jaw, neck, arms, and shoulders. The pain is almost always set off by physical exertion or emotional upset. The reason for this is that the heart muscle is forced to work harder in such circumstances than when the person is calm and at rest. His disease-narrowed coronary vessels are then unable to deliver enough oxygenated blood to meet the increased demands of the myocardium. The heart muscle *ischemia* and *hypoxia* that result from this imbalance between oxygen supply and oxygen demand are believed to be the cause of the characteristic chest pains.

Drugs that relieve anginal pain do so in two main ways:

1. By dilating the coronary vessels and thus increasing the flow of oxygen-containing blood to the hypoxic heart muscle.

2. By reducing the work that the heart has to do, and, in this way, decreasing its demand for oxygen.

One group of antianginal drugs, the organic nitrates and nitrites (Table 30-1), is particularly effective for relief and prevention of pain in angina pectoris.

The Nitrates

PHARMACOLOGICAL ACTIONS. Chemicals of this class can relax all kinds of smooth muscles, but they are especially effective for relaxing the walls of blood vessels. This leads to a local vasodilation of arterioles, venules, and capillaries that results in an increased flow of blood to the tissues served by these vessels. Administered to patients suffering from angina pectoris, nitrate-type drugs tend to dilate large coronary arteries. This is thought to produce a better flow of blood to ischemic heart muscle tissues and thus to relieve the local

TABLE 30-1 *Drugs Used for Treating Angina Pectoris*

Nonproprietary Name	Trade Name or Synonym	Single Dose Range	Remarks
Nitrates and Nitrites			
Amyl nitrite	Aspirols; Vaporoles	0.18–0.3 ml by inhalation	Very rapid onset of action vs. acute attacks
Erythrityl tetranitrate	Cardilate	5 to 15 mg sublingually; 10 to 30 mg orally	For prevention of attacks rather than for relief
Isosorbide dinitrate	Isordil	5 to 10 mg sublingually; 5 to 30 mg orally; or 40 mg for sustained action over 6–12 hours	Rapid relief (2 to 3 minutes); moderately long prophylaxis (4 to 6 hours); longer with sustained action capsules
Mannitol hexanitrate	Maxitate; Nitranitol	15 to 60 mg orally	Moderate duration of action
Nitroglycerin U.S.P.	Glyceryl trinitrate	0.2–0.6 mg sublingually; also administered orally and by application to the skin	See *Drug Digest*
Pentaerythritol tetranitrate	Peritrate; and others	10 to 30 mg orally; 30 to 80 mg for sustained action over 12 hours	See *Drug Digest*
Trolnitrate phosphate	Metamine; Nitritamin	10 mg orally for sustained action	Slow onset, prolonged duration for long-term prophylaxis
Nonnitrate Vasodilators			
Dipyridamole	Persantin	50 mg	For long-term preventive therapy
Ethaverine HCl	Ethaquin	100–200 mg	Smooth muscle antispasmodic
Papaverine HCl N.F.	Pavabid	100–200 mg	Smooth muscle antispasmotic
Theophylline N.F. and derivatives, including aminophylline and oxtriphylline		100–200 mg	Bronchodilator (Chapter 19)

myocardial hypoxia that may be the cause of the patient's anginal pain.

In addition to acting as coronary vasodilators, the nitrates may also help by reducing the heart muscle's oxygen requirements. The drugs do so indirectly through their actions on peripheral arterioles and venules. Dilation of the veins results in a pooling of blood peripherally and a reduced return of blood to the heart. Thus, the heart has less of a load of blood to pump into a more dilated arterial system. This combination of reduced venous return and reduced resistance to the flow of blood results in the patient's heart working with less difficulty. This, in turn brings the heart's oxygen demand back into balance with the supply of oxygen that the patient's diseased coronary vessels are able to deliver.

TYPES OF NITRATES

These drugs are used in two ways:

1. For *rapid* effects *to abort an acute attack* of angina pectoris or to prevent an expected attack.

2. For *long-term* effects that are intended to *reduce the total number of attacks* and to lessen the severity of their pain.

To achieve the first objective, certain nitrates with relatively rapid onset of action are administered sublingually or by inhalation. *Amyl nitrite* and *octyl nitrate* are the two most rapid acting compounds. However, even though their effects come on within seconds after they are inhaled, these drugs are not widely used to abort an acute attack because of their relative inconvenience compared to other nitrates that can be simply slipped under the tongue. *Glyceryl trinitrate+* (nitroglycerin), *erythrityl tetranitrate* (Cardilate), and *isosorbide dinitrate* (Isordil) are examples of nitrates that act rapidly when taken sublingually for relief of an attack or for immediate preventive purposes.

The same three drugs and several other nitrates, including *pentaerythritol tetranitrate+* (PETN, Peritrate, and others) are also administered orally in larger doses. Taken in this way, their onset of action is slower and less dramatic but more prolonged. Often, the duration of action of these drugs is lengthened still further by their slow release from special sustained-release pharmaceutical forms. The usefulness of oral nitrates for long-term prophylaxis is still uncertain. It has been hard to prove that these drugs are actually any better than a placebo. However, doctors continue to prescribe these sustained-action oral nitrates, presumably because they consider these products safe, and they hope that even a positive placebo effect may be beneficial.

MANAGEMENT OF ACUTE ATTACKS. Glyceryl trinitrate (nitroglycerin) is the drug most widely used for aborting an acute attack. It is usually effective in about two minutes after the patient places a soluble tablet under his tongue. However, the patient often has to be instructed in how to use this drug to get its desirable effects with a minimum of adverse reactions. It is important, for example, to tell the patient to sit down or to lie down when he takes nitroglycerin. Otherwise, he may feel faint, dizzy, and weak because of a tendency of his blood pressure to fall as a result of peripheral vasodilation. Such postural hypotension may also set off a reflex racing of the heart. The resulting cardiac palpitations may be dangerous as well as discomforting because the heart is made to work harder instead of having its work load reduced, as happens when the patient sits down and rests.

The nurse should also observe how the patient responds to nitroglycerin. The fact that he may complain of a throbbing headache— the most common side effect of early treatment with nitrates—is, at least, an indication that the drug is still active as a vasodilator. Sometimes as the patient stops getting headaches, he may also get less relief of anginal chest pains. This is because *tolerance* to nitrates tends to develop rapidly. Thus, the nurse should report any signs she sees of developing tolerance, so that the doctor will raise the dose to a more effective level. (A patient's poor response is occasionally caused by deterioration of the drug itself. The nurse should check to see that the patient's nitroglycerin tablets are kept at all times in a tightly-sealed glass vial and should instruct the patient to store them in this way.)

The nurse should also be aware of the anginal patient's emotional state, as anxiety tends to trigger attacks and increases the patient's need for nitroglycerin. Thus, it is desirable for the doctor and nurse to try to win and keep the patient's confidence and to avoid alarming him unnecessarily. Patients sometimes express concern over their dependence upon nitroglycerin for relief of attacks. This drug does not, of course, cause the kind of psychological and physical dependence that is associated with narcotics and other addicting drugs.

The nurse can reassure the patient on this point. It is essential that the nurse and the doctor work collaboratively in explaining the patient's condition and treatment to him.

Anginal patients who are hospitalized often feel less apprehensive when they are allowed to keep a supply of nitroglycerin at their bedsides. Nurses sometimes have misgivings about leaving drugs in the hands of patients for self-administration and may tend to indicate that they disapprove of the practice. However, there is no reason why an anginal patient who has been using nitroglycerin for years should be deprived of the security of knowing that he can get rapid relief when an acute attack strikes.

The nurse is, of course, not relieved of her own responsibilities when a patient has received permission to take his own medication as needed. She needs to know, for instance, how much nitroglycerin the patient requires for relief of an attack and how often he has to take a dose of any prescribed drug. She can best find this by discussing these points with the patient. If the nurse feels that a particular patient shows signs of impaired judgment or memory, she should talk to the doctor and give him a careful report of the patient's behavior. He may then decide that the patient should no longer be allowed to take his own medication.

PROPHYLACTIC USE OF NITRATES. Nitrates are used in two ways that are intended to prevent attacks:

1. For *immediate prophylaxis* the drug is taken either sublingually or orally just before the patient expects to perform physical activity of a kind that he knows can cause an attack.

2. For *sustained prophylaxis,* the drug is taken regularly in oral doses that (as indicated previously) are intended to reduce the total number of attacks.

The usefulness of these drugs for the first purpose seems to be well established. A patient who has to go outdoors in cold weather may, for example, avoid an acute anginal attack by using a sublingual tablet of nitroglycerin shortly before leaving. The drug's effects may increase the patient's ability to tolerate the extra exertion during the next half hour. *Isosorbide dinitrate* may also be taken sublingually for an even longer protective effect. *Erythrityl tetranitrate* (Cardilate) tablets that are taken sublingually or chewed have a somewhat de-layed but even longer-lasting protective effect during exercise or emotional excitement.

The effectiveness of *pentaerythritol tetranitrate*+ (PETN; Peritrate; and others) and other drugs (Table 30-1) for sustained prophylaxis is a matter of current controversy. Despite the fact that they are widely used in the long-term management of angina pectoris, these drugs have not been proved effective by controlled clinical trials. Their use in forms that permit around-the-clock effects is supposed to be safe and is claimed to reduce the patient's daily need for nitroglycerin tablets to abort acute attacks. Yet, if these long-lasting drugs induce nitrate tolerance, their continued use may make it even *more* difficult to terminate acute attacks with sublingually administered nitroglycerin.

Actually, reduction in the number of anginal attacks during the long-term management of this condition depends more upon the patient's learning to live with his condition than upon vasodilator drug therapy. Patients have to learn to avoid excessive exertion, particularly in cold weather. Their physical activity should not, however, be too severely restricted. It is also important for these patients to keep calm, as their emotional responses to the stresses of daily life can set off attacks. The doctor may prescribe a barbiturate or an antianxiety agent such as chlordiazepoxide for this purpose (Chapter 6). The nurse should also do whatever she can to help the patient accept the fact that even when he faithfully follows all instructions, he may still continue to suffer painful attacks. For if he feels frustrated and angry, his cardiac condition may be made worse.

OTHER ANTIANGINAL DRUGS (TABLE 30-1)

Most other vasodilator drugs that have been employed for long-term treatment of angina pectoris have not proved useful for reducing the number and severity of seizures. *Papaverine,* an opiate derivative, does not seem to have any value when administered orally. Neither do the chemically related synthetic compounds *ethaverine* and *dioxyline.* The xanthine derivatives, such as *theophylline* and *aminophylline,* are much more effective for relaxing spasm of bronchial smooth muscles than for dilating constricted coronary arteries. Thus, they are rarely effective in treating angina pectoris, though they may be useful in the management of bronchial asthma. *Dipyridamole* (Persantine) is said to produce an increase in blood flow through the coronary arterioles. However, it has not yet been proved to benefit patients with angina pectoris when used in long-term therapy.

Propranolol+ (Inderal), a beta adrenergic blocking agent, is being employed experimentally for treating angina pectoris. This drug is *not* a vasodilator but is believed to produce beneficial effects by its ability to reduce the demands of the patient's heart for oxygen. It does this by blocking the effects of sympathetic nervous system stimulation of the patient's heart, when physical exertion or emotional upset cause an increased outflow of sympathetic cardioacceleratory impulses. This keeps the anginal patient's heart from being driven to do more work and to consume more oxygen.

Propranolol is approved officially only for treating cardiac arrhythmias but not yet for the long-term prophylactic management of angina pectoris, except when the patient's chest pain is caused by a heart condition called *hypertrophic subaortic stenosis.* It is best employed in combination with nitroglycerin, as the two drugs seem to have supra-additive antianginal effects and also tend to counteract some of each other's adverse effects on the heart (see also Chapter 29).

Acute Myocardial Infarction (A.M.I.)

Attacks of angina pectoris are painful and often terrifying. However, they do not last very long, nor do they damage the heart muscle. A more severe and longer lasting type of attack called *acute coronary insufficiency* also leaves the patient with no permanent myocardial damage, except for persistent electrocardiographic abnormalities in some cases. Both of these types of attacks may, however, be warnings that these patients are likely to suffer the most serious kind of coronary vessel disorder, an *acute myocardial infarction* (A.M.I.).

This kind of coronary attack is caused by the complete obstruction of a blood vessel. A piece of the fat deposits lining the atherosclerotic vessel may, for example, break off and be carried to an even narrower arterial channel where it blocks the further flow of blood to the heart muscle tissues that are fed by that artery. Another cause of such a coronary occlusion may be the sudden formation of a blood clot, or thrombus, that supplies an important area of myocardial or conducting tissue with the oxygen and nutrients it needs in order to function.

A *coronary thrombosis* of this kind can cause an occlusion that deprives the cardiac tissues of their blood supply so completely that they are permanently damaged or even destroyed. The area of dead tissue is called a *myocardial infarction.* It is gradually replaced by scar tissue, and—provided the patient survives the complications that often follow a coronary attack—his heart may recover its previous ability to pump enough blood to meet the body's needs. However, if the infarcted area is relatively large, the patient's cardiac output may never again be adequate, unless he receives a drug such as digitalis to increase the contractile strength of the remaining muscle tissue.

In this section of the chapter, we shall discuss the drugs that are used to treat patients who have suffered an acute myocardial infarction. Details concerning the individual drugs of different classes may be found in various other chapters of this text, including the *Drug Digests* that appear there. Here, however, we shall emphasize aspects of these drugs that pertain to their use in the emergency management of these patients by nurses working in the intensive coronary care unit (I.C.C.U.).

ANTIARRHYTHMIC DRUGS IN CARDIAC DYSRHYTHMIAS

The most common and most dangerous complication of an A.M.I. is the development of an irregularity in cardiac rhythm.* Patients who develop either very rapid or very slow dysrhythmias may suffer sudden cardiac arrest. This is the most common cause of death during a coronary attack and in the first few hours or several days following an infarction. This fatal outcome can often be prevented by early detection of the abnormal rhythm on the patient's electrocardiogram, followed by prompt treatment with heart rhythm-regulating drugs.

RAPID VENTRICULAR ARRHYTHMIAS. The most common cardiac rhythm irregularity following

* It should be noted that the terms "arrhythmia" (an absence of rhythm) and "dysrhythmia" (a disordered rhythm) are both used to describe cardiac rhythm irregularities. The drugs that are used to treat these conditions have traditionally been called "antiarrhythmic," "antifibrillatory," or "cardiac depressant" drugs. They are now also occasionally referred to as "antidysrhythmic" agents.

an A.M.I. is the occurrence of *premature ventricular contractions* (PVCs), or extrasystoles. The nurse in the I.C.C.U. monitors the patient's EKG periodically and charts his PVC pattern. The appearance of certain types of patterns indicates that the patient may be about to develop dangerous ventricular tachycardia or even fatal ventricular fibrillation.*

In such situations, the nurse may administer the antiarrhythmic drug *lidocaine+* (Xylocaine) which usually supresses the rapid runs of PVCs within about half a minute when injected intravenously. Single doses of the same size (between 50 and 100 mg) may be repeated in about five minutes and again a little later, if the abnormal rhythm persists. Occasionally, a patient whose arrhythmia is not controlled by lidocaine will respond to *procainamide+* (Pronestyl) administered by slow intravenous infusion. With both drugs, constant monitoring of the patient's EKG and frequent measurement of his blood pressure are required to detect signs of depression of cardiac impulse conduction and any tendency of the blood pressure to fall too steeply.

To prevent recurrences of rapid ventricular irregularities, lidocaine is also infused continuously until the patient's cardiac rhythm becomes stabilized.† Later, the drug's dosage is

reduced by gradually slowing the rate of infusion and finally discontinuing it altogether. If any further treatment is needed after 24 hours, the use of orally administered *quinidine+* or procainamide may be preferred.

SLOW CARDIAC ARRHYTHMIAS. Sometimes patients who have suffered a coronary attack may develop a very slow heart rate. Bradycardia below 60 beats per minute can cause a drop in cardiac output that further reduces blood flow through the coronary circulation. This may lead to more myocardial damage. It may also cause congestive heart failure and interfere with functioning of the kidneys or affect the brain.

Slow rhythms of this kind, including sinus bradycardia and heart block, are best treated with *atropine+* and *isoproterenol+* (Isuprel). Atropine is injected by vein in doses of 0.4 to 1 mg to reduce excessive vagus nerve impulses that may be slowing the heart. Isoproterenol is infused intravenously as a very dilute solution when repeated doses of atropine fail to speed up the heart or produce typical adverse effects. The patient's pulse rate and electrocardiogram are closely monitored during infusion of isoproterenol, and the I.V. drip is adjusted to keep the heart from beating too rapidly. If the patient complains of chest pains, or if PVCs develop and persist this adrenergic drug is discontinued.

CARDIAC ARREST. The sudden loss of pumping power that occurs when a patient's ventricles stop beating (asystole), or begin to fibrillate, deprives the brain of blood. The patient immediately becomes unconscious, and he will die within a few minutes unless oxygenated blood is kept flowing to his brain by prompt treatment measures. This is usually accomplished by immediate mouth to mouth breathing, closed-chest cardiac massage, and electrical shocks applied to the patient's chest. If these measures fail to restore his heartbeat, certain drugs may be injected directly into the chambers of the heart.

Epinephrine+ (Adrenalin) and *isoproterenol+* (Isuprel) are occasionally effective when administered in such cases. Using a 1:1,000 solution of epinephrine, 0.5 to 1 ml is diluted to 10 ml with saline solution and injected into the ventricles. This, together with external pressure on the chest and electrical shock, sometimes succeeds in getting a heartbeat started. Intravenous infusion of isoproterenol

---

* Electrocardiographic signs of electrical instability of a type that often precede serious ventricular arrhythmias include:

(1) More than six PVCs per minute.
(2) Salvos of two or more repetitive PVCs.
(3) PVCs originating at several different sites (that is, multifocal PVCs).
(4) PVCs that fall on the previous T wave.

† A 2 percent solution of lidocaine is used for treating cardiac arrhythmias. To administer the single large doses ("bolus" doses), a 5-cc ampule is employed. It contains a total of 100 mg of the drug (20 mg per cc). For continuous infusion, a much more dilute solution must be prepared to permit easier dosage adjustment. One way to do so is as follows:

1. Add the contents of a single 50-cc vial of the 2 percent solution to a 500-ml bottle of dextrose solution, from which 50 cc has been removed and discarded. The 500-cc dextrose solution bottle then contains a total of 1,000 mg of lidocaine (there are 2 mg in each cc of the diluted lidocaine solution.)

2. A flow rate from a microdrip set adjusted to deliver 60 drops (1 cc) per minute then gives the patient 2 mg per minute of lidocaine. Reducing the flow rate to 30 drops, of course, delivers a dose of 1 mg per minute. Dosage may be adjusted to between 1 to 4 mg per minute, not only by altering the rate flow, but also by preparing solutions that are more or less concentrated than the one described above.

1:5,000 solution diluted in 500 ml of dextrose solution is also successful sometimes in restoring the pumping action of the stopped heart. These adrenergic drugs are most likely to prove effective when systemic alkalinizers such as sodium bicarbonate, sodium lactate, or tromethamine (THAM-E) are first infused to counteract metabolic acidosis.

VASOPRESSORS FOR TREATING CARDIOGENIC SHOCK

Almost four out of five patients who go into shock following an A.M.I. die of this complication. However, very carefully controlled administration of adrenergic drugs sometimes succeeds in overcoming the state of shock that occurs following an infarction. The nurse's observations of the patient's vital signs during the infusion of these very potent drugs is essential for the patient's safety and the success of treatment.

During infusion of the adrenergic vasopressor drugs *levarterenol*+ (Levophed) and *metaraminol*+ (Aramine), the patient's blood pressure is measured frequently. The infusion flow is adjusted to keep the patient's systolic pressure at about 95 to 100 mg of Hg. When *isoproterenol*+ (Isuprel) is employed to increase the cardiac output, the patient's heart rate is closely monitored and the drip is adjusted to keep the heart from beating too rapidly (see Chapter 23 and *Drug Digest*). It is also important to monitor the patient's central venous pressure (C.V.P.) as a guide to the amount of fluid that can safely be infused in order to fill the patient's blood vessels without overloading the left ventricle of the heart.

DRUGS FOR TREATING HEART FAILURE FOLLOWING AN A.M.I.

Failure of the left ventricle following an A.M.I. may lead to rapid development of acute pulmonary edema. To strengthen the heartbeat and to keep fluid from collecting in the lungs, patients are usually treated with a rapid-acting digitalis glycoside such as *digoxin*+ (Lanoxin), *deslanoside*+ (Cedilanid-D) or *ouabain* in combination with a fast-acting diuretic drug such as *ethacrynate sodium*+ (Edecrin) or *furosemide* (Lasix).

These drugs must be administered with extreme caution to avoid complications caused by digitalis intoxication or by excessive diuresis.

The nurse notes the rate and character of the patient's apical and radial pulse and also observes him for extracardiac signs of digitalis overdosage such as loss of appetite and visual disturbances. She carefully records the patient's fluid intake and urine output and weighs him daily, so that the doctor can adjust dosage of the potent diuretic drugs accurately. Patients who require I.V. *aminophylline*+ for pulmonary edema must have their blood pressure measured frequently during the infusion. Those who receive isoproterenol instead of digitalis must be monitored as indicated above.

ANTICOAGULANT THERAPY FOR A.M.I. PATIENTS

Most patients are treated with anticoagulant drugs in the days immediately following an acute coronary attack, when they are most likely to develop thromboembolic complications. *Heparin*+ is injected for immediate action, and oral doses of *warfarin sodium*+ (Coumadin) or *bishydroxyocoumarin*+ (Dicumarol) are also ordered. After about a week, heparin is discontinued but the patient is kept on the orally administered drugs. These are given in doses that maintain the patient's blood clotting factors at a low level (between 20 and 30 percent of normal).

Doctors disagree on how long anticoagulant therapy should be continued following recovery from an A.M.I. Some feel that the routine long-term use of these potentially dangerous drugs is not desirable. Others believe that certain selected patients can benefit by being kept on an oral anticoagulant for many months or even several years. The results of some studies suggest that this treatment has helped to reduce recurrences of myocardial infarctions and has cut the death rate in younger male patients.

CORONARY VASODILATOR DRUGS FOLLOWING AN A.M.I.

The value of vasodilator drugs for A.M.I. patients is also disputed. The administration of the rapid-acting nitrates, papaverine, and similar drugs (see above) in the period immediately following a coronary attack may have adverse effects on the patient's unstable circulation. The long-term use of longer-acting nitrates such as pentaerythritol tetranitrate has been advocated for building up the patient's circulation, during convalescence as well as after full recovery. However, there is no proof that administration of these drugs to postcoronary patients is effective for preventing further coronary attacks or even for reducing the number of anginal attacks.

ANALGESICS AND SEDATIVES

Morphine or meperidine+ (Demerol) is usually administered to relieve the severe chest pain following an A.M.I. Morphine also helps to calm the anxious patient and thus avoid emotional stress that might adversely affect the rate and rhythm of his damaged heart. After a few days, the patient may be maintained on meperidine in combination with a sedative such as *promethazine* (Phenergan) or *phenobarbital*. Finally, a sedative alone, or an antianxiety agent such as *chlordiazepoxide+* (Librium) is administered for a while and then gradually withdrawn.

SUMMARY

Patients who have suffered an acute myocardial infarction receive many kinds of drugs while under intensive care and during convalescence. The nurse who administers antiarrhythmic agents, cardiotonic and diuretic drugs, vasopressors, vasodilators, anticoagulants, and potent analgesics has important responsibilities. She should be able to recognize the therapeutically desired and toxic effects of these drugs. By closely observing how the A.M.I. patient responds to drug therapy and then discussing her findings with the physician, she can help these dangerously ill patients get the benefit of today's valuable drugs while minimizing their various adverse effects.

S U M M A R Y of Nitrate and Nitrite Adverse Effects, Cautions, Contraindications

Vasodilation

Headache of vascular (throbbing) type.

Flushing due to cutaneous vasodilation.

Intraocular pressure rise is possible; caution in patients with glaucoma.

Postural hypotension (generalized vasodilation leading to cerebral ischemia) may cause episodes of dizziness, weakness, and faintness. (Alcohol may intensify these adverse effects.)

Idiosyncrasy manifested by extreme sensitivity to the hypotensive effect is a contraindication, as it may lead to pallor, perspiration, and collapse (nitrite syncope).

Reflex cardioacceleration in response to systemic vasodilation may make these drugs unsafe during the acute phase of a myocardial infarction.

Miscellaneous

Gastrointestinal disturbances, including epigastric distress nausea, and vomiting.

Drug rash is common; exfoliative dermatitis rare.

S U M M A R Y of Some Points Concerning the Care of Patients Receiving Drug Treatment for an Acute Myocardial Infarction*

Observe the patient and his electrocardiogram continuously to detect changes in his condition that may require the immediate administration of various kinds of drugs. (For example, the development of dysrhythmias such as PVCs for which lidocaine is injected to suppress the extrasystoles before they progress to more serious heartbeat irregularities.)

Observe the patient for adverse effects of the various potent drugs. (For example, patients receiving potent diuretics are watched for signs of dehydration and neuromuscular manifestations of electrolyte imbalances; patients receiving adrenergic vasopressors and cardiac stimulants must have their blood pressure, central venous pressure, and heart rates monitored frequently; take the apical pulse of patients who are being digitalized.)

Observe the patient's emotional state, as his general condition and his response to drug therapy are affected by pain and environmental stress. Promptly administer drugs for relief of severe chest pain following an A.M.I., as this is emotionally and physically draining at a time when his primary need is for rest.

* Details concerning points to remember about the various kinds of drugs are summarized in the chapters that deal with each type of drug.

SUMMARY of Points for the Nurse to Remember about Drugs for Treating Angina Pectoris

Advise the patient to sit down or lie down after he places a nitroglycerin tablet under his tongue to treat an anginal attack. (This keeps the patient from feeling weak, faint, and dizzy as a result of the fall in blood pressure that may occur if he remains standing.)

Remind the patient for whom sublingual nitroglycerin is prescribed for the first time that the tablets are placed under the tongue until dissolved, and that they should *not* be swallowed. (The tablets and capsules containing nitroglycerin combined with other drugs that are available for long-term prophylactic treatment *are* intended to be swallowed. However, these contain much larger amounts of the drug for slow absorption rather than emergency use.)

Watch the patient's reaction when he takes a nitroglycerin tablet. Report whether the drug gives prompt relief or whether tolerance is developing. Note the presence or absence of headache and other complaints, and, particularly, any unusual cardiovascular reactions such as nitrate syncope.

If the patient's chest pain is not relieved in 15 or 20 minutes after one or more sublingual tablets have been taken, his doctor should be notified and the patient kept at complete rest until the physician arrives. (The patient may have suffered a coronary occlusion rather than an anginal attack.)

If the patient is used to taking nitroglycerin whenever he needs it, the tablets should be available to him at all times even when he is hospitalized, so that he can use them when he decides that he requires this drug. (The tablets are kept in tightly sealed glass—*not* plastic—vials to keep the drug from deteriorating and becoming ineffective.)

Be aware of the patient's emotional state and avoid alarming him unnecessarily, as anxiety tends to set off anginal attacks. Be alert for any signs of mental impairment that might make self-medication with a potent drug like nitroglycerin hazardous.

Help the patient to learn to live within the limits imposed by his coronary disability. He will accept advice about how he should change his life style and follow your instructions, if you have gained his confidence and trust while caring for him.

Clinical Nursing Situation: I

The Situation: Mr. Friedenberg, an energetic, hard-driving, 50-year-old business man, experienced severe crushing substernal pain, dyspnea, and severe apprehension. He broke out in a sweat and felt faint and nauseated.

His physician was called and had him admitted to the intensive coronary care unit of the hospital. Here, his electrocardiogram was continuously monitored, and he was given 100 mg of Demerol I.M. to lessen the severe chest pain. The nurse took his blood pressure every 15 minutes. She and the doctor noticed that Mr. Friedenberg's EKG showed periodic premature ventricular complexes indicating extrasystoles arising in multiple ectopic foci.

The physician administered an initial bolus dose of lidocaine 50 mg I.V. This seemed to suppress the patient's PVCs. However, the doctor then decided to order a continuous infusion of lidocaine to be dripped into the patient's vein with a microdrip administration set. Before leaving the patient, the physician conferred with the nurse. He suggested that the patient be started on a flow of 1 mg of lidocaine per minute but that the rate of flow could be increased to 2 mg per minute, if PVCs kept recurring.

A few minutes after the doctor left, Mrs. Friedenberg, who had been called by her husband's secretary, arrived at the hospital looking very alarmed.

The Problem: Assume that you are the nurse caring for Mr. Friedenberg. Describe the observations you would make concerning his condition and his response to drug therapy, including, particularly, Demerol and lidocaine.

Describe how you would prepare the proper concentration of lidocaine for infusion by means of the microdrip administration set.

Describe how you would approach Mrs. Friedenberg to try to help her feel less apprehensive.

Clinical Nursing Situation: II

The Situation: Mrs. Walcott is a 62-year-old widow with angina pectoris. Her first attack occurred two years ago, shortly after her husband died suddenly from a massive myocardial infarction. (He died before arrival of the ambulance.) Her doctor feels that Mrs. Walcott's anginal attacks are related to her unhappiness over the death of her husband and her fear that she will die suddenly as he did.

This patient has followed her doctor's advice that she not continue to live alone. She has sublet her apartment and entered a convalescent home. She takes phenobarbital 30 mg t.i.d. to reduce her anxiety and has received a supply of nitroglycerin tablets 0.4 mg for sublingual use when anginal attacks occur.

The Problem: Assume that you are the nurse at the convalescent home who has the responsibility for Mrs. Walcott's care. Outline a nursing care plan for this patient, considering such matters as the following: (1) her treatment with nitroglycerin and phenobarbital; (2) nursing measures to reduce her anxiety and apprehension; and (3) specific measures that may help to stabilize her condition and permit her return home to her own apartment, where she will be responsible for her own care. (This is the goal for all patients in the convalescent home.)

DRUG DIGEST

NITROGLYCERIN U.S.P. (Glyceryl trinitrate)

Actions and Indications. This rapid-acting nitrate is effective for terminating acute attacks of angina pectoris. It also often prevents attacks when taken just before anticipated physical activity or emotional stress. The drug acts in part by dilating coronary arterioles, and also, possibly, by indirectly reducing the work of the heart and the demands of the myocardium for oxygen.

Side Effects, Cautions, and Contraindications. The drug may cause feelings of faintness, weakness, and dizziness. This can be largely avoided if the patient sits or lies down after taking it. Headache is a common early side effect, but this becomes less severe and less frequent as the patient develops tolerance to the drug's effects on the cerebral circulation. Caution is required in patients with glaucoma. The drug is contraindicated in patients with a history of idiosyncracy to nitrates marked by severe drops in blood pressure. Patients should not drink alcohol, as this tends to intensify hypotensive reactions. The drug's use following a recent acute myocardial infarction is not desirable.

Dosage and Administration. This drug is usually administered sublingually in individualized doses that may range from 0.15 to 0.6 mg or more. It is sometimes administered orally in sustained action dosage forms containing 2 to 6 mg or more. A 2 percent ointment is also available which is said to produce prompt and prolonged effects when applied to the skin in amounts of 1 or 2 to 4 or 5 inches.

PENTAERYTHRITOL TETRANITRATE N.F. (Peritrate; and others)

Actions and Indications. This drug is used for long-term prophylactic treatment of angina pectoris to reduce the number of daily attacks and their severity by improving the patient's coronary circulation. It may also be used for short-term prevention of attacks—that is, before engaging in physical activity of a kind that the patient knows may set off an anginal attack. It does *not* act fast enough to abort an acute attack, and it is not available in sublingual form for this purpose.

Side Effects, Cautions, and Contraindications. Throbbing headache is common at the start of treatment but tends to lessen as tolerance develops. Feelings of faintness, weakness, and dizziness may occur. These side effects may be more severe if the patient has been drinking, so alcohol should be avoided. Patients may complain of epigastric distress and nausea. Caution is required in patients with glaucoma, and the drug is contraindicated in patients who are known to be sensitive to nitrates.

Dosage and Administration. The usual oral dose of 10 to 20 mg is taken t.i.d. or q.i.d. times daily on an empty stomach. Timed-release tablets or capsules (containing 30 to 80 mg) are taken before breakfast for full absorption. This dose is repeated 12 hours later for sustained prophylactic effects during the night.

References

Di Palma, J.R. Precautions with anticoagulants. *RN*, 34:57, 1971 (Oct.).

Friend, D.G. Angina pectoris therapy. *Clin. Pharmacol. Ther.*, 5:385, 1964.

Killip, T. Management of the patient with acute myocardial infarction. *Med. Clin. N. Amer.*, 52:1061, 1968 (Sept.).

Koprowicz, D.C. Drug interactions with coumarin derivatives. *Amer. J. Nurs.*, 73:1042, 1973 (June).

Lemberg, L., et al. The treatment of arrhythmias following acute myocardial infarction. *Med. Clin. N. Amer.*, 55:273, 1971 (March).

Lown, B., et al. The coronary care unit. *JAMA*, 199:188, 1967

Melville, K.I. The pharmacological basis of antianginal drugs. *Pharmacol. Physicians*, 4:1, 1970 (March).

Myerberg, R.J. Diagnostic and therapeutic aspects of stable angina pectoris. *Med. Clin.* N. Amer., 55:421, 1971 (March).

Rodman, M.J. Drugs used in managing cardiac emergencies. *RN*, 36:71, 1973 (March).

———. Drugs used in the C.C.U. *RN*, 32:53, 1969 (Dec.).

Sharp, L., and Rabin, B. *Nursing in the Coronary Care Unit.* Philadelphia: J.B. Lippincott, 1970.

Smith, D.W., Germain, C.P.H., and Gips, C.D. *Care of the Adult Patient*, 3rd ed. Philadelphia: J.B. Lippincott, 1971, pp. 1052-1070.

31

Drugs for Reducing Elevated Plasma Lipids

Hyperlipidemia

Lipids are fats or fatlike substances that are insoluble in water. Certain types of lipids are carried in the blood in combination with plasma proteins. People whose plasma shows persistently elevated levels of these lipoproteins often tend to develop lipid deposits in various body tissues. Sometimes, for example, these take the form of *xanthomas,* yellowish-orange growths that erupt like a rash or as nodules on the skin of the elbows, eyelids, and elsewhere. Some authorities suggest that certain types of hyperlipidemias are also the cause of the *atherosclerotic plaques* that form within the walls of arteries and lead to ischemic vascular diseases.

There is still no *direct* proof that atherosclerosis results from abnormally high levels of circulating cholesterol and other lipids such as triglycerides (neutral fat). However the results of many studies do indicate *indirectly* that hyperlipidemia is one of several factors that increase the risk of disability and death from coronary heart disease. Thus, just as it is considered desirable to counteract such other high risk factors as high blood pressure and obesity, it may also be useful for certain selected patients to have their high plasma lipid levels lowered to normal.

Dietary measures, including the substitution of foods high in polyunsaturated fats for foods rich in saturated (animal) fat, are often effective for reducing cholesterol levels. In people with other types of elevated plasma lipids, a diet low in carbohydrates and calories may succeed in normalizing the lipoprotein pattern (Table 31-2). Sometimes, when dietary treat-

TABLE 31-1   *Properties of Plasma Lipoproteins**

Type of Lipoprotein	Characteristics
Chylomicrons	The largest lipoprotein complexes. Low protein and very high triglyceride content. Formed in the intestinal mucosa during absorption of dietary fat.
Pre-beta-lipoproteins	Made up mainly of triglycerides biosynthesized in the liver from dietary fatty acids and carbohydrates. They are larger in size and less dense than beta-lipoproteins. (They are also called very low density lipoproteins.)
Beta-lipoproteins	These carry the highest content of cholesterol. They are smaller and more dense than the chylomicrons and pre-beta-lipoproteins. (They are also called low density lipoproteins.)
Alpha-lipoproteins	These are the smallest and most dense ("high density") lipoproteins because of their relatively high protein content and low triglyceride content. (They contain about 20-25 percent cholesterol.)

* The different lipoproteins carry varying amounts of the lipids cholesterol, triglyceride or neutral fat, and phospholipids. The greater the lipid content, the lower is the density; the higher the protein content, the greater the density of the lipoprotein. Free fatty acids are bound to albumin rather than transported as lipoproteins.

ment measures alone fail to bring the patient's blood lipid levels back to normal or to keep it there, the doctor may also order certain drugs to be added to his dietary regimen (Table 31-3). In this chapter, we shall briefly discuss the current status of the drugs now available for lowering plasma lipid levels.

Antihyperlipidemic (Antilipemic) Agents

There is still no direct proof that reducing the amount of fatty substances circulating in the blood prevents or reverses atherogenesis. Nationwide studies at many medical centers are attempting to find out whether taking these drugs regularly will really prevent the complications of atherosclerosis or reduce the death rate from acute myocardial infarction, strokes, and other ischemic vascular disorders. However, the clinical usefulness of these drugs has *not* really been firmly established as of yet. Thus, it is particularly important that these agents themselves do no harm.

None of the available antilipemic drugs is free of discomforting side effects, and some may even prove dangerous in certain patients if they are not employed with adequate precautions. Because these drugs do not relieve any symptoms, patients may want to stop

taking them and save the money being spent on drugs that bring no obvious benefits. They will certainly want to discontinue a drug if it makes them feel *less well* instead of better. Fortunately, the side effects of these drugs tend to diminish with continued treatment.

The nurse can help to get the patient through this period by explaining carefully why it may be beneficial for him to continue taking these drugs even though he is experiencing no direct benefits that might compensate for the drug-induced discomfort. The nurse should help the high-risk patient to understand that taking these drugs might help to lengthen his life. Without upsetting the patient, he can be told that these drugs and other measures that the doctor may also have ordered may make the difference between his living in good health or having a heart attack. Similarly, patients who are unhappy about giving up cigarettes or switching from such foods as beef, butter, milk, and cheese to a diet of fish, fowl, and vegetables should be encouraged to stick to their programs. Although the benefits of drugs, diet, giving up smoking, avoiding stressful life situations, and exercising regularly have not been proven beyond doubt, there is now very strong evidence that all such measures are likely to lengthen the lives of many people and prevent disabling complications.

T A B L E 3 1 - 2 *Dietary and Drug Treatment of Hyperlipidemia**

Type of Hyperlipoproteinemia	Type of Lipid Abnormality	Preferred Treatment
Type I A rare disease induced by dietary fat. It is marked by abnormal accumulations of chylomicrons, dietary fat particles that make the plasma cloudy or milky. It causes xanthomatosis, but not necessarily atherosclerosis.	Triglycerides are very markedly elevated, but cholesterol is normal or only slightly elevated (that is, hyperthiglyceridemia without hypercholesterolemia).	No drug is effective. A low-fat diet and treatment of such underlying disorders as diabetes and hyperthyroidism is often effective.
Type II This common disorder is marked by high levels of beta-lipoproteins. Patients with a family history also often suffer from severe atherosclerosis and premature deaths from coronary artery disease.	Cholesterol levels are abnormally high, but triglycerides are normal or only slightly elevated (patient's plasma is clear) because of hypercholesterolemia without hypertriglyceridemia.	Diet high in polyunsaturated fats may be effective alone or with addition of drugs such as nicotinic acid, dextrothyroxine, or cholestyramine (clofibrate alone is not effective).
Type III An uncommon disorder marked by an accumulation of an abnormal beta-lipoprotein. Creamy fraction floats to the top of a plasma sample. It may be associated with premature atherosclerosis of the coronary and other arteries.	Both triglycerides and cholesterol are abnormally elevated (that is, hypercholesterolemia and hypertriglyceridemia).	Weight reduction with a diet low in saturated fats and cholesterol may be supplemented by clofibrate and possibly other drugs such as nicotinic acid.
Type IV A disorder in which dietary carbohydrates are converted to fat that is transported in the form of very low density (pre-beta) lipoproteins. Marked by xanthomas and possibly by premature atherosclerosis.	Triglyceride levels are high; cholesterol levels normal or only moderately elevated (that is, hypertriglyceridemia without hypercholesterolemia).	Diet low in carbohydrates with calories restricted mostly to polyunsaturated fats. Drugs such as clofibrate and possibly nicotinic acid may be added.
Type V A mixed hyperlipemia with combined Type I and Type IV patterns (that is, both chylomicrons and endogenously-produced *pre*-beta (very low density) lipoproteins, induced by both dietary fat and carbohydrate).	Triglyceride levels are always high, and cholesterol levels are sometimes very high (that is, hypertriglyceridemia and sometimes hypercholesterolemia).	Diet higher in protein than in fat or carbohydrate. Drugs such as clofibrate and possibly nicotinic acid may be added.

* These conditions are marked by abnormally high blood levels of lipids, including triglycerides (or neutral fats) and cholesterol. They are classified in accordance with the type of lipoprotein (lipid-protein complex that predominates in the patient's plasma. The lightest (very lowest density) lipoproteins carry mainly triglycerides; less light (low density) lipoproteins carry primarily cholesterol.

INDIVIDUAL DRUGS

Patients differ in the response of their high lipoprotein patterns to treatment with diet and various antilipemic drugs. Recent studies suggest that therapeutic results are most satis-factory when treatment is tailored to fit each patient's specific plasma lipid disorder. However, the expensive equipment required for precise diagnosis based upon differences in plasma lipoprotein patterns is not yet generally available. Thus, the doctor may select the type of diet and drugs that he thinks is best suited for his patient on the basis of whether cholesterol, triglycerides, or both types of lipids predominate in relatively simple to perform laboratory tests.

In the following discussion of individual antilipemic drugs, we shall indicate whether the main effect of each is upon serum cholesterol, triglycerides, or both, rather than which specific lipoprotein patterns are altered. In each case, we shall make a brief statement about each drug's current status without attempting to review the many speculations about the complex ways in which each agent is thought to act in lowering plasma lipids.

Clofibrate (Atromid-S) is considered the most widely useful lipid-reducing drug. It reduces elevated levels of triglyceride-type lipids more effectively than any of the other available antihyperlipidemic drugs. This makes it particularly useful for *Type III* and *IV* hyperlipoproteinemias, in which *hypertriglyceridemia* predominates (Table 31-2). It is less effective for treating the *Type II pattern*, in which cholesterol *alone* is elevated. However, it is often administered in combination with one of the other drugs that are more effective for treating *hypercholesterolemia*.

Clofibrate also has another property that may account for recent reports that its use has resulted in a reduction in the expected rate of heart attacks. It tends to counteract the tendency of blood to form clots within the arteries of patients with a history of coronary thrombosis. Thus, the drug's ability to keep blood platelets from sticking together may be a more important protective factor in these patients than its lipid-lowering effect. Nevertheless, patients with xanthomas have also benefited from continuous treatment with clofibrate, which has caused these yellow lipid deposits to disappear from their eyelids, elbows, knees, and elsewhere. The drug has also reportedly caused lesions in the eyes of diabetic patients with exudative retinopathy to regress.

Side effects of clofibrate include early nausea, abdominal distress, loose stools, and headache. Liver function tests occasionally show abnormalities, but the drug has not had to be discontinued because of hepatic toxicity. However, its use is undesirable in patients with a history of liver damage that has impaired hepatic function. In general, this seems to be a relatively safe drug that has *not* caused serious skin or blood disorders, despite reports of occasional skin eruptions and reductions in the

TABLE 31-3   *Antihyperlipidemic (Hypolipidemic) Agents*

Nonproprietary Name	Trade Name or Chemical Name	Usual Daily Dosage	Remarks
Cholestyramine U.S.P.	Cuemid; Questran	4 g, 3 or 4 times daily	Used also for relief of pruritus in partial biliary obstruction.
Clofibrate	Atromid-S	500 mg, 3 to 5 times daily	More effective for reducing plasma levels of triglycerides than of cholesterol.
Dextrothyroxine sodium	Choloxin	1 to 2 mg, daily to start; later 4 to 8 mg daily	Used to reduce cholesterol levels in patients with normal thyroid function.
Estrogens (1) Conjugated estrogens U.S.P.	(1) Premarin	(1) 2 to 5 mg daily	Claimed to protect male patients and postmenopausal women against coronary artery disease.
(2) Ethinyl estradiol U.S.P.	(2) Estinyl, and others	(2) 1 mg daily	
Nicotinic acid N.F. (and (2) aluminum nicotinate)	(1) Niacin	1–2 g, 3 or 4 times daily	Large doses of this B-complex vitamin lower plasma cholesterol levels.
	(2) Nicalex	1.25–2.5 3 or 4 times daily	
Sitosterols suspension N.F.	Cytellin	15 ml before each meal	Large doses bind dietary and other cholesterol in the intestine.

number of white blood cells (leukopenia). Occasionally, patients taking clofibrate complain of muscular aches, cramps and weakness.

The doctor often orders a reduction in the dosage of anticoagulant drugs by one third to one half when he adds clofibrate to a patient's treatment regimen. He also has the laboratory make more frequent tests of the patient's prothrombin time. This is because the *interaction* between these drugs may potentiate the action of the anticoagulant and cause unexpected bleeding.

Nicotinic acid (niacin), a vitamin of the B-complex group, is also effective for reducing serum lipids. Administered orally in relatively large doses, this drug lowers plasma levels of *both* cholesterol and triglycerides. Thus, it may be useful for treating *Types II, III,* and *IV* hyperlipoproteinemias. However, the drug's ability to correct the serum lipid abnormalities in these disorders that are said to make people more susceptible to atherosclerosis development has *not* been correlated with a corresponding drop in deaths from cardiovascular disease.

Side effects of the large daily doses needed for effective treatment include heartburn, flatulence, and other gastrointestinal symptoms. A derivative, *aluminum nicotinate* (Nicalex), is claimed to lessen gastrointestinal distress, but the administration of antacid buffers may also be needed by patients with peptic ulcer. Both these nicotinic acid products make the patient's skin become flushed and itchy at first, but these symptoms tend to lessen after a while, as do skin dryness and occasional underarm eruptions. The nurse should encourage patients to bear these discomforts and assure them that these side effects are likely to lessen and disappear. She should remind them to take their tablets *after* meals and with plenty of water to lessen gastrointestinal irritation.

Dextrothyroxine (Choloxin) is a form of the thyroid hormone that reduces serum cholesterol when administered in doses that do not stimulate general metabolism as much as do other thyroid derivatives. It is considered particularly useful for treating patients with pure hypercholesterolemia—that is, the Type II pattern of hyperlipidemia (Table 31-2) whether they also have a hypothyroid condition or not.

The main advantage of dextrothyroxine over levothyroxine and other thyroid hormones is that it is less likely to increase the body tissues' demands for oxygen. Such an increase in oxy-

gen consumption makes the heart work harder and is undesirable for patients with organic heart disease and cardiac irregularities. Despite this advantage over other thyroid products, dextrothyroxine must be used only with considerable caution in patients with coronary artery disease, particularly if their thyroid function is normal. This is because only slight overdosage might set off an attack of angina pectoris or even precipitate cardiac arrhythmias or congestive heart failure.

To avoid this danger, the drug's use is limited largely to patients who have *both* hypothyroidism and hypercholesterolemia, and patients begin treatment with very low daily doses that are raised only gradually. If a patient begins to get heart palpitations or shows signs of nervousness and tremors, the drug is withdrawn and later begun again at a lower dose level. Recently, some doctors who have had considerable experience with this drug and learned to use it safely have also advocated its use for lowering cholesterol levels in patients with heart disease whose thyroid function is normal.

Like clofibrate, dextrothyroxine tends to potentiate the effects of anticoagulant drugs such as dicumarol and warfarin. The doses of these drugs must be reduced when dextrothyroxine is added to the patient's treatment regimen. Diabetic patients are closely watched, because dextrothyroxine administration may increase their need for insulin or the oral antidiabetic drugs.

Cholestyramine resin (Cuemid; Questran) is a drug marketed mainly for relief of pruritus in patients with primary biliary cirrhosis and cholestatic jaundice. It relieves the itching in this condition by removing irritating bile salts that have accumulated in the patient's skin. This ability to bind bile salts has led to the experimental use of this drug in treating hypercholesterolemia. Taken orally, this resin ties up bile salts in the patient's intestine into insoluble complexes. These are then excreted in the feces instead of being reabsorbed and carried back to the liver and gall bladder.

The body then tries to replace the missing bile salts by breaking liver cholesterol down to form these substances that are essential for absorbing fatty substances from the intestine. This leads to a lowering of blood cholesterol by about 20 percent in the average patient over a six-week period. Some patients with very high serum cholesterol have had drops of as much as 80 percent in the levels of this lipid.

The main drawback of cholestyramine is that the drug tastes bad and yet must be taken in large amounts. It also causes heartburn, nausea, and either constipation or diarrhea. The nurse should encourage the patient to continue taking the drug until the early gastrointestinal upset no longer occurs. Patients are told not to swallow the dry powder as this might irritate or block the esophagus. Instead, it is mixed with liquids such as orange or apricot juice or with pulpy foods— applesauce, for instance. Patients may require supplements of fat-soluble vitamins, which are poorly absorbed. Because cholestyramine can also keep acidic drugs from being absorbed, it should not be given at the same time. Instead, patients taking anticoagulant drugs, phenylbutazone and other antiarthritic agents, phenobarbital, thyroxine, and other drugs should do so at the longest possible interval before or after administration of cholestyramine.

Estrogens, female sex hormones, were first used for reducing cholesterol because of the observation that premenopausal women have a lower rate of heart attack than men in the same age group. However, when administered in doses high enough to lower serum lipids in men with a history of a prior heart attack, the estrogenic hormones have feminizing effects. That is, they tend to cause gynecomastia (enlarged painful growth of the breasts), loss of libido, and sometimes mental depression.

These drugs may be of value when taken by women past the menopause. However, according to recent reports, the high doses of estrogens that reduce cholesterol levels may also increase the amount of triglycerides. This may account for the higher than normal incidence of thrombophlebitis and complications such as pulmonary embolism that have been noted in some studies.

Sitosterols (Cytellin) is a product made up of natural plant sterols. Taken orally in large daily doses, it ties up dietary and bile-secreted cholesterol in the intestine and removes it by fecal excretion. This leads to a moderate drop in blood cholesterol, particularly when patients also eat a diet in which foods containing polyunsaturated fats have been substituted for foods containing saturated fats. Patients tend to lose their appetite when taking large amounts of this lipid-lowering product. The nurse may suggest that patients mix the suspension with beverages to make it easier to take. Although this product is safe, it is not often considered effective enough to be worth the expense of long-term treatment.

SUMMARY

There is still no direct proof that the life expectancy of patients with abnormally high levels of plasma lipids will be lengthened by lowering the amount of fatty substances in their circulation. However, indirect evidence suggests that patients considered to have a high risk of developing atherosclerotic complications may profit from measures that reduce blood cholesterol and triglycerides. It is possible that if high-risk patients are recognized in the early stages of their disease, the atherogenic process may be stopped and reversed by putting them on a long-term preventive diet.

If diet alone is not enough, the addition of an antilipemic drug or drugs may help the patient's prognosis. For best results, the doctor should choose the drugs that are best suited to each individual patient's pattern of lipoprotein and lipid abnormality. The nurse should advise the patient about how these drugs are best taken to minimize their side effects, and she should encourage him to continue with the medication when he wants to quit because he sees no immediate gains that warrant the expense or the possible drug-induced discomfort.

S U M M A R Y of Adverse Effects of Antihyperlipidemic (Hypolipidemic) Agents*

Cholestyramine

Gastrointestinal upset — nausea, heartburn, constipation, or diarrhea.

Possible interference with absorption of fat-soluble vitamins and acid drugs.

* The nurse's main concern is to encourage patients to continue taking these drugs despite the discomforting side effects and to teach patients how best to take these drugs to minimize gastric upset.

Clofibrate

Gastrointestinal upset—nausea, epigastric distress, vomiting. Muscular aches and cramps, occasionally.

Dextrothyroxine sodium

Stimulation of metabolism may set off attacks of angina in patients with coronary disease.

Estrogens

Feminizing effects in male patients, including gynecomastia. Loss of libido and mental depression may also develop.

Nicotinic acid

Gastrointestinal upset—heartburn flatulence, nausea, and vomiting.

Sitosterols

Flushing and itching of the skin. Looseness of stools.

SUMMARY of Points for the Nurse to Remember Concerning Antilipemic Drugs

The patient may be reluctant to take a drug that produces no dramatic benefits but which, instead, tends to cause discomforting side effects. The nurse can suggest that these may decrease in severity with continued use of the drug. She can also help by reviewing the possible benefits of this type of drug therapy. (However, once he has been fully informed of the desirability of continuing with this medication, the decision to do so or not depends upon the patient himself, and not on the wishes of his doctor or nurse.)

Teach the patient measures that may help to relieve side effects. For example, the patient should be told to take certain drugs such as nicotinic acid after meals and with plenty of fluids to avoid heartburn, flatulence, and other symptoms of gastrointestinal irritation.

Teach patients who are taking several drugs simultaneously to avoid undesirable drug interactions within the gastrointestinal tract. For example, cholestyramine can interfere with absorption of other drugs, and thus it should not be given at the same time as these drugs but only after a long interval. Be aware of possible drug interactions between such drugs as dextrothyroxine and clofibrate with anticoagulants, and observe the patient's responses.

Clinical Nursing Situation

The Situation: Mr. Marcus, a 55-year-old business man, is overweight and has a high blood cholesterol level. He is a heavy smoker and a hard-driving, energetic worker. His physician has advised him to make changes in his life style, following a physical examination that revealed certain cardiovascular abnormalities, and on the basis of a family history of premature coronary disease and death in both his parents.

Mr. Marcus has succeeded in cutting his cigarette smoking from two packs to one pack a day, but he has not lost much weight or significantly reduced his plasma cholesterol levels in his first few weeks on a low calorie, low fat diet. (Possibly, he has been occasionally having favorite foods such as a steak and french-fried potatoes, scrambled eggs and bacon.) So the doctor has decided to add *dextrothyroxine* to his daily regimen.

After a few days, Mr. Marcus calls the office to complain that he is nervous, not sleeping well, and may even be having some heart palpitations. He wonders whether or not he should go on taking his medication.

The Problem: You are the nurse working in close collaboration with Mr. Marcus's physician. In this capacity you do a good deal of health counseling and teaching by telephone and on home visits. In this case, the doctor is away at the hospital and won't be back at his office until later in the day.

What would you advise Mr. Marcus to do about taking his daily dose of the drug? How would you assess his progress when you visit him at his home the following evening as previously planned? That is, what factors would you consider in evaluating Mr. Marcus's adaptation to the overall treatment plan that has been designed to reduce the likelihood of his suffering a myocardial infarction as his parents did?

References

Bagdale, J.D., and Bierman, E.L. Diagnosis and dietary treatment of blood lipid disorders. *Med. Clin. N. Amer.*, 54:1383, 1970 (Nov.).

Berkowitz, D. Drug treatment of hyperlipidemia. *Mod. Treatm.*, 6:1341, 1969 (Nov.).

Bricker, L.A. A clinical approach to the hyperlipidemias. *Med Clin. N. Amer.*, 55:403, 1971 (March).

Connor, W.E. Measures to reduce the serum lipid levels in coronary heart disease. *Med. Clin. N. Amer.*, 52:1249, 1969 (Sept.).

Kuo, P.T. Hyperlipidemia in atherosclerosis. *Med. Clin. N. Amer.*, 54:657, 1970 (May).

Rodman, M.J. Drugs that reduce blood cholesterol. *RN*, 32:77, 1969 (Feb.).

32.

Drugs for Peripheral Vascular Disease

Arterial Diseases

Diseases that interfere with the flow of blood through the arteries are the leading cause of disability and death. We have already discussed how narrowing of the coronary vessels by atherosclerosis causes the severe ischemic pain of angina pectoris. We have also seen that the sudden closing off (occlusion) of a vessel in a vital organ can be rapidly fatal—for example, following an acute myocardial infarction or after pulmonary embolism or a stroke.

In this chapter, we shall deal mainly with drugs that are used in less dramatic but still severely disabling circulatory disturbances—the chronic diseases of the *peripheral*, or outlying, blood vessels. We shall limit our discussion largely to drugs that dilate the peripheral arteries, even though several other classes of drugs that are discussed elsewhere are also important in the management of these peripheral vascular diseases. For example, while we shall confine our observations almost entirely to peripheral vasodilator drugs, doctors often also employ anticoagulant and thrombolytic agents, analgesic-antiinflammatory agents, and antiinfective drugs in the management of these disorders.

Because many of the same drugs that are used mainly to widen disease-narrowed vessels in the skin and skeletal muscles are also claimed to improve blood flow through the brain, we shall say something, too, about the current status of some of these same drugs in the management of patients with chronic cerebrovascular disease. (Drugs used for dilating the *coronary* arterioles are taken up separately in Chapter 30.)

PATHOLOGIC PHYSIOLOGY OF PERIPHERAL VASCULAR DISEASE

The poor flow of blood to fingers, toes, and other parts of the extremities in these disorders has two main causes: (1) *organic damage* to the walls of the blood vessels; and (2) *vasospasm*—constriction of the vessels as a result of excessive stimulation by nerve impulses reaching the vascular smooth muscle by way of the sympathetic nervous system.

In both kinds of peripheral vascular diseases, it is an insufficiency in the flow of blood reaching the involved tissues that leads to discomfort or even to severe pain. This, in turn, is the result of failure of the circulation to meet the demands of the tissues for oxygen and nutrients, while metabolites that should have been removed are accumulating locally. That is, the pain in the skin and skeletal muscles, like that which arises from the myocardium in angina pectoris, is set off by local ischemia and hypoxia.

Pain, numbness and tingling, pallor, and cyanosis of the skin are only part of the problem posed by poor peripheral circulation. In some conditions, the end result of damage done to tissues that are deprived of their blood supply may be so severe that amputation of digits or even of limbs becomes necessary. This is most likely to occur in vessels that have become progressively narrowed by atherosclerosis.

In such cases, blood flowing sluggishly over the vessels' damaged inner walls tends to clot very readily. Thus, a thrombus may form suddenly in a channel already narrowed by lipid deposits and completely block blood flow. The tissues beyond the obstruction are then deprived of the oxygen and nutrients they need for survival. This soon leads to tissue necrosis and development of gangrenous ulcers*

TREATMENT OF ARTERIAL DISEASES

Increasing the blood supply to the poorly perfused tissues is an important objective of treatment—that is, to bring the tissues enough

oxygen and to remove metabolic waste materials. In theory, drugs that dilate constricted blood vessels and increase the total amount of blood reaching the ischemic tissues should be capable of correcting the imbalance between the amounts of oxygen that the tissues need and the insufficient quantities that they are actually receiving.

In some situations, this does seem to happen. In *Raynaud's disease,* for example, and in other conditions in which blood flow to the patient's skin has been reduced because the smooth muscle walls of the vessels have gone into spasm, drugs that relax the contracted muscles seem to open up the constricted channels and bring a better flow of blood to the patient's skin. During the vasodilator drug's peak action, the skin often becomes flushed and warm, and numbness, tingling, and pain—if it was present—are relieved. Such relief is often relatively brief, because the action of most drugs is not of long duration.

Unfortunately, vasodilator drugs do not help much in arterial disorders in which the vessels have been damaged by degenerative atherosclerotic disease. This is so because blood vessel walls made rigid by deposits of lipid plaques do not respond readily to the muscle-relaxing action of these drugs. Thus, for example, in *Buerger's disease,* a condition in which the vessel walls have been damaged and hardened by arteriosclerosis and the vascular channels have been narrowed by organic obstructions bulging out from the walls, the administration of vasodilator drugs usually does little to increase blood flow to the patient's ischemic tissues.

Some doctors suggest that these drugs may be of benefit by dilating *collateral* blood vessels—alternate channels—that then deliver the needed blood. On the other hand, others argue that the dilating action of these drugs on undamaged blood vessels may sometimes actually serve to shunt blood away from the tissue areas that need it most. Thus, doctors treating patients with chronic arterial diseases often depend, not primarily upon drugs, but mainly upon hygienic measures for maintaining a better arterial blood supply and for preventing breaks in the skin and other injuries that may allow microorganisms to enter.

---

* The treatment of decubital and other ulcers of the extremities is not discussed in this text. Healing of ulcerated areas may be hastened by the topical application of creams or ointments containing proteolytic (protein-splitting) *enzymes.* These biological

catalysts aid healing by speeding the removal of tissue debris from the damaged area. Following elimination of necrotic tissue in this way, granulation and epithelialization proceed more readily.

The nurse can play an important part in teaching these patients how to follow personal hygiene programs. In addition to encouraging the patient to continue with regular drug therapy, she should emphasize ways in which these patients, who are most often at home rather than in the hospital, can care for themselves. Among the practical points that can be suggested are these:

1. *Keep the entire body warm at all times*, as chilling tends to cause reflex constriction of the peripheral blood vessels.

2. *Avoid applying local heat directly* to the affected parts. For example, the patient should never try to relieve ischemic foot pain by using a hot water bottle or a heating pad, as this can result in gangrenous ulcers.

3. *Avoid damage* to delicate ischemic tissues *by caustic chemicals* such as iodine or salicylic acid (in corn remedies). Instead, feet should be protected from chemical and mechanical injury by various means, such as gentle massage with lanolin or soaking in potassium permanganate solution 1:5,000.

4. *Light exercise, particularly walking* (within the limits recommended by the doctor), is desirable for maintaining muscle tone, developing additional circulatory flow pathways, and keeping one's weight down.

5. *Resting in positions that aid blood flow* is important. For example, patients with arterial disease should have the head of the bed raised so that blood will flow more readily to their lowered legs. Those with venous difficulties should keep their legs elevated, as this tends to reduce edema and local tenderness.

6. *Clothing that constricts* the legs and thighs should be avoided by patients with circulatory disorders. Round garters and girdles that reduce arterial flow and cause excessive congestion of superficial veins are also undesirable.

7. *Smoking should be stopped,* as nicotine tends to make blood vessels constrict and thus reduces local tissue perfusion. Drug products containing vasoconstrictive adrenergic drugs such as ephedrine and amphetamines should be avoided, as should headache remedies containing ergotamine.

TYPES OF PERIPHERAL VASODILATOR DRUGS

Drugs of several different types have the ability to relax vascular smooth muscle. In theory, the widening of the arterioles that then results should bring a flow of fresh blood to the poorly perfused tissues. In practice, this does not always happen—at least, not to a degree that results in a definite increase in tissue oxygenation and a better ability to perform physical functions without suffering ischemic pain. Nevertheless, despite the lack of proof that these drugs have more than limited value, vasodilator drugs are widely promoted and prescribed. This may be because patients often *feel* that the drugs are doing some good, and, perhaps, because their doctors try to take advantage of even a placebo response in these chronic vascular conditions.

In general, vasodilator drugs act in one of two main ways: (1) *by altering sympathetic nervous system control* of blood vessel caliber; and (2) *by directly depressing the contractile mechanism* of the blood vessels' smooth muscle walls.

In both cases, the vascular walls relax, and with the reduction in vasomotor tone and in resistance to blood flow through the vessels, local perfusion increases and ischemic symptoms are relieved. Drugs that block transmission of sympathetic vasoconstrictive impulses to arterioles of the *skin* are fairly effective in bringing about a transient increase in blood flow in those disorders that are characterized by *cutaneous reflex vasospasm*—Raynaud's disease, frostbite, and acrocyanosis, for example.

Drugs that stimulate the beta adrenergic, or vasodilator, receptors in the vessels that carry blood to skeletal muscles may be more effective in such peripheral vascular diseases as *intermittent claudication*. In this condition, which is characterized by attacks of calf muscle pain brought on by walking, certain of the direct-acting vasodilators are also claimed to be useful for relief of lameness and pain in some patients.

In the following discussion, we shall briefly review the status of each of the classes of vasodilator drugs currently available.

SYMPATHETIC BLOCKING AGENTS. The sympathetic nervous system plays an important part in regulating the tone of vascular smooth muscle. Two types of drugs can block transmission of vasoconstrictor impulses to these blood vessel walls. These are: (1) the *alpha adrenergic blocking agents*; and (2) the *ganglionic blocking agents*. Although drug-induced blockade of these kinds does tend to reduce transmission of excessive vasoconstrictor impulses, these drugs often produce a variety of adverse effects that limit their usefulness. This is particularly true when attempts are made to employ these blocking agents in those chronic vascular diseases in which the vessels are partially blocked by physical obstructions to blood flow.

Phenoxybenzamine+ (Dibenzyline) is one of the best of the alpha adrenergic blockers, because it tends to produce a relatively prolonged peripheral vasodilator effect when taken by mouth. Administered in gradually increasing doses until full vasodilator effects are produced, this drug sometimes relieves vasospasm in patients with Raynaud's disease, acrocyanosis, and other disorders that mainly involve the skin rather than skeletal muscles. The resulting dilation of dermal arterioles may raise skin temperature and possibly prevent ulceration of fingertips, toes, and other parts in which blood vessels are abnormally constricted.

The reason for raising dosage of this drug only slowly is that higher doses can cause *generalized* vasodilation and a drop in blood

pressure. Overdosage that produces postural hypotension is even more likely to occur with drugs of the ganglionic blocking class (Table 32-1). That is why blocking drugs of that type are now used only rarely for treating peripheral vascular disease but are employed more often for managing high blood pressure (Chapter 26).

Elderly patients with generalized atherosclerosis, as well as peripheral vascular disease, must be carefully observed while taking sympathetic blocking drugs. Generalized vasodilation may not only cause dizziness, weakness, and fainting, but may even precipitate a stroke or a myocardial infarction in patients with severe cerebral or coronary atherosclerosis. Reflex tachycardia in response to a steep drug-induced fall in blood pressure might also set off an episode of congestive heart failure in a patient barely on the borderline of cardiac compensation.

Tolazoline (Priscoline), a drug with adrenergic blocking and other pharmacological ef-

T A B L E   3 2 - 1   *Drugs that Dilate Peripheral (and Cerebral) Vessels*

Nonproprietary Name	Proprietary Name	Usual Dosage	Remarks
Sympathetic Blocking Agents			
ALPHA ADRENERGIC BLOCKERS			
Azeptine phosphate	Ilidar	25 mg initally; 50–75 mg later three times a day	Also has direct muscle relaxing action
Dihydroergotoxine mesylate	Hydergine	4–6 sublingual tablets	Also said to depress the vasomotor center of the brain
Phenoxybenzamine HCl	Dibenzyline	10 mg initially; later, after gradual increase, between 20–60 mg daily	See *Drug Digest*
Phentolamine mesylate U.S.P.	Regitine	5 to 10 mg in 10 ml saline injected into area of norepinephrine extravasation	See *Drug Digest* (Chapter 24)
Tolazoline HCl	Priscoline	100–300 mg daily orally or 160 mg of sustained action form; 40–200 mg parenterally	Also has direct muscle relaxing action and histamine-like effects
GANGLIONIC BLOCKERS			
Chlorisondamine chloride	Ecolid	10 mg orally; 2.5 mg parenterally	
Mecamylamine HCl U.S.P.	Inversine	2.5 mg initially; later 25 mg daily	Drugs of this subclass have hypotensive effects; injections are sometimes useful in treating acute
Pentolinium tartrate	Ansolysen	20 mg orally initially; later 60 mg or more; parenterally 2.5–3.5 mg	

TABLE 32-1 *Drugs that Dilate Peripheral (and Cerebral) Vessels (continued)*

Nonproprietary Name	Proprietary Name	Usual Dosage	Remarks
Trimethaphan camsylate U.S.P.	Arfonad	Controlled continuous intravenous infusion	occlusions of a major blood vessel
Trimethidinium methosulfate N.F.	Ostensin	20–40 mg orally initially; later larger individualized dosage	
Beta Adrenergic Stimulants			
Isoxuprine HCl N.F.	Vasodilan	10–20 mg orally; 5–10 mg I.M.	Also has a direct vasodilating effect
Nylidrin HCl N.F.	Arlidin	3–6 mg orally; 2.25–5 mg parenterally	Also said to act directly on cerebral vessels
Parasympathetic (Cholinergic) Drugs			
Methacholine bromide N.F.	Mecholyl Br	200 mg orally	Iontophoresis does not cause the cholinergic side effects of systemic administration
Methacholine chloride N.F.	Mecholyl Cl	20 mg s.c; or by iontophoresis with 0.2–0.5% solution	
Direct-Acting Vasodilators			
Cyclandelate	Cyclospasmol	400–800 mg daily oral maintence doses	Improvement, if any, is said to develop gradually
Dioxylline phosphate	Paveril	100–400 mg orally, several times daily	Synthetic analogue of papaverine
Ethaverine HCl	Ethaquin	30–100 mg orally	Analogue of papaverine
Nicotinyl alcohol tartrate	Roniacol	50–100 mg orally t.i.d., or 150 mg b.i.d.	Derivative of nicotinic acid
Papaverine HCl N.F.	Cerespan; Pavabid, and others	150 mg of sustained action oral form every 12 hours; 30–100 mg parenterally, including intra-arterial	Prototype smooth muscle relaxant more effective when injected than by oral administration

fects, is also employed sometimes to relax vascular spasm and thus increase peripheral blood flow. It is relatively short-acting but is now available in an oral pharmaceutical form that releases the drug slowly so that it may act continuously all through the night. A drawback is this drug's tendency to stimulate secretion of gastric acid and thus cause epigastric distress, nausea, or vomiting. It also tends to cause more tachycardia than most drugs of this class, and so is contraindicated in patients with coronary artery disease, including angina pectoris.

Tolazoline is most likely to prove effective when administered by a parenteral route. In addition to injection intravenously, intramuscularly, or subcutaneously, the intraarterial route is sometimes employed. Administered directly into the femoral, radial, or brachial artery by a special technique, the infused drug often causes flushing of the skin and a feeling of warmth, or even a burning sensation, all through the involved limb.

Although this vasodilator effect may sometimes be useful following frostbite or for relief of pain in causalgia, it is of little use for increasing blood flow through the leg muscles of patients with intermittent claudication. Patients with Buerger's disease and advanced arteriosclerosis obliterans may actually suffer a further decrease of blood flow in the ischemic area. The reason for this is that tolazoline, like other potent blocking drugs, may relax the smooth muscles of other arterioles more readily than the walls of damaged vessels. As a result, blood flow may be diverted into these newly opened channels and away from the tissues that need it most.

Phentolamine+ (Regitine) is an alpha adrenergic blocker that is now used for diagnosis and treatment of pheochromocytoma rather than in peripheral vascular disease. However, its ability to dilate extremely constricted blood vessels is utilized in counteracting the local vaso-constrictor effect of *levarterenol*+ (Levophed), when an infusion of that vasopressor drug accidentally leaks into the skin during treatment of a patient in shock. For that purpose the affected area is infiltrated with phentolamine to prevent local tissue necrosis and ulceration.

BETA ADRENERGIC STIMULANT DRUGS. The arteriolar walls of the vessels that carry blood to the skeletal muscles contain mainly adrenergic receptors of the beta type. These receptors react to the neurohormone norepinephrine in a way that results in relaxation of the vascular smooth muscle. This results in vasodilation and an increased blood flow through the skeletal muscles. Certain synthetic sympathomimetic amines that also stimulate such beta adrenergic receptors are advocated for clinical use for relief of leg cramps and pain in patients with peripheral vascular diseases.

Two drugs of this class, *nylidrin* (Arlidin) and *isoxuprine* (Vasodilan), are claimed to bring about a marked increase in the amount of blood passing through the calf muscles of patients with intermittent claudication and other occlusive vascular diseases. Both drugs are also said to increase cerebral blood flow and thus relieve symptoms that stem from insufficient flow of blood to brain areas served by atherosclerotic arterioles. Nylidrin has also been tried for the relief of ringing in the ears, hearing difficulties, and vertigo—symptoms that are thought to be caused by spasm of inner ear arterioles. There is little proof that this drug and others (see below) are really effective for relief of symptoms that are the result of cerebral or labyrinthine arterial insufficiency. Fortunately, oral doses of these drugs have relatively few side effects (see *Summary*, p. 392).

PARASYMPATHOMIMETIC (CHOLINERGIC) DRUGS. Autonomic drugs of this class that mimic the effects of the neurohormone acetylcholine have also been employed occasionally in certain peripheral vascular diseases. *Methacholine* (Mecholyl) has been administered orally to dilate cutaneous vessels of patients with Raynaud's disease. However, oral or subcutaneous doses capable of benefitting patients by improving blood flow, are likely to cause undesirable side effects such as diarrhea (see *Summary*, p. 392). Such symptoms do not occur when methacholine is administered by

iontophoresis, a method for introducing drug solution into the skin by means of an electric current.

DIRECT-ACTING VASODILATOR DRUGS. Certain substances relax excessively constricted vessels by acting directly on their walls to reduce the tone of the smooth muscles and thus widen the arterial channels. The prototype of direct-acting muscle relaxants is *papaverine*, a non-addicting opium alkaloid. Newer drugs of this kind include derivatives of the B-complex vitamin nicotinic acid, such as *nicotinyl alcohol* (Roniacol), and *cyclandelate* (Cyclospasmol), a drug of a different chemical class.

Drugs of this type do not seem to be very effective when administered orally for peripheral vascular disorders. However, because facial flushing is seen with some of these agents, patients may *feel* that the drugs are doing some good. Later, when flushing no longer occurs, patients may stop taking the drug. The nurse should encourage the patient to keep on taking his medication for as long as the doctor continues to order it, as short-term vasodilator drug therapy is of little use in these chronic conditions.

Papaverine, administered parenterally, does dilate arterioles by relaxing reflex spasm. However, large doses administered in this way may cause cardiac arrhythmias. In acute block of a major vessel by a blood clot, papaverine may sometimes be injected directly into the artery. However, most doctors now prefer to meet this emergency by blocking spinal ganglia with regional anesthetics; if this is effective in increasing local blood flow, surgical sympathectomy may also be employed for long-term relief of vascular spasm.

All of the direct-acting vasodilator drugs are also claimed to be useful for increasing blood flow to the brain. This, in turn, is said to improve mental function in elderly patients and others with encephalopathy (brain damage) stemming from cerebral atherosclerosis and thrombosis. Actually, there is little proof that these drugs can dilate atherosclerotic and other blood vessels in the brain beyond the degree of dilation brought about naturally by the body's own response to poor local circulation. (Underoxygenation and accumulation of carbon dioxide in ischemic areas cause local vascular dilation and a maximal increase in brain blood flow.)

Despite lack of proof of their effectiveness, products containing papaverine and similar drugs are widely promoted and prescribed for treating elderly patients with cerebral atherosclerosis. These drugs are claimed to improve the patients' memory, mood, and behavior, and to relieve such symptoms as mental confusion and dizziness. Probably, any temporary improvement of this kind is the result of a placebo effect, as oral doses of these drugs have little effect, and elderly patients often respond favorably to the unusual attention they receive when they are part of a clinical study.

Venous Diseases

PHYSIOLOGY, PATHOPHYSIOLOGY, AND TREATMENT

The veins contain one-way valves that keep blood from flowing backward when it is making its way back from the venous capillaries toward the heart. However, when these valves are stretched and become incompetent, gravity tends to pull some of the blood backwards. This, in itself, does not interfere significantly with the venous return of blood to the heart, as there are so many venous pathways available. However, the increasing pressure within the distended veins tends to make their walls bulge outward in a way that may be disfiguring and painful.

VARICOSE VEINS. Excessively engorged, dilated veins often cause discomfort—aching, cramping, and feelings of fullness, itching, and burning in the affected limbs. This common condition often stems from hereditary weakness of the venous walls. This may be aggravated by obesity or by the nature of a person's work —for example, standing for long periods at a job or lifting heavy loads. Pregnancy is another common cause, because distention of the uterus puts increased pressure upon the veins of the woman's lower limbs.

 Treatment. Drugs are of only limited usefulness for treating varicose veins, and surgery is considered superior in most cases. Occasionally, however, chemicals may be employed to close off small superficial veins. The irritating substances used for this purpose are called *sclerosing agents.*

Sodium morrhuate injection (Morusul) and *sodium tetradecyl sulfate* (Sotradecol) are among the most common chemicals used for obliterating segments of distended veins. They are injected carefully into a part of the vein that has been closed off from the general circulation, and the area is then kept clamped with compression bandages. The chemicals subsequently damage the inner lining of the collapsed veins, and this in turn leads to blood clot formation. Finally, after several weeks in which the patient walks around and even sleeps wearing elastic stockings over the bandages, the blood clots are converted to connective tissue. Once the inner surfaces become "glued" together by fibrous tissue, the varicose vein is firmly occluded or obliterated.

Care is required to avoid leakage of the sclerosing solution into the surrounding tissues, as extravascular spillages can cause pain, abscesses, and sloughing of necrotic tissues. Sometimes, the doctor first administers a small test dose of these drugs to determine whether the patient is sensitive to them. Hypersensitization developing during a course of treatment can lead to allergic reactions, including anaphylaxis.

For phlebitis and venous thromboses, doctors employ *anticoagulant* and *thrombolytic agents.* Prompt treatment with these drugs can prevent such serious and potentially fatal complications as pulmonary embolism.

In summary, the status of vasodilator drugs is uncertain. Although medication may offer symptomatic relief in some cases, other measures may be even more important for improving the patient's circulation and preventing serious complications. The nurse must be willing to work with patients whose poor circulation makes them prone to develop skin damage and ulcerations. Attentive care of these patients to prevent breaks in the skin and to control fungal and other infections is very important, as is teaching the patient to care for himself at home to avoid developing the complications of peripheral vascular disease. Although these chronic conditions often improve very slowly, if at all, proper patient care can be rewarding when it helps to lessen pain, heal ulcers, and keep a limb from being lost.

SUMMARY of Clinical Indications for Peripheral and Cerebral Vasodilators*

Peripheral Vasodilation

Acrocyanosis and acroparesthesia
Arteriosclerosis obliterans
Buerger's disease (thromboangiitis obliterans)
Causalgia
Diabetic arteriosclerosis
Embolism and thrombosis, arterial
Endarteritis
Frostbite sequelae
Gangrene
Intermittent claudication
Nocturnal leg cramps
Raynaud's disease and phenomenon

Thrombophlebitis sequelae
Ulcers of extremities (and other types, such as: decubital, diabetic, thrombotic, arteriosclerotic)
Venous or varicose ulcerations

Cerebral Vasodilation

Cerebral arteriosclerosis marked by mood, memory, and behavioral changes
Inner ear disturbances marked by vertigo, dizziness, deafness, secondary to spasm or obstruction of labyrinthine circulation
Meniere's syndrome

*The lengthy list of proposed clinical uses for vasodilator drugs does not indicate that these are effective therapeutic agents. On the contrary, their true clinical usefulness in most of these circulatory disorders is quite limited.

SUMMARY of Adverse Effects, Cautions, and Contraindications of Vasodilator Drugs

Alpha Adrenergic Blocking Agents

Nasal congestion and occasional bronchoconstriction may aggravate respiratory infection or bronchial asthma.

Gastrointestinal irritation and increased motility leading to diarrhea and peptic pain require caution in patients with peptic ulcer or gastroenteritis.

Possible interference with male sexual function.

Postural hypotension and reflex tachycardia:
Feelings of fatigue, weakness, dizziness.
Caution in patients sensitive to steep drops in blood pressure; contraindicated in patients with severe cerebral or coronary atherosclerosis, compensated heart failure, and renal damage.

Shock and circulatory collapse:
Adrenergic vasopressors such as levarterenol may be employed if necessary, but epinephrine is contraindicated.

Beta Adrenergic Receptor Stimulants

Heart palpitations and hypotension occur *infrequently* with oral doses.

High doses, particularly by parenteral administration, should *not* be administered to patients with a history of recent myocardial infarction.

Drug rash is rare but requires discontinuation.

Nervousness and muscle tremors are rare reactions.

Parasympathomimetic (Cholinergic) Vasodilators

Diarrhea, flushing, sweating and other muscarinic effects (see *Summary* pp. 276-277).

Direct-Acting Vasodilator Drugs

Gastrointestinal symptoms, including anorexia, epigastric distress, nausea, diarrhea or constipation.

Cardiovascular effects, including flushing, dizziness, vascular headache, diaphoresis (sweating), feelings of fatigue, weakness, drowsiness. Hypotension, tachycardia, and occasional cardiac arrhythmias make caution necessary in patients with severe coronary artery or cerebral artery disease.

SUMMARY of Points for the Nurse to Remember Concerning Drug Treatment of Peripheral Vascular Diseases

Treatment for many patients consists of careful attention to details; one of these important details involves administration of the prescribed drug and careful observation of its effects. Is the

patient able to walk farther without pain? Is his foot warmer?

Instructing the patient and his family in measures that promote improved circulation and lessen the possibility of complications is essential. Nurses can carry out such instructions in the hospital, home, and industry. Particular nursing vigilance is required in settings where there are many elderly people, such as in nursing homes. For example, the nurse should promptly report any tiny ulcer, or any change in the temperature of an extremity, to the doctor.

Relief of pain is an important problem. Ideally, pain is relieved by improving the blood supply. Actually, analgesics may be required if blood supply cannot be sufficiently improved. Since

pain tends to be chronic, be especially vigilant in noting it and in using prescribed measures to relieve it. If these measures are not effective, be sure to discuss this with the physician. Opiates are avoided, not because the pain is trivial, but because of the danger of addiction.

When applying any medicine locally to an ulcer, use careful aseptic technique. Because of impaired blood supply, the patient is particularly hampered in fighting infection which can then lead to gangrene and necessitate amputation.

Clinical Nursing Situation

The Situation: Mr. Chesterson is a 67-year-old widower who lives alone on the third floor of a building in a deteriorating section of a large city. Lately he has had increasingly troublesome symptoms when walking, such as cramping, pain, and fatigue. The doctor diagnosed his condition as being due to arteriosclerosis of the blood vessels of the legs and prescribed Priscoline 50 mg t.i.d.

Mr. Chesterson, who lives on an extremely limited budget, has little money for recreation,

medication, or even maintaining a fully nutritious diet. He has given up smoking for reasons of health and economy. You are the nurse who sees him every week either at home or in the neighborhood health clinic and decides whether he should be seen by the doctor more often than at his usual once-a-month appointment.

The Problem: Describe how you would plan and carry out Mr. Chesterson's nursing care, for which you are responsible.

DRUG DIGEST

PHENOXYBENZAMINE HCl (Dibenzyline)

Actions and Indications. This alpha adrenergic blocking agent produces dilation of blood vessels in the skin. The better flow of blood to the skin of patients with certain peripheral vascular disorders may provide some symptomatic relief. Among vasospastic conditions benefited are frostbite, Raynaud's syndrome, acrocyanosis, and causalgia. It is *not* useful for treating thromboangiitis obliterans (Buerger's disease) or other disorders in which vessel walls are damaged.

Although this drug is also not

very useful for reducing blood pressure in essential hypertension, it can help prevent pressure rises in patients with pheochromocytoma when administered before and during surgery. The drug is being used experimentally to improve circulation in shock cases resistant to other treatment measures.

Side Effects, Cautions, and Contraindications. Minor side effects of blockade of sympathetic nerve impulses include nasal congestion, bronchoconstriction, and miosis. More serious effects of overdos-

age are postural hypotension and reflex tachycardia, as these effects can lead to a heart attack, congestive heart failure, stroke, or kidney failure in patients with coronary or cerebral atherosclerosis or renal damage.

Dosage and Administration. Treatment is started at a dose level of 10 mg daily. This is increased gradually to levels high enough to offer symptomatic relief without causing discomforting or dangerous side effects. The usual individually adjusted optimum daily dosage is between 20 and 60 mg.

References

Bartels, C.C. Occlusive arterial emergencies. *Med. Clin. N. Amer.*, 53:335, 1969 (March).

Beck, L., and Brody, M.J. The physiology of

vasodilation. *Angiology*, 12:202, 1961.

Friend, D. Drugs for peripheral vascular disease. *Clin. Pharmacol. Ther.*, 5:666, 1964.

Hecht, A.B. Self medication inaccuracy and

what can be done. *Nurs. Outlook*, 18:30, 1970 (April).

Le Fevre, F. Management of occlusive arterial diseases of the extremities. *JAMA*, 147:1401, 1951.

Lippman, H.L. Intra-arterial Priscoline (tolazoline) therapy for peripheral vascular disturbances. *Angiology*, 3:69, 1952.

Moser, M., et al. Clinical experience with sympathetic blocking agents in peripheral vascular disease. *Ann. Intern. Med.*, 38:1245, 1953.

Rodman, M.J. Vasodilator drugs in peripheral vascular disease. *RN*, 26:39, 1963 (March).

———. Drug management in peripheral vascular disease. *RN*, 29:61, 1966 (Aug.).

Spittell, J.A., Jr., Ed. Symposium on treatment of venous disorders. *Mod. Treatm.*, 2:1061, 1965 (Nov.).

Wright, I.S. Treatment of occlusive arterial disease. *JAMA*, 183:186, 1963.

Wilson, S. Chronic leg ulcers. Nursing management. *Amer. J. Nurs.*, 67:96, 1967 (Jan.).

33.

Drugs that Affect Blood Coagulation

Blood Coagulation

Blood has the ability to flow freely within healthy veins and arteries. Yet this fluid can swiftly form a solid plug at the point of any break, cut, or tear in a vessel. Such changes from a liquid to a solid state soon stop further loss of blood from the damaged vein or artery. This property of the blood—staying fluid most of the time but being able to clot and thus stop bleeding following an injury—is the result of a complex ever-ready coagulation mechanism that exists in the circulating blood.

Blood clotting factors (Table 33-1) and anticlotting factors take part in a never-ending series of reactions that ordinarily stay in a delicate balance. Any change that shifts this equilibrium excessively creates an imbalance that can: (1) cause uncontrolled bleeding, or, at the other extreme, (2) lead to the formation of clots within the vessels that can then cut off the blood supply to the tissues.

In this chapter, we shall discuss two main kinds of drugs that affect blood coagulation: first, the *anticoagulant* and *thrombolytic* agents that are used in treating blood clotting, or *thromboembolic*, disorders; and then various substances called *hemostatic agents* that are employed in the management of ailments marked by excessive bleeding, the so-called *hemorrhagic* disorders.

BLOOD CLOTTING REACTIONS

The reactions that keep blood in the vessels always liquid yet always ready to clot and close a wound are extremely complex. In fact, although some of the steps are now quite clear,

TABLE 33-1 *Blood Clotting Factors*

Factor Number	Synonym and Comments
I	Fibrinogen—a soluble plasma protein synthesized in the liver that serves as the precursor of *fibrin*, the solid strands or filaments that form the framework of the clot.
II	Prothrombin—a plasma protein produced in the liver in reactions involving vitamin K. It serves as the precursor of *thrombin*, the proteolytic enzyme that acts upon *fibrinogen (factor I)* to form *fibrin*.
III	Thromboplastin—a lipoprotein released by injured body tissues. It triggers reactions in the *extrinsic system* that convert *prothrombin (factor II)* to *thrombin* (Fig. 33-1).
IV	Calcium—ions required for various reactions that result in the activation of *prothrombin (factor II)* to generate *thrombin* and finally in the formation of *fibrin*.
V	Proaccelerin—a plasma protein (globulin) that speeds the rate at which *prothrombin (factor II)* is converted to *thrombin*.
VII*	Proconvertin—a plasma protein produced in the liver in reactions that require vitamin K. It speeds the extrinsic system reactions involving *thromboplastin (factor III)* and *factor X* that result in the conversion of prothrombin *(factor II)* to thrombin.
VIII	Antihemophilic Globulin (AHG), or Factor, (AHF)—a plasma protein that functions together with *factor IX* and a phospholipid released by blood platelets *(platelet factor 3)* in the intrinsic pathway reactions that activate prothrombin *factor II)*. It is absent in cases of classic hemophilia (hemophilia A).
IX	Christmas Factor; Plasma Thromboplastin Component (PTC)—one of the vitamin K-dependent factors that work together with *factor VIII* and platelet *factor 3* in the presence of calcium ions in the *intrinsic pathway* reactions that speed the reaction of *prothrombin (factor II)* to *thrombin*.
X	Stuart-Prower Factor—plasma factor produced in the liver in the presence of vitamin K. It takes part in *both* intrinsic and extrinsic pathway reactions to produce a prothrombin-converting principle.
XI	Plasma Thrombolastin Antecedent (PTA)—a plasma globulin that is activated by *factor XII* and then helps to speed the production of *thrombin*.
XII	Hageman Factor—a plasma factor that helps to trigger intrinsic system reactions. It activates *factor XI* and may take part in inflammatory as well as clotting reactions.
XIII	Fibrin Stabilizing Factor—a plasma component, which, when activated by *thrombin*, makes *fibrin* fibers stronger and able to form the gel that seals breaks in blood vessels.

* Factor VI may be an unstable form of factor V, a labile accelerator globulin found in blood serum.

others are still not very well understood. However, for our purpose—understanding how the various drugs do their work—the several steps in the sequence of clotting reactions can be stated rather simply (see also Fig. 33-1 for a more detailed, but still oversimplified, schematic outline of the steps in blood clotting):

STAGE I: THROMBOPLASTIN FORMATION. Injury to the inner lining of the blood vessels activates a precursor of thromboplastin. (Thrombocytes, or blood platelets, play an important part here as do various factors in the plasma and tissues.)

STAGE II: THROMBIN FORMATION. The thromboplastin formed in the first step reacts with the plasma protein *prothrombin*, converting it to an active enzyme called *thrombin*. (Prothrombin and other related circulating clotting factors come from the liver, where their molecules are constantly being biosynthesized.)

STAGE III: FIBRIN FORMATION. The thrombin formed in Stage Two then catalyzes a chemical reaction that converts the soluble plasma protein *fibrinogen* to an insoluble substance called *fibrin*, which precipitates out as fine filaments or threads. These threads then form a mesh that trap blood cells to form a gelatinous clot or *thrombus*. (Enzymes capable of digesting the fibrin framework of the clot can shift the balance of biochemical reactions back toward breakup of the clot a bit later.)

The anticoagulant, thrombolytic, and hemostatic drugs discussed in the rest of this chapter all act in one way or another to affect the various complex chemical reactions involved in each of the above blood clotting stages and in the process of clot destruction.

Anticoagulant Drug Therapy

Blood clots that block the further flow of blood in major vessels are a common cause of disability and death. More than a million Americans die each year of complications caused by thromboembolic disorders. Some blood clots begin in veins that are injured or inflamed. Such thrombi can break off and be carried to the lungs, for example, as potentially fatal pulmonary emboli. Traveling clots of this kind can also reach the brain, where they cause strokes by occluding cerebral blood vessels. Occlusions of major arteries also occur when blood platelets stick together in the area over a break in the inner lining of an atherosclerotic vessel. The closing off of a coronary artery in

this way, for example, is the usual cause of an acute myocardial infarction.

Drugs are now available for preventing clots from forming or—if they have already formed —from completely closing off a portion of the vascular channel and then growing even greater by extending up and down the vessel in both directions. Two main types of anticoagulant drugs are used for this purpose: (1) *heparin*, a drug that acts *directly* upon several kinds of circulating clotting factors to exert immediate effects in preventing the extension of thrombi that are already formed; and (2) *coumarin* and *indanedione* derivatives, chemicals that act in the liver in a way that *indirectly* reduces the amount of clotting factors that circulate in the blood. These drugs usually take a day or longer to begin exerting their anticoagulant effects.

We shall now consider the similarities and differences of these kinds of anticoagulants and then discuss their current status in the management of various kinds of thromboembolic disorders.

HEPARIN

Heparin+ is the preferred anticoagulant for treating acute thromboembolic emergencies. Injected directly into a vein, it acts quickly to block the chain of blood clotting reactions at several points. By keeping thrombin from forming, heparin permits fibrinogen to stay in the liquid state instead of precipitating out as fibrin.

Prompt treatment with heparin is particularly useful for patients with blood clots in deep veins. Venous thrombosis is usually marked by tenderness or pain, swelling, and other signs of inflammation (*thrombophlebitis*). However, even when such signs are not seen (as in *phlebothrombosis*), the main danger comes from clots that become dislodged from the femoral, iliac, and other veins. Such clots, or fragments from them, may be carried to the right side of the heart and then into the arteries of the lung where they cause *pulmonary embolism*.

To *prevent* pulmonary embolism in patients with phlebitis and in others whose history indicates a high risk, heparin is injected immediately and continued for from several days to more than a week. Patients may be started at the same time on one of the oral anticoagulants (see p. 399) that begin to act more slowly but

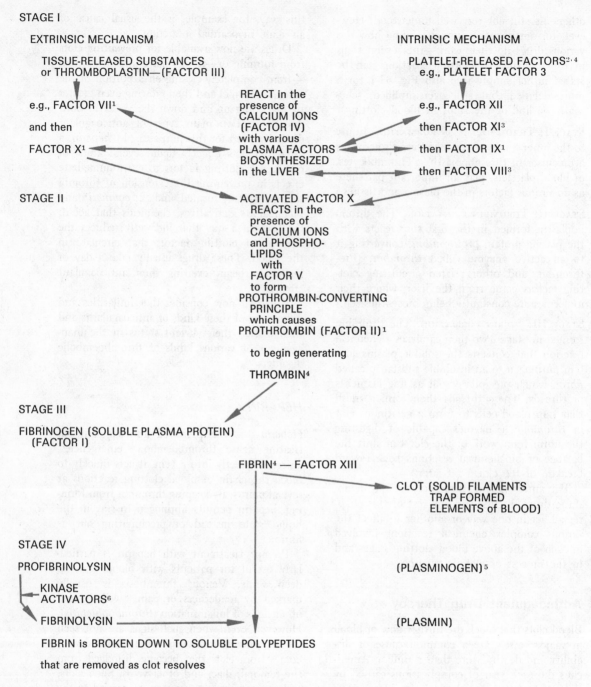

STAGE I

EXTRINSIC MECHANISM

 TISSUE-RELEASED SUBSTANCES
 or THROMBOPLASTIN—(FACTOR III)

e.g., FACTOR VII[1]

and then

FACTOR X[1]

REACT in the
presence of
CALCIUM IONS
(FACTOR IV)
with various
PLASMA FACTORS
BIOSYNTHESIZED
in the LIVER

INTRINSIC MECHANISM

 PLATELET-RELEASED FACTORS[2,4]
 e.g., PLATELET FACTOR 3

e.g., FACTOR XII

then FACTOR XI[3]

then FACTOR IX[1]

then FACTOR VIII[3]

STAGE II

ACTIVATED FACTOR X
REACTS in the
presence of
CALCIUM IONS
and PHOSPHO-
LIPIDS
with
FACTOR V
to form
PROTHROMBIN-CONVERTING
PRINCIPLE
which causes
PROTHROMBIN (FACTOR II)[1]

to begin generating

THROMBIN[4]

STAGE III

FIBRINOGEN (SOLUBLE PLASMA PROTEIN)
 (FACTOR I)

FIBRIN[4] — FACTOR XIII

CLOT (SOLID FILAMENTS
TRAP FORMED
ELEMENTS of BLOOD)

STAGE IV

PROFIBRINOLYSIN

 KINASE
 ACTIVATORS[6]

FIBRINOLYSIN

(PLASMINOGEN)[5]

(PLASMIN)

FIBRIN is BROKEN DOWN TO SOLUBLE POLYPEPTIDES

that are removed as clot resolves

Fig. 33-1. Blood clotting pathways

[1] Dependent upon presence of Vitamin K for synthesis in the liver and thus is decreased by coumarin and indanedione drugs.

[2] Platelet deficiency (thrombocytopenia) can cause purpura; drugs such as aspirin can cause bleeding by their effects on platelets.

[3] Lack of factor VIII causes classic hemophilia A; lack of factor IX causes hemophilia B (Christmas disease).

[4] Among the several sites of action of heparin.

[5] Site of action of thrombolytic (fibrinolytic) agents that activate plasminogens (for example urokinase; streptokinase).

[6] Site of action of antifibrinolytic agents that compete with natural activators (kinases) of plasminogen (such as aminocaproic acid).

are more convenient for long-continued treatment. Even after heparin is discontinued, prophylactic anticoagulation with the oral drugs may be ordered during the remainder of the patient's stay in the hospital. Nursing measures may also help to prevent thrombophlebitis, pulmonary embolism, and the other life-threatening thromboembolic complications mentioned earlier, and patients often need to be encouraged to exercise their legs during periods of enforced inactivity in order to avoid venous stasis.

Treatment of pulmonary embolism requires the use of high doses of heparin—60,000 units a day or more—to keep the clot from enlarging, while the body's own sludge-dissolving mechanisms become activated and gain control. (Heparin and other anticoagulants do *not* break up clots that are fully formed, but the drugs do favor solution of the early soft stages and thus keep the clot from enlarging and forming emboli.) The doctor controls heparin dosage by checking the patient's clotting time at the start of treatment and at frequent intervals during the drug's administration. He tries to maintain a clotting time between two and three times the normal control time of five or ten minutes—usually between 20 and 30 minutes.

Overdosage can ordinarily be avoided by simply delaying administration of the next dose, or omitting it entirely, whenever the patient's clotting time becomes excessively prolonged. If signs of bleeding are seen, the excess heparin in the patient's circulation can be neutralized by making a slow intravenous injection of *protamine sulfate*, a specific chemical antagonist of heparin. Rarely, bleeding may be dangerous enough to require transfusion of whole blood for rapid replacement of the clotting factors that have been inhibited by heparin.

The main drawback of heparin is that it must be injected rather frequently. The effect of heparin may be prolonged by injecting it in the form of a gelatin-dextrose depot suspension that is only absorbed slowly from subcutaneous fatty tissues or intramuscular sites. However, this may cause local irritation or hematomas, and one or two daily injections are still required. Thus, heparin is employed only in hospitalized patients and for periods of no more than two or three weeks. Patients who seem to need long-term maintenance therapy to prevent recurrences of thromboembolic episodes are switched to one of the more convenient oral anticoagulants.

COUMARIN AND INDANEDIONE DERIVATIVES (TABLE 33-2)

Drugs of two different chemical types are active anticoagulants when taken by mouth. Those of the coumarin class, including *warfarin+*, *bishydroxycoumarin+*, and *acenocoumarol*, are the ones most widely used in this country. The indanedione drugs act in essentially the same way but seem more likely to cause hypersensitivity-type toxic reactions.

The oral anticoagulants take some time to reduce the blood's ability to clot. Unlike heparin, these agents do not act upon already formed clotting factors in the circulating blood. Instead, they interfere with the biochemical reactions that result in the liver's synthesis of such clotting factors as prothrombin, and factors VII, IX, and X. They do this by keeping vitamin K from carrying out its metabolic function.

Because the circulating clotting factors stay active during the time these drugs are beginning to inhibit hepatic biosynthesis, the clinical effects of these anticoagulants come on slowly as compared to those of heparin. It may take from one to four days or more for full therapeutic activity to be attained. However, once the effects of these drugs begin to be felt, they may last for several days after the drugs are discontinued. These properties account for physicians' preferences for heparin in acute thromboembolic conditions and the coumarin-type agents in chronic cases. (In emergencies, drugs of both types are given together; then the heparin is withdrawn, and treatment is continued with the coumarin drugs to maintain more stable, long-lasting therapeutic effects.)

PROTHROMBIN TIME TESTING. Treatment with drugs of this type is intended to reduce the activity of the patient's circulating clotting factors to between 20 and 30 percent of normal. Patients with too much clotting activity are, of course, not being fully protected against clots and emboli; and doses of these drugs that cause a drop in clotting activity down to below 15 percent can set off episodes of spontaneous bleeding. To avoid both these dangers, the doctor makes frequent checks of the patient's prothrombin time, a test that tells him how much the drugs have affected the activity of the clotting factors.

The nurse administers each day's dosage of anticoagulant only after the doctor has seen the results of the patient's prothrombin time tests. She should not go on giving these drugs routinely when such tests are not being regularly carried out and evaluated—at least during the period when the hospitalized patient is being stabilized on an anticoagulant drug. Patients who are being maintained on long-term therapy need to be tested only once or twice a month or so. In such cases, nurses who are in contact with these patients emphasize that they must make and keep appointments for their periodic prothrombin time blood tests.

VARIATION IN RESPONSE

Patients differ very widely in the amount of anticoagulant drugs they need to keep their clotting factor levels within the safe therapeutic range. Elderly people, those in a poor state of nutrition, and patients with liver disease tend to be most susceptible to the effects of these drugs. Thus, the doctor starts treatment with a smaller dose than he would order in most cases. On the other hand, some patients may metabolize these drugs very rapidly and require high doses to reach a therapeutic anticoagulation level and to maintain it during prolonged prophylactic treatment. Diarrhea may also reduce the amount of orally administered drug that is absorbed.

TABLE 33-2 *Anticoagulant Drugs of the Hypoprothrombinemic Type**

Nonproprietary or Official Name	Trade Name or Synonym	Total Daily Initial and Maintenance Doses†	Remarks‡
Coumarin Derivatives			
Acenocoumarol	Sintrom	Initial loading dose: 16–28 mg first day; 8–16 mg second day. Maintenance dose range: 2–10 mg daily	Onset and duration: intermediate (36–48 hours). Occasional hypersensitivity reactions
Bishydroxycoumarin U.S.P.	Dicumarol	Initial loading dose: 200–300 mg first day 100–200 mg second and third days. Maintenance dose range: 50–100 mg daily	Onset: intermediate (24–72 hours). Duration: long (4–6 days). See *Drug Digest*
Ethyl biscoumacetate N.F.	Tromexan	Initial loading dose: 900–1200 mg. Maintenance dose range: 150–900 mg	Onset: rapid (18–30 hours). Duration: intermediate (48 hours). Occasional G.I. upset; hypersensitivity reactions; alopecia
Phenprocoumon N.F.	Liquamar	Initial loading dose: 21 mg first day, 3–9 mg second and third days. Maintenance dose range: 1–4 mg daily	Onset: slow (48–72 hours). Duration: long (seven days or more). Few side effects
Warfarin sodium U.S.P.	Coumadin; Panwarfin	Initial loading dose: 40–60 mg average adult; 20–30 mg elderly patients. Maintenance dose range: 5–10 mg daily	Onset: intermediate (24–36 hours). Duration: intermediate (2–4 days). See *Drug Digest*
Warfarin potassium N.F.	Athrombin-K	Same as for sodium salt	Same as for sodium salt

T A B L E 3 3 - 2 *Anticoagulant Drugs of the Hypoprothrombinemic Type* (continued)*

Nonproprietary or Official Name	Trade Name or Synonym	Total Daily Initial and Maintenance Doses†	Remarks‡
Indanedione Derivatives§			
Anisindione N.F.	Miradon	Initial loading dose: 300–500 mg first day, 200–300 mg second day 100 mg third day. Maintenance dose range: 25–250 mg daily	Onset: intermediate to long (48–72 hours). Duration: intermediate (24–72 hours). Dermatitis only side effect reported, but others of this chemical class are possible
Diphenadione N.F.	Dipaxin	Initial loading dose: 20–30 mg first day, 10–15 mg second day. Maintenance dose range: 7–15 mg daily	Onset: intermediate to long (48–72 hours). Duration: very long (up to three weeks). No adverse effects beside bleeding, but others of this chemical class are possible
Phenindione	Danilone; Eridione; Hedulin	Initial loading dose: 200–300 mg first day, 100–200 mg second day. Maintenance dose range: 50–100 mg daily	Onset: rapid (18–24 hours). Duration: short (24–48 hours). Hypersensitivity reactions include leukopenia and agranulocytosis;‖ hepatitis and jaundice; nephropathy with albuminuria and edema; dermatitis, and others.

* Drugs listed are of the hypoprothrombinemia-producing type that act in liver as competitive antagonists of vitamin K. *Heparin* (see *Drug Digest*) is an anticoagulant of a different type.

† All doses are by *oral* administration; warfarin sodium is also available in form for parenteral administration. Maintenance dosage is determined by periodic prothrombin time determinations.

‡ Onset refers to time needed to reduce prothrombin activity to the therapeutic range (20-30 percent of normal). Duration refers to time required for prothrombin time to return to normal after the drug is discontinued.

§ Patients should be told that drugs of this class may sometimes turn their urine orange, so that they will not be worried. This occurs when the urine is alkaline. Thus, a simple test to differentiate chromaturia from hematuria is to acidify the urine; the color then disappears.

‖ Patients are told to report sore throat, fever, fatigue, jaundice, or other symptoms of illness since those may signal the development of those hypersensitivity-type reactions.

DRUG INTERACTIONS (TABLE 33-3)

Another important factor in increasing or decreasing the patient's responsiveness to anticoagulant drug therapy is the simultaneous administration of other drugs. For example, a patient with thrombophlebitis who is receiving the antiinflammatory agent, phenylbutazone, may begin to bleed from ordinary doses of an anticoagulant such as *warfarin*+ (Coumadin, Panwarfin) administered simultaneously. Similarly, patients taking the lipid-lowering drugs clofibrate or dextrothyroxine during convalescence from a coronary attack require a reduction in dosage of anticoagulant drugs to avoid suffering episodes of spontaneous bleeding.

On the other hand, patients taking phenobarbital and certain other sedative-hypnotic agents may need more than ordinary amounts of anticoagulant drugs to produce therapeutically desirable effects. This occurs because these drugs stimulate the enzyme systems that destroy *bishydroxycoumarin*+ (Dicumarol), and the other coumarin-type anticoagulants. Even more serious is the problem of what may happen when such metabolism-stimulating drugs are withdrawn, and the patient continues to receive the extra-high doses of anticoagulant drugs on which he was stabilized. As the level of drug-destroying enzymes drops, the level of anticoagulant drug in the liver rises. The resulting reduction in clotting factor synthesis

T A B L E   3 3 - 3   *Some Drugs that Affect the Response to Anticoagulants (AC)*

Drugs that Increase the Response (Potentiation)

Drug	Remarks
Chloral hydrate	A metabolite of this drug, trichloroacetic acid, may intensify AC activity.
Cholestyramine (Questran; Cuemid)	May interfere with absorption of vitamin K and thus potentiate AC drug activity.
Clofibrate (Atromid-S)	Dosage of AC is reduced by about one third to one half until patient is restabilized.
Dextrothyroxine (Choloxin)	Reduce AC drug dosage by about one third to one half until prothrombin times stays in the therapeutic range.
Phenylbutazone (Butazolidin)	Potentiation of AC drug can cause upper G.I. tract bleeding.
Quinidine sulfate	May prolong prothrombin time of patients taking AC drugs.
Salicylates	Large doses that affect prothrombin complex factor synthesis and release of platelet lipids may potentiate AC drug effects and cause bleeding. (Acetaminophen may be a safer analgesic in some patients.)
Steroids, anabolic type	Reportedly prolong the prothrombin time in some patients.
Sulfonamides, and broad spectrum antibiotics with bowel-sterilizing effects	May inhibit growth of the colonic bacteria that produce vitamin K. Patient's failure to absorb this vitamin may potentiate the effect of AC drugs.

Drugs that Reduce the Response (Antagonism)

Drug	Remarks
Antacids (for example, sodium bicarbonate)	Reduced absorption of oral AC drugs results in lessened effectiveness.
Barbiturates (such as amobarbital, secobarbital, phenobarbital) and *Non*barbiturate sedative-hypnotics* such as ethchlorvynol (Placidyl) and glutethimide (Doriden)	These drugs may induce increased synthesis of liver enzymes that metabolize AC drugs. This requires raising the dose of the AC drugs to attain therapeutic effects. If sedatives are discontinued, dosage of AC drugs may have to be adjusted downward.
Estrogens (in oral contraceptives, and others)	May increase amounts of plasma clotting factors, thus requiring an increase in AC drug dosage.
Griseofulvin (Fulvicin; and others)	May cause a reduction in prothrombin time, thus requiring a rise in daily AC drug dosage.
Meprobamate (Equanil; Miltown)	Enzyme-induction may decrease AC drug activity. Antianxiety agents such as chlordiazepoxide (Librium), diazepam (Valium), and oxazepam (Serax) are claimed not to affect prothrombin time and may thus be preferred for patients on AC drugs.
Steroids, corticoid type	Reported to decrease effects of AC drugs, possibly by increasing plasma clotting factor concentrations.
Thiazide, and other diuretics	Reported to antagonize AC drugs, possibly by improving liver function.

---

* Chloral hydrate, a drug of this type, has been reported to act in the same way to reduce the level of certain AC drugs in blood and liver. However, see above concerning possible potentiation by its metabolite, trichloroacetic acid.

can lead to sudden episodes of bleeding in the brain and elsewhere that could prove fatal.

The possibility of dangerous drug interactions does not mean that patients receiving anticoagulant therapy can take no other drugs. It does mean that, whenever the doctor adds a new drug to the patient's treatment regimen, or discontinues one, he must make more frequent prothrombin time tests. Then, if he detects changes in the patient's response to the anticoagulant, the doctor adjusts his dosage upwards or reduces it in order to keep the patient's clotting factors within the safe therapeutic range.

The nurse should also advise patients not to treat themselves with *non*prescription medications but, instead, to consult their physician. Aspirin, for example, can intensify the action of anticoagulant medication. Multiple vitamin products that contain vitamin K may reduce the effectiveness of anticoagulant drug treatment. Patients should also be told not to make any drastic changes in their diet nor to drink alcoholic beverages to excess, as unexpected changes in response to anticoagulant therapy may then develop.

OTHER PRECAUTIONS

Hospitalized patients must be checked for signs of hemorrhage during the time when dosage of these drugs is being adjusted. The nurse looks for signs of even minor bleeding and instructs auxiliary personnel to do so also. Thus, for example, the contents of bedpans, urinals, and emesis basins are checked for signs of blood. Hematuria, tarry stools, and other such signs are promptly reported to the patient's physician. Of course, nothing is said or done to worry the patient while he is being watched in this way.

Similarly, in instructing patients who are taking anticoagulants prophylactically, care is taken not to alarm them. This takes tact and good judgment, as the patient and his family should know what signs to look for without being frightened into thinking that the appearance of a drop of blood on a toothbrush or towel means that the patient is about to bleed to death.

They should be told to report nosebleeds, discolored urine, skin discoloration or "bruises," "black" stools, or excessive menstrual bleeding. In order to avoid giving the patient conflicting information or suggestions, his nurse and doctor should confer informally quite often to exchange information that each has gained in observing the patient. Collaborative planning of this kind about what to teach the patient will help him to care for himself more effectively while taking anticoagulant drugs at home. (See *Summary of Instructions for Patients Taking Anticoagulant Drugs,* p. 409.) The use of printed instruction sheets, along with verbal explanation, is helpful.

Many patients today are well-informed about the dangers of both postoperative embolism and the fact that anticoagulant drugs can cause bleeding. In such cases, it is often desirable to discuss these hazards frankly and to explain the reasons for various procedures and suggested precautions. The patient's natural alarm and apprehension can be reduced by reassuring him about his safety. Often, however, the best kind of reassurance comes from letting the patient know that he is receiving intelligent attention from a nurse who cares enough to check carefully for signs of possible danger.

Patients are also advised to carry with them at all times a suppy of vitamin K_1 tablets that they should take in accordance with the doctor's instructions, if excessive bleeding occurs. Vitamin K_1, or *phytonadione*, is the specific antidote for overdosage of oral anticoagulants. The hospital nurse should see to it that an injectable form of it (and of the heparin antidote, *protamine sulfate*) is always on hand in the ward medicine cabinet whenever any patient on her floor is receiving anticoagulant therapy.

INDICATIONS AND CONTRAINDICATIONS

The thromboembolic disorders and other clinical conditions in which anticoagulants are employed are listed in the *Summary* (p. 408). The concurrent disorders that may make the use of these drugs contraindicated are summarized on p. 409. Whether or not to employ these drugs is a difficult decision that the patient's doctor must make after weighing the possible risks and benefits in each case individually. The nurse's chief concern is that these patients be kept under close observation to detect any early signs that might help the doctor prevent complications of both the bleeding and clotting types.

STATUS OF THERAPY. The use of anticoagulants is generally recognized as indicated in some clinical conditions and absolutely contraindicated in others. The desirability of their employment in other disorders is still quite controversial.

Anticoagulants are considered most effective when used to treat patients with thrombophlebitis or pulmonary embolism. Their usefulness in patients whose cerebral blood vessels are being blocked off by clots varies depending upon how far advanced the patient's condition has become (see *Summary*, p. 408). Anticoagulant therapy for patients with coronary artery disease remains controversial. These drugs may help to prevent thromboembolic complications in some cases of acute myocardial infarction, and their long-term use for several years after a coronary occlusion may prevent recurrences in some categories of cardiac patients.

Patients with rheumatic disease of the heart valves, enlarged left atrium, and chronic atrial fibrillation may be less prone to produce emboli that pass to the brain and cause strokes when they are protected by the prophylactic use of anticoagulants. Similarly, patients with artificial valves following heart surgery have fewer embolic episodes during long-term treatment with oral anticoagulants.* Herapin helps to keep blood from clotting while it is being pumped outside the body during open-heart surgery and hemodialysis procedures.

Anticoagulant therapy is clearly contraindicated in patients who have a tendency toward bleeding. This is obvious in patients with blood dyscrasias of the kind that cause bleeding. Patients with a stroke caused by bleeding from a broken cerebral vessel should also, of course, not receive these drugs. In fact, any patient who has recently suffered intracranial bleeding as a result of a head injury or a neurosurgical operation must not be treated with anticoagulants. Cases of acute peptic ulcer or active colitis can be set into uncontrollable bleeding by these drugs.

Other patients who are not prone to bleeding and who could profit from long-term anticoagulant drug treatment may, nevertheless, not be able to take these drugs. For example, chronic alcoholics cannot be trusted to follow

---

* Some patients of this type are today also receiving treatment with aspirin or with dipyridamole (Persantin), as these drugs may act to help prevent formation of arterial blood clots.

instructions. Similarly, senile or mentally unstable patients are not good candidates for treatment with these drugs, unless, of course, they are under the care of a nurse (or a dependable member of the family) who can see to it that they take their medication and come in for the required blood tests.

Thrombolytic Agents

As we have noted, the anticoagulant drugs do *not* dissolve blood clots. However, by keeping fresh clots from enlarging, these drugs allow the body's own mechanisms for breaking up the fibrin framework of the clot to operate. This process, called *fibrinolysis*, is brought about by an enzyme called *plasmin*, or *fibrinolysin*. This enzyme is formed within the clot by the action of certain activators upon a precursor substance, called *profibrinolysin* or plas*minogen*.

FIBRINOLYTIC AGENTS

Recently, two partially purified plasminogen activators have been employed experimentally in attempts to speed the rate at which freshly formed clots can be broken up in the treatment of certain serious thromboembolic disorders. One of these substances, called *streptokinase*, an enzyme obtained from certain bacteria, is sometimes effective for this purpose when injected directly into the patient's circulation. However, it has various drawbacks, including a frequent tendency to cause allergic reactions and fever.

Urokinase, a substance found in traces in human urine, has recently been purified and made available in large amounts for clinical trials. It is claimed to be nontoxic, except for increasing the incidence of bleeding. Administered by vein together with heparin to patients with pulmonary embolism, urokinase has helped to accelerate lung clot breakdown. It has not, however, succeeded in bringing about complete clot dissolution.

Clinical trials with urokinase are continuing at present to determine how this plasminogen activator can be used with the greatest safety and effectiveness in patients with the various kinds of thromboembolic complications that are by far the most common cause of disability and death among Americans. A truly effective, nontoxic thrombolytic agent would prove lifesaving, not only for treating pulmonary embolism (which still causes about 30,000 deaths annually), but also for patients who have suffered a coronary or cerebral thrombosis. An effective drug of this kind could also help to save the limbs of patients with peripheral vascular diseases and others who suffer a sudden complete occlusion of a major artery in a limb.

Drugs to Control Bleeding (Hemostatic Agents)

Bleeding in a person with normally functioning clot-forming mechanisms stops soon after a blood vessel has been broken or cut. Trauma to the vessel and surrounding tissues sets into motion a swift sequence of events:

(1) *Platelets* flowing along the vessel wall tend to stick together to form a platelet plug at the site of injury.

(2) A *substance released by the platelets*, acting together with tissue thromboplastin, starts off the series of steps (p. 398) that results in fibrin formation.

(3) The *fibrin clot* becomes anchored to the platelet plug and contracts to form a firm ball that stops the further flow of blood from the torn blood vessel (*hemostasis*).

Drugs are normally not needed to accelerate this hemostatic mechanism. Mechanical measures, such as sutures, ligatures, and gentle pressure are ordinarily enough to help hasten the clotting sequence and halt hemorrhage. However, certain substances are sometimes applied locally when blood continues to ooze steadily from broken capillaries. Patients who are lacking in one or more of the natural clotting components are also sometimes treated, either by replacing the missing factor or by the systemic administration of drugs that help the body bring its hemostatic mechanism back to normal.

In this section, we shall discuss briefly: (1) *locally active hemostatic agents*; and (2) *systemically active substances* that are being used in the current management of some of the more common bleeding disorders caused by defects in the hemostatic mechanism.

LOCALLY ACTIVE HEMOSTATIC AGENTS (TABLE 33-4)

Bleeding from soft tissues is sometimes hard to stop. Blood may continue to ooze from capillaries in the brain, liver, or kidney and elsewhere that are too tiny to be tied off by ligatures. In such cases, certain natural clotting factors such as *thromboplastin, thrombin,* or *fibrin* may be applied topically to form a clot, or other substances that form a mechanical barrier may be employed.

Thrombin, applied topically as a powder or in solution, reacts with fibrinogen in the blood to form a fibrin clot very quickly in most cases. It is used in nose, throat, and dental surgery, and in skin grafting or plastic surgery. Thrombin may also be taken internally to control bleeding from peptic ulcers. In such cases, the patient may swallow a small quantity of milk containing the hemostatic agent, or it may be administered by means of a Levine tube, dissolved in a phosphate buffer solution to neutralize excess stomach acid. Thrombin must not, of course, ever be injected as it could cause widespread clotting within the vessels.

Oxidized cellulose (Hemo-Pak; Oxycel) is a form of specially treated surgical cotton that reacts with blood to form an artificial clot. It can be packed into the abdominal cavity to control capillary bleeding following surgery on the liver, gall bladder, spleen, pancreas, or bowel. In such cases, it is absorbed in a few days. On the other hand, it must not be implanted in fractures, as it interferes with bone regeneration and can cause cysts to form.

Absorbable gelatin may be employed as sponges that are left in place when a surgical wound is closed. A film made of this material may be left in the brain following removal of a tumor or used to fill in defects of the dural membrane caused by a depressed skull fracture. A powder form has sometimes been used together with thrombin for control of massive bleeding within the G.I. tract. A sterile form of the powder has also been employed in treating skin ulcers that are slow to heal.

These and similar substances seem to be free of adverse effects when applied topically to control capillary bleeding in the various surgical situations and medical conditions for which they are recommended.

SYSTEMICALLY ACTIVE HEMOSTATIC SUBSTANCES

Some people suffer repeated episodes of bleeding. Minor nose bleeds or bruise marks in the skin are most commonly caused by weakness of the capillary walls. Sometimes, however, serious bleeding may be caused by a lack of one of the blood factors required for normal clotting. Hemorrhagic disorders that develop during childhood are usually congenital—*hemophilia*, for example; other clotting factor deficiencies may occur in adults secondary to various medical disorders or as a result of drug reactions—for example, drug-induced *thrombocytopenia*.

Transfusions of fresh whole blood or plasma help to replace the elements missing from the blood of patients with congenital or acquired bleeding disorders. Recent advances in separating specific clotting factors from blood have made it possible to administer only the substance that the patient lacks. Certain drugs can also be given that help to build up clotting proteins or to prevent their destruction.

In this section, we shall discuss the treatment of a few important hemorrhagic disorders with specific blood components and drugs. We shall not, of course, take up the total management of patients suffering from these clinical conditions. Instead, we shall indicate the kinds of illnesses caused by a lack of platelets,

prothrombin, fibrinogen, and other clotting factors and discuss the substances that are employed to counteract these deficiencies.

Platelet deficiency as a result of an abnormally rapid rate of thrombocyte destruction or reduced production leads to bleeding episodes. The best treatment for thrombocytopenic bleeding is the *transfusion of concentrated platelets* separated from whole blood. *Corticosteroid* drugs such as prednisone are sometimes employed as an aid to platelet therapy in counteracting acute bleeding of this kind. *Immunosuppressive agents* such as *azathioprine* have occasionally proved effective in chronic cases of thrombocytic purpura.* However, drug therapy is generally ineffective for stopping

* *Purpura* is a general term for hemorrhage into the skin. The term, *petechiae*, refers to pinpoint- to pinhead-sized bleeding spots in the skin. Another term—*ecchymoses*—refers to the black-and-blue or purplish bruises seen when petechiae run together to form larger skin spots.

TABLE 33-4 *Hemostatic Agents*

Nonproprietary or Official Name	Synonym or Trade Name	Dosage	Remarks
Systemically Active Agents			
BLOOD PLASMA CLOTTING FACTORS			
Antihemophilic globulin, human	AHG; AHF; factor VIII	250 ml I.V.	Less volume required than with whole blood or plasma
Antihemophilic factor, human	Hemofil; Method Four; AHG; AHF factor VIII concentrate	10–30 ml I.V.	Highly concentrated; low volume for hemophilia A
Factor IX complex, human	Konyne; (factors II, VII, IX, and X)	20 ml I.V. (500 units)	Concentrated; for treating hemophilia B
Fibrinogen, human U.S.P.	Parenogen	1–2 g I.V.	Plasma fraction for use in hypofibrogenemia
PROTHROMBOGENIC SUBSTANCES			
Menadiol sodium phosphate U.S.P.	Kappadione; Synkayvite	3–6 mg daily orally or parenterally	Water-soluble form of vitamin K; does *not* need bile salts for absorption
Menadione N.F.	Kappaxin; Kayquinone	2–10 mg daily, orally	Insoluble Vitamin K requires bile salts for absorption
Menadione sodium bisulfite N.F.	Hykinone	0.5–10 mg parenterally	Water soluble injectable form of vitamin K.
Phytonadione U.S.P.	Aqua Mephyton; Konakion	1–25 mg orally; 10–50 mg I.V.; and other parenteral routes	Vitamin K_1 fat-soluble form more effective than water-soluble
Vitamin K_5	Synkamin	2–5 mg	Synthetic water-soluble form

TABLE 33-4 *Hemostatic Agents (continued)*

Nonproprietary or Official Name	Synonym or Trade Name	Dosage	Remarks
ANTIHEPARIN (HEPARIN ANTIDOTE)			
Protamine sulfate injection U.S.P.		50 mg I.V., repeated as necessary	1 mg neutralizes 100 units of heparin
ANTIFIBRINOLYSIN			
Aminocaproic acid N.F.	Amicar	5 g orally or I.V., followed by 1 g every hour up to 30 g daily	Inhibits plasminogen activators and plasmin
MISCELLANEOUS			
Carbazochrome salicylate	Adrenosem	5–10 mg (1–2 ml) I.M.	Claimed to decrease excessive capillary permeability
Conjugated estrogens for injection U.S.P.	Premarin Intravenous	25 mg, I.V. or I.M.	Claimed to reduce capillary oozing following surgical procedures
Locally Active Hemostatics			
Absorbable gelatin sponge U.S.P.	Gelfoam	Topical	Can be left in place when wound is closed
Absorbable gelatin film	Gelfilm	Topical to brain, eye, and elsewhere	Absorbed in one week to six months
Fibrin foam		Wet with thrombin and applied to the area	Initiates clot formation by furnishing a natural network
Thrombin N.F.	Oxycel; Surgicel	Apply minimal amount topically	Forms an artificial clot
Thromboplastin	Thrombokinase	Applied locally	Used also in making prothrombin tests

bleeding due to platelet deficiency, and, in fact, drug-induced thrombocytopenia is a common cause of hemorrhage.

Hemophilia is a chronic hemorrhagic disorder that results from a lack of certain clotting factors. The most common complication is hemarthrosis—bleeding into the joints that can cause pain and disabling deformities. Fatal hemorrhage may occur following serious injuries and surgical operations. In such emergencies, patients until recently received transfusions of blood plasma containing *antihemophilic globulin* (AHG; factor VIII). However, the large quantities often required could overload the patient's circulation.

This danger has been reduced by preparation of concentrates of the missing clotting factors. One such product, antihemophilic factor, human (Hemofil), containing about 60 times more factor VIII than blood plasma, is used in the management of classical hemophilia (type A). Patients with hemophilia B (Christmas disease) can now also be treated with a potent concentrate called factor IX complex, human (Konyne), which contains factors IX—the missing factor in this bleeding disorder—combined with factors II, VII, and X (see Tables 33-1 and 33-4 and Fig. 33-1).

Hypoprothrombinemia is a general term for a lack of circulating clotting factors, including not only prothrombin (factor II) but also the related substances factors VII, IX, and X. These substances are made in the liver by biochemical reactions that require vitamin K. Bleeding disorders caused by a deficiency of the prothrombin complex are the result of either a lack of vitamin K or of a failure to utilize the vitamin, even though it may be available. Hypoprothrombinemic bleeding that is caused by a deficiency of this vitamin responds to treatment with any one of the several forms of it that are available as medications.

Vitamin K compounds come in two forms—fat-soluble and water-soluble. The water-soluble salts of *menadione* (Table 33-4) are preferred for oral administration to patients with disease of the biliary tract who lack the bile needed to absorb the natural fat-soluble form of vitamin K. However, *phytonadione* (fat-soluble vitamin K_1, Table 33-4) is considered more effective in other situations. Thus, it is preferred, for example, for treating bleeding caused by overdosage of coumarin- and indanedione-type anticoagulant drugs and for newborn babies who bleed because of lack of vitamin K.

Vitamin K deficiency is rarely the result of poor nutrition, because bacteria in a person's colon produce this substance, which is then absorbed in small but usually adequate quantities. However, people with various intestinal disorders may be deprived of this source of the vitamin. In such cases, as well as during long-term treatment with antibiotic drugs that eliminate the vitamin K-producing bacteria, both types of vitamin K products can be administered by injection. Thus, the parenteral administration of either type of prothrombigenic substance—phytonadione or menadione—helps to counteract hypoprothrombinemic bleeding.

Hypofibrinogenemia, a lack of the clotting factor fibrinogen, can, of course, cause bleeding by keeping enough of the fibrin framework of clots from being formed. Deficiencies of fibrinogen and fibrin occurs most commonly in certain clinical situations in which these substances are too rapidly destroyed. That is, the balance between clotting and anticlotting factors shifts too far in favor of fibrinolysin (plasmin), the fibrin-dissolving enzyme.

Fibrinogen and other clotting factors can be replaced by transfusing whole fresh blood or fresh frozen plasma, or the fibrinogen fraction of human plasma (Table 33-4) may be administered alone. However, a drawback of all these natural substances is the hazard of hepatitis. *Aminocaproic acid* (Amicar), a synthetic antifibrinolytic substance, is also often effective in cases of bleeding caused by breakdown of both fibrin deposits and circulating fibrinogen. This chemical counteracts hemorrhaging caused by overdoses of the experimental thrombolytic drugs that are being tried for treating pulmonary embolism and other serious thromboembolic disorders. It is also often useful for control of bleeding in various medical, obstetrical, and surgical conditions in which excessive fibrinolytic activity occurs.

Oozing from fragile capillaries sometimes occurs when blood leaks through weak spots in the thin walls of these vessels. Various substances are claimed to stop such bleeding by strengthening the capillaries. Ascorbic acid (vitamin C) may do so when bleeding from the gums is the result of a deficiency of this vitamin. However, it has no hemostatic activity against other kinds of bleeding. Similarly, estrogenic substances can control uterine bleeding caused by a hormonal imbalance. However, the usefulness of conjugated estrogens (Premarin) for stopping capillary oozing following tonsillectomies and other surgical procedures has not been proved. Application of local hemostatics and gentle pressure is probably best. Replacing platelets in deficiency states may also help to strengthen fragile capillaries, as platelets help to fill spaces between the cells of the weakened walls.

SUMMARY of the Clinical Indications for Anticoagulants

Both Heparin and Hypoprothrombinemic Agents

Venous thrombosis treatment, or for prevention in patients with thrombophlebitis.

Pulmonary embolism treatment, or for prevention in patients with thrombophlebitis or phlebothrombosis.

Acute myocardial infarction, for prevention of thromboembolic complications following an acute coronary occlusion; and for long-term use to reduce recurrences in selected cases.

Atrial fibrillation prior to attempts to convert to a normal rhythm, and for long-term prophylaxis in patients who tend to produce emboli; also in patients with rheumatic mitral valve disease and enlarged left atrium or congestive heart failure to prevent cerebral and systemic emboli.

Cerebral thrombosis and embolism, particularly in transient ischemia attacks; possibly in progressing or evolving strokes; *not* immediately following a completed stroke but for possible prevention of recurrences in selected cases.

Surgical procedures, particularly vascular and cardiac surgery, but also in selected surgical and gynecological cases involving injury to or infection of the lower limbs and pelvic organs. *Acute* thrombotic or embolic occlusion of peripheral (leg) arteries and possibly in certain peripheral vascular diseases, particularly selected cases of thromboangiitis obliterans (Buerger's disease), and other arterial and venous disorders, including severe varicosities.

Heparin Only

(1) During surgery in which vessels are kept clamped.

(2) Disseminated intravascular coagulation (DIC syndrome or "consumption coagulopathy").

(3) Prevention of coagulation of blood drawn during transfusions and as laboratory blood samples.

S U M M A R Y of Conditions and Situations in which Anticoagulants Are Absolutely or Relatively Contraindicated

Patients in whom dosage cannot be carefully controlled by periodic prothrombin time determinations (coumarin and indanedione drugs), or periodic determinations of venous clotting time (heparin).

Patients who cannot or will not cooperate in long-term treatment because of mental and emotional factors that make them unreliable (for example, chronic alcoholics; unstable, senile, or psychotic patients, unless under the close care of others who take responsibility for treatment).

Patients with blood dyscrasias or other hemorrhagic disorders (for example, thrombocytic purpura; hemophilia; marked polycythemia).

Patients with ulcerations of the gastrointestinal tract (for example, acute peptic ulcer; active colitis); or other G.I. disorders (for example, visceral carcinoma; diverticulitis); or with continuous tube drainage of the upper G.I. tract; or indwelling g.u. catheters.

Patients with open wounds from surgery or trauma, particularly when large areas of skin have been lost; or during and following prostatectomy.

Patients who have had recent surgery on brain, spinal cord, or eyes; recent trauma to the C.N.S.; or suspected intracranial bleeding (hemorrhagic stroke); and patients who require spinal, regional, and lumbar block anesthesia.

Patients with threatened abortion and possibly in other pregnant and postpartum patients and during menstruation.

Patients with severe liver, kidney, or biliary tract disease which might interfere with the absorption of vitamin K.

Patients with such disorders as dissecting aneurysms; severe degrees of uncontrolled hypertension or congestive heart failure; subacute bacterial endocarditis or infectious pericarditis; active tuberculosis or severe diabetes.

Patients requiring intensive therapy with salicylates, phenylbutazone, and many other drugs that may act to intensify or counteract the effects of coumarin-type anticoagulants or that might be affected by the presence of these drugs.

Patients with a prior history of allergic hypersensitivity to heparin or to the coumarin and indanedione derivatives.

S U M M A R Y of Some Instructions for Patients Taking Anticoagulant Drugs

Ask questions to make certain that you understand how much of the medication to take and when to take it.

Keep all appointments for the periodic blood tests that are scheduled for you at the doctor's office or the clinic.

Call the doctor if you get sick, especially if you suffer from fever or diarrhea, or have to undergo minor surgery or even have a tooth extracted.

Avoid activities, including contact sports, that can lead to injury and bleeding. If possible, do not work at a job in which the chances of getting hurt are high.

Do not take any new medications and do not stop taking any previously prescribed drugs without first telling the doctor who ordered anticoagulants for you. This means that you should not even medicate yourself with aspirin or cold products containing antihistamines; and, if a physician treating you for another illness offers to prescribe a drug for relief of pain or other symptoms, both doctors should be informed that you are taking anticoagulants.

Continue to eat a nutritious diet and try to stay at your normal weight. Do not skip meals or go on any crash diet without consulting your doctor. Do not overeat or indulge in foods that may cause an upset stomach or diarrhea.

Carry an identification card indicating that you are taking an anticoagulant which gives your name and the name, address, and telephone number of your doctor. (Cards and emblems of this kind that can help assure proper treatment in case of accident are available from nonprofit organizations, such as local branches of the American Heart Association or Medic Alert Foundation).

Report to the doctor any signs of what seems to be excessive bleeding from the mouth, nose, rectum, vaginal tract, or in the urine and stools. Also call if what seem to be skin discolorations or bruises appear on the ankles, legs, arms, or elsewhere on the body. (If the doctor has prescribed vitamin K tablets or capsules for you, always carry them with you so that they are available for prompt use when needed.)

SUMMARY of Points for the Nurse to Remember about Anticoagulant Drug Therapy

The nurse has an important role in preventing venous stasis and possible complications such as thrombophlebitis. Encouraging postoperative patients to exercise their legs is one example.

Patients receiving anticoagulant drugs should be observed carefully for signs of bleeding, including epistaxis (nosebleed), hematuria, and tarry stools. Report signs promptly to the patient's physician.

Observations are made unobtrusively in order not to alarm the patient. However, many patients are aware that both bleeding and embolism are hazards of their condition. In such situations, it is preferable to talk frankly to the patient about what you are looking for. This may help to reassure him that he is being carefully and intelligently observed by a professional person who is concerned with his safety and well-being.

Be aware that heparin acts very quickly, while the oral anticoagulants may take several days to reach their peak effectiveness. Thus, when a doctor orders both drugs to be started simultaneously in emergency situations, this does not constitute a double dose. Instead, one drug is given for its immediate effect, while the other is begun in order to start building up to therapeutic levels.

Prothrombin time is checked carefully when patients are taking oral anticoagulants such as warfarin and Dicumarol. Such checks are usually carried out daily during the acute phase of the illness. During long-term anticoagulant therapy at home, the prothrombin time is also checked regularly but less often—usually at intervals of one or two weeks. (If such safeguards are not being employed, discuss the matter with the doctor or your supervisor before continuing to administer the medication.)

In the hospital, it is important to keep protamine sulfate and injectable vitamin K_1 readily available whenever patients are being treated with anticoagulants. Patients taking these drugs at home are instructed to keep a bottle of vitamin K_1 tablets on hand to take if any bleeding should occur.

The patient who is receiving anticoagulant therapy at home is given instructions to help him avoid bleeding episodes or to detect early signs. The family is also often given this information. They should realize the importance of keeping appointments for having their prothrombin time taken at regular intervals. They should also understand the importance of noticing and reporting any signs of bleeding.

To avoid potentially hazardous drug interaction, patients are instructed not to take *any* medication without the physician's knowledge. Even aspirin can intensify the patient's response to anticoagulants. (See also the *Summaries of Drug Interactions* and of *Instructions to Patients*.)

Clinical Nursing Situation

The Situation: Mrs. Caruso developed thrombophlebitis one week after she had a cholecystectomy. This complication kept her in the hospital a week longer than expected. During that time she was treated with warm wet soaks to the leg, bed rest, and Dicumarol.

When she returned home one week ago, the doctor prescribed a maintenance dose of

Dicumarol and continued rest. Activity is restricted to using the bathroom and sitting at the table for meals. Since Mr. Caruso is away at work all day, a home health aide comes in every day for four hours to assist his wife. The aide is supervised by a visiting nurse who comes to the house every other day.

The Problem: 1. Assume that you are the visiting nurse. What observations would you make of Mrs. Caruso's condition at each visit? What instructions would you give to the home health aide? What points would it be important to teach Mrs. Caruso?

2. One day as you are about to leave her home, Mrs. Caruso bursts out bitterly, "Why did this have to happen to me? Other people have operations, and they're fine. And here I'm laid up for a month already and who knows how much longer?"

"And those pills I'm taking. I'm afraid to keep taking them here at home. I'm alone most of the day, and even for the four hours someone comes in, it's a terrible expense. What happens if I begin to bleed when I'm all alone?"

How would you reply to Mrs. Caruso?

DRUG DIGEST

BISHYDROXYCOUMARIN U.S.P. (Dicumarol)

Actions and Indications. This prototype oral anticoagulant takes a few days to reduce prothrombin activity to therapeutic levels (20 to 30 percent of the initial activity). Thus, in emergencies such as acute pulmonary embolism, heparin is also administered for more immediate action until this drug reaches its peak effect. The drug's relatively long duration of action makes it useful for maintaining stable effects in patients on longterm treatment for preventing recurrences of thromboembolic episodes. Acute and chronic disorders in which this drug is used for a few weeks or indefinitely include venous thrombosis, myocardial or cerebral infarction, atrial fibrillation, and rheumatic heart valve disorders that produce emboli.

Side Effects, Cautions, and Contraindications. The drug should be discontinued at the first sign of bleeding as its effects tend to be cumulative and relatively prolonged. Its use is contraindicated in patients with blood dyscrasias, gastrointestinal ulcers, intracranial bleeding, recent operations on the brain, spinal cord or eye, threatened abortion, and subacute bacterial endocarditis. Caution is required in patients with liver or kidney disease, moderate hypertension, and severe diabetes.

Dosage and Administration. Doses of 200 or 300 mg are administered on the first day and then adjusted in accordance with the results of daily prothrombin time determinations. Doses required to keep prothrombin activity in the therapeutic range vary from 25 to 200 mg, depending upon the individual's response. The effects on dosage of possible interactions with other drugs should be considered.

HEPARIN SODIUM INJECTION U.S.P. (Panheprin; and others)

Actions and Indications. This anticoagulant acts immediately within the bloodstream to interfere with clotting reactions. Thus, it is preferred for first use in: acute thromboembolic emergencies, including venous and arterial thrombosis; pulmonary and peripheral arterial embolism; coronary artery occlusion in myocardial infarction; cerebral thrombosis in evolving stroke; atrial fibrillation with emboli formation; and during surgery of the arteries and heart to prevent clotting.

Side Effects, Cautions, and Contraindications. Bleeding is the most common complication in case of overdosage or administration to patients with a tendency to bleed readily. It should not be administered to patients with blood dyscrasias, threatened abortion, gastrointestinal ulceration or intubation, and subacute bacterial endocarditis. Intracranial hemorrhage is a contraindication, as are recent neurological and ocular surgical procedures. Caution is required during pregnancy and post partum.

Dosage and Administration. A diluted solution may be administered by I.V. drip adjusted to deliver 20,000 to 40,000 units a day, or it may be injected I.V. intermittently in doses of 5,000 to 10,000 units every four to six hours.

Heparin may be injected into subcutaneous fatty tissues in doses of 10,000 units every eight hours. Similar doses may be administered I.M., but hematoma and tissue irritation are most common by this route.

Clotting time is determined before each injection or every four hours during continuous intravenous infusion. The aim of therapy is to keep the clotting time at about 2½ times the control value of five to ten minutes.

WARFARIN SODIUM U.S.P. (Coumadrin; Panwarfin)

Actions and Indications. This drug's anticoagulant activity is attained in about 24 to 36 hours after administration of a single large therapeutic dose. Thus, in emergencies such as acute pulmonary embolism, myocardial infarction, or atrial fibrillation with embolization, it is usually given together with heparin which begins to act immediately. Other conditions in which warfarin is indicated include thrombophlebitis and other venous disorders in which it is desired to prevent the formation or extension of blood clots.

Side Effects, Cautions, and Contraindications. Patients must be carefully selected and their dosage of this drug closely individualized in order to avoid the ever-present danger of spontaneous bleeding as a result of overdosage.

This drug is contraindicated in patients with bleeding tendencies because of blood dyscrasias, threatened abortion, gastrointestinal ulceration, and subacute bacterial endocarditis. The drug is not administered to patients with cerebral hemorrhage or recent neurological or ocular surgery.

Caution is required in patients with poor liver or kidney function, elderly or disease-weakened patients, and those who may be emotionally disturbed or mentally incompetent. Patients should not take other drugs that may interact with the anticoagulants to change the expected response.

Dosage and Administration. Dosage is adjusted for each patient individually on the basis of prothrombin time tests. Initial oral or injectable administration of 40 to 60 mg produces a therapeutic effect, but only one half that dose is used in elderly patients. Most patients may then be maintained on daily doses ranging between 2 and 10 mg daily.

References

Borden, C.W. The current status of therapy with anticoagulants. *Med. Clin. N. Amer.*, 56:235, 1972 (Jan.).

Dalen, J.E., and Dexter, L. Pulmonary embolism. *JAMA*, 207:1505, 1969.

Di Palma, J.R. Precautions with the anticoagulants. *RN*, 34:57, 1971 (Oct.).

Eipe, J. Drugs affecting therapy with anticoagulants. *Med. Clin. N. Amer.*, 56:255, 1972 (Jan.).

Hiss, R.G., and Penner, J.A. The before and after of blood clotting. *Med. Clin. N. Amer.*, 53:1309, 1969 (Nov.).

Howard, F.A. The anticoagulants. *Clin. Pharmacol. Ther.*, 2:423, 1961.

Koprowicz, D.C. Drug interactions with coumarin derivatives. *Amer. J. Nurs.* 73:1042, 1973 (June).

McDowell, F.H. Initial treatment of cerebrovascular disease. *Mod. Treatm.*, 2:15, 1965 (Jan.).

Rodman, M.J. Drugs that affect blood coagulation. *RN*, 32:55, 1969 (June); 32:65, 1969 (July).

Sasahara, A., and Foster, V. Pulmonary embolism, recognition and treatment. *Amer. J. Nurs.*, 67:1634, 1967 (Aug.).

Udall, J.A. Recent advances in anticoagulant therapy. *GP*, 40:117, 1969 (July).

Wright, I. Anticoagulant therapy. *Drug Ther.*, 1971 (Jan.).

34.

Drugs for Treating Deficiency Anemias (Antianemic Drugs)

The Blood

Blood is a life-sustaining fluid that serves many important functions. The two main components of this liquid tissue are: (1) the *plasma*, a light yellow liquid containing proteins that play significant roles in protecting against infections and in fluid balance regulation; and (2) the *formed elements* of the blood—red blood cells, white blood cells, and platelets which float suspended in the plasma.

The platelets, or thrombocytes, help to set off the series of reactions that results in formation of clots for plugging breaks in blood vessels. The white cells, or leukocytes, make up one of the body's major defense mechanisms against invading microorganisms. In this chapter, we shall be concerned mainly with the red cells, or erythrocytes, which transport oxygen from the lungs to all the tissues of the body. We shall study some of the substances that are administered when red blood cells are reduced below normal in number and when they become abnormal in their shape and size—disorders called *deficiency anemias*.

ERYTHROCYTE PRODUCTION

The bone marrow manufactures enormous numbers of red blood cells to make up for the millions of erythrocytes that are destroyed every second. By using the chemical elements released from the disintegrated red cells along with added substances supplied in the diet, the marrow factory builds new erythrocytes at a rate that keeps the blood count at a normal level. The complicated processes of biosynthesis and maturation are aimed at building up the blood pigment *hemoglobin* and *the stroma*, the supporting structure that contains the hemoglobin molecules.

To make hemoglobin, the marrow requires dietary amino acids and other nutrients including vitamins and metals, of which the most important is *iron*. To form a stromal structure strong enough to resist too early destruction, the marrow requires minute amounts of the blood-building B-complex vitamins, B_{12} and *folic acid*. Ordinarily, adequate amounts of all these essential substances are present in the diet and can be absorbed from the gastrointestinal tract. These elements are then utilized in the various steps of hemoglobin biosynthesis and for the several stages through which red cells are brought to maturity in the marrow before being released into the bloodstream.

The Anemias

In some circumstances, a person's diet may not supply enough of a nutrient to meet his needs, or a substance present in adequate dietary quantities may not be absorbed in large enough amounts. Sometimes, abnormal losses of a nutrient may raise a person's requirements above what can be supplied by his diet alone. In all such cases, continued deficiency of the nutrients needed for synthesis of hemoglobin and manufacture of healthy red blood cells results in an anemia of the *nutritional* or *deficiency* type.

People who take in less dietary iron than they lose each day suffer a gradual *depletion* of their *total body stores of iron*. Eventually, they form fewer red cells, and these erythrocytes are smaller and paler than normal and contain less hemoglobin. Patients with this type of *hypochromic microcytic anemia* may complain of feeling tired and weak and of having little appetite. Their relative lack of tissue oxygen may lead to headaches, dizziness, and even dyspnea (difficulty in breathing) after only mild exertion.

Other people may suffer the same symptoms, but their blood and bone marrow looks quite different when examined under the microscope. The bone marrow of these patients is filled with large, immature red cells, called *megaloblasts*. The circulating blood also contains an unusual number of these red cell precursors together with the abnormally large erythrocytes that they form, called *macrocytes*.

(Anemias of this kind are called *megaloblastic*, or because each of the reduced number of red cells is crammed with the red respiratory pigment, hemoglobin, they are also sometimes called *hyperchromic macrocytic*.) These abnormal red cells that have a relatively short life span are produced as a result of a deficiency of vitamin B_{12} or of folic acid.

These two types of anemia almost never occur together. Thus, each type need be treated by supplying only the specific, missing blood cell-producing substance. Once the anemia is correctly diagnosed, it can be quickly corrected by administering adequate doses of iron, *or* vitamin B_{12}, *or* folic acid in forms that can be absorbed and utilized in blood cell production. In the rest of this chapter, we shall discuss the causes and treatment, first of iron deficiency (hypochromic microcytic) anemia and then of the megaloblastic (hyperchromic macrocytic) anemias.

IRON DEFICIENCY ANEMIA

Iron deficiency develops when a person takes in less iron from his diet than he needs to meet his needs. However, the wide variation in the requirements of different people makes it difficult to know exactly who needs supplemental iron. In addition, the symptoms of developing iron deficiency are vague and resemble those of various other disorders. These include feelings of weakness and fatigue, irritability, headache, dizziness, and loss of appetite.

IRON METABOLISM. In order to understand how iron deficiency develops, we should briefly review how the body gets its iron and how it handles this essential element. Only about five to ten percent of the iron contained in foodstuffs is normally able to be absorbed into the bloodstream from the gastrointestinal tract. This means that most people take up only 0.5 to 1 mg of the 9 to 18 mg of iron contained in the average daily American diet. Yet this iron intake is enough to meet the needs of adult men and most children. This is because the body ordinarily loses no more than 0.5 to 1 mg daily.

Individuals whose iron requirements are increased during periods of rapid growth, because of pregnancy, or as a result of abnormal blood loss have an increased capacity to absorb iron. Menstruating women, who may in a few days lose an amount of iron equal to that lost during the rest of the month, tend to absorb twice as much of the available dietary iron. However, even with this metabolic mechanism for combatting tendencies toward iron deficiency, some people require more iron than they are likely to obtain from ordinary foodstuffs.

Some nutritionists have suggested that common foods such as milk, cereals, and bread should be fortified with extra iron. However, iron-fortified milk has not proved practical, and cereals with added iron are too expensive for use by those families most likely to develop dietary deficiencies of iron. The amount of iron that can be added to enriched bread is limited by law, and some authorities oppose lifting these limits. They argue that adult men, most children, and others who have enough iron stored in their bone marrow, liver, and spleen may build up excessive levels of iron in these organs and suffer ill effects from iron overloading if they eat iron-fortified foods that they do not really need.

It has been suggested, instead, that people who need iron should take medicinal iron prescribed for them by a physician, after a diagnosis of iron deficiency has established the fact that iron is indicated for the individual. The doctor also determines the cause of the patient's iron deficiency and tries to correct it if possible.

INDICATIONS FOR MEDICINAL IRON. The uncertainty as to which individuals need more iron than their diet can supply, together with the vagueness of the symptoms of iron deficiency, has been exploited by promoters of iron-containing products that people can buy without prescription. Advertisements directed at the public often lead people to diagnose and treat themselves with expensive mineral-vitamin supplements. This is undesirable because many such products often offer inadequate amounts of iron at unnecessarily high cost. More important is the fact that this disorder should not be treated without first determining what is causing the patient's anemia.

Blood loss is the most common cause of iron deficiency anemia in most types of patients. In adult men, the most common cause of an unusual increase in their iron requirements is occult (hidden) hemorrhage from the intestinal tract. Thus, these patients need to see a doctor who can find the source of their pathologic bleeding and correct it. Obviously, taking an advertised iron product can be dangerous if the patient has bleeding hemorrhoids,

a gastroduodenal ulcer, or even early, undetected cancer of the stomach or colon.

Women of child-bearing age are often anemic. Even normal menstrual periods cause a loss of iron that must be made up by increasing the daily iron intake. Women with *menorrhagia* (an unusually heavy menstrual flow) are particularly likely to become iron deficient. Often such women fail to consult a physician because they think that their bleeding is normal. Thus, the nurse who learns about the woman's condition in a casual conversation should suggest that she see a doctor and have her hemoglobin level and red cell count checked.

Women who eat a diet containing meats, dairy products, cereal grains, green and yellow vegetables, citrus fruits, and tomatoes can often absorb enough extra iron to meet the demands made by menstruation. However, if (as is often true with teenage girls) they neglect to eat an adequate diet, young women may readily become deficient in iron. *Adolescent girls* (and boys) double their need for iron during the years of rapid growth, beginning with puberty. Thus, even if she eats well, a growing girl may not get quite enough dietary iron to meet her needs.

Pregnant women cannot expect to meet their extra iron needs by dietary means alone. The growing fetus takes iron from the mother's stores, particularly during the last half of pregnancy. In addition, the mother herself needs more iron because her red blood cell volume increases by about one third at the same time. Finally, of course, there is a further loss of iron during bleeding at the time of delivery. Thus, a woman who has had several pregnancies within a relatively few years may have markedly depleted her iron stores. The prophylactic use of iron during the second and third trimesters of all pregnancies seems desirable.

Infants between about six months and two years are particularly prone to developing iron deficiency. For the first few months of life, newborn babies can draw upon the iron that they accumulated from their mothers' stores while in the uterus. However, because they triple their birth weight and blood volume during the first year of life, infants cannot meet their bodies' demands for iron for very long. Full-term babies often develop symptoms of iron deficiency at about six months, and premature infants show signs of deficiency in about half that time.

In summary, supplemental iron seems to be definitely needed by infants and women in the latter half of pregnancy. Adolescents, particularly teenage girls, and many women with normal or heavy menses are probably in borderline iron balance. Men who are suffering blood loss from a bleeding lesion in the gastrointestinal tract or elsewhere may also profit from iron therapy.

IRON THERAPY. Once the underlying cause of a patient's anemia is determined the doctor does what he can to correct it, if possible. At the same time he treats the anemic symptom itself with an iron-containing hematinic—in most cases, an orally effective product. Such treatment has two purposes: first, bringing the patient's hemoglobin and red blood cell levels back to normal; and second, restoring the patient's reserves of storage iron bound in bone marrow, liver, and spleen. Even though signs of improvement are usually seen within a couple of weeks, it may be two or three months before the first goal is fully reached, and it may take many more months to bring the level of bone marrow iron back to normal, especially if bleeding recurs. Thus, the patient on long-term hematinic therapy may be put to much expense if the doctor employs a costly product.

SELECTION OF A PRODUCT. Patients can be encouraged to ask questions about their therapy, including questions about medications that are similar to the one prescribed but are less costly. The nurse, too, can raise such questions with the physician should she observe that the cost of medication is a problem to the patient. Also, because many people medicate themselves with *non*prescription iron preparations, the nurse can advise them about which products are preferred. The most important point of information that the nurse can offer is this: *the most effective iron products available are also the least expensive ones.* Simple inorganic iron salts such as ferrous sulfate, ferrous fumarate, and ferrous gluconate (Table 34-1) furnish all the iron an anemic patient needs, often at a cost of less than two cents a day. Some heavily promoted *non*prescription products cost ten to twenty times as much, or more, and often do not supply the necessary 180 to 240 mg a day of elemental iron.

Products are available containing complex iron compounds that are claimed to be less irritating to the gastrointestinal tract than the simple inorganic salts. Some are presented in sustained-release or enteric coated form. The iron in such products is often not absorbed well enough by the mucous membranes lining the upper intestinal tract. Products containing various vitamins and trace metals also cost considerably more than simple iron salts, without increasing the absorption of iron or the effectiveness of this element for building up the patient's hemoglobin level and red blood cell count. Thus, because most patients are able to tolerate the simple salts when they are properly administered, the doctor and nurse should suggest such products and tell the patient how to take them for best effects.

ADMINISTRATION OF ORAL IRON. Iron salts are best absorbed when taken on an empty stomach. However, they are also most irritating to the gastrointestinal tract when administered in this way. Patients who experience epigastric distress, nausea, or vomiting at the start of treatment may stop taking their medication. Thus, the doctor may begin treatment with small doses taken right after meals. Then the dosage is gradually raised, and the amount of food taken together with iron is reduced. If the patient does not complain of abdominal discomfort, diarrhea, or constipation, he may then take his medication between meals for most complete absorption.

The nurse encourages patients who have difficulty tolerating iron at first. She should let the patient know that his stool may be colored red or black by an iron preparation so that he will not be alarmed by the thought that this is a sign of gastrointestinal bleeding. To protect patients' teeth from staining by liquid iron preparations, the concentrated drops are placed well back on the tongue, or the solution is well diluted and sipped through a straw or drinking tube. Care is taken to scheduling iron administration in relation to meals.

ADMINISTRATION OF PARENTERAL IRON. Most anemic patients tolerate oral iron well, and their hemoglobin rises at a steady rate. However, some types of patients may require iron by injection. These include the following kinds of cases: (1) patients who refuse to take oral iron or cannot be depended upon to do so; (2) those who have had extensive bowel surgery, suffer from ulcerative colitis or regional enteritis; or (3) suffer from diseases that keep oral iron from being absorbed. Although parenteral administration of iron does not result in more rapid correction of anemia, the patient's

TABLE 34-1 *Drugs for Treating Deficiency Anemias*

Nonproprietary Name	Synonym or Trade Name	Total Daily Dosage	Remarks
Selected Oral Iron Compounds			
Ferrocholinate	Chel-Iron; Ferrolip	1–2 g equal to 120–240 mg elemental iron	Chelate form of iron, less toxic in overdosage
Ferrous fumarate U.S.P.	Ircon; Toleron	0.6–0.8 g equal to 200–260 mg elemental iron	Readily absorbed, but irritating to G.I. tract
Ferrous gluconate N.F.	Fergon	0.960–2.0 g equal to 120–240 mg elemental iron	Readily absorbed, but irritating to G.I. tract
Ferrous sulfate U.S.P.	Iron sulfate hydrated	0.3–1.2 g equal to 60–240 mg elemental iron	See *Drug Digest*
Ferrous sulfate, exsiccated U.S.P.	Feosol; Fer-In-Sol	Dosage of this dried salt is about two-thirds of the above	
Polyferose	Jefron	0.6–1.2 g equal to 100–200 mg elemental iron	A carbohydrate chelate of iron less toxic in overdosage
Parenteral Iron Products			
Dextriferron N.F.	Astrafer; iron-dextrin	I.V.; 1.5–5 ml equal to 30–100 mg elemental iron	Administered I.V. only
Iron dextran injection U.S.P.	Imferon	I.M.; 2–5 ml equal to 100–250 mg elemental iron	See *Drug Digest* (I.V. admin. also)
Iron sorbitex N.F.	Jectofer	I.M.; 2–4 ml equal to 100–200 mg elemental iron	Never administered I.V.

stores of reserve iron may be built up at a faster rate. This may be desirable for the rare patient with chronic bleeding that cannot be readily corrected.

Two parenteral products, *iron dextran injection*+ (Imferon) and *iron sorbitex* (Jectofer) may be administered intramuscularly; another, *dextriferron* (Astrafer) is given only by vein. These products are reserved for patients whose iron deficiency anemia cannot be treated with oral iron, because both chronic and acute toxicity are possible when iron is administered by parenteral routes. The doctor must calculate the total dose of iron that must be injected and then administer it in fractional daily doses. This is done to avoid overloading the patient's tissues with iron, a chronic disorder called *hemosiderosis*. Acute toxicity may be caused by an anaphylactic reaction or from overdosage leading to severe falls in blood pressure—sometimes to shock levels.

ACCIDENTAL IRON POISONING. Oral iron products do not ordinarily cause acute toxicity. However, young children who ingest overdoses of iron may suffer a shocklike state and die of cardiovascular collapse. A specific antidote called *deferoxamine* (Desferal) is now available for binding excess iron and removing it from the body. However, it is better to prevent iron poisoning than to have to treat the potentially fatal poisoning. Patients should be warned that iron preparations are not harmless and should be kept where children cannot get at them. The container should be one of the "child-proof" type that children cannot readily open, and it should be labeled "Keep out of the reach of children."

MEGALOBLASTIC ANEMIAS

We have seen above (p. 414) that people who lack vitamin B_{12} or folic acid tend to develop anemia marked by the presence of abnormally immature bone marrow and red blood cells. As in the case of patients with iron deficiency anemia, those with megaloblastic, or marcrocytic, anemias often complain of feeling weak and tired, and they may have headaches and lose their appetite. However, they may also have other complaints, such as a sore tongue (glossitis) and other gastrointestinal symptoms—diarrhea in patients with folic acid deficiency and either diarrhea or constipation in the case of those who are lacking vitamin B_{12}.

These symptoms occur because the cells that line the gastrointestinal tract (like those of the bone marrow) need these B-complex vitamins for making the nucleic acids required for their rapid growth and reproduction. The only cells that do not seem to need folic acid are the nerve cells (neurons do not reproduce). However, vitamin B_{12} is required for synthesizing the myelin sheath of neurons. Thus, a deficiency of *this* vitamin results in damage to central and peripheral nerve cells. Patients deficient in vitamin B_{12} have not only a megaloblastic anemia but also signs and symptoms that stem from neurological damage—for example, numbness and tingling in the hands and feet, poor motor coordination, and even mental illness symptoms, in some cases.

VITAMIN B_{12} DEFICIENCY. Vitamin B_{12} is the most potent known vitamin. Adults require less than one *micro*gram—a millionth of a gram—a day. The daily diet of most Americans offers many times that amount, contained mainly in animal protein foodstuffs. Thus, people whose diet includes muscle meats, seafood, milk, eggs, and especially liver, rarely develop a dietary deficiency of vitamin B_{12}. This occurs mainly in people who eat nothing but vegetable foods. Even in such strict vegetarians, it usually takes several years for body stores of B_{12} to drop enough for signs of deficiency to develop.

Failure to absorb enough of the dietary B_{12} to replace the tiny amount that is lost each day is the main cause of vitamin B_{12} deficiency. Thus, megaloblastic anemia from this cause is sometimes seen in patients with stomach cancer and in others who require surgical removal of the stomach or other parts of their upper gastrointestinal tract. The most common condition associated with B_{12} deficiency is *pernicious anemia*, a disorder that stems from an abnormality of the stomach lining. The gastric mucosal cells of people with pernicious anemia fail to secrete a substance called the *intrinsic factor*. Without this stomach secretion, dietary B_{12} cannot be absorbed from the intestine.

(*Response to treatment.* Patients with pernicious anemia and others who fail to take in or absorb enough dietary B_{12} can have their symptoms completely reversed by receiving B_{12} by injection (see Table 34-2). The form most commonly employed is a solution of the dark red crystals called *cyanocobalamin injection*+ (Rubramin, and others). Injected deep into the subcutaneous tissues or intramuscularly, the vitamin, of course, bypasses the mucosal barrier to its intestinal absorption. It is carried by the bloodstream to such sites as the bone marrow, intestinal mucosa cells, the nervous system, and all the other cells that need the vitamin in order to function normally.

The pernicious anemia patient begins to feel better within a day or so. Soon red cells of normal appearance begin to enter his bloodstream and the abnormally enlarged cells (macrocytes) begin to disappear. In addition to this favorable hematologic response, remission is marked by improvement in gastrointestinal tract and neurological symptoms. The patient's appetite is restored, his inflamed tongue and disordered bowel activity become normal, and such neurological symptoms as paresthesias (numbness and tingling) are relieved. (Of course, atrophied stomach cells and degenerated neurons do not recover their ability to function.)

Patients who respond so remarkably tend to think themselves cured after a few weeks of treatment. Often, they continue to feel so well—even when they miss appointments with their physician—that they see no reason to return for further injections. Actually, the cyanocobalamin injections do not overcome the underlying defect—the inability to absorb dietary vitamin B_{12}. For this reason, unless the patient continues to receive cyanocobalamin injections every month, he may suffer insidious irreversible damage of the spinal cord and other parts of the nervous system. Thus, the nurse and doctor must make it very clear to the patient and his family that he has to keep on getting his periodic injections for the rest of his life.

(*Other types of treatment.* Another cobalamin derivative, *hydroxocobalamin* (vitamin B_{12a}), is claimed to produce higher and longer-lasting blood levels following parenteral admin-

T A B L E   3 4 - 2   *Hematopoietic Vitamins and Related Substances*

Nonproprietary Name	Synonym or Trade Name	Total Daily Dosage	Remarks
Cobalamin concentrate N.F.		Very variable	Reference standard
Cyanocobalamin injection U.S.P.	Berubigen; Rubramin; and others; vitamin B_{12}	Parenterally and orally in variable doses from 30–1000 μg	See *Drug Digest*
Folic acid U.S.P.	Folvite; pteroylglutamic acid	Parenterally and orally 0.5–1.0 mg daily	See *Drug Digest*
Folinic acid	Citrovorum factor; Leucovorin calcium injection	1 mg daily I.M.	Antidote for overdosage with antifolic compounds
Hydroxocobalamin	AlphaRedisol; and others; vitamin B_{12a}	50–1000 μg I.M.	Claimed longer-lasting than vitamin B_{12}
Intrinsic factor concentrate N.F.	In various panhematinic products	300 mg	Aids oral absorption of vitamin B_{12}
Liver injection	Pernaemon	Variable	Contains vitamin B_{12} in crude form; may cause allergic reactions
Vitamin B_{12} with intrinsic factor concentrate	In various panhematinic products	Variable	Orally effective but not as desirable as injections of B_{12} in pernicious anemia

istration. However, it has not proved to have any practical advantages over cyanocobalamin; nor does *aquocobalamin* (vitamin B_{12b}) offer therapeutic properties preferable to those of the prototype B_{12} compound. Certain new pharmaceutical forms of cyanocobalamin that release the vitamin only very slowly from tissue reservoirs or depots into which they are injected are now under study. These may provide more convenient maintenance treatment, as patients may require injections only about every three months.

Oral treatment with vitamin B_{12} *alone* is effective only in the rare cases of megaloblastic anemia caused by a dietary deficiency of B_{12}. Patients with pernicious anemia require an oral preparation that also contains the intrinsic factor which they lack. However, even though tablets and capsules containing vitamin B_{12} combined with intrinsic factor concentrate are available, the use of such oral products for maintenance therapy in these patients is not considered desirable. Many patients who respond at first to oral products of this kind tend to become resistant after awhile and will relapse unless they receive injections.

Other indications for cyanocobalamin. Patients with various neurological and G.I. disorders with symptoms similar to those of pernicious anemia are often treated with massive doses of cyanocobalamin. However, there is no proof that this substance is effective for treating peripheral neuritis, multiple sclerosis, or any clinical condition other than a proven deficiency of vitamin B_{12}. Fortunately, cyanocobalamin is one of the safest substances available for use in therapeutics. Even when injected in doses of 1,000 μg or more, it causes no local or systemic toxicity. Thus, doctors who order injections of such large doses of this vitamin may be employing it as a harmless placebo while they seek the real cause and cure of the patient's condition.

Dosage schedules. Doctors administer cyanocobalamin in many different doses and at varying intervals. Although injections of as little as 1 μg daily are effective for bringing about remissions of uncomplicated pernicious anemia, some doctors order injections of 1,000 μg for patients with neurological complications. Most of this large a dose is excreted without having been used by the bone marrow for making red cells or stored in the liver for later use. Patients whose symptoms have been relieved by daily injections of between 30 and 100 μg for about a week or two can be kept in remission by maintenance doses of only about 100 μg once or twice a month. Patients who do not respond to these smaller doses of vitamin B_{12} probably do not have a vitamin B_{12} deficiency, and thus they will not respond even to massive doses. Injections of 1,000 μg do not have effects that are significantly longer-lasting than 100-μg doses.

FOLIC ACID DEFICIENCY. Most people have no difficulty in meeting their daily requirements for this B-complex vitamin—about 50 μg daily for adults. Leafy green vegetables such as lettuce, spinach, and asparagus, and foods such as milk, eggs, and liver, contain many times that much folate. However, deficiency may develop during malnutrition or in periods of increased demand for the vitamin, and in patients suffering from malabsorption syndromes such as sprue or celiac disease.

《 *Deficiency states.* Malnutrition as a cause of folate deficiency is common in alcoholics and is often a factor in poor and elderly patients and in food faddists. Sometimes, megaloblastic anemia occurs in women who have had several successive pregnancies because of the increased demands on their folic acid stores by the growing fetuses. Infants fed on diets lacking in food folate sometimes develop megaloblastic anemia and diarrhea, particularly during periods of infection.

《 *Response to treatment.* Once a patient's megaloblastic anemia is definitely diagnosed as the result of folate deficiency, it can be readily reversed by oral or parenteral administration of crystalline folic acid. Patients who are not severely ill respond rapidly to as little as 1 mg administered by mouth. In practice, however, most hematologists start all patients on much higher doses of this *non*toxic substance. Orders for 5 to 15 mg daily are common, and although such large oral doses of *folic acid+* (Folvite) are adequately absorbed even in the presence of intestinal disease, the injectable sodium salt is often employed by the intramuscular or deep subcutaneous route.

Patients improve promptly both in how they feel and in their blood picture. Changes in the bone marrow from megaloblastosis to normoblastosis are seen within a couple of days, followed shortly by disappearance of macrocystosis in the peripheral blood that then begins to contain more and more normal red cells. Such symptoms as soreness of the mouth and tongue and diarrhea disappear, and the patient's improved appetite soon leads to a gain in weight. Improvement can be maintained with daily doses of 1 mg or less, but relapses are best prevented by providing a diet containing adequate quantities of food folates.

Folic acid is an entirely safe substance. However, its misuse by people who do not need it is not only unnecessarily expensive but also potentially dangerous for patients with pernicious anemia. This is so because small amounts of folic acid may bring the blood picture of these patients back to normal, while their neurological disorder continues to progress. (Folic acid cannot correct the neuronal myelin sheath damage that occurs as a result of vitamin B_{12} deficiency.) Thus, the doctor performs diagnostic tests to exclude the presence of pernicious anemia before he prescribes folic acid for a patient with megaloblastic anemia.

SELF-MEDICATION

The nurse should always advise patients not to try to treat themselves with *non*prescription antianemia products that contain mixtures of many different minerals and vitamins, including folic acid. The Food and Drug Administration now forbids the inclusion of more than 0.1 mg (100 μg) in *non*prescription products, as larger amounts may mask the presence of pernicious anemia and make its diagnosis difficult in patients whose real difficulty is a lack of vitamin B_{12}. The small amount of oral vitamin B_{12} that is offered in such so-called "shotgun" type multivitamin and panhematinic products is not likely to protect the patient against progressive neurological complications. The nurse who functions as provider of primary health care, in such settings as housing projects for the elderly, must be alert to symptoms of iron and vitamin deficiency, so that she will be able to refer patients to a physician for further study and treatment.

SUMMARY

Most patients with deficiency anemias can be treated successfully. However, the key to successful treatment is a correct diagnosis of the cause of the anemia. When the doctor has determined the nature of the deficiency, he can then employ the specific missing substance—iron, folic acid, or vitamin B_{12}.

In the process of studying the patient, he can also learn whether the cause is merely poor diet or possibly one of the kinds of disorders that cause an excessive loss of iron, or failure to absorb folic acid or B_{12}. In either case, he may sometimes be able to correct the underlying cause—for example, stopping the excessive blood loss that may have led to iron deficiency as well as supplementing the patient's diet with the necessary nutrient.

Self-medication should be avoided, because it may succeed in bringing about a normal blood picture and thus tend to mask such serious defects as still undetected internal bleeding or progressive neurological deterioration.

S U M M A R Y of Side Effects, Cautions, and Contraindications of Iron Salts

Side Effects

Oral therapeutic doses

Irritation to mucosa of stomach and intestinal tract tends to cause epigastric distress (with possible nausea and vomiting); abdominal cramps (with either diarrhea or constipation). Caution is required in patients with peptic ulcer, ulcerative colitis, regional enteritis, and other chronic gastrointestinal inflammatory disorders.

Oral toxic doses (Acute poisoning in children)

Nausea, vomiting, abdominal pain, diarrhea, with stools greenish and tarry as a result of mucosal damage and hemorrhage.

Lethargy, fast, weak pulse, low blood pressure, with possible circulatory collapse, pulmonary edema, coma, and death.

Parenteral therapeutic doses and overdoses

Local: Soreness, swelling, and brownish or bluish staining of skin at I.M. injection sites; possible pain, venous spasm, and phlebitis at I.V. injection sites.

Systemic: Headache, dizziness, flushing, nausea; possible joint pain and swelling in arthritic patients or generalized pain in others; anaphylactic and hypotensive reactions.

Contraindications

In hypersensitive patients and in those with any kind of anemia *not* caused by iron deficiency because of the danger of hemosiderosis (iron overload disease). *Extreme caution* in patients with impaired liver function.

S U M M A R Y of Points for the Nurse to Remember About Drugs Used for Treating Anemia

The nurse should advise people to have a doctor diagnose their problem instead of buying advertised hematinic products for self-medication. Taking such products is not only often an unnecessary expense but also potentially dangerous. If the patient is actually anemic, the cause, which is often loss of blood, should be sought. Besides, certain products may mask the presence of pernicious anemia without counteracting the most dangerous effects of this disease.

If a patient complains that he "can't take iron" because it causes gastrointestinal upset, the nurse should advise him to consult his physician as to whether a change in the dosage or method of administration of the drug might be possible, or even as to whether a less irritating product might not be prescribed.

Do not suggest the likelihood of nausea, vomiting, cramps, diarrhea, or constipation, but instruct the patient to report any symptoms he may experience while taking the drug. Do let the patient know that a darkening of the stool is to be expected and that this does not mean that he is bleeding but is quite harmless. (The nurse, too, should check on whether any patient with a dark stool is taking iron before deciding that this is a sign of bleeding.)

For most rapid and complete absorption, soluble iron salts are sometimes taken in orange juice. Remember that liquid iron sometimes stains the teeth and have the patient take it through a straw or a drinking tube. Drops should be placed well back on the patient's tongue.

Remember that iron-containing products are potentially toxic when taken in large quantity, and alert parents to the need for storing such substances out of the reach of young children.

Patients should be urged not to forget to visit their physician for B_{12} injections when the symptoms of pernicious anemia and similar deficiency disorders are in remission. Often it is helpful to teach the patient and/or his family to administer B_{12} injections periodically at home, in order to reduce the high cost of long-term treatment of this lifelong illness.

Clinical Nursing Situation: I

The Situation: Miss Swenson, age 52, has just learned that she has pernicious anemia. Her doctor has prescribed vitamin B_{12} 1 cc I.M. weekly, indicating that later it may be possible to decrease the frequency of injections to 1 cc every other week. He explained to Miss Swenson, however, that she would continue to require vitamin B_{12} injections for the rest of her life. The public health nurse visits weekly to give the injections.

The Problem: One day, while the nurse is preparing the injection, Miss Swenson says, "I know that you are giving me a vitamin. The doctor explained to me why I need it, but I've forgotten a lot of what he said. I've always eaten a good diet. Why is it that I'm not getting the vitamin from my food?"

Later, she says, "I have to keep taking this medicine all my life. Could it have harmful effects on me after a while?"

Miss Swenson then asks, "Would it be possible for my sister to learn to give me the injection? That would be more convenient and less expensive for me."

How would you reply to Miss Swenson's questions?

Clinical Nursing Situation: II

The Situation: Mary Ann, 14 years old, lives in a shack that has no plumbing or electricity. Her father died in an accident in the nearby mine two years ago, leaving a large family that gets meager support from public welfare. She is thin, pale, and listless when she comes to the recently opened clinic with a note from her teacher. The note states that Mary Ann had fainted in class that morning.

The nurse, who sees all patients who seek care, questions the girl. She says that she eats no breakfast and that vegetables and meat are rarely served in her home. She never has had much pep, and has been having such fainting spells for the past six months. Her menses had begun about a year ago. The nurse decides that Mary Ann should see the doctor when he comes on his next weekly visit.

The Problem: 1. Assume that you are the nurse. Make an outline of the main points in this patient's health history. Describe the instructions that you would ask her to follow until the doctor can see her. Describe the planning and teaching that you would do with Mary Ann's mother and teacher.

2. After the doctor examines Mary Ann and finds her severely anemic, he prescribes ferrous sulfate 0.2 g t.i.d. He also writes to the welfare agent asking for additional funds for the more nutritious diet that he wants her to have. She will see the doctor again in a month and will be back to the clinic each week. Describe what you will teach Mary Ann about taking the iron and following her diet.

DRUG DIGEST

CYANOCOBALAMIN INJECTION N.F. (Vitamin B_{12})

Actions and Indications. This potent blood-forming substance is effective for reversing the signs and symptoms of pernicious anemia and other megaloblastic anemias caused by a deficiency of vitamin B_{12}. It acts promptly to improve the bone marrow and blood picture and to relieve weakness, fatigue, appetite loss, glossitis (sore tongue), and other gastrointestinal disturbances. Symptoms of neurologic complications such as feelings of numbness and tingling are relieved, but there may be no change in function when the controlling neurons of the spinal cord, cerebrum, or peripheral nerves have been irreversibly damaged. Cyanocobalamin is of no value in neurological or psychiatric disorders that do *not* stem from a deficiency of vitamin B_{12}.

Side Effects, Cautions, and Contraindications. There are no known contraindications to this substance, which is remarkably free of local or systemic toxicity.

Dosage and Administration. The solution is injected intramuscularly or deep into the subcutaneous tissues in dosages that vary from 1 to 1,000 μg, depending upon the severity or duration of the deficiency. Ordinarily, uncomplicated cases of pernicious anemia are treated with daily doses of 30 to 100 μg for one week, followed by 100 μg once or twice a week until remission is complete. Patients must then receive 100 μg at regular intervals, such as once a month, *for the rest of their lives.*

FERROUS SULFATE U.S.P. (Feosol; Fer-In-Sol; and others)

Actions and Indications. This inexpensive inorganic iron salt offers elemental iron in a form that is readily absorbable from mucosal sites in the upper intestine. It is useful for supplying iron required for the synthesis of hemoglobin in iron deficiency anemia. It also restores depleted iron stores in simple iron deficiency.

Side Effects, Cautions, and Contraindications. Gastrointestinal irritation symptoms include epigastric distress with possible nausea and vomiting, and abdominal cramps with either diarrhea *or* constipation. Caution is required in patients with peptic ulcer, ulcerative colitis, regional enteritis, and other chronic inflammatory disorders of the gastrointestinal tract.

Massive overdosage may cause local corrosion of the mucosa of the stomach and intestine leading to diarrhea with black, tarry stools. Pulse may become weak and rapid with blood pressure falling to shock levels.

Dosage and Administration. The usual daily dosage is one to four 300-mg tablets, each containing 60 to 240 mg of elemental iron. These are administered after meals to avoid gastrointestinal irritation, but for better absorption in patients who tolerate iron well, this salt may be administered between meals. Liquid forms, including an elixir, syrup, and drops, are also available.

FOLIC ACID U.S.P. (Folvite; Pteroylglutamic Acid)

Actions and Indications. This B-complex vitamin is effective for treating megaloblastic anemias caused by a deficient intake of food folates. These occur as a result of nutritional lack—for example: in alcoholics; in malabsorption syndromes such as sprue and celiac disease; or when increased folate requirements are a factor, as in the megaloblastic anemias of pregnancy and infancy.

Side Effects, Cautions, and Contraindications. No toxic effects occur even with high parenteral doses. However, folic acid is contraindicated in patients with pernicious anemia, because it can counteract the megaloblastosis, macrocytosis, and gastrointestinal symptoms of this disorder without favorably affecting its neurological complications. Thus, folic acid may mask pernicious anemia and make its diagnosis difficult, while nerve damage may be progressing. This form of folate should also *not* be used for treating toxicity caused by antifol drugs, which requires *folinic* acid as an antidote to overdosage.

Dosage and Administration. Oral doses of 5 to 20 mg daily or parenteral administration of 5 to 15 mg by the deep s.c. or I.M. routes are customarily employed, although doses of only 1 mg daily are effective for treatment and prophylaxis of folate deficiency.

IRON DEXTRAN INJECTION U.S.P. (Imferon)

Actions and Indications. This injectable iron complex is effective for treating patients with iron deficiency anemia in whom oral iron therapy is undesirable. These include patients who cannot tolerate gastrointestinal irritation, or are unable to absorb iron adequately through the intestinal mucosa. Patients who cannot be depended upon to take oral iron, or who have continued chronic bleeding and require rapid replenishment of storage iron, may also require parenteral iron.

Side Effects, Cautions, and Contraindications. Minor side effects include headache, nausea, shivering, rash, and itching. Joints of rheumatoid arthritis patients may become red and swollen. Patients who have a history of hypersensitivity to parenteral iron or who react adversely to a small test dose should not be treated, as fatal anaphylactic reactions have resulted. Patients with impaired liver function require extreme caution.

Dosage and Administration. To avoid iron overloading (hemosiderosis), the total dosage is calculated in terms of the patient's body weight and hemoglobin level. The daily maximum dosage for average-sized adults is 5 ml (250 mg of iron) and proportionately less for smaller individuals and children. Intramuscular injections are made into the upper outer quadrant of the buttocks by a technique intended to avoid leakage into subcutaneous tissues with soreness, staining, and inflammation at the injection site. Intravenous administration may also be employed in some selected cases.

References

Brown, E.B. Clinical pharmacology of drugs used in the treatment of iron deficiency anemia. *Pharmacol. Physicians*, 2:1, 1968 (Nov.).

Council on Foods and Nutrition. Iron deficiency in the United States. *JAMA*, 203: 119, 1968.

Di Palma, J. R. Vitamins—facts and fancies. *RN*, 35:57, 1972 (July).

Giorgio, A.J. Current concepts of iron metabolism and the iron deficiency anemias. *Med. Clin. N. Amer.*, 54:1399, 1970 (Nov.).

Hecht, A. B. Self medication inaccuracy and what can be done. *Nurs. Outlook*, 18:30, 1970 (April).

Kahn, S.B. Recent advances in the nutritional anemias. *Med. Clin. N. Amer.*, 54:631, 1970 (May).

Lowenthal, W. Factors affecting drug absorption. *Amer. J. Nurs.*, 73:1391, 1973 (Aug.).

Rodman, M.J. Drugs for treating nutritional anemias. *RN*, 35:61, 1972 (June).

SECTION **8**

Drugs for Treating Endocrine Disorders

35.

Pituitary Gland Hormones

The pituitary gland, or *hypophysis*, is a tiny organ located deep in the head just below the brain. Actually, the pituitary body consists of two separate parts with different embryologic origins and functions. The *anterior lobe*, or forward portion, is made up of true glandular tissue. Its cells secrete several different types of hormones—chemical messengers that are carried by the blood to various other endocrine glands* to affect their functioning. The *posterior portion* of the pituitary does not make its own secretions but stores and releases hormones that are made in the *hypothalamus*, a part of the brain to which it remains connected by nerve fibers. The target tissues for its secretions are not other glands, but rather such structures as the uterus, breast, and certain kidney tubule cells.

The pituitary gland hormones have a profound influence over many metabolic functions. Through its connections with the brain by blood vessels and nerve fibers, this gland works together with the nervous system to regulate the activities of all the body's countless cells. Thus, even though human pituitary hormones have had relatively few uses in treatment up to now, we should understand their physiologic effects. This will help us to understand the functioning of the other endocrine glands that are discussed in the following chap-

* The term *endocrine* refers to glands that release their secretions into the bloodstream. These hormones then influence the functioning of specific target tissues to which they are carried. In contrast to these glands of internal secretion, the *exocrine* glands secrete substances such as sweat, or saliva and other digestive juices, directly onto body surfaces such as skin and mucous membranes.

ters of this section—the testes and ovaries, the pancreas, the thyroid gland, and the adrenal cortex.

The Anterior Pituitary Gland and Its Hormones

The anterior pituitary gland, or *adenohypophysis*, is the master gland of the entire endocrine system. It contains several different types of cells, each of which secretes specific hormones. Each kind of cell is stimulated to release its secretions by so-called releasing factors that are produced by nerve cells of the hypothalamus at the base of the brain. These controlling nerve cells are themselves influenced in turn by hormones carried back to the brain from various of the other endocrine glands (Fig. 35-1). We shall now discuss each of the anterior pituitary hormones and indicate how its functions affect other endocrine glands and metabolic processes.

THE ADRENOCORTICOTROPIC* HORMONE (CORTICOTROPIN; ACTH)

This hormone, which influences the functioning of the adrenal glands, is produced, stored, and secreted by specific pituitary gland cells. Its release is stimulated by chemical signals from the hypothalamic portion of the brain. The hypothalamus secretes a neurohormone called the corticotropin releasing factor (CRF) that is channeled directly to the pituitary cells. The *corticotropin* that is then released is carried to the outer coat, or cortex, of the adrenal glands, where its action increases the production of the several kinds of adrenocortical steroid hormones (Fig. 17-1).

These adrenal steroids, when they reach certain levels in the bloodstream, tend in turn to regulate the further secretion of corticotropin by the pituitary gland. When the circulating steroids reach the brain, they suppress the secretion of CRF. Deprived of this stimulus, the pituitary cells stop secreting stored corticotropin. This *negative feedback mechanism* from the adrenal glands, in turn, shuts off adrenocortical hormone production.

* The suffix *tropic* (or *trophic*) indicates that the anterior pituitary hormone influences the functioning of the endocrine gland that is referred to in the prefix portion of the name.

In times of physical and emotional stress, the hypothalamic-pituitary secretion mechanism is *not* turned off by the usual amounts of adrenal hormones reaching the brain by way of the bloodstream. The continued outpouring of pituitary and adrenal hormones then helps the body to meet and to overcome the stressful situation. However, patients who have been treated for various diseases (Table 17-1) with high doses of adrenocortical steroids may suffer suppression of pituitary production of corticotropin. This then can result in atrophy of the adrenal glands and thus subject the steroid-treated patient to the danger of adrenal insufficiency and failure.

The therapeutic uses of corticotropin+ (ACTH) and its current clinical status are discussed in Chapter 17 and elsewhere.

THE GONADOTROPIC HORMONES

The anterior pituitary gland produces two hormones that affect the functioning of the male and female sex glands, or gonads. These are: (1) the follicle-stimulating hormone (FSH); and (2) the luteinizing or interstitial cell-stimulating hormone (LH or ICSH). A third pituitary hormone, called *prolactin* or *luteotropin* (LTH), which stimulates the ovaries of some animal species, acts in humans on the female breasts rather than on the sex glands (Fig. 35-1).

THE FOLLICLE-STIMULATING HORMONE. FSH is first secreted at puberty, when a preset "biological clock" within the brain makes the hypothalamus increase its secretion of a neurohormone that stimulates certain pituitary cells to produce this gonadotropic hormone. In boys, this hormone stimulates the seminiferous tubules of the testes to develop and to produce spermatozoa, the male reproductive cells. In girls, FSH stimulates growth of the ovarian follicles, or egg sacs.

Stimulation of the follicles by FSH not only causes ripening and release of an ovum or ova but also results in the secretion of a type of female sex hormones called *estrogens*. These ovarian hormones act at puberty to turn an immature girl into a woman capable of bearing children. In addition, the monthly ebb and flow of FSH and the estrogens continue to influence the woman's menstrual cycle all through the reproductive years of her life.

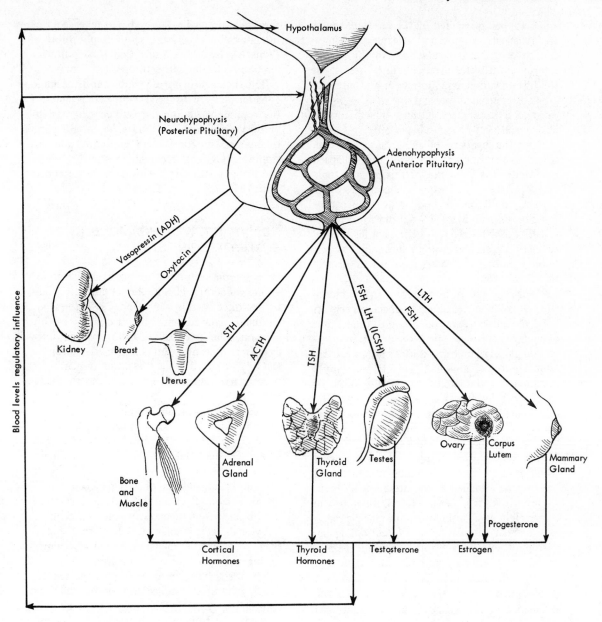

Fig. 35-1. The pituitary gland and its interrelationships with the brain and peripheral target tissues.

THE LUTEINIZING HORMONE. The production of the second gonadotropic hormone, LH, is influenced by ovarian estrogens. As the level of these female hormones rises during the first half of the menstrual cycle, they act: (1) to suppress the production and secretion of FSH by a negative feedback mechanism on the hypothalamus, and the pituitary gland; and (2)

to increase the pituitary's production of LH, which then exerts its special gonadotropic action on the ripening ovarian follicle.

Under the influence of the rising tide of LH, the wall of the follicle becomes thinner and thinner. Then, midway in the average 28-day cycle, the combined action of a sudden added spurt of LH and the small amount of

FSH still being secreted by the pituitary causes the follicle to rupture and release an ovum—the process called *ovulation*. Anything that interferes with the precisely timed release of the hypothalamic neurohormones and pituitary gonadotropins may prevent the release of the ovum and thus affect fertility (see discussion of oral contraceptives in Chapter 36).

After the ovarian follicle breaks, LH continues to act upon the cells of the collapsed sac. Under the influence of this gonadotropic hormone, the follicle capsule is converted into a thick bright orange body called the *corpus luteum* (Fig. 36-2). The continuing secretion of LH stimulates the cells of the corpus luteum to secrete a second ovarian hormone, *progesterone*, during the latter two weeks of the menstrual cycle.

The rising level of progesterone in the bloodstream exerts a negative feedback effect on the hypothalamus and on pituitary production of gonadotropins. Suppression of pituitary secretion of LH, in turn, causes the corpus luteum to shrivel and die. This then deprives the lining of the uterus, or *endometrium*, of its support by the ovarian sex steroids. The deteriorated endometrium and the unfertilized ovum leave the body during the process of *menstruation* that then begins.

However, if the ovum has been fertilized while in the oviducts, or fallopian tubes, and has become attached to the uterine wall, menstruation does not occur. This is because the corpus luteum continues to produce progesterone under stimulation by a *luteotropic* gonadotropin. This gonadotropic hormone is produced *not* by the anterior pituitary gland but by the early pregnancy tissues, or trophoblast, that eventually form the placenta, or *chorion*. (Detection of this gonadotropic hormone in a woman's urine is the basis of a pregnancy test.)

This *non*pituitary gonadotropin, called *human chorionic gonadotropin (HCG)*, is obtained from the urine of pregnant women and purified. It is used clinically to aid in bringing about ovulation in some infertile women by means of its luteinizing action. HCG is also used in treating some *male* patients with testicular failure that is caused by a deficiency of the pituitary gonadotropin LH. Ordinarily, LH is released by the anterior pituitary gland of boys at puberty and begins to stimulate the testes to produce the male hormone, *testosterone*. Specifically, this gonadotropin stimulates

the cells of Leydig, located in the spaces (or interstices) between the seminiferous tubules. (This is why LH is also called *ICSH*, the interstitial cell-stimulating hormone.)

The therapeutic use of pituitary and chorionic gonadotropins with FSH and LH activity in the treatment of infertile women who fail to produce ova is discussed in Chapter 36. The therapeutic use of human chorionic gonadotropin (HCG) in secondary testicular failure and in boys with cryptorchism, or undescended testicle, is taken up in Chapter 37.

HUMAN GROWTH HORMONE (HGH; SOMATOTROPIN; STH)

One anterior pituitary hormone acts, not on other endocrine glands, but upon all body tissues directly. This substance, *somatotropin*, stimulates growth, and when a child lacks this hormone, he may suffer from *hypopituitary dwarfism*. Recently, human growth hormone (HGH) extracted from the pituitary glands of corpses has become available in small quantities.

The injection of small doses of HGH three times weekly for several years has helped several hundred dwarfed adolescents develop to the height of small but normal adults. The main side effect of this substance is its tendency to antagonize the effects of the pancreatic hormone, *insulin*. Because this antiinsulin action may bring about diabetes in some susceptible individuals, all patients must have their blood sugar and glucose tolerance tested frequently during the course of HGH treatment.

Scientists have been trying to determine which part of the molecule is responsible for stimulating growth. They might then be able to separate it from the diabetes-producing component. If the growth-producing fragment can then also be synthesized, it would be available for clinical use in unlimited amounts.

THYROID-STIMULATING HORMONE (THYROTROPIN; TSH)

The anterior pituitary gland secretes a tropic hormone that affects the function of the thyroid gland. This thyrotropic hormone increases the thyroid's ability to take up iodine from the blood and to use this element in making thyroid hormones. Released into the bloodstream, these thyroid secretions then stimulate the metabolism of almost all body cells.

The thyroid hormones also exert an effect upon the pituitary's production of the thyroid-stimulating hormone (TSH). When their blood level rises even slightly above normal, these thyroid hormones tend to suppress further secretion of thyrotropin by their negative feedback effect. The reverse is also true: if the blood level of thyroid hormones drops below a certain point, the hypothalamus signals the anterior pituitary gland to increase its production and secretion of thyrotropin.

Thyrotropin has been prepared in a highly purified form from the pituitary glands of animals (cows and bulls). Although it has only limited therapeutic uses, such a preparation can be quite useful diagnostically in determining whether a hypothyroid person's thyroid gland has the ability to respond to stimulation by the TSH produced by his own pituitary. If his thyroid gland does, indeed, respond to injection of the bovine pituitary gland preparation by increasing its production of thyroid hormones, his hypothyroid condition may be caused by the decreased secretion of thyrotropin by his pituitary gland (*secondary* hypothyroidism), rather than by a *primary* thyroid gland deficiency.

The clinical status of thyrotropin in diagnosis and treatment is discussed in Chapter 38.

The Posterior Pituitary Gland and Its Hormones

The posterior lobe of the pituitary body, or *neurohypophysis*, stores secretions that are made by certain nerve cells of the hypothalamus. The same hypothalamic nerve fibers that transport these neurosecretions to the pituitary storage sites also send down the signals that release these hormones into the bloodstream. The two main types of posterior pituitary hormones that then affect the functioning of peripheral target tissues are: (1) the oxytocic hormone, *oxytocin* and (2) the antidiuretic hormone (ADH), *vasopressin*.

Oxytocin causes smooth muscle fibers in the uterus and breast to contract. The application of these actions in clinical therapeutics is discussed in Chapter 47.

Vasopressin that is released by the posterior pituitary is carried by the bloodstream to the kidneys, where it acts upon certain renal tubular cells to increase their ability to reabsorb water from the glomerular filtrate. Those who lack this hormone suffer from a disorder called *diabetes insipidus*, which is marked by the loss of large amounts of dilute urine. This condition may be treated with several available preparations with *antidiuretic hormone* (ADH) activity.

Extracts of the posterior pituitary glands of animals have been employed to keep patients with diabetes insipidus from becoming dehydrated. Patients with a relatively mild form of this disease may keep it under control by inhaling a powdered form of the extract through the nose for systemic absorption from the nasal mucous membranes. The more potent *posterior pituitary injection* (Pituitrin) is needed for more severe cases. However, when injections are necessary, most specialists now prefer to use the purer form of the hormone, *vasopressin injection* (Pitressin), or a longer-lasting preparation, *vasopressin tannate injection* (Pitressin tannate) (see Table 35-1).

Administered in proper dosage at optimal intervals, all these forms of the antidiuretic hormone are effective for reducing the large volume of urine voided daily (*polyuria*). However, overdosage can lead to *fluid retention* and excessive loss of sodium (*hyponatremia*). Patients are watched for such signs of water intoxication as drowsiness and mental confusion. If this occurs, the hormone is withheld until the patient's production of urine rises again to abnormal levels. Treatment is resumed at reduced dosage and less frequent intervals.

Other adverse effects of posterior pituitary extracts, including vasopressin, may occur as the result of contraction of the smooth muscles of the intestine (cramps and diarrhea), uterus, and blood vessels. Constriction of arterial smooth muscle may cause a mild rise in blood pressure. More serious is constriction of the coronary arteries of patients with angina pectoris, as it may set off chest pains or even cause an acute coronary attack. Thus, these preparations are administered cautiously in the smallest dose effective for control of diabetes insipidus when the patient also suffers from disease of the coronary arteries.

Patients occasionally become allergic to the foreign protein in even purified extracts of animal glands. This can be avoided by use of a recently introduced synthetic substance with

TABLE 35-1   *Pituitary Gland Hormones and Synthetic Substitutes*

Official or Generic Name	Trade Name or Synonym	Dosage and Administration	Remarks
Anterior Pituitary Hormone Activity			
Corticotropin injection U.S.P.	Acthar; ACTH	25–40 units I.M., or s.c. t.i.d. 10–25 units I.V. infusion in 500 ml of 5% glucose	See *Drug Digest* (Chapter 17)
Corticotropin injection, repository U.S.P.	H.P. Acthar Gel	25–40 units I.M., or s.c. every 24–72 hours	Long-acting form
Corticotropin zinc hydroxide, sterile suspension U.S.P.	Cortrophin-Zinc	20–60 units I.M., or s.c. every 24–72 hours	Long-acting form
Chorionic gonadotropin for injection U.S.P.	Human chorionic gonadotropin; HCG	1,000–10,000 units, depending upon the indication for its use	Has LH, or ICSH activity
Growth hormone, human	HGH; somatotropin; STH	2–5 mg s.c. three times a week	Used for treatment of pituitary dwarfism
Menotropins	Pergonal; HMG; human menopausal urinary gonadotropin	75 units of FSH and 75 units of LH daily for 9–12 days	Follicle-stimulating hormone from the human pituitary. Used in treatment of female sterility as an ovulatory agent (Chap. 36)
Thyrotropin N.F.	Thytropar	10 units I.M., or s.c. daily for one to eight days, depending upon the indication for its use	Thyrotropic activity; used to stimulate the thyroid gland in diagnostic and therapeutic procedures
Posterior Pituitary Activity			
Lypressin	Diapid Nasal Spray	One or two sprays to one or both nostrils	Synthetic lysine-8-vasopressin
Oxytocin injection U.S.P.	Pitocin; Syntocinon; Uteracon	2 to 10 units I.M., I.V., or by I.V. infusion depending upon the specific indication	Used for its oxytocic effect in the induction and management of labor and postpartum hemorrhage
Oxytocin, synthetic	Syntocinon Nasal Spray	One spray into one nostril	Used for its galactokinetic effect to make breast milk more readily available
Posterior pituitary injection N.F.	Pituitrin injection	5–10 units I.M.	Contains the activity of the antidiuretic hormone (ADH)
Posterior pituitary N.F.	Pituitrin powder	Variable	(Same as above)
Vasopressin injection U.S.P.	Pitressin	5–10 units I.M. or s.c. or by intranasal application, three or four times daily	Purified antidiuretic hormone (ADH) for treating diabetes insipidus
Vasopressin tannate U.S.P.	Pitressin tannate	1.25–5 units I.M. every one to three days, or at other required intervals	Long-acting form of the antidiuretic hormone for treating diabetes insipidus

antidiuretic activity called *lypressin* (Diapid). This is applied to the nasal mucosa as a liquid nasal spray that is less irritating than the dry posterior pituitary powder. These properties tend to prevent the sneezing, and asthmatic wheezing and dyspnea, sometimes seen when the natural product is employed. However, the synthetic substance may cause some running of the nose, nasal itching, congestion, and even rare ulceration of the mucosa. Overdosage can also cause systemic effects, including fluid retention, abdominal cramps, and chest pain.

References

Randall, R.V. Treatment of diabetes insipidus. *Mod. Treatm.*, 3:180, 1966 (Jan.).

Rodman, M.J. The pituitary hormones. *RN*, 31:55, 1968 (June).

Rosenbloom, A.L. Growth hormone replacement therapy. *JAMA*, 198:364, 1966.

36.

The Female Sex Hormones

Estrogens and Progestins

The female sex glands, or ovaries, synthesize
and secrete hormones mainly of two types: (1)
the *estrogens*, and (2) the *progestins*. These
sex steroids, which are first produced in significant amounts at puberty, can be said to
control the continuation of the human species.
The estrogens bring about the changes that
turn immature girls into women and, together
with the progestins, set the stage for pregnancy
and childbearing. In addition to their direct
effects on the reproductive system, these steroids affect the functioning of other body tissues
and even possess subtle psychological actions.

These hormones and certain synthetic substances now available that share many of their
properties are widely used in gynecology and
other areas of medicine. In order to understand
their many clinical uses, it is essential that we
know what effects the natural ovarian secretions have on the various tissues that serve
as their targets. Once we have seen how the
hormones produced by the gonads of women
influence the reproductive system and the metabolism of other body tissues, we may better
comprehend the reasons for their administration as medications in the management of various clinical conditions.

We shall discuss first the physiological functions of the *estrogens*, since these are the first
female hormones produced at puberty and
are the ones secreted during the earliest part
of each monthly ovulatory cycle. Then, after
we have related various of the natural actions
of the estrogens to their therapeutic uses, we
shall examine in the same manner the *progestational steroids* that are produced in the

latter half of the ovulatory cycle and during pregnancy.

Estrogens

PHYSIOLOGICAL EFFECTS

The estrogens—principally *estradiol* and its metabolites *estrone* and *estriol*—are first produced at puberty, when the ovaries are stimulated by the pituitary gonadotropin, FSH. The estrogens released at that time stimulate the growth and development of the uterus, oviducts, vagina, and breasts. In addition, these ovarian hormones influence the metabolism of other body tissues in addition to those involved in reproductive processes.

REPRODUCTIVE TISSUES. The *uterus* grows to adult size under the influence of the flow of estrogens from the ovary at puberty. In addition to their effects on the *myometrium*, or uterine smooth muscle mass, these hormones affect the inner lining of the uterus, or *endometrium*. This tissue changes in response to the varying amounts of estrogens that reach it at different times during each monthly ovulatory cycle (Fig. 36-1).

The endometrium is most significantly affected by estrogens during the first half of the menstrual cycle. During this so-called *proliferative phase*, this inner lining of the uterus, which had been destroyed and sloughed off during the previous menstrual period, is rebuilt under the influence of follicular estrogenic hormones. The endometrial epithelium increases tenfold in thickness at this time and

its initially short glands grow into long narrow tubes. The glands in the inner lining of the *cervix*—the endocervical glands—are also stimulated to secrete a thin watery fluid, which is most profuse at the midcyclic estrogen peak.

The vaginal tract mucosa is kept thick by the action of ovarian estrogens upon its epithelium, and a reduction in the glandular secretion of these hormones at the menopause is accompanied by a thinning of these epithelial layers and an increased susceptibility to vaginal infections (see below).

The breast tissues are affected by estrogens both at puberty and during pregnancy, as well as in each ovulatory cycle. Through the complicated interactions between these and other hormones, the mammary gland ducts and alveoli (the secreting sacs) grow and develop to full functional maturity.

OTHER EFFECTS OF ESTROGENS. These female hormones also affect the skin, skeleton, fat distribution, and other metabolic functions, as well as womanly behavior. For example, estrogens seem to increase the elasticity of the skin, and the falling off of ovarian production of these hormones at the menopause may result in skin changes, including wrinkling. Similarly, the postmenopausal woman's bones tend to become thinner and weaker without the supporting actions of estrogens upon the deposit of minerals in the protein bed of the bones. Estrogens also help to retain nitrogen and turn it into body protein—*an anabolic effect* similar to that of the androgens but less potent than that of the male hormone (Chapter 37).

Pituitary gonadotropin production is subject

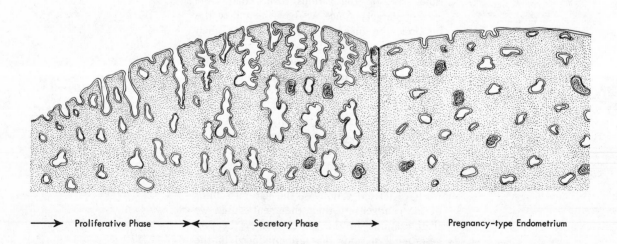

Proliferative Phase ———►◄——— Secretory Phase ———► Pregnancy-type Endometrium

Fig. 36-1. The endometrium. (*Left*) Alterations during normal ovulatory cycle. (*Right*) During pregnancy or treatment with exogenous estrogens and progestins the endometrium shows signs of secretory exhaustion.

to the negative feedback effects of estrogens (and also of *progesterone*, see p. 440). As indicated in Chapter 35, these effects upon FSH and LH play a part in such processes as ovulation and menstruation. In addition, the level of circulating estrogens has an effect upon milk production (lactation) at childbirth. All these effects of estrogens upon pituitary function have important clinical applications—for example, in the use of potent synthetic estrogens to prevent ovulation and pregnancy (see discussion of oral contraceptives, p. 445), and in their use to prevent painful breast engorgement in mothers who do not intend to nurse their newborn infants (p. 439).

THERAPEUTIC USES OF THE ESTROGENS

THE MENOPAUSE OR FEMALE CLIMACTERIC. This syndrome, which women often call "the change of life," is a physiological process that occurs most often during a woman's middle to late forties. It is set in motion by a gradual reduction in ovarian function. The resulting deficiency in estrogen secretion is accompanied by menstrual irregularities and by a variety of other more or less discomforting physical complaints and emotional symptoms.

Some women go through the menopause with relatively few symptoms and thus may not need *estrogen replacement therapy*. However, most women profit from treatment with small, physiologic doses of drugs with estrogenic activity—at least for the few months, or at most the year or two, when menopausal discomforts are at their peak. Properly individualized doses provide prompt relief of such physical symptoms as hot flushes, heart palpitations, sweating, headaches, and dizziness. Signs of mental and emotional imbalance such as sleeplessness, crying spells, and anxiety can also be controlled by estrogens administered alone or together with tranquilizer or antidepressant drugs.

When a woman discusses menopausal symptoms with the nurse, the latter should suggest consultation with a physician. The nurse can help the woman to understand the physiologic changes occurring and help her develop ways of coping with her reactions to this experience. Some women seem reluctant to visit a doctor —perhaps because they do not want to admit that they are undergoing the "change." Others are afraid that these hormones will cause toxic effects, including cancer. Actually, the side effects of estrogens are relatively few, minor, and readily controllable (see p. 439). Similarly, there is no evidence that these hormones cause cancer of the breasts or uterus in human beings. In fact, recent studies suggest that the administration of these sex steroids actually protects these tissues against the malignant changes that sometimes develop in older women. Thus, the nurse should convey this and other factual information to menopausal women in order to counteract various kinds of old wive's tales.

POSTMENOPAUSAL USE OF ESTROGENS. Some doctors advise women to continue taking estrogens indefinitely following the menopause. The reasoning behind this advocacy of prolonged postmenopausal estrogens is that these hormones exert *nonsexual* metabolic effects which play an important part in protecting the well-being of practically every tissue, organ, and system in the body. Thus, doctors claim that continued estrogenic therapy not only will help to keep breasts firm and skin supple, but may help to avoid serious disorders such as osteoporosis and coronary atherosclerosis.

Osteoporosis. This skeletal disorder, which sometimes thins the bones of elderly men as well as women, is often treated with either estrogens or androgens, or sometimes with combinations of sex steroids of both types. It is believed that the anabolic effects of the two kinds of hormones are helpful for providing the protein framework into which calcium is laid down by bone cells. Patients are also often put on a diet high in protein and milk, with supplementary calcium salts and perhaps vitamin D and fluorides.

Estrogens seem to relieve back pain caused by weakened vertebrae, even though there seems to be no clear-cut x-ray evidence that these bones are thickened or that compression fractures are less likely to occur. Nevertheless, the continued use of these hormones for preventive purposes during the postmenopausal period has been recommended as a means of keeping the bones strong and hard and less liable to fracture. Prophylactic therapy with estrogens or other anabolic steroids is considered especially desirable during treatment of menopausal or postmenopausal patients with corticosteroids.

Coronary atherosclerosis. The prophylactic use of estrogens for preventing heart attacks in both men and women has been advocated recently. The theoretical basis for this therapy is the fact that *pre*menopausal women are relatively free of coronary artery disease, whereas women who have had their ovaries removed show a sharp rise in atherosclerosis. Similarly, postmenopausal women have about the same rate of myocardial infarctions as men in the same age range (see also Chapter 30).

Actually, there is little evidence that estrogens lower plasma lipid levels or delay the development of atherosclerosis in coronary vessels. In fact, recent studies suggest that some dose levels of estrogen may actually cause an increase in blood vessel lesions and complications, with a resulting reduction in the survival time of some patients with a previous heart attack history.

Despite the uncertain status of this treatment, some doctors now prescribe estrogens for postmenopausal women not only to maintain physical and mental well-being, but also with the thought that replacement of these hormones will lessen their chances of suffering from coronary vascular disease. Estrogens employed for this purpose are probably harmless to women; however, such hormone therapy may create problems for some male patients, including such physical changes as gynecomastia (breast enlargement) and mental effects, including depression and loss of libido.

⟨ *Vaginal mucosa.* A reduction in estrogen production by the ovary is quickly reflected in a thinning of the cell layers lining the vaginal tract. A continued lack of stimulation by the female sex hormone leads to atrophic changes. This tends to increase the older woman's susceptibility to vaginitis. Thus, estrogens are often administered orally and by local application to help thicken the vaginal epithelial layers of women with *senile vaginitis.*

The nurse can help make the use of local estrogenic medications more convenient by suggesting measures for proper use of vaginal creams and suppositories. For example, it should not be assumed that patients will be aware of how to use suppositories. The nurse should suggest that this medication be refrigerated to avoid its melting in warm temperatures. She should instruct the patient to wash her hands before and after inserting the suppository and explain that the foil must be peeled off prior to insertion.

Similarly, when creams are to be applied intravaginally, or on the external genitalia for relief of itching in *pruritus vulvae* and *kraurosis vulvae*, the patient should be told how to use a perineal pad to avoid soiling clothing. The small pads with adhesive backing are espe-

cially useful. Patients treated in the doctor's office should be provided with a pad before they get dressed. Such attention to the patient's comfort and esthetic sensibilities will make it easier for her to follow through with a treatment that often seems tedious and messy.

⟨ *Skin.* Administration of estrogens to postmenopausal women has recently been claimed to produce regenerative changes in aging skin. This is part of the widely publicized and emotionally appealing claim that estrogen replacement therapy can keep women young and attractive indefinitely. Women who ask questions about such still unestablished assertions are best advised to consult their physicians concerning the desirability of long-term estrogens for them.

The doctor has to decide whether such therapy is desirable on an individual basis, following a complete physical examination and in the light of each patient's medical history.

⟨ *Female hypogonadism.* We have seen that estrogen replacement therapy is desirable during the menopause and probably all through the *post*menopausal period. The indefinitely continued use of these hormones is also desirable for maintaining the femininity and general health and well-being of young women whose ovaries have had to be removed for medical reasons.

Even more dramatic than their effects in such ovariectomized (that is, castrated) women is the response to estrogen administration in girls of adolescent age or older who have failed to develop sexually. This condition may be the result either of congenital absence of the ovaries or of the failure of the ovaries to respond to pituitary gonadotropin secretion at the time for normal onset of puberty. In either case, patients with such *sexual infantilism* are best treated with estrogens. Hormone administration induces growth and development of the accessory sex organs and development of the female secondary sex characteristics.

Such girls cannot, of course, bear children if ovaries are absent from birth, or if a normal ovulatory cycle cannot occur. They can, however, marry and have normal sexual relationships. Their *primary amenorrhea* can best be overcome by adding progestational steroids to the estrogens for a few days each month and then withdrawing both hormones for a brief period (see p. 444 for further discussion of the uses of estrogen-progestin combinations in the management of various menstrual disorders).

OTHER USES OF ESTROGENS.

❨ *Suppression of lactation.* Synthetic estrogens, such as *diethylstilbestrol+*, for example, are commonly used to overcome painful postpartum engorgement of the breasts with milk. Once the woman's breasts have been first freed of milk by pumping or by the use of oxytocin, high doses of estrogens are administered for several days to suppress production of prolactin by the pituitary gland and thus inhibit further lactation. The doctor also often has the mother wear a breast binder during these days and orders some reduction in her daily fluid intake (see also Chapter 47).

❨ *Control of height.* One of the effects of the increased flow of estrogens at puberty is to bring growth in height to a halt after a final spurt of increased growth. This happens because the sex hormones cause the cartilage at the ends of the long bones (the *epiphyses*) to be invaded by bone cells. Closure of the epiphyses stops further growth, and the girl's final adult stature is attained. However, a *lack* of female hormones as a result of ovarian failure may allow her to keep on growing. Thus, high doses of estrogens are sometimes administered well before puberty to stop expected excessive growth in girls whose personal or family history suggests this possibility.

Children who require estrogen therapy prior to puberty run the risk of having their adult height shortened. Thus, when estrogen therapy seems indicated—in treating *juvenile vaginitis,* for example—girls are treated with locally acting estrogens rather than with the systemically administered hormones. This converts the vaginal mucosa into the thicker infection-resistant adult type without setting off precocious pubertal changes or interfering with the girl's further growth in height.

❨ *Antiandrogenic effects.* Estrogens are sometimes used to counteract the effects of the male hormone on various body tissues. The use of female hormones for treating men with advanced prostatic carcinoma, a type of malignant tumor that grows under the influence of the male hormone, is discussed in Chapter 48.

Acne and growth of hair on the face and body (*hirsutism*) have also been related to excessive androgens in women as well as in male patients. The use of female hormones as a treatment measure for acne is discussed in Chapter 46.

ADVERSE EFFECTS (SEE ALSO SUMMARY, P. 448)

GASTROINTESTINAL. The most common complaint of women taking large doses of estrogens (especially the synthetic type such as diethylstilbestrol) is a tendency toward loss of appetite, nausea, and even vomiting and diarrhea. Such symptoms are similar to those of early pregnancy, and, like the latter, they tend to disappear as the patient becomes tolerant of the gastrointestinal side effects of the female hormones. These symptoms or the headaches and dizziness of which a few patients sometimes complain rarely require permanent withdrawal of estrogen therapy.

Breakthrough bleeding, or spotting, sometimes occurs in women taking relatively low doses of estrogens. This can often be prevented by raising the dose. However, high doses of estrogens administered for long intervals can also cause irregular uterine bleeding. This is best avoided by withdrawing estrogenic medication for a week or so after several weeks of treatment. Often, a normal menstrual period occurs during such a rest period. (Predictable *cyclic bleeding* of this kind can be assured by taking a progestational steroid together with the estrogen for the last few days before both sex hormones are withdrawn, as described below.

Postmenopausal women who are placed on cyclic estrogen therapy should understand that they will have a menstrual period when the hormones are withdrawn every few weeks. It should be explained that this is actually *pseudo-menstruation* and that they have not been made fertile once more and likely to become pregnant. They should, of course, be cautioned to report any bleeding that occurs while the drug is being administered, so that the doctor can make a pelvic examination and rule out the possibility of bleeding from an organic lesion.

CANCER. Estrogens are not known to cause cancer in human patients. However, if a breast or cervical tissue tumor is already present, these hormones may stimulate their growth. Thus, caution is required in women with a personal or family history of malignancies. Estrogens are *contraindicated* in *pre*menopausal women with breast or genital cancer. However, as indicated in Chapter 46, estrogens are sometimes useful for symptomatic relief of advanced mammary carcinoma in women who are at least five years past the menopause.

TYPES OF ESTROGENS (SEE TABLE 36-1)

All available estrogens exert the same effects but vary in their potency, onset and duration of action, and method of administration. Those that are effective upon oral administration, including *conjugated estrogens+* (Premarin) and the synthetic *nonsteroid* estrogenic chemical, *diethylstilbestrol+*, are preferred for most purposes because of their convenience and the ease with which their effects can be predicted and controlled. The injectable esters of the natural hormone *estradiol valerate+* have a very prolonged duration of action. This makes them useful for treating cancers that respond to estrogen therapy. However, they are a suitable substitute for oral medication in only a relatively few special situations.

Progesterone and the Synthetic Progestins

Progesterone is an ovarian hormone that is secreted by the corpus luteum in the last half of each menstrual month under the influence of the pituitary gonadotropin, LH. Its effects upon the endometrium prepare the uterine lining for pregnancy. If pregnancy does occur, the corpus luteum, and later the placenta, continue to pour out progesterone, which plays an essential part in maintaining the pregnancy.

Progesterone and various synthetic steroids with progestational activity—called *progestins* or *progestogens*—have important therapeutic applications. Before discussing the uses of these substances in treating many kinds of menstrual disorders and for dealing with problems related to female fertility, we shall first briefly review the physiological effects of the natural hormone, *progesterone*.

PHYSIOLOGICAL EFFECTS

ACTIONS ON THE UTERUS. Progesterone acts upon both the thick muscle mass of the uterus and on its inner mucous lining in ways that are significant for the survival of the fertilized ovum and the embryo. The endometrial actions of progesterone prepare the uterine mucosa for reception and implantation of the egg, and the quieting effect of this luteal secretion on the

TABLE 36-1 *Natural and Synthetic Estrogens*

Nonproprietary or Official Name	Proprietary Name	Usual Dosage
Natural Steroid Estrogens and Derivatives		
Estradiol N.F.	Aquadiol; Diogyn; Ovocyclin; Progynon; and others	250 μg
Estradiol benzoate N.F.	Diogyn B; Progynon B; and others	1 mg I.M.
Estradiol cypionate N.F.	Depo-Estradiol	1–5 mg I.M., every four weeks
Estradiol dipropionate N.F.	Dimenformon dipropionate, and others	1 mg I.M.
Estradiol valerate U.S.P.	Delestrogen	10–40 mg
Estriol	Theelol	240 μg
Estrogenic substances, conjugated, U.S.P.	Premarin; and others	0.3–2.5 mg
Estrone N.F.	Theelin; and others	1 mg I.M.
Ethinyl estradiol U.S.P.	Estinyl; and others	0.01–0.5 mg
Mestranol	Ethinyl estradiol-3-methyl ether	100 μg
Piperazine estrone sulfate	Sulestrex	1.5 mg
Nonsteroid Synthetic Estrogens		
Benzestrol N.F.	Chemestrogen	2.5 mg
Chlortrianisene N.F.	Tace	24 mg
Dienestrol N.F.	Synestrol; and others	0.5 mg
Diethylstilbestrol U.S.P.	Stilbestrol; Stilbetin; DES	0.1–25 mg
Diethylstilbestrol dipropionate N.F.	Stilbestrol D.P.	0.5–5 mg
Hexestrol	Esta-Plex; and others	0.2–3 mg
Methallenestril	Vallestril	3–20 mg
Promethestrol dipropionate	Meprane	1 mg

myometrium keeps the embryo from being dislodged by muscular contractions of the uterus.

The *endometrium*, which has been previously primed by the proliferative effects of the estrogens, undergoes so-called *secretory* changes under the influence of progesterone. Its glands multiply rapidly and secrete large amounts of glycogen, a carbohydrate that will serve as the first source of energy for the rapidly dividing fertilized ovum. The accumulating secretions fill the glands and make them swell and twist into corkscrew shapes that give the pregravid endometrium a characteristic lacelike appearance in microscopic cross-section (Fig. 36-1).

The *myometrium* tends to relax under the influence of progesterone. Such suppression of rhythmic uterine contractions favors implantation of the fertilized egg and, later, protects the placenta from being dislodged and, with the embryo, expelled prematurely. Throughout fetal development progesterone continues to counteract uterine spasms that could lead to spontaneous abortion. Finally, a falling off in progesterone production late in pregnancy is thought to play a part in initiating labor, since lack of this hormone may sensitize the myometrium to the contractile effects of oxytocin (Chapter 47).

PITUITARY ACTIONS OF PROGESTERONE. Like the estrogens, progesterone acts to suppress the secretion of pituitary gonadotropins. Late in the menstrual month, the progesterone produced by the corpus luteum reaches levels that inhibit the hypothalamic cells which control pituitary secretion of the luteinizing hormone. This, in turn, causes regression of the corpus luteum, a fall in further production of progesterone and finally, the failure of the secretory endometrium, which leads to its desquamation during menstruation (Fig. 36-2).

If the ovum is fertilized, the corpus luteum is stimulated by chorionic gonadotropin and later by the placenta. It continues to produce progesterone, and the high levels of this hormone keep the secretion of the pituitary gonadotropins FSH and LH suppressed. This negative feedback effect of progesterone stops production of ova by the ovaries during pregnancy, a fact that first led scientists to study

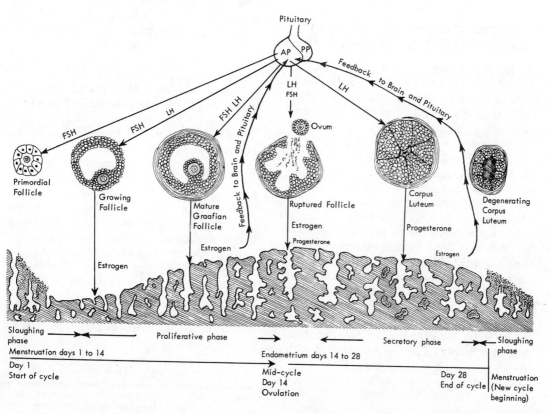

Fig. 36-2. Changes in the endometrium and ovary during the menstrual cycle.

the possibility that administration of this "pregnancy supporting" hormone might have contraceptive effects.

OTHER EFFECTS OF PROGESTERONE.

《 *The breasts*. During pregnancy this hormone acts upon the secretory sacs of the mammary glands, causing them to grow and to fill with fluid. However, when milk production (*lactation*) occurs at the time of the baby's birth, progesterone and estrogen levels are relatively low. In fact, the postpartum administration of these sex steroids in pharmacological doses *suppresses* lactation. This may occur because these ovarian hormones inhibit production of the pituitary hormone, *prolactin*, or because of their direct antisecretory effects upon the postpartum breasts.

《 *Body temperature*. Progesterone plays a part in producing an increase in body temperature at the time of ovulation midway in the menstrual cycle. Women who want to be aware of when they ovulate, in order to know the time when they are most fertile, are often instructed in how to chart their daily temperature and thus detect the rise that indicates the release of an ovum.

THERAPEUTIC USES OF PROGESTERONE AND THE PROGESTINS

When progesterone first became available, gynecologists tried to employ it in the treatment of menstrual and reproductive difficulties that stemmed from a lack of the natural hormone. They reasoned that many women failed to menstruate, or bled excessively, because a deficiency of endogenous progesterone led to endometrial abnormalities. Similarly, many women with no organic defects of the reproductive tract remained childless as a result of deficient production of this hormone.

In practice, progesterone proved disappointing. Although the hormone seemed useful in some menstrual disorders and in certain selected cases of endocrine infertility and habitual or threatened abortion, the need to administer either massive oral doses or frequent painful injections put severe practical limitations upon the use of the natural hormone. Many of these difficulties seem to have been eliminated with the advent of the synthetic progestins.

Some of these progestins are preferred to others for various clinical uses because they possess properties that make them superior for particular purposes. Thus, few of the synthetic progestins are purely progestational. Some have, in addition, slight estrogenic or androgenic (male hormone) actions, which affect their suitability for treating various conditions. However, all these compounds are sufficiently similar to permit certain generalizations about their utility in the clinical situations we shall discuss here.

MENSTRUAL DISORDERS. The menstrual cycle requires the sequential production of estrogens and progesterone by the ovary under the influence of the pituitary gonadotropins, FSH and LH. The two sex steroids, in turn, affect the endometrium in ways that prepare it for pregnancy or result in menstruation. If any link in the timed production and release of the gonadotropins or the ovarian hormones fails, various kinds of menstrual disturbances may result. These include: (1) *hypermenorrhea* (excessive uterine bleeding);* (2) *amenorrhea* (the absence of menstruation); and (3) *dysmenorrhea* (painful menstruation).

In all of these conditions, and in others such as *endometriosis* and *premenstrual tension*, the introduction of convenient, orally effective synthetic progestins has led to better control. Combined with estrogens, or administered alternately with them in accordance with the principles of menstrual cycle physiology, the progestins seem to help correct many of the hormonal imbalances responsible for menstrual abnormalities.

《 *Uterine bleeding*. Hemorrhage from the uterus may be the result of an organic lesion. The gynecologist always makes an examination to rule out this possibility before employing estrogens or progestins. These medications are used only for controlling bleeding that is the result of glandular disturbances. *Dysfunctional bleeding* of this kind occurs most commonly at puberty and at the menopause, when the ovaries are most likely to secrete sex hormones irregularly and in less than normal amounts.

Acute bleeding can often be controlled by estrogens or androgens, but hemostasis is best accomplished today by administering an oral progestogen such as *norethindrone*+ (Norlutin). When given by mouth several times a day for a week or two, this drug (and other progestins)

---

* It is important to distinguish between two types of uterine hemorrhage: (1) *menorrhagia*, which is marked by excessive blood loss during a normal menstrual period; and (2) *metrorrhagia*, a term which refers to bleeding at irregular intervals at times other than menstrual periods.

repairs the necrotic endometrial areas. Then, the withdrawal of the progestational steroids at the end of that time is followed by shedding of the endometrium, with what appears to be essentially normal bleeding. Such a hormone-induced removal of the uterine mucous membrane frequently does away with the need for dilatation and curettage, a procedure considered undesirable in young unmarried women. Often after several such intermittent "medical curettage" treatments with a progestin or with combined estrogens and progestins, the woman's normal cycles are reestablished and excessive bleeding episodes no longer occur.

To prevent recurrences, it is desirable to use the sex steroids in ways that imitate their release by the ovary in a normal ovulatory cycle. Often, bleeding is the result of the ovary's failure to produce enough progesterone in proportion to estrogen secretion. This may occur when there is no ovulation and consequently no formation of a corpus luteum (Fig. 36-2). In such an *anovulatory* cycle, the proliferative endometrium is not converted to the secretory form. This leads to irregular and, often, prolonged and excessive bleeding from an endometrium that fails to slough off. Regular menstrual bleeding can be brought about by the administration and withdrawal of a progestin in such cases.

❮[*Amenorrhea* may have many causes. Failure to menstruate can be entirely physiological—in pregnancy, for example, or following the menopause; absence of menstruation may, on the other hand, be secondary to many systemic diseases and endocrine malfunctions. Once the cause has been determined by a variety of diagnostic tests, treatment to establish normal menstrual bleeding can be undertaken. The new and potent synthetic progestins are often useful for both the diagnosis and treatment of amenorrhea.

In a normal menstrual cycle, female sex hormones of both types must be secreted in adequate amounts and exert their sequential proliferative and secretory effects upon the endometrium. Then, when ovarian secretion drops off late in the menstrual month, the mucous membrane breaks down and menstruation occurs.

❮[*Diagnostic test for endogenous estrogen production.* To determine whether the ovaries of a patient with amenorrhea are capable of producing estrogens, the doctor may administer a progestational steroid (see Table 36-2). Since this produces a secretory endometrium and withdrawal bleeding only when the endometrium has first been primed by estrogens, failure to menstruate indicates that the patient's ovaries are not producing enough natural estrogen. Bleeding a week or so after withdrawal shows that her ovaries *can* secrete enough estrogen to produce a proliferative endometrium.

❮[*Diagnostic test for endogenous progesterone production (pregnancy test).* If a patient is producing estrogen, the administration and withdrawal of a progestin will produce menstrual bleeding. Failure to menstruate means that the corpus luteum is still producing

---

TABLE 36-2 *Progestational Steroids*

Nonproprietary Name	Proprietary Name or Synonym	Dosage Range
Chlormadinone acetate N.F.	Lormin	2–20 mg
Dydrogesterone N.F.	Duphaston	5–30 mg
Ethisterone N.F.	Ethinyl testosterone; Pranone; Progesterol; and others	25–100 mg
Ethynodiol diacetate U.S.P.	In Ovulen	1 mg
Hydroxyprogesterone acetate	Prodox	25–50 mg
Hydroxyprogesterone caproate U.S.P.	Delalutin	250 mg I.M.
Medroxyprogesterone acetate U.S.P.	Provera	2.5–40 mg
Norethindrone U.S.P.	Norethisterone; Norlutin	5–30 mg
Norethindrone acetate N.F.	Norlutate	2.5–15 mg
Norethynodrel U.S.P.	In Enovid	2.5–30 mg
Progesterone N.F.	Colprosterone; Lipo-Lutin; Lucorteum; Lutocylin; and others	10–25 mg

progesterone. This occurs because the corpus luteum is still being stimulated by a gonadotropic hormone, the *chorionic* gonadotropin that is released by the trophoblastic tissues. Thus, when a woman who receives a combination of estrogen and a progestin fails to menstruate a few days after withdrawal of the hormones, she is most probably pregnant.

(*Amenorrhea treatment.* In both *primary* amenorrhea—the kind seen in a *hypo*gonadal girl who has never menstruated—and in *secondary* amenorrhea, which occurs in women who have previously menstruated, the two types of female hormones may be administered cyclically to bring about menstruation. In girls and women who do not have functioning ovaries, combination therapy of this kind must be continued indefinitely. In secondary amenorrhea, however, several such artificial cycles are often followed by a return of normal cyclic function and menstruation.

(*Dysmenorrhea.* Many women with no evidence of organic pelvic disease suffer disabling uterine cramps during their menstrual periods. Numerous drugs, including analgesics, sedatives, and antispasmodics are employed for symptomatic relief, and a variety of hormones including thyroid, insulin, and even the male hormone have been tried. However, all drug treatments and even the ovarian uterus-relaxing hormones, lututrin and progesterone, have offered only inconsistent relief.

Progesterone injections just prior to the menstrual period were first employed as replacement therapy on the assumption that the uterine contractions in this condition are the result of a lack of this myometrium-quieting hormone. This *premenstrual* progesterone treatment did not help many patients. However, the oral administration of either synthetic progestins or estrogens, or a combination of the two steroids, *early* in the menstrual month, has recently been reported to be followed by painless menstruation after withdrawal.

(*Premenstrual edema and tension.* Many women tend to retain fluid as their menstrual periods approach. Weight gain, painful breast fullness, backache, and headache are some of the physical complaints in this premenstrual condition. In addition, some women suffer from emotional upsets of varying intensity. Although its cause is uncertain, some physicians have suggested that this syndrome results from inadequate production of progesterone by the corpus luteum and a resulting relative excess of fluid-retaining estrogens.

The new oral progestins have been administered as replacement therapy, alone or combined with oral diuretics and sedatives, during the latter half of the menstrual month. This regimen has been claimed to be effective for relief of premenstrual crankiness and irritability as well as for removal of retained fluid.

Progestin-estrogen combinations administered early in the menstrual cycle have also proved effective for counteracting premenstrual distress. As in the dysmenorrhea treatment mentioned above, the benefits may stem from suppression of ovulation.

(*Endometriosis.* Until recently, severe endometriosis was treated mainly by surgical removal of the ovaries and uterus. Such hysterectomy and castration, of course, halted the disease but also ended the woman's childbearing years and brought about a premature menopause. Today, this serious condition is being successfully treated by the continuous administration of progestins, alone or combined with estrogens, for many months. Such a regimen not only prevents the painful menstruation of this condition but also often leads to regression of the growths within the abdomen.

(*Spontaneous abortion.* This occurs in about 10 percent of all pregnancies and thus accounts for the termination of very many desired pregnancies. Some women abort repeatedly, and those who have had three or more consecutive miscarriages are termed "habitual" or "recurrent" aborters. Progesterone has been employed in such cases for many years, on the assumption that at least some abortions result from a failure of the placenta to secrete enough of the hormone to keep the uterus quiet. Administered in large and frequent doses all through pregnancy, progesterone is claimed to counteract the contractile effects of estrogens on the myometrium and thus to prevent premature expulsion of the embryo or fetus from the uterus.

Some of the synthetic progestins are claimed to be even more effective than progesterone itself for maintaining pregnancies in patients who have aborted habitually and for other women when staining and uterine cramps indicate that abortion is a threat. For example, daily administration of oral doses of medroxyprogesterone acetate during pregnancy is claimed to have helped to salvage fetuses. A long-acting ester derivative, *hydroxyprogesterone acetate*+, which requires less frequent injection than the natural luteal hormone, is also claimed to be helpful for maintenance of pregnancies. Thus, although there is still some controversy as to whether treatment with progesterone and its derivatives is truly more effective in threatened abortion than bed rest and sedation alone, many doctors now feel that the use of the new synthetic progestins is worth a trial when a woman who badly wants her baby seems in danger of losing it.

INFERTILITY. Progestins have been employed in attempts to increase the fertility of women who have failed to become pregnant. The new synthetic steroids seem to have proved most effective in those women whose infertility can be traced back to a poorly functioning corpus luteum that fails to produce enough progesterone to maintain an adequate secretory endometrium. The administration of small daily oral doses of synthetic progestins (combined with estrogens) during the *post*ovulatory phase of the menstrual cycle is claimed to have helped some women with luteal phase defects to conceive and bear children.

In such cases of infertility, the progestins serve as *substitutional therapy.* That is, when administered daily from the time when a rise in the woman's body temperature indicates that ovulation has occurred, these synthetic hormones supplement the patient's own inadequate progesterone production. Under their influence, the woman's proliferative endometrium is converted into the secretory type that is capable of receiving and nourishing a fertilized egg. Repetition of such steroid replacement therapy during several menstrual cycles eventually leads to pregnancy, provided that the woman with luteal phase deficiency is capable of producing an ovum, and that viable sperm reach it during its descent through the oviduct.

ANOVULATION. Progestins have also been used to treat women whose infertility stems from failure to ovulate. This may seem strange, since the ovarian sex steroids themselves *suppress* ovulation (see discussion of oral contraceptives, below). However, it has been suggested that, after withdrawal of progestin therapy, there may be an increased production of the pituitary gonadotropins FSH and LH that stimulate the ovaries to produce ova.

Recently, infertility resulting from anovulation has also been treated with products containing gonadotropins obtained from the urine of women. In one type of treatment, the infertile woman is first treated with *menotropins* (Pergonal), a product rich in gonadotropins (including FSH), which is obtained from the urine of postmenopausal women. After these injections have stimulated the patient's ovarian follicles to mature, she also receives injections of *human chorionic gonadotropin* (HCG). This hormone, which is obtained from the urine of pregnant women, is high in the activity of the gonadotropin LH. This causes the ripened follicle of the ovary to rupture and release its ovum (Fig. 36-2), which may then be fertilized during its passage down the oviduct.

Clomiphene citrate (Clomid), an orally effective drug, has also been used to treat infertility by inducing ovulation. This agent is *neither* a female sex steroid *nor* a gonadotropic hormone. It is thought to act by stimulating the patient's own pituitary gland to produce the gonadotropins necessary for ovulation.

Both these types of treatment have helped some women to conceive and to bear children. However, undesirable effects may result from overstimulation of the patient's ovaries. There has been, for example, an unusually high number of multiple births in these patients. Another complication has been the development of painfully enlarged ovaries and ovarian cysts. Thus, patients should receive frequent pelvic examinations to determine whether treatment must be discontinued in order to prevent ovarian enlargement and cystic rupture.

Oral Contraceptives

Progestins and estrogens are employed most commonly in combinations that are intended to prevent conception. Taken daily in one of two types of course schedules (see below), these steroids come close to being 100 percent effective for pregnancy prevention. Because of its ability to regularize the menstrual cycle, this treatment even permits more effective utilization of the so-called rhythm method of birth control by women with highly irregular cycles.*

MANNER OF ACTION

These sex steroids produce their contraceptive effects by suppressing ovulation, brought about by their ability to inhibit gonadotropic hormone release by the pituitary gland. The presence of the progestin, in addition to producing menstrual bleeding upon withdrawal, has other effects that would tend to prevent conception even if ovulation were to occur. Like the natural hormone progesterone, these synthetic steroids stimulate production of a thick secretion by the endocervical glands that prevents passage of sperm cells into the uterus, and its continued use causes atrophic changes in the endometrium, which would make it difficult for a fertilized egg to be implanted (Fig. 36-2).

PREPARATIONS AND THEIR ADMINISTRATION

The various products listed in Table 36-3 consist of: (1) a potent estrogen, either *ethinyl estradiol* or its derivative, *mestranol*; and (2) any one of many progestins. These are administered in one of two types of courses. (1) Most commonly a single tablet containing both steroids is taken for 20 or 21 days consecutively beginning on the fifth day of the menstrual cycle (day one is the first day of menstruation). Then, for the final seven days of the cycle, the patient takes *no* tablet or one containing therapeutically inert material. (2) Products may be taken which consist of two types of tablets—one containing only an estrogen, which the woman takes for from 14 to 16 days beginning on the fifth day of the cycle, and a second containing the same estrogen *combined* with a progestin that is taken for the following five to seven days (the *sequential method*).

With both the combined and sequential products, menstruation usually occurs within a few days after withdrawal of the active medication. Both types of products come in convenient packages containing color-coded tablets to help patients keep track of tablet taking. Patients are told to follow the recommended dosage schedule very closely, and it is suggested that the medication be taken at the same time daily.

ADVERSE EFFECTS (SEE SUMMARY, P. 449)

The most common undesirable effects resemble those of early pregnancy, and, like the latter, they tend to diminish or disappear after several monthly cycles. These include nausea and vomiting, headache and dizziness, weight gain, breast fullness and discomfort and, occasionally, acne and *chloasma* (an increase in skin pigmentation). Another reaction that some women find frightening and confusing is the occurrence of breakthrough bleeding, or spotting, during their cycle, or, on the other hand, failure to menstruate upon withdrawal of the drugs at the end of the cycle.

Despite these distressing symptoms, many women continue taking oral contraceptives through the first few cycles, after which—as in pregnancy—nausea and other discomforts lessen. Most side effects are, in any case, controllable. Nausea, for example, can be reduced by taking the tablet at bedtime with a glass of milk. Breakthrough bleeding can be overcome by *increasing* the steroid dosage to prevent premature endometrial breakdown.

LONG-TERM SAFETY. Although no truly toxic effects have been traced to these steroid combinations, serious concern has often been expressed as to the possible adverse results of prolonged administration of these drugs. Doctors are still studying the long-range effects of these medications on glandular function and reproductive capacity, and on the blood vessels, among other organs. In certain situations, it is felt that the risk of using these substances for contraceptive purposes is not warranted.

The results of several studies suggest that use of oral contraceptive products *raises the risk of developing thromboembolic disease.* Apparently, products with relatively high doses of estrogen are the ones most likely to cause an increased incidence of *thrombophlebitis, pulmonary embolism, and cerebral thrombosis.* Although of statistical significance, the actual increased risk is said to be extremely small for most women. Nevertheless, this birth control method should *not* be used by women with a

---

* The Catholic church recognizes only the rhythm method as a means of limiting family size. *Temporary* use of oral contraceptive products in an attempt to regularize the menstrual cycle rhythm is considered acceptable for facilitating family planning.

TABLE 36-3 *Steroid Combinations* Used as Oral Contraceptives, Etc.*

Synthetic Progestin	Synthetic Estrogen	Product Name
Chlormadinone, 2 mg	Mestranol, 0.08 mg + Mestranol, 0.08 mg	C-Quens (S)†
Dimethisterone, 25 mg	Ethinyl estradiol, 0.1 mg + Ethinyl estradiol, 0.1 mg	Oracon (S)
Ethynodiol diacetate, 1 mg	Ethinyl estradiol, 0.05 mg	Demulen
Ethynodiol diacetate, 1 mg	Mestranol, 0.1 mg	Ovulen; Ovulen 21
Medroxyprogesterone acetate (Provera), 10 mg	Ethinyl estradiol, 0.05 mg	Provest
Norgestrel, 0.5 mg	Ethinyl estradiol, 0.05 mg	Ovral
Norethindrone, 2 mg	Mestranol, 0.1 mg	Norinyl; Ortho-Novum
Norethindrone, 2 mg	Mestranol, 0.08 mg + Mestranol, 0.08 mg	Norquen; Ortho-Novum SQ (S)
Norethindrone acetate (Norlutate), 2.5 mg	Ethinyl estradiol, 0.05 mg	Norlestrin
Norethynodrel, 2.5 mg	Mestranol, 0.1 mg	Enovid E

* Various other formulations containing the same synthetic progestins and estrogens in amounts other than those indicated here are also available.
† (S) = Sequential

history of thromboembolism, and the drugs should be immediately discontinued should any signs of a thrombotic disorder appear.

Another question that has disturbed some doctors is whether these synthetic sex hormone combinations might cause cancer when taken for long periods as contraceptives. Careful studies of thousands of patients have revealed no evidence of genital tract cancer, and there is instead some indication that these drugs may have some protective action against uterine carcinoma. However, the presence of estrogens tends to increase the growth of uterine fibroid tumors, and these hormones might also stimulate growth of an undetected mammary or genital carcinoma. Thus, the use of oral contraceptives is *contraindicated* in patients with a previous *history* of such *cancers,* and the steroids are discontinued if enlargement of fibromas is detected.

Caution is also required in patients with a history of liver disease, mental depression, and various disorders that might be adversely affected by steroid-induced fluid retention—for example, epilepsy, migraine headaches, asthma, or cardiovascular disease. Patients with thyroid disease, diabetes, and other endocrine disorders must be closely watched for signs of worsening of their conditions while taking these drugs.

Products of this kind are quite effective when used correctly. Most women have found this contraceptive method safe and convenient. However, the use of any measures that interfere with fertility often produce emotional reactions in many of the women who employ them. Thus, for example, some women resist the temporary suspension of their reproductive capacity by "forgetting" to take their tablets. In others, side effects may be made worse by emotional responses to the medication.

Other methods of using sex steroids for contraception are being employed experimentally. *Diethylstilbestrol (DES),* for example, is sometimes administered in large daily doses as an emergency *postcoital* measure for preventing pregnancy. The drug has proved highly effective for preventing conception when used soon after intercourse in such situations as rape or incest. It is not, however, to be used routinely, because nausea often occurs with the two daily doses of 25 mg. of diethylstilbestrol that are required, and because there may be some danger to the fetus in case this postcoital treatment is tried too late to prevent pregnancy.

A repository form of *medroxy-progesterone acetate* called Depo Provera provides long-lasting protection against pregnancy following its injection. This drug, which had previously been employed mainly in the management of endometrial cancer (Chapter 48), is injected at intervals of three months as a pregnancy-preventing agent. However, because this form of contraception is sometimes followed by months of infertility after treatment has been discontinued, its use is recommended at present only under special circumstances. Women must be warned that they may not be able to become pregnant when they want to.

The nurse is now the professional person from whom women most often seek advice about contraceptive measures. It is essential to listen to the patient's expression of her concerns and to be sensitive to her emotional reactions to taking oral contraceptives. The nurse can be most helpful by providing factual information. This in itself can often help to lessen the patient's apprehension.

SUMMARY of Clinical Indications for Estrogens and Progestins, Alone and in Combination

Estrogens

Menopause—relief of discomforting symptoms.

Postmenopausal (senile) osteoporosis.

Senile vaginitis, kraurosis vulvae, pruritus vulvae.

Dysfunctional uterine bleeding.

Female hypogonadism and primary amenorrhea.

Secondary amenorrhea.

Dysmenorrhea.

Contraception and postcoital pregnancy prevention.

Postpartum breast engorgement (suppression of lactation).

Mammary carcinoma (in women at least five years past the menopause).

Prostatic carcinoma.

Acne and hirsutism.

Coronary atherosclerosis and occlusion prevention.

Prevention of excessive growth in height.

Progestins

Dysfunctional uterine bleeding.

Amenorrhea, primary and secondary.

Endometriosis.

Dysmenorrhea.

Premenstrual edema and tension.

Infertility with luteal phase insufficiency.

Contraception.

Habitual and threatened abortion.

Chronic cystic mastitis.

Postponement of menstruation in patients with anemia.

Diagnosis of ovarian function (estrogen secretion).

Pregnancy testing.

SUMMARY of Adverse Effects, Cautions, and Contraindications of Estrogens

Adverse Effects

Women
Nausea, anorexia, vomiting; abdominal cramps, diarrhea.

Breakthrough bleeding (spotting) and withdrawal bleeding.

Headache, dizziness, irritability, fatigue.

Breast enlargement and tenderness.

Male Patients
Gynecomastia (breast enlargement and tenderness).

Loss of libido.

Testicular atrophy.

Cancer Patients
Hypercalcemia (may require drug withdrawal).

Children
Precocious puberty.

Premature bone maturity (closure of the epiphyses), leading to shortness of stature.

Cautions and Contraindications

Premenopausal women with suspected early mammary carcinoma or genital malignancies.

Abnormal vaginal bleeding for which all organic causes have not been ruled out by pelvic examination, Pap smear, and other tests.

Patients with thromboembolic disorders, including thrombophlebitis, retinal thrombosis, pulmonary embolism, and cerebrovascular disease.

Patients with cardiac or kidney diseases, epilepsy, migraine, and other disorders that might be adversely affected by fluid retention.

Patients with severe liver disease.

Observe diabetic patients for decrease in glucose tolerance and need for adjustment of medication.

S U M M A R Y of Adverse Effects, Cautions, and Contraindications of Oral Contraceptives (Estrogen-Progestin Combinations)

Adverse Effects

Nausea, vomiting, abdominal cramps, and bloating.

Breakthrough bleeding (spotting) and changes in menstrual flow, including amenorrhea during treatment and delayed return of menses after treatment.

Fluid retention leading to edema and weight gain.

Breast tenderness and enlargement.

Hypertension (blood pressure rise in susceptible patients).

Headaches, including migraine.

Mood changes, including irritability, mental depression, and premenstrual tension-type symptoms.

Chloasma (melasma)—irregular brown spots on skin in susceptible women.

Altered tests of liver and thyroid function.

Blood coagulation test altered in favor of increased prothrombin complex proteins. (This may require increased doses of anticoagulant drugs, if these are being employed.)

Increased susceptibility to thromboembolic disorders is possible in some patients.

Cautions and Contraindications

Patients with a history of thromboembolic disorders, including thrombophlebitis, pulmonary embolism, and cerebral thrombosis, should not receive these drugs.

Discontinue medication if retinal vessel lesions develop with sudden loss of vision.

Do not administer to patients with known or suspected breast or genital cancers dependent upon sex hormones for growth.

Do not administer to patients with irregular bleeding from vagina until the cause has been determined by adequate diagnostic tests.

Administer only after pretreatment pelvic, breast, and Pap smear examinations, and periodic exams thereafter.

Carefully observe patients with a history of disorders affected by fluid retention, including cardiac and kidney disease, epilepsy, migraine, and asthma.

Carefully observe patients with a history of mental depression and discontinue if symptoms occur.

Carefully observe diabetic patients for signs of a decrease in glucose tolerance.

Severely impaired liver function is a contraindication to the use of these drugs.

S U M M A R Y of Points for the Nurse to Remember Concerning the Female Sex Hormones

Be alert for comments and complaints that indicate distress over normal physiological processes (such as the menopause) and encourage the women to seek medical advice.

Help male patients who require estrogen therapy for coronary atherosclerosis or cancer to cope with their emotional reactions to feminizing side effects. Show that you recognize the patient's essential manliness despite such changes as gynecomastia induced by these female sex hormones.

Instruct women carefully in how to insert suppositories and apply creams containing estrogens. Suggest ways to store suppositories and to avoid soiling clothing after use of such medications.

Make certain that all girls—or the parents in the case of children—who are being treated with female sex hormones in doses high enough to bring about changes in secondary sex characteristics know in advance what to expect from the physiological actions of these substances. Give them an opportunity to ask questions about the significance of such changes.

If a woman raises questions concerning the possibility of estrogens causing cancer, help her to explore her concerns, provide her with factual information, and suggest that she discuss the matter further with her physician. He will assure her of the safety of these hormones for women who first have a full physical examination and continue to take the drug under medical supervision.

Indicate the desirability of regular visits to the physician during prolonged estrogen therapy, since the only established hazard in such therapy is failure to follow treatment with regular examinations.

Women should be told that the occurrence of bleeding when estrogens are withdrawn is natural. It should be carefully explained that such bleeding in *post*menopausal women is *pseudo*menstruation and does not, of course, mean that they have regained fertility and are capable of becoming pregnant. Bleeding at other times is *not* natural and should be reported to the doctor so that he can rule out any organic causes.

Encourage the woman who it taking oral contraceptives to report any discomforting side effects to her physician, so that he can seek their cause and deal with them.

Recognize that the same sex steroids can be used for widely different purposes. Thus, estrogen-progestin combinations can be used both to promote fertility and to prevent conception.

Remember that it is essential to respect the decision of the patient in regard to the desirability of employing contraceptive drugs, regardless of one's personal religious views.

Clinical Nursing Situation

The Situation: Mrs. Johansen, who is 46 years old, visited the gynecologic clinic because of nervousness, sweating, and a feeling of depression. Her menstrual periods had become irregular, and Mrs. Johansen told the clinic doctor that she thought her symptoms were due to "change of life." After talking with her and examining her, the doctor stated that he, too, believed her symptoms were due to menopause. He prescribed Premarin 2.5 mg daily, for 3 weeks, followed by a one-week rest period. As Mrs. Johansen was leaving the clinic, she said to the nurse, "The doctor says I must take female hormones. I've heard that they cause cancer—is that true?"

The Problem: How would you reply to Mrs. Johansen?

DRUG DIGEST

CONJUGATED ESTROGENS U.S.P. (Premarin)

Actions and Indications. These natural estrogens are used as replacement therapy in various disorders marked by estrogen deficiency, including the menopause and the years following it. Its use relieves such symptoms as hot flashes and heart palpitations, and it may help to prevent postmenopausal osteoporosis and senile vaginitis.

The oral preparation may also be employed to bring about development of secondary sex characteristics in girls with hypogonadism and primary amenorrhea. It is also useful in the management of various menstrual disorders marked by secondary amenorrhea or functional uterine bleeding. Male patients with prostatic carcinoma may receive this hormone for symptomatic relief.

Side Effects, Cautions, and Contraindications. Nausea, breast fullness and tenderness, abdominal bloating, and cramps may occur early in treatment of menopausal women. Breakthrough bleeding may result from underdosage, but the presence of organic lesions must be ruled out by diagnostic examination before raising the dosage. Use of estrogens is contraindicated in patients with suspected breast or genital tissue cancer.

Male patients may develop gynecomastia and testicular atrophy with a loss of libido and mental depression. Susceptibility to thromboembolism may be increased.

Dosage and Administration. The most common dose range is between 1.25 and 3.75 mg daily for three weeks followed by a one-week rest period. Higher doses (3.75–10 mg) are employed to control uterine bleeding and in cancer treatment. Conjugated estrogens are also administered as an intravaginal cream for juvenile or senile vaginitis or topically for pruritus vulvae or kraurosis vulvae.

DIETHYLSTILBESTROL U.S.P. (DES; Stilbestrol; Stilbetin)

Actions and Indications. This synthetic estrogen offers effective replacement therapy in the menopause and postmenopausal periods and in various disorders resulting from a deficiency of ovarian secretion of the natural hormone. Oral administration is employed together with adjunctive suppositories for relief of itching in senile vaginitis. It is often combined with male hormone anabolic agents for prevention or control of postmenopausal osteoporosis. Postpartum administration relieves painfully engorged breasts and suppresses lactation. Prostatic cancer in men and mammary cancer in women at least five years past the menopause may be treated with DES for symptomatic relief.

Side Effects, Cautions, and Contraindications. Nausea, vomiting, and sometimes abdominal distress or diarrhea may occur at the start of treatment. Breast tenderness, headache, and irritability may also occur. Fluid retention and electrolyte imbalance must be watched for, especially in patients with cardiac or kidney disease or with migraine or epilepsy. Estrogens are contraindicated in women with breast or genital cancer or with thromboembolic disorders. In men, gynecomastia, testicular inhibition, loss of libido, and mental depression may develop.

Dosage and Administration. Doses for menopausal patients range from 0.1 to 1 mg depending upon the response. Control of uterine bleeding may require 5 mg several times daily. Postmenopausal breast cancer patients receive 15 mg daily by mouth. For more long-acting intensive therapy, the diprorionate ester and phosphate salt may be administered intravenously or intramuscularly, as well as orally, in mammary and prostatic cancer treatment.

ESTRADIOL VALERATE U.S.P. (Delestrogen)

Actions and Indications. This ester of estradiol produces prolonged estrogenic effects. The fact that injections are required only every two or three weeks makes this form of the female hormone useful for treating cancers such as prostatic carcinoma in men and advanced mammary carcinoma in women who are at least five years past the menopause. It is also employed for suppression of lactation and relief of postpartum engorgement of the breasts. It is recommended for cyclic use with a long-acting progestational preparation in the management of various menstrual cycle disorders and ovarian deficiency syndromes.

Side Effects, Cautions, and Contraindications. Patients with prostatic or mammary carcinoma are observed for hypercalcemia, which requires discontinuation of the medication. They are also watched for signs of thromboembolic disorders, such as thrombophlebitis, and for irregular uterine bleeding. Caution is required in patients with heart, kidney and liver disease, and in those with epilepsy, migraine, diabetes, or a history of cerebrovascular disease. Male patients may develop gynecomastia and suffer a loss of libido.

Dosage and Administration. This preparation is injected deep into the upper outer quadrant of the gluteal muscle in doses of 10 to 40 mg, depending upon the condition being treated. A single injection of 10 to 25 mg is used for suppressing lactation, while the treatment of prostatic carcinoma requires 30 mg every week or two. For menstrual and ovarian deficiency syndromes, 20 mg is administered alone on the first day of the cycle, and 5 mg is administered two weeks later in combination with a long-acting progestational steroid.

HYDROXYPROGESTERONE ACETATE U.S.P. (Delalutin)

Actions and Indications. This ester derivative of progesterone exerts long-acting hormonal activity upon the estrogen-primed endometrium, the myometrium, breasts, and pituitary gland. It is employed in a cyclic therapy schedule that includes a long-acting estrogen in the management of dysfunctional uterine bleeding and amenorrhea in order to convert a proliferative endometrium to the secretory form, which sloughs off following discontinuance of this drug's action. Failure to bleed may indicate pregnancy.

It is used alone in large doses in efforts to prevent threatened abortion and all through pregnancy in patients with a history of habitual and recurrent abortion. Other therapeutic uses include relief of postpartum afterpains, dysmenorrhea, premenstrual tension, and breast disorders such as chronic cystic mastitis.

Side Effects, Cautions, and Contraindications. Prolonged use during pregnancy carries a slight risk of masculinizing the female fetus. This sex steroid should not be used in patients with genital bleeding until organic causes have been ruled out. It is contraindicated in breast cancer patients and in those with impaired liver function. Caution is also required in patients with heart and kidney disorders and in those with histories of migraine, epilepsy, or asthma. Allergic reactions have occurred in some patients.

Dosage and Administration. In cyclic therapy, 250 mg is injected intramuscularly midway in a 28-day cycle and repeated every four weeks. Single injections of 125 or 250 mg are used in diagnostic tests, including a pregnancy test and in the treatment of various painful disorders. Repeated daily doses of 25 mg are given to control threatened abortion, after which injections are repeated weekly until two weeks before delivery is expected.

NORETHINDRONE ACETATE AND ETHINYL ESTRADIOL TABLETS N.F. (Norlestrin)

Actions and Indications. The acetate ester of the progestational steroid norethindrone is used alone in conditions marked by a deficiency of progesterone, including abnormal uterine bleeding, amenorrhea, and endometriosis. Ethinyl estradiol is a potent estrogen employed in management of the menopause and other conditions for which estrogen therapy is indicated. However, a combination of this kind is used mainly as an oral *contraceptive* for prevention of pregnancy. Employed properly in accordance with the recommended course schedule, the progestin-estrogen mixture is close to 100 percent effective for this purpose.

Side Effects, Cautions, and Contraindications. The most common side effects resemble the discomforts of early pregnancy such as nausea, vomiting, loss of appetite, and abdominal bloating. These and other side effects such as headache, dizziness, breast tenderness, and weight gain tend to lessen after the first one or two cyclic courses. Brownish skin blemishes appear occasionally, and some susceptible patients may have a small rise in blood pressure.

Products of this kind are contraindicated in patients with thromboembolic disorders, undiagnosed vaginal bleeding, suspected breast or genital cancer, or severely impaired liver function. Patients with a history of heart or kidney disease, diabetes, mental depression, migraine, epilepsy, or asthma are watched closely for any worsening of these disorders during treatment.

Dosage and Administration. The combination is taken daily for three weeks (21 days) beginning on the fifth day of the menstrual cycle. During the final seven days of the menstrual cycle, the patient takes no pill, or—in some forms—an inert tablet, or one containing therapeutically inactive amounts of an iron salt. Tablets should be taken at a regular time—at bedtime or with a meal.

References

Berczeller, P.H., Young, I.S., and Kupperman, H.S. The therapeutic use of progestational steroids. *Clin. Pharmacol. Ther.*, 5:216, 1964.

Cole, M. Strokes in young women using oral contraceptives. *Arch. Intern. Med. (Chicago)*, 120:551, 1967 (Nov.).

Council on Drugs, American Medical Association. Oral contraceptives: Current status of therapy. *JAMA*, 214:2316, 1970.

Davis, M.E., et al. Estrogens and the aging process. *JAMA*, 196:219, 1960.

Goldzieher, J.W. Newer drugs in oral contraception. *Med. Clin. N. Amer.*, 48:529, 1964.

Rodman, M.J. The oral contraceptives. *RN*, 29:51, 1966 (March).

———. The female sex hormones. *RN*, 31:57, 1968 (May).

37.

The Male Sex Hormones and Anabolic Agents

The Male Sex Hormone

The male sex glands, or testes, secrete a hormone called *testosterone*. This substance is responsible for the development and maintenance of the male sex organs and secondary sex characteristics. Even primitive peoples were well aware that castration (removal of the testes) was accompanied by the loss of male physical features and mental attitudes. However, the extraction and purification of the testicular hormone and the preparation of more potent, longer-acting derivatives for use in therapy did not occur until earlier in this century.

Now available for use in treating men and boys who lack the natural hormone are several esters, including *testosterone cypionate+*, that have a much more prolonged action when injected than testosterone itself. Also available are *fluoxymesterone+* and other synthetic substances that are effective when taken by mouth —unlike the natural hormone, which is largely destroyed in the liver after oral ingestion. However, all the available substances with male sexual (*androgenic*) activity and with tissue-building (*anabolic*) effects upon metabolism (Table 37-1) are essentially similar to the testicular hormone in their physiological effects. Thus, before we discuss the clinical situations for which doctors order the use of these compounds, we shall review briefly the physiology of the male hormone.

PHYSIOLOGY OF THE MALE HORMONE

As indicated in Chapter 35, the functions of the testes are under the control of anterior

T A B L E   3 7 - 1   *Androgenic and Anabolic Agents*

Nonproprietary or Official Name	Trade Names	Usual Dose
Preparations Used Mainly for Their Androgenic Effects		
Fluoxymesterone U.S.P.	Halotestin; Ora-Testryl; Ultandren	2 to 20 mg
Methyltestosterone N.F.	Metandren; Neo-Hombreol M; Oreton Methyl	Buccal, 5 mg
Testosterone N.F.	Androlin; Neo-Hombreol F; Oreton; Testryl	Buccal, 10 mg, I.M. 25 mg; pellet implantation, 300 mg
Testosterone cypionate U.S.P.	Depo-Testosterone cypionate	I.M. 50 to 100 mg every 7 to 14 days
Testosterone enanthate U.S.P.	Delatestryl	I.M. 200 mg every two to four weeks
Testosterone phenylacetate	Perandren phenylacetate	I.M. 50 mg
Testosterone propionate U.S.P.	Neo-Hombreol; Oreton propionate; Perandren	I.M. 25 mg daily or three times a week
Preparations Used Mainly for Their Anabolic Effects		
Dromstanolone propionate	Drolban; Masterone	100 mg three times weekly
Ethylestrenol	Maxibolin	8 to 16 mg oral
Methandrostenolone N.F.	Dianabol	5 mg oral
Nandrolone decanoate	Deca-Durabolin	I.M. 50 to 100 mg every three or four weeks
Nandrolone phenpropionate	Durabolin	I.M. 25 mg once a week
Norethandrolone	Nilevar	10 to 30 mg I.M. or oral
Oxandrolone	Anavar	5 to 20 mg oral
Oxymetholone	Androyd; Anadrol	5 to 10 mg oral
Stanozolol	Winstrol	2 mg oral three times a day

pituitary gonadotropins. The pituitary hormone FSH, which, in women, stimulates the ovarian follicles to bring their ova to maturity, has an analogous function in the male; that is, it influences sperm development (spermatogenesis) by its stimulating action on the seminiferous tubular tissues of the testes. FSH does *not*, however, simultaneously stimulate testicular secretion of the male hormone in the way in which it prods the ovaries to produce estrogens.

Testosterone production is, instead, under the influence of another anterior pituitary gonadotropin. This hormone, known in the female as the luteinizing hormone (LH), acts upon the cells of Leydig, located in the spaces or interstices between the seminiferous tubules of the testes. Thus, in the male, it is called the interstitial cell-stimulating hormone (ICSH). The testosterone secreted by these cells, in turn, plays a part in regulating pituitary gonadotropin production. That is, high levels of androgens (male hormones) in the blood tend to suppress the secretion of FSH and ICSH. This is why the administration of testosterone derivatives in doses high enough to reduce pituitary gland production of FSH can actually cause a reduction in sperm cell production by the seminiferous tubules of the testes (see the discussion of oligospermia treatment, p. 456).

FUNCTIONS OF TESTOSTERONE. The functions of testosterone may be broadly classified as: (1) *sexual* and (2) *metabolic*. These actions become dramatically evident at puberty when previously suppressed gonadotropic hormones are released in large amounts upon a signal from the hypothalamus. The outpouring of testosterone that follows such gonadotropic stimulation of the boy's testes produces effects of the two types (sexual and metabolic) upon all the tissues of the body. That is, the testicular secretions act as a growth hormone not only to the boy's sex organs but also to such structures as the skeletal muscles and the bones. The skin and hair are also affected, and protein metabolism in general is stimulated, so that dietary nitrogen is retained in the tissues in larger amounts (an *anabolic* action).

❨ *Sexual function.* The accessory sex organs—the penis, prostate gland, seminal vesicles, and vas deferens—grow in size and functional capacity under the influence of pubertal testosterone. The testes themselves grow in size as does the scrotal sac in which they are contained. The seminiferous tubules of the testes share in this growth and, under the combined influence of testosterone and FSH, spermatogenesis begins. Sperm production is maintained throughout the man's reproductive life by the balanced effects of these testicular and pituitary hormones.

The *secondary sex characteristics* of the male also make their appearance at puberty under the influence of testosterone. At this time, the boy's high-pitched voice deepens as his vocal cords thicken under the influence of this hormone. Hair begins to grow, not only in the axillary and pubic areas, but also on his arms, legs, and trunk. Interestingly, some young people predisposed to baldness by heredity begin to show the first signs of future loss of hair at this time. Apparently, testosterone plays a part in producing so-called male pattern baldness. Facial hair makes its first appearance at this time, and the beard continues to come in gradually over the next few years. Testosterone also stimulates the skin's sebaceous glands to grow in size and secretory capacity. As indicated in Chapter 46, this plays a part in the pathogenesis of acne, a condition very common in adolescence.

❨ *Metabolic function.* The greater growth of the male's skeletal structures is also attributable to testosterone. This hormone somehow stimulates tissue-building processes by aiding retention of the dietary protein nitrogen needed for formation of the amino acids from which new muscle is built. At the same time, less nitrogen is lost from the pool of chemical fragments formed in the constant breakdown of body tissues. This hormone-regulated combination of increased anabolism and decreased catabolism of protein helps to produce the larger, more powerful muscles of the male.

The boy's bones also begin to grow in thickness and in length. However, after stimulating a sudden spurt of growth at puberty, this action of testosterone finally puts an end to any further growth in height. This happens because the hormone converts the cartilaginous tissues at the ends of the long bones (the *epiphyses*) into bone. The shafts of the limb bones can then no longer lengthen.

The Therapeutic Uses of the Androgens

ANDROGEN THERAPY IN MEN

Testosterone and its derivatives are used in medicine mainly as replacement therapy in males who lack the hormone. Such hypogonadism may become apparent at puberty when the boy fails to develop normally, or it may occur in men at some time after the masculinizing changes of adolescence have taken place. *Eunuchism*, as a result of castration, or *eunuchoidism* from testicular hypofunction or failure, can also be successfully treated with testosterone preparations of various kinds.

EUNUCHOIDISM. *Male hypogonadism* caused by various diseases of the testicles or of the pituitary gland (see *Summary*, p. 458) is usually treated by the administration of testosterone. In theory, testicular failure secondary to failure of the pituitary gland to produce the gonadotropic hormone ICSH could be treated with human chorionic gonadotropin (HCG), a substance that stimulates testicular function. In practice, however, HCG is used only in the differential diagnosis of primary and secondary hypogonadism.

Even when the patient's testes do respond to administration of HCG by secreting endogenous testosterone, the doctor probably employs testosterone for treating the patient's secondary testicular failure. This is mainly because use of a long-lasting male hormone preparation is much less expensive for long-term maintenance therapy than is use of the gonadotropic hormone obtained from the urine of pregnant women.

The effects of male hormone replacement therapy upon the patient's physical and psychic development are often truly dramatic. Administered in doses and intervals intended to imitate the natural rate of testicular hormone secretion, these preparations almost literally make a man of a boy. Some of these changes —in height, depth of voice, size of sex organs, and pattern of hair distribution, for example —are permanent. However, hypogonadal patients must continue to receive hormone replacement therapy indefinitely in order to maintain muscular strength, physical vigor and libido, or sex drive.

Men who develop a hormone deficiency after sexual development has occurred naturally at puberty do not need as intensive treatment as does the young eunuch or eunuchoid. Thus, treatment may begin with injections of testosterone esters, and then these patients may often be maintained with oral therapy, using methyltestosterone or its synthetic derivative, fluoxymesterone+. The latter agent is somewhat more potent and is claimed unlikely to cause the jaundice that sometimes occurs with methytestosterone.

THE MALE CLIMACTERIC. This condition is analogous to the menopause in women. The symptoms also—hot flashes, heart palpitations, nervous irritability, or fretting over minor matters, failure of concentration and memory, and insomnia—are somewhat similar. They are often so vague and subjective that some doctors tend to feel that the condition is psychogenic rather than the result of an endocrine imbalance stemming from testicular failure. Differential diagnosis is important, since symptoms resulting from a true hormone deficiency will respond readily to replacement therapy, whereas a depressive neurosis or psychosis may require psychotherapy, antidepressant drugs, or even electroshock if—as sometimes happens—the patient develops suicidal tendencies.

The doctor may order laboratory studies of the hormone levels in the patient's blood and urine to help determine whether the patient actually is suffering from the relatively rare male climacteric. If these tests indicate that the patient's urine is low in testosterone metabolites and that his blood is correspondingly high in pituitary gonadotropins, the doctor may start the patient on testosterone propionate injections for a trial period. Often dramatic improvement follows one or two weeks of treatment. Not only do the patient's cardiovascular and mental symptoms clear up, but he often gains in physical vigor, sense of well-being, and restoration of lost libido and potency. The doctor may then decide to put the patient on long-term therapy with one of the testosterone esters with a long duration of action.

PRECAUTIONS. Before proceeding with such maintenance treatment with exogenous male hormone, the doctor tries to rule out the presence of prostate gland growths, which are not uncommon in men of late middle age and might be stimulated into more rapid activity by hormone treatment. Similarly, such men are examined frequently during treatment to detect any signs of possible prostatic carcinoma, since such a hormone-dependent neoplasm might grow rapidly and spread to other sites in the body.

Other adverse effects of excessive amounts of testosterone which must be guarded against are: (1) a steroid-induced retention of salty fluids, that may tend to raise the patient's blood pressure or send a person with previous cardiovascular difficulties into congestive heart failure; and (2) psychological and physical changes, including an unseemly increase in libido that might prove socially embarrassing to a middle-aged man. Both of these reactions, including increased sex drive, are unlikely with carefully regulated replacement therapy.

CRYPTORCHISM. Undescended testicle is a condition caused either by an obstruction of the inguinal canal or a lack of testosterone. In the latter case, it is customary to treat the boy with a course of human chorionic gonadotropin (HCG) injections. Even if this ICSH-containing substance fails to stimulate enough secretion of endogenous testosterone to let the testes descend from the abdomen into the scrotum, it helps to facilitate the surgery that may be required later. If the doctor decides to try testosterone from an outside source, he must regulate the dosage very carefully to avoid precipitating premature puberty in the youngster. For, as when HCG is used in such patients, the sex hormone may cause too-early development of accessory sex structures and secondary sex characteristics.

OLIGOSPERMIA. A lack of viable, motile sperm in the semen is commonly a cause of male infertility. It is unlikely to be corrected by testosterone treatment alone, because high doses of the hormone are likely to suppress pituitary secretion of FSH, the gonadotropin that ordinarily stimulates the seminiferous tubules. Occasionally, however, when testosterone is withdrawn, the temporarily suppressed pituitary gland may respond with a rebound secretion of FSH in greater amounts than before. This may then result in a rise in sperm production. (See also the discussion of the treatment of *female* infertility, p. 444.)

ANDROGEN THERAPY IN WOMEN

GYNECOLOGIC DISORDERS. Women are sometimes treated with the male hormone because:

(1) it antagonizes the effects of excessive amounts of estrogens; and (2) it suppresses the secretion of pituitary hormones. These effects sometimes help to control uterine bleeding and relieve dysmenorrhea, premenstrual tension, and postpartum breast engorgement. However, most doctors now prefer to use oral estrogen-progestogen combinations for treating these gynecologic conditions.

APLASTIC ANEMIA. Women (as well as men and children) suffering from certain serious anemias are sometimes treated with testosterone derivatives. Patients with aplastic anemia or bone marrow depression produced by treatment with anticancer drugs sometimes respond with an increase in red blood cell production, when an androgen-anabolic agent is added to the standard antianemia regimen. To lessen the likelihood of producing masculinizing effects in women who require long-term treatment, the less virilizing anabolic agents (see below) are often preferred for stimulating erythropoiesis in such cases.

METASTATIC MAMMARY CARCINOMA. Cancer of the breast that has spread beyond the reach of surgery or radiation therapy is a condition in which large doses of androgens are administered to women. The symptomatic relief sometimes obtained in such cases is occasionally accompanied by masculinizing effects. Thus, these patients are watched for early signs, such as growth of facial hair and development of acne. Withdrawal of hormone treatment results in clearing of these skin symptoms and prevents permanent signs of virilization, such as deepening of the voice and clitoral enlargement. The patient is often willing to endure such virilizing effects in order to obtain the feeling of well-being and the relief of pain that hormone treatment often offers.

The nurse should, of course, be sensitive to the woman's emotional responses to the physical and psychological effects of hormone therapy. For example, the woman may discuss such matters as her hormone-induced increase in libido with the nurse rather than the doctor, and the nurse can then bring such subjective responses to the doctor's attention.

HYPERCALCEMIA. Cancer patients being treated with the male hormone are also watched for signs and symptoms of hypercalcemia. This condition requires prompt withdrawal of androgen therapy and the forcing of fluids to avoid formation of kidney stones. Because the action of the long-acting esters still in the intramuscular depots cannot be turned off, these forms of the hormone can cause hypercalcemia to continue even after their further administration is stopped. Thus, the short-acting ester, *testosterone propionate*, is often preferred for treating cancer patients. *Fluoxymesterone*+ and certain other new synthetic derivatives that are discussed in Chapter 48 are also claimed less likely to cause hypercalcemia in cancer patients or to produce masculinizing effects in women patients (see *Summary of Adverse Effects*, p. 459).

The Actions and Therapeutic Uses of Anabolic Agents

Doctors often want to stimulate the flagging appetites of debilitated patients and to reverse the processes responsible for protein wastage and subsequent weight loss. When it was found that testosterone possessed anabolic activity that could produce positive nitrogen balance in patients who were in negative balance, physicians tried administering the hormone in such cases. Although it often brought a return of appetite and a feeling of well-being, the hormone's sexual effects limited its usefulness for women and children and caused mental and physical changes undesirable even in male patients.

Chemists have tried to modify the testosterone molecule in attempts to devise compounds free of sexual effects, yet capable of stimulating muscle growth and strength in the manner of the hormone. Several synthetic anabolic steroids which are now available (Table 37-1) are capable of increasing protein anabolism when administered in doses that are less likely to cause undesired masculinizing activity than are doses of testosterone that cause comparable anabolic activity. However, a complete separation of the sexual effects from the anabolic effects has not yet been achieved. Thus, patients taking any of these drugs must be watched for possible development of virilizing and other toxic effects of testosterone.

CLINICAL USES

The clinical uses of these anabolic steroids with reduced androgenic activity are potentially very varied. These substances might prove useful in any of many conditions marked by inadequate protein biosynthesis or excessive protein breakdown. However, it has been hard to prove that patients actually do better on these drugs, which tend to stimulate the appetite, than they would by simply eating a diet adequate in proteins and other food factors. This difficulty, as well as the possibility of causing undesired side effects, particularly in women and children, has limited the acceptance of these agents.

Patients being treated with *corticosteroid drugs* sometimes receive adjunctive anabolic steroids. The catabolic, or protein breakdown, effects of the corticosteroids are especially dangerous for patients with arthritis who are confined to bed or inactive. These patients are subject to *osteoporosis* resulting from disease of their limbs. Like elderly patients with senile osteoporosis, they may suffer bone fractures as a result of calcium loss from the protein matrix of osseous structures. Administration of anabolic steroids in such cases is said to help prevent osteoporosis (see also Chapter 17).

Convalescent patients sometimes receive a course of treatment with an anabolic agent. Patients who have suffered the stress of surgery or other trauma are often in negative nitrogen balance. Administration of anabolic agents in such cases or in patients who have suffered fractures, deep extensive burns, or weakening virus infections such as influenza sometimes helps to retain nitrogenous compounds that would otherwise be lost to the body, and to convert them into the amino acids from which new tissues are built. Here too, however, it has been hard to prove that patients actually recover more rapidly than they would with good nursing care and an adequate diet only.

Some patients with wasting diseases such as tuberculosis and cancer are claimed to benefit from the protein-building action of these drugs. They cannot, of course, be used in patients with prostatic carcinoma, because the retained androgenic component, although less potent than that of testosterone, may be sufficient to stimulate the growth and spread of the hormone-dependent cancer.

Some patients with *refractory anemias*— aplastic anemia and other blood disorders that do not respond readily to treatment with iron alone, or B-complex vitamins such as folic acid and B_{12}—sometimes recover when maintained on anabolic steroids. As indicated above, these substances may stimulate production of erythrocytes by the bone marrow when administered in doses that are less likely than testosterone to produce undesirable masculinizing effects.

Children whose growth is retarded or who eat poorly and are weak and anemic may sometimes respond to small doses of these drugs. However, most doctors do not lightly undertake such therapy, since children may be especially sensitive to the androgenic component in all these drugs. This could, of course, have adverse effects on the child's ability to achieve his full height. That is, an initial increase in weight and a spurt in growth might be bought at the expense of early closure of the epiphyses.

To avoid this, the doctor may consult an authority on growth and development before beginning treatment with anabolic drugs. Then, in the intervals between courses, the ends of the long bones are examined by x-ray to detect any early changes which might indicate the start of premature ossification that could keep the child from further growth. The child is also watched for signs of premature puberty, which would require withdrawal of the anabolic agents.

Perhaps further research in this field will succeed in entirely separating the sexual from the metabolic effects of these compounds. Such drugs could then be used with greater safety in children, women with senile or disuse type osteoporosis, and men debilitated by metastatic prostate cancer.

S U M M A R Y of Clinical Indications for the Use of Androgens and Anabolic Agents

Male Patients

Male Hypogonadism (Eunuchism and Eunuchoidism)

Eunuchism—complete functional failure of the testes (prepubertal, or in surgically castrated adult males).

Eunuchoidism—partial *primary* testicular failure caused by diseases affecting the testes directly (for example, following severe mumps, orchitis, or trauma); also *secondary* to a deficiency of gonadotropin as a result of pituitary or hypothalamic disease (for example, pituitary tumor or insufficiency; following head injuries).

Male Climacteric
Gradual reduction in hormone secretion by Leydig cells of aging men.

Oligospermia
Discontinuing male hormone administration may result in rebound recovery of spermatozoa production.

Cryptorchism
Undescended testicle may move from the abdomen under the influence of testosterone administered from an outside source or produced endogenously by the patient's testes following stimulation with human chorionic gonadotropin (HCG).

Anemias
Caused by defective production of erythrocytes by the bone marrow (for example, aplastic anemias).

Osteoporosis
Of the senile type or occurring during long-term treatment of inactive rheumatoid arthritis patients with corticosteroid drugs.

Female Patients

Metastatic Mammary Carcinoma
Relief of pain and discomfort of advanced inoperative breast cancer between one and five years postmenopausal.

Gynecologic Disorders
Menorrhagia, metrorrhagia, dysmenorrhea, premenstrual tension; also for suppression of postpartum breast engorgement.

Negative Nitrogen Balance

In convalescence following surgical operations, severe injuries, burns, or infections.

During chronic illnesses marked by tissue wastage (for example, tuberculosis; carcinosis).

In children with dwarfism or other forms of retarded growth, weakness, or anemia.

S U M M A R Y of Adverse Effects, Cautions, and Contraindications of Androgens and Anabolic Agents

Virilizing (Masculinizing) Effects

Adult Men
Chronic priapism (persistent erections).
Inappropriate behavioral manifestations of increased libido (excessive sex drive).
Oligospermia (reduction in sperm count).
Prostate growth requires caution in patients with prostatic hypertrophy; prostatic carcinoma is a contraindication.

Prepubertal Boys
Precocious puberty (for example, growth of accessory sex organs and development of male secondary sexual characteristics at a too early age).
Premature closure of the epiphyses. (This may result in a reduction of adult height below what would be normally reached by the individual.)

Women
Growth of facial hair (hirsutism).
Acne as a result of increased sebaceous gland growth and secretion.
Baldness of male pattern type (hair recedes at temples and thins at crown).
Deepening of the voice (hoarseness).
Amenorrhea and other menstrual irregularities.
Enlargement of the clitoris.
Increased libido.

Cardiovascular-Renal Effects

Edema as a result of steroid-induced retention of sodium and water may be dangerous for elderly patients and those with severe kidney or heart disease, including nephritis, nephrosis, and incipient failure.

Hypercalcemia from large doses in women with advanced breast cancer.

Liver dysfunction* (hepatitis of cholestatic type). Jaundice and liver function test abnormalities. (Caution in patients with preexisting liver disease.)

Drug Interactions

Anticoagulants of the coumarin type may have their actions intensified. (Dosage is adjusted downward if the more frequently performed prothrombin time tests indicate potentiation of the anticoagulant action.)

Phenylbutazone-type drugs may also require a reduction in dosage when administered with some anabolic agents.

---

* This does *not* occur with testosterone and its esters but may develop during treatment with *methyltestosterone* and certain synthetic androgens with a particular chemical structure.

S U M M A R Y of Points for the Nurse to Remember About Male Hormone Therapy

Instruct the patient to report any symptoms which may be attributed to the use of testosterone therapy: weight gain, a feeling of bloatedness, and increased libido. In women, look for signs of masculinizing effects, such as growth of facial hair and deepening of the voice.

Remember that patients with conditions such as eunuchism and the male climacteric are usually under considerable emotional stress, since a person's self-esteem and his acceptance by others are often related to maintenance of his sexual potency and the adequacy of his sexual development.

The woman patient with metastatic carcinoma who is receiving male sex hormones as palliative therapy usually has many severe physical symptoms. The advantages of androgen therapy must be evaluated in the light of their side effects, which may be very disturbing. The attitude of others toward the patient is important in helping her cope with masculinizing side effects.

Clinical Nursing Situation

The Situation: Mrs. Johnson had a radical mastectomy a year ago for carcinoma of the breast. Her disease has metastasized, and she now has severe weight loss, pain in her spine as well as in the operative area, anorexia, and pronounced weakness. Mrs. Johnson has been started on a course of testosterone therapy. This has improved her appetite, made her stronger, and markedly reduced her pain. However, she has a very obvious growth of facial hair, her voice has grown deeper, and her facial features have become somewhat masculine. Mrs. Johnson shares a room with a teen-age girl who, with her young visitors, has made some cruel jokes within the older woman's hearing about her mannish appearance.

The Problem: Describe how you would work with both of these women in order to lessen the tension which is apparent between them, and to foster their helping one another.

Do you view this nursing intervention as helping only the older woman or both women? Explain your viewpoint.

DRUG DIGEST

FLUOXYMESTERONE U.S.P. (Halotestin; Ora-Testryl; Ultandren)

Actions and Indications. This is a synthetic derivative of testosterone that has male hormone effects when taken by mouth. It is used for replacement therapy in male patients with an androgen deficiency. In such cases it brings about maturation of the sex organs or prevents atrophic changes in them. It has also been used for relief of symptoms of the male climacteric.

This drug is also used in treating women with metastatic breast cancer, following a beneficial response to prior removal or destruction of their ovaries at least one year previously.

Side Effects, Cautions, and Contraindications. Excessive effects in adult males may include persistent erections with reduced sperm production. Boys may show signs of premature pubertal changes and of developing secondary sex characteristics. They must be watched for signs of skeletal system maturation, as this may cause their growth in height to stop prematurely. The masculinizing effects in women may be marked by deepening of the voice, growth of facial hair, menstrual irregularities, and other physical and psychological changes.

This drug's tendency to cause edema requires caution in its use in patients with kidney or heart disease; it is contraindicated in those with severe nephritis and nephrosis. It is also contraindicated in patients with severe liver disease and is discontinued if jaundice develops.

Dosage and Administration. Daily oral doses of 2 to 10 mg are administered to eunuchoid adult male patients. Prepubertal boys are begun on 2 mg daily and dosage is raised only very cautiously. Women with advanced breast cancer receive 20 to 30 mg daily.

TESTOSTERONE CYPIONATE U.S.P. (Depo-Testosterone Cypionate)

Actions and Indications. This ester of testosterone produces long-lasting masculinizing and anabolic effects—from two to four weeks following a single injection. It is a preferred form of the hormone for treating eunuchoidism in order to develop and to maintain the accessory sex organs and secondary sexual characteristics. It is also used for symptomatic relief of the male climacteric and for its adjunctive anabolic effect in both male and female patients with senile or postmenopausal osteoporosis.

Side Effects, Cautions, and Contraindications. Overdosage in adult males may cause persistent erections. Sperm production may be markedly reduced (oligospermia), but because the suppressed spermatogenesis may rebound after the drug is discontinued, this hormone has sometimes actually been used to treat this condition. Young boys may show signs of too early puberty, and caution is required to avoid premature maturation of the bones, as this may result in reduced adult height. Women may show physical and mental signs of masculinization, including irreversible deepening of the voice, growth of facial hair, and baldness.

The drug is contraindicated in patients with severe cardiac and kidney disease because of its tendency to cause fluid retention. It is also contraindicated in patients with prostatic carcinoma, severe hypercalcemia, or pregnancy.

Dosage and Administration. The usual dose is 200 to 400 mg administered intramuscularly every two to four weeks. A weekly dose of 200 mg may first be used in treating oligospermia to suppress spermatogenesis prior to inducing a rebound of that testicular function.

References

Berczeller, P.H., and Kupperman, H.S. The anabolic steroids. *Clin. Pharmacol. Ther.*, 1:464, 1960.

Bishop, P.M.F. The male sex hormones. *Brit. Med. J.*, 167:184, 1960.

Frohman, I.P. The steroids. *Amer. J. Nurs.*, 59:518, 1959.

Fruehan, A.E., and Frawley, T.H. Current status of anabolic steroids. *JAMA*, 184:527, 1963.

Heller, C.G., and Myers, G.B. Male climacteric, its symptomatology, diagnosis, and treatment. *JAMA*, 126:472, 1944.

McGavack, T.H. The male climacterium. *J. Amer. Geriat. Soc.*, 3:639, 1955.

Rodman, M.J. The male sex hormone and anabolic steroids. *RN*, 30:41, 1967 (May).

Werner, A.A. Male climacteric. *JAMA*, 132:188, 1946.

38.

The Thyroid Hormones and Antithyroid Drugs

The Thyroid Gland

The thyroid gland regulates the rate of metabolism in almost all body cells. That is, the thyroid gland secretes hormones that control the speed of the combustion processes by which body tissues burn food to derive the energy needed for normal function and for growth and development.

We still do not know precisely how thyroid hormones control the rate of cellular metabolic processes. However, we are very much aware of what happens to a person when his thyroid gland fails to function properly. In this chapter, we shall discuss the drugs that are used to treat clinical conditions caused by the underfunctioning and the overactivity of the thyroid gland.

Thyroid gland disorders may be broadly classified as (1) *hypothyroidism*—conditions marked by a decrease in the production and secretion of thyroid hormones; and (2) *hyperthyroidism*—conditions in which the thyroid gland produces and secretes excessive amounts of its hormones into the systemic circulation. In hypothyroid conditions, body metabolism slows down to subnormal levels, rates of growth and development are reduced, and the effects of sluggish metabolism are apparent in many body systems, including the central nervous system. In hyperthyroidism, on the other hand, the metabolic rate is abnormally elevated, with far-reaching effects on many systems, particularly including the cardiovascular system. (The signs and symptoms accompanying full-blown hypo- and hyperthyroidism are summarized in Table 38-1.)

Simple nontoxic goiter is a thyroid disorder

TABLE 38-1 *Signs and Symptoms of Thyroid Dysfunction*

	Hypothyroidism	Hyperthyroidism
Central nervous system	*Functions depressed*: hypoactive reflexes (hyporeflexia), lethargy, emotional dullness, sleepiness, slow speech, stupid appearance.	*Functions stimulated*: hyperactive reflexes, anxiety, nervousness, restlessness, insomnia, tremors.
Cardiovascular-renal	*Functions depressed*: bradycardia, hypotension, increased circulation time, oliguria, anemia, decreased secretion of catecholamines, and decreased sensitivity to catecholamines and to adrenergic drugs.	*Functions stimulated*: tachycardia, palpitations, decreased circulation time, increased pulse pressure, systolic hypertension, increased secretion of catecholamines, and increased sensitivity to catecholamines and to adrenergic drugs.
Skin and other epithelial structures	Skin pale, coarse, dry, thickened, especially on hands and face which is puffy about the eyelids, cheeks, and elsewhere; hair coarse and thinned on scalp and in eyebrows; nails thick and hard.	Skin flushed, thin, warm, moist due to vasodilation and sweating; hair fine and soft; nails soft and thin.
Metabolism rate	*Decreased*, with body temperature reduced, intolerance of cold, decreased appetite, with more of food intake converted to fat, including cholesterol (that is, tendency toward weight gain and definite hypercholesterolemia).	*Increased*, with body temperature raised (low-grade fever), intolerance of heat, increased appetite, but with tendency toward weight loss, which may be severe sometimes and accompanied by muscle wasting and weakness (thyrotoxic myopathy).
Generalized myxedema	Including accumulation of mucopolysaccharides in heart (cardiomegaly), tongue and vocal cords (hoarseness and thickened speech), periorbital areas.	Localized, with accumulations of mucopolysaccharides in the orbits, eyeballs, and ocular muscles; periorbital edema, puffiness of eyelids, lid lag, and exophthalmos; occasional pretibial edema.
Ovarian function	*Decreased*, with tendency toward menorrhagia, possible habitual abortion, or sterility.	Altered, with tendency toward oligomenorrhea or amenorrhea.
Goiter	Relatively rare and of simple, nontoxic type.	Diffuse, highly vascular, and murmurous (bruit), is very frequent.

of another type. The thyroid gland is enlarged but the secretion of its hormones may be more or less normal. This so-called *euthyroid*, or essentially normal, state occurs because the gland has grown enough to compensate for conditions which would otherwise result in deficient secretion. The most common cause of simple goiter is a lack of dietary iodine, which tends to reduce thyroid hormone production. However, the compensatory increase in the size of the gland and its greater blood supply helps the thyroid to extract maximal amounts of iodine from the circulation. As a result, enough thyroid hormones are usually produced to maintain normal metabolism. Nonetheless, such thyroid enlargement indicates an abnormal functional state which requires correction.

Biosynthesis and Release of Thyroid Hormones

Before undertaking our discussion of the treatment of hypothyroidism, hyperthyroidism, and simple goiter, it is desirable to review the way in which the production and secretion of thyroid hormones are controlled and carried out. The reason for this is that nearly every kind of thyroid function disorder stems fundamentally from some defect that alters the normal rate of thyroid hormone synthesis and release.

BIOSYNTHESIS OF THYROID HORMONES

The thyroid gland produces two types of thyroid hormones: (1) *thyroxine*, or tetraiodothyronine, which contains four atoms of iodine; and (2) *liothyronine*, or triiodothyronine, a molecule with three iodine atoms. Both are made in three biosynthetic steps: (1) iodine trapping; (2) attachment of iodine atoms to the amino acid tyrosine; and (3) coupling of two types of iodotyrosine molecules.

IODINE TRAPPING. The thyroid gland removes iodine from the blood that passes through it. The element is concentrated within the gland in much higher amounts than are present in the plasma. A dietary deficiency of iodine, resulting in reduced synthesis of thyroid hormones and in simple goiter, was once common in some parts of the world, including the midwestern United States. Now, however, people who cannot get this element from seafood, drinking water, or leafy vegetables grown in soil that contains it can avoid iodine-deficiency diseases by using table salt to which iodine salt supplements (iodides) have been added.

IODINATION. The thyroid tissue that takes up iodide from the blood contains enzymes that oxidize it to active iodine atoms which are then attached to the amino acid tyrosine. Some of the drugs that are used in treating *hyper*thyroidism (Table 38-2) act by inhibiting the enzymes responsible for this oxidative reaction. Thus, even though the overactive gland continues to trap large amounts of iodide, hormone production is reduced, as are the signs and symptoms of *thyrotoxicosis* (see hyperthyroidism, Table 38-1).

COUPLING. In the final biosynthetic step, oxidative enzymes cause two molecules of diiodotyrosine to couple and to form *tetra*iodothyronine, or one molecule of *di*iodotyrosine may couple with one molecule of *mono*iodotyrosine to form *tri*iodotyrosine. Both hormones are then stored in the thyroid gland in a mucoprotein molecule called *thyroglobulin*, from which they are split off and secreted into the bloodstream when needed.

THYROID-PITUITARY RELATIONS

The secretion of stored thyroid hormones into the bloodstream is regulated by the anterior pituitary gland hormone *thyrotropin*. This thyroid-stimulating hormone (TSH) also regulates the thyroid gland's ability to extract iodine from the blood for building the thyroid hormone molecules. Under the influence of this tropic pituitary hormone, the thyroid gland grows in size, and it contains greater numbers of blood vessels.

A delicate balance exists between the pituitary and thyroid gland hormones. Ordinarily, if the level of thyroid hormones in the blood rises even slightly above normal, this suppresses the secretion of TSH by the pituitary gland. This negative feedback effect leads in turn to a reduction in thyroid hormone production. The reverse is also true: if the blood level of thyroxine is reduced, the pituitary gland increases its secretion of TSH. This then causes the thyroid to synthesize and to secrete more of its hormones. It is the failure of these reciprocal mechanisms to operate properly that often results in goiter and other thyroid gland disorders.

Hypothyroidism

A lack of thyroid hormone leads to two clear-cut deficiency syndromes: (1) *cretinism*, which is the result of glandular failure in infancy; and (2) *myxedema*, which is a condition that sometimes develops in adults and older children (juvenile myxedema).

In addition to these obvious deficiency states, some patients apparently suffer from a partial or *borderline* type of hypothyroidism. These patients, who often seem to have more or less normal thyroid activity, complain of various vague symptoms which are often dramatically improved by the administration of thyroid.

CRETINISM

Cretinism, or congenital hypothyroidism, may result from an inborn enzymatic defect that interferes with iodine uptake and utilization. More commonly, the child is born without a thyroid gland (athyreosis) or with one that has failed to develop properly. The routine use of iodized salt has largely eliminated endemic goiter in this country, but a lack of iodine in the mother's diet may still account for cases of cretinism in certain isolated mountainous regions elsewhere in the world.

Growth and development of the nervous and skeletal systems are retarded in congenitally hypothyroid infants. If the pediatrician recognizes the condition early and treats it with adequate doses of thyroid hormones, the child may develop normally. However, in those who are hypothyroid during fetal development and in infants whose condition goes unrecognized and untreated for more than a few months, the likelihood of permanant mental retardation is very high.

Once the cretinous condition is recognized, thyroid replacement therapy is promptly instituted. Doctors may differ in regard to the particular thyroid product that they prefer, but all agree that it is desirable to administer full doses of any preparation from the start. Infants apparently require relatively large doses and are able to tolerate them. After thyroid treatment has been initiated, the doctor determines the maintenance dose which will be required, through frequent checks of the levels of protein-bound iodine (PBI) (see *Summary of Tests for Thyroid Function*, p. 472) and by periodic x-ray films intended to follow the baby's bone development.

MYXEDEMA

Myxedema, the adult form of thyroid hormone deficiency, is marked by characteristic signs and symptoms (see Table 38-1). The condition most often develops slowly, as the person's thyroid gland gradually atrophies and functioning cells are replaced by fibrous connective tissue. Occasionally, myxedema follows acute or chronic inflammatory destruction of the gland—as in Hashimoto's (chronic) thyroiditis, for example. Overtreatment of hyperthyroidism with antithyroid drugs, excessive radiation therapy, or excessive tissue removal by surgery may also cause this severe form of hypothyroidism.

Some cases of myxedema are secondary to pituitary gland failure following childbirth complications or tumor development. Patients with pituitary myxedema have a thyroid gland that is capable of functioning, but which does not because of a lack of thyroid-stimulating hormone (TSH). Primary and secondary myxedema can be differentiated by administering the tropic pituitary hormone, *thyrotropin*. A normal thyroid gland then markedly increases its uptake of radioactive iodine despite the pituitary gland disorder. Patients with primary myxedema continue to show low iodine uptake despite administration of thyrotropin.

TREATMENT OF MYXEDEMA. The administration of adequate doses of thyroid hormones has a remarkable effect upon the mental and physical condition of the myxedematous patient. Even small amounts of thyroid quickly make a great difference in the patient's appearance and behavior. Puffiness disappears as most of the retained fluids are removed from the tissues by way of the kidneys. The dull, expressionless look is replaced by an alert, interested appearance, and physical sluggishness gives way to normal activity. Once the patient achieves normal hormonal balance, he can be kept in such functional equilibrium indefinitely by maintenance thyroid therapy.

The aim of treatment in primary myxedema is to bring about the greatest possible improvement with the lowest dosage of thyroid. That is, the patient is returned to as close to normal a state as possible without pushing him into a *hyper*thyroid state. Ordinarily this is done by administering relatively small doses which are raised gradually to exert a cumulative effect over a period of several weeks. Special care is taken to avoid overdosage in elderly patients and in those with a history of cardiac complications.

In myxedema that arises secondary to pituitary gland damage—as in hemorrhagic postpartum necrosis—thyroid treatment is helpful. Here, however, and in the case of hypophysectomized patients, the doctor may also order sex hormones and adrenal corticosteroids to make up for the lack of these secretions following the loss of the gonadotropic and adrenocorticotropic hormones of the pituitary. Replacement of corticosteroids is especially important when thyroid hormones are being administered, because the increased tissue metabolism brought about by the latter may send the patient into a state of adrenal insufficiency.

BORDERLINE HYPOTHYROIDISM

Hypometabolism is a term sometimes used to describe the state of a group of patients who do *not* show the multiple symptoms of full-blown myxedema but who nonetheless complain of various vague symptoms, traceable to a thyroid gland that is functioning at only a low normal level. When symptoms such as muscle weakness and pain, fatigue, lethargy, headaches, and emotional upsets are recognized to be the result of a mild, or borderline, hypothyroidism and thyroid therapy is administered, the patient may respond with a remarkable improvement.

NONTHYROID-DEFICIENCY CONDITIONS

Thyroid medication has long been advocated for treating many *non*myxedematous conditions which are marked by the presence of one or more signs and symptoms found in hypothyroidism. Obviously, since inadequate thyroid secretion can affect the functioning of nearly every body tissue, there are a great number of signs and symptoms that might in theory respond to thyroid replacement therapy. There is no reason to believe, however, that thyroid treatment will be effective for these conditions in the absence of hypothyroidism. Nonetheless, the fact that patients with seemingly normal thyroid gland activity sometimes respond well to thyroid administration has encouraged the *misuse* of thyroid drugs as a panacea.

OBESITY. Thyroid medication has often played a part in weight reduction regimens. Its use for this purpose seems unjustified and potentially dangerous. Although thyroid replacement therapy often reduces the flabbiness and puffiness of a myxedematous patient, it will speed neither fat metabolism nor removal of fluids from the tissues of a patient whose thyroid function is normal.

High doses of thyroid products may accelerate the patient's metabolism enough to cause some loss of weight. However, overdosage not only is dangerous (see below), but also may stimulate the patient's appetite. This, of course, makes it difficult for him to carry out the most effective weight-reducing measure —lowering his caloric intake.

The nurse can explain to women who ask whether thyroid would help them to lose weight that this hormone medication is prescribed by the doctor for those whose own glandular secretion is inadequate. She can help them understand that the overweight individual should consult her doctor for proper diagnosis and for whatever treatment he may order, including thyroid if he decides that replacement therapy is needed. The same advice applies in female reproductive disorders, in relation to which women sometimes inquire about thyroid therapy.

OBSTETRICAL-GYNECOLOGICAL DISORDERS. The reproductive system tissues are adversely affected by a lack of thyroid secretion. Frequently, hypothyroid women may suffer (for example) from a secondary deficiency of ovarian hormones. This lack of estrogens or progesterone often leads to menstrual irregularities, including menorrhagia. The fact that the administration of thyroid hormones sometimes helps to regularize the menstrual cycle of such *hypothyroid* patients does *not* mean that thyroid drug administration will be useful for treating abnormal menses in *euthyroid* women. Yet thyroid has often been administered routinely in *unselected* cases of amenorrhea, dysmenorrhea, premenstrual tension and other gynecological disorders, including sterility and habitual abortion.

OTHER CONDITIONS. The use of thyroid seems much less justified—even in theory—in dermatological, musculoskeletal, and other conditions marked by signs and symptoms similar to some found in hypothyroidism. Thus, although the myxedematous patient's skin may be dry and scaly, thyroid is no panacea for such symptoms when they occur in *euthyroid* individuals. Similarly, thyroid often relieves muscular cramps and joint pains in overt hypothyroidism, but it is no cure-all in arthritis and myositis; nor does the reversal of anemia by thyroid treatment of hypothyroidism mean that thyroid is ever a substitute for the adequate diagnosis and specific treatment of anemia with iron salts or other hematinics (Chapter 34).

Suppression of thyrotropin by the administration of a thyroid product has several uses in treatment and diagnosis. In *simple goiter* (p. 463), for example, giving thyroid often helps to reduce the size of the gland that has grown in size in response to stimulation by the pituitary hormone, TSH. Similarly, in hyperthyroid patients whose glands have undergone compensatory enlargement as a result of successful treatment with antithyroid drugs (see discussion of *goitrogens*, p. 470), the addition of thyroid medication in doses that suppress the thyroid-stimulating pituitary hormone sometimes stops further growth of the gland. The growth of thyrotropin-dependent thyroid cancer may also be slowed by administering thyroid. (The use of thyroid products in the diagnosis of hyperthyroidism and for evaluating the patient's response to antithyroid drugs is discussed below.)

ADVERSE EFFECTS (SEE SUMMARY, P. 472)

Overdosage with thyroid products results in the appearance of adverse cardiac effects and other signs and symptoms similar to those of hyperthyroidism or thyrotoxicosis (Table 38-1). The heart muscle is forced to work harder to meet the demands of the rapidly metabolizing peripheral tissues for blood. As a result, the rapidly beating heart may tend to outrun the capacity of its own coronary

vessels to supply the myocardium with oxygenated blood. Anginal chest pains then occur as a result of such myocardial ischemia. Older patients with some prior degree of coronary insufficiency may be precipitated into congestive heart failure if they receive too high a dose of a thyroid preparation. Patients taking thyroid should not be treated with catecholamines or other adrenergic drugs because of the possible adverse cardiac effects of the combination.

THYROID PRODUCTS

Several types of thyroid products are available (see Table 38-2). Opinions differ as to which

---

TABLE 38-2 *Drugs Used in Treatment and Diagnosis of Thyroid Disorders*

Official, Generic, or USAN Name	Proprietary Name	Daily Dosage
Drugs Used in Hypothyroidism		
Liotrix	Euthroid; Thyrolar	Initially one tablet daily containing 25–30 mg of levothyroxine and 6.25–7.5 μg liothyronine. Later, maintenance with mixtures of levothyroxine 50 to 180 μg and liothyronine 6.25 to 45 μg daily
Sodium dextrothyroxine	Choloxin	Initially 1 to 2 mg daily; maintenance 4 to 8 mg
Sodium levothyroxine U.S.P.	Synthroid; Letter	Initially 100 μg daily; maintenance 150 μg to 400 μg
Sodium liothyronine U.S.P.	Cytomel; triiodothyronine	Initially 5 μg daily; maintenance 5 to 100 μg
Thyroglobulin	Proloid	60 to 180 mg
Thyroid U.S.P.	Desiccated thyroid	15 to 180 mg
Drugs Used in Hyperthyroidism		
ANTITHYROID DRUGS (THIOCARBAMIDES)		
Methimazole U.S.P.	Tapazole	5 to 20 mg
Methylthiouracil N.F.	Methiacil; Thimecil	50 to 200 mg
Propylthiouracil U.S.P.	Propacil	50 to 500 mg
IODIDES AND IODINE		
Sodium iodide U.S.P.		300 mg to 1 g
Sodium iodide I 131 U.S.P.	Iodotope; Oriodide; Radiocaps; Theriodide; Tracervial	Oral or I.V. Diagnostic: the equivalent of 1 to 100 *microcuries*. Therapeutic: the equivalent of 1 to 100 *millicuries*
Strong iodine solution U.S.P.	Lugol's solution	0.1 to 1 ml
IODINE UPTAKE INHIBITORS		
Potassium perchlorate		200 to 400 mg every six to eight hours
Potassium thiocyanate		1 g daily
ANTERIOR PITUITARY HORMONE (for Diagnosis and Treatment)		
Thyrotropin	Thyroid-stimulating hormone; TSH; Thytropar	10 international units

preparation is preferable, and each kind has its advocates. Actually, all exert the same kind of metabolic effects and differ mainly in potency and in the time they take to act and to stop acting.

Thyroid+ and *thyroglobulin* (Proloid) are dried defatted powders prepared from the thyroid glands of animals. They are, of course, less potent than the pure hormones that they contain. However, when given in adequate dosage, these products are capable of producing all the desired effects of the purified or synthetically prepared hormones. The official thyroid powder is relatively cheap and serves as entirely satisfactory replacement therapy in most cases of hypothyroidism.

Sodium liothyronine+ (Cytomel; triiodothyronine) is the faster-acting of the two natural hormones. This makes it most useful for emergency treatment of myxedema coma. However, the relatively short duration of its action may be a drawback during long-term maintenance therapy of hypothyroidism. The fact that it is the most potent preparation available means only that it may be given in the lowest milligram dosage, but this in itself offers no significant advantage.

Thyroxine is now available in two forms: (1) the levo isomer, *sodium levothyroxine*; and (2) the dextro isomer, *sodium dextrothyroxine* (Choloxin)—the preferred form for reducing plasma cholesterol levels in patients with hyperlipidemia. *Sodium levothyroxine+* (Letter; Synthroid) produces its effects more slowly than liothyronine, but its effects, once fully attained, are longer-lasting.

Liotrix (Euthroid; Thyrolar) is a mixture containing four parts of levothyroxine to one part of liothyronine. This four to one ratio of the two hormones is claimed to imitate closely the effects of the natural thyroid gland secretions. Its advantage over powdered thyroid gland is said to lie in the constancy of its unvarying strength. The advantage of administering this mixture, instead of either hormone individually, is that its use permits better interpretation of the laboratory tests employed to determine the patient's response to treatment (see *Summary of Tests*, p. 472).

Hyperthyroidism

This condition is characterized by the excessive secretion of thyroid hormones, which increase the rate of oxidative metabolism in almost all the tissues of the body. This results in signs and symptoms (Table 38-1) which are distressing and dangerous. The basic cause of thyrotoxicosis is not known, but a thyroid-stimulating antibody is now believed to be involved.

This substance—also called the long-acting thyroid stimulator, or LATS—continues to act on the thyroid gland for many years. Unlike the thyroid-stimulating hormone of the pituitary gland (TSH), production of LATS is *not* shut off by an abnormally high plasma level of thyroid hormones. This is demonstrated in the so-called thyroid-suppression test.

In this test, *sodium liothyronine* is administered daily for a week. This reduces radioactive iodine uptake of *euthyroid* individuals to less than 20 percent of normal by suppressing pituitary production of thyrotropin (p. 467). In the *hyperthyroid* patient, on the other hand, such suppression of pituitary TSH by the thyroid hormone does not keep the thyroid gland from continuing to take up the radioactive iodine.

TREATMENT OF HYPERTHYROIDISM

Even though its exact cause is not known, the symptoms of hyperthyroidism can now be readily controlled, and, in many cases the condition can actually be cured. The main forms of treatment are: (1) the administration of one or more of the so-called *antithyroid drugs*; (2) *radiation therapy* employing the radioactive iodine isotope, I 131; and (3) subtotal *surgical excision* of the gland (*thyroidectomy*).

Radiation and surgery permanently eliminate the mass of thyroid gland tissue that has been excreting hormones in excessive amounts. Antithyroid drugs, on the other hand, are also effective for bringing about permanant remissions of hyperthyroidism, without damaging the gland beyond repair as do radiation and surgery. It is often possible to determine during the course of treatment with antithyroid drugs whether further treatment is likely to result in a cure. The patient is given a thyroid-suppression test (see above) after six months of drug treatment. If the test dose of liothyronine now suppresses the uptake of radioactive iodine, the chance of a permanent remission is good; if uptake is not suppressed, remission is unlikely, and surgery or radioactive isotope therapy will probably be required.

ANTITHYROID DRUGS (GOITROGENS)

Drugs of several different kinds act in one way or another to interfere with the biosynthesis of hormones by the thyroid gland. The most widely used are the thiocarbamides listed in Table 38-2. These chemicals inhibit the oxidative enzymes that catalyze the iodination and coupling steps in the synthesis of thyroxine and liothyronine. As a result, the gland soon stops secreting the excessive amounts of hormones responsible for the signs and symptoms of hyperthyroidism. Even though the thyroid then undergoes compensatory enlargement, the patient's condition improves over a period of weeks. (Further enlargement of the thyroid gland can often be halted by administration of thyroid medication to suppress pituitary production of thyrotropin; see p. 467).

More than half the patients who take a drug such as *methimazole*+ (Tapazole) or *propylthiouracil* (Propacil) faithfully for a year or more may never again have a recurrence of hyperthyroidism. It is important to encourage patients to take the drug regularly and exactly as directed since, if they neglect to continue taking the drugs daily for many months and at the proper times of day until control is established, the condition may recur. They should also be urged to report any symptoms of illness immediately; sore throat, fever, rash, or jaundice may be signs of drug reactions calling for prompt withdrawal of these drugs. Only a small minority of patients develop adverse reactions. However, these may include serious disorders such as agranulocytosis and hepatitis.

PREPARATION FOR SURGERY. Although a third or more of hyperthyroid patients cannot be cured with drugs alone, the administration of *propylthiouracil* or one of its relatives is useful in preparing patients for subtotal thyroidectomy. After taking daily doses of an antithyroid drug for several weeks, the patient's metabolism is brought back closer to normal and his cardiovascular system is stabilized. The only difficulty with such drug therapy is that the patient's gland tends to grow larger and is more likely to bleed excessively during the operation. To prevent this, the surgeon has the patient take a few drops of an iodide solution such as Lugol's solution (Table 38-2) daily for a week or ten days before the surgical procedure is to be done.

IODIDES

In addition to their preoperative use for reducing the size and fragility of the enlarged thyroid gland, iodine salts are sometimes effective for control of mild cases of hyperthyroidism. More severe cases are not permanently controlled by iodides alone and may even be made worse. However, when administered following *methimazole*+, iodides are sometimes helpful for treating *thyroid crisis*.* The small amounts of Lugol's solution or of saturated solution of potassium iodide that are ordered for this purpose must be accurately measured, and the drops should be added to fruit juice or milk to disguise the unpleasant taste.

RADIOACTIVE IODINE. The iodine isotope I-131 is trapped by the thyroid gland in the same manner as ordinary iodides. Reaching very high concentrations there, it gives off beta and gamma radiations in amounts that are useful for both the diagnosis of thyroid disorders and the treatment of some cases of hyperthyroidism. Tiny tracer doses are administered to determine the thyroid gland's capacity to store iodine; much larger amounts are administered deliberately to destroy thyroid tissue—for example, in patients for whom surgery does not seem safe and whose hyperthyroidism has not responded to drugs.

The *diagnostic use* of sodium radioiodide solution is based on the measurable differences in retention and excretion of iodine. In myxedema only a small proportion of any administered dose is taken up by the patient's thyroid gland, and the rest is excreted in the urine. In the hyperthyroid patient, on the other hand, the thyroid retains a high percentage of the amount administered, and relatively little radioactivity is detected in the urine. The small doses of radioiodide give off enough gamma rays so that such determinations may readily be made; the beta rays are so few that there is little danger of damage to the patient's thyroid or other tissues.

The *therapeutic use* of sodium iodide I 131 involves the administration of perhaps a thousand times as high a dose of the radioisotope.

---

* *Thyroid crisis*, or *thyroid storm*, is a dangerous reaction marked by high fever and a very rapid heart rate that can lead to congestive heart failure. Among drugs used to control the tachycardia are the beta adrenergic blocking agent, *propranolol*,+ and the adrenergic neuron blocking drugs, *guanethidine*+ and *reserpine*+ (Chapters 26 and 29).

The drug is given either as a single large dose or in a series of smaller cumulative doses. In either case, the iodine isotope accumulates in the patient's thyroid in amounts as much as 10,000 times as high as that in other body tissues. The very short-range beta rays that are then given off thus destroy thyroid tissue without harming other cells. As a result of the gradual reduction in hormone secretion, the symptoms of hyperthyroidism are gradually reduced, and the patient's metabolic rate may become normal in about 12 weeks.

The main difficulty with radioactive iodine is that the beta rays may destroy too much thyroid tissue. Therefore, the patient is examined periodically for signs of *hypo*thyroidism and, if any tendency toward myxedema is noted, thyroid therapy is instituted. Just as in hypothyroidism caused by surgical removal of too much thyroid tissue, the patient who is made myxedematous by too great a destructive action of radioactive iodine may require replacement thyroid therapy for the rest of his life.

In caring for patients who are taking radioactive iodide, the nurse should check on what precautions are necessary. The doses employed for diagnostic purposes are so small that special care is not required, but therapeutic doses can result in potential dangers. Thus, the nurse should read the product literature and other references in regard to current practices in radiation therapy, so that she can then work more closely with personnel in the hospital's radiation therapy department. The nurse also has a role in explaining to the patient the use of radiation precautions, should these be necessary.

Other goitrogenic chemicals, such as *potassium perchlorate,* have found a place in the treatment of hyperthyroidism. Administered in several small daily doses with food to reduce gastric irritation, this drug quickly reduces the signs and symptoms of thyrotoxicosis. Like the thiocarbamide-type goitrogens, this chemical has sometimes caused blood dyscrasias. Unlike the latter group of antithyroid drugs, perchlorate can*not* be used preoperatively along with iodides to prepare the person for thyroid gland surgery. The reason for this lies in this drug's manner of action: the perchlorate ion competes with the iodide ion and keeps it from being taken up from the blood by the patient's thyroid gland. This, of course, accounts for its clinical utility in reducing the synthesis of excessive amounts of hormones in hyperthyroid individuals, but it also keeps these patients from profiting from the ability of iodides to shrink a hyperplastic, brittle thyroid gland before thyroidectomy.

S U M M A R Y of the Clinical Uses of Thyroid Preparations

Hypothyroidism (Replacement Therapy)

Myxedema (adult and juvenile).

Cretinism (after very early diagnosis).

Gynecological disorders (amenorrhea, dysmenorrhea, habitual abortion, and so forth, when these are the result of thyroid hormone deficiency).

Male infertility (as a result of oligospermia stemming from reduced thyroid function).

Hypometabolism as a result of borderline hypothyroid deficiency, with signs and symptoms such as dry skin and hair, loss of scalp hair, brittle nails, intolerance to cold, feelings of fatigue and sluggishness, and obesity.

Other Uses (Suppression of thyrotropin)

Simple nontoxic goiter in the following:
(1) Euthyroid patients (normally functioning thyroid gland).
(2) Hypothyroid patients (for example, chronic thyroiditis).
(3) Hyperthyroid patients treated with antithyroid drugs.

Treatment of thyrotropin-dependent thyroid gland malignancies.

Thyroid suppression test (using sodium liothyronine):
(1) Differential diagnosis of response of hyperthyroid and euthyroid patients to radioactive iodine uptake test.
(2) Evaluation of response of hyperthyroid patients to treatment with antithyroid drugs.

S U M M A R Y of Adverse Effects, Cautions, and Contraindications with Thyroid Products

Signs and Symptoms of Overdosage

Tachycardia, cardiac arrhythmias, elevated pulse pressure, anginal-type chest pains, dyspnea, possible precipitation of congestive failure; excessive sweating, intolerance to heat, fever, flushing; nervousness, irritability, insomnia, headache; increased gastrointestinal motility, abdominal cramps, diarrhea, nausea, increased appetite.

Cautions and Contraindications

Caution in patients with a history of angina pectoris, recent myocardial infarction or congestive heart failure, and hypertension.

Contraindicated in adrenal insufficiency, or in hypopituitarism, unless adrenal deficiency is first corrected by administration of adequate doses of cortisone or hydrocortisone.

Drug Interactions

Patients taking anticoagulants such as warfarin and bishydroxycoumarin may require a one-third reduction in dosage when thyroid preparations are added to their regimen.

Patients taking insulin or oral hypoglycemic agents should also be closely observed when thyroid treatment is begun.

S U M M A R Y of Adverse Effects, Cautions, and Contraindications of Antithyroid Drugs

Thiocarbamides (Methimazole; Propylthiouracil; and others)

Skin rashes—mild hives, papules, purpura.

Gastrointestinal upset—nausea, epigastric distress.

Arthralgia—pain and stiffness in joints of wrists and hands.

Nervous system—headache, dizziness, drowsiness.

Blood dyscrasias—mild leukopenia and rarely agranulocytosis, signaled by severe sore throat and fever. (Patients are advised to report such illness immediately. Differential blood counts are done periodically.)

Iodine (Potassium iodide; Sodium iodide; Strong iodine solution)

Mouth—brassy taste; burning sensation; gum soreness, salivary gland swelling, and excessive salivation.

Respiratory tract—irritation resembling common cold and sinusitis with frontal headache, and also conjunctivitis.

Skin—acnelike lesions; rarely, bulbous lesions.

Gastric—irritation with nausea and vomiting.

Radioactive Iodine (Sodium iodide I-131)

Thyroid gland—early soreness or tenderness and swelling with rare asphyxial reactions; late hypothyroidism.

Late development of acute leukemia or thyroid carcinoma is possible but considered unlikely.

Contraindicated in pregnant women and nursing mothers.

Potassium perchlorate

Gastric irritation, nausea, and vomiting.

Hypersensitivity reactions—skin rashes, fever.

Lymphadenopathy; nephrotic syndrome.

Agranulocytosis and, rarely, aplastic anemia.

S U M M A R Y of Tests for Thyroid Function*

The Basal Metabolic Rate (B.M.R.)

This test is intended to measure the extent to which the patient's tissues are using up oxygen in carrying out combustion processes when the patient is in the resting state. When properly performed, it not only helps to differentiate euthyroid from hyperthyroid and hypothyroid individuals, but also aids the doctor in following his

* All of these laboratory diagnostic tests are often useful when evaluated simultaneously. However, all are subject to error and serve best when the doctor uses the results to supplement his clinical judgment as based upon the patient's history and physical examination.

patient's response to circulating thyroid hormones administered as replacement therapy, or the drop in tissue response to such hormones under the influence of antithyroid drugs.

Radioactive Iodine Uptake (R.A.I. 131)

This test is intended to measure the thyroid gland's capacity for trapping and concentrating radioiodide. The gland of hypothyroid patients takes up only a small fraction of the orally administered tracer dose of the isotope, whereas hyperthyroid patients show accumulation of a large percentage of the amount of I-131 that was taken 24 hours before. (The iodine uptake of a normal gland is suppressed by prior administration of the hormone sodium liothyronine; in Graves' disease, the patient's hyperplastic gland continues to concentrate radioactive iodide even after thyroid suppression of pituitary TSH production.)

Protein-Bound Iodine (PBI)

This test is intended to determine the amount of thyroid hormone circulating in loose combination with plasma carrier proteins. The PBI is high in hyperthyroidism and low in hypothyroidism. A more accurate modification, the *Butanol-Extractable Iodine (B.E.I.)* test, measures only the thyroxine content of the plasma and *not* other circulating iodine-containing compounds that may also be present in addition to the hormone.

SUMMARY of Points for the Nurse to Remember About Thyroid Preparations

Thyroid preparations sometimes cause unpleasant side effects. Observe the patient for signs and symptoms such as nervousness and insomnia; report the symptoms to the physician if they should occur, and teach the patient to do so.

Misconceptions concerning the appropriate use of thyroid preparations are widespread. The nurse can help to clarify the legitimate use of thyroid preparations and encourage patients to seek medical advice for conditions such as fatigue and weight gain.

Regular and persistent drug therapy are especially important in the treatment of patients with hyperthyroidism. Because many of these patients continue drug treatment at home for extended periods, it is particularly important to instruct them in the importance of regular and continued drug therapy as prescribed by the physician.

Particular care should be taken in accurate measurement of the small amounts of liquid iodide preparations ordinarily prescribed. The disagreeable taste of these drugs can be disguised by placing them in milk or fruit juice.

Special precautions are ordinarily not required when radioactive iodide is administered for diagnostic purposes. However, the nurse should confer with personnel of the radiation therapy department of the hospital in regard to necessary precautions when using any radioactive isotope.

Clinical Nursing Situation

The Situation: Mrs. Larsen is a 32-year-old woman who has hyperthyroidism. The first signs of her condition were the development of weight loss, increased appetite, nervousness, and insomnia. Her doctor has prescribed methimazole, and has outlined a program of ample nutrition and adequate rest. Both are difficult for Mrs. Larsen to follow, since she has four small children and a very limited budget. Her husband is a truck driver who is periodically unemployed. Mrs. Larsen's symptoms grow worse whenever her husband is out of work.

The objective in caring for Mrs. Larsen is to help her maintain a regimen of methimazole, adequate food intake, rest, and relief from some of the stress in her life situation. The physician will see Mrs. Larsen once every six weeks. It is your responsibility to visit the patient at home at the intervals that you think necessary, to help her establish and maintain her treatment program.

The Problem: Describe the observations you would make to guide you in caring for Mrs. Larsen and in evaluating her condition and response to treatment. Describe some measures you believe may be useful in assisting Mrs. Larsen to carry out her treatment.

DRUG DIGEST

METHIMAZOLE U.S.P. (Tapazole)
Actions and Indications. This antithyroid drug is used in the treatment of hyperthyroidism to reduce the rate of biosynthesis of thyroid hormones. Continued treatment for up to a year or more often brings about remission of thyrotoxicosis. Patients who require thyroid surgery or radioisotope treatment often benefit from pretreatment with methimazole. It is also used as part of the management of thyroid crisis, or storm.

Side Effects, Cautions, and Contraindications. Minor side effects that occur in a small proportion of patients include skin rash, gastrointestinal upset, headache, and joint pain. The potentially most serious adverse effect is the development of blood dyscrasias such as agranulocytosis and thrombocytopenia. Although this is not common, all patients are cautioned to report such signs as severe sore throat and fever, so that differential blood counts can be made and the drug discontinued if necessary. Further treatment is contraindicated in patients who have shown signs of hypersensitivity.

Care is also required in administering this drug during pregnancy, as it can cross the placenta and induce goiter and cretinism in the fetus. To avoid this in treating hyperthyroidism, dosage of this drug is kept at minimal effective levels and supplemented with a thyroid preparation to prevent hypothyroidism from developing in the newborn infant.

Dosage and Administration. This drug is taken by mouth in three daily doses at intervals of eight hours. Mild cases in adults can often be controlled with a daily dose of 15 mg. More serious cases may require a rise in dosage to 30 or 40 mg daily, and 60 mg may be required for the most serious cases. Dosage can later be reduced to maintenance levels of 5 to 15 mg daily. The latter is also the dose used for initiating treatment of children aged 6 to 10.

SODIUM IODIDE I 131 U.S.P.
(Iodotope; Radiocaps; and others)
Actions and Indications. This radioactive isotope of iodine is taken up by the thyroid gland and concentrated there. With small doses, the amount taken up serves as an index of thyroid function, as the gamma radiation that is given off is low in hypothyroidism and abnormally high in hyperthyroidism.

High doses are used to destroy glandular tissue in hyperthyroidism. This (and the resulting reduction in secretory activity) is brought about by the beta rays that are given off by the iodide that has accumulated in the gland.

Side Effects, Cautions, and Contraindications. Use of this isotope is contraindicated during pregnancy and in nursing mothers. It is given only with caution to children and young adults, as the question of whether this compound can cause thyroid cancer, leukemia, or chromosome damage is not yet considered resolved.

Pain in swallowing and soreness in the neck often follows treatment, but severe swelling and thyroiditis are relatively rare. Hypothyroidism may develop as a late result of treatment. Large doses may cause bone marrow depression or set off thyroid storm.

Dosage and Administration. The solution may be administered orally or by vein in doses that depend upon the intended use and the size of the gland. Doses of 1 to 100 *micro*curies are used for diagnostic tracer purposes. Doses for treatment of hyperthyroidism are 1,000 times as high—that is, 1 to 100 *milli*curies.

SODIUM LEVOTHYROXINE U.S.P.
(Letter; Synthroid)
Actions and Indications. This synthetic salt of the natural thyroid hormone L-tetraiodothyronine produces a gradual but long-sustained stimulation of tissue metabolism, growth, and development. This makes it effective for long-term replacement therapy of patients with hypothyroidism. It is useful as substitution therapy in cretinism and other pediatric cases, in myxedema, and in hypothyroidism without myxedema in other adults, including pregnant women and elderly patients. It also reduces the size of the enlarged thyroid gland in simple, nontoxic goiter.

Side Effects, Cautions, and Contraindications. Patients are watched closely for the gradual development of signs of hypermetabolism and thyrotoxicosis. These include: loss of weight; abdominal cramps, diarrhea, and vomiting; nervousness, tremors, sweating, and heart palpitations. Caution is required in patients with cardiovascular diseases, including angina pectoris and hypertension. The drug is con-

traindicated in patients with uncorrected adrenal insufficiency.

Dosage of anticoagulant drugs is reduced by one third because of possible potentiation of their hypoprothrombinemic effects by the action of this drug. The dosage of insulin or oral hypoglycemic agents may have to be increased when this thyroid hormone is added to the regimen of a patient with diabetes mellitus.

Dosage and Administration. Dosage is individualized in accordance with clinical response and laboratory tests. Treatment is usually started with a single dose of 0.025 mg, which is very gradually raised to the usual maintenance dose of 0.1 to 0.3 mg daily. In myxedematous coma, 200 to 400 μg may be injected by vein.

SODIUM LIOTHYRONINE U.S.P.
(Cytomel)
Actions and Indications. This synthetic salt of the natural thyroid hormone L-triiodothyronine has a rapid onset and short duration of action. These properties may make it more useful in emergency situations than other thyroid preparations but less useful than forms with a longer action for long-term maintenance therapy of hypothyroidism.

It may be most useful for patients in coma from myxedema and for patients made suddenly hypothyroid as a result of overtreatment of hyperthyroidism. This hormone is also useful in the differential diagnosis of borderline hyperthyroidism from euthyroidism. In this situation and in the treatment of simple (nontoxic) goiter, it acts by suppressing the production of thyrotropin by the anterior pituitary gland.

Side Effects, Cautions, and Contraindications. Overdosage produces signs and symptoms of hyperthyroidism including nervous irritability, sweating, headache, diarrhea, menstrual irregularities, and tachycardia. These adverse effects can be quickly controlled and the dosage readjusted because of this drug's short action. Caution is required in patients with cardiovascular diseases such as angina pectoris and in patients with hypopituitarism and others with adrenal insufficiency. It should not be administered until supplemental adrenal steroids have corrected any tendency toward adrenal insufficiency.

Dosage and Administration. Treatment is usually initiated with oral doses of only 5 μg because of the sensitivity of myxedematous patients. Dosage is then gradually increased to maintenance amounts between 50 and 100 μg daily, administered as a single dose. For thyroid suppression tests 75 to 100 μg is administered daily during the week between the two tests of radioactive iodine uptake.

THYROID U.S.P.

Actions and Indications. This preparation, a dried powder made from animal thyroid glands, contains the natural hormones. Thus, it exerts the same therapeutic effects as the pure compounds when administered in adequate dosage as replacement therapy in hypothyroidism, myxedema, cretinism, and nontoxic goiter. In such cases the full effects of thyroid administration come on slowly but are then relatively prolonged.

Side Effects, Cautions, and Contraindications. Overdosage causes cardiac palpitations and rapid rhythmic irregularities, sweating, nervousness, headache, tremors, and insomnia. Thyroid is used only with caution in patients with a history of hypertension or angina pectoris, and it is contraindicated in patients with an acute myocardial infarction. In patients who also suffer from Addison's disease, hypothyroidism should be treated only after hypoadrenalism is first corrected with corticosteroid drug therapy. The same is true in cases of hypothyroidism that occur secondary to hypopituitarism. Patients taking anticoagulant drugs of the coumarin type may require a reduction in dosage of about one third when thyroid is added to their regimen.

Dosage and Administration. Dosage of thyroid varies widely, depending upon the degree of hypothyroidism that requires correction. Treatment may be begun with 15 to 60 mg daily, depending upon pretreatment PBI values. Dosage is then gradually increased until the desired effect is attained. The usual maintenance dose is between 100 and 200 mg daily but may range from 30 to 600 mg daily depending upon the individual patient's response.

References

Asper, S.P. Physiological approach to correction of hypothyrodism. *Arch. Intern. Med. (Chicago)*, 107:112, 1961.

Astwood, E.B. Management of thyroid disorders. *JAMA*, 186:585, 1963

Clark, D., and Rule, J.H. Radioactive iodine or surgery in treatment of hyperthyroidism. *JAMA*, 159:995, 1955.

De Groot, L.J. Therapy of thyrotoxicosis. *Mod. Treatm.*, 1:176, 1964.

Greer, M.A. The treatment of myxedema. *GP*, 22:123, 1960.

Lerman, J. Treatment of hypothyroidism. *Mod. Treatm.*, 1:146, 1964.

McGirr, E.M. Sporadic goitrous cretinism. *Brit. Med. Bull.*, 16:113, 1960.

Rodman, M.J. Drugs used in thyroid diseases. *RN*, 25:61, 1962.

———. The thyroid and antithyroid drugs. *RN*, 31:55, 1968 (Feb.).

Selenkow, H.A., and Collaco, F.M. Clinical pharmacology of antithyroid compounds. *Clin. Pharmacol. Ther.*, 2:191, 1961.

Zellmann, H.E. Hyperthyroidism. *Med. Clin. N. Amer.*, 56:717, 1972 (May).

39.

Drugs Used in Diabetes

Diabetes Mellitus

Diabetes is the most common of all the metabolic diseases. About two million people in this country are known diabetics, and an estimated million more have not yet come to medical attention. The number of diabetics is expected to increase as more people live to middle and old age—the age at which four out of five cases are first recognized.

Diabetes first manifests itself as *hyperglycemia* (fasting sugar levels of over 110 mg per 100 ml of venous blood) and *glycosuria* (the presence of *any* sugar in the urine). However, despite this focusing of attention on sugar (the term *mellitus* means "honeyed"), diabetes is a disease not only of carbohydrate metabolism but also of protein and fat metabolism. In fact, even though screening tests and diagnostic techniques for detecting diabetes are based upon finding evidence of defects in carbohydrate metabolism, the most dangerous of both the acute and the chronic complications of diabetes are the result of abnormalities in fat and protein chemistry.

The *metabolic abnormalities of diabetes stem from a lack of effective insulin activity.* Insulin is a hormone secreted into the bloodstream by the endocrine portions of the pancreas. These are the so-called *beta cells* located in tiny islets of tissue scattered through the rest of the pancreas, an organ which also produces exocrine digestive juices. (The Latin word *insula* means "island.")

In diabetes, the patient's metabolism seems to function as though he were fasting, even when he is actually eating and absorbing the products of digestion. This occurs either because his pancreas fails to produce adequate amounts of insulin or because the hormone which is produced does not carry out its metabolic functions effectively.

The Role of Insulin in Regulating Metabolism

The relationship between the pancreas and carbohydrate metabolism was first recognized late in the last century, when dogs whose pancreases had been surgically removed developed diabetes-like signs. In 1922, the Canadian scientists Banting and Best gave an extract of pancreatic islet tissue to a boy dying of diabetes. His dramatic recovery demonstrated the ability of insulin to correct the metabolic abnormality responsible for his severe illness.

Later, insulin was prepared in pure crystalline form from extracts of the pancreatic tissues of animals. This led to its use as replacement therapy in patients with diabetes mellitus whose own pancreatic beta cells failed to secrete enough active insulin. Before discussing the use of insulin in diabetes, we must first review the physiological functions of this hormone and the metabolic abnormalities that develop when there is a lack of insulin.

THE ACTION OF INSULIN

Body cells burn fragments of digested foodstuffs to produce energy. The products of the digestion of carbohydrates, fats, and proteins must first be absorbed into the blood from the intestine. They are then transported to the tissues and released into the extracellular fluids. Finally, they make their way through the membranes of the cells of all the various tissues. Only after it gets inside the cell can a molecule of a substance such as glucose enter the metabolic mill—the series of enzymatically catalyzed intracellular oxidation-reduction reactions—and be converted into energy.

One of the main metabolic actions of insulin is to influence the rate at which glucose molecules move through cell membranes. Under the influence of this hormone, muscle cell membranes, for example, permit rapid entry of glucose from the extracellular fluid surrounding the cells. Without insulin's action in springing this trap door in the membrane, glucose levels of the blood stay high (*hyperglycemia*).

Glucose molecules that move into muscle cells may be burnt immediately or stored as glycogen. The liver also keeps glucose in this storage form, until the cells need this sugar for producing more energy. The reconversion of glycogen to glucose is brought about by the action of the adrenal medulla hormone, *epinephrine*, and by another pancreatic hormone, called *glucagon*. A lack of insulin also causes liver glycogen and muscle protein to be converted to glucose, thus increasing hyperglycemia and causing a muscle-wasting effect.

Insulin secretion by the pancreatic beta cells is stimulated when glucose begins to enter the blood during the digestion of food. The hormone then helps to remove the excess glucose by aiding entrance of the sugar into muscle and fat cells and by keeping liver glucose in the glycogen storage form. As the blood sugar level returns to normal, insulin secretion stops.

Insulin deficiency leads not only to a rise in blood sugar levels but also to other metabolic abnormalities. A lack of insulin causes muscle protein to break down to amino acids. These are carried to the liver where some are converted to glucose, while others form fatty acids and ketone bodies such as acetone, acetoacetic acid, and beta-hydroxybutyric acid. Another source of these substances is the burning of fat by the body as a source of energy, when the absence of adequate amounts of insulin interferes with glucose metabolism. The excess keto acids are combined with alkali and excreted by the kidney.

SIGNS AND SYMPTOMS OF INSULIN DEFICIENCY

The onset of acute diabetes in a person who had previously shown no overt signs may be slow and insidious, or it may occur with dramatic suddenness. At one extreme, the patient may complain only of being chronically tired; at the other, the first sign may be a swift slide into diabetic coma. In general, however, acute diabetes of moderate severity is marked by a classic clinical picture. It is essential that the nurse be alert to early symptoms of diabetes as she gives primary health care. Older people, especially, require vigilance, particularly if their family history shows the disease. Prompt referral to a clinic or a physician is necessary.

In addition to feelings of fatigue and complaints of *pruritus* (itching of the skin and genital area), the patient may become aware of being excessively thirsty and hungry. These symptoms persist even when he drinks large amounts of fluid and eats heavily. Weight loss is common in young patients; obesity frequently occurs in older ones. The patient produces large amounts of urine, which tests reveal to be loaded with sugar and, often, with acetone or other ketones. Blood tests also show the presence of high glucose and ketone levels.

All of these features of this phase of diabetes can be explained in terms of the underlying metabolic defect. The hyperglycemia, as we have indicated, stems from the lack of effective insulin for shunting blood glucose into muscle cells, adipose tissues, and liver glycogen. The patient's *polyuria* and *glycosuria* develop when the amount of sugar filtered by the glomeruli of the kidneys is greater than the renal tubules can reabsorb. Because the sugar dissolved in the tubular fluid drags water along with it by osmotic action as it drains out into the ureters, the diabetic patient tends to become dehydrated.

DIABETIC KETOACIDOSIS AND COMA. This acute complication resulting from a lack of insulin is most dangerous. It occurs most frequently in youngsters with *juvenile-onset* diabetes—that is, diabetes diagnosed between birth and about age twenty. However, older people, in whom so-called *maturity-onset* diabetes usually manifests itself after age forty in a relatively mild form, sometimes go suddenly from an asymptomatic state into severe acidosis and coma. This condition, which is a medical emergency requiring prompt diagnosis and vigorous treatment, is the result of a vicious cycle of events set in motion by the absence of insulin. Patients whose condition had previously been controlled by insulin from an outside source may be precipitated into acidosis and coma when they develop an acute infection.

The process that finally results in uncontrolled diabetes is initiated when the patient's insulin lack and consequent failure to utilize glucose leads to the breakdown of tissue proteins and fats for use as fuel. The fatty acids formed in this way flood the liver with metabolic fragments that are converted to ketones. When these pile up to levels higher than the tissues can handle by burning for energy, they accumulate in the blood (*ketonemia*) and are carried to the kidneys for excretion in the urine (*ketonuria*).

Some of these ketones are carried to the lungs for elimination and account for the fruity odor on the patient's breath. Other ketoacids are excreted by the kidneys combined with bicarbonate, sodium, and potassium ions. This reduces the body's alkaline reserves and leads to a loss of fluids and electrolytes that may send the dehydrated patient into shock. The patient's respiratory center is at first stimulated (Kussmaul-type hyperpnea) and then depressed.

Insulin in the Treatment of Diabetes

The injection of insulin obtained from the pancreatic tissues of animals is the most important measure in the management of diabetes. All patients whose condition cannot be adequately controlled by diet and weight reduction must receive properly adjusted doses of insulin, unless various complications make its use impractical. In some such cases, oral hypoglycemic agents can be substituted for insulin.

Various forms of insulin are available for use in different clinical situations. Some are rapid in onset and relative short in duration of action. Others exert long-lasting effects following a single subcutaneous injection. A third group of preparations produces effects intermediate between these two extremes (see Table 39-1).

The doctor selects the insulin preparation best suited to each patient. One type must never be substituted for the particular kind of preparation that was ordered. The dosage and duration of action of all products varies from patient to patient. Dosage adjustments must be made only under the doctor's direction.

INITIAL THERAPY

The nurse often plays an important part in instructing the diabetic patient in important points about storing insulin products and preparing them for administration. Thus, for example, patients are advised to keep insulin in a cool place. Most often this is a refrigerator, but patients should be warned not to put a vial in the freezer compartment. The patient should learn to look for the expiration date stamped on the package and not use an outdated preparation. He should discard medication that shows sign of deterioration or contamination. Instruction in the use of insulin

TABLE 39-1   *Insulin Preparations Used in the Treatment of Diabetes*

	Proprietary Name or Synonym	Dosage	Onset and Duration of Action
Rapid-Acting Preparations			
Insulin injection U.S.P.	Regular insulin; regular Iletin	5–100 U.S.P. units s.c. as needed	1 hour onset; 6–8 hours duration
Prompt insulin zinc suspension U.S.P.	Semilente Insulin; Semilente Iletin	10–80 U.S.P. units s.c.	1 hour onset; 12–18 hours duration
Intermediate-Acting Preparations			
Isophane insulin suspension U.S.P.	NPH Insulin	10–80 U.S.P. units s.c.	2 hours onset; 24–28 hours duration
Insulin zinc suspension U.S.P.	Lente Insulin; Lente Iletin	10–80 U.S.P. units	2 hours onset; 24–28 hours duration
Globin zinc insulin		10–80 U.S.P. units	2 to 4 hours onset; 10–22 hours duration
Long-Acting Preparations			
Extended insulin zinc suspension U.S.P.	Utralente Insulin; Ultralente Iletin	10–80 units s.c.	5–8 hours onset; 2–36 hours duration or more
Protamine zinc insulin suspension U.S.P.	Protamine Zinc Iletin	10–80 U.S.P. units s.c.	7 hours onset; 24–36 hours duration

is but one aspect of a teaching program designed to help the patient to care for himself.

Regular insulin, for example, should be water-clear and not discolored or turbid. Insulin suspensions should not appear to have clumps of granules or solid deposits. They should be rotated and inverted several times to assure even distribution, but the vials should not be vigorously shaken. The different kinds of modified preparations must never be mixed together.

Many patients with newly diagnosed diabetes should be hospitalized to have their exact needs for insulin determined. Most internists start the patient on doses of about 10 units of regular *insulin+* administered before breakfast. Further doses may be added before other meals and at bedtime. The patient's response is observed to determine whether his condition requires insulin at all or can be managed by diet and weight reduction.

Patients whose blood sugar tends to rise during the night may do best on a long-acting insulin, such as *protamine zinc insulin+*, which continues to dissolve slowly from the depot injection site into the bloodstream all through the night. Unfortunately, those patients who are most likely to suffer nocturnal hyperglycemia are also the ones whose unstable, or brittle disease makes them prone to suffer hypoglycemic reactions also. Thus, these pa-

tients usually need to take bedtime and between-meal snacks to prevent recurrent drops in blood sugar.

INSULIN IN KETOACIDOSIS

Various kinds of stressful conditions may increase a diabetic patient's need for insulin. Most commonly the occurrence of an acute infection and fever raises the patient's insulin requirements. However, the patient may think that he does not need insulin because he has not eaten on account of nausea and vomiting. Patients are instructed not to neglect taking their insulin in such circumstances. They should, in fact, administer an additional dose of rapid-acting regular insulin if their tests of urine specimens reveal a rising glucose content or persistent ketonuria. It is desirable that a member of the family be instructed to call the doctor and handle the testing of the patient's urine and the necessary adjustments in insulin dosage, since the acutely ill patient may become too drowsy or confused to do so.

The patient with definitely diagnosed ketoacidosis or diabetic coma requires prompt and vigorous treatment. He receives injections of relatively large doses of rapid-acting insulin together with fluids and electrolytes. The nurse must see to it that these and other needed supplies are available. She takes and records data such as the patient's pulse, blood pressure, body temperature, fluid intake, and urinary output, and makes careful observations of his general condition and response to therapy. The patient in diabetic coma requires meticulous care and must be protected from injury (by side rails, for example).

HYPOGLYCEMIC REACTIONS TO INSULIN

Too much insulin may also cause coma, which must be differentiated from diabetic coma by determination of the patient's blood sugar and ketone levels. It is better, however, to *prevent* such dangerous reactions by carefully observing the patient for signs of hypoglycemia and administering some food containing readily absorbed glucose. The nurse can help here also by teaching the patient to recognize the symptoms of hyperinsulinism and to take appropriate actions when he detects hypoglycemic symptoms typical of his own pattern.

Signs and symptoms (see *Summary*, p. 484) vary from patient to patient. The patient's response to insulin overdosage depends in part upon the type of preparation that he has been using. Thus, for example, the more dramatic signs seen with an overdose of regular insulin do not ordinarily occur with the more slowly absorbed insulins that cause blood sugar to fall gradually to excessively low levels.

Most patients first show the effects of falling blood sugar in the brain, which largely burns glucose alone as its source of energy. Drowsiness and irritability or confusion are often the first signs that the patient and his family should be alerted to look for. If the patient realizes what is happening when he finds it suddenly difficult to concentrate or to think clearly, he can often clear up the condition at this stage by taking some candy, orange juice, or other quick source of carbohydrate that he carries with him.

Other signs that should alert the patient are the result of autonomic nervous system reflex responses to development of hypoglycemia. Signs of sympathetic stimulation include cardiac palpitations, profuse sweating, anxiety, and tremors. Parasympathetic hyperactivity often causes gastrointestinal contractions that feel like hunger pangs. An increase in secretion of acid and digestive enzymes may also cause nausea and epigastric distress.

Severe reactions are most likely in patients who fail to recognize hypoglycemic symptoms or who do nothing to counteract them. This sometimes happens with long-acting insulin preparations, not only because the changes in the patient's personality and mental efficiency may come on more slowly and subtly, but also because these products often reach their peak action during the night while the patient is asleep. As a result, the patient may feel no muscular weakness and fatigue before the sudden onset of motor symptoms such as twitching, athetoid (twisting) movements, clonic spasms, and, finally, full-blown tonic seizures. Repeated episodes of continuing convulsions followed—as they often are—by coma may result in permanent cerebral cortical damage.

Treatment of even severe hypoglycemic reactions is simple enough, once the condition is recognized. It involves, mainly, giving glucose by vein if the patient is unable to swallow. Often, simply the injection of an ounce or two of a concentrated (50 percent) solution of glucose will produce dramatic recovery. Occasionally, when it is difficult to find a good vein or the patient is thrashing about in delirium, drugs such as epinephrine, hydrocortisone, or glucagon may be administered subcutaneously.

Glucagon, a purified polypeptide extracted from pancreatic alpha cells, acts to speed conversion of the liver's glycogen stores to glucose. It may be useful when no one capable of injecting glucose intravenously is available. Members of the family can readily be taught to give glucagon subcutaneously or I.M. while awaiting the arrival of the doctor, thus avoiding the danger to the patient of delayed awakening. Ordinarily, the patient responds in five to twenty minutes, provided that his liver glycogen has not been previously depleted.

Once the patient recovers consciousness, he should take more carbohydrate by mouth to avoid lapsing into unconsciousness as the effects of the glucagon injections wear off. If the patient's hypoglycemia was caused by a long-acting agent that continues to enter the blood, sources of rapidly available sugar, such as corn syrup or Coca-Cola syrup, should be supplemented by a more slowly digestible form of carbohydrate, such as bread and honey. The doctor should always be informed of any hypoglycemic reaction so that he can examine and question the patient and take measures to prevent future episodes of the same kind.

Prevention of hypoglycemic reactions requires careful adjustment of insulin dosage. The doctor, of course, works out a schedule of injections suited to the needs of each individual. In addition, however, it is necessary to teach the patient how to keep his insulin dosage and food intake in proper balance. The nurse can help to reinforce the physician's instructions for control of hyperglycemia and prevention of hypoglycemic reactions.

Thus, the nurse can help the patient remember the need for adjusting the times of his main meals to the peak activity of the type of insulin preparation that he is taking. He is told to replace any meals not eaten with amounts of food containing the missing carbohydrates, fats, and proteins. Snacks between meals and at bedtime may also be suggested as a means of neutralizing the amounts of insulin being absorbed at certain hours.

The nurse can also help the patient become aware of the effect of exercise on his insulin requirements. She can point out that sudden strenuous exercise of an unusual nature is undesirable for diabetics taking insulin (regular moderate exercise is, of course, considered desirable). The importance of compensating for the carbohydrate that is burned up in unaccustomed physical activity must be made clear to the patient. He is told that this can be done by taking extra sugary snacks up to a point, and that it may also be necessary to reduce his next insulin dose after unusually prolonged exercise.

Children with diabetes—and their parents—require special instruction. When youngsters are told to carry candy or some other source of quick carbohydrates, they are likely to consume these sweets and then not have them when needed for combating a hypoglycemic reaction. They should be warned against this practice and be taught the importance of not missing meals and of not changing their exercise patterns suddenly from day to day, if sudden drops of blood sugar are to be avoided.

Patients with diabetes of long duration sometimes require reeducation if their condition becomes unstable. Patients with juvenile-onset type diabetes who have grown older may suddenly become "brittle" in their responses to insulin. They may suffer sudden episodes of severe hypoglycemia that seem to come on with little warning. This calls not only for reevaluation of their therapeutic program by the physician but also for reminders that they be constantly on the alert for any unusual feelings that may signal the onset of a reaction that requires quick carbohydrate ingestion.

The Oral Hypoglycemic Drugs

The need to administer insulin by injection has various disadvantages. Scientists have not yet succeeded in preparing a practical oral insulin. However, two classes of synthetic chemicals have been developed that are effective for reducing high blood sugar when taken by mouth. These chemicals—the *sulfonylureas* and the *biguanides* (Table 39-2)—offer some patients the convenience of symptomatic control of diabetes without the need for repeated daily injections.

These kinds of drugs are, however, useful only for certain selected patients. They are

TABLE 39-2   *Oral Hypoglycemic Agents*

Official or Nonproprietary Name	Proprietary Name	Usual Daily Dosage Range	Remarks
Sulfonylurea Compounds			
Acetohexamide N.F.	Dymelor	250 mg–1.5 g	Relatively long duration of action (12–24 hours)
Chlorpropamide U.S.P.	Diabinase	100–250 mg	See *Drug Digest*
Tolazamide U.S.P.	Tolinase	100 mg–1.0 g	Moderate duration of action (10–14 hours)
Tolbutamide U.S.P.	Orinase	500 mg–2.0 g	See *Drug Digest*
Biguanide Compound			
Phenformin HCl U.S.P.	DBI; Meltrol	25–50-mg tablets; 50–100 mg timed-release capsules	See *Drug Digest*

used almost entirely for patients whose diabetes has developed during adult life—the *maturity-onset* type. The drugs are never used alone in cases that were first diagnosed during childhood—the *juvenile-onset* type of diabetes—nor are they employed in patients likely to develop ketoacidosis or other complications of this disease.

The clinical indications for these drugs are now even more severely limited, following the finding that patients taking them for long periods tended to develop cardiovascular complications more often than those diabetics who were treated in other ways. These orally effective drugs are *not* indicated in any case that can be controlled by diet and a weight-reducing regimen alone, or by these measures together with insulin. They are, however, useful for control of mild to moderately severe but nonketotic cases of the maturity-onset type, when insulin cannot be employed for any reason.

Among the cases of maturity-onset diabetes in which oral hypoglycemic agents can often be substituted for insulin are the following: (1) patients allergic to insulin; (2) patients unwilling to take insulin because they find the frequent injections painful or a cause of disfiguring skin lesions; (3) patients who fail to follow directions for correct use of insulin; and (4) patients with physical disabilities such as blindness or other visual difficulties, or arthritis and other neuromuscular disorders that make self-administration of the hormone difficult.

THE SULFONYLUREAS

Patients for whom oral hypoglycemic agents seem indicated are most often started on either *tolbutamide+* (Orinase) or *chlorpropamide+* (Diabinase). Tolbutamide, the shorter-acting of the two, is said to be somewhat safer, mainly because hypoglycemic reactions tend to occur less often and are easier to treat than those that develop during treatment with the longer-acting chlorpropamide. However, reactions are also relatively rare with the latter drug when dosage is carefully regulated. The need for taking only a single daily dose of chlorpropamide is an advantage of that compound.

Most patients taking properly selected doses of these drugs or of the newer sulfonylurea compounds *acetohexamide* and *tolazamide* can have their condition satisfactorily controlled with little risk of hypoglycemic reactions or sulfonamide-type hypersensitivity reactions (see *Summary*, p. 485). However, hypoglycemia may occur in patients with kidney disorders who take ordinary doses of chlorpropamide, a drug that depends upon renal excretion for elimination. Similarly, caution is required when tolbutamide and other drugs that must be metabolized by the liver are employed by patients with hepatic disease.

Other patients who are prone to suffer reactions are the elderly and those who are careless in following their prescribed diet. Adverse reactions have also been reported in patients taking certain other drugs together with the sulfonylureas. Thus, for example, caution is required in patients taking coumarin-type anticoagulants or antiinflammatory agents such as phenylbutazone, as both of these types of drugs tend to increase the hypoglycemic effects of these drugs. On the other hand, patients taking thiazide-type diuretics may show reduced responsibilities to the usual therapeutic doses of sulfonylurea drugs.

THE BIGUANIDES

Phenformin+, the only drug of this group in current use in this country, differs from the sulfonylureas in the way in which it produces hypoglycemia. It does *not* stimulate endogenous production of insulin by the patient's pancreatic beta cells but instead tends to increase passage of glucose into muscle cells. Some doctors claim that this is an advantage for middle-aged overweight patients, in whom insulin tends to stimulate the appetite and cause fat formation.

Generally, however, phenformin is used for treating the same kinds of patients as those in whom the sulfonylureas are more commonly employed—those whose condition cannot be controlled by diet and a weight-reducing regimen alone or combined with insulin, or those who cannot or will not take insulin. Like the sulfonylureas, it is contraindicated in patients with unstable or "brittle" diabetes who tend to suffer frequent acute complications, including ketoacidosis.

Patients who have failed to respond to the sulfonylureas or those whose condition responded at first and then became resistant are sometimes switched successfully to phenformin. Sometimes administration of the two drugs in combination—for example, phenformin and chlorpropamide—brings about better control than either drug alone. This is carried out by adding small daily doses of phenformin to the patient's sulfonylurea drug regimen. The dose of his drug is then gradually raised until control is achieved or gastrointestinal upset develops. Phenformin frequently causes a metallic taste and nausea. Development of vomiting or diarrhea may require withdrawal of this drug.

Complications of Diabetes

Complications of long-standing diabetes include arteriosclerosis, resulting in retinopathy and blindness, nephropathy, coronary, and cerebral vascular disease, and neuropathy. Diabetic patients are also prone to infections of the skin and deeper tissues, which may become gangrenous, particularly in the extremities, and consequent amputation of the foot or the leg may be required.

It is not yet known whether treatment of diabetes can prevent vascular complications. Recent evidence suggests that long-term treatment with oral hypoglycemic agents may even increase the risk of death from circulatory disorders in some diabetic patients. However, it is still thought that occurrence of late complications is less likely in patients who keep their condition under control. Thus, part of the nurse's responsibility is to teach the diabetic patient to take the best possible care of himself. This, of course, includes advising him, not only about drug and dietary therapy, but also about such self-care measures as protecting the skin of his feet from injury and infection.

Instruction of the patient is intended to help him play his own part—and an important one —in the control of his illness. Without unduly alarming the patient, it must be made clear to him that diabetes is a serious disease and that he must follow the doctor's instructions carefully, so that the possible complications of his condition can be kept to a minimum. Among the points that must always be emphasized are the following:

1. *The need for the patient to store his insulin properly, measure the required amount accurately, and inject it correctly*: The patient should not only be taught what to do; he should also be observed to see how he actually carries out the instructions given him. (One nurse explained that insulin must be injected rather than swallowed. She then proceeded to demonstrate the technique of giving oneself an injection by making an injection through the skin of an orange. Later that day, when she asked the patient to show her how he would go about taking his insulin, he injected the insulin into an orange, which he then began to eat!)

2. *The need for the patient to know the early signs and symptoms of hypoglycemia, hyperglycemia, and acidosis, and the measures to take to counteract these potentially dangerous conditions*: The patient must be taught to test his own urine routinely and to realize the significance of abnormalities about which the doctor must be notified.

3. *The need for the patient to pay attention to personal hygiene, diet, and exercise*: The patient should know that what he eats, how he eats, and the hour at which he eats, as well as the type and amount of physical activity in which he indulges, in order to help determine his response to the insulin he injects. He should know how to minimize chances of acquiring infections of the skin or other tissues that could lead to serious complications for diabetics.

S U M M A R Y of Signs and Symptoms of Insulin-Induced Hypoglycemia

Sympathetic and parasympathetic nervous system reactions.

Profuse sweating; facial pallor; paresthesias.

Cardiac palpitations; tachycardia (occasionally, bradycardia); rise in blood pressure (occasionally, fall).

Nausea; hunger pangs, hyperventilation.

Central nervous mental, motor, and other reactions.

Headache; blurring of vision, and diplopia.

Drowsiness; yawning; difficulty in concentrating; feelings of fatigue and weakness.

Muscle spasms, twitching; choreiform movements; athetosis; ataxia; clonic or tonic convulsive seizures.

Nervous irritability; delirium; occasionally, psychotic reactions and late mental retardation. Unconsciousness, stupor, and coma.

Note: Cause and contributory factors in "insulin shock" are:

Overdosage, resulting from:

Error in calculation of dose

Unpredictable response in patient with labile, or "brittle," diabetes

Failure to eat

Unusually vigorous exercise

Stress due to infection or surgery

SUMMARY of Signs and Symptoms, Cautions, and Contraindications with Oral Hypoglycemic Agents of the Sulfonylurea Class

Hypoglycemic reactions.
These are relatively rare but can sometimes be severe in cases of overdosage, or unexpectedly high sensitivity during the period of conversion from insulin (that is, while the latter is still being given).

Allergic dermatological reactions.
Itching, redness, wheals, measles-like and maculopapular eruptions have been reported.

Blood dyscrasias.
Leukopenia, agranulocytosis, thrombocytopenia, and pancytopenia are rare occurrences.

Liver disorders.
Both the hepatocellular and the cholestatic jaundice types of liver disorders have occurred; tests of liver function are made upon initiation of therapy and periodically during treatment.

Gastrointestinal upset.
Anorexia, nausea, vomiting, epigastric distress, diarrhea.

Nervous system side effects.
Headache, tinnitus, paresthesias (tingling), weakness, alcohol-like intoxication. (*Note:* An intolerance to alcohol similar to that seen with disulfiram has been observed.)

Contraindications.
In diabetic acidosis, coma, gangrene, pregnancy, infection with fever, and other conditions for which insulin is required; also in *non*diabetic patients with renal glycosuria.
In patients with liver disease.

Cautions.
Watch for possible drug interactions that can intensify the effects of oral hypoglycemic drugs —for example, with coumarin-type anticoagulants, phenylbutazone-type antiinflammatory agents, probenecid, salicylates, and sulfonamide-type antibacterial agents.
Be aware that patients taking thiazide-type diuretics may require an increase in dosage of oral hypoglycemics.

SUMMARY of Points for the Nurse to Remember Concerning Diabetes Drug Treatment

Carefully observe the patient for signs of hypoglycemia—for example, nervousness, pallor, tremors, and sweating. If you observe such symptoms, administer some readily absorbed food which serves as a quick source of glucose, such as lump sugar, candy, or orange juice. Teach the patient and family to be alert to symptoms of hypoglycemia and how to relieve the symptoms.

Watch for signs of hyperglycemia and ketoacidosis. For example, the patient may become thirsty, drink a great deal, void copiously, become drowsy, and dehydrated. Instruct the patient and family concerning the significance of such symptoms and the need to continue taking prescribed insulin, and to notify the physician immediately, should such symptoms occur.

Insulin should be properly cared for (and the patient should be instructed in these measures) in the following manner:

1. It should be kept in a cool place.
2. Solutions containing particles in suspension should be gently rotated just before the medication is drawn into the syringe, to make certain that an even suspension has been attained.
3. Care must be taken to use the correct scale on the syringe for measuring insulin. U-40 insulin, for example, should be measured using the U-40 scale on the syringe. Currently, efforts are underway to supply syringes with only one measuring scale, and to encourage patients to use these syringes. Such may lead to a decrease in the number of errors that result from the patients' selecting the wrong scale for measuring insulin.
4. The patient should be taught never to switch from insulin of one type to another except on orders from his doctor.

When injecting insulin, be certain to rotate the injection sites and teach the patient to do so, in order to minimize trauma to tissues, and to facilitate absorption. Demonstrate the technique of injection, and supervise the patient as he commences giving his own injections.

Recognize the relationship between duration of the action of the type insulin the patient is receiving, and the timing of his meals, and teach the patient to do so. Be alert to any changes in the timing of the patient's meals—which may be necessitated, for example, by diagnostic tests—and adjust the timing of insulin administration as necessary. For instance, if your patient is fasting for a determination of blood sugar, do not give him regular insulin until you are certain that he may have his breakfast within 10 or 15 minutes.

Include the family in your teaching. However, whenever feasible, the patient should be encouraged to assume responsibility of his own care, rather than delegating it to a member of the family.

Clinical Nursing Situation

The Situation: Miss Jordan, age 22, has newly diagnosed diabetes mellitus. She takes 20 units of N.P.H. Insulin daily. One week after discharge from the hospital, Miss Jordan experienced anorexia and nausea. She was unable to eat, but she took her insulin as usual in the morning. That afternoon, Miss Jordan experienced profuse sweating and was tremulous and apprehensive, and she went to the hospital emergency room. The physician's diagnosis was insulin reaction, brought about when Miss Jordan omitted her usual food intake, owing to her gastrointestinal upset. Miss Jordan was treated at the emergency room with intravenous glucose to relieve hypoglycemia, and chlorpromazine to relieve nausea. After she had rested for an hour, Miss Jordan was ready to return home.

The Problem: What instructions would you, as the emergency room nurse, give Miss Jordan before she leaves the hospital?

DRUG DIGEST

CHLORPROPAMIDE U.S.P. (Diabinase)

Actions and Indications. This sulfonylurea-type oral hypoglycemic compound is similar to tolbutamide and other drugs of the same chemical class. That is, it stimulates pancreatic beta cells to synthesize and release endogenous insulin. As a result, its use may be indicated in selected cases of maturity-onset diabetes that do not respond to a regimen of diet and weight reduction alone or to the use of these measures together with insulin. Its use may be necessary in mild to moderately severe cases, in which insulin cannot be employed for various reasons.

Side Effects, Cautions, and Contraindications. Like other oral hypoglycemic agents, this one is contraindicated in juvenile or growth-onset type diabetes, in severe unstable or "brittle" cases, and in those complicated by ketoacidosis or coma, severe infection or injury, and conditions that require major surgery.

Hypoglycemic reactions may be prolonged and require close observation of the patient for several days because of this drug's long duration of action. The drug is slowly excreted unchanged by the kidneys, and its use is consequently contraindicated in patients with chronic kidney disease. The drug is discontinued if jaundice develops as a result of hepatic tissue hypersensitivity, allergic dermatologic reactions, or blood dyscrasias. Gastrointestinal and neurologic side effects are usually reversible when dosage is reduced.

Dosage and Administration. A single daily dose of 250 mg is usually adequate for control of symptoms. Elderly patients are started on smaller doses, such as 100 mg. Patients who do not respond to high doses of this drug alone (up to 500 mg) can sometimes have their condition controlled by combining it with up to 150 mg of phenformin in the timed-release form.

INSULIN INJECTION U.S.P. (Iletin; Regular Insulin)

Actions and Indications. This form of insulin is the most prompt-acting of the available insulin preparations that act to aid diabetic patients to utilize dietary carbohydrate and fat in a manner that controls hyperglycemia, glycosuria, and ketosis.

It is often used alone for stabilizing newly diagnosed cases and later as a supplement to various of the longer-acting modified insulin products. (It may, for example, be employed in the morning when use of an intermediate-acting product does not prevent prelunch glycosuria.) It is particularly useful in unstable cases of diabetes in which glucose tolerance fluctuates widely, and for patients with severe infection, injuries, or surgical trauma and shock who are likely to develop ketoacidosis or coma.

Side Effects, Cautions, and Contraindications. Overdosage can cause the rapid onset of hypoglycemic reactions. Thus, frequent blood sugar determinations are desirable, and patients should be watched for such early signs as sweating and anxiety reactions. Failure to detect and to treat these and other early manifestations of insulin shock may result in more severe reactions that include coma and convulsions, and even death.

Dosage and Administration. Dosage varies very widely, ranging from as little as 5 units to as much as 100 units. Treatment is usually initiated with 10 to 20 units administered subcutaneously about half an hour before breakfast. The intravenous route is used in patients in diabetic coma and with circulatory collapse.

INSULIN ZINC SUSPENSION U.S.P. (Lente Insulin; Lente Iletin)

Actions and Indications. This mixture has a duration of action midway between that of the prompt zinc insulin suspension and protamine zinc insulin, preparations of rapid and prolonged duration. Like isophane insulin suspension, with which it can be used interchangeably, this preparation has its onset of action in over two hours, exerts its peak effects between 8 to 12 hours after administration, and lasts over 24 hours. It is not suited for intravenous administration in emergencies.

Side Effects, Cautions, and Contraindications. Hypoglycemic reactions may not have a dramatic onset but tend to be prolonged and recurrent, as any overdose continues to be absorbed from the injection site. To assure withdrawal of a uniform suspension of particles and thus avoid dosage irregularities, the vial is inverted several times from end to end. It should not, however, be shaken vigorously, nor be exposed to freezing or warm temperatures. Local sensitivity reactions do not occur with this preparation, which contains no protamine or other modifying protein.

Dosage and Administration. This preparation is administered subcutaneously in initial doses of 10 units, but final dosage may range up to 80 units in some cases. It is best given before breakfast to counteract the expected rise in blood sugar after that meal. During the later hours of the morning, it may have to be supplemented by injection of a more rapid-acting insulin and, during the night, the addition of a long-acting insulin may be necessary.

PHENFORMIN HCl U.S.P. (DBI; DBI-TD; Meltrol)

Actions and Indications. This oral hypoglycemic agent differs from those of the sulfonylurea type in its manner of action. It lowers blood sugar without stimulating the release of insulin. This may be an advantage in the management of obese patients with adult-type diabetes in whom insulin tends to stimulate the appetite and to increase fat formation.

Like the sulfonylurea compounds, use of this drug is now recommended mainly for patients whose condition is not controlled by diet and weight reduction alone, or by these measures plus insulin. It is sometimes combined with a sulfonylurea derivative such as chlorpropamide for control of cases that do not respond to the latter alone. It is also occasionally added to insulin to aid in the control of unstable cases of both the adult and juvenile types.

Side Effects, Cautions, and Contraindications. The most common side effects include loss of appetite, nausea, vomiting, and diarrhea. This is often preceded by an unpleasant metallic taste that may serve as a warning sign for reducing dosage. This drug does not ordinarily cause hypersensitivity-type reactions of the kind sometimes seen with the sulfonylurea drugs, and hypoglycemic reactions are also less likely to occur. However, use of this drug is sometimes associated with development of lactic acidosis and ketosis, particularly in patients with severe kidney disease and sustained hypotension.

Dosage and Administration. Dosage must be adjusted individually, starting with 25 mg daily, and gradually increased up to 150 mg in divided doses taken with meals. Later, patients may be maintained with 50 or 100 mg timed-disintegration capsules administered with breakfast and, if necessary, with the evening meal for an effect lasting at least 12 to 14 hours.

PROTAMINE ZINC INSULIN SUSPENSION U.S.P. (Protamine Zinc and Iletin)

Actions and Indications. This preparation possesses a prolonged duration of action. Its effects come on only after four to six hours but may last 36 hours or longer. It is most useful for treating cases in which the patient's condition is stable, and timing is not of primary importance. Its use is desirable in patients whose blood sugar begins to rise at night and stays high during sleep. This form is never used in diabetic emergencies, nor is it ever substituted for other ordered insulin preparations except when the patient's doctor directs such a change.

Side Effects, Cautions, and Contraindications. Dosage adjustment is necessary to avoid long-lasting and recurrent episodes of hypoglycemia. If such reactions occur they are counteracted by administering a combination of a soluble, rapidly utilized source of carbohydrate, such as orange juice, together with a more slowly digestible food substance. It is desirable for patients to take snacks between meals and essential that they eat something before going to sleep. Presence of the protein protamine may lead to development of local sensitivity reactions.

Dosage and Administration. Subcutaneous injections ranging from 10 to 80 units are made once daily about one-half to one hour before breakfast. It is never injected by vein.

TOLBUTAMIDE U.S.P. (Orinase)

Actions and Indications. This oral hypoglycemic agent lowers blood sugar by stimulating the synthesis and release of insulin by beta cells of the pancreas. Its use is now limited largely to cases of adult or maturity-onset type diabetes mellitus that are not adequately controlled by diet and weight reduction alone, or by these measures plus insulin. Its use is also justified in mild to moderate cases of adult-onset diabetes in which insulin cannot be used for any of various reasons.

Side Effects, Cautions, and Contraindications. This drug is contraindicated in juvenile- or growth-onset diabetes, or in cases complicated by ketosis, acidosis, or the presence of infection, fever, severe injury, or major surgery. Hypoglycemic reactions may occur with overdosage or in patients with severe liver disease that interferes with metabolic degradation of the drug. Caution is necessary when other drugs such as the coumarin-type anticoagulants, salicylates, or phenylbutazone are also employed in order to prevent potentiation of the hypoglycemic effect. Other adverse effects include gastrointestinal disturbances and allergic skin reactions.

Dosage and Administration. Dosage is individualized in accordance with the patient's response. Treatment is usually begun with 1 to 2 g daily administered in divided dosage. This is adjusted downward to as little as 0.5 g or upward to as much as 3 g daily. The usual maintenance dose is 2 g daily administered in several divided amounts.

References

Boshell, B.S., and Barrett, J.C. Oral hypoglycemic agents. *Clin. Pharmacol. Ther.*, 3:705, 1962.

Bradley, R.F. Treatment of ketoacidosis and coma. *Med. Clin. N. Amer.*, 49:961, 1965.

Bressler, R., et al. Insulin treatment of diabetes. *Med. Clin. N. Amer.*, 55:861, 1971 (July).

Di Palma, J.R. Drugs for diabetes mellitus. *RN*, 30:71, 1967 (Oct.).

Fajans, S.S. What is diabetes? Definition, diagnosis, and course. *Med. Clin. N. Amer.*, 55:793, 1971 (July).

Gorman, C.K. Hypoglycemia, a brief review. *Med. Clin. N. Amer.*, 49:947, 1965.

Martin, M.M. The unconscious diabetic patient. *Amer. J. Nurs*, 61:92, 1961.

Moss, J.M., and De Lawter, D.E. Oral agents in the management of diabetes meillitus. *Amer. J. Nurs.*, 60:1610, 1960.

Rodman, M.J. Drugs for diabetes treatment. *RN*, 24:51, 1961 (June).

————. Oral drugs for diabetes. *RN*, 26:35, 1963 (Dec.).

Root, H.F., et al. Diabetic coma. *Amer. J. Nurs.*, 55:1196, 1955.

Shuman, C.R., ed. Symposium or treatment of complications of diabetes. *Mod. Treatm.*, 4:13, 1967 (Jan.).

SECTION **9**

Drugs

for

Treating

Infections

40.

Infection Treatment and Prevention

In this section we shall discuss the drugs that are employed for treating infections. Among the pathogenic microorganisms that can be controlled by drug treatment today are most bacteria, many fungi, and a very few viruses. Drugs are also available for treating diseases caused by parasitic invaders such as protozoa and worms.

Ideally, antimicrobial and antiparasitic drugs should strike selectively at the invading pathogenic organisms within the body without harming their human hosts. Drugs of this kind are called *chemotherapeutic agents*. The term "chemotherapy" is often limited to the clinical use of synthetic chemicals that kill or otherwise eliminate disease-causing organisms. It may also be broadened to include the use of *antibiotics*, which are chemical compounds of natural origin.

The first clinically useful antibiotics were chemicals produced biosynthetically by certain species of bacteria, fungi, and other microorganisms. Today, several semisynthetic antibiotics are also available. These are chemotherapeutic agents that are prepared by chemically treating a naturally produced substance to obtain a modified product with different antiinfective properties.

In this chapter, we shall summarize some of the *general principles of antiinfective chemotherapy* that have evolved during the years in which antibiotics and other antimicrobial and antiparasitic drugs have been in clinical use. The nurse should understand the concepts that underlie the proper employment of these agents, for the misuse of these drugs not only deprives patients of their valuable infection-fighting properties but may also often result in harmful reactions and toxicity.

Treatment of Systemic Infections

In order to treat an infection, the doctor first tries to select the most effective and least toxic drug. The best drug is often one which is *bactericidal*—able to kill bacteria when present in such low tissue concentrations that the patient's cells are not affected by its presence. Sometimes, however, a drug that is only *bacteriostatic* may also prove useful. That is, even though the drug only inhibits the growth and multiplication of the pathogens without killing them, the patient's own antimicrobial defenses are able to cope with the otherwise overwhelming invaders.

Identifying the pathogen responsible for the infection is the first step toward choosing the most effective antiinfective agent. Often, the doctor can do this just by examining the patient, particularly when the physician knows what is "going around." Sometimes he stains a sample of sputum, exudate, urine, or other body fluid to determine whether bacteria are *gram-positive* or *gram-negative*. If this does not provide an adequate clue to the nature of the infection, the physician takes a smear and sends it to the laboratory for culturing and susceptibility testing.

Sensitivity tests are necessary because microorganisms vary very greatly in their resistance to drugs. Some organisms are congenitally, or inherently, *resistant* to many of the available antibiotics. Other pathogens acquire the ability to resist the drugs which once were effective for controlling them. To determine which antiinfective drug is most likely to prove effective, the laboratory technician streaks a culture containing the organism over agar and then places paper drug-diffusing discs on the plate. If the organisms fail to grow in the area around a disc containing a particular drug, the doctor then chooses that active agent for initiating treatment.

Sometimes, of course, treatment cannot be delayed while waiting for the laboratory results. In such cases the doctor may select an antiinfective agent on the basis of its *antimicrobial spectrum*. He may choose a *broad spectrum* antibiotic because of its ability to interfere with vital metabolic processes common to a wide variety of pathogenic organisms. The *tetracycline-type* antibiotics, for example, are effective not only against many strains of both gram-positive and gram-negative bacteria, but also against rickettsiae and even large viruses. Similarly, *ampicillin*, a broad-spectrum penicillin derivative, is often injected in large doses for treating meningitis in children even before the specific causative pathogen has been isolated.

Once the laboratory has reported on the exact nature of the organism, it is often possible to treat the infection with a *narrow-spectrum* antibiotic. *Penicillin G*, for example, strikes at relatively few types of microbes and not at all on most others, yet it remains remarkably effective for treating infections caused specifically by streptococcal organisms of the Group A beta-hemolytic type. Similarly, if an infection is found to be caused by a fungus, *amphotericin B*, an antibiotic not effective against bacteria but specific for attacking fungal organisms, often proves effective. For treating sepsis traced to a specific gram-negative bacillus, the doctor may select *gentamycin* or *kanamycin*, the antibiotics currently considered most effective in such cases.

Administering the drug in adequate dosage and for a long enough period of time is important for successful infection therapy. Most minor infections respond to orally administered doses, which are usually best taken between meals to assure complete absorption. Severe infections require parenteral treatment for maintaining high drug concentrations in the blood and tissues.

The intravenous route is preferred for treating life-threatening infections such as bacterial endocarditis, meningitis, and sepsis produced by gram-negative bacteria. I.V. injections may be made intermittently to attain peak levels in blood and tissues periodically, or the drug may be infused steadily to maintain a continuously high level. Because thrombophlebitis may develop during prolonged I.V. drip of irritating antibiotics, the patient is placed on oral maintenance therapy as soon as the infection seems to have been brought under control.

The *length of treatment* is also very important in avoiding relapses or the development of resistance or adverse reactions. Once an antiinfective drug is selected and administered, it should be continued until such signs of infection as fever and abnormally high white blood counts are absent for at least several days to a week or more. Thus, most bacterial pneumonias require seven to ten days of treatment, and staphylococcal pneumonia must often be treated continuously for a month or more to avoid recurrences.

Patients with a sore throat that stems from a streptococcus infection sometimes become symptom-free following a single injection of penicillin or just a day or two of oral drug treatment. Nevertheless, in such cases a child's parents should be urged to continue penicillin treatment for a full ten days to avoid relapses. Such recurrences of streptococcal pharyngitis can sometimes result in rheumatic fever or glomerulonephritis that lead to cardiac or kidney damage.

Most cases of tuberculosis require at least two years of treatment with the chemotherapeutic agents found most effective for each case. Although this favors the emergence of resistant organisms, this risk is warranted in tuberculosis treatment. In other conditions, however, excessively prolonged antibiotic treatment is undesirable because of the danger of drug-induced tissue toxicity, allergic reactions, and secondary superinfections caused by the emergence of resistant strains (see below).

Combination therapy with two or more antiinfective agents is sometimes desirable. In tuberculosis treatment, for example, the simultaneous employment of two or three antibiotic and chemotherapeutic agents is a standard procedure. The main reason for this is that striking at the tuberculosis bacillus simultaneously with several effective drugs tends to slow the development of resistant organisms.

On the other hand, the administration of other antibiotic mixtures may actually favor the emergence of resistant strains. This is most likely to happen with use of commercial combination products in which one of the antibiotics is present in too small a quantity. The reason for this is that inadequate treatment kills off only some of the pathogens that are present but leaves alive many microorganisms of the kinds that are capable of producing resistant strains.

Recently, the Food and Drug Administration has required certain fixed dosage combination products to be withdrawn from the market. The FDA has called the use of two or more antibiotics together "irrational" when the patient's infection could be cured by only one of the agents. The patient not only pays for an unnecessary antibiotic substance, but he is also unnecessarily exposed to its possibly toxic effects.

In addition, as we have already indicated, the presence of a drug in doses inadequate for effective treatment tends to result in the emergence of pathogens that will later be resistant to treatment with even massive doses of the drug.

Prevention of Infection

The employment of antiinfective drugs for preventing infections is sometimes a very useful measure. More often, such attempts at prophylaxis of infection are not effective and may, indeed, even be harmful. In still other situations, the question of whether attempts at prevention are worthwhile is still unsettled and controversial.

The long-term administration of penicillin G for preventing repeated streptococcal infections in patients judged likely to suffer recurrent attacks of rheumatic fever is an example of a well-established use of a prophylactic antiinfective regimen. Similarly, the short-term use of penicillin prior to oral surgery in certain heart disease patients is a recognized means of reducing the chance that these susceptible patients may develop bacterial endocarditis following dental procedures or throat surgery.

On the other hand, the usefulness of common cold products containing prophylactic doses of antiinfective agents has been questioned. The antibiotics and sulfonamides that are added to the decongestants and analgesics in such products have no effect at all on the common cold virus. However, the manufacturers of such combinations sometimes suggest that the addition of a penicillin, tetracycline, or sulfonamide-type agent may help to prevent development of a secondary bacterial infection. Actually, clinical studies indicate that these antibiotics are no more effective for this purpose than they are for controlling the virus that caused the primary infection in the first place.

Most authorities also agree that the routine addition of an antistaphylococcal or an antifungal antibiotic to products containing tetracycline-type antibiotics, in order to prevent development of infections by tetracycline-resistant organisms, is wasteful and ineffective. If, on the other hand, symptoms of such antibiotic-induced superinfections actually occur, treatment of the secondary infection with a properly selected antistaphylococcal or antifungal drug is justified.

Adverse Reactions to Antiinfective Agents

All the available antibiotics are capable of causing adverse effects. These fall into three general classes:

1. *Direct toxic effects* upon such organs as the gastrointestinal tract, kidneys, and liver, or the auditory, optic, and other peripheral nerves.

2. *Allergic reactions* and other kinds of hypersensitivity affecting the skin and other organs and structures, including the bone marrow and circulating blood.

3. *Superinfections* as a result of drug-induced overgrowths by resistant bacterial strains or fungal organisms.

DIRECT TISSUE TOXICITY

This is rarely a problem with the penicillins, even when these antibiotics are administered in massive doses. On the other hand, other antibiotics, including *kanamycin* and *colistimethate*, can cause *kidney damage*. Drugs of this kind are particularly dangerous in patients whose kidney function is already impaired. They must be administered in low doses and at least frequent intervals in order to prevent their accumulating to toxic levels in other tissues, including the auditory nerve. These drugs and others such as *streptomycin* may cause *deafness* in such cases.

ALLERGIC REACTIONS

These are particularly common with *penicillin-*type antibiotics. Patients who take these valuable antibiotics for self-treatment or trivial infections may become sensitized to them. Then, if they later develop a severe infection, these patients may not be able to receive the required penicillin treatment. Thus, it is important to warn patients against casual self-medication with antiinfective drugs that may be left over from an earlier illness or with a drug that was prescribed for a friend or another member of the family.

SUPERINFECTIONS

These occur most frequently in patients receiving tetracyclines or other broad-spectrum-type antibiotics. By eliminating susceptible pathogens, these drugs permit organisms that are resistant to them to grow rapidly. Yeast-like fungi of the *Candida* type, for example, may then cause localized infections in the mouth, vagina, and elsewhere. Overgrowths of penicillin-resistant staphylococci in the gastrointestinal tract can cause severe diarrhea. Superinfections by *Pseudomonas* species and other gram-negative bacilli cause the most serious superinfections, particularly in disease-weakened patients and in those receiving corticosteroid and anticancer drugs.

MISUSE OF ANTIBIOTICS

The nurse should know that the misuse of antibiotics has various undesirable consequences, and she should make patients aware of the fact that these valuable drugs should be taken only when prescribed by a doctor and only exactly as ordered. The main reasons may be summarized by the following:

1. *Indiscriminate use* of antiinfective drugs may lead to development of microbial strains that have become *resistant* to these agents. Thus, a valuable drug may become worthless for treating infections of a kind that it once readily controlled. Patients who could have profited from treatment are then deprived of the drug's benefits.

2. *Taking a drug for a trivial infection* that really requires no treatment at all, or that does not, in any case, respond to treatment with that particular antiinfective agent, may serve only to *sensitize* the person who tries to treat himself in this way. Then, if he later really needs treatment with the same drug for a serious infection against which it could be very effective, he may be unable to take it because of the allergy that he has developed through its earlier misuse.

3. *Self-medication* for relief of infection symptoms may lead to flare-ups of the infection, if the drug is taken in too small doses for too short a period of time. On the other hand, taking antiinfective drugs in too high doses for too long a time can cause various kinds of adverse reactions that are often more dangerous than the original infection.

References

Bryson, V., and Demerec, M. Bacterial resistance. *Amer. J. Med.*, 18:723, 1955.

Dowling, H. F. Present status of therapy with combinations of antibiotics. *Amer. J. Med.*, 39:796, 1965.

Feingold, D. S. Antimicrobial chemotherapeutic agents: The nature of their action and selective toxicity. *New Eng. J. Med.*, 206:900, 957, 1963.

Finland, M. The new antibiotic era: For better or worse? *Antibiotic Med. Clin. Ther.*, 4:17, 1957.

Hall, J. W. Drug therapy in infectious diseases. *Amer. J. Nurs.*, 61:56, 1961.

Jager, B. V. Untoward reactions to antibiotics. *Amer. J. Nurs.*, 54:966, 1954.

Rodman, M. J. The status of the antibiotics. *RN*, 23:51, 1960 (Aug.); 23:51, 1960 (Sept.).

Sabath, L. D. Drug resistance of bacteria. *New Eng. J. Med.*, 280:91, 1969.

Spink, W. W. Clinical problems related to the management of infections with antibiotics. *JAMA*, 152:585, 1953.

Weinstein, L. Superinfection, a complication of antimicrobial therapy and prophylaxis. *Amer. J. Surg.*, 107:704, 1964.

41.

The Antibiotics

The introduction of penicillin into clinical medicine during the 1940s revolutionized the treatment of bacterial infections. The successful use of this substance obtained from strains of certain molds stimulated studies of other antibacterial agents of natural origin, Today, scores of antibiotics are available, including some that are prepared synthetically.

In this chapter, we shall discuss the clinically important properties of the several major classes of antibiotics. We shall indicate which pathogenic microorganisms are most sensitive to antibiotics of each type (*Summary*, p. 512). This will help us to understand why doctors tend to select certain antibiotics for treating particular kinds of infections. We shall also take up the potential toxicities of each type of antibiotic, in order to understand why these valuable drugs must often be employed with caution or even discontinued despite their effectiveness.

The Penicillins

The first penicillin products were obtained from mold cultures of the *Penicillium* species. The most important of these *natural* penicillins is penicillin G, or benzylpenicillin; another is the phenoxymethyl derivative known as penicillin V. Today, many chemically modified forms of penicillin have been prepared semisynthetically, starting with the natural penicillin nucleus, 6-aminopenicillanic acid (Table 41-1).

All of the natural and semisynthetic penicillins share certain properties such as, for example, their ability to kill microorganisms instead of simply slowing their rate of growth.

However, chemical modification of natural penicillin has resulted in production of penicillin products with different properties. These differences account for the greater suitability of certain semisynthetic penicillins in some clinical situations. Thus, we shall discuss the several subgroups of penicillins separately.

PENICILLIN G PREPARATIONS

Penicillin G+ is the preferred form for use against organisms sensitive to treatment with penicillin (Table 41-2). Although its spectrum is relatively narrow, the pathogens against which it is effective are those that are the cause of some of the most common infections. These include such gram-positive cocci as streptococci, pneumococci, and some strains of staphylococci, and also the gonococcus and *Treponema pallidum*, the organisms responsible for the most common venereal diseases.

Streptococcal infections are very well controlled by penicillin G preparations. Acute pharyngitis caused by *Streptococcus pyogenes* (the group A beta-hemolytic streptococcus) is often promptly improved following a single injection. However, if a throat culture taken at that time reveals the presence of this organism, treatment should be continued for ten days to eradicate the streptococcus.

This is important, because failure to eliminate this organism may lead to a recurrence of the infection. Frequent recurrences are a cause of such serious complications as rheumatic fever and carditis, and acute glomerulonephritis. Thus, people with a sore throat should be warned against taking a few tablets of penicillin left over from an earlier prescription. Haphazard treatment of this type may give temporary relief but leave them exposed to serious complications.

People with a history of rheumatic fever are often maintained on long-term penicillin prophylaxis. By preventing streptococcal infections, penicillin protects these patients against possible development of rheumatic

TABLE 41-1   *Penicillin Preparations*

Generic or Official Name	Trade Name or Synonym	Dosage and Administration	Remarks
Penicillin G Preparations			
Benzathine penicillin G U.S.P.	Bicillin, Permapen	500,000 units orally, or 600,000 units I.M. at various intervals	Longest-lasting penicillin (see *Drug Digest*)
Potassium penicillin G U.S.P.	Pentids, Pfizerpen, Sugracillin	400,000 units orally, or I.M. every six hours, or I.V. 10 million units daily	First choice for severe infections by sensitive organisms (see *Drug Digest*)
Sodium penicillin G N.F.	. . . .	400,000 units orally or I.M. q.i.d., or I.V. 10 million units daily	High doses can cause an electrolyte imbalance
Procaine penicillin G U.S.P.	Crysticillin, Duracillin, Wycillin, and others	I.M. 300,000 units every 12–24 hours	Long-lasting penicillin (see *Drug Digest*)
Procaine penicillin G with aluminum stearate suspension U.S.P.		I.M. 300,000–600,000 units daily, or 600,000 –1.2 million units for more severe infections	Oily suspension for long duration of action
Penicillinase-Resistant Penicillins			
Sodium cloxacillin U.S.P.	Tegopen	500–1,000 mg every four to six hours	Semisynthetic penicillin for oral use
Sodium dicloxacillin	Dynapen, Pathocil, Veracillin	125 mg orally every six hours, or 250 mg for more severe infections	Congener of oxacillin and cloxacillin

TABLE 41-1 *Penicillin Preparations (continued)*

Generic or Official Name	Trade Name or Synonym	Dosage and Administration	Remarks
Penicillinase-Resistant Penicillins			
Sodium methacillin U.S.P.	Staphcillin	1–1.5 g every four to six hours	Injectable only (see *Drug Digest*)
Sodium nafcillin U.S.P.	Unipen	250–1,000 mg every four to six hours	Oral and injectable forms available
Sodium oxacillin U.S.P.	Prostaphlin	500 mg every four to six hours for five or more days	Oral and injectable forms available (see *Drug Digest*)
Flucloxacillin	Floxapen	Oral or I.M. 125–250 mg every six hours	Long duration of action
Other Penicillins			
Ampicillin U.S.P.	Alpen, Amcill, Omnipen, Polycillin, Principen	250–500 mg every six hours	Effective against certain gram-negative bacteria
Carbenicillin	Geopen, Pyopen	I.V. or I.M. 200–500 mg/kg per day, up to a maximum of 40 g per day (I.M. no more than 2 g per injection)	Effective against *Pseudomonas* and other gram-negative bacteria
Carbenicillin indanyl sodium	Geocillin	1–4 tablets orally (equivalent to 382 mg–1,528 mg of carbenicillin) daily	Oral form effective for urinary tract infections
Hetacillin	Versapen	225 mg orally q.i.d.	Converted to ampicillin in the body
Phenoxymethyl penicillin U.S.P.	Pen-Vee, V-Cillin	125 mg (200,000 units) q.i.d.	More acid-resistant than penicillin G
Potassium phenethicillin N.F.	Darcel, Maxipen, Syncillin, and others	125 or 250 mg t.i.d.	Synthetic oral penicillin with same spectrum as penicillin G
Potassium phenoxymethyl penicillin U.S.P.	Compocillin-VK, Ledercillin VK, Pen-Vee K, V-Cillin K	200,000–600,000 units every six to eight hours	Oral form of penicillin, more acid-resistant than penicillin G

heart disease. For this purpose, some children take daily oral doses of penicillin G for many years. A more convenient way of maintaining protective levels of penicillin in the patient's tissues is by periodic injection of a long-lasting repository preparation of penicillin G.

Benzathine penicillin G+ (Bicillin; and others) is a product that provides very prolonged protection. A single injection of 1.2 million units is absorbed so slowly from an intramuscular tissue depot that the patient need visit the doctor only about once a month. Thus, the physician may prefer this preparation for use in patients whom he feels may fail to take daily oral doses of penicillin G tablets. The nurse should make it clear to the patient

receiving repository penicillin, or to his family, that he must return on schedule for each injection. The importance of not missing a visit must be emphasized, and the patient should be made to realize the seriousness of letting his protection against infection lapse. Then, if the patient should find it impossible to come on the day of the scheduled visit, he may remember the nurse's warning and call for an alternate appointment instead of skipping the monthly or bimonthly dose of penicillin entirely.

Prompt penicillin G treatment of streptococcal sore throat or the related illness, scarlet fever, accounts for the rarity of such once common complications as acute middle ear

T A B L E   4 1 - 2   *Antibacterial Spectrum of Some Penicillin Products*

Penicillin G (benzylpenicillin); Phenoxymethyl penicillin; Phenethicillin

Streptococci, including group A beta-hemolytic type

Staphylococci, except penicillinase-producing strains

Pneumococci (*Diplococcus pneumoniae*)

Gonococci (*Neisseria gonorrhoeae*)

Meningococci (*Neisseria menigitidis*)

Corynebacterium diphtheriae

Clostridium tetani

Clostridium welchii

Bacillus anthracis

Listeria monocytogenes

Enterococci

Spirochetes (for example *Treponema pallidum*, *T. pertenue*)

Actinomycetes (for example, *Actinomyces bovis*, *A. israeli*)

Methacillin; Oxacillin; Cloxacillin; Dicoxacillin; and others

Penicillinase-producing strains of staphylococci and most other gram-positive cocci

Ampicillin; Hetacillin

Gram-negative bacilli, including *Hemophilus influenzae*, *Proteus mirabilis*, and strains of *Salmonella*, *Shigella*, and *Escherichia coli*

Gram-positive cocci, except for penicillinase-producing staphylococci

Gram-negative cocci, such as gonococci and meningococci

Carbenicillin

Gram-negative bacilli, such as *Pseudomonas aeruginosa*, *Proteus* species, and certain *E. coli* strains

Gram-positive cocci, except for penicillinase-producing staphylococci

---

infections (otitis media) and mastoiditis. The drug also aids in preventing infections by *Streptococcus viridans*, an organism capable of causing endocarditis. Patients with certain types of heart disease should receive prophylactic injections of *procaine penicillin G+* (Duracillin; and others) before and for a couple of days after undergoing dental procedures or surgery of the mouth or throat.

Bacterial pneumonia caused by the common gram-positive organisms are also responsive to prompt treatment with penicillin G preparations. The most common lung invader, the *pneumococcus*, is very sensitive to prompt treatment with parenterally administered procaine penicillin G or benzathine penicillin G. Usually, the patient's fever breaks dramatically within 48 hours. However, even though the patient often improves remarkably, penicillin treatment is continued for at least a week and even longer in cases of pneumococcal pneumonia that are complicated by other illnesses.

Venereal diseases still responsive to treatment with penicillin G include syphilis and gonorrhea. The *spirochete* responsible for syphilis infections is very sensitive to this antibiotic. Most early cases are managed by repeated injections rather than with orally administered penicillin. Benzathine penicillin G is given

intramuscularly in a dose of 2.4 million units at weekly intervals. In late syphilis, including neurosyphilis, larger doses of the same drug are given a greater number of times.

Gonorrhea treatment requires higher tissue levels of penicillin than are needed in treating syphilis. In fact, higher doses are now required than was once necessary because of the emergence of strains of the gonococcus that are much more resistant than previously. Current recommendations call for administration of 4.8 million units of aqueous procaine penicillin G at a single session. It is also suggested that these patients take probenecid in tablet form about one half hour before the injections. This substance delays the elimination of penicillin by the kidneys, resulting in a rise of penicillin levels in the infected tissues.

OTHER PENICILLIN PREPARATIONS

Phenoxymethyl penicillin (Penicillin V) and *phenethicillin* (Syncillin; and others) have the same range of antibacterial activity as penicillin G. However, they are more stable in acid gastric juice, and so more of any administered oral dose escapes destruction and is systemically absorbed. This does *not* mean that these drugs are superior to penicillin G, which is much cheaper and reaches equally effective blood levels when administered in somewhat larger oral doses. Severe infections should, in any case, be treated by parenteral forms of penicillin G rather than with these products that are available for oral administration only. (Injectable penicillin is also preferred for treating patients who are vomiting or who have intestinal hypermotility.)

All oral penicillins are best administered about one hour before meals or two hours afterward to assure more rapid and complete absorption and higher blood levels. Penicillin V is claimed to be better absorbed *after* a meal than on an empty stomach. If the nurse is doubtful about this, it is best to check with the physician to find out whether he wants a particular penicillin preparation given well before meals (as is usual) or after them.

Penicillinase-resistant pencillins (Table 41-1) are employed for treating infections by strains of staphylococci and other pathogens that are resistant to treatment with penicillins G and V, phenethicillin, and ampicillin. The reason for this resistance is that these organisms produce an enzyme called *penicillinase* that is capable of breaking these penicillins down to inactive fragments. The newer semisynthetic penicillins can not be split apart by this action of bacterial penicillinase. Thus, when sensitivity studies and cultures indicate that an infection is caused by organisms resistant to penicillin G, the doctor selects one of these newer penicillin products.

Staphylococci are a common cause of skin and soft tissue infections. These may be so mild that they need no penicillin treatment at all. However, organisms that get into the blood and spread to the nervous system, bones, and lungs can cause extremely severe infections. Staphylococcal pneumonia, for example, requires prompt and vigorous treatment to avoid fatalities, which are fairly frequent in infants and the elderly.

When the doctor suspects the presence of a resistant staphylococcal strain, he does not delay treatment while waiting for the results of bacteriologic studies. He begins treatment immediately with an injectable form of a penicillinase-resistant penicillin such as *methicillin+*, *oxacillin+*, or *nafcillin*. This is because staphylococcal toxins cause abscesses and rapid tissue necrosis. The accumulating pus and destroyed tissue may then make it difficult for penicillin to penetrate and reach the bacteria lurking in pus-filled tissue pockets.

These narrow-spectrum penicillins are not as effective as penicillin G against other kinds of gram-positive organisms. Thus, the doctor may also administer injections of aqueous penicillin G, in case the infection turns out to be caused by a pneumococcus, streptococcus, or a *non*penicillinase-producing staph. If he thinks it possible that the severe infection is caused by a gram-negative organism, he may even combine *kanamycin+* or *gentamycin+* (p. 509) with the penicillinase-resistant penicillin.

Once the laboratory report establishes which pathogen is responsible, treatment is continued with only the antibiotic to which the organism is most sensitive, and the others are withdrawn. Injections are also stopped, and the patients are switched to oral forms of these penicillins or of *cloxacillin* (Tegopen; and others) or *dicloxacillin* (Dynapen; and others). This spares the patient the pain of tissue irritation from injections during the four weeks or more required for treating complicated staphylococcal infections.

Ampicillin+ (Omnipen; and others) is a semisynthetic penicillin with a wider antibacterial spectrum than other penicillins. Although it is not quite as effective as penicillin G against most gram-positive organisms and is ineffective against penicillinase-producing staphylococci, ampicillin has proved remarkably useful against infections by certain strains of gram-negative bacilli. It is particularly useful for treating urinary tract infections caused by *E. coli* and *Proteus mirabilis*, and meningitis and respiratory tract infections caused by *Hemophilus influenzae*.

Ampicillin and a related broad-spectrum penicillin, *hetacillin* (Versapen), which is rapidly converted to ampicillin in the body, have some advantages over other previously available broad-spectrum antibiotics. These penicillins do not, for example, have the drawback of potential toxicity that limits the usefulness of *chloramphenicol+* (p. 508), and they provide blood and tissue levels that are bactericidal, while the tetracycline-type broad spectrum antibiotics (p. 506) are only bacteriostatic. However, ampicillin is not as widely effective as the tetracyclines, and does *not*, for example, control infections by rickettsial organisms or by *Mycoplasma pneumoniae*. Ampicillin is also *not* effective against such gram-negative bacilli as *Klebsiella*, *Enterobacter*, or *Pseudomonas aeruginosa*.

Carbenicillin (Geopen; Pyopen) is another

new semisynthetic penicillin that is effective against gram-negative as well as gram-positive organisms. However, unlike ampicillin, it *is* effective for treating infections caused by *Pseudomonas aeruginosa*. It is particularly useful for urinary tract infections because of the high concentrations reached as the drug is being excreted in the urine.* Unlike other antipseudomonal antibiotics, including polymyxin B, colistimethate, and gentamycin, carbenicillin is not toxic to kidney tissues. Thus, it can be used to treat patients with chronic kidney disorders whose condition would be made worse by administration of these other nephrotoxic antibiotics.

Patients with pseudomonal infections that have spread from the urinary tract to the systemic circulation and to such sites as the C.N.S. require treatment with very large doses of carbenicillin administered by the I.M. or I.V. routes. Since carbenicillin is available as the disodium salt, heart patients have to be watched for signs of sodium retention in such situations. Patients with impaired kidney function may suffer central nervous system toxicity (see below) from the high levels that this drug reaches in the blood and brain when its renal excretion is interfered with. It should be injected in smaller doses at less frequent intervals in such cases.

THE ADVERSE EFFECTS OF PENICILLIN

The penicillins are capable of causing all three of the general types of adverse reactions that occur during antiinfective drug treatment (p. 516). However, direct tissue toxicity and superinfections occur less often than with various other antibiotics. Hypersensitivity reactions, on the other hand, often complicate the treatment of patients with infections that require penicillin therapy.

HYPERSENSITIVITY REACTIONS. Allergic reactions to penicillin occur in about 1 to 10 percent of patients, according to various estimates. Reactions are most common with parenteral

* An ester derivative, carbenicillin indanyl sodium, which is not destroyed by gastric acid, is now available. When it is taken by mouth, it is well-absorbed and then converted in the body to carbenicillin, which is then excreted by the kidneys. The antibiotic reaches high enough concentrations in the urine to eradicate susceptible bacteria, including not only strains of *Pseudomonas*, but also *Proteus mirabilis* and *E. coli*, pathogens which often cause acute and chronic pyelonephritis and cystitis.

products such as procaine penicillin G. However, severe reactions can occur even when penicillins are taken by mouth. Sensitization occurs so commonly from topically applied penicillin preparations that this antibiotic is now rarely applied directly to the skin.

Reactions may be mild or so severe as to cause death within a few minutes. Thus, it is important to ask each patient whether he has ever had a reaction to penicillin and whether he has a history of asthma, hay fever, or allergy to other drugs or foods. When the physician is uncertain whether to risk using penicillin he may employ skin tests in an effort to determine the patient's sensitivity.

Skin tests in which penicillin itself is scratched into the skin surface or injected intradermally are used clinically to predict a patient's response to a therapeutic dose. If a red flare and wheal develop rapidly, penicillin should probably not be administered. However, because highly sensitive patients may have a severe systemic reaction rather than a local one, safer tests have been sought. Whenever the nurse administers an injection of penicillin to a patient whose response to the drug has not previously been observed, she should observe him closely for at least 20 minutes following the injection. Thus, outpatients are asked to remain for 20 minutes following injection, and hospitalized patients are observed at frequent intervals for 20 minutes following injection.

Two experimental substances being tried as substitute antigens are: (1) penicilloyl-polylysine (PPL) and (2) minor determinant mixture (MDM). Both are claimed safer and more reliable for determining which patients with a past history of penicillin allergy are likely to have rapid adverse reactions if treated again with this antibiotic.

Treatment of anaphylactic reactions to penicillin is similar to that for other severe reactions in which histamine and other chemical medicators are released. Epinephrine injection is the most important measure. Soluble corticosteroids, parenteral antihistamines, and oxygen must also be available for emergency use. The administration of aminophylline, vasopressors, and I.V. fluids may also be necessary. (See also Chapters 17, 18, 19, and 23.)

The place of *penicillinase* (Neutrapen) in penicillin allergy treatment is still uncertain. This purified enzyme is sometimes injected to seek out and destroy the molecules responsible for the reaction. However, it works too slowly to affect anaphylactoid reactions. It may help to lessen the severity of delayed serum-sickness type reactions. Allergy to penicillinase products of the penicillase-resistant type (p. 501) cannot be expected to respond to treatment with this product.

Direct tissue toxicity may occur when very large doses lead to development of high concentrations of penicillin in the nervous system. Carbenicillin (p. 501), for example, has sometimes caused convulsive seizures. Similarly, the injection of penicillin solutions into the spinal fluid for treating meningitis has sometimes set off seizures. Actually, however, penicillin has remarkably low direct tissue toxicity. The potassium and sodium content of the penicillin salts constitute a greater danger to some severely ill patients when large doses are administered than does the penicillin part of these salts.

Superinfection from treatment with this narrow-spectrum antibiotic is less common than with the tetracyclines (p. 506). However, the prolonged use of ampicillin may lead to the emergence of resistant staphylococci and *non*susceptible gram-negative bacteria. Similarly, bacilli resistant to carbenicillin may emerge to cause serious secondary infections following treatment with that penicillin.

The nurse can play an important part in detecting early signs of allergy and other reactions to penicillin. If she notes development of hives or other rashes in a patient who has been given penicillin, she should withhold further doses of the drug until she has checked with the doctor. This should be done promptly so that the patient is not deprived of required antiinfective medication.

The nurse can also help *prevent* reactions to penicillin by listening to the patient. For example, the patient sometimes fails to inform the doctor about previous minor reactions to penicillin. Yet when the nurse is about to inject the antibiotic, he may suddenly say "If that's penicillin, I'm allergic to it." In such a situation, never proceed without consulting the doctor.

Alternatives to Penicillin

One or another of the various types of penicillins now available is likely to prove effective against most bacterial pathogens. However, many patients who are allergic to penicillin cannot be treated safely with these drugs. In such cases, the doctor may order an alternative drug that is also effective against the organism. Drugs of this kind and others that sometimes strike at strains of organisms that are not sensitive to penicillin are listed in Tables 41-3 and 41-4.

TABLE 41-3 *Antibiotics Used as Alternatives to the Penicillins*

Nonproprietary or Official Name	Trade Name or Synonym	Dosage and Administration	Remarks
Cephalosporins Cefazolin sodium	Ancef; Kefzol	250–500 mg every eight hours I.M. or I.V., or higher doses more often for more severe infections	Claimed less irritating to tissues than cephalothin and not to cause kidney toxicity like cephaloridine
Cephalexin monohydrate	Keflex	1 to 4 g daily in divided doses of 250–500 mg usually for adults	Stable in stomach acid and absorbed to produce effective levels in the tissues
Cephaloglycin dihydrate	Kafocin	250–500 mg q.i.d.	Acid-stable and absorbed to reach effective concentrations in the urine
Cephaloridine	Loridine	500 mg–1 g t.i.d. or q.i.d. I.M. or I.V.	Causes less pain by I.M. injection than cephalothin, but kidney toxicity is more likely
Cephalothin sodium U.S.P.	Keflin	500 mg–1 g every four to six hours I.V. or by deep I.M.	For serious infections by susceptible gram-positive and gram-negative organisms

TABLE 41-3 *Antibiotics Used as Alternatives to the Penicillins* (continued)

Nonproprietary or Official Name	Trade Name or Synonym	Dosage and Administration	Remarks
Erythromycin and its Derivatives			
Erythromycin U.S.P.	E-Mycin, Erythrocin, Ilotycin	2–4 g daily in divided doses every six hours for adults	Administer before meals or as acid-resistant tablets
Erythromycin estolate N.F.	Ilosone	250 mg orally every six hours	May cause jaundice in sensitive patients upon continued administration
Erythromycin ethylsuccinate	Erythrocin ethyl-succinate, Pediamycin	200 mg orally five times daily for adults, 30–50 mg/kg for children, I.M. 100 mg every 8–12 hours	I.M. injections are irritating and painful and should be avoided in small children
Erythromycin gluceptate U.S.P.	Ilotycin glucceptate	250–500 mg by slow I.V. injection every six hours or by continuous infusion	For severe infections, including primary atypical pneumonia, pneumococcal pneumonia, and diphtheria
Erythromycin lactobionate U.S.P.	Erythrocin lactobionate	1–4 g daily by continuous I.V. infusion or in divided doses every four to six hours	For severe infections by susceptible organisms
Erythromycin stearate	Erythrocin stearate	250 mg orally every six hours	Administer before meals
Miscellaneous			
Clindamycin HCl and palmitate	Cleocin	8–25 mg/kg per day in three or four divided doses, depending upon severity of infection	Less likely to cause diarrhea, and other G.I. distress than is its relative, lincomycin
Lincomycin HCl U.S.P.	Lincocin	500 mg t.i.d. or q.i.d. orally; or 600 mg I.M. or I.V. every 8–24 hours	Oral form may cause diarrhea; parenteral form may cause hypotension
Novobiocin sodium N.F.	Albamycin	250–500 mg orally or parenterally every six hours	Causes frequent skin reactions; little used today
Oleandomycin N.F.	Matromycin	250–500 mg orally every six hours	Less potent than erythromycin
Troleandomycin N.F.	Cyclamycin, TAO	250–500 mg orally every six hours	Derivative of oleandomycin with spectrum similar to that of erythromycin
Vancomycin HCl U.S.P.	Vancocin	500 mg every six hours by slow I.V. infusion	Nephrotoxic and ototoxic but lifesaving in some infections by bacteria resistant to other antibiotics

Erythromycin+ is similar to penicillin G in its effectiveness against the common gram-positive and gram-negative cocci. Thus it may, for example, be substituted in the long-term prevention of streptococcal pharyngitis in children with a history of rheumatic fever, or in the short-term prophylaxis against streptococcal endocarditis in similar patients before mouth and throat operations.

Other patients who are allergic to penicillin may receive erythromycin for the treatment of gonorrhea or primary syphilis. Parenteral forms are available for treating pneumococcal pneumonia in patients unable to tolerate large oral doses. Erythromycin ethylsuccinate may be administered parenterally, but because repeated deep I.M. injections are painful and irritating to the tissues, they should not be used in children. Instead, the soluble glueceptate or lactobionate salts may be administered by slow I.V. infusion in this and other severe illnesses caused by organisms susceptible to erythromycin.

This antibiotic is most commonly administered by mouth before meals in buffered forms with acid-resistant coatings that protect it from being inactivated. One form, the estolate ester of erythromycin, may be administered with meals because it is stable in gastric acid. However, unlike the erythromycin base or its stearate salt, which cause few adverse effects, this form has occasionally caused cholestatic jaundice, a form of allergic hepatitis.

Lincomycin (Lincocin) is also effective against the same gram-positive organisms as erythromycin and can, like the latter, be substituted for penicillin in allergic patients. Although it is not a first choice for any infection, this antibiotic is sometimes effective against strains of staphylococci resistant to other agents. Unlike the penicillins and erythromycin it is not useful for treating gonorrhea.

The oral form of this drug sometimes causes severe persistent diarrhea and even acute colitis. The parental form employed for attaining high levels of the antibiotic in patients with pneumococcal pneumonia and other severe infections has sometimes caused falls in blood pressure and, rarely, cardiac arrest when injected too rapidly. Intramuscular administration is safer and relatively free of pain.

Clindamycin (Cleocin) is a derivative of lincomycin with the same antibacterial spectrum. Administered by mouth, is less likely than lincomycin to cause gastrointestinal upset, and it is more readily absorbed even when taken with food. Although it is not a first choice drug, clindamycin may be useful for eradicating streptococci, when the patient does not tolerate penicillin, or for treating selected cases of staphylococcal or pneumococcal respiratory tract infections.

Troleandomycin (Cyclamycin; TAO) is another antibiotic with the same spectrum as all the above antibiotics. However, it is recommended for use only against bacterial strains that prove insensitive to the other agents. This is because of the drug's tendency to disrupt liver function, and, occasionally, to cause cholestatic jaundice. This is not likely to occur, however, when the drug is used for no more than ten days to two weeks, as in the treatment of beta-hemolytic streptococcal infections. Large doses are employed for control of the rare case of acute gonococcal urethritis that fails to respond to treatment with ordinarily more effective and safer drugs.

Novobiocin (Albamycin) is another drug effective against the common gram-positive organisms. However, it is rarely employed, because it causes more side effects than most of the other penicillin substitutes. This antibiotic has been added to tetracyclines to prevent the emergence of resistant staphylococci during tetracycline treatment. However, the presence of novobiocin is not now believed to be effective for this purpose.

Vancomycin (Vancocin) is an antibiotic that has occasionally proved lifesaving when injected by vein to penicillin-sensitive patients who were seriously ill with severe staphylococcal pneumonia, septicemia, or other infections resistant to safer drugs. Although it is not absorbed when taken orally, it may sometimes be administered by mouth for its local effects in treating staphylococcal enterocolitis. Streptococci of the enterococcal group are also sometimes sensitive to vancomycin.

Vancomycin is very irritating and must be well diluted to minimize thrombophlebitis. Kidney function must be monitored, as this drug is nephrotoxic. It should not be administered to patients with poor kidney function, as its accumulation in the blood and auditory nerve tissue can cause deafness, particularly in patients with some previous loss of hearing.

CEPHALOSPORINS

Antibiotics of this family resemble the penicillins chemically and in manner of action. *Cephalothin* (Keflin), the first to be introduced, was suggested for use in patients allergic to penicillin. However, this and related drugs can also cause hypersensitivity reactions, particularly in patients with a history of penicillin allergy. This antibiotic and the related drug *cephaloridine* (Loridine) are reserved for use in serious infections caused by susceptible gram-positive and gram-negative pathogens, including both penicillin-sensitive and penicillinase-producing staphylococci.

Cephalothin sometimes causes local reactions when administered repeatedly by I.M. or I.V.

injections. Cephaloridine is less likely to do this, but it is more likely to cause kidney toxicity. Thus, during treatment, the patient's kidney function is closely observed, and this antibiotic is discontinued if adverse renal effects begin to develop. A new member of the cephalosporin family, cefazolin (Ancef; Kefzol), is said to cause little or no local irritation or nephrotoxicity when administered parenterally for treating moderately severe infections.

Two oral cephalosporins are now available. *Cephalexin* (Keflex) is rapidly absorbed when taken by mouth and reaches effective anti-infective concentrations in the respiratory tract, skin and soft tissues, and urinary tract. It may be used for maintenance therapy of a severe infection that has first been brought under control by one of the parenterally administered cephalosporins. *Cephaloglycin* (Kafocin) reaches effective concentrations only in the urine after its absorption from the gastrointestinal tract. It is recommended for use in cases of acute and chronic pyelonephritis caused by susceptible uropathogens, but it is *not* used for treating infections of other tissues.

The Tetracyclines

The antibiotics, *chlortetracycline* (Aureomycin) and *oxytetracycline* (Terramycin) were among the first broad-spectrum antibiotics introduced into medicine. The newer drugs of this class, including demeclocycline, methacycline, doxycycline, and minocycline do not differ significantly in the types of pathogens that they can control. However, they do produce longer-lasting antimicrobial activity. Thus, the newer tetracyclines can maintain effective tissue concentrations when administered in lower and less frequent doses. (See Table 41-4.)

THERAPEUTIC USES

Although the tetracyclines are effective against many different types of microbes (Table 41-5), they are only rarely the best antibiotic for treating most kinds of infections (*Summary*, p. 512). One reason for this is that they exert a bacteriostatic effect, rather than a bactericidal action such as that which the penicillins and other more potent antibiotics bring to bear upon susceptible bacteria. In addition, many strains of microorganisms have emerged that have acquired resistance to the tetracyclines. Thus, while patients are often started on these antibiotics, their administration is continued only when laboratory tests have indicated that the invading organism is still sensitive to tetracyclines.

The tetracyclines are, no doubt, effective for treating infections by many of the gram-positive and gram-negative cocci and bacilli that cause the most common respiratory and urinary tract infections and venereal diseases. However, they are best reserved for treating patients who are allergic to the penicillins or who do not tolerate erythromycin or the more toxic antibiotics, kanamycin and gentamycin.

On the other hand, the tetracyclines are almost uniquely effective for treating rickettsial infections, including Rocky Mountain spotted fever, a frequently fatal disease. Only chloramphenicol compares with the tetracyclines in quickly controlling this tick-borne form of typhus. Similarly, the tetracyclines are the best antibiotics for treating infections by the agents responsible for such disorders as psittacosis, trachoma, and lymphogranuloma venereum. These antibiotics also often produce dramatic results in primary atypical pneumonia that is caused by *Mycoplasma pneumoniae*, a microorganism that is susceptible only to the tetracyclines and to erythromycin.

ADVERSE EFFECTS

The tetracyclines are relatively safe antibiotics, but reactions of all three kinds (p. 516) can occur, some of which are occasionally serious. The most frequent complaint from the first few doses is *abdominal discomfort*, with *nausea and vomiting*. This is less likely to occur with the newer tetracyclines, doxycycline and minocycline, which are administered in smaller daily doses (100-200 mg) than is the case with tetracycline+ itself and other prototype drugs of this class that are taken in much larger amounts (1-2 g daily).

When large oral doses must be administered, gastrointestinal irritation is best minimized by dividing the total daily dose into small doses that are then administered more often. It is *not* desirable to give the patient milk or a snack, because food interferes with the absorption of tetracyclines. The administration of antacids is also undesirable, because ions such as calcium, magnesium, and aluminum tend to bind tetracyclines and to impair their ability to get into the bloodstream.

Diarrhea that develops during *later* treatment may be the result of a superinfection

TABLE 41-4 *Tetracyclines and Chloramphenicol Preparations*

Generic or Official Name	Trade Name or Synonym	Dosage and Administration	Remarks
Tetracyclines			
Chlortetracycline HCl N.F.	Aureomycin	250 mg q.i.d. oral or parenteral	First drug of this class to be introduced
Demeclocycline HCl N.F.	Declomycin	150 mg q.i.d. or 300 mg b.i.d	Relatively long duration of action
Doxycyline hyclate and monohydrate	Vibramycin (Oral and I.V. forms are available)	200 mg (100 mg every 12 hours) on the first day, followed by 100 mg a day as a single dose, or as 50 mg every 12 hours	Requires smaller doses, less frequently administered
Methacycline HCl N.F.	Rondomycin and others	Oral 600 mg daily, either 150 mg q.i.d. or 300 mg b.i.d.	Relatively low doses are effective
Minocycline	Minocin and others	200 mg initially, followed by 100 mg every 12 hours	Claimed effective against some strains of staphylococci resistant to other tetracyclines
Oxytetracycline HCl U.S.P.	Terramycin	Oral 250 mg q.i.d. I.V. 500 mg daily	One of the first drugs of this class to be introduced
Rolitetracycline N.F.	Syntetrin	I.M. 150 mg every eight hours, I.V. 350–700 mg every 8–12 hrs.	Parenteral form claimed less likely to cause G.I. superinfection
Tetracycline HCl U.S.P.	Achromycin, Bristacycline Panmycin, Sumycin, Steclin, Tetracyn	Oral 500 mg q.i.d., I.V. 500 mg b.i.d.	See *Drug Digest*
Tetracycline phosphate complex N.F.	Tetrex	1 g per day in four doses of 250 mg each	Buffered form claimed to be more completely absorbed
Chloramphenicol Preparations			
Chloramphenicol U.S.P.	Chloromycetin	50–100 mg/kg daily, oral or I.V., in four doses at six-hour intervals	Broad spectrum, but with blood dyscrasia danger (see *Drug Digest*)
Chloramphenicol palmitate U.S.P.	. . . .	50–100 mg/kg daily, oral or I.V. in four doses at six-hour intervals	For children mainly
Chloramphenicol sodium succinate U.S.P.	. . . .	50–100 mg/kg daily, I.V., in four doses every six hours	Injectable form

rather than a direct irritating effect. Most serious is staphylococcal enterocolitis, which can cause severe dehydration unless quickly controlled by oral vancomycin (p. 505) or a penicillinase-resistant penicillin (p. 501) and parenteral administration of replacement fluids and electrolytes.

Overgrowths of the yeastlike fungus, *Candida albicans*, may cause inflammation of the mouth, tongue, and throat. Monilial over-

TABLE 41-5 *Antimicrobial Spectrum of the Tetracyclines**

Gram-Positive Cocci
Streptococcus (anaerobic type)
Streptococcus pyogenes (Group A beta-hemo-
lytic type)
Streptococcus viridans (alpha-hemolytic type)
Streptococcus faecalis (enterococcus group)
Staphylococcus aureus*
Diplococcus pneumoniae
  Gram-Negative Cocci
Gonococcus (*Neisseria gonorrhoeae*)
Meningococcus (*Neisseria meningitidis*)
  Gram-Positive Bacilli
Bacillus anthracis
Clostridium tetani
Listeria monocytogenes
  Gram-Negative Bacilli
Escherichia coli
Enterobacter (*Aerobacter aerogenes*)
Hemophilus influenzae
Hemophilus ducrei (chancroid)

Hemophilus pertussis (whooping cough)
Klebsiella pneumoniae
Shigella species
Pasteurella pestis (bubonic plague)
Brucella species (brucellosis)
Bacteroides species
Fusobacterium fusiforme (Vincent's infection)
Vibrio comma (cholera)
  Spirochetes
Treponema pallidum (syphilis)
Treponema pertenue (yaws)
Borrelia recurrentis (relapsing fever)
  Miscellaneous
Rickettsia (typhus, Rocky Mountain spotted
fever, Q fever, and others)
Mycoplasma pneumoniae (Eaton agent; PPLO)
Lymphogranuloma venereum agent
Granuloma inguinale agent
Psittacosis and ornithosis agents
Actinomyces species

* Although infections caused by these and other organisms are often responsive to treatment with the broad-spectrum antibiotics of this class, many strains have become resistant to the tetracyclines. Thus, these drugs are indicated for treating clinical infections by these pathogens only after the results of culturing and bacteriologic testing indicates that the responsible organism is sensitive to them.

growths of this kind in the anogenital areas may cause itching. Washing the patient's perineum several times daily is said to reduce drug-induced pruritus. Topical application of the antifungal antibiotics nystatin or amphotericin B is a more specific treatment for vulvovaginitis of this kind.

Allergic reactions to tetracyclines are relatively rare, but skin rashes of various kinds have been reported. Demeclocycline and other tetracyclines sometimes set off *phototoxic reactions* in patients who are exposed to sunlight. Patients should be advised to stay out of direct sunlight while taking these drugs. If signs of sunburn develop, the tetracycline treatment may have to be discontinued.

Teeth discoloration may occur when these drugs are taken during the period of a child's tooth development—that is, during the last months of pregnancy, in infancy, and up to eight years old. The yellow, gray, or brown stains are believed caused by formation of a tetracycline-calcium complex. Similar deposits in the bone-forming tissues may slow the rate of skeletal growth temporarily. Thus, these antibiotics are best avoided in very young children, unless other antiinfective agents prove ineffective.

Patients with impaired kidney function may show signs of *nitrogen retention* when taking tetracyclines. These drugs do not cause kidney damage, although this has been reported in patients who received products that had deteriorated as a result of improper storage. The nurse should check the expiration date of all antibiotic packages and look for any evidence of physical change that may make the drug ineffective or dangerous.

Liver damage has occurred in patients with pyelonephritis or other kidney diseases that interfere with the excretion of tetracyclines. *Hepatotoxicity* of this kind has occurred most often in pregnant women who were receiving large daily doses by I.V. injection of parenteral tetracycline products. However, even orally administered doses can accumulate to toxic levels in the tissues of patients with impaired kidney function.

Chloramphenicol+ (Chloromycetin)

This antibiotic also has a broad antimicrobial spectrum. However, it is used only for treating certain serious infections that do not respond as well to treatment with other antiinfective agents. This is because this drug can cause bone marrow depression leading to blood dyscrasias, including fatal *aplastic anemia*.

It is now never ordered routinely for treating minor infections but is best reserved for use against organisms that are shown to be especially sensitive to this antibiotic. These include: *Salmonella typhi*, the cause of typhoid fever; *Rickettsia*; agents of the lymphogranuloma-psittacosis group; *Hemophilus influenzae*; and other gram-negative bacilli. (See Table 41-4.)

Antibiotics for Special Uses

The antibiotics discussed in this section are not as widely useful as the penicillins and tetracyclines. However, they are often useful in clinical situations in which other antiinfective agents are less effective or not well tolerated. Although these antibiotics have more limited usefulness and are, in some cases, quite toxic, they have an important place in the antiinfective therapy of a variety of disorders.

THE GENTAMYCIN-KANAMYCIN-NEOMYCIN GROUP

These antibiotics are effective against various gram-negative and gram-positive bacteria when applied topically, taken orally for local effects in the G.I. tract, or administered parenterally for treating serious systemic infections. *Neomycin* is rarely injected any longer because of its toxicity. *Kanamycin*+ is injected for only short periods, usually, because it tends to cause cumulative auditory nerve toxicity. *Gentamycin*+ is now the most commonly used antibiotic of this group because of its relative safety and somewhat wider antibacterial spectrum. (See Table 41-6.)

TABLE 41-6   *Antibiotics Used Mainly Against Gram-Negative Organisms*

Nonproprietary or Official Name	Trade Name or Synonym	Dosage and Administration	Remarks
Colistimethate sodium U.S.P.	Coly-Mycin M Intramuscular; Polymyxin E	2.5 mg/kg daily I.M. in two divided doses. No more than 300 mg daily	Useful for treating *Pseudomonas* infections
Colistin sulfate N.F.	Coly-Mycin S Oral Suspension	3–5 mg/kg orally in three divided doses for children	Used for local effect in G.I. tract in treating diarrhea
Gentamycin sulfate U.S.P.	Garamycin	0.8–5 mg/kg daily I.M. in two to four divided doses for seven to ten days. Also, administered orally and applied topically	Drug of choice for gram-negative sepsis (see *Drug Digest*)
Kanamycin sulfate U.S.P.	Kantrex	6 to 8 g daily by mouth; 250–500 mg every six hours; I.M. or I.V.	Useful for treating serious infections but nephrotoxic and ototoxic (see *Drug Digest*)
Neomycin sulfate U.S.P.	Mycifradin, Myciguent	4 to 8 g daily by mouth; 250 mg I.M. every six hours; also applied topically	Same spectrum as kanamycin, but even more toxic
Polymyxin B sulfate U.S.P.	Aerosporin	75 to 100 mg orally q.i.d.; 1.5–2.5 mg/kg daily I.M. or I.V.; also topically	Effective for treating *Pseudomonas* infections, but irritating to tissues and nephrotoxic
Streptomycin sulfate U.S.P.		1 to 2 g daily I.M. in two divided doses	Effective against many gram-negative organisms and in tuberculosis

Gram-negative bacilli, including *E. coli*, *Pseudomonas aeruginosa*, and species of *Proteus* are a cause of acute urinary tract infections. Often these pathogenic invaders then enter the blood stream to produce septicemia. Pneumonia caused by *Klebsiella* species is difficult to treat, as is pseudomonal meningitis. Sometimes such infections are the result of the overgrowth of these resistant bacteria following treatment with tetracycline-type antibiotics, which eliminate the natural competitors of these pathogens. Such infections are particularly likely to spread and get out of control in elderly and other disease-weakened patients whose natural defenses are lowered as a result of blood disorders or diabetes.

Gentamycin+ is particularly effective for treating cases of gram-negative sepsis that sometimes develop in hospitalized patients. It is considered to be as effective as *kanamycin+* for treating *Klebsiella* (Friedlander's) pneumonia and as dependable as the polymyxins (see below) against kidney infections caused by *Pseudomonas*. Its main advantage over these other antibiotics is that it is less toxic. (Only *carbenicillin*, p. 501, with which gentamycin is sometimes administered, is safer for use against gram-negative bacillary infections of this kind.)

Polymyxin B sulfate and its close chemical relative, *colistimethate sodium*, are also useful for treating urinary tract infections by *Pseudomonas* species and other gram-negative pathogens. Colistimethate is not as irritating as polymyxin when injected intramuscularly. However, both drugs are equally likely to cause kidney damage, particularly in patients whose renal function is already impaired. Failure to eliminate these antibiotics then results in their accumulation in body tissues, including the eighth cranial nerve. This can lead to dizziness, vertigo, and deafness.

Applied topically to the skin and eyes, all of the above-mentioned antibiotics are free of the nephrotoxicity and ototoxicity that can occur when they are injected for treating systemic infections. Thus, gentamycin+, neomycin, and polymyxin are commonly applied as creams, ointments, or ophthalmic solutions in the treatment of dermatological and ocular infections. They are effective not only against gram-negative organisms but also against such common gram-positive causes of skin infections as staphylococci and streptococci.

Orally administered, kanamycin, colistin, and neomycin are also relatively safe. These drugs are taken by mouth to exert their antibacterial effects against microorganisms within the gastrointestinal tract. Little is absorbed, and that which is is readily excreted by the kidneys. However, patients with poor kidney function can accumulate toxic amounts of neomycin and kanamycin if treatment is continued for more than a few days.

Diarrhea caused by enteropathogenic strains of *E. coli* (and, in the case of colistin, *Shigella*) responds to treatment with these antibiotics. Administered alone, or combined with locally acting adsorbents and demulcents such as kaolin, pectin, and attapulgite, these antibiotics often eliminate the bacteria responsible for enteritis within a few days. Longer use is not recommended, as it may lead to overgrowths of fungal organisms.

Hepatic coma is treated with oral kanamycin and neomycin, which act to suppress the intestinal bacteria that produce ammonia. Administered by mouth as an adjunct to other measures, these antibiotics sometimes bring about improvement by reducing the level of ammonia in the patient's blood.

Preoperative preparation of the bowel before abdominal surgery by the oral administration of kanamycin or neomycin is claimed to reduce the risk of peritonitis. If time permits, the patient receives large oral doses for several days, together with cathartics and enemas. Sometimes, if fecal spill occurs during surgery, a solution of kanamycin may be instilled into the abdominal cavity. This is done only after the patient has recovered from anesthesia, and the effects of skeletal muscle relaxants such as succinylcholine or tubocurarine have worn off. This is because drugs such as kanamycin and neomycin have neuromuscular blocking properties that could add to the patient's respiratory depression.

OTHER ANTIBACTERIAL ANTIBIOTICS (SEE TABLE 41-7)

Other antibacterial antibiotics with narrower spectrums include two of the earliest agents to be introduced—*bacitracin* and *tyrothricin*—which are active against gram-positive pathogens, and a recent addition, *spectinomycin* (Trobicin), which is employed only in the treatment of gonorrhea.

Bacitracin and *tyrothricin* are now used

T A B L E   4 1 - 7   *Miscellaneous Narrow-Spectrum Antibiotics*

Nonproprietary or Official Name	Trade Name or Synonym	Dosage and Administration	Remarks
Amphotericin B U.S.P.	Fungizone	I.V. 0.05 to 1 mg/kg; Intrathecal 0.5 to 0.75 mg; topical application	For systemic fungal infections and topically in moniliasis
Bacitracin U.S.P.	Baciguent	Ointment 500 units/g	Bactericidal for gram-positive organisms.
Candicidin	Candeptin	Topical vaginal tablets and ointment	For vaginal moniliasis
Griseofulvin U.S.P.	Fulvicin; Grifulvin; Grisactin	500 mg–1 g orally in divided doses	Effective against dermatophytes that cause ringworm (tinea) infections
Nystatin U.S.P.	Mycostatin	0.5–1 million units orally, t.i.d.; also topically	Active against *Candida albicans* and other monilial organisms
Paromomycin	Humatin	25 to 75 mg/kg daily in divided oral doses	For intestinal amebiasis
Ristocetin	Spontin	I.V. 0.5–1 gram every 8 to 12 hours	Effective against resistant staphylococci, and others
Spectinomycin dihydrochloride pentahydrate	Trobicin	Male patients 2 g I.M.; female patients 4 g I.M. in single doses	For treating acute gonorrheal urethritis, proctitis, and cervicitis
Tyrothricin N.F.*	Soluthricin	Topically as a spray solution or ointment	Bactericidal mainly against gram-positive organisms and some gram-negative bacilli
Zinc bacitracin U.S.P.	. . . .	Topically in ointments, troches, and tablets	Bactericidal for gram-positive organisms

* Contains two polypeptide components, *tyrocidine* and *gramicidin*; the latter is available for topical application in combination with other antiinfective agents.

only by topical application to the skin and the mucosa of the eye and throat. Like neomycin and polymyxin, with which bacitracin is often combined, this antibiotic and the tyrothricin derivative, gramicidin, are used to treat impetigo (after first gently removing the crusts) and for control of other pyodermas. They are also—like colistin—ingredients of the otic-type preparations employed locally in ear infections.

Spectinomycin is administered as a single large intramuscularly injected dose for treating cases of acute gonorrheal urethritis, cervicitis, or proctitis resistant to treatment with penicillin, tetracyclines, or other antiinfective agents. It is not effective against syphilis, and so patients should be checked serologically for several months if the presence of syphilis is also suspected.

ANTIFUNGAL ANTIBIOTICS

Antibiotics are now available for control of infections caused by fungal organisms rather than by bacteria. *Amphotericin B*+ (Fungizone), for example, is effective both against *Candida*, a yeastlike fungal organism that affects mainly the skin and mucous membranes, and against various systemic fungal invaders. Another antifungal antibiotic, *nystatin*+ (Mycostatin), is too toxic for systemic administration, but is useful when applied *topically* to treat *Candida* infections.

Neither of these antifungal antibiotics can control infections caused by dermatophytic fungi. However, these ringworm-type infections can now be treated by an orally administered antifungal antibiotic, *griseofulvin*+

SUMMARY of Antibiotic Drugs of Choice

Pathogenic Microorganisms	Types of Infections	First-line Antibiotic Treatment	Alternative Antibiotics (in approximate order of effectiveness)
GRAM-POSITIVE COCCI Staphylococcus aureus Nonpenicillinase producers	Skin, subcutaneous tissues, eyes, ears, lungs, gastrointestinal tract, bones, joints, blood and meninges (for example, abscesses, burns, decubiti, surgical and traumatic wounds, pneumonia, enterocolitis, osteomyelitis, bacteremia, endocarditis, meningitis)	Penicillin G	Penicillinase-resistant penicillins, cephalosporin-type antibiotics, erythromycin, lincomycin, clindamycin, chloramphenicol, tetracyclines
Penicillinase-producing strains		Penicillinase-resistant penicillins (for example, oral cloxacillin or dicloxacillin, parenteral nafcillin, oxacillin, methicillin)	Same as above, but also vancomycin, kanamycin, gentamycin, novobiocin
Streptococcus pyogenes Group A beta-hemolytic, and others	Upper respiratory infections, including pharyngitis, tonsillitis, sinusitis, otitis media, and pneumonias, bacteremias, scarlet fever	Penicillin G, ampicillin, hetacillin	Penicillinase-resistant penicillins, cephalosporin or tetracyline-type antibiotics, chloramphenicol, novobiocin
Streptococcus viridans	Dental procedures, endocarditis, meningitis, urinary tract infections	Penicillin G (alone or with streptomycin)	Cephalosporin-type antibiotics, erythromycin alone or with streptomycin, vancomycin
Enterococcus (sensitive strains)	Endocarditis, meningitis, septicemia, peritonitis, urinary tract infections	Penicillin G, ampicillin, hetacillin (alone or with streptomycin)	Erythromycin or tetracyclines with streptomycin, vancomycin, kanamycin, gentamycin
Streptococcus anaerobius	Abscess (brain, and others), endocarditis, peritonitis	Penicillin G	Tetracyclines, erythromycin
Pneumococcus	External and middle ear, respiratory tract (for example, pneumonia), meningitis, endocarditis, arthritis	Penicillin G	Erythromycin, lincomycin, clindamycin, cephalosporin or tetracycline-type antibiotic, penicillinase-resistant penicillin

Organism	Disease	Drug of first choice	Alternative drugs
GRAM-NEGATIVE COCCI			
Meningococcus (*Neisseria meningitidis*)	Meningococcal meningitis, septicemia	Penicillin G	Ampicillin, chloramphenicol, cephalosporin or tetracycline-type antibiotics (sulfonamides may also be employed)
Gonococcus (*Neisseria gonorrhoeae*)	Gonorrheal urethritis, salpingitis, vaginitis, arthritis, etc.	Penicillin G	Ampicillin, tetracyclines, spectinomycin, erythromycin, kanamycin
GRAM-POSITIVE BACILLI			
Bacillus anthracis	Anthrax ("malignant pustule"), pneumonia, meningitis	Penicillin G	Erythromycin, lincomycin, tetracycline or cephalosporin family antibiotics, chloramphenicol
Listeria monocytogenes	Meningitis, endocarditis, septicemia	Penicillin G	Erythromycin, cephalothin, tetracyclines, chloromycetin
Corynebacterium diphtheriae	Pharyngitis, laryngitis, tracheitis, pneumonia, etc.	Penicillin G	Erythromycin, cephalothin, tetracyclines, lincomycin, etc.
Clostridium tetani	Tetanus	Penicillin G	Tetracyclines
Clostridium welchii (*Bacillus perfringens*)	Gas gangrene	Penicillin G	Tetracyclines
GRAM-NEGATIVE BACILLI			
Escherichia coli	(a) Gastrointestinal tract infectious diarrhea due to enteropathogenic strains	Oral neomycin	Oral colistin and other polymyxins, kanamycin
	(b) Urinary tract infections, septicemia, peritonitis, meningitis	Ampicillin, kanamycin	Gentamycin, carbenicillin, cephalosporins, colistimethate, tetracyclines, chloramphenicol
Klebsiella pneumoniae	Pneumonia, urinary tract, biliary tract, and bone infections	Gentamycin, kanamycin, cephalosporins	Tetracyclines or chloramphenicol with streptomycin, colistimethate, polymyxin B sulfate
Enterobacter (*Aerobacter aerogenes*)	Urinary tract infections, septicemia	Gentamycin	Kanamycin, colistimethate, chloramphenicol, tetracyclines, carbenicillin
Proteus mirabilis, and other species	Urinary tract infections, septicemia	Ampicillin, kanamycin	Gentamycin, carbenicillin, tetracyclines, chloramphenicol
Pseudomonas aeruginosa	Urinary tract, septicemia, skin and subcutaneous tissues	Carbenicillin, gentamycin	Colistimethate, polymyxin B sulfate

SUMMARY of Antibiotic Drugs of Choice (continued)

Pathogenic Microorganisms	Types of Infections	First-line Antibiotic Treatment	Alternative Antibiotics (in approximate order of effectiveness)
GRAM-NEGATIVE BACILLI (continued)			
Mima, Herellea species	Endocarditis, meningitis, urethritis, septicemia	Gentamycin, kanamycin	Colistimethate, polymyxin B sulfate, tetracyclines
Bacteroides Respiratory strains	Pharyngitis (ulcerative), gingivitis, lung abscess, female genital infections	Penicillin G, ampicillin	Tetracyclines, chloromycetin, erythromycin, lincomycin, clindamycin
Intestinal strains	Septicemia, abscesses (Brain, and others)	Tetracyclines	Chloramphenicol
Shigella species	Acute gastroenteritis or bacillary dysentery, or shigellosis	Ampicillin	Oral neomycin, kanamycin, colistin, or paromomycin, tetracyclines, cephalosporins
Salmonella species	Salmonellosis gastroenteritis, typhoid, and paratyphoid fevers, septicemia	Ampicillin for milder and chloramphenicol for more severe cases	Tetracyclines, cephalosporins
Vibrio comma	Cholera	Tetracyclines	Chloramphenicol, streptomycin, erythromycin
Pasteurella pestis	Bubonic plague	Streptomycin	Tetracyclines, chloramphenicol
Pasteurella tularensis	Tularemia	Streptomycin	Tetracyclines, chloramphenicol
Hemophilus influenzae	Respiratory tract infections, including pneumonia, meningitis	Ampicillin	Chloramphenicol, tetracyclines, streptomycin
Hemophilus ducreyi	Chancroid	Tetracyclines	Chloramphenicol, streptomycin
Brucella species	Brucellosis (undulant fever)	Tetracyclines, with or without streptomycin	Chloramphenicol, with or without streptomycin
Bordetella pertussis	Whooping cough	Ampicillin	Tetracyclines, erythromycin
ACID-FAST BACILLI			
Mycobacterium tuberculosis	Infections of lungs, bones, kidneys, meninges, and all body surfaces (miliary)	Streptomycin	Rifampin, cycloserine, viomycin, kanamycin (with chemotherapeutic agents, see Chap. 46)

Organism	Disease	Drug of choice	Alternatives
SPIROCHETES			
Treponema pallidum	Syphilis	Penicillin G	Tetracyclines, erythromycin
Treponema pertenue	Yaws	Penicillin G	Tetracyclines, erythromycin
Borrelia recurrentis	Relapsing fever	Tetracyclines	Chloramphenicol, penicillin G
Leptospira	Weil's disease	Penicillin G	Tetracyclines
Spirillum minus	Rat-bite fever	Penicillin G	Tetracyclines
RICKETTSIA	Typhus fever, murine typhus, Brill's disease, Q fever, Rocky Mountain spotted fever, and others	Tetracyclines	Chloramphenicol
FILTRABLE PATHOGENIC AGENTS (LARGE "VIRUSES")			
Mycoplasma pneumoniae	Atypical pneumonia	Tetracyclines	Chloramphenicol, erythromycin
Psittacosis (ornithosis) agent	Parrot fever pneumonia	Tetracyclines	Chloramphenicol
Lymphogranuloma venereum	Venereal disease	Tetracyclines	Chloramphenicol
Trachoma	Blinding eye disease	Tetracyclines	Erythromycin (orally), chloramphenicol topically, (with sulfonamides)
FUNGI			
Aspergillus, Blastomyces, Cryptococcus, Coccidioides, Histoplasma, Mucor, Candida albicans	Disseminated (systemic) mycoses in skin, lungs, bones, brain, etc.	Amphotericin B	No antibiotic alternative, but a chemotherapeutic agent, Flucytosine, is effective in some kinds of systemic fungal infections
Candida albicans	Skin and mucous membranes	Amphotericin B	Nystatin, candicidin
Dermatophytosis	Ringworm of skin, scalp, nails	Griseofulvin	No antibiotic alternative, but various chemicals may be applied topically
ACTINOMYCETES			
Actinomyces israeli (actinomycosis)	Granulomas of jaw, brain, lungs, etc.	Penicillin G	Tetracyclines, erythromycin
Nocardia asteroides	Nocardiosis of lungs, brain, etc.	Streptomycin with a sulfonamide	Tetracyclines with cycloserine

(Fulvicin U/V; Grifulvin V; Grisactin), as well as by the topical application of various chemicals effective against dermatophytes (see Chapter 46 for further discussion of the treatment of fungal infections of the skin).

Other antibiotics are available for treating tuberculosis. These will be discussed separately in the next chapter, together with the synthetic chemotherapeutic agents that are used to treat that infectious disease. No antibiotics are effective for treating virus infections. The few available antiviral chemicals will be briefly discussed in Chapter 41 together with the immunologic agents that are employed in the prevention and treatment of viral and bacterial infections.

S U M M A R Y of Adverse Effects of Antibiotics

The Penicillins

Allergic reactions can occur, mainly skin rashes of all kinds, including urticaria, but also more serious angioedema and potentially fatal anaphylactoid-type reactions. Serum-sickness type reactions with fever, rash, and arthritis can also occur.

Direct toxicity is rare, but includes pain at injection sites; C.N.S. irritation with possible muscle twitching and convulsions (from intrathecal injections or after very high parenteral doses of carbenicillin); bone marrow depression has been reported with methicillin. The potassium or sodium of the penicillin salts may be hazardous for patients with kidney impairment who receive large doses.

Superinfections are rare but are most likely to occur with ampicillin; these may take the form of stomatis and glossitis (black, "hairy" tongue) and diarrhea.

The Tetracyclines

Allergic reactions of various kinds may occur, including photosensitivity reactions, particularly with demeclocycline.

Direct toxicity includes epigastric distress early in treatment and tooth discoloration in infants and children. Liver damage has occurred in patients with impaired kidney function and in pregnant women receiving high daily doses.

Superinfection as the result of overgrowths of nonsusceptible microorganisms may cause discomforting moniliasis and serious staphylococcal enterocolitis.

Chloramphenicol

Blood dyscrasias, including fatal aplastic anemia, develop occasionally.

Infants may suffer cardiovascular collapse as a result of the so-called *gray syndrome*.

Gastrointestinal disturbances may result from *superinfections*.

Cephalosporins

Allergic reactions may occur in patients with a history of penicillin allergy. Hypersensitivity of this type may result in urticaria, maculopapular rash, serum sickness, and anaphylaxis.

Direct toxicity includes pain and tenderness at sites of I.M. injections (cephalothin), and nephrotoxicity with renal tubular necrosis (cephalordine).

Superinfections as the result of overgrowth of *Pseudomonas* species or other pathogenic microorganisms may occur.

Gentamycin-Kanamycin-Neomycin Group, and Polymyxins, including Colistimethate sodium

Nephrotoxicity and *neurotoxicity* are possible, especially in patients with renal disease or in those receiving other drugs that adversely affect the eighth cranial nerve. Drug-induced kidney damage is usually reversible, but damage to the auditory nerve may be irreversible, and ototoxicity involving the vestibular nerve may also lead to permanent difficulties.

Lincomycin and Clindamycin

Gastrointestinal disturbances including diarrhea may be severe with lincomycin, but are much less frequent with the related drug, clindamycin.

SUMMARY of Points for the Nurse to Remember About Antibiotic Therapy

Always ask whether the patient has ever had reactions to drugs before administering any antibiotic, and penicillin in particular. Do not give him the drug but consult the physician, if the patient indicates that he may be allergic to the antibiotic.

Observe the patient for any signs or symptoms of an allergic response such as urticaria or other skin eruptions, or itching, wheezing, and so forth, following the first doses of the antibiotic.

Gastrointestinal irritation and epigastric distress follow administration of some antibiotics. Giving the medication with food may reduce its irritating effect. However, food may interfere with the absorption of some antibiotics; thus, these are best administered between meals.

Inform the physician if a patient cannot take an antibiotic by mouth because of nausea, or if he vomits an orally administered antibiotic. The doctor may then decide to administer the antibiotic parenterally to assure its attaining therapeutic levels in the area of the infection.

It is essential to administer antibiotics at the prescribed intervals in order to maintain the anti-infective agent at therapeutic levels. This means that sleeping patients must be awakened to take a dose of a drug that is ordered on such schedules as "six times daily, every four hours" or "three times daily, every eight hours."

Teach the patient not to take antibiotics left over from a previous illness of some member of the family. Taking an antibiotic unnecessarily to treat a trivial illness can lead to sensitization that may make it impossible to use the drug for treating a serious illness at a later time.

Teach patients not to rely solely on antibiotic therapy. These drugs do not substitute for other health measures. Thus, for example, the patient with a respiratory infection for which an antibiotic was prescribed should not continue with his usual routine—going to work, and so forth. He should rest, force fluids, and employ other supportive hygienic measures in addition to taking the drug.

Discussion Topics: Dealing with Antibiotics

The Situation: Miss Jones was admitted to the hospital for treatment of pneumonia. A few minutes after she was given an injection of 300,000 units of penicillin intramuscularly, she became restless, developed urticaria, and then fainted. Her roommate observed these symptoms and called the nurse.

The Problem: Discuss the following questions:

What is the probable reason for Miss Jones's symptoms?

What actions could you take in this situation? Indicate the order in which you would carry out each task. What equipment and supplies would you prepare for the physician's use?

What nursing actions are indicated for Miss Jones's roommate?

DRUG DIGEST

AMPHOTERICIN B U.S.P.
(Fungizone)

Actions and Indications. Administered parenterally, this antifungal antibiotic is effective for treatment of most serious systemic fungal infections. Among the disseminated mycotic infections that often respond to treatment with this drug are: blastomycosis, coccidiomycosis, cryptococcosis, histoplasmosis, and candidiasis.

It is also effective against can-

didiasis when applied topically to the skin and nails, or to the mucous membranes of the mouth. Taken internally in oral dosage forms, amphotericin B is sometimes employed to prevent the overgrowth of intestinal fungi that occurs during treatment with tetracyclines and other broad-spectrum antibiotics.

Side Effects, Cautions, and Contraindications. The topical application

of this antibiotic causes little irritation and few allergic reactions. However, toxic effects are frequent during intravenous administration, and efforts must be made to minimize toxicity. For example, administration of this drug in the lowest effective dose together with antipyretic, antihistamine, and antiemetic drugs may help to reduce reactions.

Patients' renal function must be carefully monitored to detect increases in blood urea nitrogen (BUN) and nonprotein nitrogen (NPN). If these levels rise, the drug is discontinued for a time. Kidney excretion of the antibiotic is increased by alkalinizing the urine.

Dosage and Administration. Dosage is adjusted individually, but should not ordinarily be more than 1 mg/kg/day or 1.5 mg/kg every other day. Solutions for slow intravenous infusion must be freshly prepared and protected from light.

AMPICILLIN U.S.P. (Alpen; Amcill; Omnipen; and others)

Actions and Indications. This semi-synthetic penicillin possesses a wider antibacterial spectrum than most penicillins. It is effective, for example, against such gram-negative bacilli as *E. Coli, H. influenzae, Proteus mirabilis,* and strains of *Shigella* and *Salmonella,* including *S. typhosa (typhi),* the cause of typhoid fever:

Because ampicillin is effective against the pathogens most commonly involved in meningitis (pneumococcus, meningococcus, and H. influenzae), it may be injected I.V. even before the results of bacteriologic studies are obtained. It is also useful for treating urinary tract infections, including gonorrhea. Bacillary dysentery caused by tetracycline-resistant strains responds to treatment, as does salmonellosis. It is, however, used mainly for mild *Salmonella* infections and for treating known carriers rather than for use in acute systemic infections such as typhoid fever.

Side Effects, Cautions, and Contraindications. Allergic reactions similar to those caused by other penicillins occur, so this drug is contraindicated in patients with a history of penicillin allergy, and it is used only with caution in patients known to have many allergies.

It is ineffective against staphylococci (and other organisms) that produce penicillinase, and its use is contraindicated in cases of infection by these strains. Ampicillin can produce changes in the bacterial flora that may result in superinfections by *non*susceptible pathogens, including gram-negative bacilli.

Dosage and Administration. Oral doses of 250 to 500 mg q.i.d. are effective for most infections in adults. For more severe infections such as meningitis or septicemia, sodium ampicillin is administered I.M. or I.V. in doses of 8 to 14 g daily. Children receive 150–200 mg/kg/day by I.V. drip for three days,

followed by I.M. injections every three or four hours for these serious infections.

BENZATHINE PENICILLIN G (Bicillin; Permapen)

Actions and Indications. This form of penicillin G is administered in the form of an aqueous suspension that is only very slowly absorbed into the bloodstream from the depot left at the injection site. It produces much lower plasma levels than other parenteral penicillins, but these provide very long-lasting effects against pathogenic organisms that are sensitive to low concentrations of penicillin G.

It is used in the treatment of streptococcal pharyngitis and other mild to moderate respiratory tract infections caused by this organism. It is also used for long-term prophylaxis against recurrences of rheumatic fever, chorea, and acute glomerulonephritis.

This drug is administered in the management of all stages of syphilis and in other spirochetal infections. However, it is *not* recommended for treating gonorrhea.

Side Effects, Cautions, and Contraindications. The only type of toxicity is the occurrence of allergic reactions in patients previously sensitized to penicillin. Since such reactions can be serious and even fatal, use of this product is *not* recommended in patients with a history of hypersensitivity to penicillin. It is used with caution in patients known to be allergic to other substances. Superinfections may occur as a result of prolonged use that promotes overgrowth of fungi and other organisms not susceptible to penicillin G.

Dosage and Administration. A single injection of 900,000 to 1.2 million units is used for treating streptococcal pharyngitis. For prophylaxis against recurrences, injections of 600,000 units may be made every two weeks, or 1.2 million units once a month.

Currently recommended treatment for primary, secondary, and latent syphilis is 2.4 million units, which may be repeated in one week. For late (tertiary) syphilis and neurosyphilis a dose of 3 million units is administered at weekly intervals, to a total of 6 to 9 million units.

CHLORAMPHENICOL U.S.P. (Chloromycetin)

Actions and Indications. This antibiotic has a broad spectrum of antimicrobial activity. However, it is now recommended for use only in certain severe infections caused by pathogens that are particularly sensitive to it. These include: acute

typhoid fever and other serious *Salmonella* infections; Rocky Mountain spotted fever and other rickettsial infections that do not improve upon treatment with tetracyclines; infections by agents of the lymphogranuloma-psittacosis group that do not respond to tetracycline treatment; and serious infections such as bacteremia and meningitis caused by gram-negative bacteria that are not susceptible to treatment with less potentially dangerous antiinfective drugs.

Side Effects, Cautions, and Contraindications. This antibiotic has caused fatal blood dyscrasias, including aplastic anemia. Thus, it is never used routinely for treating trivial infections, for prophylactic purposes, or for conditions in which it is ineffective such as the common cold, influenza, or other viral infections.

Treatment of newborn and, particularly, premature infants is carried out with low doses and with careful control of serum levels to avoid toxic reactions of the kind called the "gray syndrome." This disorder can cause fatal vasomotor collapse and respiratory failure within a few hours as a result of the accumulation of unmetabolized and unexcreted chloramphenicol.

Dosage and Administration. Doses of 50 mg/kg per day are administered in four divided doses at intervals of six hours. Occasional severe infections may require 100 mg/kg/day. However, in newborn infants, only 25 mg/kg/day is employed for the first two weeks of life. The serum concentration of chloromycetin is checked chemically.

ERYTHROMYCIN U.S.P. (AND ITS SALTS AND ESTERS; Erythrocin; Ilotycin; and others)

Actions and Indications. This antibiotic has a spectrum similar to that of penicillin and is used as an alternative for treating infections in patients allergic to penicillin. It is effective for treating respiratory infections caused by streptococci pneumococci, and susceptible strains of staphylococci and *H. influenzae.* It is also useful in treating primary atypical pneumonia caused by *Mycoplasma pneumoniae.* It is employed sometimes in the management of intestinal amebiasis.

Side Effects, Cautions, and Contraindications. The most common side effects are those affecting the gastrointestinal tract—abdominal discomfort and cramps, and occasionally nausea, vomiting, and diarrhea. The estolate ester of erythromycin has occasionally caused jaundice, fever, and other signs of allergic hepatitis of the cholestatic type.

Overgrowths of bacteria and fungi sometimes cause superinfections, and skin rashes or, rarely, anaphylactic reactions have been reported.

Dosage and Administration. Adult dosage is usually 250 mg every six hours, but this may be raised to 4 g or more per day depending upon the severity of the infection. The drug is usually administered orally but the rectal route may also be employed. Erythromycin ethylsuccinate is available for deep intramuscular administration in doses of 100 mg at four to eight hour intervals. The gluceptate and lactobionate forms are suited for intravenous administration in severe infections when large oral doses are not tolerated.

GENTAMYCIN SULFATE U.S.P. (Garamycin)

Actions and Indications. This wide-spectrum antibiotic is effective against various gram-negative bacilli, including *Pseudomonas aeruginosa* and *Proteus* species. Strains of gram-positive pathogens such as streptococci, staphylococci, and pneumococci are also sensitive to its bactericidal action.

The perenteral form is injected for treating serious, life-threatening systemic infections that do not respond to less toxic antiinfective drug treatment. This antibiotic has proved effective against septicemia caused by gram-negative bacilli including, the *Klebsiella-Enterobacter-Serratia* group. It is also useful in meningitis and acute urinary tract infections caused by resistant strains of *E. coli* and other uropathogens.

Side Effects, Cautions, and Contraindications. Although this antibiotic is considered safer than others of the same chemical class, care is required because of its potential toxicity to the kidney (nephrotoxicity) and to the eight cranial nerve (ototoxicity). Renal function should be closely checked for signs of nitrogen retention during its administration to patients with impaired kidney function. Functioning of the eighth nerve should also be monitored, as this drug can cause damage leading to loss of hearing and vertigo. This drug should not be administered together with potent diuretics, as this may intensify its neurotoxicity.

Dosage and Administration. Intramuscular or intravenous injection of 3 mg/kg/day, divided into three equal doses, is the usual treatment for adult patients with normal kidney function. This may be adjusted

upward in life-threatening infections or downward for patients with impaired kidney function.

This antibiotic is also available in cream and ointment form for treatment of skin infections, and as an ophthalmic ointment and solution for use in eye infections by susceptible bacteria. In impetigo, crusts should be removed before applying the dermatological preparations gently. The eye drops are administered every four hours, or more frequently.

GRISEOFULVIN U.S.P. (Fulvicin U/V; Grifulvin V; Grisactin)

Actions and Indications. This antifungal antibiotic is effective for treating tinea (ringworm) infections of the skin. Taken orally, it is absorbed into the bloodstream and deposited in new skin and nail keratin, which can then resist invasion by species of *Trichophyton, Microsporum,* and *Epidermophyton.* Among the infections that respond to treatment are tinea pedis (athlete's foot), tinea capitis (scalp ringworm), tinea cruris (groin ringworm), and tinea ungvium (onychomycosis, a fungal disease of the nails).

Side Effects, Cautions, and Contraindications. Skin rashes of the hypersensitivity type sometimes occur, as do photosensitivity-type reactions in some patients exposed to sunlight. Since this drug is not effective against *Candida,* overgrowths of *Monilia* may cause oral thrush. Gastrointestinal distress with nausea, vomiting, and diarrhea, and central effects such as headache, dizziness, and mental confusion may occur. This drug is contraindicated in patients with acute porphyria or liver damage.

Drug interactions with warfarin-type anticoagulants may result in reduced responsiveness to the anticoagulants, which then requires an upward adjustment of their dosage. The effectiveness of griseofulvin may be reduced when barbiturates are taken at the same time. Thus, dosage of the antibiotic may have to be raised.

Dosage and Administration. Daily oral doses of 0.5 or 1 g are taken after meals. The length of treatment may vary from several weeks in skin infections to several months for nail infections. The adjunctive use of topically applied antifungal chemicals is also often desirable.

KANAMYCIN SULFATE U.S.P. (Kantrex)

Actions and Indications. This antibiotic is active against strains of gram-negative bacilli such as the *Klebsiella-Enterobacter-Serratia* group, the *Mima-Herellea* group,

and others; it is also active against some strains of gram-positive cocci, including *Staphylococcus aureus.*

The injectable form is used in the short-term treatment of serious systemic infections including Friedlander's pneumonia, gram-negative infections of the urinary tract, and septicemia. The oral form acts locally within the gastrointestinal tract to control infections caused by enteropathogens, including diarrhea-inducing strains of *E. coli.* It is also used to suppress intestinal bacteria as an adjunct to other therapeutic measures in the management of hepatic coma, and for sterilizing the bowel prior to surgery.

Side Effects Cautions, and Contraindications. This drug is not used parenterally for prolonged periods because of its potential for damaging the auditory nerve and causing deafness. Even when used for five days or more, it is desirable to monitor the patient's hearing with audiograms. If these show loss of high frequency perception, treatment is stopped. Otoicity of this type is most likely to occur in patients with impaired kidney function, and the drug is itself potentially nephrotoxic. The risk of hearing loss is increased when this drug is administered together with other ototoxic drugs (such as the diuretic, ethacrynic acid) or nephrotoxic antibiotics such as the polymyxins and gentamycin.

Dosage and Administration. The usual total daily dose for adults is 1.0 g I.M., and no more than 1.5 g should be administered. This is usually given in four injections at intervals of six hours. The I.V. route is only rarely used, and the drug is administered intraperitioneally only if peritonitis is present or possible. Oral administration of 1.0 g every four hours is usual, but as much as 8 to 12 g may be given daily in hepatic coma.

NYSTATIN U.S.P. (Mycostatin; Nilstat)

Actions and Indications. This antifungal antibiotic is effective against candidal infections (moniliasis), when it is applied topically to the skin or to the mucous membranes of the mouth (in thrush) or of the vagina. It is also often taken orally to prevent superinfections by overgrowths of intestinal fungi in patients who are being treated with tetracyclines or other broad-spectrum antibacterial drugs.

It is doubtful that the small amounts of this antibiotic contained in commercial fixed dosage combinations can serve a useful prophylactic purpose. However, the administration of adequate oral doses may be desirable for preventing intestinal moniliasis during antibacterial treatment of diabetics and other high-risk patients, such as those receiving corticosteroids for systemic lupus or antineoplastic drugs for leukemia, lymphoma, and so forth.

Side Effects, Cautions, and Contraindications. Large oral doses sometimes cause epigastric distress and diarrhea. However, the drug is not absorbed and does not cause systemic toxicity. Topical application rarely causes irritation or hypersensitivity-type reactions.

Dosage and Administration. This drug may be administered orally in doses of 0.5 to 1 million units t.i.d. daily for suppression of yeast-like intestinal fungi. Tablets may be deposited in the vagina by applicator in doses of 100,000 to 200,000 units daily. Other dosage forms for topical application include: an oral suspension that is dropped into the mouth four times daily to treat thrush in infants and children; a dusting powder for fungal infections of the feet; and a cream and ointment that are applied twice daily to cutaneous areas affected by candidiases.

POTASSIUM PENICILLIN G U.S.P. (Pentids; and others)

Actions and Indications. This form of penicillin is the first choice for treating and preventing infections by susceptible pathogens, as it is more effective and less expensive than the semisynthetic derivatives. Its antibacterial spectrum includes gram-positive and gram-negative cocci, certain gram-positive bacilli, and spirochetes.

Penicillin G is used for prophylaxis and treatment of streptococcal pharyngitis, pneumococcal respiratory tract and meningeal infections, and infections by *non*penicillinase-producing strains of staphylococci. It is also effective for treating meningococcal infections, gonorrhea and syphilis, tetanus, and diphtheria.

Side Effects, Cautions, and Contraindications. Penicillin causes little direct tissue toxicity, except when it is injected into the spinal canal in too high concentration. Such intrathecal injection can cause central nervous system stimulation and convulsions. The administration of very large I.V. doses of the potassium salt may also cause convulsions and hyperkalemia, particularly in patients with kidney damage.

Allergic reactions are common and potentially very serious. Thus, all patients must be questioned concerning any previous reactions to penicillin, the use of which is

contraindicated in those with a history of hypersensitivity to it. The drug is ordinarily discontinued if skin reactions develop during treatment. Caution is required in patients with a history of asthma or other significant allergies.

Dosage and Administration .Oral doses for adults range between 600,000 and 1.6 million units daily, in most cases. Children may receive 400,000 units daily for prophylaxis. I.M. or I.V. doses of 5–20 million units or more may be administered daily for treating severe infections.

PROCAINE PENICILLIN G SUSPENSION, STERILE U.S.P. (Crysticillin; Duracillin; Wycillin; and others)

Actions and Indications. This preparation of penicillin in combination with the local anesthetic procaine is only slowly absorbed into the systemic circulation when deposited in depot sites by intramuscular injection. Thus, both the aqueous suspension and the oily aluminum stearate suspension produce long-lasting plasma-tissue levels of the antibiotic (15 to 20 hours).

These concentrations are adequate for treating moderately severe infections. However, when high penicillin levels must be maintained in the treatment of severe infections such as bacteremia, meningitis, pericarditis, and peritonitis, aqueous penicillin G itself (rather than this poorly soluble procaine derivative) should be injected I.M. or I.V. during the acute stages.

This form of penicillin G is recommended for the one-day treatment of uncomplicated gonorrheal infections and for prophylaxis against gonorrhea. Follow-up treatment may be required if clinical signs and laboratory tests indicate that the infection is still present. For such severe complications of gonorrhea as septic arthritis or endocarditis, intensive treatment with aqueous penicillin G (*not* this procaine preparation) should be employed.

Side Effects, Cautions, and Contraindications. Hypersensitivity reactions similar to those with other penicillin G preparations may occur. Some patients are also sensitive to the procaine component.

Dosage and Administration. Because of its procaine content, I.M. injections are almost entirely pain-free, but because of the presence of suspending agents, it is particularly important to aspirate to be sure that the needle has not accidentally entered a vein.

Dosage varies with the sensitivity of the organism and severity

of the infection. In syphilis, for example, doses of 1.2 to 2.4 million units repeated at three-day intervals are employed; in gonorrhea, a single 4.8 million-unit dose is given. For prophylaxis against bacterial endocarditis, doses of 300,000 to 600,000 units are administered on the day before dental or oropharyngeal operations and for two days after these procedures. (On the operative day, aqueous penicillin G is employed.)

SODIUM METHICILLIN U.S.P. (Staphcillin)

Actions and Indications. This semisynthetic penicillin is highly effective against strains of staphylococci that produce penicillinase, an enzyme that inactivates natural penicillin G and V. It is less effective than the latter penicillins in infections caused by other organisms, including streptococci, pneumococci, and *non*penicillinase-producing staphylococci and, consequently, should not be used in such cases. Among the resistant staph infections that often do respond to this antibiotic are lobar or bronchial pneumonia and lung abscesses, septicemia, endocarditis, osteomyelitis, and infections of the skin and soft tissues.

Side Effects, Cautions, and Contraindications. Hypersensitivity reactions of the kind common to all penicillins have been reported. These range from minor skin rashes to fatal anaphylactoid reactions. Staphylococci and other organisms resistant to methicillin have caused serious superinfections. This drug has occasionally caused bone marrow depression and nephritis. The latter disorder may lead to sodium retention.

Dosage and Administration. Methicillin is instable in stomach acids and poorly absorbed from the intestine, so it must be administered parenterally. It is injected I.M. fairly frequently (every four to six hours) in relatively large doses (1 to 1.5 g). Because I.M. injections are somewhat painful, the I.V. route is often preferred, in which case 1 g is injected slowly in the form of a freshly prepared dilute solution (50 cc in five minutes) every six hours.

SODIUM OXACILLIN U.S.P. (Prostaphlin)

Actions and Indications. This semisynthetic penicillin is useful against infections by staphylococcal strains resistant to penicillin G or V. Its molecule resists destruction, not only by bacterial penicillinase, but also by stomach acids. Thus, it is effective orally as well as parenterally. While it may be used to begin treatment in various skin, soft tissue, and respiratory infections believed to be caused by resistant staph organisms, it should be discontinued in favor of penicillin G if sensitivity tests prove the organism to be susceptible to treatment with that natural penicillin.

Side Effects, Cautions, and Contraindications. Allergic reactions typical of other penicillin products have occurred with this one, especially in patients with a history of previous hypersensitivity to penicillin. The drug should be discontinued if such reactions, or the development of superinfections by nonsusceptible microorganisms, are seen to develop.

Dosage and Administration. The injectable form is preferred for use in serious infections. However, once the infection is brought under control, the oral form, which is effective for mild to moderate infections, may be employed. The oral form should be taken on an empty stomach, one or two hours before meals, for maximal absorption. Oral dosage of 500 mg, every four to six hours, is recommended for mild staph infections, and 1 g for more severe infections. For staphylococcal septicemia or other deep-seated infections, doses as high as 500 to 1,000 mg may be administered by intramuscular or slow intravenous injection.

TETRACYCLINE HCl U.S.P.
(Achromycin; and others)

Actions and Indications. The broad-spectrum antibiotic is most commonly employed as an alternative to the penicillins in patients who are hypersensitive to antibiotics of that type. However, it is effective not only against gram-positive and gram-negative bacteria, but also against the rickettsial organisms responsible for Rocky Mountain spotted fever, Q fever, and typhus. It is also effective against *Mycoplasma pneumoniae*, a cause of atypical pneumonia, and against the agents that cause trachoma, psitta-cosis, and certain relatively rare venereal diseases.

Side Effects, Cautions, and Contraindications. Gastrointestinal side effects including epigastric distress, nausea, vomiting, and diarrhea are the most common adverse effect of this relatively safe antibiotic.

Overgrowths of candidal organisms may cause superinfections of the mouth and the anogenital region. Staphylococcal superinfections of the gastrointestinal tract are rare but may be very serious.

Photosensitivity reactions resembling sunburn may occur in patients exposed to sunlight while taking this drug. Infants and young children may suffer discoloration of the teeth. Patients with kidney damage may accumulate toxic amounts of this drug in the liver when they receive ordinary doses.

Dosage and Administration. The usual daily dose for adults is 1 to 2 g divided into two to four doses. Children's dosage is 10 to 20 mg per pound of body weight.

References

Best, W.R. Chloramphenical-associated blood dyscrasias. *JAMA*, 201:181, 1967.

Di Palma, J.R. The antifungal drugs and their use. *RN*, 30:35, 1967 (June).

Fishman, L.S., and Hewitt, W.L. The natural penicillins. *Med. Clin. N. Amer.*, 54: 1081, 1970 (Sept.).

Friend, D.G. Penicillin therapy—newer semisynthetic penicillins. *Clin. Pharmacol. Ther.*, 7:706, 1966.

Martin, W.I. Newer penicillins. *Med. Clin. N. Amer.*, 51:1107, 1967.

Rodman, M.J. New drugs for fighting infections. *RN*, 30:55, 1967 (June).

————. Drugs for treating bacterial pneumonias. *RN*, 34:55, 1971 (Nov.).

Sparling, P.F. Antibiotic resistance in Neissceria gonorrhoeae. *Med. Clin. N. Amer.*, 56:1133, 1972 (Sept.).

Sweeney, F. J., and Rodgers, J.F., Therapy of infections caused by gram-negative bacilli. *Med. Clin. N. Amer.*, 49:1391, 1965.

Van Arsdel, P.P., Jr. Allergic reactions to penicillin. *JAMA*, 191:240, 1965.

West, R.I. The staphylococcus—approach to therapy. *Med. Clin. N. Amer.*, 49:1403, 1965.

42.

Chemotherapeutic and Biologic Control of Bacterial and Viral Infections

Long before the first antibiotics came into clinical use in the 1940s, doctors attempted to control infections by means of chemicals and with products of natural, animal origin. Chemical treatment of infectious diseases dates back to the use of mercury for treating syphilis in the 1500s. Biological substances obtained from cows infected with cowpox were first employed successfully for smallpox prevention in the 1700s.

The modern use of *synthetic chemicals* to treat infection stems from the work of Paul Ehrlich early in this century. This scientist synthesized hundreds of chemicals for use in treating diseases caused by protozoa and spirochetes. The present status of chemotherapy in malaria and other protozoal and parasitic diseases is discussed in Chapter 43. In this chapter we shall take up the use of *non*-antibiotic synthetic chemicals in the treatment of bacterial and viral infections.

The first significant antibacterial chemicals for treating *systemic* infections were the *sulfonamides*. The current status of this class of chemotherapeutic agents will be reviewed in this chapter. Here, we shall also discuss the *chemotherapy of tuberculosis, leprosy*, and *bacterial infections of the urinary tract*.

Virus infections have been most resistant to chemotherapy, and we have, until recently, been entirely dependent upon vaccines for protection against diseases of this kind. However, recent breakthroughs in molecular biology have resulted in advances in antiviral chemotherapy, and the first few antiviral drugs have now become available. We shall briefly discuss a couple of these agents here and also summarize the status of the *biological agents* that are currently available for prevention and treatment of viral and bacterial infections.

The Sulfonamides

HISTORY AND CURRENT STATUS

The introduction in the 1930s of sulfanilamide for treating bacterial infections marked the start of a new era in antiinfective chemotherapy. Up to that time, no drugs had been available for treating serious infections by streptococci, staphylococci, pneumococci, meningococci, and other pathogenic bacteria. Reports of the lifesaving effects of this sulfonamide stimulated chemists to synthesize many more antibacterial chemicals of this class.

The sulfonamide drugs that are now available (Table 42-1) are safer and more effective than sulfanilamide and its first successors, sulfapyridine and sulfathiazole. Yet the sulfonamides as a class are now not nearly as important as they once were, and they are not often the physician's first choice for treating most common infections. This is because most bacterial infections can now be better controlled by antibiotics than by these synthetic chemotherapeutic agents.

One reason for this is that the antibiotics are often more dependable than the sulfonamides. Penicillin, for example, exerts a bactericidal effect when administered in small safe doses. The sulfonamides, on the other hand, are only bacteriostatic, and thus they may not prove effective for treating a patient whose own natural defenses against bacterial invaders have been lowered by disease or age. Another important reason for the change in status of the sulfonamides is that various kinds of bacteria that were once sensitive to sulfonamides are now resistant to treatment with these drugs.

Resistance to sulfonamides has resulted mainly from their administration for prophylactic purposes in subtherapeutic doses. Thus, the sulfonamides at first produce dramatic cures in cases of gonorrhea. Later, after the sulfonamides had been widely used for prophylaxis of venereal disease during World War II, most gonorrheal infections encountered in many areas were no longer susceptible to sulfonamide treatment. Apparently, the low-dose regimens employed for preventing this disease had fostered the survival of sulfonamide-resistant strains of the gonococcus. Similarly, the routine use of sulfonamides to protect army recruits from respiratory infections soon produced sulfonamide-resistant strains of staphylococci, and the continued careless use of sulfa drugs seems even to have resulted in some resistance among the once very sensitive meningococci.

ANTIMICROBIAL SPECTRUM AND CLINICAL USE

Although the clinical usefulness of the sulfonamides is now relatively limited, these drugs are still effective against a broad spectrum of pathogenic microorganisms (see *Summary*, p. 544). The sulfonamides are, in fact, still considered the best treatment for a few important infections. They are also often useful in situations that do not permit use of the antibiotic of choice—for example, in patients who are allergic to penicillin. The sulfonamides may also serve as useful adjuncts to antibiotic therapy in certain infections by difficult to control bacteria.

Urinary Tract Infections. *E. coli*, the gram-negative organism responsible for about 85 percent of acute cases, can often be controlled by treatment with sulfonamides. Infections by more resistant uropathogens of the *Proteus* and *Klebsiella-Aerobacter* groups also sometimes respond to treatment with these drugs. However, it is impossible to predict in advance whether the strain of the organism that is the cause of any particular infection will be susceptible. Thus, before beginning treatment, it is essential to have laboratory tests done to determine whether the specific bacterial strain responsible for the infection is actually sensitive to sulfonamides.

The *preferred sulfonamides* for treating acute, chronic, and recurrent urinary tract infections by susceptible bacterial strains are those that quickly reach high levels in the urine as they are being rapidly excreted by the kidneys. *Sulfisoxazole+* (Gantrisin), *sulfamethizole*, and *sulfisomidine*, for example, are said to reach such high concentrations in the urine that they become bacteri*cidal* rather than just bacteriostatic. This accounts for their effectiveness in treating *acute* bladder infections (cystitis) and urethritis. These drugs also reach antibacterial levels in the blood and tissues, including the kidneys. Thus, they are also effective for treating prostatitis and acute pyelonephritis, conditions in which the organs as well as the urinary passages are infected.

TABLE 42-1 *Sulfonamide Drugs*

Nonproprietary or Official Name	Proprietary Name	Usual Dosage Initially	Usual Dosage Maintenance	Remarks
Acetyl sulfameth-oxypyridazine	Midicel; Kynex Acetyl	250–1,000 mg orally	125–500 mg once daily as a suspension	Tasteless form of a slowly excreted drug suitable for children
Acetyl sufisoxazole N.F.	Lipo Gantrisin	270–1,010 mg orally	270–1,010 mg twice daily as a suspension	Tasteless, slowly absorbed form for use in pediatrics
Mafenide acetate	Sulfamylon	Applied topically as a cream containing 85 mg of the base, once or twice daily in a layer 1–16-inch thick		For use on second- and third-degree burn surfaces to prevent sepsis
Para-nitro-sulfathiazole	Nisulfazole	Rectally, 10 ml of a 10% solution		Used as an adjunct to other treatments of ulcerative colitis and proctitis
Phthalyl-sulfacetamide N.F.	Enterosulfon; Thalamide	200 mg/kg orally	50 mg/kg q.i.d.	Poorly absorbed sulfonamide for use to alter intestinal flora
Phthalyl-sulfapyridine	Sulfathalidine	125 mg/kg orally	30 mg/kg q.i.d. pre- and postoperatively	Poorly absorbed sulfonamide for local effect in the intestine prior to and after bowel surgery and for infections
	Azulfidine	4 g orally	1 g four times daily	Poorly absorbed sulfonamide for use in ulcerative colitis
Silver sulfadiazine		0.1% ointment for topical application		Used on burn surfaces to control sepsis by gram-negative and gram-positive pathogens
Succinyl-sulfathiazole U.S.P.	Sulfasuxidine	250 mg/kg orally	60 mg/kg q.i.d. five to seven days pre-operatively	Poorly absorbed sulfonamide for use prior to surgery of the colon and in treating bacillary dysentery
Sulfacetamide sodium U.S.P.	Sulamyd sodium	Ophthalmic solution 10–30%	Ophthalmic ointment 10%	For use locally in eye infections
Sulfacetamide N.F.	Urosulfon	4 g orally	1 g every four hours	Rapidly excreted sulfonamide
Sulfachlor-pyridazine	Sonilyn	1–4 g orally	1 g three to six times daily	Highly soluble in urine; rapidly excreted; short duration of action
Sulfadiazine U.S.P.		4 g orally	1 g every four hours	Low solubility requires forcing of fluids; available in combination with other sulfonamides
Sulfadiazine sodium U.S.P.		100 mg/kg I.V. or s.c. up to a total dose of 5 g	30–50 mg/kg I.V. or s.c. every six to eight hours	Parental form for use in serious infections

TABLE 42-1 *Sulfonamide Drugs (continued)*

Nonproprietary or Official Name	Proprietary Name	Usual Dosage Initially	Usual Dosage Maintenance	Remarks
Sulfadimethoxine N.F.	Madribon	1 g orally	0.5 g once daily	Slowly eliminated, long-acting, low dosage drug
Sulfaethidole N.F.	Sul-spansion; Sul-Spantab	1.3 g orally	1.3 g b.i.d., every 12 hours	Short-acting but presented in sustained-release form to achieve high levels in blood and urine for prolonged periods
Sulfamerazine U.S.P.		2–3 g orally	1 g t.i.d.	Used mainly in fractional doses in combination with other sulfonamides
Sulfameter	Sulla	1.5 g orally	0.5 g once daily	Slowly excreted, long-acting, low-dose sulfonamide
Sulfamethazine U.S.P.		2–3 g orally	1 g. t.i.d.	Used mainly in combination with other sulfonamides
Sulfamethizole N.F.	Thiosulfil	2–3 g orally	0.5 g four to six times daily	Rapidly excreted, highly soluble in urine
Sulfamethoxazole N.F.	Gantanol	2 g orally	1 g b.i.d. or t.i.d.	Absorbed and excreted more slowly than its congener sulfisoxazole
Sulfamethoxy-pyridazine	Kynex	1 g orally	0.5 g once daily	Slowly excreted, long-acting low-dose drug
Sulfapyridine		0.5 g orally	0.5–5 g daily in doses gradually raised	Not used as an antiinfective but as a specific for dermatitis herpetiformis
Sulfathiazole		Now used only topically in vaginitis		Ingredient of vaginal creams and tablets
Sulfisomidine	Elkosin	2 g orally	1 g four to six times daily	Rapidly absorbed and excreted; highly soluble in urine
Sulfisoxazole U.S.P.	Gantrisin	4 g orally	1 g four to six times daily	See *Drug Digest*
Sulfisoxazole diolamine U.S.P.	Gantrisin diolamine	I.V. or s.c. 100 mg/kg initially and same for 24-hour maintenance		Injected and applied topically to eye; contains equal parts of sulfadiazine, sulfamerazine, and sulfamethazine
Trisulfapyrimidines U.S.P.		3–4 g orally	1 g every six hours	

Most acute urinary tract infections respond promptly to sulfonamides, and their use can usually be discontinued after two or three weeks. However, *bacteriuria* sometimes persists in patients with stones or structural abnormalities of the genitourinary tract. In such *chronic* cases, some physicians prefer to maintain the patient on one of the slowly excreted sulfonamides. *Sulfamethoxypyridazine*+ (Kynex; Midicel), *sulfadimethoxine*, and *sulfameter*, for example, are claimed to reach adequate concentrations for control of bacteriuria when administered in a single daily maintenance dose.

The main disadvantage of these long-lasting drugs is that their effects can last for several days after an allergic or other toxic reaction occurs (see p. 529). Therefore, most authorities now claim that the convenience of these long-acting sulfonamides does not justify the danger of their use in preference to the shorter-acting drugs of this class. In any case, the usefulness of all the sulfonamides and certain other chemotherapeutic agents (see p. 529) in treating chronic and recurrent urinary tract infections is limited by the frequent development of resistant strains of uropathogenic organisms. *Sulfamethoxazole* (Gantanol) is now available in combination with another antibacterial chemical, *trimethoprim*. The two drugs given together are said to be more effective for treating *chronic* urinary tract infections than is either drug alone. The combination is recommended for preventing recurrent infections by uropathogenic strains resistant to other antiinfective agents.

Meningitis is still responsive to treatment by sulfonamides when this central nervous system infection is caused by strains that are still susceptible to these drugs. These include group A strains of meningococci and the gram-negative organism, *Hemophilus influenzae*. The parenteral forms of *sulfadiazine*+ and *sulfisoxazole*+ are preferred for initiating treatment of such infections. These drugs readily penetrate the inflamed meninges to reach therapeutic levels in the cerebrospinal fluid. Later, if the meningitis patient is conscious and is able to swallow, he is switched to oral sulfonamide treatment, which is also often supplemented by ampicillin, streptomycin, or other appropriate antibiotices.

Intestinal infections by *Shigella* species and other gram-negative bacteria are not as readily treated or prevented by sulfonamides as they once were, before the emergence of the many resistant strains now prevalent. However, cases of bacillary dysentery caused by sensitive organisms can still be treated successfully, by *sulfadiazine*, *sulfisoxazole*, or, occasionally, by the poorly absorbable sulfonamide, *succinylsulfathiazole*+ (Sulfasuxidine).

The latter drug and a similar *nonsystemic* sulfonamide, *phthalysulfathiazole* (Sulfathalidine) are mainly used *prophylactically* prior to intestinal surgery. These poorly absorbable drugs reach high antibacterial concentrations locally within the intestinal tract. This lessens the number of gram-negative organisms that could cause peritoneal cavity contamination during colonic surgery. However, the value of this procedure for preventing complications postoperatively is uncertatin. Similarly, it is doubtful that taking these drugs routinely while traveling is effective for preventing development of bacterial diarrhea, or that sulfonamides bring about sustained improvement in patients with ulcerative colitis.

Respiratory tract infections by gram-positive organisms are *not* now ordinarily treated with sulfonamides. Although the first sulfonamides were often used to cure cases of pneumococcal pneumonia, this condition is now treated almost entirely with antibiotics, except for an occasional case caused by some strain that is found to be highly sensitive to sulfonamides. Similarly, streptococcal infections are not now ordinarily treated with these drugs, which once provided curative effects that had not been previously available for such infections.

However, *sulfadiazine*+ and *sulfisoxazole*+ are still recommended for *prophylactic use* against infections by group A beta-hemolytic streptococci in patients who are allergic to penicillin. Taken daily for long periods, these drugs seem to be as safe and effective as penicillin for preventing recurrences of rheumatic fever and strep throat (pharyngitis) in such patients. Patients who develop an *actual* infection are best treated with antibiotics, as sulfonamides do not eradicate the streptococci in such cases, and thus, these drugs will not prevent such complications as rheumatic fever or glomerulonephritis.

Topically applied sulfonamide ointments and creams were once used indiscriminately in prevention and treatment of skin infections. These drugs are rarely used in this way today because it has become clear that topical application of the sulfonamides is a common cause of *allergic sensitization* and that these drugs are not very effective in the presence of pus and tissue debris on the skin and mucous membranes.

However, sulfonamides are sometimes applied topically to the eye, ear, vaginal tract and rectum, as well as to burned or traumatized skin areas. *Sulfacetamide sodium+* and *sulfisoxazole diolamine+* are commonly employed for treating conjunctivitis, lid infections (blepharitis), and corneal ulcers. Sulfanilamide is still available in an otic solution for topical treatment of external and middle ear infections. Products containing several sulfonamides in combination (including sulfathiazole) are available in cream, ointment, or tablet form for treating vaginal and cervical infections, including vaginitis caused by *Hemophilus vaginalis*.

Mafenide acetate (Sulfamylon) possesses properties that have made it particularly useful for topical application to second- and third-degree burns. This sulfonamide retains its antibacterial activity even in the presence of pus, serum, and necrotic tissue, and it is often effective for preventing infections by the usually resistant pathogen, *Pseudomonas aeruginosa*. The application of a cream containing this sulfonamide has helped to prevent the spread of sepsis and thus reduced mortality in severely burned patients.

Silver sulfadiazine has also been employed experimentally to prevent sepsis in burned skin surfaces. It is claimed effective for control of pseudomonal, staphylococcal, and other gram-negative and gram-positive organisms. However, the place of this sulfonamide in burn therapy is still unsettled.

MISCELLANEOUS USES. The antimicrobial spectrum of the sulfonamides is not limited to bacteria. These drugs are also sometimes effective for treating infections by fungal, protozoal, and other pathogens. The systemic fungal infection *nocardiosis*, for instance, is best treated by a sulfonamide administered alone or combined with the broad-spectrum antibiotics, tetracycline or chloramphenicol, or with streptomycin.

Cases of chloroquine-resistant *Plasmodium falciparum* malaria have responded to treatment with sulfonamides combined with pyrimethamine+. A similar combination is said to be the most effective treatment for toxoplasmosis, another serious sporozoite (protozoal) infection. Sulfonamides are also sometimes effective for preventing blindness from infections by the pathogenic organisms responsible for trachoma and inclusion conjunctivitis.

Sulfapyridine, a drug largely discarded since the development of safer sulfonamides, is employed empirically by dermatologists in the treatment of dermatitis herpetiformis. For reasons as obscure as the cause of the condition itself, administration of sulfapyridine often stops vesiculation, itching, and burning within a few days. Because it must be administered daily for months in smaller doses for maintenance of the improvement, some doctors have tried transferring patients to treatment with the more convenient long-acting agent, *sulfamethoxypyridazine+*.

ADVERSE EFFECTS OF SULFONAMIDES (SEE SUMMARY, PP. 545-546)

Most patients receiving sulfonamides suffer no ill effects. However, these drugs are capable of causing severe and potentially fatal reactions in some patients. Thus, patients taking sulfonamides should be closely watched for early signs of toxicity, so that the drug may be withdrawn while the reaction is still in a mild stage.

Reactions to sulfonamides occur most commonly in patients who are allergic or otherwise sensitive to these drugs. Another cause of toxicity, less common today than with the first sulfonamides, is *crystalluria*, the formation of drug crystals in the urinary tract.

Renal damage and injury to other urinary tract tissues results mainly from the formation of sulfonamide drug crystals in the kidneys, ureters, or bladder. It may be manifested by hematuria, oliguria, and, finally, anuria, azotemia, and a sometimes fatal uremia. Because some of the earlier sulfonamides and their acetyl derivatives tended especially to precipitate in acid urine, it became customary to try to alkalinize the patient's urine by having him take a teaspoonful of sodium bicarbonate or some other systemic alkalinizer with each dose of sulfa drug.

This is rarely necessary today with drugs such as sulfamethizole, sulfisomidine, and sulfisoxazole+, which are much more soluble in acid urine than the older drugs. Nevertheless, even with these drugs, the other measure that became routine—that is, maintenance of a high fluid intake—must never be neglected. Patients should be encouraged to drink enough fluids to produce at least 1,200 ml of urine daily, and, of course, the amount of urine eliminated should be measured and recorded.

The mixture of three sulfonamides called *trisulfapyrimidines* also produces a relatively low incidence of crystalluria. It contains one third of the therapeutic dose of each of three drugs—*sulfadiazine+*, *sulfamerazine*, and *sulfamethazine*. The total sulfonamide dosage is capable of controlling susceptible bacteria. Yet this mixture is only about one third as likely to cause crystalluria and kidney complications as an equally effective dose of a single sulfonamide administered alone.

Sensitization and idiosyncratic reactions to sulfonamides may take many forms. Among the most serious are those that affect the blood, skin, and liver. Some blood dyscrasias are the result of bone marrow depression. Thus, the doctor may order frequent laboratory tests to check for early signs of agranulocytosis, thrombocytopenia, or aplastic anemia. Acute hemolytic anemia is another rare complication that tends to occur in patients whose red blood cells are deficient in a protective enzyme.

Dermatological reactions of various kinds have been reported. Sometimes urticaria has occurred as part of an anaphylactoid reaction in sensitized individuals. Eruptions of various other types also are seen, often in patients who have exposed themselves to sunlight during treatment (photosensitivity). Most serious of all has been the development of severe exfoliative dermatitis and of bullous (blistery) eruptions, which have occurred both with and without episodes of drug fever.

The *Stevens-Johnson syndrome*, erythema multiforme, is a serious nonspecific reaction. It may take the form of blisters on the skin or mucous membranes. Bleeding into the center of the blister causes a characteristic bull's eye lesion. If the drug is not withdrawn, the respiratory tract and other organs may be so seriously damaged that death may result. Thus, sulfonamides must be discontinued as soon as skin eruptions are seen.

Because the long-acting sulfonamides often continue to exert their toxic effects for several days after they are withdrawn, they are considered more dangerous than the more rapidly excreted drugs. Thus, as indicated earlier, use of the short-acting sulfonamides is preferred for treating most of the infections that are responsive to chemotherapy with this class of antiinfective agents. Patients who have previously shown signs of hypersensitivity to sulfonamides should not, of course, be treated with any drugs of this class.

Sulfonamide Substitutes

As we have noted, the usefulness of therapy with sulfonamides is sometimes limited by: (1) the emergence of resistant strains of previously susceptible bacteria; and (2) the development of sensitization and subsequent allergic or idiosyncratic reactions that require withdrawal of these drugs.

The need to discontinue long-term therapy with sulfonamides may be especially serious for patients with chronic urinary tract infections that were at first well-controlled by daily doses of these drugs. Fortunately, in addition to the antibiotics discussed earlier, several *non*-sulfonamide antibacterial chemicals are also particularly effective for preventing relapses of urinary tract infections. These chemotherapeutic agents are not as useful as sulfonamides and antibiotics for checking infection within kidney tissues and thus stopping systemic symptoms such as chills and fever. However, they have effective local actions in the urinary passages.

Methenamine mandelate+ and *nitrofurantoin+* are broad-spectrum urinary antiseptics that continue to exert their antibacterial effects during long-term treatment of chronic or recurrent infections such as cystitis, pyelitis, or pyelonephritis. These drugs sometimes control infections by organisms resistant to sulfonamides and to some antibiotics. Uropathogens that are sensitive to treatment at first do not ordinarily become resistant.

This makes these antiinfective agents especially suitable for patients who are prone to suffer recurrent flare-ups of urinary tract infection. Bacteriuria tends to persist in patients with stones or various structural abnormalities, such as prostatic obstruction or ureteral constriction. In such cases, urine backing up behind the blockage tends to act as a culture medium for bacterial growth. These locally acting antiseptics help to inhibit growth and reproduction of *E. coli* and other organisms in such cases of recurrent bacteriuria.

Two similar salts of *methenamine*, the *hippurate* and *sulfosalicylate* (Table 42-2) act similarly. That is, their molecules break down into two major components: (1) an *acidifier* such as hippuric acid or sulfosalicylic acid; and (2) *methenamine*, a substance that breaks

TABLE 42-2 *Miscellaneous Nonsulfonamide Urinary Tract Antiinfectives*

Official or Nonproprietary Name	Proprietary Name	Usual Daily Dosage	Remarks
Mandelic acid		3 g q.i.d.	Restrict fluid intake to one liter
Methenamine N.F.	Urotropin; Uritone	300–600 mg q.i.d.	Often combined with sodium biphosphate for urinary acidification
Methenamine hippurate	Hiprex	1 g b.i.d. to q.i.d.	Keep urine acid with supplemental acidifiers
Methenamine mandelate U.S.P.	Mandelamine	1 g q.i.d.	See *Drug Digest*
Methenamine sulfosalicylate	Hexalet	1 g q.i.d.	Claimed not to require separate acidification ordinarily
Methylene blue U.S.P.	Urolene Blue	60–120 mg t.i.d.	Not very effective as a urinary antiseptic
Nalidixic acid N.F.	NegGram	1 g q.i.d.	Disc sensitivity testing is recommended before use
Nitrofurantoin U.S.P.	Furadantin Macrodantin	50–100 mg q.i.d.	See *Drug Digest*
Phenazo-pyridine HCl N.F.	Pyridium	200 mg t.i.d.	Weak antiseptic and topical anesthetic

down in acid urine to form the bactericidal substance *formaldehyde*.

When the patient's urine is difficult to acidify—during infection by urea-splitting pathogens that produce ammonia, for example —methenamine and its salts must be supplemented by other acidifiers such as ammonium chloride, ascorbic acid, the amino acid methionine, or sodium biphosphate. Patients should be taught to test their urinary pH regularly, using nitrazine paper to check that the pH stays at or below 5.5 If a rise above this level is not corrected by taking acidifying salts, urinary antiseptics of this type will fail to form formaldehyde and a relapse will occur.

Nalidixic acid (NegGram), another agent effective against gram-negative uropathogens, was at first considered particularly effective for treating urinary infections by *Proteus* species. However, resistant strains have emerged rapidly. Thus, this drug, which has occasionally caused some serious side effects, is now employed only after the uropathogen responsible for the infection has been proved sensitive to this drug by disc testing.

Phenazopyridine (Pyridium) is a substance with only weak antiseptic action. However, it is often combined with sulfonamides, methenamine mandelate, and other urinary antibacterials, because it is thought to have a soothing *topical anesthetic* effect upon the urinary tract mucosa when excreted in the patient's urine. This tends to relieve the burning pain and the feeling of urgency which lead to the patient's frequent desire to void; it thus helps to reduce the patient's restlessness and wakefulness. (Anticholinergic drugs also are often administered in cystitis to relieve the reflex bladder muscle spasm of cystitis, which is a cause of pain, urgency, and frequency.) Patients taking preparations containing this azo dye are warned that their urine may be colored orange or red, lest they worry about "blood" in the urine.

The Chemotherapy of Tuberculosis

Tuberculosis has long been one of the most prevalent of all infectious diseases. During the last century, pulmonary tuberculosis was the greatest killer of young men and women. Even though the death rate has dropped remarkably during this century, tuberculosis is still one of the three most common causes of death worldwide.

In this country, there has been a steady decrease in new cases of active tuberculosis. This may be because of generally good sanitation and living conditions—factors that help to reduce the spread of infection. However, the disease is still a serious problem among poor people, particularly those who live in substandard, inner-city housing, and whose resistance to bacterial invasion has been reduced by inadequate nutrition.

Recent statistical reports indicate that over 100,000 Americans still had active tuberculosis early in the 1970s. This may not seem great when compared to the 50 million people estimated to be infected elsewhere in the world. Actually, however, several hundred thousand more Americans may have active tuberculosis that has not yet been diagnosed. Thus, it is important to discover these cases before they become an active reservoir for further spread of the infection. These people and those with whom they come in contact could then be cured by treatment with the excellent chemotherapeutic agents now available for treatment and prevention of tuberculosis.

DRUG TREATMENT

The modern chemotherapy of tuberculosis is so successful in arresting or curing tuberculosis that the vast majority of patients need no longer be sent to a sanitarium or undergo lung surgery. Most new cases can now be treated as outpatients after an initial, relatively brief period of hospitalization. If the patient continues to take his oral medication at home faithfully and returns to the clinic for frequent check-ups, his condition can usually be cured even when his housing and diet are not optimal.

The available drugs can be classified broadly in terms of their effectiveness and safety as *primary*, or first-line, and *secondary*, or second-line, chemotherapeutic agents (Table 42-3). The first group has until recently consisted of *isoniazid+* (INH), *aminosalicylic acid+* (PAS), and *streptomycin+*. Two newer drugs, *rifampin+* and *ethambutol+*, can now be added to this class on the basis of reports of excellent results obtained with relatively safe doses.

COMBINED THERAPY

The antituberculosis drugs are not administered singly but are instead ordered in combinations of two or three chemotherapeutic agents. The main reason for this is that combination treatment slows the rate at which drug-resistant strains of tubercle bacilli develop. Thus, isoniazid, the single most effective drug, is ordinarily given in combination with PAS or with ethambutol. In certain situations (see below), streptomycin is used as the second or even third drug in such chemotherapeutic combinations.

RESPONSE. Patients with pulmonary tuberculosis who are treated with combinations of INH and PAS, or of INH and streptomycin, for example, frequently follow the following response pattern:

1. Temperature returns to normal; coughing is less severe; appetite improves and there is a gain in weight and a general feeling of well-being.

2. Sputum is reduced in amount, and the number of bacteria that can be cultured is steadily reduced until, finally, all cultures are negative.

3. X-ray findings indicate improvement of an objective type, as lesions regress in size, stabilize, and undergo gradual healing.

Clinical improvement of this kind does not mean that the patient is cured. Although sputum conversion occurs rapidly and the caseous (cheesy) lesions begin to clear up, the natural healing process proceeds quite slowly. Patients who become symptom-free often fail to continue taking their medication for the many months that are required for completion of repair of pulmonary damage.

Often, in such cases, the bacilli still alive in the unhealed lesions break loose and enter the bronchi and sputum. As a result, the patient is not really cured but becomes able to spread the disease again, and he himself may suffer a relapse. That is, his fever, cough, and feelings of weariness return, he begins to lose weight again, and, worst of all, tissue destruction and caseation begin again. Chest x-rays then reveal a widening of the open pulmonary cavities and the spread of lesions to new lung areas.

The nurse can help prevent such relapses by encouraging the patient to continue with his drug regimen and other aspects of his therapy. Patients who feel remarkably better may want to stop taking the drugs, especially if—as with PAS—these agents cause stomach upset or other discomfort. It must be made clear to the patient that dropping his chemotherapeutic regimen can lead to a flare-up of infection by lurking microorganisms. The patient must be made to understand that he is compromising not only his own welfare but the welfare of others whom he could infect.

Thus, the nurse's teaching should stress the value of the treatment both in hastening the patient's recovery and preventing tubercular

TABLE 42-3   Tuberculostatic Chemotherapeutic Agents

Official, Generic, or USAN Name	Synonym or Proprietary Name	Dosage	Remarks
Primary, or First-Line Drugs			
Aminosalicylic acid U.S.P.	Para-aminosalicylic acid; PAS; and others	12 g daily in four divided doses after meals	1. PAS, its salts, and related compounds are used in combination with isoniazid and streptomycin
Calcium aminosalicylate N.F.	Pasara Calcium	3 g q.i.d. with meals	2. PAS and its congeners are less potent than the other primary agents, but their use reduces the rate of development of resistant strains of tubercle bacilli
Phenyl aminosalicylate	Pheny-PAS-Tebamin	4 g t.i.d. with meals	
Potassium aminosalicylate	Paskalium; Neopasalate-K; Parasal potassium Potaba; and others	12 g daily in divided dosage	3. Potassium salts are preferred for patients in whom sodium is restricted
Sodium aminosalicylate U.S.P.	Pamisyl sodium; Para-Pas; Pasem; Pasmed, Pasna; and others	12 g daily in four divided doses	4. Calcium and phenyl derivatives are claimed to cause less gastric irritation
Ethambutol HCl	Myambutol	15 mg/kg daily in a single dose	Often substituted for aminosalicylic acid in combinations with isoniazid and streptomycin
Isoniazid U.S.P.	INH; Nydrazid; and others	*Treatment:* Orally, 5 mg/kg a day (up to 300 mg) for adults, and 10–30 mg/kg for children depending on severity of infection. *Prevention:* Adults, 300 mg a day in single or divided oral doses; children, 10 mg/kg a day (up to 300 mg total) orally in single or divided doses	The safest, most effective, inexpensive, and convenient drug for treatment and chemoprophylaxis of all forms of tuberculosis

Drug	Trade names	Dosage	Remarks
Rifampin	Rifamycin; Rifadin; Rimactane	Adult single daily dose 600 mg orally on empty stomach; children 10–20 mg/kg up to 600 mg daily	Best given in combination with isoniazid
Streptomycin U.S.P.		1 g daily I.M.	Combined with isoniazid and aminosalicylic acid or ethambutol for treating advanced active cases of pulmonary and extrapulmonary types.
Secondary or Second-Line Drugs			
Capreomycin	Capastat	1 g daily by deep I.M. injection for 60–120 days; then two or three times weekly up to 18–24 months	Always administered with one or more tuberculostatic agents to which the patient's strain of tubercle bacilli are still susceptible
Cycloserine U.S.P.	Seromycin	500 mg to 1 g daily in divided oral doses; initially only 250 mg twice daily at 12-hour intervals	Excessively high blood levels result in central nervous system toxicity
Ethionamide U.S.P.	Trecator	500 mg to 1 g daily in divided oral doses	Related to isoniazid but less effective and more toxic
Pyrazinamide U.S.P.	Aldinamide; Tebrazid	20 to 35 mg/kg daily in three or four divided oral doses, up to a total of 3 g daily	Potent tuberculostatic agent but with risk of hepatotoxicity at higher dose levels
Viomycin sulfate	Vinactane; Viocin	1 g I.M. in two equal doses 12 hours apart; repeat every three or four days	Antibiotic similar to streptomycin, kanamycin, and neomycin in bacteriostatic action and toxicity

complications, but also the importance of protecting his family—including especially susceptible children—his coworkers and others. If there is reason to believe that the patient is not taking his drugs, periodic checks of his urine should be made for the presence of the medication and its metabolites.

The nurse plays an important role in helping the patient and his family to develop more healthful ways of living. Although health instruction is useful, other very fundamental social and economic changes are required to assist these families in breaking out of the pattern of poverty, crowding, unemployment, and despair. When these issues are recognized and help is provided toward their resolution, the patient and his family are more likely to attend to and profit from health teaching.

INDIVIDUAL DRUGS

Detailed data concerning the drugs of primary importance for treating tuberculosis appear in each of the *Drug Digests* concerning these agents. The toxic effects that limit the long-term usefulness of all the *second-line* tuberculostatic drugs are summarized on p. 533. Thus, we shall offer here only a few additional points of practical significance concerning the clinical use of the various individual drugs.

Isoniazid+ is the basic drug with which all other major agents are combined in beginning treatment of any new case of active tuberculosis. It is also employed to prevent subclinical and healed cases from flaring up. This drug is effective when taken orally in small daily doses that do not usually cause disturbing side effects. Its low cost and ease of administration are important factors in keeping patients on the drug.

However, despite these advantages and its generally low toxicity, hepatitis has been reported in a small percentage of patients hypersensitive to isoniazid. Thus, it is now recommended that all people taking isoniazid for preventive purposes be carefully tested for the presence of developing liver disease. If signs of liver dysfunction are seen, the doctor must then decide whether the risk of continuing with isoniazid chemoprophylaxis outweighs the danger of the patient's developing active tuberculosis.

Chemoprophylaxis is particularly desirable for children under six years old who have been exposed to tuberculosis. The risk of tuberculous meningitis or of generalized (miliary) infection is greatest in the very young. Daily administration of isoniazid can now prevent these once nearly 100 percent fatal extrapulmonary complications of tuberculosis infection. Palatable liquid preparations are available but parents should be warned to store this drug in a safe place out of reach of the family's children. Accidental overdosage has caused acute poisoning marked by coma and convulsions.

Protective daily doses of isoniazid are also recommended for all other cases of infection that are identified, as well as for the members of their households. Most of those who take a single daily dose of this drug for one year will avoid the danger of having a reactivation of infection later in life. The drug is often ordered not only for people whose skin test has recently changed from negative to positive (*recent converters*), but also for those who have had an inactive untreated infection for many years. (Some middle-aged or elderly people whose primary infection first occurred before modern chemotherapy was available may suffer sudden reactivation of the disease.)

The exact reason for reactivation of most such cases of *post*-primary tuberculosis is not known. However, certain clinical situations are known to reduce people's resistance to tuberculosis infection. Thus, isoniazid chemoprophylaxis is now often employed in positive reactor patients who are receiving prolonged treatment with corticosteroid drugs, or in those who are being treated for leukemia or Hodgkin's disease. Patients with poorly controlled diabetes, and children with measles or whooping cough who are tuberculin reactors, should also take a daily dose of isoniazid.

Aminosalicylic acid+ (PAS) is not nearly as active against tubercle bacilli as are the other first-line drugs. Yet, it is still often combined with isoniazid or streptomycin because of its ability to help prevent resistance to these other major drugs. Patients who complain of heartburn, nausea, and other gastrointestinal discomforts caused by this drug should be encouraged to continue taking the large number of tablets needed daily. Successful treatment with the more potent tuberculostatic drug often depends upon PAS supplementation.

Ethambutol+ (Myambutol) is now often employed as a substitute for PAS. Although this supplement to isoniazid and streptomycin also causes some gastrointestinal upset and other side effects, most patients seem to find it more acceptable than PAS. A potentially serious drawback is the possible development of optic neuritis in patients taking high doses. However, visual defects seldom occur with ordinary doses, and these can be readily detected in early stages by frequent ophthalmological examinations.

Streptomycin is now often reserved for use in cases marked by large cavities in the lungs or as part of a triple-drug regimen for *extrapulmonary* tuberculosis. In such advanced cases of cavitary tuberculosis and in tuberculous meningitis and miliary, or disseminated, disease this antibiotic is always combined with isoniazid and often also with PAS or ethambutol. Otherwise, resistance to streptomycin develops very rapidly. Resistance also often results when streptomycin is administered intermittently. Thus, when it is used together with isoniazid, daily injections of streptomycin are now recommended as long as the patient's sputum stays positive.

Rifampin+ has been recently found as effective in combination with isoniazid as the three-drug combinations containing streptomycin. This two-drug combination, which now comes packaged together, is claimed to be ideal for both hospital and outpatient use, because neither drug needs to be injected, and both cause fewer side effects than the other major tuberculostatic agents. Since the success of tuberculosis chemotherapy depends upon the patient's willingness to take his medication regularly, such *rifampin-isoniazid combinations* may well replace earlier regimens—at least for treating outpatients with noncavitary disease.

Some authorities prefer to reserve rifampin for hospital use at present. This is in part due to its relatively high cost, but also because resistance may develop if its use becomes too widespread. They suggest that this relatively new antibiotic is best employed for treating patients who have developed resistance to one or more of the other major drugs. It is best combined with other drugs to which the patient's bacilli are still susceptible, including secondary drugs.

Second-line, or *minor, tuberculostatic drugs* are added to the patient's regimen mainly when his infection fails to respond to steady treatment with combinations of the primary, or major, agents. The main drawback of all the secondary drugs is their relatively small safety margin. All are capable of causing serious toxicity, and so patients must be carefully watched for signs of damage to such organs as the liver, kidneys, peripheral nerves, and the central nervous system.

Antibiotic substitutes for streptomycin and the other first-line drugs most commonly employed are *viomycin, cycloserine,* and *capreomycin,* a relatively new agent. Other antituberculosis antibiotics, such as kanamycin, neomycin, and the tetracyclines are now rarely used for this purpose. Instead, doctors sometimes turn to certain *synthetic chemicals* not obtained from natural microbial sources. *Pyrazinamide* and *ethionamide* are examples of secondary drugs of this kind.

Viomycin is an antibiotic similar to streptomycin and kanamycin in its antibacterial spectrum. It is sometimes effective in treating severe infections by streptomycin-resistant tubercle bacilli when administered in combination with PAS, isoniazid, or other chemotherapeutic agents. Its toxic effects are similar to those of streptomycin but occur more frequently. Patients must be watched for signs of kidney damage, hearing loss, and allergy to this drug.

Cycloserine (Seromycin) is an antibiotic that is effective against a broad spectrum of bacteria. However, it is used clinically only in difficult cases of tuberculosis and in some stubborn urinary tract infections by *E. coli* and the *Aerobacter* group that do not respond to sulfonamides and other safer antiinfective agents. The main limitation of this drug is its tendency to cause toxic central nervous system effects when administered in adequate doses for treating tuberculosis.

Patients receiving cycloserine must be observed for early signs of central toxicity including headache, drowsiness, and confusion. Tremors may precede convulsive seizures, and a period of increasing anxiety and disorientation may be followed by a psychotic episode of mental depression. The drug is contraindicated in tubercular patients who also have epilepsy or a history of psychosis or chronic alcoholism.

Capreomycin (Capastat) must be administered by deep intramuscular injection to minimize pain and to prevent sterile abscess development. Like other polypeptide-type antibiotics it is potentially toxic to the kidneys and the eighth cranial nerve. Thus, tests of hearing, balance, and renal function are made before and during treatment. Despite these drawbacks, this new tuberculostatic drug is valuable in cases no longer controllable by first-line drugs to which the tubercle bacilli have developed resistance.

Pyrazinamide (Aldinamide) is a highly active synthetic chemotherapeutic agent, but its clinical utility in tuberculosis treatment is limited by its potential hepatotoxicity. It is used only in a hospital setting in which the patient can be carefully observed. This drug has been recommended for a short-term use in advanced cases prior to pulmonary surgery. It is thought to help prevent the spread of infection by bacilli no longer sensitive to any of the first-line drugs, especially when combined with ethionamide.

Ethionamide (Trecator) is claimed to be less toxic than most of the other second-line drugs when administered orally in combination with other tuberculostatic agents. However, it is capable of causing a wide variety of adverse effects, including liver damage. More common side effects include gastrointestinal disturbances, drowsiness, dizziness, evidence of endocrine imbalance, and allergic skin eruptions.

The Chemotherapy of Leprosy

Leprosy is believed to be caused by an acid-fast bacillus, *Mycobacterium leprae*, which is related to the organism responsible for tuberculosis infections. Because it was isolated by Dr. Hansen from the lesions of patients during an outbreak in Norway in the last century, the condition is often called Hansen's disease. Although the organism is found in infected humans in any climate, the disease is today seen mainly in the warmer parts of the world. In the United States, it is endemic mainly in Hawaii and in the states bordering the Gulf of Mexico.

Drug treatment of leprosy with chemotherapeutic agents that have bacteriostatic effects upon the pathogenic organism can now cure all forms of this disfiguring disease. Some signs and symptoms improve soon after treatment is begun; other manifestations may take several years to improve. Drug reactions are frequent during long-term treatment.

The sulfones, a class of drugs chemically related to the sulfonamides, are the most effective chemotherapeutic agents for control of leprosy. *Dapsone*+ (Avlosulfon; DDS), one of the first drugs of this class to prove effective, is still considered the most useful leprostatic drug. Most of its derivatives (Table 42-4) break down this chemical in the body, and none has been shown to be superior to the parent compound. Taken by mouth in small doses, these drugs stop any further advance of the leprous lesions that can destroy the nose, cause blindness, damage nerves, and turn hands into claws. Healing of skin and nasal mucous membrane lesions is usually complete in two or three years, if the condition is caught early. Maintenance therapy to prevent relapse is probably desirable in most cases, even after the lesions are bacteriologically negative.

Adverse reactions can often be avoided by beginning treatment with a small dose of a

TABLE 42-4 *Leprostatic Chemotherapeutic Agents**

Official, Generic, or USAN Name	Synonym or Proprietary Name	Dosage
Acetosulfone sodium	Promacetin	500 mg daily initial oral dose; increase every two weeks by 0.5–1.5 g up to total daily doses of 3 to 4 g
Dapsone U.S.P.	Avosulfon	10–25 mg initial oral doses are increased gradually up to 400 mg several times weekly
Glucosulfone sodium	Promin	Orally or I.V. 1 g daily, increasing gradually to 5 g
Sulfetrone sodium	Cimedone	1.5 to 6 g daily in three divided oral doses
Sulfoxone sodium U.S.P.	Diasone	330 mg orally twice weekly, increasing gradually to 990 mg twice weekly
Thiazolesulfone	Promizole	1.5 to 6 g daily in three divided oral doses

* The listed drugs are all in the *sulfone* chemical class. *Non*sulfone leprostatic agents of various chemical classes include: long-acting sulfonamide drugs (sulfadimethoxine); thiosemicarbazones (amithiozone); dibenzopyrazines (clofazimine); thioureas (thiambutosine); and others, including thalidomide.

sufone and then gradually increasing the weekly drug intake. Often, the only side effects of carefully controlled drug administration schedules are some gastrointestinal upset or allergic skin rashes. On the other hand, high doses commonly cause hemolysis of red blood cells, particularly in people who lack a protective enzyme in their red blood cells.

The sulfones sometimes set off a severe form of the disease—so-called lepra reactions. When the disease worsens suddenly in this way, the drug is discontinued, and the patient receives high doses of a corticosteroid drug for a few days. Once the inflammatory skin reactions and systemic symptoms have been brought under control, the sulfones may be begun again in very small doses and dosage even more cautiously than before.

Nonsulfone drugs of various classes are also effective against the bacteria that cause leprosy. Those that are also effective clinically are usually reserved for treatment of the relatively few cases of infection that are caused by organisms resistant to the sulfones. One such agent, *clofazimine*, has sometimes been effective in such cases. A drawback is its tendency to cause red and black pigmentation of the skin of light-colored patients. *Thalidomide*, the drug responsible for deforming the fetuses of women who took it for its sedative effects, has recently been reported to be remarkably effective in bringing about rapid improvement of leprosy (Chapters 1 and 3).

Antiviral Chemotherapy

Virus diseases are difficult to treat with drugs. Only two antiviral agents are available in this country at present for the prevention and treatment of specific virus infections. Two other drugs used for treating leukemia and cancer have also been shown to exert antiviral effects. Several other kinds of chemicals offer promise of opening new pathways to successful control of viruses.

Influenza, the *common cold*, and other *respiratory virus infections* are difficult to control by immunization. This is because these viruses mutate so frequently that the vaccines that are developed against them quickly become ineffective. Thus, for example, the influenza vaccine developed for protecting against the Asian A_2 form of influenza in 1957 was not very useful against the Hong Kong strain of virus prevalent in 1968. The London flu strain of 1972-73 was a variant which was not well controlled by the vaccines then available. One approach to influenza prevention has been biological, and another has involved the development of an antiviral chemical.

A vaccine recently developed by "forcing" the evolution of the influenza virus in the laboratory is aimed at protecting against strains of the influenza virus that have not yet even evolved in nature. Scientists hope that this new vaccine will provide protection against future flu viruses, including the kinds that are expected to cause an influenza epidemic in 1978. However, even if the vaccine prepared by forcing the formation of virus mutations in the laboratory proves effective, it will probably protect only about 75 percent of those who are vaccinated.

Amantadine (Symmetrel) is a drug that has proved effective for preventing influenza caused by certain strains of the A_2 type virus. It is not very useful for treating the illness after symptoms appear. However, if taken for ten days or more during an epidemic year, amantadine may have prophylactic value for people who are exposed to this flu virus strain —for example, when one member of a family comes down with the disease and others are in daily contact with him.

Ill effects from prophylactic doses of this drug that have been occasionally reported include difficulty in concentrating, ataxia, and complaints of a lightheaded, giddy, or drunken feeling. Patients whose vision becomes blurred or whose speech is slurred while taking this drug are warned against driving or working with dangerous machinery. More serious reactions reported in experimental subjects taking somewhat higher doses include insomnia, nervousness, depression, feelings of depersonalization, hallucinations, and convulsions.

Reactions of these kinds are most likely to occur in patients with a history of epilepsy or with cerebral arteriosclerosis. Since protection against influenza is particularly important for elderly patients, some of whom may have organic brain disease, the possibility of inducing psychotic reactions may limit the usefulness of amantadine for this patient population. When this drug is administered to patients with Parkinson's disease, the dosage of anticholinergic drugs or of levodopa may have to be reduced in order to avoid C.N.S. toxicity (see also Chapter 11).

Idoxuridine+ (Dendrid; Herplex; Stoxil) is an antiviral chemotherapeutic agent that is applied topically for treating eye infections caused by the herpes simplex virus. It seems most effective in acute cases of keratitis in which invasion of the cornea by viral particles is still only superficial. Recent reports indicate that strains of virus resistant to idoxuridine develop readily and that this may reduce the drug's usefulness for treating herpes simplex keratitis.

Methisozone (Marboran) is a synthetic antiviral compound effective for protecting against smallpox. *Cytarabine* (Cytosar; see Chapter 48), a drug available for treating leukemia, is also effective for control of herpes zoster in patients with low resistance to spread of this virus infection. *Floxuridine* (FUDR; see Chapter 48), an anticancer drug that interferes with the formation of deoxyribonucleic acid (DNA) and ribonucleic acid (RNA), has been used experimentally to inhibit the synthesis of these same substances in viruses.

All the above antiviral agents are potentially quite toxic, because drugs that damage viruses within invaded human cells are also likely to interfere with the metabolism of the cells. Because the body's cells produce a natural antiviral protein termed *interferon*, scientists have been searching for substances capable of stimulating cells to produce this safe, natural defender against virus invaders. Several chemicals, including one called *statolon*, have been discovered that speed up the rate of cellular formation of interferon. However, none are available at present for therapeutic use against virus infections.

Biologicals for Producing Immunity

Substances obtained from biological sources are often employed to protect people against infectious diseases. These immunizing biologicals are *not* drugs, and so we can not discuss them in detail in this pharmacology textbook. Yet the value of these biological preparations in preventing infections or for modifying the course of some diseases is so great that we shall briefly review the concepts and terms connected with their use and then list the most common *vaccines*, *toxoids*, *antitoxins*, and other substances available for *immunoprophylaxis* and *treatment*.

Immunology has made remarkable contributions to public health. Epidemic and endemic diseases that have caused millions of deaths during recorded history can now be almost completely controlled by immunization. In this country, where more than 200 million people are protected against smallpox and other diseases, doctors are hopeful that immunization will soon help to eliminate certain infections completely.

Immunoprophylaxis has been one of the most important of the medical advances that have lengthened life expectancy from about 35 to 70 years during the last hundred years. Children have been the chief beneficiaries, for infectious diseases killed two out of five born in this country late in the last century. Today, routine immunizations in infancy against smallpox, diphtheria, tetanus, and whooping cough have caused deaths from these diseases to drop to the vanishing point.

ACTIVE AND PASSIVE IMMUNITY

Immunity is a state of relative resistance to disease that develops after exposure to the specific agent responsible for an infection. Some individuals or species are born with an innate ability to resist certain diseases. Most people, however, are not congenitally immune to the common infectious diseases. Instead, they *acquire* immunity in the process of fighting off the foreign microbial invaders.

Active immunity of this kind is brought about by the body's response to proteins and polysaccharides in the invading viruses and bacteria. These chemicals foreign to the individual's tissues act as an *antigen*. That is, they stimulate the gradual formation of immune *antibodies* by the reticuloendothelial and lymphoid tissues. These specifically structured protective protein molecules then circulate in the serum, particularly in its gamma globulin fraction. Then, whenever the same foreign substance enters the body in the future, the antibodies of the immune serum combine with the antigen and neutralize it.

Artificial active immunity can be induced without a person's having to suffer an actual clinical infection. The person is purposely exposed to biological products that have the ability to stimulate the production of antibodies against pathogenic viruses, rickettsia, and bacteria (or their toxins). These immunizing agents do not cause the natural disease because the microorganisms have been killed or weakened by special production techniques.

Artificial immunity is not as long-lasting as natural active immunity. This is because inoculation with killed or attenuated microbes does not stimulate the primary production of as great a quantity of antibodies. However, the level of antibodies can be kept high enough to protect the person by administering so-called "booster" doses of the immunizing biologic product at periodic intervals.

Passive immunity is the transfer of immune serum from an animal or a human who has been actively immunized to a person who has not been previously exposed to the pathogen and thus must borrow antibodies in order to combat or ward off an infection caused by that organism. These borrowed antibodies begin immediately to attack the invaders or to neutralize their toxins exactly as would antibodies made by the patient's own tissues, if there had been time enough for them to have been formed in adequate amounts.

Antibodies against infectious microbes and bacterial toxins fight infection equally well, whether they are acquired as the result of an actual infection (active immunity), or by injection in the form of serum globulins obtained from an outside source (passive immunity). The main difference is that in a state of active immunity the antibodies remain in the body much longer and are reinforced by still larger numbers after later exposure to the same antigen. Borrowed antibodies, on the other hand, are destroyed and readily removed from the body within a few weeks (see below).

Actively or passively acquired antibodies act in the same ways. They may make bacteria clump together (agglutinate), precipitate, or break up before they can gain a foothold in the body and begin to grow and multiply. Some antibodies (antitoxins) keep the poisons produced by tetanus or diphtheria bacilli from becoming fixed to body tissues, thus forestalling the worst effects of infections by these pathogens.

BIOLOGICAL PRODUCTS FOR ACTIVE IMMUNIZATION

Antigenic products employed for conferring active immunity artificially are mainly of two types. *Vaccines* are made from the microorganisms—viruses, bacteria, and rickettsia—responsible for various diseases. *Toxoids* are made from the toxins, or poisons, secreted by certain bacteria. It is the toxins that are responsible for the most devastating effects of diseases caused by these organisms, such as diphtheria and tetanus.

VACCINES. These may contain either killed or live organisms. In both types, the activity of antigenic protein is preserved, even though the bacteria may be dead, or the live virus has been made very weak in pathogenic potency by special treatments. Depending upon how many different types of antigens they contain, vaccines are called *monovalent*, *bivalent*, or *polyvalent*. Poliomyelitis vaccine, for example, is a polyvalent vaccine, as it contains three types of weakened live strains of poliovirus.

Bacterial vaccines for cholera, pertussis, plague, and typhoid all contain killed organisms. The vaccine for tuberculosis, BCG vaccine, contains a live but weakened strain of tubercle bacilli. *Rickettsial vaccines*—for typhus, for example—are prepared by culturing the organism in the living cells of embryonated eggs. This can make them dangerous when administered to people who are allergic to eggs.

Virus vaccines are also often made by growing the virus particles in chick or duck embryos, and so the same risk is present for sensitive individuals. Other living cells sometimes employed as culture media include monkey kidney and rabbit kidney tissue. Recently, a poliomyelitis vaccine has been marketed that is made from polio virus grown in cultures of human cells. It is said to be safer because it is free of animal protein. However, *all* tissue cultures are treated with antibiotics to prevent contamination by bacteria. Thus, they may cause allergic reactions in patients sensitive to penicillin or other of the antibiotics employed.

Reactions to vaccines are really not very common, and authorities agree that the risk of a reaction is much smaller, in most cases, than the risk of *not* being immunized against a disease for which protection is available. This is particularly true of virus vaccines since, as we have seen, very few antiviral chemotherapeutic agents are available. Thus, although there is more illness in this country from smallpox vaccination than from the disease itself, the U.S. Public Health Service advocates its continued use.

TOXOIDS. These are vaccines made by modifying the toxins secreted by certain bacteria so that they are no longer poisonous but are still able to stimulate production of antibodies by the tissues of the inoculated individual. That is, careful treatment with heat or chemicals such as formaldehyde destroys their poisonous qualities without affecting their capacity to act as antigens that confer long-lasting immunity.

The two most important products of this type employed for inducing artificial active immunity are *tetanus toxoid* and *diphtheria toxoid*. The fluid toxoids are made more effective and less likely to cause local reactions by special methods of preparation that involve precipitation or adsorption with aluminum compounds. This procedure also helps to slow the systemic absorption of the two toxoids from the intramuscular or subcutaneous injection sites. As a result, the antigens are said to stimulate longer-lasting plasma levels of protective antibodies against diphtheria and tetanus.

BIOLOGICAL PRODUCTS FOR PASSIVE IMMUNIZATION

Products containing preformed antibodies manufactured by the bodies of animals or people include *antitoxins, antiserums*, and immune *serum globulins*. Antitoxins and antiserums are usually made by injecting animals —horses, most commonly—with bacteria, bacterial toxins, or toxoids, or with virus vaccine particles. The hyperimmunized horse reacts to the antigen by producing high plasma levels of antibodies. These are then removed by special purification procedures for use in treating patients who have been exposed to, or are actually suffering from, such diseases as tetanus, diphtheria, or botulism.

The chief advantage of these products is that their antibodies begin to react with the bacterial toxin or other antigen as soon as they are injected. This may help a person who has not previously been actively immunized to recover from his infection. However, the passive immunity conferred by these products lasts for only a few weeks, as the antibodies are broken down and eliminated.

The animal protein in these antiserums can cause serious allergic reactions. These may be of the anaphylactoid type, which can occur immediately upon injection of the antitoxins, and so forth, in an individual previously sensitized by exposure to horse serum. Reactions of the serum sickness type may be delayed for several days after injection. Such delayed reactions are marked by fever, joint pains, hives, and swollen glands.

Patients who require passive immunization must be closely questioned about possible previous exposures to horse serum or past allergic reactions. To avoid setting off serious serum reactions, the doctor may decide to withhold the immune serum from patients with a history of earlier allergy episodes, particularly when they show a strong positive reaction to skin or ophthalmic tests for sensitivity to horse serum. If the seriousness of the patient's infection warrants the risk of treatment with antisera, the materials required for managing an acute allergic reaction must be kept readily available. These include epinephrine, oxygen, corticosteroids, and antihistamines, and the equipment for administering these agents.

Human blood serum also serves as a source of immune globulins containing antibodies against various bacterial and viral infections. Such *homologous sera* have the advantage of being free of the foreign allergenic proteins that are responsible for horse serum reactions. *Immune serum globulin*, a product obtained from the pooled plasma of human donors, contains antibodies against various common infectious diseases including measles, German measles, poliomyelitis, and infectious hepatitis.

The administration of *human* immune serum globulins to a person exposed to infection is a safe and effective emergency procedure. However, such passive immunization is never a substitute for active immunoprophylaxis when a vaccine is available for use *before* a person is ever exposed to the disease. Thus, despite the value of tetanus immune globulin, everyone should be urged to seek prior active immunity by tetanus toxoid inoculations.

Similarly, although a pregnant woman who has been exposed to German measles may profit from treatment with immune serum globulin, it is preferable to immunize young children or adolescent girls with the rubella vaccine that is now available for conferring active immunity. This procedure is preferred because the fetus of a pregnant woman who is infected with wild rubella virus can suffer congenital malformations and sensory defects before immune globulin can be administered. In addition, by the active immunization of all young children, it may be possible to wipe out the reservoir of rubella virus infection and so completely eliminate German measles in the entire population.

The immunologic products available for producing active or passive immunity in various infectious diseases are listed in Table 42-5.

TABLE 42-5 *Immunologic Agents*

Disease	Organism	Products Employed for Prevention or Treatment	Dosage and Administration
Botulism	*Clostridium botulinum*	Botulism antitoxin U.S.P. (passive immunizing agent)	I.M. or I.V. Prophylactic: 2,500 u. Therapeutic: 10,000 to 50,000 u.
Cholera	*Vibrio comma*	Cholera vaccine U.S.P. (active immunizing agent)	S.C. or I.M. 0.5 ml; then 1 ml at least seven days later
			Repeat 0.5-ml dose every six months if necessary
Diphtheria	*Corynebacterium diphtheriae*	Diphtheria antitoxin U.S.P. (passive immunizing agent)	I.M. or I.V. Prophylactic: 1,000 to 10,000 u. Therapeutic: 10,000 to 80,000 u.
		Diphtheria toxoid U.S.P. (active immunizing agent)	S.C. injections of 0.5 to 1 ml, at least four weeks apart
		Adsorbed diphtheria toxoid U.S.P. (active immunizing agent)	S.C. or I.M., two injections of 0.5 to 1 ml at least four weeks apart; a third, reinforcing dose six to 12 months later
		Diagnostic diphtheria toxin (for Schick test)	Intracutaneous 0.1 ml
German Measles	Various strains of rubella virus	Rubella virus vaccine, live	S.C. injection into outer aspect of upper arm, of the total volume of the reconstituted vaccine
Influenza	Various strains of influenza virus	Influenza virus vaccine U.S.P. (active immunizing agent)	S.C. two injections of 1 ml, at least two months apart
Measles	Various strains of rubeola virus	Measles virus vaccine, live, attenuated (Edmonston B strain)	S.C. 0.5 ml for active immunization
		Measles virus vaccine, live, attenuated (Schwarz strain)	S.C. 0.5 ml for active immunization
		Measles virus, inactivated	I.M., 0.5 or 1 ml in three doses at monthly intervals for active immunization
		Measles immune globulin U.S.P. (passive immunizing agent)	Prophylactic: I.M., 0.22 ml per kg of body weight. Modification of measles: 0.022 to 0.045 ml per kg
		Immune serum globulin U.S.P. (passive immunizing agent)	Prophylactic: I.M. 0.22 ml per kg for measles (0.02 ml per kg for infectious hepatitis). Modification of measles: 0.045 ml per kg
Mumps	Various strains of epidemic parotitis virus	Mumps virus vaccine, live, attenuated (active immunizing agent)	S.C. a single dose of not less than 5,000 TCID$_{50}$ for active prophylaxis
		Mumps vaccine, inactivated virus for active prophylaxis (active immunizing agent)	S.C. or I.M. two injections of 1 ml each administered at intervals of one to four weeks
		Mumps immune globulin human (passive immunizing agent)	1.5 ml to 4.5 ml, depending on body weight

TABLE 42-5 Immunologic Agents (continued)

Disease	Organism	Products Employed for Prevention or Treatment	Dosage and Administration
Pertussis	Bordetella pertussis	Pertussis vaccine U.S.P. (active immunizing agent) Pertussis immune globulin U.S.P. (passive immunizing agent)	S.C. three injections, usually of 0.5 ml at least four weeks apart Prophylactic: one or two I.M., injections at one-week intervals in amounts recommended by manufacturer. Therapeutic: two injections at one-day intervals
Plague	Pasteurella pestis	Plague vaccine U.S.P. (active immunizing agent)	S.C. two injections of 0.5 to 1 ml at least seven days apart
Poliomyelitis	Various strains of polio virus	Poliomyelitis vaccine U.S.P. (Salk vaccine) (active immunizing agent) Live oral poliovirus vaccine, monovalent U.S.P. (active immunizing agent) Live oral poliovirus vaccine, trivalent U.S.P. (active immunizing agent)	S.C. two injections of 1 ml, four to six weeks apart, then 1 ml at least seven months later. Each of the monovalent vaccines is given separately at intervals of six to eight weeks Two drops to 2 ml, depending upon the concentration used are administered for primary immunization in three doses at intervals of eight weeks
Rabies	Various strains of rabies virus	Rabies vaccine U.S.P. (active immunizing agent) Antirabies serum (passive immunizing agent)	S.C. 2 ml of a 5% suspension or its equivalent daily for 14 to 21 days for postexposure immunoprophylaxis I.M. 20 u. per lb of body weight
Smallpox	Variola virus	Smallpox vaccine U.S.P. (active immunizing agent)	Percutaneous injection (into the skin) of the contents of one capillary tube by the multiple puncture method

Tetanus	*Clostridium tetani*	Tetanus toxoid U.S.P. (active immunizing agent)	S.C. three injections of 0.5 ml at least four weeks apart
		Adsorbed tetanus toxoid U.S.P. (active immunizing agent)	I.M. or S.C. two injections of 0.5 ml at least four weeks apart
		Tetanus antitoxin U.S.P. (passive immunizing agent)	I.M. or S.C. Prophylactic: 1,500 to 10,000 u. Therapeutic: 10,000 to 100,000 u.
		Tetanus immune globulin U.S.P. (passive immunizing agent)	I.M. Prophylactic: 250 u. Therapeutic: 1,500 u. (or more)
Tuberculosis	*Mycobacterium tuberculosis*	BCG vaccine U.S.P. (active immunizing agent)	Intradermal, 0.1 ml Percutaneous, one drop on surface of skin, administered by multiple puncture method
		Old tuberculin U.S.P. (diagnostic aid)	Intracutaneous 0.00001 to 0.001 ml
		Purified protein derivative of tuberculin U.S.P. (diagnostic aid)	Intracutaneous, 0.02 to 5 μ
Typhoid	*Salmonella typhosa*	Typhoid vaccine U.S.P. (active immunizing agent)	S.C., three injections of 0.5 ml at least seven days apart
		Typhoid and paratyphoid vaccine U.S.P. (active immunizing agent)	S.C. three injections of 0.5 ml at least seven days apart
Typhus	*Rickettsia prowazekii*	Typhus vaccine U.S.P.	S.C., two injections of 1 ml at least seven days apart
Yellow fever	Virus	Yellow fever vaccine U.S.P. (active immunizing agent)	S.C. 0.5 ml

SUMMARY of Current Status of Sulfonamides in the Treatment of Infections

Microbial Susceptibility*

Therapeutic Effectiveness

Gram-positive cocci
Streptococcus pyogenes, group A beta-hemolytic type

No longer used for treating an active infection by this organism, but may be used for prophylaxis against pharyngitis and recurrences of rheumatic fever in patients allergic to penicillin

Staphylococcus aureus

Occasionally effective in urinary tract infections by susceptible strains of these organisms

Enterococcus
Pneumococcus

May occasionally be effective in cases of pneumonia or meningitis by susceptible strains

Gram-negative cocci
Meningococcus

I.V. administration of sulfadiazine sodium or of sulfisoxazole diolamine may be very effective in meningitis infections by susceptible strains. An oral sulfonamide may also be administered to the patient's contacts, particularly if a sensitive group A strain is the known cause of infection

Gram-positive bacilli
Bacillus anthracis

Anthrax infections may occasionally respond to sulfonamides, but various antibiotics are considered superior

Listeria monocytogenes and other gram-positive rods, including clostridia
Gram-negative bacilli
E. coli

Penicillin and various other antibiotics are superior to the sulfonamides

Acute urinary tract infections by most strains of this organism are still very susceptible to treatment with sulfonamides. The drugs are also effective in chronic bacteriuria for suppressing this pathogen

Proteus mirabilis

May be effective in urinary tract infections by this and other *Proteus* species

Klebsiella and *Enterobacter* (*Aerobacter*) species

Only occasionally effective in urinary tract infections by strains shown to be susceptible by laboratory studies

Hemophilus influenzae

Sometimes effective for acute and chronic otitis media and respiratory infections by this organism when combined with streptomycin or tetracyclines for patients who are allergic to ampicillin

Hemophilus ducreyi

Chancroid, a venereal disease, is quite responsive to treatment with sulfonamides administered alone or with tetracyclines or streptomycin

Pasteurella pestis

Sulfonamides alone or preferably combined with streptomycin are effective for treating bubonic plague

Shigella

Some strains of this pathogen are still sensitive to sulfonamides, but these drugs, preferably sulfadiazine or sulfisoxazole, are used for treating bacillary dysentery only when the organism is proved to be sensitive to them and not to antibiotics

Filtrable Agents, including Large Viruses
Lymphogranuloma venereum agent

Sulfonamides are effective in this venereal disease when administered alone or combined with a tetracycline or chloramphenicol

S U M M A R Y of Current Status of Sulfonamides in the Treatment of Infections *(continued)*

Microbial Susceptibility*	Therapeutic Effectiveness
Chlamydia trachomatis (trachoma agent)	Effective in this eye disease when taken orally and applied topically together with tetracyclines or chloramphenicol
Inclusion conjunctivitis agent (blenorrhea)	Topical application of ophthalmic preparations of sulfacetamide sodium or of sulfisoxazole diolamine may be effective in this eye disease
Fungi *Nocardia asteroides*	Effective against lung and brain lesions of this disseminated fungal infection, particularly when combined with tetracyclines, chloramphenicol, or cycloserine
Actinomyces	Possibly effective when combined with penicillin in some cases of this systemic fungal infection
Blastomyces brasiliensis	Occasionally effective when amphotericin B can not be employed in cases of South American blastomycosis
Protozoa Toxoplasmagondii	An effective adjunct to pyrimethamine in treating toxoplasmosis
Plasmodium falciparum	An effective adjunct to quinine and other antimalarial drugs in chloroquine-resistant cases of malaria

* Many strains of previously susceptible species are now resistant to sulfonamides. Thus, these drugs are now best used for treating certain serious infections only after the causative organism has been proved sensitive to sulfonamides in laboratory tests.

S U M M A R Y of Sulfonamide Toxicity

Urinary Tract Disorders

Crystalluria in the kidneys and other genitourinary tract organs may lead to pain, obstruction, and tubular necrosis, with hematuria, oliguria, anuria, azotemia, and uremia.

Sensitization-type Reactions

Stevens-Johnson syndrome (erythema multiforme exudativum), a condition marked by crops of blisters on the skin and mucous membranes of the mouth, nose, and other parts of the respiratory tract, has occurred during administration of both long- and short-acting sulfonamides.

Other skin reactions are marked by eruptions of the urticarial, morbilliform, or scarlatiniform types. Severe exfoliative dermatitis, petechiae, pupura, and photosensitivity sometimes occur. Sulfonamide therapy should be discontinued upon development of skin rashes and pruritus.

Drug fever sometimes develops during the second week of treatment, along with headache, chills, and general malaise. Discontinuation of sulfonamide therapy results in return to normal temperature. Joint pains, bronchospasm, conjunctivitis, and other indications of serum sickness reaction may occur.

In addition to maintaining adequate fluid intake, the doctor may order renal function tests, especially if these drugs must be administered to patients whose renal function is already impaired.

Blood and Bone Marrow Disorders

Acute hemolytic anemia, thrombocytopenia, agranulocytosis, and aplastic anemia have occurred. Periodic blood tests are desirable, with discontinuance of sulfonamide therapy if changes in hematopoietic function or peripheral blood components are noted.

Gastrointestinal Side Effects and Toxicity

Anorexia, nausea, vomiting, abdominal pain, diarrhea, jaundice, liver enlargement; rarely, hepatitis and fatal acute yellow atrophy of the liver.

Neurological and Psychiatric Complications

Psychiatric disturbances, including confusion, depression, drowsiness may occur with or without signs of ataxia and vertigo, as a result of electrolyte imbalances, vasculitis, or direct drug effects. Peripheral neuritis has occasionally developed.

SUMMARY of Cautions and Contraindications in the Use of Sulfonamides

Patients with a history of sulfa sensitivity should not be treated with sulfonamides.

Advanced kidney disease manifested by elevated blood urea nitrogen levels is a contraindication to the use of sulfonamides.

Caution is required in patients with liver disease, blood dyscrasias, and impaired liver function.

Sulfonamides should not be administered to infants under one month of age, since they lack the detoxifying enzymes required for elimination of sulfonamides.

Pregnant women near term should not receive sulfonamides because of possible placental transmission to the fetus.

Caution is required in all women who are or may become pregnant.

SUMMARY of Points for the Nurse to Remember Concerning Sulfonamide Therapy

Although crystalluria resulting from sulfonamide therapy is less common now than formerly, fluid intake should be encouraged in order to prevent its occurrence. The amount of urine excreted should be noted, and the urine should be examined for signs of hematuria. Nonhospitalized patients should be instructed to drink large quantities of fluids and to promptly report any urinary tract problems.

Observe the patient for other toxic effects of sulfonamides, such as skin rash, fever, chills, sore throat.

Remember that the dosage of the slowly excreted sulfonamides is much less than that of the more rapidly eliminated drugs. Be aware of the usual dosage range of each sulfa drug that is administered.

Patients receiving drugs containing the azo dye, phenazopyridine, will have an orange-red hue to their urine. This should not be mistaken for blood, and the patient should be reassured that the unusual color of his urine is a harmless result of drug therapy.

SUMMARY of Toxic Effects of Antituberculosis Drugs

Aminosalicylic Acid, and Its Salts

Gastrointestinal upset—nausea, vomiting, diarrhea

Hypersensitivity reactions—skin eruptions, fever, sore throat, blood dyscrasias

Rarely, liver damage and goiter

Capreomycin

Nephrotoxicity—rise in blood urea nitrogen and changes in other tests of kidney function

Ototoxicity—some hearing loss, ringing in the ears, vertigo.

Liver function test abnormalities

Hypersensitivity reactions—fever, skin eruptions

Cycloserine

C.N.S. toxicity—convulsions, headache, drowsiness, confusion, disorientation, hallucinations, coma

Peripheral neuropathy—paresthesias, paresis

Ethambutol

Optic neuritis—loss of visual acuity, peripheral vision, and color discrimination

Peripheral neuropathy—numbness and tingling

Hypersensitivity—pruritic skin rashes

Ethionamide

Gastrointestinal—anorexia, unpleasant metallic taste, epigastric burning and discomfort, nausea, vomiting, and diarrhea

Peripheral neuropathy, including rare optic neuritis

C.N.S. and endocrine abnormalities—depression, amenorrhea, impotence

Isoniazid

Peripheral neuropathy—numbness, tingling, burning pain, muscle weakness, rarely optic neuritis

C.N.S. effects—hallucinations, mental depression, convulsive seizures

Liver damage—jaundice, abnormalities in liver function tests

Autonomic blockage—postural hypotension, difficulty in micturition.

Pyrazinamide

Hepatotoxicity—liver function test abnormalities, jaundice

Hyperuricemia—gout symptoms

Hypersensitivity—fever, joint pains

Rifampin

Liver dysfunction—abnormalities in tests, high serum bilirubin, jaundice

Gastrointestinal—anorexia, epigastric distress, nausea, vomiting, cramps, diarrhea

Blood—thrombocytopenia, leukopenia

Streptomycin

Eighth nerve damage—vertigo, headache, tinnitus, deafness.

Hypersensitivity reactions—skin eruptions, anaphylactoid shock

Blood dyscrasias—occasional agranulocytosis, thrombocytopenia, aplastic anemia

Viomycin

Eighth nerve damage:
(a) Vestibular—headache, vertigo
(b) Auditory—tinnitus, deafness

Nephrotoxicity—albuminuria, hematuria, electrolyte imbalance and fluid retention, nitrogen retention

---

SUMMARY of Points for the Nurse to Remember Concerning Tuberculosis Drug Therapy

Administer these drugs in ways which minimize the likelihood of unpleasant side effects that may make the patient reluctant to keep taking the medication. For example, see that PAS is given after meals in divided dosage to lessen gastric irritation.

Observe the patient carefully for signs and symptoms of potentially severe reactions. Some of the tuberculostatic drugs may be highly toxic when taken over the long periods that are required. Streptomycin, for example, can cause deafness; therefore, watch for any sign of hearing loss.

Report promptly to the doctor any condition that may make it difficult or impossible for the patient to continue taking his medication with the essential regularity. Thus, if the patient becomes nauseated and tends to vomit an orally administered medication, the physician should be made aware of this. Also, advise the patient to report promptly any unusual symptoms to his physician.

Encourage the patient, who often is being treated at home for prolonged periods, to continue taking his medication despite discomforts such as gastric distress. Stress the value of drug treatment which shortens the period of his disability, prevents possible complications and reduces substantially the chance of his transmitting his infection to others in the family or at work.

Advise the patient, who may feel remarkably better after an initial course of therapy has reduced his fever and coughing and helped him regain his strength and appetite, not to exceed the limits of the physical activity prescribed by his physician.

Clinical Nursing Situation
Related To Tuberculosis Drug Therapy

The Situation: Mr. Leslie, 52 years old, has been admitted to the hospital with a diagnosis of pulmonary tuberculosis and chronic alcoholism. He is receiving streptomycin 0.5 g. I.M. twice weekly, isoniazid 50 mg q.i.d., and pyridoxine 25 mg q.i.d. Mr. Leslie has gastritis resulting from alcoholism, and experiences periods of nausea and vomiting.

The Problem: What observations would you make for toxic reactions Mr. Leslie may have, related to the prescribed drug therapy?

What nursing actions are indicated when Mr. Leslie is unable to take his oral medications, because of nausea and vomiting?

It is anticipated that Mr. Leslie, who lives alone, will recover sufficiently to continue his treatment on an outpatient basis. What factors will have to be considered when teaching Mr. Leslie to take isoniazid and pyridoxine at home? (If injections of streptomycin are still required, they will be administered at the clinic.)

DRUG DIGEST

AMINOSALICYLIC ACID U.S.P. (Para-Aminosalicylic Acid; PAS; and others)

Actions and Indications. This drug is effective in the treatment of tuberculosis when administered in combination with isoniazid or streptomycin, or both. Although its own tuberculostatic effect is relatively weak, it adds to the effectiveness of the other drugs and slows the rate at which drug-resistant strains tend to emerge.

Side Effects, Cautions, and Contra-indications. The main side effects are the result of irritation of the gastrointestinal tract and include anorexia, nausea, vomiting, cramps, and diarrhea. These may be reduced by administering the drug in divided doses after meals or with antacid-absorbent drugs. Its use in patients with peptic ulcer is contraindicated, and it is withdrawn if gastric bleeding or other indications of developing ulceration occur.

The main types of hypersensitivity reactions reported may involve the skin and blood-forming organs. Sudden development of prolonged high fever, headache, and skin eruptions may require withdrawal of the drug to prevent more serious reactions, including fatal blood dyscrasias and liver damage. Goiter and signs of hypothyroidism developing during prolonged treatment may require administration of thyroid supplements.

Dosage and Administration. A daily dose of 8–12 g is usually adminis-

tered in four equally divided doses after meals. Sodium, potassium, and calcium salts, as well as the phenyl ester and an amide derivative, are also available for oral administration. All are claimed to cause less local gastrointestinal irritation.

DAPSONE U.S.P. (Avlosulfon; DDS)

Actions and Indications The most important use of this prototype sulfone derivative is as a leprostatic agent in the control of leprosy, or Hansen's disease. Administered over long periods, this drug gradually brings about variable degrees of improvement in most leprous patients. New lesions do not develop during treatment, and healing of skin nodules is adequate enough to make possible the return of some patients to their communities.

Side Effects, Cautions, and Contra-Indications. Toxicity is related to dosage and the subsequent blood levels of the drug. Side effects of low doses affect mainly the gastrointestinal tract—anorexia, nausea, and vomiting—and the central nervous system—headache, nervousness, sleeplessness.

More serious are effects on the circulating red blood cells, resulting in hemolysis, particularly in people with a deficiency of the protective enzyme, glucose-6-phosphate dehydrogenase (G-6PD) These untoward effects are less likely to occur if dosage is built up gradually, and blood levels of the drug are checked periodically to

avoid accumulation of the slowly excreted drug to toxic levels.

The drug must be discontinued and corticosteroids administered if acute lepra reaction develops.

Dosage and Administration. Initially the drug is administered in oral doses of 25–50 mg twice a week for four or five weeks. It is then increased by 100 mg at monthly intervals until a maximum dose of 400 mg two times a week is reached. Doses of 100–200 mg daily are occasionally employed to suppress acute flare-ups of dermatitis herpetiformis.

ETHAMBUTOL HCl (Myambutol)

Actions and Indications. This relatively new tuberculostatic drug is being used increasingly as a substitute for aminosalicylic acid in chemotherapeutic combinations for control of active pulmonary tuberculosis. It is administered both with such standard drugs as isoniazid and streptomycin in the initial treatment of primary tuberculosis and—for retreatment of relapsing chronic cases—together with one of the second-line drugs that had not been previously employed. This drug is not administered alone, as resistance to it develops rapidly.

Side Effects, Cautions, and Contra-indications. The most serious adverse effect of high dosage for long periods is the possible development of optic neuritis. Patients must have their vision thoroughly examined before treatment is begun and at periods of one month or less during therapy to detect decreases in visual acuity. If such tests show significant progressive changes, the drug must be discontinued. Recovery then takes place over a period of several weeks or months.

Other side effects include gastrointestinal disturbances, headache, dizziness, and mental confusion, and allergic skin eruptions, joint pains, or anaphylactoid reactions. Abnormalities may be noted in liver function tests, and serum uric acid levels may rise. The drug is not recommended for use in children under 13 years old, and it is given only in reduced dosage to patients with kidney impairment.

Dosage and Administration. A single oral dose of 15 mg/kg is taken daily together with isoniazid in initiating treatment. The retreatment dosage is 25 mg/kg daily, taken together with one or more drugs not previously employed to which the organism has been shown to be susceptible.

IDOXURIDINE U.S.P. (Dendrid; Herplex; Stoxil; IDU)

Actions and Indications. This is an antiviral chemotherapeutic agent specifically indicated in the treatment of herpes simplex keratitis. Topical application in infections that are limited to the corneal epithelium often checks such infections. Responses are less favorable in more deeply localized infections.

Idoxuridine may be combined with antibiotics to control secondary infections by bacteria. Its use in combination with corticosteroids is ordinarily contraindicated in superficial keratitis, for such steroids may accelerate the spread of the herpes simplex virus to deeper structures. However, some ophthalmologists employ such combinations of topical idoxuridine and systemic steroids cautiously for treating deep-seated virus infections of the eye.

Side Effects, Cautions, and Contraindications. Some local irritation and edema of the eyes and lids has been reported after instillation of solutions of idoxuridine, but these may be manifestations of the condition being treated rather than side effects of the drug. The simultaneous use of boric acid solutions is undesirable since it can cause irritation in the presence of idoxuridine.

Dosage and Administration. Idoxuridine is available in ophthalmic solutions and ointments. One drop of the solution is placed in each infected eye every hour during the day and every two hours at night,

until definite improvement occurs. The ointment need be instilled only about every four hours. Treatment with these ophthalmic products is continued at reduced dosage for several days after the corneal lesions seem healed.

ISONIAZID U.S.P. (INH; Nydrazid; and others)

Actions and Indications. This effective antituberculosis agent is commonly combined with aminosalicylic acid (PAS) or streptomycin for treating all forms of active tuberculosis.

It is also employed alone in the preventive treatment of people considered to run a high risk of developing active infection. These include: (1) household contacts of active cases; (2) individuals whose tuberculin test has recently converted to positive; (3) other positive reactors, including those under 20 years old and those with chest x-ray abnormalities; and (4) cases that are inactive but that have never had adequate chemotherapy.

Side Effects, Cautions, and Contraindications. This drug is contraindicated in those who develop severe hypersensitivity reactions, including hepatitis. Patients are watched for signs, symptoms, and laboratory tests that suggest liver damage, and the drug is discontinued in such cases. Other hypersensitivity-type reactions include various kinds of skin eruptions that require stopping the drug promptly. (It may be started again with very small, gradually increasing doses.)

Peripheral nerve symptoms may appear, particularly in malnourished and diabetic patients. (The administration of *pyridoxine* is recommended in such cases and in adolescents taking this drug.) Caution is required in patients with seizure disorders who may be prone to develop convulsions.

Dosage and Administration. The usual adult dosaeg is 5 mg/kg daily in single or divided oral dosage up to 300 mg. Children receive 10 to 30 mg/kg per day for treatment or 10 mg/kg daily (up to a total of 300 mg) for prophylaxis.

METHENAMINE MANDELATE U.S.P. (Mandelamine)

Actions and Indications. This compound breaks down in the urinary tract to two components, mandelic acid and methenamine, both of which act as urinary antiseptics in an acid urine. Methenamine is then converted to formaldehyde, which exerts a bactericidal effect upon both gram-positive and gram-negative bacteria, including *E. coli* and

certain staphylococci and streptococci.

This drug is used mainly in chronic infections to suppress bacteriuria in patients with recurring cystitis, pyelonephritis, or pyelitis. It is *not* effective against acute kidney infections that cause such systemic symptoms as chills and fever. Organisms originally sensitive do not develop resistance.

Side Effects, Cautions, and Contraindications. Irritation caused by gastric distress is minimized by administering this drug after meals or in enteric-coated form. Skin rash is a relatively rare sign of hypersensitivity. High doses cause occasional painful urination (dysuria).

This drug is not toxic to the kidney but is contraindicated in patients with renal insufficiency. It should not be administered when the patient's urine can not be acidified.

Dosage and Administration. One gram is administered orally after each meal and at bedtime for adults and fractions of this 4-gram total are taken by children. The patient's urine is tested to determine whether acidifying agents such as ammonium chloride or ascorbic acid are needed to keep the urinary pH at the necessary 5.5 or below. (Such supplementation is particularly required to control infections by bacterial strains that split urea to form ammonia.)

NITROFURANTOIN U.S.P. Furadantin; Macrodantin)

Actions and Indications. This antibacterial agent is used for treating urinary infections such as cystitis, pyelitis, and pyelonephritis. When excreted in the urine, it exerts bacteriostatic or even bactericidal effects upon susceptible gram-negative and gram-positive bacteria, including some strains resistant to sulfonamides and other urinary antiseptics. Among these uropathogens are *E. coli*, enterococci, *Staph aureus*, and some strains of *Pseudomonas*, *Proteus*, and the *Klebsiella-Aerobacter* group. Organisms that prove sensitive do not ordinarily develop resistance.

Side Effects, Cautions, and Contraindications. The most common side effect, nausea and vomiting, occurs less frequently than formerly with a new oral form made up of larger crystals. Other minor discomforts include headache, dizziness, and drowsiness. Various kinds of skin eruptions may occur as a result of hypersensitivity, including urticarial, exzematous, erythematous, or macropapular rashes.

This drug is highly soluble in urine, and crystalluria does not occur. However, it must not be administered to patients with severely damaged kidneys, as it is ineffective in such cases and may accumulate to toxic levels in nervous tissue. Severe peripheral polyneuropathy has occurred in such cases. Hemolytic anemia may occur in individuals who lack the protective enzyme, glucose-6-phosphate dehydrogenase (G-6PD), and in very young infants with immature enzyme systems. The drug is contraindicated in such cases and in pregnant patients at term. Its safety earlier in pregnancy is not established.

Dosage and Administration. Oral doses of 50 to 100 mg are taken q.i.d. with food for at least one week. The parenteral form is injected I.M. or I.V. in doses of 180 mg for individuals weighing over 120 lbs, or 3 mg/lb for those weighing less.

RIFAMPIN (Rifadin; Rimactane)

Actions and Indications. This antibiotic is used mainly as a primary drug in the treatment of pulmonary tuberculosis, but it may also prove effective in cases of infection that have spread to extrapulmonary sites. It is always used in combination with another tuberculostatic drug such as isoniazid or ethambutol, because resistant tubercle bacilli may emerge rapidly when it is used alone.

A number of other pathogens are susceptible to this antibiotic, but it is used at present only to treat asymptomatic carriers of meningococci. It is *not* used to treat meningitis infections but only to eliminate meningococci from the nose and throat of the carrier in situations in which the risk of spreading meningococcal meningitis is high.

Side Effects, Cautions, and Contraindications. This drug is said to cause fewer side effects than most other antituberculosis drugs. These include gastrointestinal disturbances, headache, drowsiness, and dizziness, skin eruptions, thrombocytopenia and leukopenia, and fever.

Caution is required in patients with liver disease and in those taking anticoagulant drugs. Jaundice and transient liver test abnormalities may occur and tests should be continued periodically during treatment to detect any further hepatotoxicity. Daily prothrombin time tests should be performed while readjusting anticoagulant drug dosage to the higher levels that may be required during treatment with rifampin.

Dosage and Administration. A single dose of 600 mg is administered

orally an hour before or two hours after a meal. Children receive 10 to 20 mg/kg but no more than 600 mg daily.

SODIUM SULFACETAMIDE U.S.P. (Sulamyd sodium)

Actions and Indications. This sulfonamide penetrates readily into ocular tissues when applied topically. It is used for treating eye infections caused by susceptible strains of various gram-positive and gram-negative bacteria.

Among the external eye infections in which it is employed are blepharitis (lid styes), conjunctivitive, and corneal inflammation and ulceration (keratitis). It is also applied topically in trachoma as an adjunct to systemic sulfonamide drug therapy.

Side Effects, Cautions, and Contraindications. This drug is contraindicated in patients with a history of hypersensitivity to sulfonamides. Its use should be discontinued if signs of a sensitivity reaction develop. Patients are observed for signs of overgrowth of nonsusceptible organisms such as fungi.

Dosage and Administration. The 10 percent ointment is applied q.i.d. and at bedtime as an adjunct to treatment with the solution forms. One or two drops of a 10 percent solution containing methylcellulose 0.5 percent are instilled into the lower conjunctival sac every two or three hours during the day. One drop of the 30 percent solution is instilled every two hours for treating acute conjunctivitis or corneal ulcer. Two drops are applied in trachoma in conjunction with systemic sulfonamides

STREPTOMYCIN U.S.P.

Actions and Indications. This antibiotic is one of the primary antituberculosis agents and is commonly administered together with isoniazid and aminosalicylic acid. These drugs help to reduce the rapid rate at which resistant organisms develop and emerge when streptomycin is employed alone.

Various other infections respond to treatment with this antibiotic alone or in combination with other antiinfective drugs. It is particularly useful against the *Pasturella* species that cause plague and tularemia. It is combined with penicillin for treating enterococcal infections of the urinary tract. A combination with chloramphenicol is effective for *Klebsiella pneumoniae* infections. It may be combined with a sulfonamide to treat nocardiosis.

Side Effects, Cautions, and Contraindications. The most common side

effect is the development of vertigo as a result of damage to the vestibular portion of the eighth cranial nerve. Disturbances in hearing may also result from dysfunction of the auditory nerve. The optic nerve and other peripheral nerves may also be adversely affected occasionally.

Allergic reactions, including skin eruptions, may occur both in patients and in personnel handling and administering the antibiotic. Blood dyscrasias develop occasionally. Kidney damage is uncommon with ordinary doses of the drug but may occur in patients with impaired kidney function who do not excrete it well.

Dosage and Administration. Streptomycin is usually administered by deep I.M. injection in daily doses of 1 to 2 g divided into two equal parts at 12-hour intervals. It is administered intermittently in dosage schedules that vary in accordance with the severity and location of the infection.

SUCCINYLSULFATHIAZOLE U.S.P. (Sulfasuxidine)

Actions and Indications. This poorly absorbable sulfonamide concentrates in the intestinal tract, where it inhibits the growth of coliform bacteria. It is used before bowel surgery to reduce the danger of secondary infections such as peritonitis that might occur as a result of contamination. It has also been employed for prophylaxis and treatment of bacillary dysentery. However, an increasing number of *Shigella* strains are proving resistant to sulfonamides and in any case soluble sulfonamides, such as sulfadiazine, which are excreted through the bowel wall, are preferred for treating actual infections.

Side Effects, Cautions, and Contraindications. Systemic toxicity is uncommon, because the small amounts of sulfathiazole that are absorbed are readily excreted. However, caution is required in patients with liver or kidney damage or urinary tract obstruction, and use of the drug is contraindicated in patients with abdominal obstruction. Typical sulfonamide hypersensitivity reactions, including various blood dyscrasias, have occurred with the use of these drugs. Patients require blood counts as well as kidney and liver function tests periodically.

Dosage and Administration. Oral dosage of 250 mg/kg of body weight is administered initially and followed by the same daily amount divided into six doses.

SULFADIAZINE U.S.P.

Actions and Indications. This sulfonamide is administered alone or combined with sulfamethazine and sulfamerazine in the combination called trisulfapyrimidines. It is used for treating acute urinary infections such as cystitis, urethritis, pyelitis, pyelonephritis, and prostatitis caused by susceptible strains of *E. coli* and other uropathogens.

This, like other sulfonamides, is also used for prophylaxis and treatment of meningococcal meningitis caused by group A strains of meningococci and for prevention of rheumatic fever (group A hemolytic streptococci) in patients sensitive to penicillin.

Among relatively rare infections for which it is useful are toxoplasmosis (in combination with pyrimethamine), chloroquine-resistant strains of *Plasmodium falciparum* malaria (in combination with quinine), nocardiosis, trachoma, and chancroid.

Side Effects, Cautions, and Contraindications. This drug must be administered with adequate quantities of fluid to avoid crystalluria. It is discontinued if hematuria develops and is contraindicated in patients with kidney failure or severe liver damage. It should not be administered during late pregnancy, to premature infants, or to newborn babies under two months old because of possible development of kernicterus in the very young child. Patients should be watched for signs of allergic reactions characteristic of sulfonamides.

Dosage and Administration. The usual initial dose administered orally to adults is 2 to 4 g; doses of 1 to 1.5 g are then administered every four to six hours. Children's dose is 100–150 mg/kg followed by one sixth of the first dose every four hours. Intravenous dosage of 100 mg/kg is administered initially and followed by 30–50 mg/kg every six to eight hours.

SULFAMETHOXYPYRIDAZINE (Kynex; Midicel)

Actions and Indications. This is an unusually long-acting sulfonamide which seems especially suited for treatment of conditions requiring prolonged sulfonamide therapy, and for long-term prophylaxis against streptococcal infections in patients with a history of rheumatic fever. Among other disorders in which this drug has been employed are: upper respiratory infections, including pneumococcal pneumonia; gastrointestinal infections, including bacillary dysentery (shigellosis); the eye infection, trachoma; and various soft tissue and surgical infections.

Side Effects, Cautions, and Contraindications. Although this drug's slow rate of excretion makes crystalluria unlikely, the difficulty in clearing it from the body in the event of development of sulfonamide reaction is a disadvantage. Thus, the severity of the Stevens-Johnson syndrome and other adverse reactions in hypersensitive individuals may continue to an irreversible state even after the drug has been discontinued. In any case, the drug should be immediately withdrawn if a skin eruption develops during therapy.

Dosage and Administration. Because of its slow excretion only one gram is administered to adults to initiate therapy, and this is followed by 0.5 g once daily thereafter. If larger doses—for example, 2 g, then 1 g daily—are required for severe infections, blood levels of sulfonamide should be checked after three days of treatment to avoid cumulative toxicity.

SULFISOXAZOLE U.S.P. (Gantrisin)
SULFISOXAZOLE DIOLAMINE U.S.P. (Gantrisin diolamine)
ACETYL SULFISOXAZOLE N.F. (Lipo Gantrisin)

Actions and Indications. These forms are all used for their bacteriostatic effects against a broad spectrum of susceptible microbial strains. This sulfonamide is employed in urinary tract infections by *E. coli* and other uropathogens. It is used for prophylaxis (but *not* for treatment) of group A beta-hemolytic streptococcal infections in patients allergic to penicillin. It is used for prevention and treatment of meningococcal meningitis and, in combination with antibiotics, for treating *Hemophilus influenzae* infections such as acute otitis media and meningitis. The cream is used in infections by *Hemophilus vaginalis*.

Side Effects, Cautions, and Contraindications. This drug is contraindicated in patients with a history of hypersensitivity to sulfonamides. It is discontinued if skin eruptions occur, as such dangerous dermatological reactions as exfoliative dermatitis and erythema multiforme (Stevens-Johnson syndrome) have occurred. Blood dyscrasias and anaphylactoid-type allergic reactions are also possible.

Nausea, vomiting, epigastric distress, and headache are among the more common, less severe reactions. Patients should drink adequate amounts of fluid to avoid crystal and stone formation. Caution is required in patients with impaired liver or kidney function. Use of this drug is undesirable late in pregnancy, as it may have adverse effects upon the child. Kernicterus may also occur in early infancy, so use of this and other sulfonamides is avoided at that time.

Dosage and Administration. The initial oral dose of 2 to 4 g is followed by 1 to 2 g every four to six hours. Children's dosage is 60 to 75 mg/kg.

References

Carroll, O.M., Bryan, P.A., and Robinson, R.J. Stevens-Johnson syndrome associated with long-acting sulfonamides. *JAMA*, 195:179, 1966.

Coriel, L.L. Smallpox vaccination. When and whom to vaccinate. Pediatrics, 37:493, 1966.

Di Palma, J.R. Status report on immunizations. *RN*, 33:69, 1970 (Sept.).

Francis, B.J. Current concepts in immunization. *Amer. J. Nurs.*, 73:646, 1973 (April).

Frenay, M.A.C., Sr. Drugs in tuberculosis control. *Amer. J. Nurs.*, 61:82, 1961.

Hilleman, M.R. Advances in control of virus infections. *Clin. Pharmacol. Ther.*, 7:752, 1966.

Pruitt, B.A. Jr., et al. Successful control of burn wound sepsis. *JAMA*, 203:150, 1968.

Rodman, M.J. Drug treatment of tuberculosis. *RN*, 22:56, 1959 (Jan.).

———. New drugs for fighting infections. *RN*, 30:55, 1967 (June).

———. Combating urinary tract infections. *RN*, 31:59, 1968 (Nov.).

Schwartz, W.S. Developments in treatment of tuberculosis, and other pulmonary diseases. *JAMA*, 178:43, 1961.

Weiss, M. Chemotherapy and tuberculosis. *Amer. J. Nurs.*, 59:1711, 1959.

Wolinsky, E. Modern drug treatment of mycobacterial diseases. *Med. Clin. N. Amer.*, 47:1271, 1963.

43.

The Chemotherapy of Malaria and Other Parasitic Infections

In this chapter we shall discuss the chemotherapy of malaria and certain other parasitic diseases. Nurses are called upon to care for patients with these conditions, not only when practicing abroad (for example, as a member of the armed forces) but sometimes in this country also. In addition to the occasional patient who may become infected with malaria in the continental United States, others, traveling by jet plane from a land in which these diseases have not yet been eradicated, may come down with this or other illnesses with an incubation period longer than the flying time.

Malaria

Malaria is a parasitic disease that has killed hundreds of millions of people and changed the course of history. Even today, when great advances have been made in the control of malaria, millions of people are infected in the many lands in which this mosquito-borne disease is still endemic.

The continued prevalence of malaria in many parts of the globe indicates the need to sustain a vigorous attack on the malaria parasite and on its insect vector, the *Anopheles* mosquito. Strains of mosquitoes that have developed resistance to DDT and other insecticides have appeared. Similarly, malaria parasites insensitive to antimalarial drugs are now a cause of disease in various parts of the world (see p. 557).

TYPES OF MALARIA

Four species of protozoa of the genus *Plasmodium* cause malaria in man. The two that are of prime importance are: (1) *Plasmodium vivax*, the cause of benign tertian malaria; and (2) *Plasmodium falciparum*, the cause of malignant tertian malaria. The term *tertian* refers to the fact that the attacks of chills and fever tend typically to recur every third day. The term *benign* indicates only that *P. vivax* infection is less severe than *P. falciparum* infection and less likely to kill quickly. The malignant disease, though relatively easy to cure in most cases with modern drugs, may start explosively and end fatally, with its victims following a rapidly progressive downhill course.

LIFE CYCLE OF THE PLASMODIUM (FIG. 43-1).

The parasites that cause clinical malaria spend part of their lives in the female *Anopheles* mosquito and part in the human host. The mosquito that bites an infected person and sucks up a drop of blood ingests *gametocytes*, which are sexual (male and female) forms

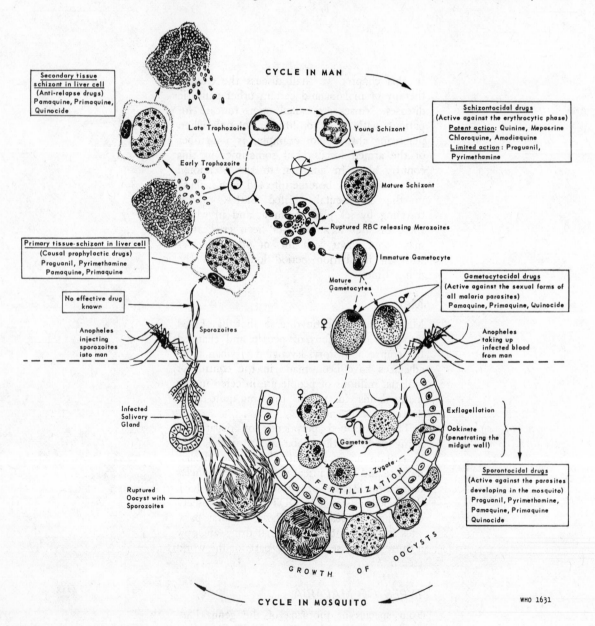

Fig. 43-1. Classification of antimalarial drugs in relation to different stages in the life-cycle of the parasite. (Bruce-Chwatt, L. J. W.H.O. Bull. No. 27, p. 287, 1962.)

of the plasmodial parasite. These gameto-cytes mate in the mosquito's stomach, and the product of this mating (the zygote) goes through several stages and finally forms *sporozoites* (spore animals) that make their way to the mosquito's salivary glands.

The next human being bitten by the mosquito gets an injection of thousands of these sporozoites. These do not linger very long in the person's bloodstream but, instead, lodge in the liver and other tissues where they undergo *asexual cell division* and reproduction.

During the next week to ten days, these *primary tissue schizonts* grow and multiply by simple division within the liver cells. Finally, *merozoites* are formed by malarial schizonts and burst forth when the liver cells that had been parasitized are ruptured. Most of the merozoites enter the circulation and invade red blood cells.

After a period of development and asexual division within the first blood cells to be invaded, a new batch of merozoites bursts forth from the ruptured red cells. These liberated spores invade still more erythrocytes, and repeat the process of division. After several such cycles, the number of organisms is so great and the number of parasitized red cells so large that the patient begins to suffer from the symptoms of an acute attack of malaria.

THE CLINICAL COURSE OF MALARIA

The sudden release of swarms of malaria parasites from millions of destroyed red cells sets off the chills and fever that mark the beginning of the clinical attack. The chill is caused by the break-up of the erythrocytes; the fever is the result of a reaction to the freed foreign protein and cellular debris.

Each time a new mass of erythrocytic schizonts bursts, releasing toxins into the circulation (about every 48 hours in the tertian malarias), the patient suffers a paroxysm of chills and fever. In *P. vivax* malaria, such attacks continue for a long time if untreated. Even after the body's defense mechanisms have brought the infection more or less under control, the patient is subject to periodic relapses.

RELAPSES. Relapses occur in *P. vivax* malaria because some of the schizonts make their way back into the liver and other tissue cells. Then these so-called *exoerythrocytic forms*, or secondary tissue schizonts, periodically send forth

more invaders of red cells. As these plasmodial spores proceed to divide, invade, and then destroy still more erythrocytes, the infected individual suffers yet another attack. Relapses of this kind can occur periodically for years, if the person goes untreated.

In the case of *P. falciparum* malaria, no such secondary exoerythrocytic schizonts persist in the tissues. Thus, provided that the patient survives the first series of attacks, he will suffer no further relapses. However, this form of malaria is often fatal, because the parasite-damaged red cells tend to clog the patient's capillaries and thus cut off the circulation in vital organs.

DRUG TREATMENT OF MALARIA

The antimalarial drugs (Table 43-1) are all capable of controlling plasmodial parasites at one or more stages in their life cycle. Thus, they should in theory be useful: (1) for the prevention and treatment of acute attacks; (2) for completely curing the patient; and (3) for breaking the chain of transmission of the disease. Actually, however, it is not always practical to use drugs on an entire population in order to keep people from becoming infected and then acting as a source of infection to others.

MASS PROPHYLAXIS. Prevention cannot be readily applied to the populations of areas where malaria is endemic. In theory, these people could routinely receive antimalarial drugs such as *primaquine+* or *pyrimethamine+*, in order to keep them from ever getting the disease or transmitting it.

Both these drugs (and *chlorguanide*) can destroy the gametocytes in the person's blood or sterilize these sexual forms before they might mate. This could break the man-mosquito-man chain of transmission by which malaria is spread. Similarly, these same drugs are *schizonticides* as well as gametocides. Thus, if taken routinely, they could kill plasmodial parasites in the tissues before they ever got a chance to move back into the bloodstream to invade and destroy red cells.

Unfortunately, these *true causal prophylactic drugs* are considered too toxic and expensive for mass administration to uninfected people in endemic areas for the purpose of protecting the population and breaking the chain of transmission. Instead of drugs, public health officials in these areas depend upon

T A B L E 4 3 - 1   *Antimalarial Drugs*

Nonproprietary or Official Name	Synonym or Proprietary Name	Oral Dosage
Amodiaquin HCl N.F.	Camoquin	Suppressive:* 400 mg once weekly. Therapeutic:† 600 mg then 400 mg for next two days
Chloroquine phosphate U.S.P.	Aralen	Suppressive: 300 mg weekly. Therapeutic: 1 g initial, then 300 mg in six hours and 300 mg on second and third days
Chloroguanide HCl	Proguanil; Paludrine	Suppressive: 100 mg daily. Therapeutic: 600 mg followed by 300 mg daily as needed
Hydroxychloroquine sulfate U.S.P.	Plaquenil	Suppressive: 300 mg weekly. Therapeutic: 600 mg initially followed by 600 mg in six hours
Primaquine phosphate U.S.P.	. . . .	26.3 mg (the equivalent of 15 mg of the base) daily for 14 days to achieve a radical cure‡
Pyrimethamine U.S.P.	Daraprim	Suppressive: 25 mg weekly. Therapeutic: Single dose of 50 mg; or for resistant strains of *P. falciparum*, 50 mg daily for three days in combination with quinine
Quinacrine HCl U.S.P.	Atabrine	Therapeutic: 0.2 g given with 1 g of sodium bicarbonate in 200 to 300 ml of fluid, after a meal, every four to six hours. Then 100 mg t.i.d. for six days
Quinine sulfate N.F.	. . . .	Therapeutic: 1 g daily for two days, then 600 mg daily for five days

* The term *suppressive* refers to the use of a single small dose periodically to prevent development of clinical signs and symptoms in a person who may have been bitten and infected with plasmodial parasites (that is, for *clinical prophylaxis*).

† The term *therapeutic* refers to the use of larger or more frequently administered doses to terminate an acute attack (that is, for *clinical cure*).

‡ The term *radical cure* refers to use of drugs of this kind to prevent relapses through their effects upon the secondary tissue forms of the parasites.

mosquito control, protective screening, and insect repellents. That is, they try to keep people from being bitten by the insect vector, rather than having them take potentially toxic and expensive drugs in an effort to eradicate the parasites when they enter the person's blood and tissues.

SUPPRESSIVE AND THERAPEUTIC MEASURES. Although it is impractical to use drugs for keeping people from becoming infected, it is possible to keep them from ever suffering clinical symptoms of the disease, and it is now also practical to eliminate secondary tissue forms of the parasite and thus achieve the complete cure of an infected individual.

Suppressive treatment refers to the routine use of small, safe doses of certain drugs in order to keep a person who has been bitten by the mosquito and infected by plasmodial parasites from suffering an actual clinical attack of malaria. Taken only once weekly, drugs such as *chloroquine+* (Aralen), *hydroxychloroquine, amodiaquine,* and others (Table 43-1) control the forms of the parasites that enter red blood cells. This protects the person's erythrocytes from destruction and thus suppresses the periodic malarial paroxysms of chills, fever, and any other signs and symptoms of an acute attack.

CURATIVE MEASURES. *Clinical cure*, the relief of an actual attack, can be brought about by the same drugs that are used for suppressive treatment. They act, of course, by stopping the cycles of erythrocytic schizogony through which more and more red blood cells are parasitized by waves of liberated merozoites. By calling a halt to the periodic release of toxins responsible for paroxysms of chills and fever, drugs such as *chloroquine+* and the other synthetic successors to *quinine+* quickly terminate the attacks. They do not, however, completely eliminate the parasite from the patient's body. Thus, although his attack is clinically cured, he himself is not truly cured and is subject to relapses of *P. vivax* malaria.

Radical cure of *P. vivax* infection *can*, however, be brought about by chemotherapy. This is accomplished with drugs such as *primaquine*, which wipe out the secondary tissue forms of *P. vivax*. By acting to kill these *exo-erythrocytic* schizonts produced by merozoites that have made their way back into liver cells, primaquine prevents the red blood cell parasitizers from ever again emerging. Simultaneous *suppressive therapy* is, of course, needed to keep blood forms from continuing to survive.

In the case of *P. falciparum*, as previously indicated, suppressive treatment alone is adequate, since this organism possesses no persisting secondary exo-erythrocytic tissue forms.

Travelers to areas where malaria is still endemic cannot usually be kept from being bitten and infected by mosquitoes that are carrying the parasites. However—as was shown with malaria prevention measures employed by the U.S. Army in Vietnam—people can be protected from developing disease symptoms, and, as was done with soldiers leaving Southeast Asia, any parasites still in their tissues when they leave the malarious lands can also be eradicated by drug therapy.

Such suppressive treatment and radical cure can be carried out most conveniently by having the traveler take a single tablet that combines *chloroquine+* or amodiaquine with *primaquine+* in small, safe doses once weekly. The first tablet is taken at least one day before arriving in the malarious area. Then this drug combination is repeated on the same day of the week at weekly intervals during the person's entire stay.

After he leaves the country, the traveler continues to take his weekly tablet for the next eight weeks. The *chloroquine+* or *amodiaquin* component of such mixtures attacks the primary tissue parasites as they emerge from the tissues and enter the bloodstream. This keeps the traveler from ever suffering any symptoms while in the area. The *primaquine+* portion of the combination tablet eradicates any secondary tissue forms that are left when he leaves, as described above in the discussion of radical cure.

TREATMENT OF RESISTANT CASES. Reports of patients with malaria resistant to treatment with *chloroquine+* have appeared in recent years. Cases caused by infection with resistant strains of *P. falciparum* have caused particular concern because of the seriousness of infections by this plasmodial parasite. The appearance of such cases in American soldiers in Southeast Asia (Vietnam, Cambodia, and Thailand) and in South America (Brazil, Colombia, and Venezuela) has led to many scientific studies aimed at discovering more effective antimalarial drugs.

Oddly, some of the oldest chemotherapeutic agents such as *quinine+* and drugs tried earlier and discarded, including certain *sulfonamides* and *sulfones*, have been among the most successful ones for treating chloroquine-resistant infections. Newer sulfonamides for this purpose include *sulforthormadine* (Fanasil) and *sulfalene* (Keifizin). The most effective sulfone is the antileprosy agent *dapsone*, but one of its derivative called DFD is said to be much safer for use in managing resistant malaria cases (see also Chapter 42).

Other Parasitic Infections

Protozoan organisms other than plasmodia are a frequent cause of infection. Amebic infections of the intestine are taken up in the next chapter, together with a discussion of treatment of most intestinal worm infections. Here we shall discuss briefly the chemotherapy of protozoan infections such as trypanosomiasis and leishmaniasis, and infections caused by trematode-type worms, or flukes, and by nematode-type filarid worms such as those that cause schistosomiasis and filariasis.

SCHISTOSOMIASIS

Schistosomiasis (bilharziasis) is one of the world's most important parasitic infections. Three species of blood flukes are involved: *Schistosoma haematobium*, *S. mansoni*, and *S. japonicum*, a resistant parasite which was

TABLE 43-2   Drugs for Miscellaneous Parasitic Infections

Nonproprietary, Generic, or Official Name	Proprietary Name, or Synonym	Chemical Category	Dosage and Administration	Remarks (see also Drug Digest)
Antimony potassium tartrate U.S.P.	Tartar emetic	Trivalent antimony compound	40 mg I.V. as a 0.5% solution on alternate days up to a total dose of 2.5 g	Treatment of *Schistosoma japonicum* infection and in leishmaniasis
Arsenamide	· · · · · · · ·	Trivalent organic arsenic compound	1 mg/kg I.V. for five days	For filariasis treatment against microfilaria and adult worms
Diethylcarbamazine citrate U.S.P.	Hetrazan	Piperazine derivative	2 mg/kg of body weight three times daily after meals for one or two weeks	For filariasis against the microfilariae and adult female worms of *Wuchereria*
Hydroxystilbamidine isethionate U.S.P.	· · · · · · · ·	Aromatic diamidine derivative	150 mg I.V. by slow drip in 5% dextrose solution	For leishmaniasis and trypanosomiasis (also in blastomycosis)
Lucanthone HCl U.S.P.	Miracil D	Xanthone derivative	10–20 mg/kg of body weight orally for one to three weeks	For schistosomiasis (esp. against *S. haematobium*)
Melarsoprol	Arsobal	Organic arsenical	2–5 ml of a 3.6% solution in propylene glycol I.V.	African trypanosomiasis caused by *Trypanosoma rhodiense* and *T. gambiense*
Melarsonyl potassium	Trimelarsen	Organic arsenical	1–4 mg/kg of body weight I.M. up to a maximum of 200 mg in a single dose. Repeat course in seven to ten days	For African trypanosomiasis and for filariasis

Drug	Trade name	Chemical nature	Dose	Use
Niridazole	Ambilhar	Complex organic compound	25 mg/kg orally for five to ten days	Experimental for schistosomiasis
Nitrofurazone	Furacin	Nitrofuran derivative	500 mg orally three times daily	Experimental for systemic use in trypanosomiasis
Pentamidine isothionate	Lomidine	Aromatic diamidine derivative	4 mg/kg of body weight I.V. or I.M.	For treatment and prevention of African trypanosomiasis by *T. gambiense*
Sodium antimony dimercaptosuccinate	Astiban	Trivalent antimony compound	30–50 mg/kg of body weight I.M. or by slow I.V. injection up to a maximum total dose of 2.5 g	For treatment of trypanosomiasis by *S. mansoni* and *S. haematobium*
Sodium antimony gluconate	Triostam	Trivalent antimony compound	40 mg/kg of body weight I.V.	For leishmaniasis and filariasis
Sodium stibogluconate	Pentostam	Pentavalent antimony compound	600 mg I.M. or I.V.	Experimental for leishmaniasis
Stibophen U.S.P.	Fuadin	Trivalent antimony compound	1.5–5 ml of a 6.3% solution I.M. or I.V. to a total of 80–100 ml	For schistosomiasis by *S. haematobium* or *S. mansoni*
Suramin sodium	Naphuride	Complex organic compound	1 g in 10 ml of water by slow I.V. injection every other day in weekly courses up to a total of 5–10 g	For African trypanosomiasis by *T. rhodiense*; also in filariasis by *Onchocera*
Tryparsamide	· · · · · ·	Organic arsenical compound	Up to 50 mg/kg of body weight I.V. or I.M. (1–3 g)	For late as well as early stages of African trypanosomiasis by *T. gambiense*

a source of infestation for American soldiers in Southeast Asia. The disease, which is spread by certain species of snails, appears to be increasing in incidence because of advances in irrigation of farmlands.

Chemotherapy of schistosomiasis involves the use of: (1) trivalent antimony compounds such as *stibophen+* (Fuadin) and *antimony potassium tartrate+* (Tartar Emetic); and (2) nonmetallic schistosomacides such as *lucanthone+* (Miracil D), and its relative *hycanthone*, or a new agent, *niridazole* (Ambilhar) (see Table 43-2).

The antimonial compounds are potentially quite toxic. They are, however, still the most effective chemotherapeutic agents, particularly for treating infestations by the most resistant species, S. *japonicum*. An advantage of the nonmetallic agents is that they can be taken by the convenient oral route without causing excessive gastrointestinal discomfort.

Patients with chronic blood fluke infestations are often debilitated and anemic. Thus, it is desirable that they be built up by dietary and antianemia treatments before being subjected to treatment with these toxic chemotherapeutic agents.

FILARIASIS

Filariasis is a parasitic disease caused by the presence of tiny roundworms in body tissues. A person becomes infected by being bitten by a mosquito (*Culex* species, especially) that deposits larvae in the skin. Later, the adult females give birth to thin threadlike microfilariae which migrate into the lymphatics and the bloodstream. Symptoms are the result of inflammatory reactions to the presence of living and dead worms. Obstruction of the lymphatic system by inflammatory lesions may lead to elephantiasis—gross enlargement of the legs, arms, scrotum, or breast by edema fluid.

Until relatively recent years no safe drug was available for treatment of filariasis, and, in fact, there is still no chemical that can be taken to prevent infection upon entering an endemic area. Prevention involves mosquito control by means of insecticides aimed at breeding places, as well as special efforts to avoid being bitten. The relatively toxic arsenical and antimony compounds once employed with only fair success have now been largely

displaced by two nonmetallic compounds, *diethylcarbamazine+*, and *suramin sodium+* (see Table 43-2).

LEISHMANIASIS

Leishmaniasis is a term used to describe several diseases caused by infection with protozoan parasites of the *Leishmania* genus. These include: kala-azar, or visceral leishmaniasis; oriental sore, or cutaneous leishmaniasis; and American mucocutaneous leishmaniasis. Kala-azar is a generalized infection with signs and symptoms involving the liver, spleen, and bone marrow and ranging from vague pains in muscles, bones, and joints to common complications such as bronchitis and pneumonia. The other leishmania infections are limited— to the skin, in oriental sore, and to the skin, mouth, nose, and throat in mucocutaneous leishmaniasis.

Once the diagnosis is definitely established treatment of kala-azar with an organic antimonial is usually undertaken. The early forms of antimony, including *antimony and potassium tartrate+* (Tartar Emetic) *and stibophen+* (Fuadin) or related trivalent antimonials, have largely been superseded by the safer and more effective pentavalent antimonial *sodium stibogluconate* (Pentostam). A course of treatment with the last-named drug is said to cure most cases of kala-azar after six injections on consecutive days. Local intralesional injection of these compounds often clears oriental sore; mucosal lesions require parenteral therapy.

Resistant cases of kala-azar, such as are often encountered in the Sudan, have recently been treated with the diamidines, *pentamidine isethionate* and *hydroxystilbamidine isethionate+* (see Table 43-2).

TRYPANOSOMIASIS

Trypanosomiasis is a protozoal infection transmitted by insects—the biting tsetse fly, in the case of African sleeping sickness, and the bedbug-like insect vector of Chagas' disease in the Americas. African trypanosomiasis is marked mainly by brain damage; American trypanosomiasis causes cardiac complications. The prognosis for patients with Chagas' disease is poor, for no satisfactory chemotherapeutic agent has as yet been discovered. Fortunately, drugs are now available for use in both the treatment and prevention of African sleeping sickness.

In general, compounds of two types are employed in African trypanosomiasis: (1) organic arsenicals such as *tryparsamide* and *melarsoprol*; and (2) nonmetallic trypanocides such as *suramin sodium+*, *pentamidine*, and *hydroxystilbamidine* (see above). The arsenicals, which pass the blood-brain barrier and penetrate into the central nervous system, are essential when there is C.N.S. involvement and urgent treatment is required. The less toxic nonmetallic compounds are employed for prophylaxis and in the treatment of early infections (see Table 43-2).

DRUG DIGEST

ANTIMONY AND POTASSIUM TARTRATE U.S.P. (Tartar emetic)

Actions and Indications. This trivalent antimony compound is toxic but effective schistosomicide. It is sometimes useful for treating infestations by *Schistosoma japonicum*, the blood fluke species most resistant to chemotherapy with other, safer agents. It has also been employed in leishmaniasis and filariasis.

Side Effects, Cautions, and Contraindications. This heavy metal often causes nausea, vomiting, abdominal cramps, and diarrhea. Toxic doses may cause liver damage, including necrosis. The drug is contraindicated in patients with severe kidney or heart disease and in those with hepatic dysfunction other than that caused by schistosomiasis.

Dosage and Administration. Treatment of *S. japonicum* infestation is started with a slow infusion of 8 ml of a fresh 0.5 percent solution. If toxicity is not severe, a second dose of 12 ml is administered after a day's rest. Each subsequent dose, administered on alternate days, is raised by 4 ml until a dose of 28 ml is reached. This dose level is continued until a total dose of 360 to 500 ml has been administered. Too rapid injection is avoided to prevent circulatory and respiratory difficulties.

CHLOROQUINE PHOSPHATE* U.S.P. (Aralen)

Actions and Indications. This is the drug most widely used for suppressive treatment of malaria and for effecting the clinical cure of an acute attack. It acts against the erythrocytic forms of the parasites, *Plasmodium vivax* and *P. falcipa-*

---

* Another salt, the *hydrochloride* (U.S.P.) is employed for parenteral administration in I.M. doses not exceeding 800 mg of the base daily.

rum. Infections by susceptible strains of *P. falciparum* are usually cured. However, chloroquine does *not* keep patients with *P. vivax* from relapsing.

Side Effects, Cautions, and Contraindications. Side effects rarely occur with the small amount of chloroquine that is needed for suppressive effects. With the large loading dose given to initiate treatment of an acute attack, epigastric discomfort and headache may occur, and the patient may also complain of pruritus, blurring of vision, and diarrhea.

Much more serious toxicity is possible during prolonged use of chloroquine for treating chronic diseases such as rheumatoid arthritis and discoid lupus erythematosus. Blindness may result from retinal damage and blood dyscrasias, and lichenoid skin eruptions have developed. The drug is contraindicated in patients with evidence of changes in the visual field or retina. It may cause severe attacks in patients with psoriasis, as it may set off the acute progressive phase of that disease.

Dosage and Administration. A single once-weekly oral dose of 0.5 g is adequate for suppressive therapy. It is administered as long as the person remains in the malarious region and for four weeks after he leaves the area in which the disease is endemic.

For clinical cure of the acute malarial attack, an initial dose of 1 g is followed by 500 mg in six hours and by additional doses of 500 mg on the second and third treatment days. These may be given with meals to allay gastric distress.

In hepatic amebiasis with liver abscess, 1 g is given daily for two days and then 500 mg is administered twice a day for at least two or three weeks.

In discoid lupus erythematosus, 250 mg is taken orally twice daily for two weeks and then followed by a maintenance dose of 250 mg daily.

Rheumatoid arthritis requires prolonged daily administration of 250 mg orally.

DIETHYLCARBAMAZINE CITRATE U.S.P. (Hetrazan)

Actions and Indications. This nonmetallic filaricide is more effective and less toxic than the antimony compounds formerly employed against filariasis caused by *Wuchereria bancrofti*, *W. malayi*, *Onchocerca volvulus*, and *Loa loa*. Taken by mouth, the drug quickly causes the threadlike microfilariae to vanish from the blood or skin of the infected person. The adult worms of some species such as *Wuchereria* are killed or sterilized, while adults are not affected and must be removed surgically.

Side Effects, Cautions, and Contraindications. Side effects of this drug include transient anorexia, nausea, vomiting, headache, and dizziness with weakness and muscular or joint discomfort in some cases. In onchocerciacis, a condition marked by ocular involvement, rapid destruction of the microfilariae may lead to fever, pruritic dermatitis, and allergic inflammatory eye reactions.

Dosage and Administration. A dose of 2 mg per kg of body weight is administered three times daily for one to three weeks. Available for this purpose are 50 mg scored tablets and a cherry-flavored syrup containing 120 mg per 5 ml. The administration of antihistaminic and corticosteroid drugs along with diethylcarbamazine is advocated to minimize allergic reactions.

HYDROXYSTILBAMIDINE ISETHIONATE U.S.P.

Actions and Indications. This diamidine is active against the invasive fungi that cause blastomycosis and against the protozoal organisms responsible for African trypanosomiasis and leishmaniasis. In each of these conditions it is reserved for cases not responsive to preferred drugs: amphotericin B in blastomycosis; the organic arsenicals and pentamidine in trypanosomiasis; and the pentavalent antimonials in kala-azar.

Side Effects, Cautions, and Contraindications. During long-term therapy, the patient's kidney and liver function are observed because of renal and hepatic reactions reported with previous drugs of this class.

It has been suggested that light causes breakdown of solutions of these chemicals to hepatotoxic substances. Thus, precautions are required to prevent exposure of the solution to sunlight during its preparation and infusion.

The solution is injected over periods of at least 30 minutes, or one or two hours, as too rapid administration may result in release of tissue histamine which causes reactions including flushing, fainting, falls in blood pressure, reflex tachycardia, and other discomforting or disabling symptoms.

Dosage and Administration. Freshly prepared solutions containing 150 to 225 mg of the drug in 5 percent dextrose are infused over a period of about one or two hours. These are repeated every day or two for a total of ten doses.

LUCANTHONE HCl U.S.P. (Miracil D; Nilodin)
Actions and Indications. This nonmetallic schistosomicide is often effective in treating infections by *Schistosoma haematobium*. Larger doses are required against *S. mansoni*, and it seems ineffective in *S. japonicum* infections. Its main advantages are its activity when given by mouth and the likelihood that it will not cause as severe toxicity as stibophen injections.

Side Effects, Cautions, and Contraindications. Gastrointestinal upset occurs frequently and confusion, restlessness, and vertigo occasionally. This may also affect the skin, which often develops a yellow discoloration. This and the common occurrence of anorexia, nausea, burning epigastric distress, and vomiting limits this drug's usefulness for prophylactic purposes. Adults seem more susceptible than children to the central effects and sometimes develop psychotic reactions.

Dosage and Administration. An oral dose of 5 mg per kg of body weight is taken three times daily for one to two weeks, but longer courses with higher doses may be employed

if the patient requires and tolerates such amounts.

QUININE SULFATE U.S.P. AND QUININE DIHYDROCHLORIDE N.F.
Actions and Indications. These salts of the main alkaloid of cinchona bark are rarely used today for treating ordinary cases of malaria. However, quinine may be lifesaving in some *Plasmodium falciparum* infections caused by strains of this species that are resistant to treatment with chloroquine and the other blood schizonticides that are considered safer and more effective in most cases.

Quinine possesses analgesic-antipyretic properties and has sometimes been used as a substitute for salicylates in the relief of headache, fever, and general malaise. Quinine is often useful for relief of nocturnal skeletal muscle cramps and for relief of muscle spasms in the rare condition, myotonia congenita.

Side Effects, Cautions, and Contraindications. Overdosage is marked by cinchonism, a syndrome similar to that seen when salicylate dosage is pushed to high levels. Ringing in the ears, blurring of vision, nausea, and headache may be followed by further digestive disturbances, impairment of hearing and sight, and confusion and delirium. Death may follow cardiac arrhythmias, collapse, convulsions, and coma when massive amounts are taken in misguided attempts to produce an abortion.

Dosage and Administration. For treating an acute malarial attack, 1 g is administered daily for two days and followed by 600 mg for the following five days. Although the oral route is preferred, the dihydrochloride salt may be given by I.V. drip to patients severely ill with *P. falciparum* malaria affecting the brain.

PRIMAQUINE PHOSPHATE U.S.P.
Actions and Indications. This drug is used for producing radical cure and thus preventing relapses in malaria. It acts to eradicate the exoerythrocytic (secondary tissue) forms of the plasmodial parasites. However, it does *not* act against an acute attack. It is always administered together with a blood schizonticide, such as chloroquine.

Side Effects, Cautions, and Contraindications. Ordinary doses of primaquine cause few side effects in most people. Complaints are limited to occasional abdominal distress, headache, itching, and blurred vision. Much more serious is the possibility of a hemolytic reaction in a hypersensitive individ-

ual. Negroes and other darkly pigmented people with a genetic enzyme defiency are most prone to develop hemolytic anemia. The drug is discontinued if darkening of the urine develops or the level of hemoglobin, red blood cells, and leukocytes drops.

Dosage and Administration. A tablet containing 26.3 mg of this phosphate salt—the equivalent of 15 mg of primaquine base—is taken by mouth once daily for 14 days together with chloroquine to produce a radical cure. For prophylaxis, a tablet containing 79 mg—equal to 45 mg of the base—in combination with 300 mg of chloroquine is taken once weekly beginning before entering the area in which malaria is endemic.

PYRIMETHAMINE U.S.P. (Daraprim)
Actions and Indications. This antimalarial drug is effective against several stages of plasmodia species. In practice, however, it is used mainly for suppressive treatment. Its action against blood-borne schizonts is too slow in onset for the drug to be useful in treating acute attacks. It may be administered in combination with other drugs in such cases in order to control the sexual forms of the parasite that are responsible for transmission of malaria.

Pyrimethamine may also be administered together with sulfonamides for treating chloroquine-resistant cases of *P. falciparum* malaria and for control of *Toxoplasma gondii*, the organism that causes toxoplasmosis.

Side Effects, Cautions, and Contraindications. The small doses administered once weekly for malaria suppression produce no side effects. However, the high doses required in toxoplasmosis may cause signs of folic acid deficiency to develop. Thus, blood counts are carried out, and the drug is discontinued if a drop in white blood cells or platelets is noted. Megaloblastic anemia and pancytopenia may also develop during treatment with large doses.

Anorexia, nausea and vomiting, and inflammation of the tongue (glossitis) may also occur with large doses. Massive overdosage may result in signs of C.N.S. stimulation including convulsions.

Dosage and Administration. For malaria prophylaxis an oral dose of 25 mg is taken once weekly. For transmission control 25 to 50 mg is taken for two days together with a faster-acting agent that controls the blood forms responsible for the acute attack. In toxoplasmosis 50 to 75 mg is administered daily for one to three weeks together with a sulfonamide drug. Treatment may then be continued for several more weeks at about one half this dose.

STIBOPHEN U.S.P. (Fuadin)

Actions and Indications. This trivalent antimonial is considered a useful chemotherapeutic agent for schistosomiasis, despite its potential toxicity. It is most effective against infestations by the blood fluke *S. haematobium*, not as reliable against *S. mansoni*; and least successful against *S. japonicum*, the most resistant species of this parasite.

Side Effects, Cautions, and Contraindications. Nausea, vomiting, and diarrhea are common reactions. Fever, persistent joint pains, and proteinuria may be signs of hypersensitivity to antimony that require discontinuance of therapy with this metal and use of a substitute schistocomicide such as lucanthone.

Patients are watched for purpura or other signs of thrombocytopenia and hemolytic anemia. The drug is contraindicated in patients with severe cardiac, kidney, or liver disease.

Dosage and Administration. The drug is administered intramuscularly in a small initial dose that is gradually raised in accordance with a variety of dosage schedules that vary with the patients' tolerance and the resistance of the pathogenic parasite. A 6.3 percent solution is available which is injected in amounts of between about 2 to 6 ml daily in courses of varying length.

SURAMIN SODIUM* (Antipyrol; Germanin; Moranyl; Naphuride; and others)

Actions and Indications. This complex urea derivative has both filaricidal and trypanocidal properties. In filariasis caused by *Onchocerca*, this drug is given to kill the adult worms after treatment with the less toxic diethylcarbamazine has caused disappearance of the microfilariae.

In the early stages of infection by *Trypanosoma gambiense* and *T. rhodiense*, suramin may eliminate the protozoal parasite. Similarly, its prolonged presence in the blood after a single dose often offers protection against infection for two or three months. However, it is not effective in cases in which this pathogen has spread to the central nervous system.

Side Effects, Cautions, and Contraindications. The most common of varied early reactions to this drug include acute urticaria and other pruritic dermatoses, nausea, abdominal pain, and fever. Rarely, circulatory collapse and coma may develop shortly after intravenous injection in highly sensitive individuals. Later reactions include lacrimation and edematous swelling of periocular tissues, skin rashes, and paresthesia or hyperesthesia.

The drug is contraindicated in patients with renal disorders, and the urine of all patients is examined for the presence of blood, protein, and casts.

* This drug is not available by proprietary name in this country but it may be obtained from the Parasitic Disease Drug Service, Atlanta, Ga.

Dosage and Administration. In trypanosomiasis and onchocerciasis 1 g is administered by slow I.V. injection of a 10 percent solution in warm distilled water. Various course schedules are suggested, but the total dose ranges between no more than 5 to 10 g.

TRYPARSAMIDE U.S.P.

Actions and Indications. This organic arsenical is capable of penetrating into the central nervous system and destroying the protozoal parasite *Trepanosoma gambiense* or the spirochete *Treponema pallida*. Thus, it has long been employed for treating African sleeping sickness with C.N.S. involvement and in cases of neurosyphilis resistant to other treatments. However, it is being replaced by less toxic drugs such as melarsoprol, which is active against *T. rhodiense* as well as *T. gambiense*, and by procaine penicillin G in central nervous system syphilis.

Side Effects, Cautions, and Contraindications. Typical organic arsenical toxicity occurs fairly frequently. Such reactions affect mainly the skin (dermatoses and angioneurotic reactions) and the gastrointestinal tract (nausea, vomiting, abdominal pain, diarrhea, and possible liver damage). Most serious is the danger of optic nerve damage which can result in blindness. The patient's vision is examined before, after, and during treatment. If signs of visual impairment are noted, or the patient complains of persistent subjective visual symptoms, the drug must be promptly discontinued.

Dosage and Administration. A dose of 2–3 g is administered by vein about once weekly up to a total dose of 20 to 45 g.

References

Bruce-Chwatt, L. J. Changing tides of chemotherapy of malaria. *Brit. Med. J.*, 1:581, 1964.

Di Palma, J. R. Drugs for malaria. *RN*, 30:77, 1967 (Jan.).

Gabriel, H. S. Beware those jet-borne diseases. *RN*, 30:37, 1967 (April).

Hoskins, D. W., and Kean, B. H. Drugs for travelers. *Clin. Pharmacol. Ther.*, 4:673, 1963.

Huff, C. G. Man against malaria. *Amer J. Trop. Med.*, 14:339, 1965.

Most, H. The pendulum in malaria chemotherapy: From quinine to chloroquine and back to quinine? *Milit. Med.*, 129:587, 1964.

Powell, R. D. The chemotherapy of malaria. *Clin. Pharmacol. Ther.*, 7:48, 1966.

———, et al. Studies on a strain of choroquine-resistant Plasmodium falciparum from Vietnam. *Bull. WHO*, 31:379, 1964.

44.

The Chemotherapy of Amebiasis and of Intestinal Helminthiasis

Amebiasis

Amebiasis, a condition caused by the protozoan organism, *Entamoeba histolytica*, is endemic in tropical lands. However, contrary to popular opinion, amebic infection is not limited to the tropics but may develop wherever sanitary conditions are substandard. In this country, the intestinal disease sometimes spreads among patients in mental hospitals or in institutions for elderly patients or children. Although the condition is most common in the rural South, epidemics also occur in metropolitan areas.

People who have been infected with this organism react in several different ways:

1. Some may show no symptoms at all. However, these *asymptomatic* individuals may sometimes serve as carriers of the disease.

2. Some may have only relatively mild intestinal symptoms such as flatulence or loose stools. Mild diarrhea episodes may develop periodically during a prolonged *chronic* course in which the disease lies largely dormant.

3. Some may develop *acute amebic dysentery* with bowel movements so frequent and severe that these patients quickly become dehydrated. Death from prostration may result in a few days from uncontrolled acute diarrhea. On the other hand, patients may survive but suffer intestinal wall ulcerations and scarring that results in a *chronic amebic colitis* which is difficult to treat.

4. Some patients may suffer *extra*intestinal amebiasis, including *amebic hepatitis* and *liver abscess*. This occurs when amebae make

their way through the intestinal wall and are carried by the blood stream to the liver, brain, lungs, and other organs, which are then invaded and damaged.

The Chemotherapy of Amebiasis

Many drugs are available that can control infection by the parasitic protozoan, *E. histolytica*. However, not all are equally effective and safe. Thus, the doctor must choose the drug or drug combination that is best for each patient. This depends, in part, upon the severity of the disease and upon the extent to which the intestinal forms of the organism have invaded the extraintestinal tissues and damaged them.

In order to understand the usefulness and limitation of the various chemotherapeutic agents available, we should know something of the nature of this pathogenic ameba and the changes that it undergoes during its life cycle in the body of the human host.

LIFE CYCLE OF THE AMEBA

The life cycle of *E. histolytica* takes place in two stages: (1) a cyst form, and (2) a trophozoite phase.

The *cyst stage* is the one in which the organism is transmitted from one person to another. This form is very resistant to the outside environment, and is able to survive for several weeks when it is passed in the feces of infected individuals. The amebic cysts may then be picked up by other individuals who ingest them in contaminated food and drink.

Infected food handlers who are themselves free of symptoms (*asymptomatic carriers*) may spread the cysts if they fail to wash their hands thoroughly after going to the toilet. Flies moving from filth to food are another common source of amebic contamination. The swallowed cysts also resist destruction by acid gastric juices and pass down to lower levels of the small intestine, where they break out of the cystic wall and divide to form trophozoites.

The *trophozite stage* is the form that is active and sometimes damaging to intestinal and extraintestinal tissues. These motile trophozoites move down into the colon and rectum where they produce large colonies. They sometimes invade the intestinal wall and even penetrate it, accounting both for the intestinal symptoms of acute amebiasis and for the damage often done to *extra*intestinal

organs. Trophozoites in the intestine may also return to the cyst stage and be passed in the patient's feces, thus continuing the chain of person-to-person transmission.

ANTIAMEBIC AGENTS

Antiamebic agents are most effective against the trophozoite stage. Even when they work to eradicate amebic cysts, these drugs do so mainly by wiping out the trophozoites in the intestine before they can change to the resistant cystic form.

Some drugs are poorly absorbed when taken orally. Thus, they reach effective chemotherapeutic concentrations in the large intestine but not in extraintestinal tissues. These drugs are useful only for treating the intestinal forms of the disease. Other drugs are absorbed almost completely from the upper part of the intestine. These reach effective concentrations in extraintestinal tissues but not in the lower parts of the intestinal tract.

Most therapeutic regimens for managing amebiasis make use of combinations of chemotherapeutic agents in order to strike at the pathogenic organism in both intestinal and extraintestinal sites. Recently, however, certain new antiamebic drugs have been tried singly for eradicating *E. histolytica* both in the intestinal tract and elsewhere in the body. *Metronidazole+* (Flagyl), an antiprotozoal chemical, which was until recently established only as a drug of choice in the treatment of vaginitis caused by the protozoan parasite *Trichomonas vaginalis*, is now also being employed for treating all forms of amebiasis.

Treatment of the various clinical stages of amebiasis differs, and doctors in different parts of the world also often prefer dissimilar drug regimens. It is therefore difficult to indicate specific treatment schedules for each stage of amebiasis that all authorities agree to be best. Nevertheless, certain principles of amebiasis chemotherapy are well established, and these will be emphasized in the following discussion of the management of amebic infections of different types of degrees of severity.

ACUTE AMEBIC DYSENTERY

This is best treated by the safest drugs capable of controlling the invasive trophozoites. Sometimes a broad-spectrum antibiotic such as *oxytetracycline*, *chlortetracycline*, or *paromomycin* affords adequate symptomatic relief for moderately severe cases. These relatively safe agents may be administered together with or in alternate courses with one of the organic iodides such as *diiodohydroxyquin+* or an arsenical such as *carbarsone+*. The two latter types of chemotherapeutic agents are effective against trophozoites in the intestine, but not enough of these drugs is absorbed to be useful elsewhere.

Emetine+ and *dehyroemetine* are reserved for treating patients whose severe dysentery does not respond to treatment with antibiotics or iodine and arsenical compounds, and for those with extraintestinal infections (see below). These drugs, which are injected and carried by the bloodstream to both the intestinal wall and the extraintestinal tissues, are very effective against trophozoites. They give quick relief of such acute symptoms as bloody diarrhea, colicky abdominal pain from intestinal spasm, and tenesmus (involuntary straining and anal sphincter spasm). However, emetine and its derivative are very toxic drugs that can cause severe heart damage and aching pain at the injection sites. Thus, patients being treated with emetine are hospitalized and kept at rest in bed.

Taking the patient's pulse and blood pressure several times daily during a course of treatment with emetine is a nursing responsibility. If tachycardia occurs or the patient's pressure falls, the nurse should report this to the doctor, who may then order electrocardiographic tracings. The appearance of ECG abnormalities together with a rise in pulse rate of over 110 beats per minute may require emetine medication to be discontinued. Sometimes the drug's ill effects on the heart develop late; therefore patients are warned not to exert themselves for weeks after a course of therapy is completed.

The nurse should discuss with the doctor his specific recommendations in regard to how much activity the patient can safely undertake following a course of emetine treatment. She can then instruct the patient on how he should plan his activities, with something more specific than a vague "you'll have to take it easy for a while." The patient should also be warned to report promptly any symptoms that he experiences during the posttreatment period.

Metronidazole+ (Flagyl) may prove to be the drug of choice for treating acute amebic dysentery. It has two main advantages over emetine: (1) its safety; and (2) its greater effectiveness in *curing* intestinal amebiasis.

(Emetine does *not* often *cure* the disease, because safe doses do not wipe out all the trophozoites in the bowel.) Metronidazole also differs from diiodohydroxyquin and other intestinal amebicides in a way that is advantageous—it is absorbed from the intestine and reaches high enough concentrations in the liver to be effective in amebic hepatitis (see below).

AMEBIC HEPATITIS AND LIVER ABSCESS

These dangerous complications of extraintestinal amebiasis were, until recently, treated with one of only two available drugs, *emetine+* and *chloroquine* (Aralen), a much safer drug than emetine. Administered by mouth, chloroquine is absorbed from the upper intestinal tract and carried to the liver, where it readily reaches amebicidal concentrations. Effective doses have so little systemic toxicity that chloroquine is often administered routinely even to *asymptomatic* patients for prophylaxis against extraintestinal amebiasis (see below). Although absorption is best from an empty stomach, chloroquine can be given with meals when patients complain of epigastric distress.

The main drawback of chloroquine is that it fails to reach the lower intestine in large enough amounts to be effective for treating intestinal amebiasis. Thus, to prevent possible recurrences, chloroquine—like emetine—must always be given together with one of the intestinal amebicides such as *diiodohydroxyquin+* or *carbarsone+* that are effective against amebic trophozoites and cysts within the colon.

Recently, the administration of *metronidazole+* (Flagyl) has been recommended as a single agent for treating amebic hepatitis. Unlike chloroquine, this antiprotozoal agent *is* effective for treating intestinal amebiasis (see above) and, unlike the intestinal amebicides, metronidazole *is* systematically absorbed. Thus, this drug reaches chemotherapeutically effective concentrations in the liver when administered in safe oral doses. Its advantages over emetine in terms of greater safety and effectiveness against intestinal trophozoites and cysts have been mentioned above.

ASYMPTOMATIC CARRIERS (TABLE 44-1)

Asymptomatic carriers and *chronic mild cases* that show only occasional flare-ups of

TABLE 44-1 *Drugs for Treating Amebiasis*

Nonproprietary or Official Name	Proprietary Name or Synonym	Chemical Class	Dosage and Administration	Remarks
Arsthinol	Balarsen	Trivalent organic arsenical	10 mg/kg orally up to 500 mg maximum daily	For intestinal amebiasis
Bialamicol HCl	Camoform	Complex organic compound	250–500 mg orally three times daily	Mainly intestinal action but possibly also effective against extra-intestinal forms
Carbarsone N.F.	. . . .	Pentavalent organic arsenical	250 mg orally b.i.d. or t.i.d. for ten days	For intestinal amebiasis (see *Drug Digest*)
Chlorbetamide	Mantomide	Dichloroacetamide compound	750 mg orally t.i.d. for one week	Experimental for intestinal forms; less toxic than the arsenicals
Chiniofon	Yatren	Iodinated hydroxyquinoline	750 mg orally t.i.d. for one or two weeks	For intestinal amebiasis it is less toxic than the arsenicals
Chloroquine phosphate U.S.P.	Aralen	4-Aminoquinoline antimalarial	250 mg orally q.i.d. for two days; then 250 mg b.i.d. for two weeks	Safe and effective for treatment, prevention, and diagnosis of hepatic amebiasis
Chlorphenoxamide	Mebinol	Dichloroacetamide compound	500 mg orally t.i.d. for ten days	Experimental drug for intestinal amebiasis
Dehydroemetine	. . . .	Analog of emetine	80 mg daily I.M. or s.c. for ten days	Alternative to emetine for acute amebic dysentery and for extra-intestinal amebiasis, including amebic hepatitis and abscess
Diiodohydroxyquin U.S.P.	Diodoquin	Iodinated hydroxyquinoline	650 mg orally t.i.d. for three weeks	For intestinal amebiasis (see *Drug Digest*)

Drug	Trade name	Chemical class	Dosage	Remarks
Diloxanide furoate	Furamide	Acetanilid derivative	500 mg orally t.i.d. for ten days	For intestinal amebiasis including carriers as well as acute cases
Emetine HCl U.S.P.	. . . .	Ipecac alkaloid	30–60 mg daily I.M. or deep s.c. for ten days	For acute amebic dysentery and extraintestinal amebiasis (see *Drug Digest*)
Erythromycin U.S.P.	Erythrocin; Ilotycin	Antibiotic	1 to 2 g orally in three divided daily doses for ten days	Intestinal amebicide (See *Drug Digest*, Chapter 43)
Fumagillin	Fumidil	Antibiotic	40 mg daily in four divided oral doses for ten days	Withdrawn from use in the U.S. because of toxicity
Glycobiarsol N.F.	Milibis	Pentavalent organic arsenical combined with bismuth	500 mg orally t.i.d. for seven to ten days (also by suppository for vaginitis)	For intestinal amebiasis treatment and prevention
Iodochlorhydroxyquin N.F.	Entero-Vioform	Iodinated hydroxyquinoline	250 mg orally t.i.d. or q.i.d. for ten days	For intestinal amebiasis treatment. Optic nerve toxicity has been reported
Metronidazole U.S.P.	Flagyl	Nitroimidazole derivative	400–500 mg orally t.i.d. for five days	Established trichomonacide employed experimentally for both intestinal and extraintestinal forms of amebiasis (see *Drug Digest*)
Paromomycin sulfate N.F.	Humatin	Antibiotic	25 mg/kg orally in three divided doses with meals for five days	For intestinal amebiasis and for bacterial diarrhea
Phanquone	Entobex	Phenanthroline-quinone compound	500 mg orally t.i.d. for seven to ten days	For intestinal amebiasis of acute and chronic types
Tetracyclines (for example, oxytetracycline)	Various (for example, Terramycin)	Antibiotic	250 mg orally q.i.d. for ten days	For intestinal amebiasis and against secondary bacterial infections

intestinal symptoms are best treated with agents that are relatively free of side effects. After a person has been found to be an asymptomatic cyst passer, it is often difficult to convince him that he should receive drug treatment. Obviously, he will be quick to discontinue any drug that causes more discomforting side effects than the symptomless disorder he is told that he has.

Diiodohydroxyquin+ (Diodoquin) is a common choice for such patients because of its relative freedom from disturbing side effects. It is sometimes alternated with a course of *carbarsone*+ or other arsenical for treating mild chronic cases of intestinal amebiasis. *Chloroquine* prophylaxis is also often administered routinely in such cases, because some people who have never had diarrhea or other intestinal symptoms may suddenly develop amebic hepatitis as a result of trophozoite invasion from the intestine. *Metronidazole*+ may, in time, also turn out to be the single agent of choice for treating such asymptomatic carriers and mild chronic cases of intestinal amebiasis.

The nurse should encourage carriers to continue with drug therapy. The benefits to the individual should be stressed, together with the need to protect his family and coworkers. The nurse employed in industry, schools, and other institutions should teach the necessity for thorough hand-washing and recommend that all washrooms—especially those used by food handlers—be equipped with plenty of soap and towels.

Travelers in areas where amebiasis and other intestinal infections are endemic often take drugs such as diiodohydroxyquine to prevent diarrhea. This practice may be unwise because its effectiveness has not been proven, and this class of drugs may occasionally cause severe toxicity. For example, recent reports indicate that *iodochlorhydroxyquin* (Entero-Vioform), a drug commonly taken as a prophylactic against "traveler's diarrhea," can cause peripheral and central nerve cell damage. Inflammation and atrophy of the optic nerve has reportedly occurred in some individuals treated with this seemingly safe drug.

Helminthiasis

Helminthiasis, invasion of the human body by parasitic worms, is prevalent throughout the world. An estimated billion human beings are believed to harbor helminths of one kind or another. In some tropical countries more than 90 percent of the population plays host to worms. Helminthiasis is not, however, limited to tropical climates. A recent survey of hospital employees in New York City revealed that nearly one in three had parasites in his intestine. The number of Americans with pinworms is estimated at some 20 million, and several million more are infected with roundworms and other helminths.

In this section, we shall discuss the drug treatment of infection by those worms that can be readily reached by drugs acting within the intestine. The treatment of certain helminthic invaders of extraintestinal tissues, such as the blood flukes, or trematodes, is taken up in Chapter 43. Here, we shall be concerned mainly with the nematodes (round, unsegmented worms) and, to a lesser extent, with the playtyhelminths (flatworms) of the tapeworm, or cestode, type.

The nematodes of medical interest are the following (1) *Enterobius vermicularis*—also called oxyuriads—which we shall call by their common name, pinworms; (2) *Ascaris lumbricoides*, the roundworm; (3) *Strongyloides stercoralis*, the cause of the infection called strongyloidiasis, or threadworm disease; (4) *Trichuris trichiura*, the whipworm, and (5) two species of hookworm, *Necator americanus* and *Ancylostoma duodenale*.

Four species of tapeworm are involved in common infestations: (1) *Taenia saginata*, the beef tapeworm; (2) *Taenia solium*, the pork tapeworm, (3) *Diphyllobrothium latum*; the fish tapeworm; and (4) *Hymenolepis nana*, the dwarf tapeworm.

Anthelmintic Drug Therapy

Anthelmintics are drugs used to treat worm infestations (see Table 44-2). Drugs that act to expel worms from the intestinal tract are available for oral use. However, the drugs differ in their effectiveness against the various species of these parasites.

Thus, in order to choose the best drug for treating a particular patient, the doctor must often first get a stool specimen to send to the laboratory. From this or from blood, urine, or other materials obtained from the patient's body, the parasitologist can usually help the doctor to arrive at a correct diagnosis.

Once the doctor determines the type of worm involved, he selects the safest and most effective anthelmintic available for eliminating that specific parasite. Sometimes, for most efficient use of this medication, other measures must also be employed before or after administration of the anthelmintic. The nurse should be aware of the various specialized procedures and other adjunctive measures that are often part of the total diagnostic and treatment regimen in managing helminthiasis.

Common worm infestations that require anthelmintic medication are pinworms, roundworms, and whipworms. Less frequent but sometimes more serious are threadworm, hookworm, and tapeworm invasions. Trichinosis has its start in the intestine but treatment is mainly centered outside of the gut. We shall discuss the drug treatment of each of these conditions.

TABLE 44-2 *Anthelmintic Drugs*

Nonproprietary, Generic, or Official Name	Proprietary Name or Synonym	Oral Dosage Schedule	Remarks Concerning Therapeutic Uses
Aspidium oleoresin	Male fern	1–5 g	Rarely used because of its toxicity and availability of safer drugs for treating beef, pork, and fish tapeworms
Bephenium hydroxynaphthoate	Alcopara	5 g b.i.d. for one to three days	Used in hookworm infections. It is especially effective against *Ancylostoma*, but is also useful for *Necator* infections. It is also useful for mixed infestations with roundworms
Dichlorophen	Antiphen	2 to 3 g every eight hours for three doses	Taenicide particularly effective in tapeworm infestations by *T. saginata*
Dithiazanine iodide	Delvex	100–200 mg t.i.d. for varying periods	A broad-spectrum anthelmintic withdrawn from use in U.S. because of its potential toxicity
Hexylresorcinal N.F.	Crystoids	1 g taken on an empty stomach; for children 600–800 mg	Mainly for roundworm infestations. Occasionally for trichuriasis (whipworms) and in mixed infestations with hookworms or dwarf tapeworms (see *Drug Digest*)
Niclosemide	Yomesan	Two doses of 1 g taken one hour apart; for children two doses of 250–500 mg	For large and dwarf tapeworm infestation especially *Taenia saginata* and *T. solium*
Piperazine salts (for example, citrate U.S.P., phosphate, tartrate, adipate, and calcium edetate)	Antepar; Perin; Pipizan; Piperate; Entacyl; and others	For pinworm, single daily doses of up to 2 g for seven days. For roundworm, single daily doses of up to 3.5 g for two consecutive days	Drug of choice for roundworms; also very effective against pinworms (see *Drug Digest*)
Pyrantel pamoate	Antiminth	1 cc of suspension per 10 lbs. of body weight	For roundworm or pinworm infestations

TABLE 44-2 *Anthelmintic Drugs (continued)*

Nonproprietary, Generic, or Official Name	Proprietary Name or Synonym	Oral Dosage Schedule	Remarks Concerning Therapeutic Uses
Pyrvinium pamoate U.S.P.	Povan; Vanquin	For pinworm, a single dose of 5 mg/kg of body weight is administered and repeated in one or two weeks; for threadworms, five to seven daily doses	Highly effective for pinworm infestations. A bright red dye that may stain clothing and stools (see *Drug Digest*)
Quinacrine HCl	Atabrine	800 mg in two, four, or eight divided doses at intervals of a few minutes; for children 400 to 600 mg in similarly divided doses	A drug of choice for tapeworm infestations. (see *Drug Digest*)
Stilbazium iodide	Monopar	50 mg/kg of body weight once daily for one to three days	On trial for broad-spectrum anthelmintic effects against roundworm, pinworm, threadworm, and whip-worm
Triclofenol piperazine	Ranestol	50 mg/kg of body weight in a single daily dose or divided into two doses administered on successive days	On trial against roundworms and hookworms, particularly *Necator americanus*
Tetramisole MCl	Anthelvet	2.5 mg/kg of body weight	On trial against roundworms
Tetrachloroethylene U.S.P.	. . . .	Single dose of 0.2 ml/kg up to a total of 5 ml	Drug of choice for *Necator americanus* infestations; also useful for other hookworms (see *Drug Digest*)
Thiabendazole U.S.P.	Mintezol	25 mg/kg of body weight twice daily after meals to a maximum total dose of 3 g	Drug of choice against *Strongyloides stercoralis* (threadworm) and cutaneous larva migrans (creeping eruption); also effective against roundworms, hookworms, and pinworms. (see *Drug Digest*)

PINWORMS

Pinworms, or seatworms, are the most common cause of intestinal helminthiasis in school children. Fortunately, they are also the worms least likely to cause serious complications. Itching in the anal area may be the only symptom. Thus, application of an antipruritic cream or ointment may sometimes be the only treatment measure employed in light pinworm infestations.

On the other hand, it is usually desirable to treat the disorder with specific anthelmintic drugs to remove the worms, as heavier infestations may lead to development of discomforting symptoms such as abdominal pain, weight loss, and insomnia. Several safe and effective drugs are available for this purpose, including particularly *piperazine citrate+*, *pyrvinium pamoate+*, and *pyrantel pamoate*.

All are easy to take, and, indeed, a single

dose of *pyrvinium* usually eradicates all the pinworms. Actually, however, most authorities still seem to favor the use of *piperazine citrate*, which requires a one-week treatment course. This may be because the need to take a dose of this drug every day for a week may help to emphasize the fact that the child is suffering from a condition requiring special treatment and prevention measures.

The main difficulty in dealing with pinworm infestations is the ease with which children become reinfected and spread the organism to others in the family. Thus, in addition to drug therapy, it is important to teach the parent hygienic measures that help to avoid reinfection. These include the following:

1. Keeping the child's nails cut short and his hands well scrubbed, since reinfection results from the worm's eggs being carried back to the mouth after becoming lodged under the fingernails during scratching of the pruritic perianal area.

2. Giving the child a shower in the morning to wash away any ova deposited in the anal area during the night.

3. Disinfecting toilet seats daily and the floors of bathroom and bedroom periodically.

The measures required to prove that the patient is completely cured involve swabbing of the anal area with Scotch tape until no eggs are found on a microscope slide for seven consecutive mornings.

ROUNDWORMS

Roundworm infestation may produce no symptoms at all in many people. Yet, they are potentially so serious that doctors feel it desirable to treat any person who passes even a single worm. Even one worm may do damage in its migrations about the body, and the masses of worms likely to be produced from fertilized eggs may cause intestinal and respiratory tract obstruction.

This is especially true in children since they are prone to become feverish, and the worms, which are sensitive to changes in body temperature, may then be stirred into activity. During such movements, the worms may block the bile duct or appendix or even occasionally break into the abdominal cavity and cause peritonitis. Thus, to avoid these and other rare but possible complications such as liver or lung abscesses, drug treatment must be promptly undertaken.

Fortunately, the roundworm is very susceptible to the paralyzing action of piperazine. Administered daily for a week, this relatively safe and easy-to-take chemical quickly clears the intestinal tract of these worms, which are readily swept out with the fecal stream even without the aid of a laxative.

Occasionally, in some areas patients are infected with other worms as well as with roundworms. In such cases, it is important that the roundworms be removed before trying to eradicate the other parasites. This is because anthelmintic medications such as *tetrachlorethylene*+, which is used against hookworms, may activate the roundworms to make the kind of migrations that can lead to dangerous complications. *Hexylresorcinol*+ is sometimes preferred in such cases, since it is capable of eliminating *both* roundworms and hookworms.

THREADWORMS

Strongyloides persistently infests the upper gastrointestinal tract and resembles hookworm in its capacity to cause weight loss and debility. Strongyloidiasis is seen in the southern United States as well as in the tropics. Light infection that results in no symptoms requires no treatment. However, heavily infected patients, such as those sometimes seen in mental hospitals and other institutions, are treated to avoid development of malabsorption syndromes as well as for relief of diarrhea and upper abdominal discomfort.

Treatment of this disorder has been difficult in the past. The dye, *gentian violet*, often gave symptomatic relief but was not satisfactory as a cure for the condition. A newer drug, *dithiazanine*, is highly effective for eliminating threadworms from the intestine. Unfortunately, its potential toxicity upon systemic absorption led to this drug's being withdrawn from use in the United States. *Thiabendazole*+ (Mintezol), a recently introduced broad-spectrum antibiotic, appears to be very promising. It is claimed to be effective in more than 95 percent of threadworm cases.

WHIPWORMS

Whipworms are tiny threadlike parasites that become engaged in the mucosa of the cecum but rarely burrow deeper. No treatment is necessary in lightly infected patients, and drugs may even be withheld in many cases marked by only mild, occasional diarrhea. However, if the infection is a heavy one with many eggs in the stool and prolapse of the rectum, the doctor may undertake treatment with dithiazanine or *hexylresorcinol+*.

Hexylresorcinol, the less toxic agent, may be given by mouth and by rectum simultaneously. Because the concentrated drug is irritating, patients are told not to chew the pills, and precautions are taken to prevent burns of the skin, buttocks, and thighs. The mucus secreted in response to the presence of masses of attached worms protects the rectal membranes from irritation by a 1:500 retention enema, to which kaolin is added to reduce colonic cramps. Petroleum jelly is applied to protect the skin from the irritating effects of any solution that may leak during the retention period of two or three hours.

HOOKWORMS

Hookworm infection, though less common in the United States than it once was, is one of the world's most common helminthic diseases. Heavy infestations are debilitating, because the worms not only damage intestinal mucosa but cause an iron-deficiency anemia, with symptoms such as chronic fatigue and apathy. Such patients require treatment with oral or parenteral iron salts or even prompt transfusion of whole blood or packed red cells. Correction of fluid and electrolyte imbalance is desirable before administration of anthelmintic drug therapy.

Infection with *Necator americanus*, the organism most common in the Western hemisphere, is readily controlled by treatment with *tetrachloroethylene+* taken in the morning following a fasting period or no more than a fat-free, largely liquid meal the night before. The drug is safe, inexpensive, and effective in four out of five cases. In cases in which the presence of roundworms is suspected, tetrachloroethylene is given only after the roundworms have been eliminated.

Tetrachloroethylene is not nearly so effective in hookworm infections caused by the so-called Old World hookworm, *Ancylostoma duodenale*. For treating infections by this organism a new agent, *bephenium hydroxynaphthoate*, is now preferred. This drug is almost equally effective in *Necator americanus* infections and can be given in cases complicated by the presence of roundworms, which it also readily removes. The new agent is nontoxic and requires no preliminary fasting or posttreatment purging.

The drug's only drawback seems to be a bitter taste which requires partial masking in order to avoid gagging and possible nausea and vomiting.

TAPEWORMS

Tapeworms are segmented flatworms, consisting of a scolex, or head, which attaches itself to the intestinal wall, and a variable number of segments that grow from the head, sometimes forming a worm several yards long. However, the presence of lengthy beef or fish tapeworms is not truly serious. The patient may have some mild abdominal symptoms and suffer some weight loss occasionally, but treatment is sought more for psychological than physical reasons. That is, the patient may be frightened by finding worm segments in his stool, even though their passage causes little discomfort.

The pork tapeworm, which is rare in this country, can, however, cause a more serious condition called cysticercosis. In such cases, the larval form of the worm makes its way into the bloodstream and may be carried to the muscles, lungs, liver, or brain. Since no specific treatment is available for cysticercosis, it is important to remove the adult worm while it is in the intestinal tract. The once widely used vermifuge, oleoresin of aspidium, has been largely replaced for this purpose by the safer synthetic chemotherapeutic agent, *quinacrine+*.

Whichever drug is employed to make the head of the worm loosen its hold on the intestinal wall, it is desirable to empty the patient's intestine first, in order to ensure contact between the chemical and the scolex. Drug treatment is followed by a saline purge and careful examination of all stool specimens until the worm is evacuated. Identification of the head of the worm is relatively easy after treatment with quinacrine, which stains the scolex a bright yellow.

TRICHINOSIS

Trichinosis is infection with the worm *Trichinella spiralis* and is caused by eating raw or poorly cooked pork containing the encysted larvae. Although the adult worms develop in the duodenum, the main damage is done by larvae that make their way through the intestine into the bloodstream to skeletal muscles where they induce inflammatory reactions.

Corticosteroid drugs have been used to counteract the acute inflammatory reactions caused by larval invasion of the tissues. No chemotherapeutic agent has proved effective for killing the larvae. *Thiabendazole+* is said to relieve symptoms in some patients, but its effect upon larvae that have already migrated to muscles remains uncertain at this time.

S U M M A R Y of the Adverse Effects of Anthelmintic Drugs

Aspidium oleoresin

Nausea, vomiting, bloody diarrhea; visual abnormalities

C.N.S. toxicity, including tremors, tonic convulsions, coma, and respiratory failure

Bephenium hydroxynaphthoate

Occasional nausea, vomiting, and diarrhea, but no serious systemic toxicity

Dichlorophen

Nausea, diarrhea and colic

Its use in Taenia solium infestations may lead to cystercercosis (larval invasion as a result of liberation of ova by the disintegrating worms)

Dithiazanine iodide

Nausea, vomiting, cramps and diarrhea

Systemic absorption, especially in patients with kidney disease, has caused death following development of acidosis and circulatory collapse

Hexylrescorcinol (see *Drug Digest*)

Gastric irritation may cause epigastric distress

Chewing the pills can release concentrated solution that may burn the mucous membranes of the mouth

Niclosemide

A few adverse effects, except for occasional nausea and abdominal pains

Piperazine salts (see *Drug Digest*)

Occasional nausea, vomiting, abdominal cramps, and diarrhea

Rarely, transient dizziness, blurring of vision, vertigo, tremors, and muscle weakness

Skin rash—redness and uticaria, rarely

Pryantel pamoate

Anorexia, nausea, vomiting, abdominal cramps, diarrhea, tenesmus

Pyrvinium pamoate (see *Drug Digest*)

Nausea, vomiting, abdominal cramps, diarrhea; rarely, photosensitization skin reactions

Quinacrine HCl (see *Drug Digest*)

Nausea and vomiting; dizziness; hallucinations and delusions (toxic psychosis)

Tetrachlorethylene (see *Drug Digest*)

Nausea, vomiting, epigastric burning, abdominal cramps, diarrhea, headache, dizziness, drowsiness, giddiness

Thiabenzadole (see *Drug Digest*)

Anorexia, nausea, vomiting, diarrhea

Drowsiness, dizziness, giddiness, and headache

S U M M A R Y of the Adverse Effects of Drugs Used in Amebiasis

Antibiotics (see *Summary*, p. 516, Chapter 41)

Carbarsone (see *Drug Digest*)

Nausea, vomiting, epigastric distress, diarrhea

Pruritic skin eruptions (rarely, arsenical exfoliation)

Visual disturbances (contractions of visual field and color changes)

Rare arsenical encephalopathy (mental changes coma, convulsions)

Rare liver function changes with possible damage and necrosis

Chloroquine (see also Chapter 43)

Loss of appetite, abdominal distress and cramps, nausea and vomiting
Headache, restlessness, sleeplessness
Skin eruptions
Visual disturbances (blurring of vision)

Diiodohydroxyquin (see *Drug Digest)* **and Iodochlorhydroxyquin**

Flatulence, abdominal distress, nausea and vomiting
Headache, dizziness
Skin eruptions and pruritus ani
Iodism and interference with tests of thyroid function
Rarely, peripheral neuropathy, including optic neuritis and atrophy; also, spinal cord demyelination

Emetine (see *Drug Digest*) **and Dehydroemetine**

Cardiotoxicity—chest pains, tachycardia, electrocardiographic changes (T wave abnormalities; prolonged Q-T interval)
Hypotension, dyspnea
Nausea, vomiting, diarrhea, epigastric distress
Muscular weakness, aching, and stiffness, especially in the region of deep subcutaneous injections
Headache, dizziness, faintness
Skin eruptions

Metronidazole (see *Drug Digest*)

Unpleasant metallic taste, loss of appetite, nausea and vomiting, epigastric distress, abdominal cramps, diarrhea

---

S U M M A R Y of Points for the Nurse to Remember Concerning Helminthiasis Treatment

Remember to instruct the patient and family in measures to help prevent pinworm reinfection, such as careful handwashing after using the toilet, and keeping the fingernails short.

Be consistent in applying necessary hygienic measures for preventing spread of worms from one person to another. However, in emphasizing the need to use such precautions, do not convey a punitive attitude nor imply that you are afraid of acquiring the infection.

Although some worm infestations are more physically harmful than others, all can be humiliating to the patient. Show the patient, by your manner when caring for him, that you ac-

cept his illness, and that you are willing to care for him.

Suggest measures for allaying itching of the anal region, such as gentle cleansing followed by application of antipruritic ointments. These are likely to prove more effective in reducing scratching than merely reminding the patient not to scratch.

Remember to warn patients to take anthelmintic drugs as directed, in order to get rid of the worms and to prevent their spread to other persons. Warn them also of any possible fecal discolorations, in order to avoid unnecessary concern, and advise them to keep these medications out of the reach of children.

S U M M A R Y of Points for the Nurse to Remember Concerning Amebiasis Treatment

Teach carriers of amebic cysts the need to wash hands thoroughly after visiting the toilet. Recommend that washrooms of schools, factories, and institutions be stocked with soap and towels as an aid to prevention of spread of infection.

Encourage carriers to continue with drug therapy by stressing the benefits to themselves, family, and coworkers rather than by adopting a punitive attitude.

Take special care in administering emetine to see that injections are made in a manner

that will prevent local and systemic reactions. For example, rotate injection sites. Aspirate carefully, to avoid intravenous injection.

See that the patient on emetine therapy stays in bed; observe him carefully for signs such as an increase in pulse rate or fall in blood pressure and inform the physician promptly of such symptoms.

Instruct the patient to rest in the weeks following a course of emetine treatment. Physician and nurse collaboratively assess the patient's activity tolerance.

DRUG DIGEST

CARBARSONE N.F.

Actions and Indications. This arsenical amebicide is active against both the trophozoite and cystic forms of *Entamoeba histolytica*. It is useful when administered in alternation with courses of diiodohydroxyquin in the treatment of mild to moderate diarrhea and other symptoms of acute and chronic intestinal amebiasis. It is *not* effective for *extra*intestinal amebiasis including hepatic amebiasis.

This antiprotozoal agent is also used topically in treating vaginitis caused by *Trichomonas vaginalis*.

Side Effects, Cautions, and Contraindications. This is a relatively safe arsenic compound. However, it may have cumulative toxic effects if taken in successive courses without long enough rest periods to permit its excretion. Toxicity is most common in patients with liver or kidney damage or sensitivity to arsenic, and the use of this drug is contraindicated in patients with such histories.

The most common side effects include diarrhea, nausea and vomiting, and skin rashes. Patients are observed for signs of pruritic skin eruptions and visual changes, which may call for withdrawal of the drug to avoid possible development of exfoliative dermatitis and arsenical encephalitis.

Dosage and Administration. This drug is administered orally, in adult doses of 25 mg b.i.d. or t.i.d. for ten days. A rest period of at least ten days should intervene between such courses of therapy. The total daily dosage for children is 7.5 mg per kg for ten days. This may sometimes be supplemented by a retention enema containing two g in 200 ml of a warm 2 percent solution of sodium bicarbonate.

A 250-mg suppository is employed in treating trichomonal vaginitis.

DIIODOHYDROXYQUIN U.S.P.
(Diodoquin; Floraquin)

Actions and Indications. This organic iodine compound has amebicidal and trichomonacidal properties. It is useful in intestinal amebiasis for the management of mild cases for eradicating cysts in asymptomatic carriers, and for prophylaxis in endemic areas.

Although it is effective against trophozoites in the intestinal tract, it is *not* useful for *extra*intestinal infections, including amebic hepatitis and abscess. Topical application is useful for treating vaginal infection caused by *Trichomonas vaginalis*.

Side Effects, Cautions, and Contraindications. This drug causes few systemic side effects, as only relatively small amounts are absorbed from the gastrointestinal tract. Local gastrointestinal effects may cause epigastric distress and diarrhea.

The drug is contraindicated in patients sensitive to iodine and in those with severe liver disease. Symptoms of mild iodism, including pruritic skin rashes, may require discontinuation of therapy. This drug, like other iodides, may affect the accuracy of thyroid function tests.

Dosage and Administration. Oral adult dosage for intestinal amebiasis is 650 mg t.i.d. for 20 days. This may be repeated after a rest period of two or three weeks, during which an arsenical compound such as carbarsone may be administered.

For trichomoniasis, a 250-mg tablet is inserted intravaginally each evening for 10 to 15 days.

EMETINE HCl U.S.P.

Actions and Indications. This ipecac alkaloid kills the trophozoites, or motile forms, of *Entamoeba histolytica*, both in the intestinal and extraintestinal tissues. These amebicidal effects make it useful both for treating amebic hepatitis and for controlling severe diarrhea in acute amebic dysentery. However, its routine use in mild cases of amebic dysentery or for treating asymptomatic carriers of amebic cysts is contraindicated on account of its high potential cumulative toxicity and low level of effectiveness against the cyst form of the organism.

Side Effects, Cautions, and Contraindications. The toxic effects of emetine vary from relatively mild and transient—for example, increased diarrhea, nausea and vomiting—to extremely severe and even fatal reactions. The most serious toxicity is the result of the drug's depressant effects on the myocardium. This may be marked by chest pains, tachycardia, and electrocardiographic (ECG) changes, as well as by hypotension and dyspnea in some cases. The drug is administered to patients with pre-existing heart or kidney disease only when the risk from extraintestinal amebiasis, unresponsive to any other therapy, seems warranted. It is also employed only with extreme caution in children, elderly, and disease-weakened patients.

Dosage and Administration. Emetine is administered in doses of 1 mg per kg of body weight, but in a total dose not exceeding 60 mg daily, during a course of five to ten days. Patients taking emetine are kept at rest in bed throughout the entire treatment period and are warned to avoid strenuous activity for some time after completion of the course of therapy. Rest periods of at least six weeks are required before further courses of emetine may be safely employed.

HEXYLRESORCINOL N.F.
(Crystoids)

Actions and Indications. This is an anthelmintic of relatively wide spectrum and low toxicity, which is active against roundworms, pinworms, whipworms, hookworms, and dwarf tapeworms. It is used mainly in the treatment of roundworm infections when patients cannot tolerate piperazine or when their condition fails to respond to the latter drug. Hexylresorcinol may also be especially useful for treating mixed infections by roundworms and hookworms.

Side Effects, Cautions, and Contraindications. This is a drug of low systemic toxicity. It may cause gastric irritation and distress, and it is contraindicated for patients with peptic ulcer.

Dosage and Administration. The adult oral dose is 1 g in the morning on an empty stomach. The gelatin-coated pills should be swallowed whole and not chewed, as concentrated hexylresorcinol is irritating to the mucosa of the mouth and may even cause ulcerations.

Two to four hours after taking the dose, the patient receives a saline cathartic to help remove the roundworms, He may finally eat food about five hours after the drug has been ingested. Treatment may be repeated at intervals of three days if required.

METRONIDAZOLE U.S.P. (Flagyl)

Actions and Indications. This antiprotozoal drug is used in treatment of trichomoniasis and amebiasis. In *Trichomonas vaginalis* infections, it is both applied topically and taken orally for its effects on the organisms in extravaginal areas. In amebiasis, the drug is effective both for acute intestinal infections such as amebic dysentery and for extraintestinal infections such as amebic liver abscess.

Side Effects, Cautions, and Contraindications. The most common side effects include an unpleasant metallic taste, anorexia, nausea and vomiting, epigastric distress, and abdominal cramps or diarrhea. Alcoholic beverages should be avoided as gastrointestinal discomfort, headache, and flushing may develop.

This drug is contraindicated in patients with a history of blood dyscrasias, active central nervous system disease, or in the first trimester of pregnancy.

Dosage and Administration. For trichomonias in women, oral doses of 250 mg are taken t.i.d. or only b.i.d. when supplemented by daily use of a 500-mg vaginal insert. Courses of ten days duration may be repeated after rest periods of four to six weeks. The dose for *male* patients shown to have trichomonads in the urogenital tract is 250 mg b.i.d.

The adult dose for treating acute intestinal amebiasis is 750 mg orally t.i.d.: for amebic liver abscess, oral dosage is 500 to 700 mg. Courses are from seven to ten days. The total daily dosage for children with amebiasis is 35 to 50 mg/kg orally in divided doses for ten days.

PAROMOMYCIN SULFATE N.F. (Humatin)

Actions and Indications. This antibiotic, which has a broad spectrum of antimicrobial activity, is used in the treatment and prevention of gastrointestinal infections by pathogenic bacteria and amebae. In amebiasis, it is used mainly in mild to moderately severe chronic cases with subacute or acute exacerbations, rather than for patients critically ill with acute amebic dysentery. It is not effective for treating extraintestinal amebiasis.

Paromomycin is helpful for controlling the secondary infections by bacteria which sometimes complicate intestinal amebiasis. Similarly, it is effective for control of gastroenteritis in shigellosis, salmonellosis, and other intestinal infections caused by pathogenic bacteria.

Side Effects, Cautions, and Contraindications. The possibility of overgrowths by candidal organisms and resistant staphylococci exists, as does potential nephrotoxicity in the event of systemic absorption. More common is the occurrence of nausea and increased gastrointestinal motility with loose stools or even moderately severe diarrhea. Skin

rash, headache, and vertigo may occur.

Dosage and Administration. For amebiasis a minimal daily dose of 25 mg per kg daily is administered in divided doses for at least five days. A two-week rest period is recommended between courses. In bacillary dysentery, 35 to 60 mg per kg is employed for six days or longer. Doses of 35 mg per kg are given for four consecutive days prior to bowel surgery. Hepatic coma patients may require as much as 75 mg per kg per day.

PIPERAZINE CITRATE U.S.P. (Antepar; Pipizan)

Actions and Indications. This anthelmintic is considered the preferred drug for treating infections by roundworms (ascariasis). It is also quite useful against infection by pinworms (*Enterobius* or *Oxyuris*). It acts to slow the movements of these worms or to paralyze them, but it does not kill them. This is a desirable feature, as it lessens the likelihood of reactions to absorbed foreign protein from dead worms.

Side Effects, Cautions, and Contraindications. Side effects are uncommon with ordinary doses, but urticaria may occur in hypersensitive patients, and some patients with epilepsy have reportedly had an increase in seizure activity. Thus, caution is required in such cases.

Overdosage may lead to nausea, vomiting, and diarrhea. Headache, blurring of vision, vertigo, tremors, and muscle weakness may also occur with ingestion of excessive amounts.

Dosage and Administration. The official usual dose in pinworm treatment is 50 mg per kg of body weight daily for seven days or a dose of up to 3.5 g daily. In practice, one half of a flavored tablet or of a teaspoon of syrup, 250 mg, is given to infants weighing up to 15 lbs, 1 g to those between 30 to 60 lbs, and 2 g daily to those over 60 lbs.

The official dose against roundworms is 75 mg per k for two days or 1 g for infants up to 30 lbs, 2 g for those weighing from 30–50 lbs, 3 g for those between 50 to 100 lbs. and, over 100 lbs, 3.5 g.

PYRVINIUM PAMOATE U.S.P. (Povan; Vanquin)

Actions and Indications. This salt of a cyanine dye has anthelmintic activity against a variety of worms, but is recommended specifically for the eradication of pinworms. It is so effective against these

worms that a single dose very often is enough to cure oxyuriasis. However, the usual hygienic precautions are required to prevent early reinfection. This drug may also be useful for treating threadworm infestation (strongyloidiasis).

Side Effects, Cautions, and Contraindications. Side effects, which are rare with the currently recommended dose of this insoluble salt, take the form of nausea, vomiting, and cramps. Like gentian violet, which it has helped to displace in oxyuriasis treatment, this dye can stain most materials. Thus, patients should be cautioned to protect underclothing and warned that their stools can be colored bright red by this drug.

Dosage and Administration. A single oral dose of 5 mg per kg of body weight of pyrvinium base (7.5 mg per kg of this salt) is taken in the form of a suspension containing 10 mg per ml or a tablet containing the equivalent of 50 mg of the base. The tablets should not be chewed but swallowed whole because they may stain the teeth.

QUINACRINE HYDROCHLORIDE U.S.P. (Atabrine)

Actions and Indications. This substance, once widely employed as a suppressive agent in malaria, is now mainly used in the treatment of infestations by beef, pork, and fish tapeworms.

Side Effects, Cautions, and Contraindications. The drug is not ordinarily toxic to most patients, but the high doses used in treating tapeworms often cause nausea and vomiting. Some individuals have had hallucinations or a toxic psychosis following administration of this drug. Thus, its use is contraindicated in individuals with a history of psychosis. Caution is also required in patients with psoriasis because this drug may set off severe skin reactions in such cases.

Dosage and Administration. Proper use of this agent requires careful pretreatment of the tapeworm-infested patient, in order to assure maximal contact of the drug with the head of the parasite. The intestine is emptied by having the patient eat only a light, fat-free lunch on the evening before treatment, followed by administration of a saline cathartic.

The next morning, the patient takes a total of 800 mg of quinacrine in four divided doses over a half-hour period. Each dose is followed by 600 mg of sodium bicarbonate to reduce nausea and vomiting. About two hours following the final dose, a saline purgative is administered. Often, the tapeworm, its head colored yellow, is recovered in the patient's stool in a few hours.

TETRACHLOROETHYLENE U.S.P.

Actions and Indications. This chemical is a relatively safe and effective agent for removing hookworms of the *Necator americanus* type from the intestinal tract.

Side Effects, Cautions, and Contra-indications. Although it is a halogenated hydrocarbon, effective anthelmintic doses administered with proper precautions do not cause toxicity of the kind brought about by such related agents as chloroform and carbon tetrachloride. This is because the drug is not absorbed into the systemic circulation unless taken with alcohol or fats. It is contraindicated in alcoholic patients or those with gastrointestinal inflammation or severe debilitation.

If tetrachlorothylene is absorbed, the patient may show some signs of central depression, including giddiness, vertigo, drowsiness, and headache. More commonly, patients may complain of the effects of local irritation, including epigastric distress, nausea, vomiting, and abdominal cramps. Roundworms should be eliminated by other means before using this drug.

Dosage and Administration. A dose of 0.12 ml/kg, but no more than 5 ml, is taken in capsule form on an empty stomach in the morning, after a period of a day or more in which no alcohol or fatty foods have been taken.

It is undesirable to administer a cathartic, as this may reduce the drug's effectiveness and also tends to dehydrate the patient. The patient should rest for at least four hours after the drug is taken, and food is withheld for four to six hours. The treatment may be repeated in about four to seven days if examination of the stool indicates the continued presence of hookworms.

THIABENDAZOLE U.S.P.
(Mintezol)

Actions and Indications. This broad-spectrum anthelmintic is claimed to be more than 95 percent effective against enterobiasis (pinworm disease) and strongyloidiasis (threadworm disease). The drug has also been employed in trichuriasis (whipworm disease), ascariasis (large roundworm disease) and in hookworm disease caused by both types of infesting organisms. It is claimed to relieve fever, reduce eosinophilia, and produce other benefits in some patients with trichinosis, and it is said to pro-vide the first successful systemic treatment for cutaneous larva migrans (creeping eruption).

Side Effects, Cautions, and Contra-indications. Side effects involving the gastrointestinal tract and the C.N.S. may occur with high doses. Anorexia, nausea, and vomiting occur frequently and epigastric distress and diarrhea less often. Drowsiness, giddiness, and headache sometimes develop, and patients should be warned against driving a car or undertaking other potentially dangerous activities requiring alertness. The drug should be used with caution in patients with impaired liver function.

Dosage and Administration. This drug is available as a pleasant-tasting suspension that is administered after meals in a dose of 10 mg/lb of body weight twice a day. The length of treatment varies in different infestations. In pinworm disease, for example, the drug is usually given for one day and then repeated seven days later to prevent reinfection. In other intestinal parasitoses, cutaneous larva migrans, and trichinosis, it is given for two successive days. In trichinosis, treatment may be continued for four successive days. The recommended maximal daily dosage is 3 g.

References

AMEBIASIS

Anderson, H.H. Newer drugs in amebiasis. *Clin. Pharmacol. Ther.*, 1:78, 1960.

Gholz, L.M., and Arons, W.L. Prophylaxis and therapy of amebiasis and shigellosis with iodochlorhydroxyquin. *Amer. J. Trop. Med.*, 13:396, 1964.

Juniper, K. Treatment of amebiasis. *Mod. Treatm.*, 3:1016, 1966 (Sept.).

Powell, S.J., et al. Single and low dosage regimens of metronidazole in amebic dysentery and amebic liver abscess. *Ann. Trop. Med. Parasit.*, 61:26, 1969.

Rodman, M.J. Antifungal and antiparasitic drugs. *RN*, 25:71, 1962 (Nov.).

———. New drugs for fighting infection. *RN*, 30:55, 1967 (June).

HELMINTHIASIS

Brown, H.W. The actions and uses of anthelmintics. *Clin. Pharmacol. Ther.*, 1:78, 1960.

Kean, B.H., and Hoskins, D.W. Treatment of trichinosis with thiabendazole. A preliminary report. *JAMA*, 190:852, 1964.

Manson-Bahr, P.E.C. Treatment of parasitic infections (excluding amebiasis). *Mod. Treatm.*, 3:1031, 1966.

Most, H. Treatment of the more common worm infections. *JAMA*, 185:874, 1963.

Rodman, M.J. Drugs in the management of worms. *RN*, 22:47, 1959 (Aug.).

SECTION **10**

Miscellaneous Therapeutic and Diagnostic Agents

45.

Drugs that Affect Gastrointestinal Function

Gastrointestinal symptoms are among the most common complaints. Sometimes the disorders that cause discomforting gastrointestinal signs and symptoms are minor and self-limiting. Other acute and chronic stomach and intestinal ailments are more serious and may even require surgical rather than medical treatment. In any case, people are quick to seek relief of such symptoms as nausea and vomiting, painful spasms, diarrhea, and other difficulties that stem from disordered gastrointestinal function.

We have already discussed several classes of drugs with gastrointestinal effects that are therapeutically useful. For example, the cholinergic drugs, which are among the most potent stimulants of gastrointestinal motility, are taken up in Chapter 21. The effects of paregoric and other opiates that reduce gastrointestinal motility are discussed in Chapter 13. The use of belladonna alkaloids and synthetic anticholinergic drugs in combination with antacid medication for treating acid-peptic diseases are discussed in Chapter 22.

In this chapter we shall summarize the status of several classes of drugs that are not discussed elsewhere, including cathartics, antiemetics, and miscellaneous other agents that are thought to affect gastrointestinal tract function in ways which offer relief of various annoying or disabling symptoms.

Drugs with Cathartic Action

Cathartics, or laxatives, are drugs used to bring about emptying of the bowel. A drug-induced increase in peristaltic activity is desirable in various clinical situations. We have seen, for example, that powerful cholinergic drugs such as *bethanechol* and *neostigmine* are sometimes employed to induce evacuation of the bowels in postoperative and postpartum patients with intestinal atony and abdominal distention. Other surgical and medical patients also sometimes profit from administration of more gently acting cathartics for overcoming constipation.

However, not all patients who have relatively few bowel movements require treatment with cathartics. A person may remain in relatively good health even though he moves his bowels infrequently. Even when better bowel motility may be desirable cathartics need not be employed to bring this about. Contrary to what most laymen have been led to believe, cathartics have little place in the management of constipation. Actually, the habitual misuse of cathartics is one of the common *causes* of chronic constipation. The nurse, in talking to patients and other people, can do a great deal to counteract the false propaganda for proprietary laxative products, which continues to foster ancient misunderstandings that lead to the abuse of these drugs.

The most common of these misconceptions is the idea that a person has to have a daily bowel movement to keep in good health. Many people still believe that failure to empty the colon results in "poisons" being absorbed into the blood. Although this myth of autointoxication was long ago laid to rest, some advertising for laxatives continues to play on the popular fear of it. Actually, the person who misses one or more bowel movements is in no dire danger.

The kind of person who gets unduly upset when he fails to move his bowels tends to treat himself with cathartics in a way that leads to chronic constipation. This is what happens: first, the person takes a cathartic that stimulates peristalsis strongly enough to empty the entire intestinal tract. This, of course, keeps the colon from filling normally for several days. Since the desire to defecate arises only when the lower colon becomes packed with a fecal mass, the normal stimulus that sets off the defecation reflex is lacking, and so a day or two may pass without a bowel movement. This alarms the bowel-oriented person and often leads him to take a still stronger cathartic to overcome his drug-induced constipation.

Instead of restoring the "normal regularity," which is so prized by those who prepare TV commercials for these products, the continued use of cathartics soon makes it difficult for the laxative abuser ever to achieve a natural movement. He comes to depend upon the drugs' action rather than on the natural defecation reflex. Such dependence is both psychic and physical and, in one sense, does not differ a great deal from what takes place when people become addicted to drugs that act on the central nervous system!

What can the nurse do to help prevent such cathartic addiction? First, of course, she should advise people with intestinal complaints to see a physician. Even though most constipation is caused by poor dietary and living habits, a sudden change in bowel function sometimes signals the presence of intestinal pathology. Once the doctor has ruled out such organic lesions, he may advise the patient to follow a program aimed at correction of the causes of chronic constipation, thus reestablishing normal bowel movements. The nurse can help here by teaching people the need to follow the rules of hygiene upon which all such regimens are based.

An important nursing function involves assisting the patient toward following a regimen useful to him in maintaining his elimination. For instance, the nurse can instruct elderly patients to take adequate fluids, set a specific time each day for defecation, and, if necessary, to use stool softeners prior to defecating (such as a glycerin suppository). Such measures can help avoid the problem of fecal impaction which is common among older persons.

TREATMENT OF CHRONIC CONSTIPATION

The first thing the doctor ordinarily does for the person whose constipation stems from habituation to cathartics is to have him stop taking laxatives. As in any other addiction, this is likely to lead to what has with some justice been termed a "withdrawal syndrome" because of the patient's complaints of discomfort. These are usually treated symptomatically, with aspirin for his headaches and general malaise, sedatives for anxiety and tension and, perhaps, mild mental stimulants to overcome lethargy, weakness, and mental depression.

More important are measures intended to replace the patient's faulty habits with habits conducive to good hygiene. These include trying to guide patients to reduce tension in their daily lives and getting them to set regular times for going to the toilet each day. The patient is put on a diet that includes foods that leave a bulky residue. These, taken together with plenty of fluids, help to build up the intestinal contents so that normal defecation reflexes can be initiated.

The attainment of this objective is sometimes aided by the judicious use of one type of nonirritating laxative. *Bulk-producing substances* such as psyllium seeds, methylcellulose, and similar *hydrophilic* (literally, "water-loving") colloids (Table 45-1) sometimes help to form a bulkier stool. Taken daily with plenty of water, they act much as do the natural fibers in foods such as carrots, beets, and cabbage. These colloid laxatives are gradually discontinued after a few weeks when the patient's bowels have begun to function normally. If the patient succeeds in learning to live under less emotional tension and in establishing proper habits and patterns, he will have no further need for cathartics.

Of course, it is not always wise or easy to try to change a patient's habits. Thus, if an elderly patient has been taking a daily mild laxative or stool softener in which he has great faith, the nurse should not be overzealous in urging him to give up his medication. Lecturing the patient or scolding him will only upset him.

Similarly, if other medical patients regularly use a mild bulk-producing laxative or stool-softener with no obvious ill effects, there is no need to subject them to stern moralistic lectures. Even in cases of obvious cathartic abuse, it is best to proceed slowly and gently. Then, if the patient senses that he has the sympathetic support of his nurse and physician, he may more willingly follow their advice for rehabilitating his misused bowel.

INDICATIONS FOR CATHARTICS

Doctors order laxatives far less frequently than they used to in the days when they shared with the layman a misguided belief in the desirability of keeping the patient's bowel "open" with a daily purge. There are, however, some clinical situations in which it is considered desirable to induce defecation with drugs or to alter the consistency of the patient's stool. The few conditions in which the use of cathartics is considered valid are as follows:

BED PATIENTS. *People confined to bed* often tend to become constipated. This is understandable, since lack of exercise, loss of ap-

petite, and the effects of the person's illness and of the drugs used to treat it—narcotic pain relievers, such as codeine, morphine, and meperidine, for example—all conspire to reduce intestinal motility. For this reason, it was once a regular practice for the doctor to order milk of magnesia, cascara, or other cathartics for all his hospitalized patients.

Recently, however, the routine use of cathartics has declined as doctors and nurses have recognized their undesirability and turned to more natural measures for maintaining bowel function. The nurse should use her influence in the situation to accelerate this trend away from regular orders for cathartic medication and toward more physiologic means of keeping the patient's bowel open. For example, she may suggest a program designed to re-establish normal bowel function and, in collaboration with the physician, work out the details of such a program for individual patients, rather than request a p.r.n. order for a cathartic.

Among the most important of the measures that help avoid the need for cathartics is seeing that the patient is taken to the bathroom or is given the opportunity to use a commode at his bedside at a regular time each day. This is often possible and permissible today because of the present emphasis on early ambulation. Freed of the need to use the bedpan, the patient can assume a more normal and comfortable position and should be encouraged to do so. He should also be left alone, if possible, since lack of privacy often inhibits defecation.

Another desirable development is the fact that patients often not only are allowed to get out of bed but also are encouraged to begin eating a regular, varied diet, including fresh fruits and vegetables, shortly after surgery if their condition permits, instead of being kept on liquids for days as they once were. Of course, to avoid constipation, it is also important to keep the patient well hydrated, by such measures as the use of intravenous fluids postoperatively when this seems desirable or necessary and encouraging oral fluid intake.

Laxatives, suppositories, and enemas still have a place in the care of patients. In such cases these medications are used not merely to relieve the patient's discomfort but also to avoid possible fecal impaction and other dangerous complications, such as those that might result if a patient with an aneurysm, embolism, or myocardial infarction were to strain at stool.

ANORECTAL LESIONS. Patients with *hemorrhoids*, or other anorectal lesions should not strain in order to remove retained feces. Thus, measures for promoting a soft stool that can be passed without pain are desirable. These include the regular use of the lubricating type of laxatives and the wetting agents (Table 45-1).

DIAGNOSTIC PROCEDURES AND SURGERY. Cathartics are employed prior to various diagnostic or surgical procedures—before bowel surgery, for example. Sometimes the entire intestine is emptied before abdominal x-rays; at other times only the colon need be cleared—for instance, for proctosigmoidoscopy.

ANTHELMINTICS. The treatment of intestinal worm infestations with anthelmintics often requires administration of a cathartic both before and after therapy. Some anthelmintics act more effectively when the bowel has first been cleared; other medications for killing worms are potentially toxic to the patient if too much is absorbed. These are often swept out of the gastrointestinal tract by a cathartic as soon as they have had time to do their work on the worms.

CHEMICAL POISONING. In cases of poisoning by ingested chemicals, poisons that have passed the pylorus and can no longer be eliminated by gastric lavage are often flushed from the intestine by purgative drugs. This tends both to reduce local tissue damage by corrosive chemicals and to limit the systemic absorption of other toxic agents. Laxatives are also sometimes given routinely with constipating drugs, including especially those that may cause dangerous systemic effects when their evacuation is delayed (for example, the potent narcotic analgesics).

CONTRAINDICATIONS

Cathartics, as we have seen, should never be used habitually as a routine measure for inducing a daily bowel movement. Such use not only leads to chronic constipation but may produce local and systemic disturbances. The habitual use of purgatives and stimulants of intestinal motility has been held responsible for many cases of chronic colitis and other intestinal disorders that are the direct or indirect result of continued irritation of the intestinal mucosa. In addition, repeated purgation can result in dehydration and cause electrolyte imbalances similar to those that result from severe diarrhea due to gastrointestinal infections.

More serious than the effects of the long-term misuse of cathartics is the damage that can be done by giving even a single dose of a cathartic to a person with acute appendicitis. The drug-induced increase in gastrointestinal motility may lead to perforation of the inflamed intestinal wall. Such rupture of the appendix then spews pathogenic bacteria into the abdominal cavity.

Before the advent of antibiotics and other modern antiinfective drugs, the death rate from peritonitis in patients who had taken cathartics for treating painful cramps was very high. Even today, peritonitis is a serious condition. Thus, people should be warned never to medicate themselves with cathartics when they have abdominal pain and cramps or are nauseated and vomiting. These drugs are never given before adequate diagnosis has ruled out appendicitis, enteritis, ulcerative colitis, diverticulitis, or the presence of organic obstructions.

THE TYPES OF CATHARTIC DRUGS

Cathartic drugs act in several different ways to speed the passage of the intestinal contents through the gastrointestinal tract. Some substances act chemically to stimulate intestinal smooth muscles to contract more forcefully and frequently. Other agents cause an increase in intestinal bulk, which acts as a mechanical stimulus to the motor activity of the gut. The effects of other laxatives are exerted less on the gastrointestinal tract itself than on its fecal contents. That is, they soften hardened masses and ease their passage through the lower portion of the large intestine.

The manner in which each class of cathartics acts and its speed and degree of thoroughness determines which type is best for each of the various kinds of indications discussed above.

IRRITANT RESINS AND OILS. Among the most powerful natural purgatives are an oil obtained from seeds of the croton plant and resinous principles from such plants as podophyllum, colocynth, and jalap. These substances stimulate peristaltic activity by irritating the mucosal lining of the intestinal tract. Their harsh irritant action is followed by colicky intestinal contractions and prompt production of abundant watery stools. However, these irritants should have no place in modern medicine, as

T A B L E 4 5 - 1   *Cathartic Drugs*

Nonproprietary or Official Name	Trade Name or Synonym	Dosage
Drugs Stimulating Motility by Chemical Irritation		
Aloe U.S.P.		0.250 g
Bisacodyl N.F.	Dulcolax	10 to 15 mg
Calomel	Mercurous chloride	120 mg
Cascara sagrada U.S.P.		
Cascara sagrada, aromatic extract U.S.P.		2 ml
Cascara sagrada, extract N.F.		0.3 g
Cascara sagrada, fluidextract N.F.		1 ml
Castor oil U.S.P.		15 to 30 ml
Castor oil, aromatic N.F.		15 ml
Danthron N.F.	Dorbane	75 to 150 mg
Phenolphthalein N.F.		60 mg
Oxyphenisatin	Acetphenolisatin; Isocrin; and others	2 to 5 mg
Senna N.F.		2.0 g
Senna fluidextract N.F.		2 ml
Senna syrup N.F.		8 ml
Senna glycosides, concentrated	Glysennid; Senokot; and others	Varied mg dosage; ordered as one or two capsules or tablets or as one or one half suppository
Drugs Stimulating Motility by Increasing Physical Bulk		
SALINE CATHARTICS		
Magnesium citrate solution N.F.		200 ml
Magnesium sulfate U.S.P.	Epsom salt	15 g
Milk of magnesia U.S.P.	Magnesia magma	15 g
Potassium sodium tartrate N.F.	Rochelle salt	10 g
Seidlitz powders	Compound effervescent powders	Contents of a white and a blue paper mixed in water
Sodium phosphate N.F.		4 g
Sodium phosphate, effervescent N.F.		10 g
Sodium phosphate, exsiccated N.F.		2 g
Sodium phosphate, solution N.F.		10 ml
Sodium sulfate	Glauber's salt	15 g
HYDROPHILIC COLLOIDS AND INDIGESTIBLE FIBERS		
Agar U.S.P.		4 to 16 g
Methylcellulose U.S.P.		1.0 g
Plantago seed N.F.	Metamucil	7.5 g
Psyllium hydrophilic mucilloid		4 to 10 g
Sodium carboxymethylcellulose U.S.P.		1.5 g
EMOLLIENT OR LUBRICANT CATHARTICS		
Liquid petrolatum emulsion N.F.		30 ml
Mineral oil U.S.P.		15 to 45 ml
Olive oil U.S.P.		30 ml
FECAL SOFTENERS (SURFACE-ACTIVE OR WETTING AGENTS)		
Dioctyl calcium sulfosuccinate	Surfak	60 mg
Dioctyl sodium sulfosuccinate U.S.P.	Colace; Doxinate; etc.	100 mg
Poloxalkol N.F.	Magcyl; Polykol	200 mg

their continued use can cause dangerous local and systemic effects.

Castor oil+, also classified as an irritant cathartic, is not irritating in quite the same sense. For one thing, unlike croton oil and the resins, it does not damage delicate tissues. As a matter of fact, it is bland enough to be dropped in a patient's eye as an emollient after removal of a foreign body. In the intestine, however, the oil is broken down by fat-splitting enzymes to release ricinoleic acid, a substance that strongly stimulates gastrointestinal motility.

The habitual use of castor oil is certainly undesirable. It causes the kind of complete evacuation of both the small and the large bowel that leads to a period during which there is no natural stimulus to defecation. Thus, its frequent use can, in the manner previously indicated, lead to production of chronic constipation.

On the other hand, the comparatively prompt and complete action of castor oil makes its occasional use desirable in some situations. Thus, it is still used in certain hospital procedures, though much less often than it once was. Castor oil is still employed prior to x-ray examination of abdominal organs, for example, to empty the intestine and thus eliminate interfering shadows. It is usually given on an empty stomach in the late afternoon so that it will not interfere with digestion or with sleep. It should never be taken at bedtime because its strong action coming on in a couple of hours or so will cause a restless night.

OTHER STIMULANT LAXATIVES

Other natural and synthetic substances also produce peristalsis by a mild irritant action on the gastrointestinal tract. However, because their stimulating action is largely limited to the large intestine, these laxatives are *not* useful for rapidly emptying the entire tract. Instead, they are used in those patients in whom a slow, steady action is desired, including those who are confined to bed.

ANTHRAQUINONES. Cathartics containing plant principles of this chemical class include cascara, senna, aloe, and rhubarb. They are best given at bedtime, because it takes six or eight hours or more for their effects to develop. *Cascara sagrada+*, for example, exerts a mild stimulating effect on the large intestine that often leads to formation of a single soft stool

about eight hours after it is taken orally in the form of the fluidextract or extract.

Phenolphthalein is a common component of many proprietary laxative preparations, including some of the most popular chocolate and gum medications. These forms of phenolphthalein are often eaten by children in large amounts, but severe toxicity is rare and is limited mainly to a dehydrating diarrhea. However, hypersensitivity reactions are not uncommon. These often take the form of a characteristically colorful dermatitis. Sometimes the itchy, burning patches blister and become ulcerated; occasionally, the involved patches of skin stay pink or purplish for many months, and, long after the condition has cleared up, identical lesions may appear in the same places on subsequent exposure to the drug—a so-called fixed eruption.

Oxyphenisatin acetate, a chemically related compound, also stimulates colonic contractions. Because its oral administration has in some rare cases caused jaundice, it is best administered rectally. An enema powder containing this chemical has been employed for cleaning the large bowel prior to abdominal and other surgery, aiding in x-ray visualization of abdominal viscera, and in other clinical situations. Administration by the rectal route limits the drug's action to the lower colon. This leads to bowel evacuation without any systemic absorption or adverse hepatic effects.

Bisacodyl (Dulcolax) is a chemically related compound with a similar action on the large intestine. It may be given by mouth at night to produce a morning bowel movement. The drug is also available in suppository form for faster action. Rectal administration brings the chemical in contact with the mucosa and stimulates contraction of the colon within a few minutes. It has been employed in this way in preparing the lower bowel for a barium enema and prior to proctoscopy.

SALINE CATHARTICS (TABLE 45-1)

Several poorly absorbed salts that are given in solution with large amounts of water bring about an increase in the bulk of the intestinal contents. The administration of such salts as *sodium sulfate* and *phosphate* or *magnesium sulfate* and *citrate* distend the colon and mechanically stimulate smooth muscle contractions, resulting in a relatively rapid evacuation of the bowel.

Because such saline cathartics sometimes act

in as little as an hour or two, their use is preferred in poisonings for clearing the entire intestinal tract quickly. They are also used whenever a complete purge is necessary—after administration of anthelmintics in intestinal worm treatments, for example. Because their effects usually come on in less than three hours, these substances are *not* administered at night but in the morning or in midafternoon.

Substances such as *Glauber's salt* or *Epsom salt* are given in cold fruit juices to mask the taste. *Magnesium citrate* solution is a pleasant-tasting, lemon-flavored, carbonated liquid. However, it is relatively expensive, as are various salts that make a palatable effervescent liquid when poured into water. Palatability is, of course, no problem when various salts such as *sodium phosphate* and *biphosphate* (in Fleet enema, for example) are administered rectally.

OTHER BULK-PRODUCING LAXATIVES

Another kind of mechanically acting cathartic is quite different from the saline type in actions and uses. This group includes the hydrophilic colloids and other indigestible fibers, mentioned earlier as useful adjuncts in the treatment of chronic constipation. Natural substances, such as psyllium seeds and agar, and semisynthetic materials, such as sodium carboxymethylcellulose, produce their desired action by forming a bulky jellyish mass in the intestine. This resembles in its effects the food residues that normally stimulate peristalsis and defecation.

These bulk-formers are the most natural and least irritating of laxatives. They should not, however, be taken habitually any more than any other cathartic. Patients should be told never to take these products without water. This is important, and not merely because their effectiveness depends in large part upon their ability to absorb enough fluid to make a gelatinous mass. When swallowed dry, these fibers, seeds, and granules may pick up just enough moisture in the esophagus to swell and obstruct that food passageway. Thus, these materials are to be both mixed with water and followed by plenty of fluid.

LUBRICATING LAXATIVES AND STOOL SOFTENERS

It is often desirable to make defecation easier, not by stimulating peristalsis but by changing the consistency of the patient's stool. Sometimes this is best done with retention enemas of olive oil or cottonseed oil, which turn hard, dry, fecal "stones" into soft, moist masses. These can then be readily passed by the patient or washed out with cleansing tap water or soap-suds enemas.

Liquid petrolatum (mineral oil), an indigestible oil that does not add to the patient's caloric intake, is much more widely used in this way for lubricating and softening the stool. It is employed mainly for patients with hemorrhoids or other painful anal lesions and for others who must avoid straining at stool. By coating the fecal contents, mineral oil also tends to reduce fluid absorption from the feces and thus prevents their becoming excessively dry.

Mineral oil may be taken orally or rectally. For people who dislike the feel of the plain oil on the tongue, flavored emulsions may be employed. However, such products are relatively expensive, and their use may lead to systemic absorption of the oil. Thus, the nurse may suggest sucking an orange slice to cut the oily aftertaste. Liquid petrolatum is best taken at bedtime, and not with meals, as it may interfere with the absorption of fat-soluble vitamins. Loss of vitamin K in this way could make a patient more sensitive than previously to treatment with anticoagulant drugs. (See drug interactions, Chapter 2, and Table 2-1.)

Occasional use of a mineral oil enema for relief of fecal impaction avoids some of the disadvantages of oral administration. Rectal use prevents possible interference with food digestion and absorption of vitamins A, D, E, and K. It avoids the possible aspiration of the liquid into the lungs by children and others with resulting lipid pneumonia, and systemic absorption does not occur (see above and below). However, following hemorrhoidectomy, healing may be delayed by excessive use of mineral oil enemas, as well as by seepage of orally administered liquid petrolatum. (Leakage leading to soiling of clothes or bedding is an adverse esthetic effect of liquid petrolatum.)

Surface-active agents, inert chemicals that act like detergents, are also used to soften the stool. *Dioctyl sodium sulfosuccinate*, the most widely used of these substances, is available for oral administration and in enemas. It is thought to act by reducing the surface tension of the fecal contents of the rectum. This permits water and fatty materials to penetrate and make a more moist and bulky mass. This action occurs when wetting agent solutions are administered as retention enemas; however, there is some doubt that small oral doses have the desired effect.

The surface-active agents, which, in themselves, seem safe enough, are sometimes offered in proprietary combinations with irritant cathartics, which are considered much less desirable for long-term use. It may also be undesirable to administer mineral oil together with these wetting agents, because they may tend to facilitate passage of the inert oil through the intestinal mucosa. Once the liquid petrolatum, which is ordinarily unabsorbable, gets into the tissues, it cannot be eliminated and may act as a foreign body in the lymph nodes, liver, and spleen.

Drugs Used in the Management of Diarrhea

Diarrhea may be a symptom of many different diseases or disorders. Most commonly, it is an acute and self-limiting condition—the result of the intestine's attempt to rid itself of an irritant. On the other hand, diarrhea caused by chronic inflammation or overstimulation of the intestine can be most persistent and difficult to treat. Besides treating the symptom, the doctor tries to determine its cause. Usually, this is easily accomplished—for example, when a pathogenic microorganism can be cultured from a stool specimen. In such cases, the doctor may order treatment with specific antibacterial or antiamebic agents (Chapters 41, 42, and 44).

In other cases, the cause of a patient's chronic diarrhea may be even more difficult to discover—for example, when it is of emotional origin. In any case, even when the cause of diarrhea cannot be readily found and rooted out, it is usually possible to give the patient some symptomatic relief. Certain systemically acting drugs often help to reduce intestinal hypermotility. These agents include the *opiates*, which act directly on the intestinal smooth muscle to slow excessive peristaltic activity, and the *anticholinergic drugs*, which relax spasm caused by parasympathetic nervous system stimulation (Chapters 13 and 22).

LOCALLY ACTING SUBSTANCES (TABLE 45-2)

Various locally acting substances are also said to provide relief of diarrhea by their physical effects on the intestine and its contents. Some doctors doubt that these chemicals actually duplicate their test tube actions within the intestinal tract. However, these substances are safe and inexpensive. Thus, they are widely employed as vehicles for the systemically active agents on the assumption that, if nothing else, they may provide desirable placebo effects for the distressed patient.

ADSORBENTS, ASTRINGENTS, AND DEMULCENTS. Among the most commonly employed of the antidiarrheal drugs are *kaolin* and *pectin*, agents often given together several times daily in acute cases of diarrhea. Kaolin, an aluminum silicate clay, is an *ad*sorbent, a substance capable of holding on its surface other chemicals with which it comes in contact. This, it is thought, is responsible for its ability to pick up, bind, and remove bacteria, toxins, and other irritants from the intestine. It is also claimed to form a coating over the mucosa which both protects it against irritation and filters out toxins that might otherwise be absorbed into the blood. The pectin component of such products is a plant derivative that is said to provide a demulcent or soothing effect on the irritated bowel lining in addition to aiding in adsorption.

Attapulgite, a silicate clay like kaolin, is claimed to be several times more effective than the latter in its endotoxin-adsorptive action. It comes in the form of an ultrafine powder said to offer a vast surface area. (The particles in one pound of powder, it is claimed, could cover 13 acres of surface!) A heat-treated form, *activated attapulgite* (Claysorb), possesses an increased adsorptive capacity. It is sometimes suspended in alumina gel, a substance with adsorbent, demulcent, and astringent properties of its own.

Other substances, including activated charcoal and salts of such minerals as magnesium, aluminum, and bismuth, are also still employed in antidiarrhea mixtures. Valuable as it is in treating drug poisonings, activated charcoal does not seem very effective for treating diarrhea. The magnesium and aluminum preparations are more effective as antacids than for control of diarrhea. Bismuth salts are said to possess protective, adsorbent, and astringent properties, but there is little proof that they are effective when taken internally for diarrhea.

HYDROABSORPTIVE SUBSTANCES. The watery, unformed stools characteristic of diarrhea are the result of the rapidity with which the

T A B L E   4 5 - 2 *Locally Acting Antidiarrheal Drugs (Adsorbents, Astringents, Demulcents, Protectives, etc.)*

Drug	Dosage
Activated attapulgite (Claysorb)	2–5 g
Activated charcoal U.S.P.	10 g
Bismuth subcarbonate U.S.P.	1–4 g
Bismuth subnitrate N.F.	1–4 g
Calcium carbonate, precipitated (Chalk) U.S.P.	1–2 g
Kaolin N.F.	2–5 g
Kaolin mixture with pectin N.F. (Kaopectate)	30 ml
Pectin N.F.	50–300 mg
Polycarbophil	0.5–1 g
Tannic acid N.F.	1 g

chyme or liquid digestive mass is rushed through the intestine. Ordinarily, most of the fluids in the intestinal contents are reabsorbed into the blood by way of the large bowel wall. However, excessive peristaltic activity permits little time for such absorption by the colon and, as a result, unusually liquid stools are passed. This loss of fluid, if severe and long-continued, can lead to serious dehydration and electrolyte imbalances which may be made even more serious if the diarrhea is accompanied by vomiting. Fatalities from the infantile diarrheas that sometimes still spread through hospital nurseries are often the result of unrelieved dehydration, alkalosis or acidosis, hemocentration, and terminal cardiac irregularities.

Such serious complications of diarrhea require intensive treatment to rehydrate the patient and replenish lost electrolytes. However, much simpler measures may be employed in most cases to increase the consistency of the stools. Various hydrophilic (literally, "water-loving") substances may be used to absorb some of the intestinal moisture. The *pectins* act, in part, in this manner, as do *methylcellulose* and *psyllium seed mucilloids* (see the section on bulk laxatives in this chapter). Another hydroabsorptive substance, called *polycarbophil*, is claimed to possess certain advantages over the latter agents. This synthetic substance does not swell in the stomach to cause an uncomfortable feeling of fullness. It is said to exert its water-binding action only upon reaching the alkaline medium of the small intestine and colon.

Antiemetic Drugs

NAUSEA AND VOMITING

Nausea is one of the most commonly reported symptoms. This feeling of being "sick in the stomach" is often followed by retching and vomiting, the complex reflex act by which the stomach's contents are ejected. Vomiting serves a useful purpose when it removes toxic irritants from the stomach before they can be absorbed into the systemic circulation. (The use of emetics to induce vomiting and thus help rid the stomach of ingested poisons is discussed in Chapter 3.)

Unfortunately, vomiting occurs most often in situations which do not require emptying of the stomach. Thus, there is no protective value in the vomiting that is part of the body's response to certain types of motion. Similarly, the nausea of early pregnancy does not serve as a useful warning signal in any way, and vomiting that persists may actually endanger the mother by causing a severe fluid-electrolyte imbalance and interfering with her nutrition.

The stimuli that set off the vomiting reflex may originate not only in the gastrointestinal tract but anywhere in the body. Such stimuli may be physical, chemical, or psychological. Thus, it is not surprising that nausea and vomiting should be part of the picture in so many clinical conditions, ranging from minor infections to metastatic carcinoma. The doctor therefore first tries to determine the *cause* of the vomiting and then takes steps to eliminate it, if possible.

Once the cause has been recognized, however, symptomatic relief is desirable to reduce the patient's discomfort and prevent the possibly dangerous consequences of persistent vomiting. Sometimes relief requires only simple nursing care measures, such as providing a quiet, restful environment and seeing that the patient gets ice to suck or a cold carbonated drink or hot tea to sip. On the other hand, effective antiemetic drugs may also be ordered, which act by dampening hyperactive vomiting reflex activity.

DRUG TREATMENT OF NAUSEA AND VOMITING

The drugs used in the management of nausea and vomiting may be classified as (1) *locally acting*, and (2) *centrally acting*. Substances of the first type include topical mucosal anesthetics, antacids and adsorbents, demulcent-protective agents, and drugs that reduce distention of the stomach by retained gases(for example, simethicone and the carminatives).

The *centrally acting antimetics* may be further subdivided into (1) the *phenothiazine* and (2) *nonphenothiazine compounds*. The former include many agents also used as major tranquilizers, as well as some chemicals of this class that are not used in mental illness. The nonphenothiazines are also often employed as antihistaminic and anticholinergic agents.

LOCALLY ACTING AGENTS. Vomiting caused by local irritation of the gastrointestinal tract is usually self-limited because, once the stomach rids itself of the troublesome irritant, the source of the person's difficulty is gone, and the mucosal receptors stop sending their distress signals centrally. In some cases of acute gastroenteritis, however, the inflamed membranes continue to bombard the vomiting center with messages that trigger nausea and emesis. Drugs that reduce the reactivity of these receptors may be helpful in overcoming these manifestations of stomach upset while the patient's condition is being gradually cleared up by other measures aimed at removing its cause.

Topical anesthetics. Various local anesthetics are sometimes administered orally in an attempt to raise the threshold of receptor responsiveness to local irritants. Among the topically active agents often taken by mouth to reduce the number of afferent impulses originating in the gastrointestinal tract are *benzocaine* and *procaine*. It is doubtful, however, that these short-acting substances have much effect on vomiting. The longer-acting local anesthetic, *lidocaine*, is available as a viscous solution which is said to control severe reflex vomiting for several hours when taken orally in tablespoon doses. Another agent, *oxethazine*, which is suspended in an antacid alumina gel, is said to afford prolonged topical anesthesia because it is present in an adherent coating that protects the irritated gastric mucosa.

Among other locally acting agents are various volatile oils, including *peppermint, clove-ginger,* and *cinnamon.* Administered as alcoholic solutions (spirits) or as waters, these carminatives often give a feeling of warmth in the stomach and sometimes seem to help expel gas by causing a reflex increase in gastrointestinal motility. It is difficult to say whether the carminatives act chemically or psychologically (that is, through a desirable placebo effect, as discussed in Chapter 2). In any case, removal of accumulated gas is thought to lessen local stimuli that lead to discomfort and nausea.

Other commonly employed antinauseants that are claimed to work for some people include *Coca-Cola syrup* and a product with essentially similar properties, *phosphorylated carbohydrate solution* (Emetrol). These liquids are taken in tablespoonful doses without any other fluids. Although there is little scientific evidence of how they act, these substances are said to relax gastrointestinal muscle spasms by a local effect, thus reducing afferent impulses to the vomiting center.

The psychological effects of some agents used for stomach upset should not be ignored. Although scientific proof of their effectiveness is usually lacking, the placebo response is often a desirable one. Thus, if a patient who takes something occasionally to "settle the stomach" gets from it the comfortable feeling that he is doing himself some good, the nurse should not shatter his confidence in the medication that he finds helpful. If, as in this case, the remedies are considered harmless, it may be wise to stay silent about the worthlessness of a "cure for sour stomach" that makes a person feel better or more comfortable.

CENTRALLY ACTING ANTIEMETICS. The most effective drugs for prevention or relief of nausea and vomiting depress passage of nerve impulses in brain pathways. The first drugs used to depress the central parts of the vomiting reflex mechanism were: (1) the *barbiturates*, and other *sedative-hypnotics*; and (2) *scopolamine (hyoscine)*, a belladonna alkaloid with central depressant effects. Because of their side effects, these drugs have been largely replaced by other more specific antiemetic agents.

❦ *The phenothiazines.* Many of the major tranquilizers, or antipsychotic agents (Table 45-3), also possess potent antiemetic activity. They seem to act mainly by reducing the responsiveness of certain brain cells to emetic stimuli. These nerve cells, located beneath the cerebral cortex, make up an area called the *chemoreceptor trigger zone (CTZ)*, which is especially sensitive to circulating chemicals that cause emesis.

The ability of the phenothiazines to block stimulation of the CTZ by drugs, hormones, and toxins, as well as nerve impulses, may account for the effectiveness of these drugs in the following kinds of conditions: (1) *hyperemesis gravidorum*, or vomiting of pregnancy; (2) *cancer patients*, particularly those being treated with irradiation and antineoplastic chemotherapeutic agents; (3) *postoperative vomiting*; and (4) *vomiting secondary to severe infections*, such as meningitis, or with uremia, hepatitis, or gallbladder disease. The phenothiazines are *not* very useful for treating the nausea, vertigo, and vomiting of motion sickness.

ADVERSE EFFECTS. Most of the adverse effects of phenothiazines that occur in treating mental illness (see *Summary* in Chapter 7) are unlikely to occur with the relatively small doses employed for relief of vomiting. However, even a single injection of a drug such as *prochlorperazine+* (Compazine) sometimes sets off muscle spasms and other signs of extrapyramidal motor system reactions. Children and young adults are especially susceptible. Thus, even a relatively safe drug such as *thiethylperazine* (Torecan) is not recommended for children under 12 years old. Doctors prescribe these drugs in the smallest doses effective for relief of vomiting, and the nurse should advise parents not to give children any more than the doctor ordered.

❦ *The nonphenothiazines.* Drugs of this kind are mainly antihistaminic drugs related to *diphenhydramine+* (Benadryl). However, their effectiveness in preventing vomiting does not stem from histamine antagonism but from their ability to block nerve impulses passing between the vestibular apparatus of the inner ear and the vomiting center located deep in the medulla oblongata. Thus, they—like the anticholinergic drug, scopolamine—are particularly effective in motion sickness and in ailments such as labyrinthitis, Meniere's disease, and the dizziness and nausea that often follow surgical procedures involving the inner ear.

ADVERSE EFFECTS. Drowsiness is the most common side effect of centrally acting nonphenothiazines such as *dimenhydrinate+* (Dramamine), a close chemical relative of diphenhydramine. The more recently introduced

---

T A B L E   4 5 - 3 *Centrally Acting Antiemetic Agents*

Nonproprietary or Official Name	Trade Name	Antiemetic Dose (Single, Oral, Adult)
Chlorpromazine HCl U.S.P.	Thorazine	10–25 mg
Cyclizine HCl U.S.P.	Marezine	50 mg
Chlorcyclizine HCl U.S.P.	Diparalene	50 mg
Dimenhydrinate U.S.P.	Dramamine	50 mg
Diphenhydramine U.S.P.	Benadryl	50 mg
Meclizine HCl U.S.P.	Bonine	25–50 mg
Perphenazine	Trilafon	4–8 mg
Prochlorperazine maleate U.S.P.	Compazine	5–10 mg
Promethazine HCl U.S.P.	Phenergan	25–50 mg
Scopolamine HBr U.S.P.	Hyoscine	0.5–1.0 mg
Thiethylperazine maleate	Torecan	10–20 mg
Triflupromazine HCl	Vesprin	10–20 mg
Trimethobenzamide HCl	Tigan	250 mg

drugs, such as *trimethobenzamide*+ (Tigan), *cyclizine* (Marezine), and *meclizine* (Bonine) are effective in doses that rarely cause drowsiness or other side effects such as mouth dryness and visual blurring. However, the latter two drugs have caused fetal abnormalities when administered to pregnant animals in high doses. Thus, it is suggested that this possible hazard be considered before these drugs are administered to pregnant women.

Drowsiness need not be a drawback in patients who do not have to stay alert to operate an automobile or machinery. In fact, the sedative effect of the nonphenothiazines and the calming or tranquilizing effect of the phenothiazines may even add to their effectiveness as antiemetics in some situations. This is because these drugs reduce the anxiety and tension that often play a part in making patients susceptible to other stimuli that set off vomiting.

The nurse should be aware of the importance of psychological factors in nausea and vomiting. Thus, in administering these drugs, she should take advantage of the power of positive suggestion by saying something like "This medication is going to make you feel better." Similarly, it is desirable to avoid upsetting the nauseated patient in any way. Noise, vibrations, and, of course, odors tend to induce vomiting in an already queasy patient; for example, the aide should be instructed not to bring a food tray into the patient's room. Later, when he feels better, the patient may be given frequent, small meals rich in nutritive

substances. In general, it is desirable to keep the patient quiet and to offer psychological and physical support. For example, help the vomiting patient assume a comfortable position, and keep his surroundings clean and odor-free.

Digestants and Related Drugs (see Table 45-4)

DIGESTION AND INDIGESTION

In order to be utilized by the body, food must be broken down into simple, soluble molecules that can be absorbed into the blood and can enter into cellular metabolic reactions. The many mechanical and chemical processes to which food is subjected in the mouth, esophagus, stomach, and intestines comprise *digestion*. The terms *indigestion* and *dyspepsia* are not as readily defined. They are usually used by laymen to describe any one of a number of vague abdominal symptoms, including feelings of flatulence or bloating, burning epigastric pain, and acidic belching.

Such symptoms may be caused by gastrointestinal inflammatory ailments, including gastritis and peptic ulcer, or they may be the result of a functional reaction to emotional tension. Only rarely are they caused by an actual lack of the chemical substances secreted into the gastrointestinal tract during the digestive processes. Yet, many pharmaceutical preparations containing digestive enzymes, bile

---

TABLE 45-4 *Digestants and Related Drugs*

Nonproprietary or Official Name	Trade Name	Dosage Range
Betaine HCl	Normacid	500–1,000 mg
Cellulase	—	2–8 mg
Cholestyramine resin	Cuemid; Questram	12–16g
Dehydrocholic acid N.F.	Decholin	250–500 mg
Diluted hydrochloric acid N.F.	—	4–10 ml, diluted
Florantyrone	Zanchol	250–1,000 mg
Glutamic acid HCl N.F.	Acidulin	300–600 mg
Ox bile extract	—	300–600 mg
Pepsin N.F.	—	500–1,000 mg
Pancreatin N.F.	—	500–1,000 mg
Pancrelipase	Cotazyme	150–300 mg
Simethicone	Mylanta; Silain	5–100 mg
Sodium dehydrocholate injection N.F.	—	2 g I.V.

salts, and sources of hydrochloric acid are marketed for the management of indigestion.

Most people who take such products do not actually have any deficiency of digestant chemicals, and the pharmaceutical digestants are usually present in amounts too small to substitute for any actual lack if it existed. However, a relatively few patients—mostly elderly or suffering from organic digestive tract ailments or the aftereffects of gastrointestinal surgery—do have a deficiency of one or more digestive chemicals. In such cases, the administration of such substances in adequate amounts constitutes a rational form of replacement therapy.

HYDROCHLORIC ACID

A deficiency of gastric acid occurs in various disorders, including pernicious anemia. The administration of *diluted (10 percent) hydrochloric acid* to patients with hypochlorhydria or achlorhydria is said to relieve various vague symptoms of stomach distress following eating. This solution must be well watered down when taken during and after meals. To protect the patient's teeth, the well-diluted solution is sipped through a glass tube, and his mouth is rinsed with a mildly alkaline solution.

Also available as a source of hydrochloric acid are *betaine hydrochloride* and *glutamic acid hydrochloride* (Acidulin). These are powders that, when taken in capsules or tablets, release hydrochloric acid in the stomach. They do not yield large quantities of free acid, but they offer a safe, convenient, and often adequate treatment in many cases of gastric achlorhydria.

DIGESTIVE ENZYMES

Pepsin. The hydrochloric acid is provided in order to furnish an optimal medium for the action of pepsin, the gastric enzyme that begins the breakdown of proteins into smaller fragments. Some patients with gastric achylia lack both acid and pepsin. Thus, this enzyme is often administered alone or combined with sources of hydrochloric acid to aid the digestion of patients with gastric hypoacidity or anacidity. Actually, however, pepsin is not ordinarily lacking, even in patients with achlorhydria, and, in any case, the proteolytic enzymes of the pancreas and intestine can break down protein, even when it has not previously been acted upon by pepsin.

Pancreatic Enzymes. The juice secreted into the duodenum by the pancreas contains enzymes capable of attacking starches (amylases) and fats (lipases), as well as the enzymes trypsin and chymotrypsin, which aid in the breakdown of the polypeptide products of peptic digestion to amino acids. Many digestant products that are available contain these enzymes in the form of *pancreatin*, a substance prepared from hog pancreas. The amounts of pancreatin usually present ordinarily are not adequate for aiding digestion.

Pancrelipase (Cotazym) is a more concentrated mixture of pancreatic enzymes that is recommended for replacement therapy in patients whose pancreas has been surgically removed. Others with an enzyme deficiency that results in the patient's failing to gain weight may profit from treatment with products of this type. These include children with cystic fibrosis and patients with chronic pancreatitis or pancreatic duct blockage secondary to neoplastic disease.

BILE SALTS AND OTHER CHOLERETICS

Bile is secreted by liver cells, stored and concentrated in the gallbladder, and released into the duodenum via the common bile duct. Bile, although it contains no enzymes, plays an important part in the digestion of fats and is essential for absorption of the vitamins—A, D, E, and K—that dissolve in fat.

Natural bile contains organic acids which are, in part, combined into complex salts—for example, *sodium glycocholate* and *taurocholate*. These bile salts have detergent properties that account for their ability to aid in fat digestion and absorption. That is, they act like soaps to lower the surface tension of the large fat globules in food and break them down into tiny droplets. This emulsifying effect exposes a much larger surface area of the lipids to attack by pancreatic lipases. By this enzymatic action the solubilized fat is rapidly converted to readily absorbable fatty acids.

Bile salts are sometimes useful as replacement therapy for patients with partial biliary obstruction or biliary fistulas, and after cholecystectomy or other surgical operations on the biliary system which have led to a deficiency of natural bile. In such patients, administration of natural bile salts in the form of *ox bile extract*, for example, aids in the digestion of fat and in absorption of fatty acids and fat soluble food factors. It is also claimed to have a mildly stimulating effect on the smooth muscle of the gastrointestinal tract that helps to keep peristaltic activity normal.

CHOLERETIC ACTIVITY. Bile salts have other pharmacological effects besides those discussed above. For example, after they have been absorbed from the gastrointestinal tract, they tend to stimulate the liver to secrete increased quantities of whole bile. This so-called *choleretic* action, which is shared by certain natural and synthetic substances, including *tocamphyl*, is believed to serve little useful purpose in therapy.

However, certain substances that stimulate an increased flow of a thin, fluid bile seem to have some clinical utility. One of the best of these *hydrocholeretics*, as the agents that promote secretion of dilute bile are called, is *dehydrocholic acid*, a semisynthetic substance produced by oxidation of natural cholic acid. It is used to help flush out the biliary tract when it is only *partially* obstructed by mucus and small stones. This is supposed to keep the bile passages free of infections and calculi.

The sodium salt of this substance, *sodium dehydrocholate*, is sometimes injected by vein to help outline the gallbladder with x-ray contrast media and to remove such chemicals after biliary tract roentgenography. Such injections are also used for an entirely different purpose —the determination of circulation time. When the solution that is injected into the patient's cubital vein reaches his tongue, he becomes aware of its bitter taste, and the time it took to travel from arm to mouth is recorded as an index of circulation time.

Chenodeoxycholic acid (CDC), a natural constituent of human bile that has been prepared synthetically, is being tried clinically in the treatment of patients with gallstones of the cholesterol type. It is thought that this substance may keep cholesterol in gallbladder bile from becoming supersaturated and crystallizing out.

RELATED DRUGS. *Cholestyramine resin* (Cuemid; Questran), an ion-exchange resin that binds bile acids in the intestine before they can be reabsorbed, is used to lower plasma bile levels of jaundiced patients. This is said to relieve pruritus in patients with partial obstructive jaundice and primary biliary cirrhosis (see also Chapter 31).

Simethicone (Mylanta; Silain) is a substance said to aid in the elimination of gastrointestinal gas. It is taken orally alone or in combination with antacids to help relieve peptic pain, and in other conditions in which retention of gas causes distress. The drug, a defoaming agent which causes small gas bubbles to coalesce, is claimed to make it easier for patients to pass gas by belching or flatus. The usefulness of this surface-active agent as a digestive aid is uncertain. However, it seems to be free of adverse effects.

SUMMARY of Indications and Contraindications of Cathartics

Indications

Prevention of fecal impaction in bedridden patients

Reduction in straining at stool: a. in patients with cardiovascular complications, such as aneurism, embolism, and myocardial infarction, b. in patients with hemorrhoids and other anorectal lesions

Emptying the gastrointestinal tract prior to diagnostic procedures such as abdominal roentgenography and proctosigmoidoscopy

Removal of ingested poisons from lower gastrointestinal tract

Adjunctive uses in anthelmintic therapy

Adjunctive use in correction of constipation

Contraindications

Habitual use for forcing bowel movements in constipation

Acute appendicitis and other causes of abdominal pain and cramps, including regional enteritis, diverticulitis, and ulcerative colitis

Pregnancy, late in third trimester

During menstrual periods, possibly

SUMMARY of Points for the Nurse to Remember Concerning Cathartic Drugs

The nurse should suggest that the person who habitually takes any cathartic seek a physician's advice about his problem.

The nurse should instruct the constipated patient in the hygienic measures that will aid in reestablishing normal bowel function.

Observe the bowel function of all patients, and particularly those whose conditions may lead to fecal impaction. Ask the patient specific questions about his bowel function when assessing his elimination. In some instances, as with very old persons, young children, and very sick persons, it is necessary to inspect the contents of bed pan or commode.

Remember that it is not enough merely to lecture the patient on the desirability of eating a proper diet, drinking plenty of fluids, learning to handle his tensions, establishing a "habit time," and so forth. It is also necessary to recognize the patient's problem in misusing cathartics and to offer him your support in changing habit patterns which may have existed for many years.

Carefully note the patient's response to any cathartic that he receives. Note, for example, how soon the drug acted and the number and character of the stools that occurred as a result of its action.

Never administer a cathartic to a patient who has abdominal pain of unknown cause.

DRUG DIGEST

BISACODYL N.F. (Dulcolax)

Actions and Indications. This substance produces peristaltic activity upon contact with the mucosa of the colon. It may be administered orally to bring about effects within six hours or rectally for rapid action—in about 15 to 60 minutes. Because the drug acts by setting off local as well as segmental reflexes, it may produce satisfactory effects even in paraplegic and other patients with spinal cord injuries.

Other clinical indications for this laxative include: acute and chronic constipation; preparation of patients for abdominal and other surgery, for delivery, and for abdominal radiography; during postoperative and postpartum care; and in other situations in which a laxative or enema is indicated.

Side Effects, Cautions, and Contraindications. As with other laxatives, this drug should not be used in patients with an acute surgical abdomen or in the presence of still undiagnosed gastrointestinal pain. The drug's action may occasionally be accompanied by cramps or by a burning sensation in the rectum following insertion of the suppository form. Continued use of that form may cause mild proctitis. The suppository is not employed in the presence of an anal fissure or ulcerated hemorrhoids.

Dosage and Administration. Two 5-mg tablets may be swallowed but not chewed, crushed, or taken with antacids, as this affects the enteric coating. One 10-mg suppository is inserted at about the time a bowel movement is desired. Combinations of tablets and suppositories are also employed.

CASCARA SAGRADA U.S.P.

Actions and Indications. This is probably the mildest of the anthraquinone class of irritant cathartics. It acts mainly in the large intestine where its active constituent is liberated. The resulting peristaltic effect results in formation of a single soft stool in about six to eight hours after it is taken orally. It is preferred for patients who do *not* require rapid, complete purgation. These include bedridden patients, and particularly those who should not strain at stool because of possible cardiovascular complications.

Side Effects, Cautions, and Contraindications. Preparations of this plant produce few adverse effects other than diarrhea if taken in excess. Nursing mothers should not take these products, as the active constituents that are absorbed into the bloodstream may then reach the mother's milk and affect the infant. Patients should be told that their urine may be colored brown or red by constituents that are excreted by the kidneys. Those taking the drug for prolonged periods may show discoloration of the colonic and rectal mucosa, but this is reversible when the drug is discontinued, as it should be after normal bowel activity is established.

Dosage and Administration. The oral dose of about 300 mg is obtainable by taking 5 ml of the official Aromatic Cascara Fluidextract U.S.P. or 1 ml of the Fluidextract N.F. A powdered preparation, Cascara Sagrada Extract N.F., is also available. All are best taken at bedtime to bring about a formed bowel movement in the morning.

CASTOR OIL U.S.P.

Actions and Indications. This is a bland oil that is believed to break down in the small intestine to form an irritant cathartic principle called ricinoleic acid. It produces a relatively prompt and complete emptying of both the small and large bowel. Thus, it is employed in various situations in which rapid evacuation of the intestinal contents is desired. These include purges in the hospital on the day prior to x-ray examinations of the abdominal viscera, and removal of drug or food poisons from the intestine.

Side Effects, Cautions, and Contraindications. This drug seems free of adverse systemic effects, and the diarrhea that may result from overdosage is self-limited, as the cathartic is itself removed from the bowel by its own action. The oil has a taste that most people find unpleasant. This can be disguised by taking castor oil with iced carbonated beverages or fruit drinks. It is also available in the form of Aromatic Castor Oil N.F. and as a pleasant-tasting pharmaceutical emulsion.

Dosage and Administration. The adult dose is from 15 to 60 ml, and that for children 5 to 15 ml. For full effects, the oil is best administered on an empty stomach. It should not be given at bedtime, as it commonly produces one or more copious watery bowel movements within two to six hours after oral administration.

DIMENHYDRINATE U.S.P. (Dramamine)

Actions and Indications. This antiemetic agent was tested originally as an antihistaminic agent for allergy but is employed mainly for its C.N.S. action against motion sickness symptoms. In addition to preventing and relieving seasickness, airsickness, and so forth, this drug is used in various medical and surgical conditions marked by vestibular dysfunction. Such conditions include Meniere's syndrome, labyrinthitis, and streptomycin toxicity. The drug is also claimed to control nausea and vomiting in pregnancy and following anesthesia.

Side Effects, Cautions, and Contraindications. Side effects are few except for drowsiness in some patients. People who intend to operate vehicles or other motorized machinery are warned that their efficiency may be impaired.

Dosage and Administration. Adults may take 50 mg every four to six hours orally. If tablet or liquid forms cannot be retained, the drug may be administered rectally as a suppository, or parenterally, especially when prompt action is desired. Children may receive from one quarter the adult dose to the full amount in some cases.

DIOCTYL SODIUM SULFOSUCCINATE U.S.P. (Colace; Doxinate; and others)

Actions and Indications. This chemical has physical properties which help to produce a softer stool that is then more readily passed. It exerts a gradual surface tension-reducing effect that permits better penetration of a hardened fecal mass by fluid in the lower intestine. It is administered alone or as an adjunct to other laxatives, such as those of the stimulant type.

Side Effects, Cautions, and Contraindications. This compound causes few side effects, but occasional cramps may develop when it is administered in combination with other cathartics. It should *not* be taken with mineral oil because its presence may possibly increase the systemic absorption of liquid petrolatum through the intestinal mucosa. High concentrations applied locally by the rectal route may be irritating and may interfere with the healing of hemorrhoids or surgical wounds.

Dosage and Administration. The usual daily dose for oral administration to adults is 50 to 200 mg, and 10 to 40 mg for children in the form of a syrup or in fruit juice or milk. Higher doses may be needed at first to hasten the drug's full effects, which often do not develop for a couple of days. For more rapid action, a 0.1 percent solution may be administered rectally in amounts equal to between 50 to 100 mg.

PROCHLORPERAZINE MALEATE U.S.P. (Compazine)

Actions and Indications. This potent phenothiazine tranquilizer is used not only in psychiatry but also as an antiemetic in medicine, surgery, and obstetrics to control nausea, retching, and vomiting. It is believed to act by blocking the effects of circulating emetic chemicals upon the chemoreceptor trigger zone (C.T.Z.) Thus, it is probably more effective than the nonphenothiazine antiemetics against vomiting due to radiation and nitrogen mustard therapy of cancer, uremia, hepatitis, infections, and drugs such as anesthetics and narcotics. It is probably not as effective against motion sickness.

Side Effects, Cautions and Contraindications. The drugs of this class are used with caution in children and pregnant women because of the high incidence and severity of side effects caused by extrapyramidal motor system stimulation. Prochlorperazine and other drugs of its class are reserved for cautious use in cases of hyperemesis gravidarum not readily controlled by other measures. It is used during labor and postpartum but is not given in eclampsia. Children receive the lowest effective dosage, and parents are cautioned not to exceed the prescribed dosage.

Dosage and Administration. Treatment is begun with the lowest dose of this drug and adjusted in accordance with the patient's response. Dosage for antiemesis is much smaller than the amounts often required by psychotic patients. The drug is administered orally, rectally, and parenterally in single doses of 5 to 10 mg, in a total daily dosage rarely exceeding 30 mg. Children's dosage is calculated on the basis of body weight, especially when the drug is to be administered parenterally (for example, 0.06 mg/lb body weight by deep intramuscular injection).

References

ANTIDIARRHEAL DRUGS

Cooke, R. E. Current status of therapy in infantile diarrhea. *JAMA*, 167:1243, 1958.

Hoskins, D. W., and Kean, B. H. Drugs for travelers. *Clin. Pharmacol. Ther.*, 4:673, 1963.

Kean, B. H., et al. The diarrhea of travelers. *JAMA*, 180:367, 1962.

Low, D. H., et al. Drug therapy of gastrointestinal disease. *Amer. J. Med. Sci.*, 238:638, 1959.

Rodman, M. J. Drugs for vacation ills. *RN*, 25:73, 1962 (June).

————. Drugs for G.I. distress. *RN*, 28:49, 1965 (June).

ANTIEMETIC DRUGS

Belleville, J. W., Bross, I. D. J., and Howland, W. S. Postoperative nausea and vomiting; evaluation of antiemetic drugs. *JAMA*, 172:1488, 1960.

Borison, H. L., and Wang, S. C. Physiology and pharmacology of vomiting. *Pharmacol. Rev.*, 5:193, 1953.

Boyd, E. M. Antiemetic action of prochlorperazine (Compazine). *Canad. Med. Ass. J.*, 76:286, 1957.

Chinn, H. I., and Smith, P. K. Motion sickness. *Pharmacol. Rev.*, 7:33, 1955.

Doyle, O. W. Evaluation of trimethobenzamide as an antiemetic in nausea and vomiting associated with neoplasms. *Clin. Med.*, 7:43, 1960.

Hoskins, D. W., and Kean, B. H. Drugs for travelers. *Clin. Pharmacol. Ther.*, 4:673, 1963.

North, W. C., et al. Factors concerned with postoperative emesis and its prevention with thiethylperazine. *JAMA*, 183:656, 1963.

Rodman, M. J. Drugs for upset stomach. *RN*, 21:56, 1958 (Sept.).

———. Drugs for gastrointestinal distress. *RN*, 28:49, 1965 (June).

Trumbull, R. et al. Effect of certain drugs on the incidence of seasickness. *Clin. Pharmacol. Ther.*, 1:280, 1960.

Winters, H. S. Antiemetics in nausea and vomiting of pregnancy. *Obstet. Gynec.*, 18:753, 1961.

DRUGS WITH CATHARTIC ACTION

Dreiling, D. A., Fischl, R. A., and Fernandez, O. Dulcolax (Bisacodyl), a new nonpurgative laxative. *Amer. J. Dig. Dis.*, 4:311, 1959.

Frohman, I. P. Constipation. *Amer. J. Nurs.*, 55:65, 1955.

Gray, G., and Tainter, M. L. Colloid laxatives available for clinical use. *Amer. J. Dig. Dis.*, 8:130, 1941.

Hecht, A. B. Self medication inaccuracy and what can be done. *Nurs. Outlook*, 18:30, 1970 (April).

Morgan, J. W. The harmful effects of mineral oil (liquid petrolatum) purgatives. *JAMA*, 117:1335, 1941.

Munch, J. C., and Calesnick, B. Laxative studies. I. Human threshold studies of white and yellow phenolphthalein. *Clin. Pharmacol. Ther.*, 1:311, 1960.

Rodman, M. J. The use and misuse of cathartics. *RN*, 21:48, 1958 (July); 21:49, 1958 (Aug.).

Steignamm, F. Are laxatives necessary? *Amer. J. Nurs.*, 62:90, 1962.

Wilson, J. L., and Dickinson, D. G. Use of dioctyl sodium sulfosuccinate (Aerosol O.T.) for severe constipation. *JAMA*, 158:261, 1955.

46.

Drugs Used in Dermatology

Skin diseases are among the most common medical disorders. Although they are only rarely life-threatening, dermatologic disorders are often painful, disabling, or embarrassing. The nurse who knows the general principles of dermatologic therapy can help to hasten the patient's recovery.

In this chapter, we shall discuss the drugs that affect the skin in various ways (Tables 46-1, -2, and -3) and then indicate how drugs of different types are employed in the management of some of the most common skin ailments. We shall also summarize the kinds of nursing care measures that are helpful aids to effective drug treatment against the main kinds of pathological reaction patterns. These include inflammatory responses to allergy, infection, and injury, and abnormal changes in the growth and functioning of skin cells and glands.

Types of Drug Action on the Skin (Table 46-1)

Many kinds of medications are employed by topical application or are administered systemically to bring about beneficial changes in the ailing skin. The most important drugs are those that are used to reduce inflammatory reactions and to protect the damaged skin from further irritation. However, some drugs that are themselves mildly or even strongly irritating to the skin also have a place in the treatment of certain skin disorders that are marked by excessive skin cell growth or function.

T A B L E 4 6 - 1   *Glossary of Terms Used to Describe the Actions of Drugs on the Skin*

Term	Definition
Antieczematic	A general term for any drug used in treating eczema, which is itself a vague term denoting almost any kind of chronic inflammatory skin condition, the cause of which is uncertain
Antihistaminic	A drug that antagonizes the effects of free histamine on the skin and its blood vessels and thus relieves signs and symptoms of skin allergy
Antiinfective	A drug used to treat or prevent skin or mucous membrane infection by pathogenic microbes (for example, antimicrobials, antibacterials, antifungal, antiseptic, and so forth)
Antiinflammatory	An agent used to reduce skin inflammation and relieve its signs and symptoms
Antiperspirant	A chemical claimed to reduce the local flow of sweat; it is usually also an astringent and deodorant
Antipruritic	An agent used to relieve pruritus, or itching; topically applied agents usually have local anesthetic properties
Antipsoriatic	A drug used in the treatment of psoriasis, including particularly skin irritants of the keratolytic and keratoplastic types
Antiseborrheic	A chemical used to reduce the activity of the sebaceous glands or to remove greasy skin scales, including those of dandruff
Antiseptic	A chemical substance that kills microorganisms on the skin and elsewhere or prevents their growth
Astringent	Chemicals that act locally to coagulate or precipitate protein; this action tends to contract tissues and thus to stop the flow of fluid secretions, including oozing, sweat, and blood
Caustic	A corrosive chemical used to destroy tissues, including warts
Counterirritant	Chemical applied topically to the skin to produce irritation in order to relieve pain stemming from skeletal muscles or from visceral organs in various systemic diseases
Demelanizing agent	A chemical employed to remove excessive skin pigment in the treatment of hypermelanosis (hyperpigmentation)
Demulcent	A substance employed to coat the skin and mucous membranes. It provides mechanical protection against irritation of these surfaces
Deodorant	A substance used to remove or mask disagreeable odors
Depigmenting agent	See *demelanizing agent*, above
Depilatory	A chemical employed to remove hair
Desquamating agent	A chemical used to cause shedding of epidermal scales (see *keratolytic*)
Detergent	An agent used to cleanse the skin; it usually also possesses antiseptic properties
Disinfectant	A chemical that destroys pathogenic microorganisms when applied to inanimate objects; in low concentration it may also be used on the skin as an antiseptic
Dusting Powder	An inert substance applied to the skin to protect the irritated surface or to absorb excessive moisture
Emollient	An oily or fatty substance used to keep the skin soft and to prevent the evaporation of water and development of dryness
Enzymes, Proteolytic	Biological materials applied to the skin to speed the breakdown of necrotic tissues in ulcerated or burned skin areas (that is, for chemical debridement of dead tissue)
Escharotic	A caustic or corrosive chemical that cauterizes or burns away tissue and causes scab or scar formation
Hemostatic	A topically applied substance that stops bleeding from skin or mucosal surfaces
Irritant	A general term for locally applied drugs that induce inflammatory responses of various degrees, ranging from warmth and redness to blister formation (see *rubefacient, pustulant, vesicant*)
Keratolytics	Substances that soften skin keratin so that epidermal scales are more readily loosened and removed (that is, peeling or desquamating agents)

T A B L E 4 6 - 1 *Glossary of Terms Used to Describe the Actions of Drugs on the Skin (continued)*

Term	Definition
Melanizing agent	An agent employed to stimulate skin pigmentation in treating disorders marked by hypopigmentation (a pigmentation stimulating agent)
Pediculocide	A chemical used to kill lice on the skin or in hair
Protectant	A substance used to protect the exposed skin or mucous membranes from irritation by mechanically covering them (see *demulcent, dusting powder, emollient*)
Pustulant	An irritant that causes formation of small pus-filled blisters
Rubefacient	An irritant that causes reddening of the skin as a result of local reflex vasodilation
Scabicide	A chemical used to kill the burrowing mite that is the cause of scabies
Sclerosing agent	An irritating substance employed to obliterate varicose veins by stimulating production of fibrous connective tissue
Styptic	A topically applied substance that stops capillary oozing of blood by its astringent action
Sunscreen	A chemical employed to absorb the burning rays of the sun and thus to protect the skin from sunburn
Trichomonacide	A chemical employed to kill trichomonal protozoans, particularly *Trichomonas vaginalis*
Vesicant	A skin-irritating chemical that causes formation of blisters

DRUGS FOR REDUCING IRRITATION AND INFLAMMATION

Medications for soothing the irritated or inflamed skin include the antiinflammatory corticosteroids and drugs categorized as emollients, demulcents, dusting powders, and skin protectants (see Table 46-1 for the definitions of these terms and Table 46-2 for specific examples of drugs in each class).

TOPICAL CORTICOSTEROIDS. These are said to account for about half of all the orders and prescriptions that doctors write today for treating skin disorders. Applied alone or in combination with various other drugs of several different classes (see below), the corticosteroids have proved both *effective* for relief of acute and chronic inflammation and *safe* from systemic steroid toxicity (see Table 46-3). Thus, when patients whose skin conditions require prolonged application of a topical steroid preparation express concern about its possible toxicity, the nurse can assure them that little of the drug is likely to be absorbed and that Cushingoid-type toxicity rarely occurs.

Triamcinolone acetonide+ (Aristocort; Kenalog) and other steroids are available in various kinds of vehicles, including creams, ointments, lotions, and aerosol sprays. The thin film left by sprayed and cream-based steroids is preferred for reducing redness, swelling, and oozing from the denuded epidermis. Lotions containing steroids counteract inflammation and itching in hairy areas and on the face. Greasy ointment bases are not used on hairy areas and are mainly reserved for dry, scaly lesions, such as those of psoriasis. In psoriasis, steroids are frequently applied under airtight dressings, in order to promote deeper penetration of these drugs. Even in such cases, systemic absorption and subsequent development of hypercorticism is unlikely.

DRUGS WITH LOCAL IRRITANT ACTION

Chemicals that cause skin irritation are often deliberately applied for various treatment purposes. The degree of irritation can be controlled by diluting these drugs in suitable vehicles. Thus, substances such as sulfur or coal tar exert only a mildly irritating effect when applied in creams, ointments, and lotions for treating acne or psoriasis in order to speed the peeling of epithelial cells.

On the other hand, some substances that are used as *desquamating agents* (see Tables 46-1 and -2) may be irritating enough to cause skin ulcers in patients with poor local circulation. Thus, the nurse warns patients with peripheral vascular diseases or diabetes never to treat corns or calluses with proprietary prod-

TABLE 46-2   *Dermatologic Drugs*

Agent	Uses
To Counteract Irritation	
Benzocaine N. F.	Anesthetic, topical
Benzoin compound tincture N.F.	Protectant
Bismuth subcarbonate U.S.P.	Protectant
Calamine U.S.P. and Calamine ointment N.F.	Protectant
Camphor, U.S.P.	Antipruritic
Cold cream U.S.P.	Emollient
Collodion, flexible U.S.P.	Protectant
Cottonseed oil U.S.P.	Emollient
Cyproheptadine N.F.	Antihistaminic-antipruritic
Dimethicone	Protectant
Glycerin U.S.P.	Emollient-humectant
Hydrophilic ointment U.S.P.	Emollient
Lanolin U.S.P. and Lanolin anhydrous U.S.P.	Emollient
Magnesium stearate	Dusting powder
Menthol U.S.P.	Antipruritic
Methdilazine N.F.	Antihistamine-antipruritic
Oatmeal	Demulcent-emollient
Olive oil U.S.P.	Emollient
Ointment, white U.S.P.	Emollient
Ointment, yellow U.S.P.	Emollient
Peruvian balsam N.F.	Protectant
Petrolatum, hydrophilic U.S.P.	Protectant
Petrolatum, white U.S.P.	Emollient
Phenol, liquified U.S.P.	Antipruritic
Polyethylene glycol ointment U.S.P.	Protectant
Pramoxine	Anesthetic, topical
Rose water ointment N.F.	Emollient
Silicone	Protectant
Starch U.S.P.	Dusting powder
Starch, glycerite N.F.	Emollient
Talc, U.S.P.	Dusting powder
Titanium dioxide U.S.P.	Protectant
Trimeprazine tartrate N.F.	Antihistaminic-antipruritic
Zinc, gelatin U.S.P.	Protectant
Zinc oxide U.S.P.	Protectant
Zinc stearate U.S.P.	Dusting powder
Zirconium oxide	Protectant
To Cause Local Irritation	Protectant
Alcohol, rubbing (ethyl and isopropyl) N.F.	Rubefacient
Alum N.F.	Astringent-antiperspirant
Aluminum acetate U.S.P.	Astringent-antiperspirant
Aluminum chloride N.F.	Astringent-antiperspirant
Aluminum subacetate U.S.P.	Astringent-antiperspirant
Anthralin N.F.	Keratolytic
Cadmium sulfide	Antiseborrheic
Calcium hydroxide U.S.P.	Astringent
Calcium sulfide	Depilatory
Calcium thioglycollate	Depilatory
Chrysarobin	Keratolytic
Coal, tar, U.S.P.	Keratolytic
Formaldehyde	Caustic; keratolytic
Icthammol	Keratolytic
Juniper tar N.F.	Keratolytic
Pine tar N.F.	Keratolytic

TABLE 46-2 *Dermatologic Drugs (continued)*

Agent	Uses
To Cause Local Irritation (continued)	
Podophyllum resin N.F.	Caustic; keratolytic
Resorcinol U.S.P.	Keratolytic
Resorcinol monoacetate N.F.	Keratolytic
Salicyclic acid U.S.P.	Keratolytic
Selenium sulfide N.F.	Antiseborrheic
Silver nitrate U.S.P.	Caustic; keratolytic
Sulfur, sublimed N.F.	Keratolytic
Sulfurated lime solution	Keratolytic
Trichloroacetic acid	Caustic
Zinc chloride U.S.P.	Astringent
Zinc oxide paste with salicylic acid N.F.	Astringent-keratolytic
Zinc and potassium sulfates (White Lotion) N.F.	Keratolytic-astringent
Zinc sulfate U.S.P.	Astringent
Miscellaneous	
Hydroquinone	Depigmenting agent
Methoxsalen	Photosensitizer; pigment producer
Monobenzone N.F.	Depigmentation agent
Para-aminobenzoic acid U.S.P.	Sunscreen
Petroleum, red, veterinary	Sunscreen
Titanium dioxide U.S.P.	Sunscreen
Trioxsalen	Pigment producer
Zinc oxide U.S.P.	Sunscreen

ucts containing salicylic acid or other potent keratolytic agents (Table 46-2).

Caustic chemicals are sometimes applied to warts in order to destroy these unsightly skin tumors. In such cases, care is required to keep corrosive chemicals such as *trichloroacetic acid* of *formaldehyde* from coming in contact with the surrounding normal tissues. This is usually done by applying petrolatum to protect the healthy tissues from the spread of the strong solutions. *Silver nitrate* (Lunar Caustic) is available in the form of sticks or pencils that may be moistened and simply touched to granulation tissue, warts, or wounds that require cauterization.

The Treatment of Specific Skin Disorders

DERMATITIS

Inflammation is the most common skin reaction, occurring in many different kinds of dermatologic disorders. The signs and symptoms of inflammatory skin reactions differ in degree of severity. Skin changes range from slight redness (*erythema*) that may need no treatment at all to reactions marked by the formation of massive blisters (*bullae*) with deep destruction of the underlying connective tissue of the skin (the *dermis*).

The general purpose of all types of treatment is to help the skin's natural healing mechanisms bring about recovery. Ordinarily, if the patient does not rub or scratch the itching areas or pick at the protective crusts that form over oozing vesicles (*blebs*) or blisters, the inflamed skin heals completely. Thus, drug therapy is used to relieve itching, release heat, dry up oozing areas, and protect the damaged skin.

In the following discussions of some representative types of dermatitis, we shall indicate how different types of dermatologic medications are best employed.

ACUTE CONTACT DERMATITIS. This results from exposure of the skin to chemical substances that elicit inflammatory responses. The reaction may range from a slight redness and itching to severe swelling and blistering of the skin. The chemical cause may be either a primary irritant or a substance to which a particular individual has become allergic through

TABLE 46-3 *Topically Applied Corticosteroids*

Official or Generic Name	Proprietary Name	Dosage Forms	
Betamethasone N.F.	Celestone	Cream	0.2%
Betamethasone benzoate	Benisone; Flurobate	Gel	0.025%
Betamethasone valerate N.F.	Valisone	Aerosol	0.15%
		Cream	0.1%
		Ointment	0.1%
Desonide	Tridesilon	Cream	0.05%
Dexamethasone U.S.P.	Decadron; Hexadrol	Cream	0.04%
		Aerosol	0.011%
Dexamethasone sodium phosphate N.F.	Decadron phosphate	Cream	0.1%
		Ointment	0.1%
Fludrocortisone acetate	Florinef acetate; F-Cortef acetate	Ointment	0.1 and 0.2%
		Lotion	0.1%
Flumethasone pivalate	Locorten	Cream	0.03%
Fluocinolone acetonide N.F.	Fluonid; Synalar	Cream	0.01% and 0.025%
		Ointment	0.025%
Fluocinonide	Lidex	Ointment	0.05%
Fluorometholone N.F.	Oxylone	Cream	0.025%
Flurandrenolide	Cordran	Cream	0.03% and 0.05%
		Ointment	0.03% and 0.05%
		Lotion	0.05%
		Tape	4 μg per sq. cm
Hydrocortamate HCl	Ulcort	Ointment	0.5%
Hydrocortisone U.S.P.	Cetacort; Cort-Dome; Cortril; and others	Creams; Ointments; Lotions; and Aerosols	0.125% to 0.5%
Hydrocortisone acetate U.S.P.	Cort-Dome acetate Cortef acetate; Hydrocortone acetate	Ointments	0.5% to 1.5%
Medrysone	HMS	Lotion	1%
Methylprednisolone acetate N.F.	Medrol acetate	Ointment	0.25% and 1%
Prednisolone U.S.P.	Meti-Derm	Cream	0.5%
Predisolone acetate U.S.P.	Metimyd	Ointment and suspension (ophthalmic)	0.5%
Prednisolone sodium phosphate U.S.P.	Optival; Hydeltrasol; and others	Solution (ophthalmic) Ointment and Lotion	0.5% 0.5%
Triamcinolone acetonide U.S.P.	Aristocort; Kenalog	Creams; Ointments; Lotions; and Sprays	0.03% to 0.1%

prior exposure and sensitization. Although almost any chemical can cause allergic contact dermatitis, some substances are relatively stronger sensitizers than others.

One of the most familiar skin sensitizers in this country is the plant we call "poison ivy." Like its relatives of the *Rhus* genus, poison oak and poison sumac, it contains a sensitizing oil, called *urushiol*, to which most Americans react positively in skin tests. Exposure of the skin to this allergen leads to a dermatitis marked by development of groups or lines of vesicles containing serous fluid.

❨ *Treatment.* Topical treatment is aimed primarily at relieving itching and thus stopping the urge to scratch. Scratching is undesirable, *not* because it "spreads the poison," but because pathogenic bacteria may enter breaks made in the skin by the fingernails. The secondary bacterial infections that frequently follow such scratching tend to prevent the skin from recovering its normal state of health.

Itching in the acute stage of contact dermatitis is best controlled with wet dressings followed by application of protective lotions. Evaporation of water from the compress has a cooling effect. Soaking the covering cloths with *aluminum acetate solution+* or *potassium permanganate solution+* adds their desirable astringent effects. This tends to aid drying of oozing areas and causes protective crusts to form over the weeping blebs and blisters.

Such solutions are applied for about 20 minutes, and then the area is daubed with a drying lotion that is shaken before use. The thin layer of skin protectant, such as zinc oxide, that is left on the denuded areas soothes the skin and relieves itching. The addition of phenol, menthol, or camphor to *calamine lotion+* adds to the antipruritic action of such preparations. In the later stages, when the skin may be dry and cracked, the doctor may switch to *calamine ointment* or some other greasy emollient substance.

Topical steroid application is not very useful until the acute stage has subsided. Steroids do not penetrate the epithelium of vesicles and bullae, and when such blisters break, the flow of serous fluid simply washes away the drug. Later, however, when applied in the periods between wet dressings, creams containing hydrocortisone or other steroids sometimes help to relieve inflammatory itching. However, topically applied steroids are not as necessary here as in other pruritic dermatoses, and may be too expensive to use if the eruption covers large areas of the body.

Systemic steroids are preferred in extensive and severe contact dermatitis. Large doses of these drugs, administered immediately and then rapidly reduced and finally withdrawn over a period of several days or a week, are indicated in the management of acute, self-limited conditions such as poison ivy. This type of steroid treatment is relatively safe, as it does not lead to hypercorticism or significantly depress adrenal cortical function, as is inevitably the case in more chronic conditions (see discussion of "step down" dosage schedules in Chapter 17).

Later, when the acute stage has subsided, topical application of a *local anesthetic* cream may be employed for relief of persisting pruritus (see discussion of topical anesthetics in Chapter 15). Some *antihistaminic* agents also exert *antipruritic* activity when applied topically—*tripelennamine+*, for example. Orally administered antihistamines such as *cyproheptadine+* (Periactin) and others (see below) may help to relieve itching by their sedative effects.

ATOPIC DERMATITIS. This is a chronic skin condition that often appears in infancy and lasts through childhood into adult life. Like other chronic dermatoses that are often lumped under the vague term "eczema," its basic cause is not known. There are indications that a predisposition to these skin lesions is inherited. Often the patient or members of his family suffer from hay fever, asthma, or a tendency toward urticarial reactions.

People who are prone to develop chronic eczematous dermatitis have an extremely sensitive skin. Slight stimuli set off an itching sensation. This, in turn, results in scratching that can cause skin damage and secondary bacterial infections.

Treatment. Treatment of atopic dermatitis is based on the need to relieve itching and inflammation by means of topical and systemic medication. The most effective agents are topical corticosteroids in creams, lotions, or ointments. *Hydrocortisone* is the least expensive of these compounds, but *triamcinolone acetonide+* and other new synthetic steroids such as *betamethasone valerate, fluocinolone* and *flurandenolone* (Table 46-3) are much more potent.

Local anesthetic creams can also provide relief of itching. However, their prolonged use in atopic dermatitis is not desirable, because these patients may become sensitized to these drugs. In fact, anything can serve as a source of irritation when smeared on the sensitive skin of such patients. Even an antihistamine drug may cause contact dermatitis when applied topically in cream or lotion form as an antipruritic in atopic individuals.

Antihistamine drugs may, however, be administered orally for relief of itching. In part, their effectiveness may stem from control of allergic reactions to the substances to which the atopic patient is hypersensitive. On the other hand, the central effects of certain antihistamine agents may also play an important part in control of itching. *Trimeprazine* (Temaril) and *methdilazine* (Tacaryl) are related to the phenothiazine tranquilizers. Thus, these and other central depressant antihistaminics such as *diphenhydramine+* (Benadryl) and *cyproheptadine+* (Periactin) may reduce the patient's awareness of itching and lessen his emotional reaction to it.

SUNBURN AND OTHER THERMAL BURNS

The skin's reaction to heat rays is similar to what occurs when dermatitis develops as a result of chemical, allergic, or mechanical injury. First degree burns are marked mainly by skin redness (erythema). This is more intense and is followed by painful blistering in second-degree burns. Destruction of both epidermis and dermis—the entire skin thickness—characterizes deep third-degree burns from fire, boiling water, steam, or high heat.

TREATMENT. Topical care is only one aspect of *acute burn care*. Severly burned patients often require measures for aid to respiratory function, close attention to balance between I.V. fluid intake and elimination, management of pain with analgesics and sedatives, and systemic steroids to fight inflammation. Wound care involves topical application of *mafenide acetate* (sulfamylon), *silver sulfadiazine, silver nitrate* (0.5 percent solution), or *gentamycin* (Garamycin) to prevent infection and reduce odor. (See also Chapters 41 and 42.)

In accordance with the general principle of treating the most severe inflammatory reactions with the mildest means, badly burned patients are kept immersed in tepid water for long periods and are transferred to talcum-powdered bed sheets. The burned parts of the body are protected, rested, and exercised only lightly to maintain the range of motion. Complete rest, rather than the use of chemical protectants, is the rule.

Sunburn that is limited largely to the epidermis can be relieved by application of other soothing substances. Taking tepid baths containing cornstarch, oatmeal, or other colloids aids the tender, smarting skin. In acute, severe sunburn with blistering, mildly astringent and cooling liquids such as *aluminum acetate solution+* or *corticosteroid* drug sprays often help to control local pain and itching. Later, *phenolated calamine lotion+, zinc oxide* ointment, or creams containing topical anesthetics or antihistaminics can be used to cover and protect the healing skin areas.

Sun-induced skin damage of a *chronic* nature often occurs in light-skinned people whose occupations require prolonged exposure to sunlight. This can lead to skin cancer or development of *pre*malignant growths called keratoses. These lesions caused by ultraviolet (actinic) light rays are called *solar*, or *actinic*, *keratoses*

—or sometimes, because of their relationship to aging—senile keratoses.

Fluorouracil (Efudex), applied topically as a cream or solution, is often effective for clearing up solar keratoses and preventing their progress to the malignant stage. During the typical two- to four-week course of treatment, the patient's skin seems, at first, to get worse. Redness, blistering, ulcer formation, and necrosis are necessary preliminaries to healing.

Thus, the nurse encourages the patient to continue treatment despite his physical discomfort and emotional distress. She assures him that the unsightly appearance of the treated lesions will lessen in a month or two. The patient is cautioned to avoid exposure to sunlight during topical fluorouracil treatment. He is also warned to wash his hands immediately after applying the medication with a gloved hand or nonmetallic applicator. Special care is needed in treating solar keratosis lesions located close to the eyes, nose, and mouth.

SUNSCREENS. Chemicals of several kinds are available for protecting the skin of sun-sensitive patients. Opaque pigments such as *zinc oxide* and *titanium oxide* are preferred for people prone to develop solar keratoses, those subject to photosensitivity-type drug reactions, and patients with lupus erythematosus or other light-sensitive skin eruptions. *Red veterinary petrolatum* is also employed for completely excluding light rays.

Para-aminobenzoic acid (PABA), or one of its ester derivatives (Table 46-2), are preferred for use by people who want to tan without burning. A 5 percent solution of PABA in ethyl alcohol (75–90 percent) is said to be more effective for this purpose than any of the commercially available products containing other sunscreen chemicals. However, none of these screeners of rays in the ultraviolet spectrum alone is enough to protect people who react adversely to any kind of visible light.

Fortunately for those who cannot stay indoors during the day or who will not wear the white or greasy materials mentioned above, various new products that are cosmetically more attractive are now becoming available for use when complete exclusion of all light rays is required. Sunscreens of this kind belong to chemical classes called benzophenones and include *oxybenzone, dioxybenzone,* and *sulisobenzone*.

Skin Pigmenting and Depigmenting Agents.
Several drugs are available for treating various
skin disorders that are the result of a lack of
melanin or an excess of this skin pigment.
V*itiligo*, a *hypo*pigmentation disorder marked
by loss of melanin in scattered patches of skin,
has been successfully treated with orally administered drugs of the psoralen type—*tri-
oxsalen*+ (Trisoralen) and *methoxsalen* (Mel-
oxine). However, full repigmentation may require several years of carefully regulated
treatment.

*Hyper*pigmentation is managed by local application of chemicals such as *hydroquinone*
and *monobenzone*. Applied locally in lotion
or ointment form to heavily freckled skin,
these substances often lighten the spots. Similarly, in *melasma* or *cloasma*, a condition that
sometimes develops during pregnancy or in
women taking oral contraceptives, these depigmenting agents may lighten the darkened skin
areas. Care is required to avoid removing
melanin from normal skin. Contact dermatitis
occasionally develops in sensitized individuals.

ACNE

Acne is one of the most common of all skin
disorders. An estimated 80 to 90 percent of all
adolescents are affected to some extent. Many
youngsters need no special treatment besides
faithful use of simple hygienic measures for
cleansing the skin. Other teenagers cannot control the spread of acne by ordinary skin care
measures. They should be urged to seek medical attention rather than use the products
widely advertised for self-medication. Severe,
uncontrolled acne causes scarring, which may
adversely affect the emotional health and developing personality structure in young people.

The lesions of acne develop during adolescence when androgens stimulate growth and
secretion of the sebaceous glands. At the same
time, the pores that open onto the skin surface
become plugged with cellular debris containing
the protein, keratin. The resulting *comedones*,
or blackheads, provoke local inflammation that
leads to lesions of varying severity.

Treatment. Cleansing of the skin well with
soap and water to remove keratin, sebum, and
bacteria is the cornerstone of all acne control
programs. Even *non*pathogenic skin bacteria
can be a cause of local irritation and inflammation. Thus, the use of alcohol sponges and
detergent liquids locally—*hexachlorophene*+,
for example—may also be useful for reducing

the bacterial flora. (This is also the basis for
oral administration of broad-spectrum antibiotics of the *tetracycline type* in some cases.)

Topical treatment with preparations containing mild keratinolytic agents such as *resorcinol*+, *salicylic acid*, and *sulfur* is employed
in the less severe grades of acne. Creams and
lotions containing these substances help to
lessen skin oiliness and clear the pores of
keratin plugs. For deeper pustules and cysts,
hot compresses made with *sulfurated lime solution* (Vleminckx solution) or a lotion of
zinc sulfate and *sulfurated potash* (White Lotion) may be employed.

Trenitoin (Retin A), an acid derivative of
vitamin A, has recently been introduced for use
in place of the traditional peeling agents. The
patient swabs his skin with a solution of this
substance at bedtime for four to six weeks. At
first his skin may look worse as it reddens,
peels, and allows hidden comedones to come
to the surface. However, after a time, the appearance of the skin often improves and the
drug need not be applied as frequently as before. This reduces the drug-induced inflammatory reaction and lets the acne lesions heal.

Estrogens, taken internally, tend to antagonize androgens and thus to decrease sebum
secretion. Small daily doses of *mestranol*+ are
often effective for control of severe acne in
some girls who have not responded to topical
treatment or to systemic antibiotics. To avoid
menstrual irregularities, a progestin may be
added and then withdrawn. (Oral contraceptive
preparations are sometimes prescribed in cases
of acne in order to regularize the menstrual
cycle while achieving improvement of the girl's
acne.)

PSORIASIS

Psoriasis is a chronic skin eruption of the
papulosquamous type. That is, its characteristic
lesions are reddish papules, or raised areas, that
are covered by dry, silvery scales, or squamae.
Although this condition often seems to respond
readily to treatment, the lesions almost inevitably tend to recur.

Topical Treatment. Various mildly irritating
materials are applied to the skin to remove
psoriatic scales and stimulate healing of the underlying lesion. Dermatologists often begin
with mild agents such as *ammoniated mercury*+ ointment and then add somewhat more
irritating substances such as *coal tar*+. Another
irritant, *anthralin*, is less likely to stain the

skin and clothing. Most of these substances tend to lose their effectiveness after a time, but tolerance can be delayed by withholding treatment while this dermatosis is in a remission stage.

Locally administered corticosteroids were relatively ineffective when merely rubbed into the skin. However, when covered with an occlusive dressing, topical corticosteroids such as *triamicinolone acetonide*+ and *flurandrenolide* (Cordran) (Table 46-3) are often quite effective. The plastic film or tape containing the medication keeps moisture from evaporating from the skin. The steroid then diffuses down into deeper skin layers to exert its therapeutic effects.

Systemic corticosteroid therapy is sometimes employed to control extensively spreading acute psoriasis. The high doses that are required often cause hypercorticism, and when the steroids are finally withdrawn, the condition may become worse than before. Continued use of corticosteroids in a chronic condition such as psoriasis is undesirable. Though the use of long-term steroids to control skin symptoms may be justified in potentially fatal conditions such as pemphigus and disseminated lupus, psoriasis is, after all, essentially benign and never fatal.

Methotrexate+, a drug ordinarily reserved for treating malignant neoplasms, has recently been employed in treating selected cases of severe psoriasis that can no longer be controlled by topical therapy or systemic steroids. Although this drug sometimes helps produce remissions in patients disabled by psoriasis, it is potentially quite toxic. Thus, the doctor adjusts oral dosage to the lowest level that is effective for clearing severe psoriatic lesions. Patients are closely supervised and carefully observed for signs of toxicity. They should be fully informed of the risks of this treatment and taught to report all adverse reactions.

Azarabine (Triazure), a derivation of another anticancer chemical, is claimed to be safer and more effective than methotrexate. Taken orally, this drug has brought about remission of severe psoriatic lesions without causing significant toxicity of the kind expected from antimetabolite drugs (Chapter 48). Nonetheless, patients must be carefully observed during treatment courses, and blood tests must be made biweekly.

SEBORRHEIC DERMATITIS

This chronic scaling skin disorder seems closer to psoriasis than to the inflammatory-type dermatoses. The most common and mildest form is dandruff of the scalp. This can be readily kept under control by frequent shampooing, particularly with a medicated detergent suspension. *Selenium sulfide*+ (Selsun) is commonly employed for this purpose, as is *cadmium sulfide* (Capsebon), which is claimed to be free of the arseniclike systemic toxicity that may develop if the selenium salt is swallowed.

The more severe forms of chronic seborrheic dermatitis are often treated with the same sort of irritant-keratolytic combinations that are employed against psoriatic scaliness. Thus antiseborrheic ointments containing coal tar, precipitated sulfur, resorcinol, and salicylic acid are often rubbed into the scalp at bedtime and kept on overnight. The head is shampooed on the following morning. When such substances are used in lotion form, care is required to keep them from running into the eyes and ears.

Prevention and Treatment of Infection

The skin acts as an effective barrier against the entrance of microbes into the body. Pathogenic microorganisms cannot ordinarily penetrate the outer protective layer of hard keratin-containing epidermal cells. These cells are low in moisture and high in organic acids and enzymes capable of destroying surface bacteria and fungi (see Fig. 46-1).

Sometimes, however, the natural resistance of the skin may be reduced. In such cases, pathogenic microbes—most commonly grampositive bacteria such as staphylococci, but also fungi and other kinds of organisms—can set off skin infections. In addition, bacteria that break through the weakened skin defenses can then enter the blood and reach other organs such as the kidneys, bones, or brain.

Topically applied antiseptics are not very effective for treating acute skin infections, and systemically administered antiinfective agents are preferred for this purpose. However, chemicals that can kill or control the growth of skin microbes are often useful for *preventing* infection or, at least, limiting its spread. Among the purposes for which such antiinfective substances are employed are: (1) reducing the numbers of pathogenic microorganisms on the hands of those responsible for patient care—surgical and nursery personnel, for example; (2) preoperative preparation of the patient's skin and postoperative care of the surgical wound; (3) prevention of infection in possibly contaminated cuts, scratches, and abrasions; and (4) treatment of superficial infections of the

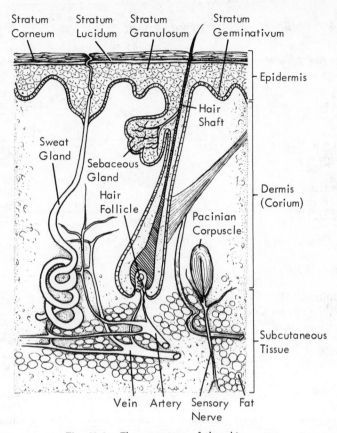

Stratum Corneum — Stratum Lucidum — Stratum Granulosum — Stratum Germinativum

Epidermis

Hair Shaft

Sweat Gland

Sebaceous Gland

Hair Follicle

Pacinian Corpuscle

Dermis (Corium)

Subcutaneous Tissue

Vein   Artery   Sensory Nerve   Fat

Fig. 46-1. The structure of the skin.

skin and the mucous membranes of such organs and structures as the eye, anorectal region, and vaginal tract (see Table 46-4).

In the following discussions of the various clinical situations in which antiseptic substances are applied topically, we shall emphasize selected aspects of individual drugs in the different chemical classes. However, these discussions will also deal with the factors that determine whether an antimicrobial agent is likely to be effective. The nurse, who often stands as the first line of defense against the spread of infection in the hospital and elsewhere, must be familiar with the *principles* of proper antiseptic use, as well as with the characteristics of the individual agents.

SKIN CLEANSING AND DISINFECTION

SURGICAL SCRUBBING. *Hand care* and *preoperative preparation* of the proposed surgical incision site is performed in many different ways and with the use of a wide variety of antiseptic chemicals. Here we shall discuss only some of the most commonly employed sub-

stances and how they are best used to assure their full effectiveness and safety. No matter what antiseptic or technique of application is employed, washing with soap and water is a standard preliminary procedure.

Soap has little effect as an antibacterial agent, but as a detergent it removes such skin debris as keratin and natural fats. At the same time most of the contaminating bacteria contained in such surface substances is removed. Soaps and certain synthetic anionic surfactants, or "wetting agents," permit water to penetrate better and thus help to float out some of the flora that reside deep in the crypts, crevices, pits, and ridges of the skin.

Alcohols, such as ethyl and isopropyl alcohols, are often used to rinse residual soap from the skin. Both can kill bacteria but not their spores. For best results, a 70 percent concentration by weight of ethyl alcohol is recommended, whereas isopropyl alcohol is used full strength. The longer these alcohols are in contact with the skin, the greater the germicidal effect. However, even briefly swabbing the skin

T A B L E 4 6 - 4 *Topical Antiinfective Agents*

Official or Nonproprietary Name	Trade Name or Synonym
Alcohols	
Ethyl alcohol U.S.P.	Ethanol
Isopropyl alcohol N.F.	. . . .
Antibiotics	
Bacitracin U.S.P.	. . . .
Chloramphenicol U.S.P.	Chloromycetin
Chlortetracycline HCl N.F.	Aureomycin
Erythromycin U.S.P.	Erythrocin; Ilotycin
Gentamycin sulfate U.S.P.	Garamycin
Neomycin sulfate U.S.P.	Mycifradin
Polymyxin B sulfate U.S.P.	Aerosporin
Tyrothricin N.F.	. . . .
Antibacterial Sulfonamides	
Mafenide acetate	Sulfamylon
Sulfacetamide sodium U.S.P.	Sulamyd
Sulfadiazine U.S.P.	. . . .
Sulfisoxazole diolamine U.S.P.	Gantrisin
Antifungal Antibiotics and Chemicals	
Acrisorcin	Akrinol
Amphotericin B	Fungizone
Calcium undecylenate	. . . .
Candicidin N.F.	Candeptin
Caprylic acid	Naprylate
Carbol-fuchsin solution N.F.	Castellani's paint
Chlordantoin	Sporostacin
Cupric sulfate N.F.	Blue Vitriol
Diamthazole HCl	Asterol
Gentian violet U.S.P.	Methylrosaniline
Haloprigin	Halotex
Hexetidine	Sterisil
Iodochlorhydroxyquin	Vioform
Nystatin U.S.P.	Mycostatin; Nilstat
Phenacridine HCl	Acrizane
Proprionic acid	. . . .
Resorcinol U.S.P.	. . . .
Resorcinol monoacetate N.F.	. . . .
Salicylanilide N.F.	Ansadol
Salicylic acid U.S.P.	. . . .
Sodium proprionate N.F.	. . . .
Tolnaftate U.S.P.	Tinactin
Triacetin N.F.	Enzactin; Fungacetin
Undecylenic acid N.F.	In Desenex
Zinc undecylenate U.S.P.	In Desenex
Antibacterials (Chemical classification)	
CATIONIC DETERGENTS (QUATERNARY AMMONIUM TYPE)	
Benzalkonium chloride U.S.P.	Zephiran
Benzethonium chloride N.F.	Phemerol
Cetylpyridinium chloride N.F.	Cepacol
Methylbenzethonium chloride N.F.	Ammorid; Diaparene
CHLORINATED COMPOUNDS	
Halazone	. . . .
Sodium hypochlorite solution N.F.	Bleach; Zonite
DYES	
Gentian violet U.S.P.	Methylrosaniline
Phenazopyridine HCl N.F.	Pyridium
IODINE COMPOUNDS	
Iodine tincture U.S.P.	. . . .

TABLE 46-4 *Topical Antiinfective Agents (continued)*

Official or Nonproprietary Name	Trade Name or Synonym
Antibacterials (Chemical classification) (continued)	
Strong iodine solution U.S.P.	. . . .
Iodoform N.F.	. . . .
Povidone-iodine N.F.	Betadine; Isodine
Undecoylium chloride-iodine	Virac
MERCURY COMPOUNDS	
Ammoniated mercury U.S.P.	. . . .
Merbromin	Mercurochrome
Mercury bichloride	
Nitromersol N.F.	Metaphen
Phenylmercuric nitrate N.F.	Phe-Mer-Nite
Thimerosal N.F.	Merthiolate
Yellow mercuric oxide N.F.	. . . .
OXIDIZING AGENTS	
Hydrogen peroxide solution U.S.P.	. . . .
Potassium permanganate U.S.P.	. . . .
Sodium perborate	. . . .
Zinc peroxide, medicinal U.S.P.	. . . .
PHENOLS AND DERIVATIVES	
Cresol U.S.P.	. . . .
Hexylresorcinol N.F.	
Hexachlorophene U.S.P.	In pHisoHex, and others
Phenol, liquefied U.S.P.	Carbolic acid
Thymol U.S.P.	. . . .
SILVER COMPOUNDS	
Silver nitrate U.S.P.	
Silver protein, mild N.F.	Argyrol
Silver protein, strong	Protargol
Silver sulfadiazine	
Toughened silver nitrate U.S.P.	Lunar Caustic
Miscellaneous Antibacterials	
Boric acid	. . . .
Nitrofurazone N.F.	Furacin
Triclobisonium chloride N.F.	Triburon
Scabicides and Pediculicides	
Benzyl benzoate U.S.P.	. . . .
Chlorophenothane U.S.P.	DDT
Crotamiton	Eurax
Gamma benzene hexachloride U.S.P.	Kwell
Isobornyl thiocyanoacetate	Bornate
Trichomonacide	
Metronidazole	Flagyl

with an alcohol-soaked cotton sponge just before inserting a hypodermic needle has some utility. This is because the solvent action of alcohol on the sebaceous secretions helps to clean the skin of surface bacteria.

Iodine+ dissolved in diluted alcohol which was introduced for use in preoperative skin preparation at the end of the last century, is widely used in preoperative preparation. The modern tincture of iodine irritates the skin less than the strong solutions that were previously employed. The iodine-stained skin site is swabbed with alcohol before the operative area is draped, for residual iodine may damage the epidermis. Some individuals are sensitive to even small amounts of iodine, and severe skin reactions may result.

Recently, iodine has been combined with various organic substances to form complexes that release elemental iodine when in contact with the skin. These so-called *iodophors* are free enough of the irritating properties of iodine to be safely used on mucous membranes as well as on skin. However, their effectiveness for preoperative preparation of the skin is controversial. Some reports state that solutions of elemental iodine in alcohol are far superior to iodophors such as *undecoylium chloride-iodine* (Virac) or *povidone iodine+*; others claim that povidone iodine is more effective for surgical scrubbing than the older, more widely used agents.

Quaternary ammonium compounds such as *benzalkonium chloride+* (Zephiran) have both antiseptic and detergent properties when used preoperatively in hand washing and for disinfection of the patient's skin. These surface-acting agents kill the common gram-positive and gram-negative pathogens, which are then removed from the skin along with sebum and keratin debris. However, it is important to remember that the antibacterial action of these *cationic* substances is almost completely neutralized by the presence on the skin of even small traces of soaps, which are *anionic* in nature. The surgical field is rinsed thoroughly with water and is then swabbed with alcohol before benzalkonium or other cationic detergent antiseptics are applied.

Phenol, the first substance to be used for preoperative skin disinfection and prevention of postsurgical infection, is no longer used for this purpose. Concentrations effective for control of skin bacteria and fungi are too irritating for safe use on human tissues. However, low concentrations help to relieve itching when added to antipruritic lotions (p. 607). Full-strength phenol is occasionally used for cauterizing tissue.

Hexachlorophene+, a phenol derivative, is an effective antibacterial agent that does not damage the skin in ordinary concentrations. The 3 percent detergent emulsion form is effective when employed regularly in surgical scrubbing. When it is to be used preoperatively, patients should be instructed to wash the area daily for four days to a week in order to build up a bacteriostatic residue on the skin. Such home scrubs with hexachlorophene-containing products are also recommended after surgery and for families infected by staphylococcal organisms. In such situations, patients should be told *not* to rinse the skin with alcohol, for this removes the hexachlorophene film from the skin that is being built up by the daily washings.

This substance was, until recently, added to many kinds of deodorants, cosmetics, and nonprescription drug products, including baby powders. It was removed from all such preparations after it was found able to damage nervous tissue when absorbed through the skin. However, hexachlorophene is still available for acne treatment programs (p. 609) or other infection-prevention uses when prescribed by a physician.

APPLICATION TO CUTS. Most of the antiseptics that are offered to the public for treating cuts have little value. Some substances used for daubing at breaks in the skin or irrigating lacerated areas may even interfere with the skin's natural defenses. Thus, most scratches and abrasions are best dealt with by washing the wound and the skin around it with soap and water.

Mercurial compounds such as mercury bichloride, an inorganic form, are not effective when applied to open wounds because they are inactivated in the presence of serum and tissue proteins. Organic mercurials such as *merbromin* (Mercurochrome), *nitromersol* (Metaphen), and *thimerosol* (Merthiolate) do not precipitate protein and are thus not as irritating as inorganic mercury. However, the tinctures, creams, and ointments containing these compounds, which are commonly used for preventing infection of cuts, abrasions, open wounds, and other denuded surfaces, are not now considered very effective for this purpose.

Silver salts, on the other hand, are highly germicidal in low concentrations. *Silver nitrate+* in a 0.5 percent solution is effective and nonirritating when applied to severely burned skin surfaces. A 1 percent solution is safe and useful for preventing ocular infection when instilled into the eyes of newborn babies. Unfortunately, this silver salt stains tissues black and it is thus not popular for routine use as a skin infection prevention measure. The non-staining colloidal silver preparations have now been largely replaced by topical antibiotics for prevention and treatment of skin infections.

Boric acid is another topical antiseptic with only weak antibacterial and antifungal effects. It is harmless in ordinary concentrations. However, applied to the abraded buttocks of babies with diaper rash as a full strength powder, boric acid has caused toxicity and death. In any case, the traditional use of this relatively ineffective antiseptic no longer seems to be desirable.

BACTERIAL SKIN INFECTIONS. These are most often caused by staphylococci and streptococci. These pus-provoking bacteria are responsible for over 90 percent of pyodermas, such as furunculosis (boils) and impetigo. Some infections occur spontaneously; others occur secondary to contact dermatitis or decubital (bed sore) ulcerations of the skin.

Boils are best allowed to localize with the aid of hot compresses or soaks. After they have "pointed" and have been incised and drained by the doctor, the skin is kept clean with alcohol swabs and is washed with hexachlorophene preparations to minimize further spread of infection. Systemic and topical antibiotic therapy is usually reserved for cases of recurrent furuncles and carbuncles. Treatment with systemic antibiotics is seldom necessary, except when the patient suffers from crops of recurring boils or carbuncles.

Impetigo, on the other hand, responds readily to treatment with antibiotics even when applied topically. First, of course, the crusts covering the skin lesions must be gently removed with soap and water washing or application of compresses. Then an ointment containing *gentamycin+*, or combinations of *bacitracin*, *neomycin*, and *polymyxin* is rubbed into the skin several times daily. This condition then usually clears within a week. (See also Chapter 41.)

FUNGAL INFECTIONS. These are caused by two main types of microorganisms: (1) *dermatophytes* that burrow into the skin to cause athlete's foot (tinea pedis) or ringworm in various areas including the scalp (tinea capitis) and the groin (tinea cruris); and (2) *Candida albicans*, a yeastlike organism.

Griseofulvin+, administered by mouth, is the most effective treatment for advanced cases of dermatophytosis affecting the skin and nails. Several kinds of topically applied antifungal chemicals are also available for treating less severe ringworm-type infections. Some are single chemicals such as the newer antifungal agents *tolnaftate*, *acrisorcin*, and *haloprigin*, or the older one *zincundecate* (Desenex).

Other topical treatments for fungal infections involve combinations of chemicals that act in various ways to relieve symptoms and to attack superficial skin fungi. *Carbol-fuchsin solution+*, for example, combines several agents that relieve pruritus, dry the area, and directly stop further fungal growth. Whitfield's ointment is a classic combination of keratolytic *salicylic acid+* with benzoic acid, an antifungal agent that reaches the microorganisms more readily as a result of the other chemical's keratin-softening action.

Candida albicans infections (moniliasis) are not limited to the skin. During treatment with tetracyclines and other antibiotics, overgrowths of this organism may develop in the mouth, anogenital region, and vaginal tract. These are best treated by applications of ointments, creams, lotions or other local dosage forms containing the antifungal antibiotics *nystatin* and *amphotericin B+*. A newer antibiotic, *candicidin*, is reserved for use in vaginal candidiasis. (See also Chapter 41.)

Vaginal infections by bacteria and protozoa can also be controlled by chemotherapeutic agents and local care. *Metronidazole+* (Flagyl) is effective against infections by the protozoan parasite *Trichomonas vaginalis*, when taken by mouth in ten-day courses. *Sulfonamides* may be applied topically to treat bacterial vaginitis. As in the case of skin infections, adjunctive measures are employed to strengthen the body's own defenses—the use of mildly acid douches, for example, or insertion of suppositories containing estrogenic substances.

Parasitic infestations by mites and lice lead to itching and to scratching that often results in secondary skin infections which cause oozing and crusting of the skin and scalp. These conditions—*scabies* and *pediculosis*—occur when people live under conditions of crowding and particularly when they have little or no opportunity or desire to bathe. Alcoholics on skid row, for instance, sometimes suffer from scabies and lousiness requiring the attention of medical personnel. These conditions are also still all too frequently seen in the slum areas of our cities.

Safe and effective insecticides, including *chlorophenothane* (DDT), *benzyl benzoate*, and *gamma benzene hexachloride+*, can quickly overcome these conditions. Scabies lesions, which are caused by the burrowing of a female mite in the stratum corneum of the skin, are found in the spaces between fingers, on the wrists, waistline, buttocks, axillae, and breasts. The tunneling mite can be seen with a hand lens when the upper layer of skin is lifted gently with a needle. Lice are not readily seen, but pediculosis is recognized by the presence of nits, or eggs, attached to the patient's hair or clothing.

Scabies and pediculosis are readily controlled by application of creams and lotions containing the new scabicides and pediculocides in regimens that also employ prolonged bathing in warm, soapy water and vigorous shampooing. It is also important, however, that clothing and bedding be laundered, sterilized, or fumigated in order to avoid prompt reexposure to the vermin.

SUMMARY of Types of Topical Skin Preparations

Type of Preparation	Physical Properties	Usefulness
Ointments	Up to 10 percent of active ingredients dispersed in fatty bases such as petrolatum and lanolin, or in nongreasy bases	Best when applied to dry, scaly, or keratotic lesions; exert a prolonged protective action when applied at night. *Not* suitable for use on hairy areas or on oozing surfaces
Pastes	Ointments into which powders are mixed, such as zinc oxide, starch, talc, and small amounts of tars, salicylic acid, and other medications	Possess a prolonged protective and occlusive action but are porous enough to permit heat to escape from the skin. *Not* suited for hairy surfaces or on oozing areas
Creams	Active ingredients are incorporated into an emulsion-type base that vanishes when rubbed in. This has cosmetic advantages	Good for daytime use, particularly with potent active ingredients that are effective when rubbed into oozing denuded areas (for example, corticosteroids)
Lotions	Suspensions or solutions of active ingredients to be applied liberally by brushing or daubing on the affected area, after shaking to disperse the ingredients	Protect and cool oozing areas in acutely inflamed dermatoses on the face and on hairy areas of the body
Liniments (Emulsions)	Have a higher proportion of oil than ordinary lotions. Various active ingredients may be added	Protect skin that is dry, cracked, or fissured
Paints	Liquids used to touch up small localized areas (for instance, anogenital) or intertriginous surfaces (such as moist lesions betwen the toes or in the axillae)	Often have a desirable drying effect on moist areas where two skin surfaces are in contact. Sometimes stain and are messy
Powders	Materials in fine particles for dusting on surfaces (for instance, inorganic substances such as talc)	Absorb moisture from large areas and exert a cooling or protective effect
Wet Dressings, Soaks, and Compresses	Watery solutions of substances with mild astringent properties (for example, aluminum acetate, potassium permanganate)	Have a soothing, cooling, antipruritic effect when applied to areas of skin containing vesicles, pustules, and oozing serous fluids and debris, which are washed away. (Hot soaks and compresses are also employed to localize boils and cellulitis)
Baths	Starch, oatmeal, and other substances are dissolved or suspended in water and added to a bath in which the patient is immersed. (Medication such as coal tar or potassium permanganate may be added)	Useful for treating generalized acute inflammatory dermatoses to stop widespread itching and to soften psoriatic or keratotic lesions

SUMMARY of Points for the Nurse to Remember Concerning Dermatologic Preparations

Note the reaction of the skin to locally applied medications and bring to the doctor's attention any signs of irritation that may indicate primary irritancy or a sensitization reaction.

Avoid applying all ointments, creams, lotions, and so forth (especially those containing corticosteroids) in too copious quantities, for this is messy and unnecessarily expensive. (Check with the physician as to whether he wants previously applied topical medication removed before applying a new layer.)

Apply liquids sparingly to the scalp for treating seborrhea, to prevent the liquid from running into the eyes or ears. (In general, products containing keratolytic agents require care to prevent contact of the medication with the eyes.)

Shake heavy lotions such as calamine before using. Apply them with a firm touch, for light dabbing can increase the sensation of itching.

Dry the skin surface before applying a powder, for caking caused by moisture may lead to irritation.

Use an emollient rather than alcohol for back care if the skin is excessively dry, for alcohol can predispose to decubitus ulcers by irritating and cracking the already dry skin.

Remove any blood or pus that might interfere with contact. When using silver nitrate sticks, apply the medication only to the area being treated. (In general, when caustic chemicals are applied to hyperkeratotic and other areas, protect adjacent areas with petrolatum or by other means.)

Know which skin lesions are infectious and take all appropriate precautions. Explain the need for such measures to the patient but avoid the gingerly touch when applying medications, which may make him feel that his condition is unacceptable to others.

In scrubbing, remember that friction is important in preoperative preparation for surgery, regardless of which germicides or regimens are employed.

Advise patients with a history of allergy against trying a variety of skin products, such as deodorants or depilatories, for they may become sensitized to new chemicals. They should stick to the few products that they know by experience cause them no adverse reactions.

Advise patients who have peripheral vascular disease against self-medication with products containing keratolytic agents, such as plasters for removal of corns and calluses. Such products may be irritating and lead to formation of skin ulcerations in persons with poor circulation.

Advise people not to worry about the possibility of systemic absorption of corticosteroids and consequent dangerous systemic reactions, for this is unlikely in most circumstances. (On the other hand, women sometimes overestimate the usefulness of cosmetic creams containing estrogens, on the erroneous assumption that these hormones are absorbed systemically to produce desirable feminizing effects, including a more youthful skin.)

DRUG DIGEST

ALUMINUM ACETATE SOLUTION U.S.P. (Burow's solution)

Actions and Indications. This solution is used as a soak and as a basis for soothing wet dressings. It is employed in the treatment of acute inflammatory reactions of the skin serving mainly as a mild astringent. In undiluted form, it exerts a mild antiseptic effect and may be used as a gargle as well as on the skin.

Applied to oozing, or weeping lesions in acute contact dermatoses (such as poison ivy), acute fungal infections of the skin, and bacterial infections, especially in intertriginous areas, this solution helps to give some relief of itching and pain. Its cleansing and

antiseptic actions also exert a favorable effect upon the local environment that helps healing after opening of vesicles.

Side Effects, Cautions, and Contraindications. The solution is said to be nonirritating and nonsensitizing. However, it should not be allowed to come in contact with the eyes. When applied topically, evaporation should *not* be prevented by plastic coverings or other impervious materials.

Dosage and Administration. The official 5 percent solution is diluted with 10 to 40 parts of water for use as a wet dressing that may be applied in cold, tepid, or warm form. Powder in packets and tablets

are also available, from which solutions of the proper strength may be conveniently prepared for application to loosely bandaged areas every 15 to 30 minutes for four to eight hours.

AMMONIATED MERCURY U.S.P.

Actions and Indications. This form of mercury is an insoluble compound which releases the free ion slowly in small amounts that have an antiseptic action on the skin without being excessively irritating. It is used in ointment form in impetigo and fungal infection of the skin, and as an ophthalmic preparation for application to the conjunctiva.

The official ointment is one of

the mildest medications for accelerating the scaling and healing of dry lesions in chronic psoriasis. It may also be useful in pediculosis, pinworms, and pruritus ani.

Side Effects, Cautions, and Contraindications. The continued use of ammoniated mercury in infants and young children is contraindicated, as toxic amounts of mercury may be absorbed through the skin in some rare circumstances.

Dosage and Administration. A 5 percent ointment is available for topical application to the skin, and a 3 percent opthalmic ointment is used topically on the conjunctiva.

BENZALKONIUM CHLORIDE U.S.P. (Zephiran)

Actions and Indications. This cationic-type detergent and antiseptic is effective against gram-positive and gram-negative bacteria. It is used preoperatively and on small wound surfaces for preventing and treating infections of the skin. Dilute solutions may be used for irrigating mucosal surfaces. Higher concentrations are employed for preserving the sterility of heat-sterilized surgical instruments and other operating room materials that are to be stored in a sterile state.

Side Effects, Cautions, and Contraindications. To avoid inactivation when applied to the skin preoperatively, benzalkonium solutions should be used only after all soap has been rinsed from the skin site, and it has been swabbed with alcohol. Dilute solutions are not ordinarily irritating, but irritation may occur if the skin is kept covered for long periods. Concentrated disinfectant solutions may have caustic effects. Absorption of irritating solutions from body cavities may result in skeletal muscle weakness.

Dosage and Administration. A 1:750 dilution is used for disinfection of the patient's intact skin and the surgeon's hands. More dilute aqueous solutions (1:5,000–1:20,000) are ordinarily preferred for use on broken skin and on mucous membranes of the eye, vaginal tract, and urinary bladder.

CALAMINE LOTION PHENOLATED U.S.P.

Actions and Indications. This lotion offers the protectant action of calamine and zinc oxide and the mild antipruritic action of a low dilution of phenol. It may be applied to the oozing lesions of poison ivy and other contact dermatoses, or in acute exudative stages of fungal and bacterial skin infections.

Other substances may be added to the basic lotion, including 1 percent camphor or menthol, which possess cooling and antipruritic actions that also relieve the discomfort of itchy, oozing eruptions. This lotion may be made more drying by the addition of alcohol, or it may be made more soothing by the addition of such emollients as glycerine and lanolin when the skin is scabby, dry, or fissured. (A petrolatum-based ointment may sometimes be preferred for such cases.)

Side Effects, Cautions, and Contraindications. The use of this lotion in the presence of infection is not desirable, and its accumulation in excessive quantities in hairy areas may cause discomfort and irritation.

Dosage and Administration. After *shaking*, the lotion is applied in small amounts to the affected areas. Frequent application with cotton pledgets or a brush is preferred to the occasional use of large amounts. A firm touch is used, as light dabbing may increase itching sensations.

CARBOL-FUCHSIN SOLUTION N.F. (Castellani's Paint)

Actions and Indications. This alcohol-acetone solution of the antiseptic dye, fuchsin, and such other antifungal agents as benzoic and boric acids and phenol, is often effective against ringworm in interdigital areas and intertriginous sites. Painted between the toes, on the axillae, or in the anogenital region, the medication tends to dry the moist tissues and relieve itching.

Side Effects, Cautions, and Contraindications. This solution is rarely irritating or sensitizing. However, it may cause excessive drying and thus add to the chronic fissuring if applied too frequently.

Administration. The solution should be applied with an applicator no more than once daily. It should be kept tightly closed to avoid evaporation and concentration of the solution. Care should be taken to avoid staining clothing. A fresh solution should be used, as deterioration occurs in a few weeks.

COAL TAR U.S.P. (In numerous proprietary preparations)

Actions and Indications. This substance, a thick fluid derived from the distillation of coal, is combined with zinc oxide paste and in various ointments and lotions. Applied to the skin in psoriasis, seborrheic dermatitis, and chronic eczematous or lichenified lesions, it is often effective for removing scales and plaques. In addition to this keratolytic action, coal tar is said to possess antiseptic, astringent, and antipruritic properties, among others.

The exfoliative effect of coal tar is increased when its aplication is followed by carefully regulated daily doses of ultraviolet irradiation. The patient then takes a long tub bath to remove the loosened scales (Goeckerman regimen).

Side Effects, Cautions, and Contraindications. Prolonged use may lead to allergic sensitization. Exposure of the skin to direct sunlight should be avoided because of the photosensitizing effect of coal tar. Application to hairy areas may result in irritation and folliculitis. This substance has an odor that some may find unpleasant, and it tends to stain the skin and darken blond hair.

Dosage and Administration. Coal tar is used in concentrations of 1 to 10 percent, and most commonly as a 1 percent dilution in zinc oxide paste (coal tar ointment), or as an alcoholic solution (Liquor Carbonis Detergens) for direct application or for use in bath water.

CYPROHEPTADINE HCl N.F. (Periactin)

Actions and Indications. This antihistamine drug is used for relief of itching in various dermatologic disorders, including atopic and contact dermatitis, acute and chronic urticaria, angioneurotic edema, and the pruritus of chicken pox, pruritus ani and vulvae, and others. It may also be useful in respiratory allergy, including perennial rhinitis and hay fever. It does not give relief of asthma symptoms but sometimes seems to bring about a gain in weight and growth in asthmatic children.

Side Effects, Cautions, and Contraindications. This drug's central depressant action may be the main source of its antipruritic activity. It is certainly the cause of the drug's most common side effect, drowsiness. The resulting loss of alertness may be dangerous in some circumstances. Thus, patients should be warned against driving a car, if they are made drowsy by this drug, and they should be cautioned against drinking alcoholic beverages while taking this medication.

Dosage and Administration. Adult dosage ranges from 4 to 20 mg daily. Children receive reduced dosage in accordance with their age, size and response. The usual dose for children aged two to six is 2 mg and for those seven to fourteen, it is 4 mg b.i.d. or t.i.d.

ETHYL ALCOHOL U.S.P. (Ethanol)

Actions and Indications. Topically applied alcohol has several properties that make it useful for skin care and disinfection. It is used preoperatively in surgical scrub procedures to dissolve sebaceous secretions and to reduce the bacterial flora of the skin. It is also rubbed on the skin over sites at which parenteral injections are to be made.

Alcohol is the basis for skin rubs because of its mild rubefacient and counterirritant effects. Its skin cleansing, drying, and hardening effects may make it useful for preventing decubital ulcerations. The solvent properties of alcohol have been used for removing the plant oils responsible for poison ivy from the skin, and also for removing concentrated phenol that has been spilled on the skin.

Side Effects, Cautions, and Contraindications. Alcohol is not very effective for disinfecting instruments, as it cannot kill bacterial spores (sterilization by heat is preferred). When applied to open wounds, it causes painful stinging, irritation, and protein precipitation. It has a dehydrating action that can cause excessive skin dryness. Allergic sensitization sometimes occurs.

Taken internally it can, of course, cause central nervous system depression leading to signs and symptoms typical of alcohol intoxication. Young children may suffer from hypoglycemia following accidental ingestion or even after absorption from burn surfaces or skin lesions.

Dosage and Administration. Alcohol is used in concentrations ranging from 50 to 95 percent. However, its antiseptic action appears to be most effective when a 70 percent solution in water is employed, as this dilution possesses the most efficient penetration.

GAMMA BENZENE HEXACHLORIDE U.S.P. (Lindane; Kwell)

Actions and Indications. This parasiticide is effective for treating scabies and lice infestations. In pediculosis, it kills the nits or eggs as well as the adult head and crab lice. This relieves itching and thus stops the scratching which is often the cause of secondary infections.

Side Effects, Cautions, and Contraindications. Skin eruptions may occur in sensitized individuals or as a result of direct irritation. This may require discontinuation of the product. Care should be used while shampooing to avoid contact with the eyes; if this occurs, the eyes should be thoroughly flushed out with water.

Repeated use should be avoided to prevent possible absorption of toxic quantities into the systemic circulation. Accidental ingestion has resulted in central nervous system stimulation and cardiac arrhythmias. In treatment of poisoning, oily gavage fluids and cathartics should be avoided and epinephrine should *not* be used.

Dosage and Administration. A 1 percent cream and lotion are available for use on the body after the patient takes a hot, soapy bath and then dries the skin. In treating scabies, a thin layer is applied to the entire body surface and kept on for 24 hours before being completely washed off. If further treatments are needed, they are carried out at weekly intervals. For pediculosis, a thin layer of cream or lotion is left on hairy infested areas for 12 to 24 hours, and 1 oz of a 1 percent shampoo is rubbed vigorously into the wet hair of the head, which is then rinsed and dried.

HEXACHLOROPHENE U.S.P. (HCP; pHisoHex; and others)

Actions and Indications. This chlorinated diphenol antiseptic possesses potent bacteriostatic action against gram-positive oragnisms, especially strains of the staphylococcus. The 3 percent detergent suspension is employed as a presurgical hand scrub and for preparing the skin of the operative field.

It is also used by hospital nursery personnel for washing the hands just before and after handling each infant. However, its routine use for total body bathing of newborn infants to prevent staphylococcal infections is controversial. Some sources condemn its use for this purpose; others feel that the benefits outweigh its risks, provided that the hexachlorophene solution is rinsed off completely following the infant's bath.

HCP is available in prescription products for treating acne, impetigo, carbuncles, cradle cap, and other infectious and allergic dermatoses. It is no longer available for use in nonprescription consumer products such as soaps, deodorants, cosmetics, and toiletries.

Side Effects, Cautions and Contraindications. Systemic absorption from burn surfaces and the vaginal mucosa has caused central nervous system toxicity and death. Absorption through the intact skin of newborn monkeys has also caused nervous system lesions, and it is possible that enough may be absorbed through human skin to cause similar toxicity.

Dosage and Administration. Detergent solutions (3 percent) are applied topically by various techniques as a surgical scrub or as an adjunct to other measures for preventing and treating skin infections. Regularly repeated use is needed to build up a residue sufficient for antibacterial action.

HYDROQUINONE N.F. (Eldoquin; Eldopaque)

Actions and Indications. This depigmenting agent is believed to act by blocking an early step in the biosynthesis of melanin. Thus, it temporarily bleaches and lightens hyperpigmented skin areas. The drug is indicated for treating severe facial freckling, bleaching skin blemishes such as liver spots, and counteracting cloasma caused by oral contraceptives, pregnancy, or age.

Side Effects, Cautions and Contraindications. The patient's possible sensitivity should be determined before treating wide areas of skin in order to avoid generalized allergic reactions. The drug is discontinued if rash or signs of irritation develop. Preparations are not applied to irritated or sunburned skin, following use of a depilatory, or in the presence of prickly heat. Occasionally, depigmentation may not be uniform with only slight hypopigmentation in some areas and excessive melanin loss elsewhere.

Dosage and Administration. A 2 percent ointment, cream or lotion is applied to the affected area twice daily at 12-hour intervals and rubbed in well. A 4 percent concentration in a base that is opaque to light is applied without rubbing in order to cover the area for cosmetic purposes and to exclude ultraviolet light during the day. More rapid and dependable bleaching occurs when the treated area is protected from sunlight in this way.

IODINE U.S.P.

Actions and Indications. This element is an effective antiseptic when applied to the skin in dilute solution. It is still often employed preoperatively to disinfect the skin of the surgical site. However, it is no longer recommended for direct application to cuts in order to prevent skin infections. Iodine, like chlorine, can be used to disinfect water that may be contaminated by bacteria or amebae.

Side Effects, Cautions, and Contraindications. Topically applied alcoholic solutions of iodine tend to irritate the abraded skin. Iodine, used preoperatively, should be removed from the skin with alcohol to prevent possible irritation by residues remaining on the skin. It should not be used on individuals known to be sensitive to iodine.

Taken internally, strong iodine solutions may have a corrosive effect on the mucosa of the mouth and other alimentary tract areas. Ordinarily, only nausea, vomiting, and diarrhea result. However, death from circulatory collapse has sometimes occurred. Thus, it may be desirable to wash out the patient's stomach with a solution of starch, which acts to precipitate iodine. (Weak dilutions of iodine (1:250) may be safely employed as a gavage fluid for precipitating alkaloidal poisons.)

Dosage and Administration. Tincture of Iodine, a 2 percent alcoholic solution, is a form preferred for preoperative preparation of the skin but not for application to open wounds. Iodine solution (2 percent aqueous) and Strong Iodine solution (7 percent aqueous) are diluted to much lower concentrations and are applied to cuts and abrasions, but soap and water cleansing is now preferred. For disinfecting water, one to three drops of the tincture may be added to one quart of water.

POTASSIUM PERMANGANATE U.S.P.

Actions and Indications. This oxidizing type antiseptic and deodorant may be applied in dilute solution to weeping skin lesions in acute, exudative dermatoses, and in fungal or bacterial skin infections. These solutions also have a mild astringent action that aids drying of oozing areas in the acute vesicular stages of contact dermatitis.

Strong solutions are bactericidal and are used to disinfect organic matter. Very much weaker solutions are sometimes used internally as a vaginal douche or as a gavage fluid for oxidizing certain ingested poisons such as strychnine, for example.

Side Effects, Cautions, and Contraindications. The purple crystals must be completely dissolved in adequate amounts of water to avoid irritant and caustic actions. Severe local trauma has occurred when undissolved tablets intended for solution have been inserted into the vaginal tract. The skin and dressings are stained by solutions of this substance.

Dosage and Administration. Solutions ranging from 1:1,000 to 1:10,000 and higher are employed for various purposes. A 1:1,000 solution is used in poison ivy. A 1:10,000 solution is applied as a soak, wetting dressing, or in compresses for acute dermatoses. Tablets or crystals totalling 5 to 15 g may be dissolved in a quart of water, which is then added to a tubful of water to serve as a bath in cases of generalized exudative dermatoses. (This makes a solution of about 1:50,000.)

POVIDONE-IODINE N.F. (Betadine; Isodine)

Actions and Indications. This topical antiseptic contains iodine in a complex with polyvinylpyrrolidone, from which it is released when it comes in contact with the skin or mucous membranes to which the solution is applied. The iodine let loose in this way is not as irritating to tissues as tincture of iodine.

This type of iodine preparation is often preferred for application to abraded or burned skin, for vaginal douching, and for mouth and throat swabbing. However, it it not considered as effective as iodine tincture as a surgical scrub for operating room personnel and for preoperative preparation of the patient's skin.

Side Effects, Cautions, and Contraindications. Patients sensitive to other iodine products are likely to prove allergic to this compound also. Treatment should be discontinued if redness, swelling, or other signs of irritation develop.

Dosage and Administration. Among the products available are: an antiseptic solution for full strength application as a soak, spray, or paint, and as a surgical scrub; an aerosol for spraying on burns, wounds, and stasis, or decubital, ulcers; an ointment applied in prevention and treatment of bacterial and fungal infections, lacerations, and abrasions; a gargle for use following oral surgery and in stomatitis and Vincent's infection; and a douche and gel for use in the management of vaginal moniliasis, trichomoniasis, and nonspecific bacterial infections.

RESORCINOL U.S.P. and RESCORCINOL MONACETATE N.F.

Actions and Indications. This phenolic substance is a constituent of many proprietary dermatological preparations. It exerts a mild irritant effect which helps to loosen and remove the outer layer of dead skin cells or scales. This keratolytic action is useful in the management of eczema, psoriasis, and seborrheic dermatitis. Its mild drying and peeling actions are also thought useful in the management of acne. Rescorcinol has also been employed as an antibacterial in pyo-

derma and for fungal infections such as ringworm and athlete's foot.

Side Effects, Cautions, and Contraindications. Higher concentrations of this chemical may cause skin irritation marked by excessive redness, dryness, and scaling. Topical use should be discontinued if signs of sensitization appear. Accidental ingestion by a child or excessive absorption through the skin may cause systemic toxicity involving the central and circulatory systems.

Dosage and Administration. Resorcinol is applied topically in ointments, pastes, and lotions varying in concentration from 2 to 20 percent. It is frequently found in combination with sulfur and with salicylic acid in lotions and soaps. Resorcinol monoacetate N.F., which releases resorcin at a slow rate, is said to exert a longer lasting effect and to be less likely to cause light hair to darken.

SALICYLIC ACID U.S.P.

Actions and Indications. Depending upon the degree to which it is concentrated or diluted, this topical irritant can produce several different effects useful in dermatological treatment. In higher concentrations it exerts a mildly caustic or strongly keratolytic action that aids in removal of warts, corns, callouses, and fungus-infested layers of skin keratin. Lower concentrations that are only mildly keratolytic may be useful in seborrheic dermatitis, psoriasis and acne, especially when combined with coal tar, resorcin, and sulfur.

Side Effects, Cautions, and Contraindications. Caution is required in applying high concentrations of this chemical to the skin of people with poor peripheral circulation, including diabetics and patients with peripheral vascular disease. Overuse may cause inflammation and skin ulceration in such cases.

It should not be applied over wide areas for prolonged periods, as enough may be absorbed through the skin to cause signs and symptoms of salicylism.

Dosage and Administration. Salicylic acid is compounded in concentrations of 1 to 40 percent in the form of ointments, powders, plasters, and lotions or solutions. Dilutions of 1 to 3 percent are used in seborrheic dermatitis, acne, and psoriasis. Somewhat higher concentrations (up to 6 percent) help to remove calloused or thickened epithelial tissue and permit penetration of the other agents with which it is combined—for example, the antifungal agent, benzoic acid, in Whitfield's ointment. Removal of corns and warts may require still higher concentrations up to 40 percent.

SELENIUM SULFIDE N.F. (Selsun)

Actions and Indications. This antiseborrheic agent, available in the form of Selenium Sulfide Detergent Suspension N.F. (a 2.5 percent suspension), is effective in the control of mild to moderately severe seborrheic dermatitis of the scalp. It is most successful against the dry form of seborrhea—that is, common dandruff marked by profuse, dry, powdery scales. It is also useful for tinea versicolor but *not* for scalp ringworm caused by *Microsporum audouini*.

Side Effects, Cautions, and Contraindications. The suspension should be kept from coming in contact with the eyes, as it may cause irritation, stinging, and conjunctivitis or keratitis. Avoid application to the genital area also. Although selenium is a toxic substance when taken internally, systemic absorption from the scalp is unlikely, except in the presence of extensive acute inflammatory lesions.

Dosage and Administration. Control chronic seborrhea of the scalp with two treatments weekly of the following type. Massage one or two teaspoonsful into the wet scalp and keep it in contact for two or three minutes Then, after, thoroughly rinsing the scalp, repeat the application.

For treating tinea versicolor, allow the suspension to remain in contact with the affected areas for five minutes and then rinse thoroughly. Repeat this procedure on each of the next three days. Further courses may be employed for treating recurrences.

SILVER NITRATE U.S.P.

Actions and Indications. This silver salt is bactericidal in low concentrations. Higher concentrations have astringent and caustic actions. A 1 percent opthalmic solution is employed routinely for preventing gonorrheal eye infections in new born babies. (Prophylaxis of opthalmia neonatorum is often required by state law.)

A highly local concentration of silver nitrate is sometimes attained deliberately by moistening a solid stick of the salt and applying it to tissues for caustic effect. This is sometimes used for removing warts and granulomatous tissues and for cauterizing wounds. Care is required to see that solutions of the proper strength are employed for the intended purposes.

Side Effects, Cautions, and Contraindications. Silver nitrate solutions often cause a chemical conjunctivitis, and accidents in their use have resulted in cauterization of delicate eye tissues with subsequent blindness.

Dosage and Administration. The official 1 percent ophthalmic solution is available in collapsible capsules containing five drops for topical application to the conjunctival sacs of the eyes of infants. Toughened Silver Nitrate U.S.P., or Lunar Caustic, comes in pencils, the ends of which are moistened just prior to topical application of the area to be treated. Solutions ranging from 1:10 to 1:10,000 concentration are sometimes ordered.

TRIAMCINOLONE ACETONIDE U.S.P (Aristocort; Kenalog)

Actions and Indications. This potent corticosteroid provides prompt relief of inflammation, allergy, and itching when applied topically in various acute dermatoses, including atopic and contact dermatitis and sunburn. It is also an effective adjunct to other measures in the management of such chronic dermatoses as psoriasis, lichen planus, lichen simplex, and chronic neurodermatitis, or the chronic eczematous type.

Side Effects, Cautions, and Contraindications. Local irritation or hypersensitivity to any of the components of a topical corticosteroid preparation may cause sensations of itching, burning, or dryness. Further use may have to be discontinued in the presence of a hypersensitivity-type reaction or of a skin infection that can not be adequately controlled by topical or systemic therapy with antiinfective agents.

Topical application is contraindicated in tuberculous, fungal, or viral skin infections, including herpes simplex, vaccinia (cowpox), or varicella (chicken pox). Preparations should not be placed in the external ear canal if the patient's drum is perforated. Care is required to keep sprays from coming in contact with the eyes or from being inhaled.

Systemic side effects are rare but possible with prolonged use of occlusive dressings.

Dosage and Administration. Ointments, creams, lotions, foams, and sprays ranging in potency from 0.025-0.1 percent to 0.5 percent are applied to the affected areas two to four times daily in small amounts and rubbed in gently with or without occlusive dressings.

TRIOXSALEN (Trisoralen)

Actions and Indications. This photodynamic drug is used to produce repigmentation in vitiligo and to increase pigmentation and tolerance to sunlight in selected fair-skinned persons who fail to tan. Taken by mouth, the drug is thought to concentrate in the melanocytes located in the basal layers of the epidermis. There, when activated by ultraviolet light, it acts to stimulate production of melanin.

Side Effects, Cautions, and Contraindications. The photosensitizing action of this drug during its first days of administration makes the patient's skin more subject to sunburn than usual. Thus, exposure to sunlight must be very carefully controlled in order to prevent severe reactions which may result in skin damage.

This drug is contraindicated in patients with porphyria, lupus erythematosus, and other disorders marked by photosensitivity. High oral doses may cause epigastric distress. If this occurs, the dose is reduced, and the drug is taken after meals or with milk.

Dosage and Administration. One or two 5-mg tablets are taken daily after a meal. The patient with vitaligo then waits two to four hours before exposing himself to a source of ultraviolet light or to fluorescent black light for a brief period to increase sunlight tolerance. The fair-skinned patient takes the drug two hours before exposure to sunlight or to ultraviolet light. The dose of the drug and the exposure time to light must be carefully controlled in order to produce a gradual increase in skin pigment and to avoid severe burning and injury to the skin.

References

Kimbrough, R.D. Review of the toxicity of hexachlorophene. *Arch. Environ. Health* (*Chicago*) 23:119, 1971.

Kretzer, M.P., and Engley, F.B. Effective use of antiseptics and disinfectants. *RN*, 32:48, 1969 (May).

Leider, M. Some principles of dermatological nursing. *RN*, 35:49, 1972 (May).

Richards, R.C. Some practical aspects of surgical skin preparation. *Arch.Surg.* (*Chicago*), 106:575, 1963.

Rodman, M.J. Drugs used in skin diseases. *RN*, 31:53, 1968 (March).

———. Preventing and treating skin-sun reactions. *RN*, 23:63, 1969 (April).

Shaw, B.L. Current therapy of burns. *RN*, 34:33, 1971 (March).

Smith, D. W., Germain, C. H., Gips, C. D. Care of the Adult Patient. 3d ed. Philadelphia: J. P. Lippincott, 1971.

47

Drugs Used in Labor and Delivery

Structure and Function of the Uterus

The uterus is a hollow organ in which the fertilized ovum develops into the embryo and fetus. Its rounded upper part, the *fundus,* is joined at its two sides by the fallopian tubes, through which ova pass from the ovary to the main body of the uterus. The lower part—the neck, or *cervix*—tapers to the *external os,* or mouth, which opens into the vaginal tract. The uterus of a nonpregnant nulliparous woman is only about three inches long, but it grows enormously during pregnancy. This organ is made up mainly of two kinds of tissue: (1) the *endometrium,* a layer of mucous membrane that lines its inner surface; and (2) the *myometrium,* a thick wall of muscle that constitutes the bulk of the uterus.

Uterine tissue of both kinds responds to circulating chemical substances. The glandular epithelium of the endometrium undergoes continual changes during the menstrual month and in pregnancy in response to steroid hormones secreted by the ovaries. The nature and significance of these changes are discussed in Chapter 36, the Female Sex Hormones. We shall limit this review to the myometrium, since the drugs discussed in this chapter act directly upon its smooth muscle cells to contract or relax them.

The *myometrium* is made up of interlacing bands of muscle fibers that circle the uterus on the inside and run lengthwise and obliquely in its outer layers. Blood vessels pass between the interwining fibers, bringing a rich flow of nutrient fluids to the placenta, the organ formed from fetal and maternal tissues in the pregnant uterus. The inner surface of the placenta sends fingerlike projections into openings, or *sinuses*, in the wall of the uterus. The blood in the sinuses bathes the placental extensions and thus transfers oxygen and nutrients to the fetal circulation. The mother's vessels and those of the developing fetus are not directly connected; materials contained in the blood supply of both—including carbon dioxide and other wastes from the fetus—diffuse across the vascular membranes of the placenta and the umbilical cord which passes from the placenta's outer surface to the fetus.

The size and weight of the uterus increase greatly during pregnancy. It grows from only a couple of ounces to two pounds or more, exclusive of its contents. The fiber bundles stretch to accommodate the rapidly growing fetus. Their contractions, which are weak in early pregnancy, become stronger and occur more often as pregnancy advances. Finally, at term, myometrial irritability is markedly increased, presumably because of sudden changes in the levels of various circulating hormones, and the contractions of labor begin.

Parturition (Labor) and Delivery

The exact nature of the complex chemical and physical changes that initiate labor is not fully established. A sudden increase in estrogen secretion and a decrease in progesterone production seem to play a part. In addition, when the uterus distends beyond a certain point, nerve impulses passing from it to the brain and the posterior pituitary gland are believed to bring about the reflex release of *oxytocin*. This hormone induces strong rhythmic contractions in the muscles of the uterus. The pressure built up in this way helps to dilate the cervix, the narrow neck of the uterus leading into the vaginal tract. Such cervical dilation increases the transmission of stimuli to the brain that cause more oxytocin to pour out of the pituitary and pass to the uterus by way of the blood stream.

LABOR OR PARTURITION. The process by which the baby is delivered is divided into three stages. The *first stage* begins with the onset of strong contractions of the fundus, the rounded upper portion of the uterus, and continues until the opening of the cervix is fully dilated. In the *second stage*, mounting contractions, becoming stronger and occurring more frequently, propel the infant's head through the open cervical mouth, or os, into the vaginal tract and continue to push the child along the

birth canal until delivery is completed. The *third stage* is marked by separation of the placenta from the wall of the uterus and the expulsion of the so-called afterbirth. This stage is followed by the *puerperium*, the period during which the uterus gradually returns to its pregravid state.

Immediately after the delivery of the baby and the placenta, the uterus becomes completely relaxed. During this period of uterine atony, the mother may lose a good deal of blood through the sinuses in the uterine wall where the placenta tore away. A pint or more of blood may be lost before the flaccid myometrium begins to contract again spontaneously and becomes firm once more. Once such contractions start, the muscle fibers clamp down on the blood vessels like living ligatures, thus halting any further significant hemorrhaging. During the next few days of the puerperium, the uterus regains much of its tone, and in the next eight or ten weeks *involution*—a reduction in size—gradually takes place. These natural processes can often be speeded by the administration of certain pharmacological agents that are widely employed in obstetrics.

Oxytocic Drugs

Oxytocics are drugs that act on the smooth muscle of the uterus to increase its tone and motility. They act most strongly late in pregnancy, particularly during labor and in the period immediately following it. The response of the myometrium to oxytocic agents is also dose-related. Very small amounts may set off contractions followed by relaxation, as in normal labor. Larger doses cause more powerful and longer-lasting contractions that come at a more rapid rate and with shorter rest periods. Excessively high doses produce sustained tetanic contractions of the uterus that can often be relaxed only by having the patient inhale a general anesthetic.

Only two of the various types of substances that can stimulate uterine smooth muscle are considered dependable enough for routine use in obstetrics. These are: (1) *oxytocin+*, one of the two main hormones secreted by the posterior lobe of the pituitary gland (actually, however, the form of oxytocin that is now used clinically is synthetic rather than a natural glandular extract); and (2) the ergot alkaloids, *ergonovine+* and *methylergonovine*. These are preferred for this purpose to ergotamine, because ordinary doses act almost entirely on the uterus rather than also on the smooth muscles of blood vessels. A third type of oxytocic agent, the plant derivative *sparteine sulfate*, is not as predictable in its effects as are the other two kinds of clinically useful uterine stimulants (see Table 47-1).

Both oxytocin and the ergot derivatives produce powerful contractions of the uterus at the time of parturition and early in the puerperium. However, they are not equally effective for use in *all* of the clinical situations in which an oxytocic agent may be indicated (see *Summary*, pp. 629-630).

Only oxytocin, for example, is administered to induce labor or to restart labor that has stalled (uterine inertia). The ergot alkaloids are *never* used before labor has begun or during the first and second stages of labor, because ergot can cause contractions of the uterus that are too prolonged and difficult to relax. This can be dangerous to both the mother and fetus. On the other hand, oxytocin, when infused intravenously in small amounts of a very dilute solution, is safer than ergot because it is more rapidly inactivated. Thus, even if the uterus responds too strongly, the excessive action of oxytocin wears off quickly after the dilute infusion is discontinued.

The manner in which each of these types of oxytocics is safely employed for the obstetrical conditions in which they are indicated will now be discussed.

OXYTOCIN+ (PITOCIN; SYNTOCINON; UTERACON)

INDICATIONS AND DANGERS. The dose of oxytocin and its manner of administration vary, depending upon the situation in which it is being employed. Thus, when it is administered late in the second stage or during the third stage of labor in order to bring about contraction of the uterine muscle fibers and thus check postpartum bleeding, oxytocin is usually injected intramuscularly in doses of 3 to 10 units. On the other hand, when the doctor uses oxytocin to induce labor or for overcoming uterine inertia, the drug is diluted a thousandfold (see below) and then dripped into a vein only very slowly and cautiously.

The reason for administering oxytocin in this way *before* delivery or early in labor is the same as that for never giving ergot at all at such times—that is, a too highly concentrated solution may produce difficult-to-control contractions of the uterus. This—as the nurse sometimes needs to explain when a patient asks why she can't be given a drug to make labor proceed more quickly—can cause serious injury to both the mother and baby.

Strong contractions that force the fetus against a hard, unyielding, and only partially dilated cervix can tear the cervical tissues or even rupture the muscles of the fundus itself. The infant's head or other parts may be damaged when shoved against the unripe cervix in this way. Sustained uterine spasms may also choke off the child's only source of oxygen—the blood that flows from the mother's arteries into the placenta during periods of relaxation. Thus, tetanic contractions of the uterus can kill the unborn baby or cause serious birth defects.

INDUCTION OF LABOR. In some situations, the obstetrician may decide that early delivery is desirable for the safety of the mother and

TABLE 47-1 *Oxytocic Agents*

Nonproprietary or Official Name	Trade Name	Dosage
Ergonovine maleate U.S.P.	Ergotrate	0.2 mg (200 μg) orally three or four times a day, or by I.M. or S.C. injection
Methylergonovine maleate U.S.P.	Methergine	0.2 mg (200 μg) orally three or four times a day, or by I.M. or I.V. injection
Oxytocin injection U.S.P.	Pitocin; Syntocinon; Uteracon	1 ml (10 units) I.M., repeated in 30 minutes if necessary
Oxytocin citrate	Pitocin citrate	200 to 3,000 units parabuccally
Sparteine sulfate	Spartocin; Tocosamine	150 to 600 mg I.M.

fetus (see *Summary of Indications*, p. 629). In such cases he may employ oxytocin to set off labor, instead of waiting until the time when the uterus would begin to contract spontaneously. This procedure is begun only after the doctor has ruled out the presence of conditions that might lead to complications caused by drug-induced labor (see *Summary of Contraindications*, p. 630).

⟨ *Administration for induction.* One of the safest ways to give oxytocin is by slow intravenous infusion of a very dilute solution. Ten units of the drug are added to 1,000 ml of a glucose solution and dripped into a vein at a rate of only about 15 drops per minute. Later, if contractions are slow in coming, the flow of the dilute solution is gradually raised to up to 2 ml per minute and continued until regular contractions begin. Too strong spasms must be avoided, lest they interfere with blood flow to the fetus. When caring for any patient who is receiving oxytocin for induction, the nurse carefully observes the frequency, strength, and duration of uterine contractions and listens to the fetal heart sounds.

Less efficient but more convenient ways of administering oxytocin are by buccal tablets and by application of a solution to the nasal mucosa. A tablet that contains pitocin citrate is placed betweeen the patient's cheek and gum. Tablets are added every half hour until labor begins, and the number of tablets needed to maintain moderate contractions is kept at that level. If contractions become too strong, the tablets may be spat out, or even swallowed, since they are inactivated in the gastrointestinal tract. All the usual precautions, including medical supervision in a hospital, are required, even when the drug is given by the buccal or intranasal routes, because tetanic contractions of the uterus and fetal heart irregularities have been reported even with this relatively safe route of administration.

UTERINE INERTIA. Oxytocin is not ordinarily injected during the first and second stages of labor. However, it has been used to stimulate labor that has stopped or that is proceeding so slowly that the mother is close to exhaustion. Infused intravenously in carefully regulated amounts, very dilute solutions of oxytocin sometimes succeed in restoring rhythmic contractions in selected cases of arrested labor. The criteria for selection of cases are the same as those employed in deciding whether oxytocin should be used for inducing labor.

INCOMPLETE ABORTION. Oxytoxin is occasionally used to rid the uterus of a fetus that has died. Because the uterus is not very responsive to stimulation in the earlier months of pregnancy, the drug must be administered in much larger doses than are employed at term. Excessive amounts of oxytocin have sometimes caused water intoxication because of an antidiuretic action similar to that of the related posterior pituitary hormone, vasopressin (ADH), which was discussed in Chapter 35.

OXYTOCIN AND THE BREAST. Oxytocin released by the posterior pituitary gland in response to a baby's suckling plays a part in the ejection of milk from the breast. This hormone is not responsible for the process by which the mammary glands make milk, but it does make it easy for the baby to obtain the mother's milk. Synthetic oxytocin is now available in the form of a nasal spray for use when the natural reflex fails. When the mother sprays the solution into her nostrils, oxytocin is absorbed and carried to the smooth muscle cells surrounding the alveoli of the breasts. This causes them to contract and to force the milk into the larger ducts, from which the baby can draw it more readily.

ERGOT ALKALOIDS

Ergot is a parasitic fungus that grows on rye and other cereal grains. It contains many potent chemical substances, including the alkaloids ergotamine and ergonovine, which are widely used in modern medicine for their dependable actions in certain clinical conditions. The use of ergotamine in the management of migraine headache is discussed in Chapter 41. *Ergonovine* and a semisynthetic derivative, *methylergonovine*, are used in obstetrics because of their relatively selective action on the uterus at term.

EFFECTS ON THE UTERUS. Small doses of these drugs, administered parenterally toward the end of the second stage or during the third stage of labor, are used in the management of *postpartum hemorrhage* and *uterine atony*. The ergot alkaloids act directly on the smooth muscle fibers of the flaccid uterus. The resulting contraction makes the fibers clamp down on the open arterioles. This keeps postpartum bleeding from the now firm uterus to a minimum.

ADMINISTRATION. Ergonovine+ and methylergonovine are usually administered intramuscularly in a dose of 0.2 mg during the third stage of labor. The drug reaches the uterus two to five minutes later, at about the time when the placenta is being expelled. This causes the uterus to become hard instead of staying relaxed, thus preventing excessive blood loss in the period of atony that ordinarily follows delivery of the afterbirth.

Some doctors prefer to give the ergot alkaloids earlier—following delivery of the infant's front shoulder but before expulsion of the placenta. The drug's action on the uterus then aids in completing the second stage and shortening the third stage of labor. A possible difficulty with this method is that—if the placenta does not separate spontaneously—the drug's action on the uterus may trap the afterbirth in the womb, from which it may then have to be removed manually.

The nurse assisting in the delivery aids in administration of the ergot alkaloids by whichever method the doctor prefers. The physician's directions for timing must be followed precisely, as it is important to administer the ergot product neither too late nor too soon. Too early injection can endanger the baby and mother; late injection can allow excessive maternal blood loss. Thus, the nurse sees to it that the oxytocic drug and the needles and syringes for injecting it are readily available.

INVOLUTION OF THE UTERUS. Ergot alkaloids are sometimes given during the puerperium to help hasten return of the normal tone of the uterus. This is thought to lessen the likelihood of infection by closing the gaping sinuses through which bacteria might enter. For this purpose, the doctor orders tablets for oral administration three or four times a day during the first week when the process of involution is normally most rapid. Longer use is undesirable because of possible chronic toxicity, or ergotism (see below).

PARTIAL ABORTION. Like oxytocin, ergot is sometimes ordered after a spontaneous partial abortion. Whereas oxytocin is often considered superior for initiation of contractions, ergonovine may be more effective for reducing the bleeding that follows expulsion of the dead fetus and the membranes. If hemorrhage persists, the doctor may have to do a dilatation and curettage of the womb. Surgical repair is necessary for control of hemorrhage from cervical tears or lacerations of the birth canal, since ergot alone does not stop bleeding from trauma to such sites.

SIDE EFFECTS AND TOXICITY. Ergonovine is a remarkably safe drug when given in proper dosage, because its effects are largely limited to myometrial smooth muscle. Occasionally, however, it may have effects on blood vessels. Sometimes, for example, when given intravenously for immediate action in an emergency, methylergovine cay cause a sudden rapid rise in blood pressure that can lead to hypertensive crisis or cerebral hemorrhage. Thus, even when I.V. injection is considered a necessary life-saving measure, the methylergonovine infusion is made slowly and with constant monitoring of the patient's blood pressure.

Even though ergonovine and methylergonovine have very little vasoconstrictor activity as compared to other ergot alkaloids, including ergotamine, their use is best avoided in patients with the obliterative type of peripheral vascular diseases. The main danger of overdosage with ergot products is that the patient's peripheral circulation may be severely impaired. Narrowing of the vessels and damage to the inner lining of the arterioles may lead to the formation of blood clots and finally to gangrene of the toes, fingers, and other parts.

Signs and symptoms of accidental ergotism are sometimes seen in women who take a prescribed ergot alkaloid for too long a time during the puerperium. Early side effects to watch for include nausea, vomiting, and complaints of abdominal cramps. Sometimes, the patient may have a headache and show signs of confusion. Most serious are signs of circulatory stasis, including itching, tingling, numbness, and cold in the fingers and toes.

Ergot poisoning is relatively rare today but may still occur as the result of attempts to produce an abortion with drugs of this type. During the early months of pregnancy, the uterus does not react as strongly to ergot alkaloids as do the blood vessels. Thus, the danger of gangrene from overdosage is great, when an abortion is rashly attempted by taking large doses of preparations such as the fluidextract, which contains vasoconstrictive alkaloids. Such efforts are misguided at best and are especially dangerous because, in the early months of pregnancy, a woman's blood vessels are much more reactive to these drugs than is her uterus.

In dealing with a patient recovering from an unsuccessful attempt at abortion, the nurse should concentrate on her care and not attempt to judge her. A kind and considerate attitude by the nurse can play an important part—

together with support from her family, the doctor, or a clergyman—in helping her to get well and go through with her pregnancy.

The nurse can also often help to prevent abortion attempts in the first place: women who want to terminate a pregnancy will often approach a nurse, rather than a doctor, for information about abortifacient drugs. It is important to listen patiently and carefully to these questions and to encourage the woman to talk about her problems. The patient may then be encouraged to seek the help of her physician or her clergyman. These measures can often help the patient to carry through with her pregnancy.

The nurse also recognizes more subtle clues that may suggest that a pregnant woman may be planning to take an oxytocic drug. In teaching a mothers' class, for example, the nurse should be alert for the occasional woman who seems upset and depressed or who asks more or less pointed questions about drugs for inducing uterine contractions. The nurse should allow time after the group session for an individual conference with such a patient, to give her an opportunity to express some of her fears or worries in regard to her pregnancy. The doctor can then be notified or an arrangement made for him to see her promptly so that the woman can get further assistance with her problems.

SPARTEINE SULFATE (SPARTOCIN; TOCOSAMINE)

The usefulness of this uterine stimulant is limited by the unpredictability of its action. Sometimes, a small dose administered after a couple of earlier injections have proved ineffective may cause sudden, rapid labor. Occasionally, rupture of the uterus has been reported.

This plant derivative is *not* used like the ergot alkaloids—during or after the third stage of labor. It is, instead, recommended for use in indications similar to those of oxytocin: the induction of labor at term, and to stimulate the hypotonic uterus in cases of arrested labor. All the precautions required with the more reliable oxytocin must be observed with this drug also (see *Summary*, p. 630).

Sparteine, it has been suggested, may be particularly effective for *elective* induction of labor in pregnancies that have been proceeding normally, rather than in cases where induction is made necessary by serious obstetrical complications (see *Summary*, p. 629). This elective use

of oxytocic drugs to induce labor at a time convenient for the physician or the patient is controversial, at best.

If employed at all, elective induction is best accomplished by the use of the much more predictable oxytocin administered very cautiously by an obstetrician experienced in the safe use of that drug in such situations. The two drugs —oxytocin and sparteine—must never be administered together, as their combined effects can cause tetanic contractions of the uterus. The patient must be kept under close observation following injection of these drugs.

PROSTAGLANDINS

Two types of pure prostaglandins, *dinoprost* (PGF_{2a}) and *dinoprostone* (PGE_2), have recently been employed experimentally in obstetrics. These members of the prostaglandin family of biologically active lipids can stimulate strong uterine contractions not only late in the third trimester but also early in pregnancy.

Dinoprost and dinoprostone have been employed in the following situations: (1) to induce labor at term; (2) to bring about therapeutic abortion; and (3) to induce menstruation when it has been delayed.

These substances are said to have various advantages over oxytocin infusion. They do not, for example, have the antidiuretic effect of the latter that sometimes causes water intoxication and convulsions (page 625). The prostaglandins are also claimed less likely to set off sudden tetanic contractions of the uterus.

Actually these new substances have not yet been proved to be more effective or safer than the standard oxytocis agents. Clinical studies are continuing with these natural prostaglandins and with certain longer-acting synthetic derivatives. Some of these may in time prove superior to present methods of inducing labor, performing abortion, and preventing unwanted pregnancy.

Uterine Relaxants

Drugs capable of relaxing the smooth muscles of the uterus as dependably as the oxytocic drugs contract them have several important clinical applications: (1) to overcome premature labor and prevent threatened abortion; (2) to relax tetanic contractions of the uterus developing during abnormal labor; and (3) to reduce severe uterine cramps in women with dysmenorrhea. In practice, only a few drugs are available for use in these situations, and none act specifically upon the uterine musculature to bring about dependable, effective relaxation.

OVARIAN HORMONES

The status of the use of estrogenic and progestational sex steroids in the management of dysmenorrhea is discussed in Chapter 36, as is the use of progestogens in preventing threatened abortion. Two other nonsteroidal ovarian principles have been employed as uterine relaxants in obstetrics. The value of these substances, *lututrin* (Lutrexin) and *relaxin* (Releasin; Cervilaxin), has not been established.

ANTISPASMODIC DRUGS

Smooth muscle relaxants of the atropine type that are useful against gastrointestinal spasm have been combined with mild analgesics in drug combinations advertised for use in treating dysmenorrhea. Such anticholinergic drugs have not, however, been proved very useful for relief of uterine menstrual cramps. *Isoxuprine* (Vasodilan), a beta adrenergic stimulant, has been employed for relaxing uterine smooth muscle in cases of premature labor and for the relief of menstrual cramps in dysmenorrhea. It has not proved dependably effective in these clinical situations.

PREMATURE LABOR

Lacking an effective drug for specifically relaxing the uterus and reducing uterine motility, the obstetrician employs various nonspecific measures for managing cases of threatened abortion and premature labor. He usually orders bed rest and attempts to sedate the patient with barbiturates or opiates. These drugs are employed, not for any specific relaxing effect on the uterus, but to keep the pregnant woman calm.

SUMMARY of Clinical Indications for the Use of Oxytocic Drugs

Oxytocin

Induction of labor at term in selected cases, for example: (1) when the mother has diabetes, or shows signs of pre-eclampsia, or when her membranes have ruptured prematurely and labor fails to begin spontaneously; (2) in some cases with Rh problems, including erythroblastosis fetalis; and (3) in normal presentations when conditions seem favorable for *elective* induction.

Uterine inertia in selected cases of arrested labor

Postpartum hemorrhage and uterine atony

Incomplete abortion management to control postabortal bleeding after spontaneous or therapeutic abortion

Expulsion of the placenta in management and control of the third stage of labor

Facilitation of breast feeding (by its galactokinetic action)

Ergonovine and methylergonovine

Prevention of postpartum hemorrhage and uterine atony after delivery of the placenta

Control of postabortal bleeding

To hasten involution of the uterus in cases of puerperal subinvolution

Sparteine sulfate

Elective induction of labor at term

Hypotonic uterine contraction treatment

SUMMARY of Adverse Effects of the Oxytocic Drugs

All oxytocics—administered under unfavorable obstetric conditions

Tetanic contractions of the uterus can interfere with placental blood flow to the fetus, resulting in fetal distress, hypoxic cardiac irregularities, or asphyxia

Laceration of the cervical tissues and perineum of the mother and trauma to the fetus

Rupture of the fundus of the uterus

Too rapid labor and precipitous delivery may damage the infant's head and cause intracranial hemorrhage

Oxytocin

Severe water intoxication with convulsions and coma following prolonged I.V. infusion

Premature ventricular contractions (PVC)

Possible increased blood loss following hypofibrinogenemia or afibrinogenemia

Nausea and vomiting

Ergonovine and methylergonovine

Elevation of blood pressure—usually transient, but possibly extreme and resulting in hypertensive crisis and cerebral hemorrhage in case of injection into a vein

Headache, dizziness, drowsiness, ringing in the ears, sweating

Nausea, vomiting, abdominal cramps, diarrhea

Cardiac palpitations, chest pains, dyspnea

Circulatory changes—itching, tingling, numbness and cold in the fingers and toes, possible thrombophlebitis with necrosis of tissue and gangrene

Sparteine sulfate

Headache, dizziness, sweating, and blurring of vision

Cardiac palpitation and irregularities

SUMMARY of Cautions and Contraindications in the Use of Oxytocic Drugs

All oxytocics (for induction or stimulation of labor during first and second stages)

Cephalopelvic disproportion of a type that would prevent normal vaginal delivery

Abnormal position of fetus (for example, transverse lie)

Abnormal presentation of fetus (for example, vertex must be presented and engaged)

Premature, or "unripe," cervix (for example, cervix should be at least 3 cm dilated and partially effaced)

Overdistended uterus

Predisposition to uterine rupture, for example: primiparous patients over 35 years old; multiparous patients (parity of four and over); previous caesarean section or other surgery of cervix or fundus of the uterus; history of previous difficult delivery with trauma or sepsis of the uterus; hypertonic pattern of labor

Predisposition to amniotic fluid embolism, for example: abruptio placentae; dead fetus

Severe toxemia

Fetal distress

Lack of trained professional personnel for keeping patient under constant observation during drug administration

Ergonovine and methylergonovine

Not given until after delivery of the anterior shoulder of the fetus, or preferably following delivery of the placenta

Peripheral vascular disease (obliterative type)

Hypertension; severe liver or kidney disease

History of allergic hypersensitivity

SUMMARY of Points for the Nurse to Remember Concerning Oxytocic Drugs

The nurse must follow meticulously the obstetrician's orders in regard to the *timing* of administration of oxytocic drugs in the delivery room. She should prepare the required drugs and equipment and acquire the knowledge needed to administer these drugs promptly and accurately, in advance, as part of her preparation for assisting in delivery.

The nurse should warn women against the use of oxytocic drugs when they approach her to discuss ways of terminating an unwanted pregnancy. She should listen to the patient's views with understanding and compassion, and arrange an opportunity for her to talk further with a physician and, perhaps, a social worker.

The nurse should be aware of the toxic symptoms of ergotism in order to be able to recognize quickly that a patient may have accidentally or deliberately taken a toxic overdose of an ergot preparation.

The nurse should concentrate her attention exclusively on the all-important aspects of the care required when a woman is suffering the effects of an attempted drug-induced abortion. She should be aware of the complex emotional and social factors which may have precipitated such an action. A helpful, nonjudgmental attitude on the part of the nurse and others is desirable for the patient's recovery, and for the sake of the unborn baby if the abortion attempt was (as is usual) unsuccessful and the fetus was not expelled.

The nurse should be able to explain to the patient in labor why her doctor has not ordered medication to make it proceed more quickly—that is, that such drugs are too dangerous to be used to speed up an otherwise normal labor as a way of lessening the normal distress and discomfort of this period.

The nurse keeps under constant observation the patient in whom labor is being induced with the aid of oxytocin. She checks the patient's blood pressure and the fetal heart sounds as well as the frequency, strength, and duration of uterine contractions. If relatively prolonged uterine contractions occur, the intravenous drip of dilute oxytoxin solution is temporarily cut off and other necessary measures are taken.

The nurse helps to calm patients with premature labor contractions who are receiving sedatives and opiates to reduce uterine motility. By staying with the patient or observing her frequently, the nurse can add to her sense of security and thus help to relax both the patient and her uterine contractions.

DRUG DIGEST

ERGONOVINE MALEATE U.S.P. (Ergotrate)

Actions and Indications. This ergot alkaloid produces prompt and prolonged contraction of the smooth muscle of the uterus. It is administered *only after* delivery of the infant and the placenta and *not* to induce labor *nor during* labor. It is, however, an oxytocic drug of choice for preventing postpartum uterine atony and hemorrhage, and it may also be used to stop postabortal bleeding. Some obstetricians also use oral doses of this drug to speed return of the uterus to normal size (that is, to hasten involution, and to reduce possible bleeding and infection during this period).

Side Effects, Cautions, and Contraindications. This drug is not ordinarily administered before the placenta is delivered because the "afterbirth" may become trapped in the persistently contracted uterus, and its use during pregnancy or in the first two stages of labor is always contraindicated. It is not administered to patients with a history of allergic hypersensitivity or idiosyncracy to ergot derivatives.

This alkaloid causes relatively little constriction of blood vessel smooth muscle as compared to ergotamine. However, its prolonged use is undesirable because of the possibility that particularly sensitive patients may suffer excessive vasoconstriction and other chronic toxic effects (ergotism). Its use is contraindicated in patients with severe peripheral vascular disease, and caution is required in patients with cardiac disease or hypertension. (The drug occasionally causes elevation of central venous pressure or of arterial blood pressure.)

Dosage and Administration. Intramuscular or intravenous injection of 0.2 mg usually controls postpartum bleeding. An additional dose of 0.2 to 0.4 mg may be given every six to 12 hours for the first two days postpartum (or longer), if uterine atony persists.

OXYTOCIN INJECTION U.S.P. (Pitocin; Syntocinon; Uteracon)

Actions and Indications. This drug's ability to raise the muscle tone of the uterus and start contractions or increase their frequency makes it useful in several obstetrical situations. These include: (1) induction of labor in carefully selected cases; (2) stimulation of slow or arrested labor in cases of true uterine inertia; (3) management of cases of incomplete abortion; and (4) management of the third (placental) stage of labor and of postpartum uterine atony and hemorrhage.

Side Effects, Cautions, and Contraindications. Oxytocin should be administered only by trained professional personnel in closely controlled dosage and to carefully selected patients. Too strong stimulation of the uterus may be dangerous to both mother and fetus. Excessive contractions that cause severe spasms may cut off the circulation to the fetus, with resulting hypoxia that causes cardiac irregularities. Rupture of the uterus can occur, especially in patients predisposed to this danger. Thus, the drug is not administered to women with a history of uterine surgery, including caesarian section, or when the uterus is already overdistended.

Unlike the natural hormone, synthetic oxytocin does not increase the tone of blood vessel smooth muscle. It may, however, occasionally cause water intoxication because of some small antidiuretic activity.

Dosage and Administration. This varies with the particular indication. For control of postpartum hemorrhage, oxytocin is usually administered intramuscularly in a dose of 3 to 10 units. For induction of labor, 1 ml (10 units) is added to one liter of a 5 percent solution of dextrose and dripped into a vein at a controlled rate— usually 10 to 15 drops per minute initially.

References

Cramer, W.C., Reeves, B.D., and Danforth, D.N. Sparteine sulfate in the conduct of labor. *Amer. J. Obstet. Gynec.*, 89:268, 1964.

Davis, M.E., Adair, F.L., and Pearl, S. The present status of oxytocics in obstetrics. *JAMA*, 107:261, 1936.

DiPalma, J.R. Prostaglandins, the potential wonder drugs. *RN*, 35:51, 1972 (Oct.).

Kobak, A.J. Intravenous pitocin infusion in obstetrics. *Amer. J. Obstet. Gynec.*, 71:1272, 1956.

Moir, J.C. The history and present day use of ergot. *Canad. Med. Ass. J.*, 72:727, 1955.

Rodman, M.J. Drugs used in labor and delivery. *RN*, 28:81, 1965 (Sept.).

———. Prostaglandins: Experimental OBG uses. *RN*, 36:63, 1973 (July).

48.

Drug Treatment of Neoplastic Diseases

Current Status of Cancer Chemotherapy

Cancer is the second most common cause of death. Treatment of malignant tumors is most successful when they are still localized. Following early diagnosis, it is often possible to eradicate the tumor surgically or with radiation. Once the neoplastic cells have metastasized, or spread to other sites in the body, surgery and radiation alone may fail to cure the condition.

Anticancer drugs are used mainly: (1) for treating advanced cases of *disseminated cancer* that can no longer be controlled by surgical removal of the localized tumor, or by destroying the neoplastic tissues with radiation; and (2) for control of *leukemia*, a condition in which the cancerous blood cells were spread through the patient's body from the start.

Until recently, chemotherapy of these conditions had only limited usefulness. In solid tumor malignancies that have metastasized, drug treatment usually decreases the size of the tumor masses only temporarily. This often results in some symptomatic relief. However, the patient's life is prolonged in only a relatively few cases. Similarly, in leukemia, drugs have often brought about temporary remissions. However, in the past, the disease inevitably returned before long in a form that could no longer be controlled by the available antineoplastic agents.

Recently, cancer chemotherapy has come closer to reaching its goal, which is to control or destroy cancer cells without damaging normal body cells. Doctors now speak cautiously of "cures," by which they mean that, in some cases, all the cancer cells have been eliminated, and the patient's life expectancy is the same as that of others in his age group. For example, children and others with acute lymphocytic leukemia, a disorder formerly always fatal, have now survived for long periods following treatment with combinations of antileukemic drugs (p. 646). Similarly, many women with choriocarcinoma, a form of fetal membrane cancer, have now remained free of the disease for ten years or more after drug treatment.

Chemotherapy seems also to have brought about cures when combined with surgery and radiation for treating Wilms's tumor and other childhood malignancies. Lymphatic tissues tumors, including Burkitt's lymphoma, lymphosarcoma, and Hodgkin's disease, have also proved responsive to attack with combinations of drugs, radiation, and surgery. Drugs have also helped to save the lives of patients with certain types of testicular tumors and lengthened the lives of women with disseminated adenocarcinomas of the breast and ovary, and of adults with chronic and other leukemias.

Before we discuss the several classes of anticancer chemicals and the kinds of neoplastic disorders for which various individual drugs are considered to give best results, we shall first discuss some of the factors that limit the usefulness of all the currently available chemotherapeutic agents. One drawback shared by almost all types of antineoplastic drugs is that their *toxic effects* are not limited to cancer cells alone. Another drawback is the fact that drugs which are at first effective for control of cancer cells later lose their activity, as new neoplastic cell strains emerge that are *resistant* to the anticancer chemicals.

THE TOXICITY OF ANTINEOPLASTIC DRUGS

Drugs that damage cancer cells or interfere with their growth and reproduction are also likely to interfere with the functioning of normal cells. This is particularly true of the healthy cells of such rapidly metabolizing tissues as the *bone marrow* and the epithelial lining of the entire *alimentary tract*. Thus, these drugs often cause a dangerous drop in the formed elements of the blood, with resulting toxic effects. Similarly, they sometimes cause ulcers in the mouth, nausea, vomiting, intestinal bleeding, and diarrhea.

To prevent severe drug-induced *hematopoietic toxicity*, the doctor orders frequent blood tests during anticancer chemotherapy. The drug is promptly discontinued when white blood cell counts fall excessively. A sudden drop in leukocytes tends to expose the patient to severe infection. Such a patient must be protected from exposure to pathogenic organisms during this period of reduced resistance. Thus, for example, the nurse who is caring for the patient puts a clean gown over her uniform and washes her hands carefully.

In some centers, such as the National Cancer Institute, patients are protected from outside infection by isolation in germ-free treatment units. Patients who are to receive intensive cancer chemotherapy are "degermed" by administration of prophylactic antibiotics before being housed in one of these "Life Islands." No one may enter the enclosed area, and medical or nursing procedures are performed from the outside through ports. This method is said to increase the number of infection-free days and to reduce deaths from infection in patients receiving intensive antileukemia drug treatment.

Drug-induced damage to bone marrow also often causes dangerous bleeding, as a result of a drop in blood platelets. Deaths from thrombocytopenic hemorrhage have recently been reduced by the routine use of transfusions of packed blood platelets. Administration of this clotting component instead of whole blood reduces the risk of serum hepatitis. Patients who receive large numbers of concentrated platelets can then be treated with quite high doses of anticancer drugs, with less danger of developing severe potentially fatal bleeding episodes.

Gastrointestinal toxicity can also lead to dangerous bleeding and infection. More often, however, it is important as a cause of discomfort that may make the patient want to stop taking medication. The nurse can encourage the patient to bear this type of toxicity by commenting on the benefits to be gained by drug therapy. She also helps lessen his discomfort by not serving food until drug-induced nausea has subsided. Then, when the patient is feeling better, the nurse finds out what he feels like eating and gets it for him. If oral ulceration develops, the patient will need special mouth care and a diet of soft, bland foods.

DEVELOPMENT OF RESISTANCE

Resistance has been a common result of continued treatment of leukemia and other neoplastic disorders with single anticancer drugs. Apparently, as these drugs eliminate the susceptible neoplastic cells, new populations of cells arise that are so different in some aspect of their metabolism that they are no longer readily destroyed. In time, strains of cancer cells take over which are unaffected by drug concentrations that are prohibitively damaging to normal tissues. The patient then no longer improves but suffers side effects if higher doses are administered.

Combinations of several drugs given simultaneously have recently proved effective for delaying the emergence of drug-resistant cancer cell strains. Giving two or more drugs together that act in different ways tends to kill a greater number of leukemic and lymphoma cells, for example. This has helped to lengthen the period in which the patient is free of disease symptoms.

Sometimes, new drugs discovered during such delaying actions help to prolong the patient's remission for a still longer time. Although the theoretical goal of reducing cancer cell population growth to zero has not yet been reached, doctors now hope that they may soon be able to destroy the last remaining pockets of resistant cells with drugs and by activating the patient's own *immunological defense mechanisms.*

Unlike what happens in bacterial infections, in which the body's own defenses destroy pathogens whose growth has been stopped by bacteriostatic drugs, cancer cells are not ordinarily attacked by the phagocytes and antibodies that fight foreign invaders. Thus, the cells left alive after intensive drug therapy are free to grow, reproduce, and establish new populations of drug-resistant cells. However, recent evidence indicates that immune systems do operate against some kinds of cancer. Thus, there is now hope that it may be possible to eradicate all the remaining cancer cells by stimulating the body's immune defenses.

Classes of Chemotherapeutic Agents

Several dozen drugs have been discovered that are effective for treating one or more types of neoplastic disease. These antineoplastic agents are commonly grouped into several classes: (1) alkylating agents; (2) antimetabolites; (3) products obtained from natural sources, such as plant alkaloids and antibiotics; (4) steroid hormones of various kinds; (5) radioactive isotopes; and (6) miscellaneous synthetic chemicals. We shall first discuss some of the clinically significant properties of individual drugs of each class and then later indicate their special uses in the treatment of various specific kinds of cancer and leukemia.

ALKYLATING AGENTS (TABLE 48-1)

Anticancer drugs of this class react chemically with cellular chemicals, including molecules of deoxyribonucleic acid (DNA). Their *cytotoxic* (cell-poisoning) action results from the alkyl groups that these compounds introduce into the biological molecules. This interferes with the ability of cancer cells to divide and multiply, and it finally leads to their death. Unfortunately, these drugs are also toxic to healthy tissues, including in particular those that reproduce rapidly, such as the cells lining the gastrointestinal tract, hair follicles, and blood-forming bone marrow cells.

Although all the alkylating agents act by the same general mechanism, individual drugs of this class differ in many ways. For example, some, such as *mechlorethamine+*, act almost immediately after a single injection and are then rapidly detoxified. Other drugs, including *cyclophosphamide+*, are slower in onset but exert a more prolonged cytotoxic effect. Both of the above drugs strike mainly at lymphocytic cancers and are most beneficial for treating Hodgkin's disease and other lymphomas (p. 646). *Busulfan+*, on the other hand, has a relatively selective action on those bone marrow cells that make myelocytes, and it is thus used mainly for treating chronic myelocytic (granulocytic) leukemia.

Individual drugs of this class are discussed in detail in *Drug Digests*, and their clinical indications are summarized in Tables 48-1, -2 and -3. Other specific points about each are made in the following brief discussions, and their clinical applications in treating various neoplastic diseases are discussed in the sections on treatment of solid tumors, leukemias, and lymphomas.

Mechlorethamine+, a nitrogen mustard, was the first drug of its class found useful for treating cancer. It is injected intravenously as a freshly prepared solution, taking care to avoid letting it leak into surrounding tissues, as the chemical can cause severe local reactions. This vesicant (blistering) agent must not be splashed on the skin or be allowed to come in contact with the eyes. Its local irritating actions in

TABLE 48-1 *Major Antineoplastic Agents for Cancer Chemotherapy*

Generic or Official Name	Synonym or Proprietary Name	Usual Daily (or weekly) Dosage Range	Clinical Indications
Alkylating Agents			
Busulfan U.S.P.	Myleran	1–6 mg orally	Chronic granulocytic leukemia
Chlorambucil U.S.P.	Leukeran	2–12 mg orally	Chronic lymphocytic leukemia; Hodgkin's disease; choriocarcinoma and other trophoblastic neoplasms
Cyclophosphamide U.S.P.	Cytoxan	40–50 mg/kg I.V. in divided doses over a period of several days, then adjusted to lower maintenance dosage; oral maintenance therapy 1–3 mg/kg	Acute lymphoblastic leukemia; Hodgkin's disease; lymphomas; multiple myeloma; solid tumor cancers
Mechlorethamine U.S.P.	Mustargen; nitrogen mustard	200–600 μg/kg I.V. in single or divided doses	Hodgkin's disease; lymphomas; lung cancer; for control of effusions
Melphalan U.S.P.	Alkeran; 1-phenylalanine mustard	6 mg orally for two to three weeks; maintenance 2 mg daily	Multiple myeloma; testicular seminoma; ovarian carcinoma
Thiotepa U.S.P.	Thio-TEPA; triethylenethiophosphoramide	Up to 200 μg/kg parenterally daily for five days	For control of effusions in breast, ovary, and lung cancer; malignant lymphomas
Triethylenemelamine N.F.	TEM	2.5 mg orally for two or three days; then 0.5–5 mg weekly for four weeks	Chronic lymphocytic and granulocytic leukemias; malignant lymphomas; retinoblastoma
Antimetabolites			
Cytarabine	Cytosar; cytosine arabinoside	2 mg/kg I.V. for ten days; raised to 4 mg/kg for maintenance, if necessary	Acute granulocytic leukemia of adults; other leukemias of children and adults
Floxuridine	FUDR	0.1 to 0.6 mg/kg by continuous arterial infusion	Carcinoma of the liver and other organs
Fluorouracil U.S.P.	5FU; Efudex	12 mg/kg I:V. for four days followed by 6 mg/kg on alternate days through the 12th day; also by topical application to the skin twice daily for several weeks	Carcinoma of the colon, rectum, breast, stomach and pancreas; also topically against solar keratoses
Mercaptopurine U.S.P.	Purinethol	2.5 mg/kg orally	Acute lymphocytic leukemia; chronic granulocytic leukemia
Methotrexate U.S.P.	Amethopterin; MTX	2.5–5.0 mg/kg orally or parenterally for leukemia: 15–30 mg orally or I.M. for five days in choriocarcinoma	Acute lymphoblastic leukemia; choriocarcinoma; mycosis fungiodes; and others, including psoriasis

TABLE 48-1 *Major Antineoplastic Agents for Cancer Chemotherapy (continued)*

Generic or Official Name	Synonym or Proprietary Name	Usual Daily (or weekly) Dosage Range	Clinical Indications
Antimetabolites			
Thioguanine N.F.	6-TG	2 mg/kg orally	Acute leukemia; chronic granulocytic leukemia
Alkaloids and Antibiotics from Natural Sources			
Dactinomycin U.S.P.	Cosmegen; actinomycin D	0.015–0.05 mg/kg I.V. divided dosage over one week; repeat for three to five weeks; repeat course after recovery	Wilm's tumor; testicular carcinoma; choriocarcinoma; rhabdosarcoma; and others
Mithramycin	Mithracin	25–30 μg/kg I.V. infused slowly over four to six hours	Testicular carcinoma; choriocarcinoma, and other trophoblastic tumors
Vinblastine sulfate U.S.P.	Velban	0.1 mg/kg increased weekly by 0.05 mg/kg, up to 0.5 mg/kg	Hodgkin's disease and other lymphomas; choriocarcinoma; reticulum cell sarcoma; breast cancer
Vincristine sulfate U.S.P.	Oncovin	2 mg/sq. m of body surface once weekly I.V. for remission	Acute lymphoblastic leukemia; lymphosarcoma; choriocarcinoma, and others
Miscellaneous Synthetic Chemotherapeutic Agents			
Hydroxyurea	Hydrea	20–30 mg/kg orally	Chronic granulocytic leukemia; melanoma
Mitotane	Lysodren	6–15 mg/kg orally	Carcinoma of the adrenal cortex
Procarbazine	Matulane	1–2 mg/kg, orally increased to 3 mg/kg and maintained for three weeks; then reduced to 2 mg/kg	Hodgkin's disease and other lymphomas; lung cancer
Hormones (Adrenocorticosteroids: Androgens; Estrogens; Progestins)			
ADRENOCORTICOSTEROID DRUGS (EXAMPLES)			
Prednisone U.S.P.	Deltasone; Meticorten; and others	10–100 mg orally	Acute and late chronic lymphocytic leukemia; Hodgkin's disease; lymphosarcoma; carcinoma of the lung or breast
Predisolone sodium succinate N.F.	Meticortelone; and others	10–100 mg orally	
ANDROGENIC DRUGS (EXAMPLES)			
Dromstanolone proprionate N.F.	Drolban	100 mg I.M. three times weekly for 8 to 12 weeks	All used for treating disseminated carcinoma of the breast in premenopausal women, often after ovariectomy and sometimes after adrenalectomy
Fluoxymesterone U.S.P.	Halotestin	20–30 mg orally for maintenance of remissions	
Testolactone	Teslac	100 mg I.M. three times weekly or 50 mg orally three times daily	Testolactone, which is claimed to be free of virilizing properties, is also recommended for use in *post*menopausal women with advanced or disseminated breast cancer, when hormone treatment is indicated
Testosterone cypionate U.S.P.	Depotestosterone	200–400 mg I.M. every two to four weeks	
Testosterone enanthate U.S.P.	Delatestryl	200–400 mg I.M. every two to four weeks	
Testosterone propionate U.S.P.	Perandren; Oreton; and others	100 mg I.M. three times weekly	

T A B L E   4 8 - 1   *Major Antineoplastic Agents for Cancer Chemotherapy (continued)*

Generic or Official Name	Synonym or Proprietary Name	Usual Daily (or weekly) Dosage Range	Clincal Indications
Female Sex Hormones			
ESTROGENS (EXAMPLES)			
Diethylstilbestrol U.S.P.	DES; Stilbestrol; and others	1.5–15 mg orally	Carcinoma of the prostate; metastatic mammary carcinoma in postmenopausal women
Ethinylestradiol U.S.P.	Estinyl; and others	3 mg orally	
PROGESTINS			
Hydroxyprogesterone caproate U.S.P.	Delalutin	500 mg–1.5 g I.M. twice weekly and divided doses for recurrences	All are used for endometrial carcinoma recurrences and metastases
Medroxyprogesterone acetate U.S.P.	Depot-Provera	400–800 mg I.M. twice weekly or 200–300 mg orally every day	
Megestrol acetate	Megace	40 mg orally in divided daily doses	
Radioactive Isotopes			
Radioactive gold solution Au 198 U.S.P.	Aurocoloid Aureotope	35–100 μc intrapleurally or intraperitoneally	For pleural effusions and ascites caused by cancer
Sodium iodide I 131 solution U.S.P.	Iodotope; Theriodide; Oriodide; Radiocaps; Tracervial	1–100 μc orally or I.V. for treatment; 1–100 μc for diagnosis	For hyperthyroidism and thyroid carcinoma
Sodium phosphate P 32 solution U.S.P.	Phosphotope	6 μc orally; 3–5 μg I.V.	For polycythemia vera

subcutaneous tissues can be counteracted by applying ice-cold compresses to the area, or by infiltrating it with a solution of sodium thiosulfate that the doctor may order. Antiemetic drugs may allay the nausea and vomiting that commonly occur. The nurse assures the patient that the severe discomfort sometimes set off by this drug will disappear in a few hours.

Cyclophosphamide+ can be given orally as well as by various parenteral routes, because it does not cause local tissue damage. However, this nitrogen mustard is converted to toxic metabolites in the liver, and these can cause severe bladder irritation when excreted in the urine. The patient is kept well hydrated to dilute these urinary drug metabolites and thus prevent cystitis. The drug is discontinued if blood appears in the urine or the patient complains of pain upon voiding. Because baldness often follows treatment with this drug, the patient is prepared for this possibility and assured that the hair will grow back. Women may wish to obtain a wig before treatment.

Thiotepa+, like mechlorethamine may be injected into various body cavities to control fluid effusions from local metastases of breast and ovarian cancer tissues. These drugs are also sometimes administered by regional perfusion, a procedure that delivers large doses of systemically toxic drugs to cancerous areas that are temporarily isolated from the rest of the body by tourniquets. A new alkylating agent, *carmustine*, crosses the blood-brain barrier by itself to attack tumor tissue within the central nervous system. It is being tried for treating brain tumors and metastases of cancer cells to the eyes and leukemic cell invasion of the meninges.

Several other alkylating agents that are active when taken orally in small, relatively safe doses, are often effective for bringing about symptomatic relief in certain specific kinds of cancer (Table 48-3). Such drugs include—in addition to *busulfan*+, mentioned above—*chlorambucil*+ for chronic lymphocytic leukemia and malignant lymphomas, including Hodgkin's disease, *melphalan* mainly for treating multiple myeloma, and *pipobroman* and *uracil mustard* mainly for polycythemia vera, and in chronic leukemias.

ANTIMETABOLITES (TABLE 48-1)

Antimetabolites are drugs with chemical structures close to those of the different dietary substances that cancer cells need in order to grow and multiply. These anticancer chemicals, which resemble various vitamins, amino acids, and other substances essential for cellular growth and reproduction, keep the cancer cells from using the natural nutrients in metabolic processes. This, in turn, interferes with cellular production of protein for enzymes and with the biosynthesis of nucleic acids, including DNA and RNA.

Methotrexate+, one of the first antimetabolites found useful for leukemia treatment, acts by keeping the cancer cells from utilizing the B-complex vitamin, folic acid. It is particularly effective when used in combination with other anticancer chemicals for treating acute lymphoblastic leukemia, the advanced stages of malignant lymphomas, and in choriocarcinoma, a swiftly spreading placental tissue tumor. It has even been used successfully for treating the *non*malignant skin disease, *psoriasis*, because of its ability to slow the growth of all rapidly reproducing body cells (Chapter 46).

This, of course, accounts for its toxicity to bone marrow, the mucosa of the mouth and gastrointestinal tract, and hair or skin cells. Patients are closely watched for signs of toxicity that require discontinuation of further therapy. An antidote, *folinic acid* (Leucovorin), may be effective for counteracting methotrexate toxicity if promptly injected parenterally.

Mercaptopurine+, another type of antimetabolite, also interferes with cancer cell synthesis of nucleic acids. Its effects upon the production of leukemic and normal blood cells account both for its usefulness in treating leukemia and for its toxic hematopoietic effects. It is used mainly for providing further periods of prolonged remission for children with acute leukemia.

Like other antineoplastic drugs, mercaptopurine often causes increased production of uric acid. To prevent high plasma levels (hyperuricemia) and to keep crystals of this chemical from causing kidney injury, the antigout drug *allopurinol* may be given. However, in such cases, it is very important to remember that mercaptopurine dosage must be reduced to only one third or one quarter of what it was. This is because allopurinol blocks the enzyme responsible for detoxifying mercaptopurine.

Thus, this drug interaction may result in the cancer drug's accumulating to toxic levels in the body (Chapters 2 and 16).

Fluorouracil+, an antimetabolite that antagnizes DNA biosynthesis in still another way, helps to relieve symptoms of breast, ovary, and gastrointestinal cancers. It has only a narrow safety margin, so patients must be hospitalized and observed closely for signs of toxicity. The drug is usually administered by vein. However, its systemic toxicity and that of its derivative, *floxuridine* (FUDR), may often be reduced by injecting them directly into the arteries that carry blood to the various visceral organs. This lessens the danger of damage to *non*malignant tissues such as the bone marrow.

Cytarabine (Cytosar), the most recently introduced antimetabolite, is effective for controlling cases of advanced leukemia, particularly when it is combined with *thioguaninine* (Table 48-1). Cytarabine is best given by *rapid* I.V. injection because it is better tolerated this way than when infused slowly. Once signs of remission appear, the patient can be maintained on subcutaneous injection. As with other drugs of this class, cytarabine administration requires close monitoring for signs of bone marrow toxicity.

ANTINEOPLASTIC ANTIBIOTICS AND ALKALOIDS (TABLE 48-1)

Natural products, including several antibiotics too toxic for use against infections and two alkaloids derived from the periwinkle plant, have proved very useful for control of some types of cancer. *Dactinomycin* is an antibiotic that is particularly effective for treating cancers that attack young children, including Wilms's tumor (p. 647). It is also sometimes combined with another antibiotic, *mithramycin*, in the treatment of metastatic testicular cancer.

Vincristine+ and *vinblastine*, plant alkaloids extracted from the periwinkle plant, have proved useful for treating several types of neoplastic disorders, including Hodgkin's disease, particularly when given in combination with other classes of cancer chemotherapeutic agents (p. 646). Both drugs cause some toxic effects that are similar to those of other neoplastic agents, but vincristine is less toxic to bone marrow.

In addition, both these drugs can cause severe nervous tissue toxicity. Patients are checked for complaints of tingling and numbness in fingers and toes, as the dosage must then be reduced or the drug discontinued in order to avoid severe psychomotor disability. Vincristine neurotoxicity can, for example, affect the patient's ability to walk normally. Vinblastine can cause convulsions, mental depression, and psychotic reactions.

HORMONES (TABLE 48-1)

Steroid hormones of several kinds are useful for symptomatic relief of several kinds of cancers and their complications. Corticosteroids, and *prednisone+* in particular, play an important part in the treatment of certain kinds of leukemia and lymphomas. These drugs are also used to reduce high blood levels of calcium—a complication of breast cancer that has spread to the bones.

Male and female sex hormones and synthetic substances with similar actions are highly effective for treating cancers of the breast and prostate that have metastasized. Such cancers are best managed by surgical removal of the glands—testes or ovaries—that secrete the sex hormones which stimulate growth of the cancerous tissues. However, sex hormones of one kind can also be used to antagonize the effects of hormones of the other class and thus slow the growth of these hormone-dependent malignancies.

Estrogens, for example, are employed to combat metastasized cancer of the prostate, and androgens are used against breast cancers that have spread to the bones and elsewhere. *Progestins* are employed to suppress the growth of endometrial tissue in uterine cancer of this type (see also Chapter 37).

MISCELLANEOUS (TABLE 48-2)

Synthetic anticancer chemicals and other natural substances that do not fall into any of the above classes have also been found useful for terating certain neoplasms. *Procarbazine* (Matulane), for example, has proved useful against advanced Hodgkin's disease (p. 646). *Hydroxyurea* (Hydrea) produces remissions in melanoma and myelocytic leukemia. The mechanisms by which these drugs act is still uncertain.

Asparaginase, an enzyme that is being employed experimentally in acute leukemia, is especially interesting. It is the first anticancer chemical to be discovered that acts by taking advantage of a basic biochemical difference between neoplastic cells and normal ones. This enzyme acts by breaking down an amino acid called *asparagine* in body fluids. Leukemic cells require this substance and starve when it becomes unavailable. Normal cells can make their own asparagine and are thus unaffected by the administration of asparaginase.

Early reports of asparaginase-induced remissions with relatively few toxic reactions have raised hopes that still more compounds will be discovered that can be used to exploit specific biochemical differences between normal and cancerous cells.

RADIOACTIVE ISOTOPES

A few radioactive elements are used to treat certain types of neoplasms. Ideally, such a substance concentrates in the cancer and selectively damages its cells without affecting normal tissues. In practice, such selective toxicity does not occur with any isotope. Thus, although some do destroy tumor tissues, they also damage normal cells.

Two official radioisotopes in common use in cancer treatment are *sodium phosphate P 32+* and *radiogold* (Au[198]). A third isotope employed to deliberately damage human tissues is *sodium iodide I 131,* which is discussed in Chapter 38. In adequate doses, all emit *beta particles* or "radiations" in amounts that destroy living tissues in the immediate vicinity. Although beta radiations penetrate only a short distance, they can damage enough erythroid or myeloid cells to produce remissions in polycythemia vera and to a lesser extent in chronic granulocytic anemia.

If overdosage permits too much radioactive phosphate to accumulate in the bone marrow, normal hematopoietic tissues may also be damaged. This can result in leukopenia, thrombocytopenia, and anemia as a result of excessive reduction in all the formed elements of the peripheral blood. Thus, the less toxic alkylating agent busulfan is usually preferred for chronic leukemia treatment, and the new alkylating agent *pipobroman* may be preferable to P[32] in polycythemia vera treatment.

Chemotherapy of Specific Kinds of Cancer (Table 48-3)

Cancer is actually not a single disease but a hundred or more different diseases. Depending upon the tissues in which they originate, neoplastic cells possess different biological properties, growth rates, and ability to invade healthy

TABLE 48-2 *Minor and On-Trial Anticancer Chemicals*

Generic Name	Synonym or Chemical Name	Usual Daily or Weekly Dosage	Clinical Indications
Adriamycin	. . . .	60–90 mg/sq. m of body surface I.V. Repeat in three weeks	Hodgkin's disease; lymphomas; sarcomas of bone and soft tissues; carcinomas of breast and lungs
Asparaginase	Elspar	200 I. U. per kg I.V. for 28 days	Acute lymphocytic leukemia
Bleomycin	. . . .	10–15 mg/sq. m of body surface weekly or twice weekly I.V. or I.M. (Maximum total dose 300–400 mg)	Hodgkin's disease; other lymphomas
Carmustine	BCNU; bischlorethyl nitrosourea	100 mg/sq. m of body surface twice daily I.V. Repeat after six weeks	Gliobastoma and other C.N.S. neoplasms; Hodgkin's disease; other lymphomas; malignant melanoma; adenocarcinoma of the gastrointestinal tract; multiple myeloma
Dacarbazine	DIC; DTIC	3–5 mg/kg I.V. for ten days. Repeat after four weeks	Hodgkin's disease; malignant melanoma
Daunorubicin	Daunomycin; Cerubidin; Rubidomycin	30–60 mg/sq. m of body surface I.V. for three days; or once a week	Acute lymphocytic and granulocytic leukemia
Hexamethylmelamine	. . . .	12 mg/kg orally for 21 days	Carcinoma of the lung and ovary
Lomustine	CCNU; cyclohexyl chlorethyl nitrosourea	130 mg/sq. m of body surface orally; repeat at intervals of six weeks	Hodgkin's disease; adenocarcinoma of the gastrointestinal tract, lung cancer; C.N.S. neoplasms
Piprobroman	Vercyte	1 mg/kg initially; 0.1–0.2 mg/kg maintenance	Polycythemia vera; chronic myelocytic leukemia
Quinacrine HCl	Atabrine	50–100 mg intrapleurally; 100–200 mg intraperitoneally. Raised gradually up to 1 g daily	For management of recurrent effusions and ascites secondary to cancer of breast, ovary, lung, and others
Streptozotocin	. . . .	1 g/sq. m of body surface I.V. weekly for four weeks	Malignant carcinoid; insulinoma
Uracil mustard	. . . .	1–2 mg orally; or 3–5 mg orally for only seven days; maintenance 1 mg daily	Chronic lymphocytic leukemia; lymphomas; polycythemia vera; mycosis fungoides

tissues. No one group of chemotherapeutic agents is effective against all kinds of cancer.

Accurate diagnosis to determine whether a patient actually has cancer is necessary before beginning treatment with these toxic drugs.

The treatment plan is based on the pathologist's report of the type of cancer cell found in a biopsy. Once he knows in what organ the neoplasm originated, the physician chooses drugs that are known to be effective

TABLE 48-3   Chemotherapy of Specific Kinds of Cancer

	Primary Drug Treatment	Other Active Drugs	Remarks
Leukemias and Lymphomas			
ACUTE LYMPHOBLASTIC LEUKEMIA			
For induction of remission	Vincristine combined with prednisone	Daunorubicin; adriamycin	Combinations of chemotherapeutic agents are employed in continued maintenance therapy. The five-year survival rate has been extended to 50% of patients
For maintenance of remission	Methotrexate; mercaptopurine; cyclophosphamide	Cytarabine; thioguanine; asparaginase; carmustine	
CHRONIC LYMPHOCYTIC LEUKEMIA			
For symptomatic relief of complications and some gain in survival time during prolonged maintenance therapy	Chlorambucil or cyclophosphamide, combined with prednisone	Triethylenemelamine; cytarabine	Drugs and radiation of lymph nodes, liver, and spleen can often control the disease and keep patients comfortable for long periods in close to 50% of cases
ACUTE MYELOBLASTIC (GRANULOCYTIC) LEUKEMIA			
For induction of remission	Cytarabine combined with thioguanine	Daunorubicin; carmustine; asparaginase; prednisone	Remission rate has recently been increased to close to 50%, but the five-year survival rate is still less than 1%
For maintenance of remission	Methotrexate; mercaptopurine; cyclophosphamide		
CHRONIC MYELOBLASTIC (GRANULOCYTIC) LEUKEMIA			
For induction of remission and long-term maintenance	Busulfan; mercaptopurine	Dibromomannitol; colcemid; hydroxyurea; melphalan	Disease can be controlled for long periods with chemotherapy and radiotherapy of spleen. No increase in survival when blast crisis occurs
HODGKIN'S DISEASE			
For complete remission in advanced cases (Stages III and IV) and long-term maintenance therapy	Combination of mechlorethamine, vincristine (Oncovin), procarbazine, and prednisone (the "MOPP" combination)	Vinblastine; carmustine; lomustine; bleomycin; cyclophosphamide; chlorambucil; thiotepa; methotrexate; adriamycin; dacarbazine	Radical radiation or sometimes surgery are best in localized (Stages I and II) diseases. Chemotherapy with several active agents in sequence or combined has controlled advanced disease for long periods (five-year survival rate about 40%)

Type of Neoplasm	Drugs of Choice	Other Drugs	Remarks
LYMPHOSARCOMA	Cyclophosphamide, vincristine (Oucovin) prednisone (the "COP" combination)	Procarbazine; vinblastine; adriamycin; bleomycin; carmustine; chlorambucil	Remission and a significant lengthening of survival time is being achieved in an increasing number of cases
BURKITT'S TUMOR — For cure of the still localized tumor and for remission of recurrences	Cyclophosphamide	Carmustine; cytarabine; vincristine; methotrexate	Chemotherapy of localized disease has led to prolonged survival in African children and others
MULTIPLE MYELOMA — For remission and for management of recurrences	Cyclosphosphamide combined with prednisone; or melphalan and prednisone combined	Chlorambucil; carmustine	Chemotherapy may increase survival time in a small proportion of patients and causes disease regression in more
POLYCYTHEMIA VERA — For suppression of erythropoiesis temporarily	Azauridine; busulfan	Sodium phosphate P 32; pyrimethamine	Irradiation with the isotope may lead to late leukemia. Drugs produce some remissions
Solid Malignant Tumors / MAMMARY CARCINOMA / (1) Breast cancer in premenopausal women	Androgens, including long-acting testosterone esters and synthetic substances, such as fluoxymesterone and dromstanolone	Prednisone; cyclophosphamide; methotrexate; vincristine; fluorouracil	Male hormone derivatives are often effective for maintaining remissions in women who have responded to ovariectomy and other surgical procedures
(2) Breast cancer and pleural effusions in postmenopausal women	Estrogens, including diethylstilbestrol and ethinyl estradiol; androgens, including testolactone	Thiotepa; mechlorethamine; radioactive gold and phosphorus; quinacrine	Alkylating agents decrease size of masses and some reduce peritoneal fluid effusion. Other drugs also help to bring about tumor tissue regression and to raise five-year survival rate, following surgery, to about 30%
OVARIAN CANCER	Cyclophosphamide; chlorambucil; melphalan	Methotrexate; fluorouracil; mechlorethamine; thiotepa; radioactive gold. Also experimentally: dactinomycin, hexamethylmelamine, and vinblastine	Alkylating agents decrease size of masses and some reduce peritoneal fluid effusion. Other drugs also help to bring about tumor tissue regression and to raise five-year survival rate following surgery to about 30%
UTERINE CERVIX	Cyclophosphamide; methotrexate; fluorouracil	Vincristine; bleomycine; methylmitomycin	Pelvic radiotherapy and surgery are preferred to drugs

TABLE 48-3 *Chemotherapy of Specific Kinds of Cancer (continued)*

	Primary Drug Treatment	Other Active Drugs	Remarks
UTERINE BODY (ENDOMETRIAL CANCER)	Progestational steroids, including hydroxyprogesterone, medroxyprogesterone, and megestrol acetate		Help to shrink size of metastases to the lungs, bones, and other sites
CHORIOCARCINOMA And other neoplasms of the trophoblastic type	Methotrexate; dactinomycin	Vincristine; vinblastine; chlorambucil; mercaptopurine	Long time survival in 75–90% of cases has been achieved even in patients with metastases to the lungs
WILMS'S TUMOR (NEPHROBLASTOMA) And other solid tumors of childhood (for example, Ewing's sarcoma, rhabdosarcoma, neuroblastoma, retinoblastoma)	Dactinomycin, vincristine, cyclophosphamide combined with extensive radiation and surgery	Adriamycin; thiotepa; methotrexate; vinblastine; Daunorubicin; prednisone	Five-year survival rate has been raised to about 80% for Wilms's tumor in some centers by a vigorous attack with drugs, surgery, and radiation combined
PROSTATIC CARCINOMA	Estrogens, including diethylstilbestrol, ethinyl estradiol, and chlortrianisene		High five-year survival rate when castration is followed by female hormones
TESTICULAR CANCER Seminomas, carcinomas (embryonal)	Melphalan is sometimes employed but irradiation and surgery alone produce a high survival rate Vincristine; vinblastine; chlorambucil; dactinomycin; methotrexate, in combinations	Mithramycin; bleomycin	Combinations of drugs sometimes produce prolonged remissions in patients with lung metastases
MALIGNANT MELANOMA	Melphalan; hydroxyurea; dacarbazine, carmustine	Vincristine; dactinomycin; cyclophosphamide; chlorambucil; thiotepa	Some newer drugs have helped to bring about remissions in carefully selected patients

ADRENOCORTICAL CARCINOMA	Mitotane	This drug suppresses hormone secretion in metastatic masses not removed by surgery
GASTROINTESTINAL ADENOCARCINOMA (colorectal, gastric, pancreatic)	Fluorouracil	Cyclophosphamide; mitomycine; carmustine; lomustine Mainly useful for symptomatic relief in some cases rather than for prolonging life
LIVER CANCER OR HEPATIC METASTASES from gastrointestinal cancer	Floxuridine, intraarterially	Fluorouracil Constant intraarterial infusion of floxuridine in low concentration may help slow growth of liver cancer with minimal systemic toxicity
LUNG CANCER (bronchogenic carcinoma)	Mechlorethamine; cyclophosphamide; methotrexate; thiotepa	Adriamycin; bleomycin combined with vincristine; lomustine; hexamethylmelamine; procarbazine Drug therapy has had little success but is used as an adjunct to early lung surgery to bring about a five-year survival rate of only about 5%
HEAD AND NECK (squamous cell)	Methotrexate; cyclophosphamide	Bleomycin; fluorouracil Occasional regression but no significant increase in survival rate
BRAIN TUMORS (PRIMARY)	Carumstine; lomustine	Vincristine; methotrexate Little significant improvement
SARCOMAS (osteogenic and soft tissues)	Dactinomycin, adriamycin, and dacarbazine in combination	Cyclophosphamide; vincristine Experimental drugs show some activity as adjuncts to surgery

against that kind of cancer. Dosage is carefully adjusted in accordance with each patient's response and ability to tolerate the treatment.

The chemotherapeutic agents that are at present considered best for treating various specific neoplastic diseases are listed in Table 48-3. In this section, we shall discuss some aspects of the drug treatment used for certain types of disorders that seem to respond especially well to treatment with combinations of antineoplastic drugs and other measures, including surgery and radiation.

THE LEUKEMIAS AND LYMPHOMAS

Cancers of the tissues that form the blood cells cannot be removed by surgery and they are difficult to treat with drugs and x-ray. Treatments intended to halt the growth of white cell neoplasms (the leukemias) also often damage the normal blood cell elements. Even when drugs succeed in producing clinical remissions, some cells survive. These then proliferate and produce drug-resistant leukemic cell strains. This, in time, results in recurrences of the disease that cannot be controlled by safe doses of the drugs that were at first effective.

Nevertheless, remarkable advances have been made recently in the treatment of *acute lymphocytic leukemia.* Children who receive the best treatment now available for this kind of leukemia often stay in good health for long periods. Patients with other kinds of leukemia also often obtain prolonged symptomatic relief when treated in centers equipped to detect drug toxicity and prevent drug-induced infection and bleeding.

These gains are, in part, the result of new tactics in the use of established and experimental antileukemic agents. Instead of using the available drugs singly in sequence, some cancer treatment centers strike at the disease with high-dosage combinations of several effective drugs (Table 48-3) at once. Intensive drug treatment of this kind is intended to eliminate every leukemic cell and thus prolong remissions and prevent recurrences.

Drug schedules for leukemia vary in different treatment research centers. The cancer nurse must be familiar with the effects of all the drugs in the protocols employed by her clinic. She observes patients closely for the expected side effects as well as for the beneficial effects of combination drug therapy. The care that the nurse gives and the emotional support that she can often offer contribute to the patient's recovery and feelings of well-being and to his family's ability to respond constructively.

Dealing with the child and his parents requires mature judgment and tact. It is important not to raise false hopes, only to have these hopes dashed later. However, nothing should be said that might discourage the parents from continuing to make the effort to help their child. Thus, when the leukemic patient goes into remission the nurse can share the parents' pleasure, but she should not contribute to unrealistic attitudes about the possibility of cure. On the other hand, she encourages the continuation of drug treatment when signs of the drug's toxicity temporarily loom larger than the eventual benefits. Working with the child is also a challenge. Often the child senses that death is near, and in his own way tries to express his fears and feelings of isolation. The sensitive nurse can show the child that she understands what he is saying, and, although she cannot change the course of the illness, she can support the child and maintain communication with him as he goes through the remissions, relapses, and the final stage of the illness. Sometimes the nurse can help the parents and the child to communicate more effectively with one another and thus face the experience more fully together.

Hodgkin's disease and other lymphomas have also been successfully treated by combinations of chemotherapeutic agents. If diagnosed while the lesions are still localized (Stages I or II), Hodgkin's disease is often curable by radical radiation therapy alone. Patients with more advanced disease (Stages III and IV) are now best treated with a battery of drugs administered in sequence or in combination (Table 48-3).

Many patients who have been treated with the four-drug "MOPP" combination— mechlorethamine, vincristine or Oncovin, procarbazine, and prednisone—have stayed in good health for several years. Authorities now believe that mortality from this disease could be sharply reduced if all patients were managed with the available drug combinations and dosage schedules. The death rate from Hodgkin's disease could also be reduced if it were more often diagnosed in its early stages while still localized. (This is, of course, true of all kinds of cancer, but irradiation therapy of localized lymphomas has been especially effective.)

SOLID TUMOR MALIGNANCIES

Most kinds of carcinoma and other solid tumors are curable by surgery and x-ray when detected before they have spread from the primary site. Cancer experts claim that half of the close to one half million persons who develop cancer each year could be cured by these means, if their condition were detected early enough. Thus, nurses and others in the health professions should educate the public about cancer. The nurse in her daily contacts with people can carry out effective teaching to promote periodic physical examinations, for cancers often can be detected before they have produced any symptoms at all. (Diagnostic measures such as the "Pap smear" test, which has helped bring about an almost 50 percent drop in deaths from uterine cancer, may also aid in detecting breast and rectal cancers in their early stages.) Similarly, if she recognizes a warning sign of cancer, she often can persuade the person to visit a physician. He may find a mass or other lesion and can confirm the presence of cancer by biopsy. The nurse who gives primary care, as in working with youngsters and with older persons to help them maintain health, has an especially important role in detecting early indications of malignancy and in referring such patients to a clinic or a physician for further study.

Metastasized tumors vary widely in their responsiveness to drug therapy. Some respond poorly, while other malignancies regress and patients show objective signs of improvement that may continue for long periods. *Choriocarcinoma*, for example, can be very well controlled, even after the tumor tissue has spread to the lungs. This placental tissue tumor was first treated successfully with *methotrexate*. Now, other drugs are also available that are effective in those patients who do not benefit from treatment with this antimetabolite. The antibiotic *dactinomycin* is most commonly administered in such cases and to patients who become resistant after an initial remission. Also effective are the plant alkaloids, *vincristine* and *vinblastine*.

Wilms's tumor is also treated with these same drugs together with extensive surgery and radiation. This growth, an embryonal tissue sarcoma of the kidneys, is one of the most common solid cancers of childhood. In some treatment centers, the survival rate has recently been raised from 40 to 80 percent by the vigorous use of all types of available treatment measures. *Dactinomycin, vincristine,* and *cyclophosphamide combinations* have also proved effective in other pediatric cancers, including *Ewing's sarcoma,* a bone tissue tumor.

Breast cancer is the most common of all malignancies in women and the greatest killer of women in middle life. Because metastatic mammary carcinoma is dependent upon female sex hormones for continued growth, surgical removal of the ovaries is the first measure employed in premenopausal women. Sometimes, an adrenalectomy is also performed to eliminate another source of growth-stimulating estrogens.

Patients who show signs of relapse may be maintained for many months on *male hormones*. The long-acting depot form androgens (Table 48-1) are often preferred for maintenance therapy because of their convenience when administered by I.M. injection. However, the short-acting oral compounds are safer in case the patient develops an attack of hypercalcemia that requires immediate withdrawal of androgen therapy. Fluids are then forced to prevent formation of calcified kidney stones that could cause renal failure. Patients often also profit from corticosteroids such as *prednisone*, which help to lower the level of calcium in the plasma and return this mineral to the bones.

Of course, the most common adverse effects seen from androgen therapy of breast cancer is *masculinization*. The patient should be advised in advance that hair may grow on her face and that her voice may deepen. Special skin care may be required to counteract oiliness and prevent acne. The nurse should be aware that the patient may show personality changes and an increase in libido. She should encourage the patient to continue sex steroid treatment and to talk about her concerns about masculinization. The nurse's role lies in helping the patient to understand and to cope with the effects of the drug, and to help the patient recognize the values of drug therapy at times when she is discouraged and is focusing primarily on the distressing side effects.

Chemotherapy of gastrointestinal cancer that has metastasized to the liver and elsewhere is not nearly as successful for producing palliation or prolonging life. In addition, *fluorouracil*, the most effective drug, is highly toxic and causes many discomforting side effects. Patients often have many questions to ask about their treatment in such situations. For example, can the patients whose primary cancer has spread from the pancreas to the liver gain enough in terms of added time and comfort to warrant possible drug-induced discomfort or toxicity that may even hasten his death?

What the patient and his family can be

told about the drug he is receiving depends on various individual circumstances. In any case, it is important that everyone—doctor, nurse, and other staff personnel—give the patient the *same* explanations concerning the purposes, advantages, limitations, and potential toxicity of the drugs employed and that everyone respects the patient's right to choose, once he has the relevant information, what therapy he is willing to accept.

Once the nurse knows what the patient and his family have been told about the nature of his condition and the reason for treating it with drugs that can cause so much discomfort, she can listen to their expressions of hope or their complaints and then help to make the difficult situation more bearable for all concerned.

It is usually desirable for the family to know that the prognosis is poor for patients with primary lesions of the liver or with hepatic metastases from cancers of the colon, rectum, or stomach. However, the patient should be allowed to cling to hope for recovery if this helps to fulfill his emotional needs. Patients who undergo the ordeal of cancer and its treatment with toxic drugs require the nurse's utmost responsiveness to their need for such support.

Special techniques for administering fluorouracil and the related antimetabolite, floxuridine, are employed to increase their effectiveness for treating liver cancer and to reduce their systemic toxicity. *Regional chemotherapy* is accomplished by inserting a small plastic catheter into the patient's hepatic artery and then pumping a solution of the drug directly into the tumor area.

The electric pump provides a high local concentration of the drug in the liver, but only small amounts of the carefully calculated dose ever enter the systemic circulation to cause adverse effects on the bone marrow and other healthy tissues. However, ambulatory patients who are discharged with such a portable pump are warned to report any early signs of drug toxicity. The development of even a very small mouth ulcer may be the first sign of severe toxicity that could lead to death from gastrointestinal bleeding.

Malignant melanoma metastases to the limbs, liver, head, neck, or pelvic area are also treated by prolonged arterial infusion of anticancer chemicals including *melphalan*, a new alkylating agent. This drug has produced good results against tumors made up of these pigment-forming skin cells while they are still confined to a single limb. In such cases, the circulation of the extremity is cut off from the rest of the patient's body, and only the cancerous region receives the intraarterially perfused solution.

Immunotherapy of selected patients has also been employed experimentally in some cases of inoperable malignant melanoma. Patients are inoculated intradermally with tumor cells grown in tissue culture to produce antibodies against melanoma. Some patients who have received a series of such injections have responded with prolonged tumor regression.

SUMMARY

Cancer chemotherapy has recently proved successful for prolonging the lives of patients with some kinds of leukemia and solid tumor cancer. Among the factors responsible for these advances are the following:

1. *The use of combinations of chemotherapeutic agents* to eliminate quickly as many cancer cells as possible and thus lessen development of drug resistance.

2. *The use of special techniques of administration* to deliver high concentrations of anticancer chemicals to the tumor with few effects on healthy tissues.

3. *The use of supportive measures to counteract* such complications of chemotherapy as infection, hemorrhage, hypercalcemia, and hyperuricemia.

4. *The discovery of new antieoplastic drugs*, some of which are relatively selective for certain specific types of cancer. (At least one experimental drug may prove to act with true selective toxicity because it affects a biochemical process that only cancer cells possess.)

5. The discovery that it may be possible to *activate* the cancer patient's *immune mechanisms* against proliferating neoplastic cells. (In the future, *immunotherapy* may aid chemotherapeutic agents in the total elimination of the residual drug-resistant cells responsible for recurrences of leukemia and cancer.)

Despite these recent advances, the drug treatment of most kinds of cancer is still difficult. Even with the most carefully calculated adjustment of dosage, toxic effects are quite common because of the narrow safety margin of most available drugs. Thus, it is important to monitor patients for signs of potential toxicity. Cancer patients require especially skillful nursing care and supportive therapy. The nurse can, for example, use special precautions to protect the patient with leukopenia from infection. She can lessen the discomfort of drug-induced oral inflammation and ulceration by providing the patient with frequent mouth care and serving him bland foods that are neither too hot nor too cold.

The nurse also has an important role in implementing and assisting with the various supportive treatments that the doctor orders, such as transfusions and administration of medications to relieve pain. The patient who receives radioisotope therapy requires special safety precautions.*

* See Chap. 19, Care of the Adult Patient, by Smith, D.W., Germain, C.P.H., and Gips, C.D. Philadelphia: J.B. Lippincott, 1971.

SUMMARY of Points for the Nurse to Remember Concerning Neoplastic Drug Therapy

Most drugs used in cancer chemotherapy are potentially toxic. Observe the patient's reaction carefully and report any new symptoms promptly to the physician, since it may be necessary to alter the dosage or to discontinue the drug.

Make every effort to lessen the discomfort brought about by drug therapy, thus helping the patient to tolerate treatment which can relieve some of the distressing symptoms of his disease and prolong his life.

Work collaboratively with the physician to help the patient understand the purpose and expected action of the drug, so that the patient is spared being given conflicting information.

Encourage the patient to take his medication, and show him that you share his satisfaction when he shows symptomatic improvement. Avoid comments that may lead the patient and his family to develop unrealistic hopes of cure by drug therapy.

Be available to the patient and his family if they wish to talk with you about the drug therapy. Often they feel caught between the ravages of the disease and the distressing effects of its treatment.

Find out what precautions are necessary when working with patients who are treated with radioisotopes, in order to protect yourself and others.

Clinical Nursing Situation

The Situation: Larry, age 4, has acute leukemia. This is his second hospital admission. He has had serious bleeding from his nose and from his rectum and is very pale and listless. Larry has been receiving maintenance doses of methotrexate, which no longer seem as effective as before. Now Larry's physician has decided to add prednisone and vincristine to his regimen.

The Problem: What observations would you make of Larry's response to these drugs? How would you reply to Larry's mother when she asks, "How much good will these drugs do for Larry? He had them before and they didn't keep him from relapsing. Is there really any chance for him ever to be completely cured?"

DRUG DIGEST

BUSULFAN U.S.P. (Myleran)
Actions and Indications. This alkylating agent has a selective action on the myeloid cells of the bone marrow. Thus, it is especially effective for bringing about remissions in many patients with chronic granulocytic (myelocytic) leukemia. Patients feel better and eat with more appetite soon after beginning treatment. Later, there is a lessening of immature white cells in the blood, and a reduction in the size of the patient's enlarged spleen. Although this drug does not cure this or the other neoplastic disorders in which it is employed, it often prolongs the patient's life.

Side Effects, Cautions, and Contra-indications. Complete blood cell counts are made regularly, and the drug is discontinued if there is any sudden drop in leukocyte count or if thrombocytopenia and bleeding develop. Careful hematologic control of this kind is necessary to avoid pancytopenia and the danger of irreversible bone marrow depression. Hyperuricemia may be controlled and kidney damage by uric acid crystals avoided by the adjunctive use of allopurinol. Skin pigmentation and other signs resembling Addison's disease may develop. Nausea, vomiting, and diarrhea occur in some cases.

Dosage and Administration. The usual daily dosage range is 4 to 8 mg orally. Treatment is usually initiated with 4 mg daily and continued until the leukocyte count drops below 10,000/cu. mm. Therapy is resumed when the WBC count rises above 50,000/cu. mm. Maintenance therapy at doses between 1 to 3 mg daily helps to prevent relapse.

CHLORAMBUCIL U.S.P. (Leukeran)

Actions and Indications. This anti-neoplastic agent acts primarily upon lymphoid tissue. Thus, it is used to bring about remissions in patients with chronic lymphocytic leukemia, Hodgkins disease, and other malignant lymphomas, including the giant follicular type and lymphosarcoma.

Side Effects, Cautions, and Contra-indications. This nitrogen mustard derivative is less toxic than other alkylating agents. Therapeutic doses cause relatively few gastrointestinal side effects or blood cell reductions other than lymphopenia and neutropenia. However, frequent blood counts are required, and dosage is reduced or the drug discontinued in the event of severe neutropenia. Excessive dosage can cause irreversible bone marrow damage.

Patients with evidence of bone marrow infiltration receive smaller doses. The drug is not administered to patients who have received full radiation therapy or other antineoplastic drugs during the previous four weeks. Its use during the first trimester of pregnancy is also avoided.

Dosage and Administration. The usual daily dose is between 4 to 10 mg administered at one time—usually an hour before breakfast or two hours after the evening meal —for three to six weeks after treatment is initiated. Dosage is adjusted to lower levels if the W.B.C. count falls abruptly. If maintenance dosage is employed, it ordinarily runs between 2 to 4

mg daily depending upon the patient's response.

CYCLOPHOSPHAMIDE U.S.P. (Cytoxin)

Actions and Indications. This antineoplastic agent is chemically related to the nitrogen mustards but does not cause local irritation while interfering with the growth of lymphatic and myeloid tissues.

It is employed in the advanced stages of malignant lymphomas, including Hodgkin's disease, lymphosarcoma, reticulum cell sarcoma, Burkitt's lymphoma, and lymphoma of the follicular type. It prolongs remissions of acute lymphoblastic leukemia in children. It may be of some use in advanced mycosis fungioides, multiple myeloma, and such solid tumor neoplasms as neuroblastoma and retinoblastoma.

Side Effects, Cautions, and Contra-indications. Alopecia is a common complication, about which patients should be warned and also reassured, as the hair will grow back following the course of treatment. Nausea and vomiting are also common, as is leukopenia. Thrombocytopenia also occurs sometimes, and caution is required in patients with these hematopoietic disorders as well as in those with impaired liver or kidney function.

Patients should force fluids and void frequently to prevent possible bladder irritation that can lead to severe sterile hemorrhagic cystitis.

Dosage and Administration. Patients initially receive a total loading dose of 40 to 50 mg/kg I.V. at a rate of 10 to 20 mg/kg daily for two to five days. The drug may also be administered orally in doses of 1 to 5 mg/kg daily both for initiation and maintenance or dosage may be raised or reduced as required.

FLUOROURACIL U.S.P. (5 FU; Efudex)

Actions and Indications. This potent antimetabolite of the pyrimidine type is thought to cause a thymine deficiency and thus to interfere with the biosynthesis of DNA and RNA. It may help to produce temporary relief in selected cases of solid tumor cancer that cannot be treated surgically or by x-ray. Among the kinds of carcinoma that may be benefited by management with this antineoplastic agent are solid tumors of the colon and rectum, stomach and pancreas, and breast and ovarian cancers. A topical form is used to treat solar keratoses—*non*malignant skin lesions that are the result of prolonged exposure to sunlight.

Side Effects, Cautions, and Contra-indications. Patients who are re-

ceiving their first treatment course with this agent are hospitalized and carefully supervised, as the drug has a low safety margin. Inflammation and even ulceration of the mouth and esophagus are common, as are vomiting and diarrhea. Skin reactions and alopecia are also frequent. Leukopenia occurs in every case treated with adequate dosage.

Patients are carefully selected to screen out those with various conditions that make them a poor risk for treatment with this toxic drug. It is contraindicated in those with bone marrow depression, serious infections, or those in poor nutrition. Extreme caution is required in patients with liver and kidney function impairment.

Dosage and Administration. The undiluted drug is injected I.V. once daily for four successive days in a dosage of 12 mg/kg. If no toxicity occurs, treatment is continued at a lower dosage level for a few more days. A cream is applied twice daily for two to four weeks in treating solar keratoses.

MECHLORETHAMINE HCl U.S.P. (Mustargen)

Actions and Indications. The first of the nitrogen mustards is still considered the most effective of the alkylating agents for bringing about rapid and prolonged remissions in patients in advanced stages of Hodgkin's disease and other lymphomas, such as lymphosarcoma. It is also used in treating some solid tumors, including carcinomas of the lung.

Side Effects, Cautions, and Contra-indications. This drug has certain drawbacks in addition to the danger of producing bone marrow depression that limits the utility of all antineoplastic agents. It can, for example, cause local tissue damage and must be administered with special care to avoid leakage which can lead to severe pain and even to sloughing of the involved tissues. Anorexia, nausea, and vomiting occur commonly, and headache, drowsiness, and weakness are other complaints.

Dosage and Administration. This drug is administered by vein in doses ranging from 200–600 μg/kg of body weight per course of treatment, which may be spread over several days or given all at once, as a freshly prepared solution. The injection is made directly into the tubing of a fast-flowing intravenous infusion in order to dilute the vesicant and thus avoid possible damage to the lining of the vein, which can result in thrombophlebitis.

MERCAPTOPURINE U.S.P.
(Purinethol)

Actions and Indications. This antimetabolite interferes with the biosynthesis of nucleic acids by preventing cells from utilizing certain precursor substances including purines. It is useful mainly for treating acute lymphocytic leukemia in children, particularly when combined with other antineoplastic drugs for maintenance of remissions. Adults with this acute condition also often respond to treatment, but it is *not* effective for treating the chronic form of lymphatic leukemia. Only a few patients with chronic myelocytic (granulocytic) leukemia get temporary relief, and the drug is ineffective in Hodgkin's disease or solid tumors.

Side Effects, Cautions, and Contraindications. The blood count is carefully observed, and the drug is discontinued at the first sign of a large drop in the number of white cells, because bone marrow depression may continue even after the drug is withdrawn. Leukopenia and thrombocytopenia are common toxic hematologic effects, but a change in the number of erythrocytes rarely occurs.

Gastrointestinal upset is uncommon in therapeutic doses, but toxic doses may cause vomiting, diarrhea, and mucosal lesions of the mouth. The drug is withheld from patients with jaundice or other signs of liver damage, and caution is required in those with impaired liver function.

Dosage and Administration. The usual first dose is 2.5 mg/kg orally each day. When allopurinol is employed with mercaptopurine to prevent hyperuricemia, this usual dose of about 100 to 200 mg daily for adults or about 50 mg for young children is reduced to about one third or one fourth, as the antigout drug interferes with the metabolic breakdown of this antineoplastic agent.

METHOTREXATE U.S.P.
(Amethopterin; MTX)

Actions and Indications. This antimetabolite of the folic acid antagonist type is used in treating various neoplastic disorders and severe cases of psoriasis. Among the conditions most responsive to treatment are: acute lymphoblastic leukemias and such complications as leukemic meningitis; choriocarcinoma and hydatidiform mole; the advanced stages of lymphosarcoma and mycosis fungoides; and various solid tumors, including carcinomas of the head, neck, and cervix.

Side Effects, Cautions, and Contraindications. Close clinical observation is required to detect early signs of toxicity, particularly by performance of blood tests to detect bone marrow damage leading to leukopenia, thrombocytopenia, and anemia.

Damage to the mucosa of the alimentary tract may cause ulcerative stomatitis, gingivitis, vomiting, and diarrhea. Alopecia and skin eruptions of various kinds may occur. Central side effects include headache and drowsiness.

This drug should not be used to treat psoriasis in patients with severe kidney or liver disease or during pregnancy, as the drug can damage these organs and the fetus.

Dosage and Administration. Dosage schedules and methods of administration vary depending upon the disorder that is being treated. Oral doses betwen 2.5 and 5.0 mg daily are most common, but the sodium salt of methotrexate is also administered I.M., by rapid I.V. injection, and intrathecally.

SODIUM PHOSPHATE P 32 SOLUTION U.S.P. (Phosphotope)

Actions and Indications. Radioactive phosphate concentrates in cells with a high reproductive rate, including the bone marrow, lymph nodes, and spleen, and then gives off beta particles which damage the cells that they penetrate. Although the range of penetration is only between 2 to 8 mm, this is enough to cause a significant drop in the number of blood cells being produced by the bone marrow.

The ionizing radiations from radiophosphorus have been utilized particularly in the treatment of polycythemia vera and to a lesser extent in treating chronic granulocytic leukemia. In these conditions the excessive numbers of cells produced by the erythroid and myeloid bone marrow elements are reduced and clinical remission follows.

Side Effects, Cautions, and Contraindications. The patient's blood is examined between courses of radioactive phosphorus in order to avoid administering too much too frequently, as this can excessively depress the bone marrow and cause leukopenia, thrombocytopenia, and anemia, and other signs of radiation sickness.

Dosage and Administration. An intravenous dose of about 3 to 5 mc or an oral dose of 6 mc is administered initially for treating polycythemia vera or chronic myelocytic leukemia. Later doses and the intervals at which they are given are determined by the patient's response.

THIOTEPA U.S.P.
(Thio-Tepa; Tespa; TSPA)

Actions and Indications. Thiotepa is mainly used to control the effusion of fluid into various body cavities containing breast or ovarian cancer metastases. Local instillation often results in relief of symptoms such as cough and dyspnea caused by pressure of fluid effusions from the growth.

The drug is also used as an adjunct to radical mastectomy to reduce the rate of recurrences and to support the palliative effect of the operation. It is also applied topically to treat papillary carcinoma of the bladder.

Side Effects, Cautions, and Contraindications. This alkylating agent does not cause tissue irritation, as nitrogen mustard does. It may, however, have toxic hematopoietic effects. Thus, white blood cell counts are employed to check the drug's effect upon the bone marrow.

Nausea, vomiting, loss of appetite, and headache may occur, particularly in patients with impaired kidney function. Caution is required in patients receiving other antineoplastic drugs or radiation therapy. The drug is not ordinarily administered during pregnancy.

Dosage and Administration. Dosage is individualized using the W.B.C. count as a guide to avoid bone marrow depression. The initial adult dose for local instillation is 45 to 60 mg weekly, intraperitoneally, intrapleurally, and elsewhere. One half of these doses is injected intravenously in treating malignant lymphomas. A solution containing 60 mg in 30 to 60 cc of water is instilled into the bladder for prolonged retention.

VINCRISTINE SULFATE U.S.P.
(Oncovin)

Actions and Indications. This plant alkaloid is used mainly in combination with a corticosteroid drug to treat acute lymphoblastic leukemia in children. It brings about remission in a high proportion of cases but seems ineffective in leukemic meningitis. It is also employed in treating Wilm's tumor, Hodgkin's disease, and other malignant lymphomas, and some solid tumors.

Side Effects, Cautions, and Contraindications. Alopecia is the most common adverse effect. More serious are the effects of this drug on neuromuscular function. These include loss of deep tendon reflexes, development of a slapping gait, and wastage of muscles. Impaired sensation and paresthesias followed by neuritic pain may precede the motor impairment and ataxia.

Vomiting, diarrhea, abdominal

cramps, and occasionally constipation with fecal impaction in the upper colon are other side effects. Leukopenia may appear early, but the platelets and erythrocytes are not affected.

Dosage and Administration. This drug is injected intravenously at weekly intervals, beginning in children with 0.05 mg/kg and raising the dose in increments up to a maximum of 0.15 mg/kg over a period of five weeks. The carefully calculated dose is injected either into a running I.V. infusion or directly into the vein with care to avoid leakage into surrounding tissues, as the drug is quite irritating and can cause pain and possible cellulitis.

References

Blake, F.G., Wright, F.W., Waechter, E.H. Nursing Care of Children. 8th ed. Philadelphia: J.B. Lippincott, 1970.

Clarkson, B.D., and Fried, J. Changing concepts in treatment of acute leukemia. *Med. Clin. N. Amer.*, 55:561, 1971.

Ellison, R.R. Treating cancer with antimetabolites. *Amer. J. Nurs.*, 62:79, 1962.

Golbey, R.B. Chemotherapy of cancer. *Amer. J. Nurs.*, 60: 521, 1960.

Hiatt, H.H. Cancer chemotherapy—present status and prospects. *New Eng. J. Med.*, 276:157, 1967.

Isler, C. The cancer nurses—How the specialists are doing it. RN, 35:28, 1972 (Feb.).

———. Care of the pediatric patient with leukemia. RN, 35:30, 1972 (April).

Krakoff, I.H. The present status of cancer chemotherapy. *Med. Clin. N. Amer.*, 55:683, 1971.

Kubler-Ross, E. On Death and Dying. New York: Macmillan, 1969.

Rodman, M.J. Anticancer chemotherapy: part 1. The kinds of drugs and what they do. RN, 35:45, 1972 (Feb.); Part 2. Against solid malignant tumors. RN, 35:61, 1972 (March); Part 3. Against the leukemias and lymphomas. RN, 35:49, 1972 (April).

Silverstein, M. and Morton, D. Cancer immunotherapy *Amer. J. Nurs.*, 73:1178, 1973 (July).

Teitelbaum, A.C. Intra-arterial drug therapy. *Amer. J. Nurs.*, 72:1634, 1972.

49.

Blood, Body Fluid, and Nutrient Replenishers

In this chapter we shall discuss several kinds of substances that are not classified as drugs. Materials such as blood and its components are, of course, physiological substances rather than pharmacological agents. Thus, pharmacology texts often do not discuss blood plasma, plasma substitutes, and solutions used for making up deficits in the body's supply of water, salts, and essential nutrients.

Nevertheless, the nurse is often called upon to administer blood and fluid-electrolyte solutions by vein, and people frequently ask her questions about vitamins and minerals. Thus, we shall offer brief discussions of some clinically significant aspects of these topics. However, the nurse whose practice requires her to make frequent use of blood and its fractions or of intravenously administered fluids for replenishing lost stores will wish to consult more specialized texts for detailed information about the administration of these *non*pharmacological therapeutic agents.

Blood, Plasma, and Plasma Substitutes

Patients in various clinical situations often require whole blood or various of its fractions, including red cells, platelets, and plasma. Administration of these substances makes up for deficiencies of these vital materials and thus helps to restore normal function (see Table 49-1). However, it is also always necessary to correct the cause of the patient's condition—for example, to stop the patient's bleeding.

T A B L E   4 9 - 1   *Blood, Plasma, and Plasma Substitutes (See also Chapter 33)*

Official or Generic Name	Trade Name or Synonym	Dosage and Administration
*Blood and Blood Fractions**		
Citrated whole human blood U.S.P.	. . . .	500–1,000 ml (1 or 2 units) I.V.
Packed human blood cells U.S.P.	Packed Red Cells	Equivalent of 1 or 2 units of whole blood I.V.
Plasma, platelet-rich	Thrombocyte Concentrate	Equivalent of 1 or 2 units of whole blood I.V.
Normal human plasma U.S.P.	. . . .	500–1,500 ml I.V.
Normal human serum albumin U.S.P.	Albuminate Albumisol Albuspan Proserum	25–75 g of protein I.V. (variable amounts of 5% and 25% solutions)
Plasma protein fraction, human	Plasmanate; PPF	50–75 g of protein I.V. (up to 1.5 liters of 5% solution)
Plasma Substitutes or Expanders		
Dextran 70	Macrodex; and others	500–1,000 ml of 6% solution I.V.
Dextran 75	Gentran 75; and others	500–1,000 ml of 6% solution I.V.
Dextran 40	Gentran 40; Rheomacrodex; and others	10–20 ml/kg of 10% solution I.V.
Gelatin solution	Plazmoid	500 ml of a 5 or 6% solution I.V.
Polyvinylpyrrolidone	Povidone	500 ml of a 3.5% solution I.V.

* Mostly available through blood banks, rather than from commercial manufacturers.

WHOLE BLOOD

In shock resulting from severe hemorrhage, the best treatment is the infusion of an adequate quantity of compatible whole blood obtained from another individual. Such transfusions correct not only hypovolemia, or low blood volume, within the vascular tree, but also the anemia resulting from red cell loss. Thus, provided that the source of the bleeding is located and repaired, whole blood transfusions usually overcome both the dangerous hemodynamic disturbances of shock and the low oxygen tension of the tissues.

Dangers. Whole blood is ordered only when a need for it is clearly demonstrated. The transfusion of blood contaminated with hepatitis virus can transmit serum hepatitis. Errors in blood typing and administration may lead to serious transfusion reactions.

The nurse can help to reduce transfusions of virus-contaminated blood by encouraging donations by volunteers, of whom only about 1 in 1000 is a carrier of the hepatitis-associated antigen (HBAg, or Australian antigen). The incidence is ten to twenty times higher in blood obtained from people who sell their blood to commercial blood banks, which, in turn, sell it to doctors and hospitals.

She cannot, of course, avert ill effects brought about by the carelessness of someone else during the collection, labeling, handling, and storage of whole blood. However, the nurse takes every precaution to avoid administering blood to any individual other than the one for whom it is intended. It is her responsibility, as well as that of the person who starts the infusion, to check the labels on the blood carefully and to identify the patient correctly, in order to avoid the very serious error of the patient's receiving mismatched blood.

During the administration of blood, the patient is watched carefully for signs of hemolytic or allergic reactions. The blood is transfused at a slow rate at first, and the patient is observed for signs such as flushing, chills, fever, restlessness, and complaints of headache, back pain, and nausea. If these signs of transfusion reactions or the itching, urticarial rashes, or bronchospastic reactions of allergy occur, the transfusion is stopped and measures are taken to prevent more serious effects from developing.

BLOOD COMPONENTS

Blood fractions are often preferable to whole blood in certain clinical situations. As we have seen previously, bleeding disorders are best treated by administration of the specific blood coagulation component that is lacking. Thus, depending upon the deficiencies, hemorrhagic disorders may be treated by transfusion of platelet-rich plasma, antihemophilic globulin, or fibrinogen (Chapters 33 and 48).

Packed red cells are preferred for counteracting anemia in patients whose blood volume must not be allowed to expand excessively. For example, elderly patients, infants, and other people with cardiopulmonary or renal disease who may be endangered by whole blood transfusions that overload their cardiovascular system should receive red cells that have been separated from plasma and other blood components.

Plasma, the cell-free portion of uncoagulated blood, is available in liquid, frozen, or dried form for use when red cells are not required or are to be avoided—for example, when the blood of a burn patient in shock is too highly concentrated. Plasma alone is adequate for replacing proteins lost from severely burned skin surfaces, or as a result of severe bleeding, malnutrition, or other disorders.

The use of plasma for treating traumatic shock (or even some cases of hemorrhagic shock) has certain advantages. It is more readily available than whole blood. There is no need for typing, since there is little risk of a reaction to the pooled plasma, which is obtained from eight or more donors.

Unfortunately, the fact that plasma is obtained from several sources tends to increase the risk of its being contaminated with the virus responsible for homologous serum hepatitis. There is still no safe way to sterilize plasma chemically. However, the hazard of hepatitis is said to be reduced somewhat by aging the prepared material through prolonged storage at room temperature.

Serum albumin is a concentrate of the main component of plasma that needs no refrigeration and has no hepatitis hazard. It is useful for rapidly restoring the blood volume of patients in shock when administered in relatively small amounts of a 5 or 25 percent solution.

The latter so-called *salt-poor* solution is preferred for edematous patients suffering from nephrosis, hepatic cirrhosis, and other disorders marked by low plasma protein levels (*hypoproteinemia*). Albumin has also been used in treating hyperbilirubinemia and erythroblastosis fetalis, as an adjunct to exchange transfusions.

Plasma protein fraction is a solution of both albumin and globulin that is also thought to be free of hepatitis virus. It is low in potassium and other electrolytes and is said to be especially useful for treating shock in infants dehydrated by infection. However, in hemorrhage, it is less useful than plasma, which contains clotting factors. Its use may lead to development of a relative degree of anemia.

PLASMA SUBSTITUTES

Plasma substitutes or expanders are often useful for improving circulatory function in shock when natural plasma products are not available. One such substance, *dextran 40,* is employed for this purpose and also as a priming fluid for pump oxygenators in heart surgery procedures that require extracorporeal circulation. A similar substance, *dextran 70,* with a higher molecular weight, is also useful for emergency treatment of shock.

These nonprotein products are cheaper than plasma and do not, of course, transmit the virus of hepatitis. However, it is important to monitor the patient's central venous pressure during their infusion to avoid overloading his circulation. The patient's urinary output should also be carefully observed. He is also watched for signs of allergic reactions. All of these potential adverse effects require discontinuation of the infusion and prompt treatment with appropriate measures.

Fluids and Electrolytes

The proper functioning of every cell in the body depends on the composition of the fluids that surround it. If the volume and composition of this internal environment are drastically altered and allowed to stay that way, severe functional disturbances soon develop. Thus, when the body's defense mechanisms fail to maintain internal homeostasis, medical measures must be taken.

Most important are measures that correct the primary causes of the homeostatic disorder— disease, trauma, and poisoning, for example. It is often necessary to correct the abnormality by supplying missing minerals, water, and nu-

trients. Some substances commonly employed to overcome fluid and electrolyte deficiencies are listed in Table 49-2.

Although a discussion of the fundamental principles of fluid and electrolyte therapy is beyond the scope of this pharmacology textbook, we shall briefly review the kinds of products available for treating various types of water, salt, and acid-base imbalances.

Simple dehydration in which the patient has

TABLE 49-2 *Fluid-Electrolyte and Nutritional Replenishers*

Agent	Remarks
Agents for Treating Abnormal Hydration States	
DEHYDRATION TREATMENT	
Dextrose injection (5% in H_2O) in U.S.P.	I.V. as required
Dextrose and sodium chloride injection U.S.P.	I.V. as required
Sodium chloride injection (isotonic 0.9%)	I.V. as required
Sodium chloride injection (3%; 5%)	I.V. as required
Balanced electrolyte injection	I.V. as required
(Isolyte; Normosol; Plasmalyte; and others)	
OTHER ELECTROLYTE DEPLETION TREATMENTS	
Potassium chloride U.S.P.	Oral 15 mEq of potassium, three or four times daily; I.V. up to 10 mEq per hour, or up to 100–200 mEq daily
(Kaochlor; Kato; Kay Ciel; and others)	
Potassium gluconate (Kaon)	Oral 20 mEq of potassium twice daily
Potassium bicarbonate; potassium citrate (in Potassium Triplex; K-Lyte; and others)	Variable oral dosage
Calcium gluconate U.S.P.	Oral 15 g daily
Magnesium sulfate U.S.P.	Up to 2 mEq/kg of magnesium every four hours
Ringer's injection U.S.P.	I.V. or S.C. as required
Lactated Ringer's injection U.S.P.	I.V. or S.C. as required
Lactated potassic saline injection N.F.	I.V. or S.C. as required
Acidosis Treatment	
Disodium hydrogen citrate (Citralka)	Oral 1–2 g as required
Sodium bicarbonate U.S.P. (tablets and injection)	Oral or I.V. as required
Sodium citrate U.S.P.	Oral 1–2 g as required
Sodium lactate injection U.S.P. (one-sixth molar solution)	I.V. as required
Tromethamine N.F. (THAM; Tris buffer)	I.V. as required
Alkalosis Treatment	
Ammonium chloride U.S.P.	Oral 4 g
Potassium chloride, sodium chloride, and others	See above
Nutritional Deficiency Treatment	
Dextrose injection U.S.P.	I.V. in various concentrations
Fructose and sodium chloride injection N.F.	I.V. as required
Fructose injection N.F. (Levugen; and others)	I.V. or S.C. as required
Invert sugar injection (Travert)	I.V. as required
High calorie solution for injection	I.V. as required
(Hi-Cal 900; Isolyte H 900; Normosol M 900)	
Protein hydrolysate injection (Amigen; Aminosol; Hyprotigen)	I.V. 230–1,500 ml of 5% solution as required

lost water and salt in equal proportion is best counteracted by administration of an *isotonic solution of sodium chloride*, preferably by mouth. However, when fluid-electrolyte loss has been severe as a result of vomiting and diarrhea, an intravenous infusion may be more rapidly effective. In addition, since other electrolytes besides sodium may have been lost, the doctor may order fluids for replacement of several salts at once.

Products that contain combinations of several electrolytes in proper isotonic balance include *Ringer's solution, lactated Ringer's solution,* and various commercial preparations of multiple salts in high, low, or intermediate electrolyte concentrations.

Other states of abnormal hydration include those in which relatively little electrolyte loss has occurred. In such cases of hypertonic dehydration, water alone is provided to make up the deficit caused by water loss. For this purpose, a *5 percent dextrose infusion* by vein is preferred for maintaining isotonicity. The dextrose also provides a source of energy, but because it is metabolized by the body in processes that require insulin, it is not administered to dehydrated patients who are in diabetic coma. Once the patient's plasma has reached normal tonicity, he can be switched to an infusion of several isotonically balanced electrolytes to bring his extracellular fluid content back to normal.

In cases of dehydration that are marked by an excessive loss of *sodium (hyponatremia)*, higher concentrations of sodium chloride (3 or 5 percent) are employed to make up the deficit. This hypotonic type of dehydration is sometimes seen in patients with Addison's disease who should, of course, also receive adequate corticosteroid replacement therapy. Hyponatremia that develops during diuretic therapy requires adjustment of the diuretic drug dosage, in addition to rehydration with one of these hypertonic sodium solutions.

Other electrolytes are also often depleted during treatment with potent diuretics. Loss of *potassium* is the most serious result of such overtreatment, particularly in patients who are also receiving digitalis. *Hypopotassemia (hypokalemia)* is best treated by administration of potassium chloride in liquid form, preferably by mouth but also by carefully monitored intravenous infusion.

In other disorders marked by severe vomiting and diarrhea, hypokalemia may be accompanied by the loss of several other electrolytes. Thus, in this and other disorders, it is often also necessary to correct loss of cations such as calcium and magnesium and anions such as chloride and bicarbonate. Solutions of *magnesium sulfate, calcium gluconate, ammonium chloride,* and *sodium bicarbonate* are available for I.V. use in such cases (Table 49-2).

Acid-base imbalances are the result of a buildup or excessive loss of hydrogen ions. *Acidosis* is, of course, best counteracted by removing the underlying cause of the disorder. However several *systemic alkalinizers* are also available for oral or intravenous administration. Administration of *sodium bicarbonate solution* is the simplest and best way to treat metabolic acidosis, in which plasma bicarbonate has fallen to a relatively low level as compared to the high hydrogen and chloride ion concentrations —for example, in salicylate poisoning.

Another systemic alkalinizer, sometimes administered alone or combined with sodium and potassium chloride salts, is *tromethamine*. It has been used to correct the metabolic acidosis that develops during cardiac arrest and in the cardiac bypass procedures used in heart surgery. Its dosage must be very carefully regulated to avoid development of metabolic alkalosis.

Metabolic alkalosis has various causes that must be corrected. This acid-base imbalance is not overcome by supplying hydrogen ions directly but by furnishing chloride ions. This is best done by administering *sodium chloride* or *potassium chloride* solutions by vein. *Ammonium chloride* is sometimes employed to counteract alkalosis caused by overtreatment with organic mercurial diuretics (Chapter 27).

Intravenous feeding of various nutrients is employed in the management of patients who cannot take food and fluids by mouth. Available products (Table 49-2) include injectable solutions of *carbohydrates* and *amino acids* (protein hydrolysates) to provide calories and permit protein synthesis. Information concerning such *hyperalimentation agents* is best obtained from textbooks on nutrition. The only nutritional aids which we shall discuss here are vitamins and minerals.

Vitamins and Minerals

THE PHYSIOLOGICAL FUNCTION OF VITAMINS

Vitamins are substances that the body requires for carrying out essential metabolic reactions. Because the body cannot biosynthesize enough of these compounds to meet all its needs, preformed vitamins must be obtained from vegetable and animal tissues taken in as foodstuffs.

The body needs only small amounts of vitamins because they function mainly as *coenzymes*—substances that activate the protein portion of enzymes. Small quantities of enzymes catalyze a great deal of biochemical activity. Thus, tiny amounts of vitamins go a long way, and any excess of these nonprotein cofactors is either rapidly excreted by the kidneys or gradually broken down to inactive fragments after storage in the tissues.

DIETARY DEFICIENCIES

Ordinarily, a person who eats a well-balanced diet takes in enough of these natural nutrients to meet the everyday needs of his body. In such circumstances, there is no need to supplement his intake with purified vitamin concentrates in pharmaceutical form. To take vitamins in amounts that exceed the body's requirements is a needless expense and, occasionally, the ingestion of excessive amounts of vitamins may prove toxic.

There are, however, various situations in which supplemental vitamins may be of value to avoid development of multiple deficiencies of these nutrients. Even people who are in good health and eat an adequate diet sometimes need extra nutrients, including vitamins, at certain periods of their lives. This is true, for example, of infants fed by formula, as well as women during pregnancy and lactation. Children often require some supplementation of their dietary vitamin intake during periods of rapid growth.

Vitamin supplementation is desirable for the many people who do not eat properly. Some have developed poor eating habits; others have never learned what foods are needed for a balanced diet containing adequate quantities of all the vitamins. Poverty keeps some people from purchasing enough of the foods needed for good nutrition.

Yet many people who can well afford to purchase a full quota of nutritionally desirable foods often fail to do so. For example, alcoholics and other emotionally disturbed people are likely to eat foods that do not supply adequate amounts of vitamins. People who adhere to faddish diets may develop deficiencies of several vitamins found together in the foods that are absent from their diets. Occasionally,

a person adheres too strictly to a religious code regulating diet.

In all such cases, patients should be helped to get adequate amounts of vitamins through better dietary planning or from supplementary vitamin concentrates. The dietitian and the doctor determines how the patient's diet should best be supplemented, while the nurse concentrates on helping the patient realize the need for a properly balanced diet and on teaching him what he should know about proper eating. Such help should be offered with due respect for the patient's religious beliefs and the practices of his ethnic group in regard to diet. When giving primary care, the nurse often assumes responsibility for instructing the patient and his family about adequate dietary intake, referring the patient, if it becomes necessary, to a clinic or a doctor.

Patients with certain types of pathology are among those most likely to develop vitamin deficiencies. In various gastrointestinal disorders, for example, vitamins may not be absorbed from food. If parenteral feeding is necessary vitamin supplementation is almost certainly required. During prolonged chronic illnesses, most patients lose their appetites and become unwilling or unable to eat well.

The nurse then does all she can to encourage the patient to eat properly, and the doctor often orders vitamins added to the patient's diet in amounts calculated to make up for those he fails to get from food. He usually prescribes high potency pills—that is, *therapeutic* vitamin formulations—when deficiencies of one or more vitamins are evident or seem likely.

Most people in normal health do not need therapeutic doses of multiple vitamins. If such a person feels the need for nutritional supplements, he should be advised that vitamin products available in low doses are much less expensive and entirely adequate for his needs.

Provided a person does not overpay for what should be available at moderate cost, such supplementation is harmless and, in view of the proved value of placebos in many medical situations, vitamins may even provide psychological benefits far beyond their actual physiological effects for those who believe in their value.

VITAMIN ALLOWANCES

When the patient requires vitamin therapy, the nurse may well advise him to look for the least expensive product that will meet his needs. She may suggest that they read the labels to compare the formulas and prices of competing products, which sometimes vary considerably in cost. The Food and Drug Administration requires that the labels of all vitamin products indicate the amounts of each ingredient and the proportion of the *Minimum Daily Requirement (MDR)* represented. The MDR is the amount of the nutrient needed to *prevent deficiency symptoms* from developing.

WATER-SOLUBLE VITAMINS

Certain vitamins are commonly considered together because they are all water soluble, and most are found in the same kind of foods. They are subdivided into vitamin C and the B-complex group. The latter include thiamine, riboflavin, nicotinic acid, pyridoxine, pantothenic acid, folic acid, cyanocobalamin (B_{12}), and possibly biotin, choline, inositol, and para-aminobenzoic acid (PABA). Two of these—

folic acid and cyanocobalamin—are discussed in Chapter 34 because they are best reserved for the treatment of macrocytic anemias resulting from deficiencies of one or another or both of these blood-building B vitamins.

THIAMINE. Thiamine was the first of the B-complex vitamin group to be isolated and chemically identified. Thus, it is also known as vitamin B_1 and—because it counteracts the neurological signs and symptoms of beriberi—as the *antineuritic* and *antiberiberi* vitamin. Its natural sources include meats, whole cereal grains, and yeast.

When ingested with foods that contain it, thiamine is converted to a coenzyme that plays an important part in carbohydrate metabolism. A lack of thiamine results in a reduction in numerous biochemical reactions that are essential to the normal functioning of all living cells. However, overt symptoms of thiamine deficiency appear most commonly in the form

T A B L E 4 9 - 3 *Vitamins and Related Substances*

Nonproprietary or Official Name	Synonym or Chemical Name	Recommended Daily Dietary Allowance*	Therapeutic Dose
Water Soluble Vitamins			
Ascorbic acid U.S.P.	Vitamin C	60 mg approximately	150 mg oral or parenteral
Biotin U.S.P.	Vitamin H	150–300 μg possibly	500 μg oral
Choline dihydrogen citrate and other salts of choline	Trimethyl-ammonium derivative	Unknown (possibly not a true vitamin)	500 mg–6 g
Cyanocobalamin U.S.P.	Vitamin B_{12}	5 μg approx.	15–1,000 μg oral or parenteral
Folic acid U.S.P.	Vitamin M; folacin pteroylglutamic acid (PGA)	0.4 mg	1–10 mg oral or parenteral
Inositol U.S.P.	Inosite; hexahydrocyclohexane	Unknown (possibly not a true vitamin)	50–500 mg oral
Niacin N.F.	Nicotinic acid	13–20 mg equivalents	10–100 mg oral or parenteral
Niacinamide U.S.P.	Nicotinamide Nicotinic acid amide Vitamin B_5	As above, depending upon intake of calories and tryptophan	10–100 mg oral or parenteral
Para-aminobenzoic acid	PABA	Unknown (probably not a true vitamin)	100–500 mg
Pantothenic acid	Vitamin B_3	5–10 mg	. . . .
Calcium pantothenate	(salt of the above)	. . . .	10–50 mg oral or parenteral
Pantothenyl alcohol	Panthenol	. . . .	10–50 mg oral or parenteral

TABLE 49-3 *Vitamins and Related Substances (continued)*

Nonproprietary or Official Name	Synonym or Chemical Name	Recommended Daily Dietary Allowance*	Therapeutic Dose
Water Soluble Vitamins			
Pyridoxine HCl U.S.P.	Vitamin B_6	2 mg/100 g of protein intake	25–100 mg oral or parenteral
Riboflavin U.S.P.	Vitamin B_2	1.5–2.0 mg	5–10 mg oral or parenteral
Thiamine HCl U.S.P.	Vitamin B_1	1.0–1.5 mg	10–30 mg oral or 25–50 mg I.M.
Fat Soluble Vitamins			
Vitamin A U.S.P.	Retinol	5,000 units	5–15,000 units orally
Vitamin D	. . . .	400 units	. . . .
Cholecalciferol U.S.P.	Vitamin D_2	. . . .	1,500–5,000 units orally; up to 500,000 units parenterally
Ergocalciferol U.S.P.	Vitamin D_3	. . . .	
Vitamin E	. . . .	25–30 units	. . . .
Alpha-tocopherol U.S.P.	. . . .		30–100 mg orally or parenterally
Vitamin K	. . . .	0.3 μg/kg of body weight	. . . .
Phytonadione U.S.P.	Vitamin K Mephyton	. . . .	5–25 mg orally; 10–50 mg parenterally
Menadione N.F.	Vitamin K_3	. . . .	As above
Menadione sodium bisulfite N.F.	Hykinone	. . . .	As above
Menadiol sodium diphosphate U.S.P. and N.F.	Synkayvite Kappadione	. . . .	5–25 mg orally; 10–50 mg parenterally

* These adult allowances, which are set by the Food and Nutrition Board of The National Academy of Science–National Research Council, are amounts recommended for maintaining good nutrition in normal people under ordinary living conditions. These are larger than the minimum daily requirements (MDR), but they may not be enough to meet the needs of some people who require therapeutic quantities.

of malfunctioning of nerve cells and as gastrointestinal and cardiovascular system disabilities.

The *neurological difficulties*—seen today in this country mostly in alcoholic patients—are manifested mainly in complaints stemming from peripheral neuritis. These include sensory nerve signs such as tingling, burning, and aching, and motor nerve disabilities leading to muscle weakness and paralysis. C.N.S. function is often disturbed by a lack of thiamine, as indicated by irritability, depression, inability to concentrate, and loss of memory.

Cardiovascular complications of thiamine deficiency include signs of congestive heart failure such as edema, dyspnea, and tachycardia, together with a variety of cardiac irregularities. Gastrointestinal ill effects include loss of appetite, vomiting, and chronic diarrhea. (See also Chapter 8, Alcoholism.)

No more than 2 mg a day is ever needed as a vitamin supplement in normally healthy people who have an ordinary diet. However, patients with diagnosed thiamine deficiency may require as much as 30 mg daily. This is best administered parenterally in the form of several spaced fractional doses. Once the thiamine stores return to normal in this way, low oral doses are sufficient.

Thiamine *replacement therapy* usually produces prompt improvement in patients suffering from beriberi, alcoholic neuritis, and the neuritic and cardiovascular complications that sometimes occur in pregnant women and others whose diets lack this vitamin. Patients with similar symptoms that, however, do *not* stem from a deficiency of thiamine cannot be expected to improve.

RIBOFLAVIN. This substance, vitamin B_2, gets its name from the presence of the sugar ribose and from its yellow color (Latin *flavus*—yellow). It is converted in the body to two coenzymes that work together with a wide variety of proteins to catalyze many of the cellular respiratory reactions by which the body derives its energy. Rich dietary sources of riboflavin include dairy products (milk and cheese), eggs, meats, green vegetables, beans, and whole cereal grains.

Deficiency of riboflavin does *not* result in a definite disease such as beriberi, but is accompanied by a variety of typical lesions. Ocular symptoms include itching, burning, photophobia, and tearing. The cornea may show signs of invasion by tiny capillaries (vascularization). A typical lesion of the lips and angles of the mouth (*cheilosis*) is characterized by development of deep fissures in the mucous membranes and skin, together with inflammation of the tongue (*glossitis*).

Riboflavin deficiency states may be treated with injections totaling up to 10 mg daily, followed by oral doses of 1 to 5 mg daily for maintenance, together with an adequate diet. Actually, ariboflavinosis rarely occurs alone, and patients who require treatment usually receive thiamine, niacin, and other B-complex vitamins simultaneously.

NIACIN (NICOTINIC ACID). This substance is available in such foods as meat, peas, cereals, and liver. It is also biosynthesized in the body from the dietary amino acid, tryptophan. Both these substances are converted into two coenzymes that play a vital role in many enzyme-catalyzed biochemical reactions.

A lack of these metabolically essential substances results finally in *pellagra*, a nutritional deficiency disorder affecting the skin, digestive tract, and nervous system. In its milder form, subclinical pellagra—as seen sometimes in chronic alcoholics, for example—is manifested by nervousness, insomnia, headache, itching-burning skin sensations, and gastrointestinal upset. The full-blown pellagra syndrome, now relatively rare as a result of niacin enrichment of diets in endemic areas, includes the following characteristic changes: (1) symmetrical *skin eruptions* resembling sunburn—on the backs of both hands, for example—tend to heal as darkened scars; (2) a characteristically bright *red swollen tongue*, together with other oral lesions and heavy salivation, and (3) *mental disturbances* ranging from confusion, depression, and memory loss to psychosis

marked by dementia, hallucinations, and delusions.

Pellagra responds readily to high oral doses of niacin (50 mg up to ten times daily); much lower doses are adequate for maintenance therapy. Occasionally, psychotic patients and those suffering from gastrointestinal malabsorption syndromes require parenteral therapy.

Niacin often causes flushing of the skin, and sometimes—especially following injections—a fall in blood pressure. The nurse should explain to the patient that the flushing is a natural reaction, so that he will not worry unnecessarily that he is suffering an allergic reaction. Patients who complain of weakness or dizziness from niacin are advised to lie down until the discomfort passes and to tell their doctor about the reaction. He may then substitute *nicotinamide*, which is the preferred form of the vitamin because it does not cause these local and systemic circulatory effects. Unlike niacin itself, however, this amide derivative cannot, of course, be used clinically as a vasodilator, nor is it effective for reducing serum cholesterol levels in the manner discussed in Chapter 31.

PYRIDOXINE (VITAMIN B$_6$). This B-complex vitamin is converted in the body to a biologically active form that plays an important part in protein metabolism. No specific disease develops as the result of a dietary deficiency of this vitamin alone. However, infants may suffer convulsions as a result of a dietary lack of pyridoxine, and some tuberculosis patients taking isoniazid have developed peripheral neuritis that can be counteracted by vitamin B$_6$ supplements. On the other hand, patients taking levodopa for parkinsonism should not receive multiple vitamin supplements containing pyridoxine, as it tends to antagonize the effects of this drug.

PANTOTHENIC ACID. This organic acid is so widely distributed in natural foods that specific deficiencies are unlikely to occur. An ordinary American diet containing about 10 mg of pantothenic acid provides an adequate intake of this vitamin. Deficiencies produced experimentally by administration of an antivitamin compound are marked by gastrointestinal disturbances, headache, and fatigue.

Although the daily requirement for this vitamin is not known, it is considered an essential substance and its salt, calcium pantothenate, is a common constituent of many multivitamin preparations, including the official Decavitamin capsules and tablets.

Biotin, choline, inositol, and *p-aminobenzoic acid* are sometimes considered to be part of the vitamin B complex. Deficiencies have not been shown to occur in humans, and no daily requirements have been set. Because choline tends to prevent fatty degeneration of the liver in experimental animals, its use has been advocated for patients with liver disease. However, its usefulness in hepatitis, cirrhosis of the liver, and chronic alcoholism has not been established.

Ascorbic Acid. This essential dietary substance is water soluble but so different in its natural distribution in foods from the vitamin B complex group that it was given the separate designation *vitamin C.* The term *ascorbic acid* stems from its ability to prevent the deficiency disease scurvy (that is, it is the antiscurvy or antiscorbutic vitamin). It is found in fruits such as oranges, lemons, and limes and in vegetables, including cabbage, tomatoes, and potatoes.

Deficiency of vitamin C interferes with the formation of the connective ground tissue substance that cements cells together. Loss of collagenous fibers from this bed of intracellular connective tissues leads to development of widespread lesions. Local bleeding, for example, is believed to be the result of excessive fragility of the capillary walls. In scurvy, the gums become red and swollen and bleed readily. The teeth are loosened and bone is lost from the jaws. Joints and growing long bones are also subject to hemorrhages. All such symptoms of vitamin C deficiency are relieved in a few days by the administration of about 200 mg of ascorbic acid daily, divided into several fractional doses. Once healing becomes apparent, dosage can be lowered gradually to 100 mg or less.

This vitamin has been advocated for use in various clinical conditions which are not caused by a clear-cut lack of ascorbic acid. Most recently, it has been touted as a preventive of the common cold when taken in quite high doses. However, its usefulness for this purpose or for any other conditions not caused by a definite deficiency of vitamin C has not been established.

FAT-SOLUBLE VITAMINS

Vitamins A, D, E, and K, the fat-soluble essential food factors, tend to stay in the body for much longer periods than the water-soluble B vitamins and ascorbic acid. Absorption of these vitamins requires the presence of adequate amounts of digestible fat and bile salts in the intestinal tract. Once absorbed, little is lost by way of the kidneys, and considerable amounts of these vitamins may be stored in body fat, muscles, and liver. Some aspects of each of these vitamins, except vitamin K (which is discussed in Chapter 33), will be briefly reviewed here.

Vitamin A. This essential dietary substance is found in the fat of milk, yolk of eggs, and in liver. Although it does not occur as such in plants, vitamin A is formed in the body from carotene, the plant pigment responsible for the color of carrots and other deep-yellow and dark-green vegetables. When carotene rather than already formed vitamin A is the **main** dietary source of the vitamin, the daily requirement of 4,000 to 5,000 units of vitamin A may double.

Signs and symptoms of vitamin A deficiency are manifested mainly in changes in ocular structure and function and in other epithelial tissue abnormalities. Night blindness, a decreased ability to adapt to darkness or dim light, is an early deficiency symptom. Dryness and then deformity of the cornea may lead to permanent visual impairment if not quickly detected and corrected by administration of vitamin A. The skin may become dry and keratinized.

Skin disorders that stem from a lack of vitamin A respond to administration of supplements that contain it. Acne, a condition unrelated to vitamin A deficiency, does *not* improve when the vitamin is taken by mouth. However, topical application of *trenitoin* (vitamin A acid or retinoic acid) is said to be an effective treatment for acne (Chapter 46).

True deficiency states are rare in this country, and most healthy individuals do not require vitamin A supplements, excessive amounts of which may even prove toxic. Its use is limited largely to people with diseases that interfere with absorption of fats and fat-soluble vitamins. Some infants on milk-free formulas or formulas made with unfortified skimmed milk may require vitamin A supplementation. Only the rare cases of severe *hypo*vitaminosis A requires high therapeutic dosage. ¶ *Treatment.* Once diagnosed, a deficiency state is treated with high daily doses—25,000 to 50,000 units—of vitamin A. Even higher parenteral doses may be administered for a few days to correct corneal and other ocular lesions quickly. The daily dose is then reduced to that employed as a dietary supplement during pregnancy, lactation, and in infants—that is, about 5,000 units daily.

Chronic overdosage can result in hypervitaminosis A. This condition is marked by loss of appetite, abdominal discomfort, joint pain, and bone changes. Changes may also occur in the skin, lips, and hair. Recovery occurs rapidly when the condition is recognized, and the very high daily doses of vitamin A are discontinued.

VITAMIN D. Rickets is a crippling disease in which the bones become deformed because of a lack of calcium deposition. It is caused by a deficiency of *calciferol*, a substance which regulates the rate at which calcium is laid down in the bones. Calciferol, or *vitamin D,* is formed in the human skin when it is irradiated by ultraviolet rays from the sun.

A person who gets enough exposure to sunlight will not suffer from rickets, as the condition results from a lack of solar irradiation. However, calciferol can also be obtained by ingesting materials from outside sources such as fish livers or substances prepared by irradiating certain plant and animal sterols.

Irradiating the plant sterol, ergosterol, with ultraviolet rays results in the formation of *ergocalciferol* (Vitamin D_2). This substance and another of animal origin, called *cholecalciferol* (Vitamin D_3), are administered as vitamin supplements. The latter is also present in irradiated milk, which is the main source of vitamin D in the American diet. (The only other food source really rich in calciferol is fish liver, or its oil—cod liver oil, for example.)

The main action of vitamin D is to aid the absorption of ingested calcium from the gastrointestinal tract. By raising the blood levels of calcium and of the phosphate that moves with it, vitamin D tends to facilitate the deposition of these minerals in bone. Thus, a deficiency of vitamin D in infants and children can quickly lead to rickets, and adults may develop osteomalacia, a deforming softening of the bones.

Once these metabolic bone disorders have developed, rapid administration of relatively high doses of vitamin D is required to heal the bone lesions and prevent permanent deformity of skeletal structures. Infants with rickets may receive about ten times the daily prophylactic dose, or about 4,000 units, each day for several

weeks or until bone x-rays reveal adequate mineralization; dosage is then reduced to 1,000 or 2,000 units daily and finally to the 400-unit maintenance level. Adults with softening and malformation of the bones (resulting from lack of vitamin D and *not* due to osteoporosis) may receive up to 50,000 units of this vitamin for a time.

❮ *Toxicity.* This is a definite threat when this vitamin is taken in excessive doses for more than a few weeks or months. *Hypervitaminosis D,* as this condition is called, results in the movement of calcium from bones to blood (*hypercalcemia*). This mineral may then be deposited in such tissues as the kidneys, heart, and blood vessels. Fatalities have resulted from impaired renal function. However, the condition is readily reversible if further administration of the vitamin is stopped and the patient is put on a low calcium-high fluid regimen.

VITAMIN E. This substance, chemically called *alpha-tocopherol,* is needed in human nutrition. However, deficiency states are very rare, as the average American diet offers enough vitamin E to meet the needs of most people. This substance is available in whole grain cereals, leafy vegetables, and various fats, and a lack occurs only in rare individuals who are unable to absorb fats, and sometimes in certain premature infants.

This vitamin has been promoted to the public as a cure for sterility and impotence, for preventing heart attacks, and as a substance that delays aging, retards arteriosclerosis, and slows the progress of multiple sclerosis. Despite the recent rise of a fad for taking vitamin E supplements, there is still no proof that this substance is of value in preventing or treating *any* clinical condition.

VITAMIN K (SEE CHAPTER 33 AND TABLE 49-3).

MULTIVITAMIN PRODUCTS. The administration of combinations of several vitamins is rational, as deficiences of only one vitamin are rare. Two useful official preparations are: (1) *hexavitamin* capsules, containing vitamins A and D, ascorbic acid, thiamine, riboflavin, and nicotinamide; and (2) *decavitamin* capsules, which contain, in addition to the latter six substances, calcium pantothenate, cyanocobalamin, pyridoxine, and vitamin E.

Commercial products differ mainly in the amounts that they contain of various vitamins.

Some that are intended to prevent development of deficiencies during brief periods contain only small but adequate doses. Others intended for patients with specific pathological states contain perhaps twice as much in order to meet the patient's increased need for vitamins or to overcome an actual deficiency.

MINERALS

Many minerals play important parts in maintaining body structure and function. *Iron*, for example, is an essential element in the manufacture of red blood cells and for the functioning of certain cellular enzyme systems. *Iodides* are required for synthesis of thyroid hormones. These are discussed in Chapters 34 and 38. Here, we shall briefly discuss only calcium and fluorides, two substances commonly employed today as supplements to a normal diet.

CALCIUM. Calcium, in the form of its phosphate and carbonate salts, makes up a major part of the skeletal system. It plays an important part in maintaining neuromuscular activity in a normal state, and in regulating the rhythm of the heart. It is an essential factor in the series of complex steps leading to blood coagulation. The body's stores of this mineral must be replenished through ingestion of foods that are high in calcium—for example, milk and products made from it. Children and pregnant women need more dietary calcium than others and their diets may have to be supplemented with calcium salts.

Hypocalcemia, a reduction in calcium levels of the blood below the normal 10 mg/100 ml, may occur as a result of a dietary deficiency of this mineral. A lack of vitamin D and of the hormone of the parathyroid glands, both of which help to regulate the body's complex calcium economy, may also lead to a drop in blood calcium. When these substances are lacking, dietary calcium is inadequately absorbed from the upper gastrointestinal tract, and calcium tends to move from bone to the blood. This can cause rickets and osteomalacia.

Despite this drain of the calcium stored in bone, blood levels may finally fall so far below normal that signs of excessive neuromuscular excitability appear. This is manifested by muscular fibrillations, twitching, tetanic spasms, and, finally, exhausting convulsions. The main treatment of *hypocalcemic tetany*, no matter what the underlying cause, is to raise the blood level of the mineral back to normal. In an emergency, this is best accomplished by a slow and careful intravenous injection of available soluble salts, such as *calcium chloride* or *gluconate*.

These salts are injected slowly in order to avoid the adverse effects of high calcium concentrations upon the heart. Care is required, especially with the acidic and highly irritating chloride salt, to avoid leakage into extravascular tissues. Calcium gluconate injection may also cause abscess formation in infants when given intramuscularly. Both these drugs may be administered by mouth for milder states of tetany, but less irritating salts such as *calcium lactate* and *levulinate* are often preferred for this purpose. When hypocalcemic tetany is the result of *hypoparathyroidism*, calcium injections may be supplemented by administering parathyroid hormone extracts parenterally.

During pregnancy and lactation, the demands of the fetus or infant may double the mother's daily requirement for calcium. Dietary calcium in milk is supplemented by preparations containing calcium salts alone or combined with vitamin D. The ordinary multivitamin and mineral supplements are relatively low in calcium. (A one-a-day capsule containing a dozen or more different vitamins and minerals but only about 250 mg of a calcium salt does not go very far toward satisfying a daily requirement of close to 2 g of elemental calcium.)

Among products available for oral use are the dibasic and tribasic salts of calcium phosphate, and calcium lactate. The nurse should suggest that patients purchase these in the cheapest forms available. These include powders that can be sprinkled on food, watery suspensions that can be prepared at low cost by a pharmacist, or flavored wafers. Expensive and often nutritionally inadequate combinations with vitamins and with several other minerals, including iron and various trace metals, should be avoided.

FLUORIDES. Fluorides have effects on dental enamel and bone that may be beneficial when these salts of the halogen element fluorine are employed as dietary supplements. The use of fluorides together with calcium salts in the treatment of osteoporosis is still experimental, as is their administration to aid in retention of calcium by the body in conditions such as multiple myeloma and Paget's disease.

The addition of fluorides to pediatric vitamin supplements in minute amounts appears justified in some circumstances because they aid the development of teeth that are more than normally resistant to dental caries. Fluoride salts are often incorporated into commercial dentifrices and their solutions are sometimes applied directly to teeth to reduce decay.

Actually, fluoridation of community water supplies to bring the fluoride concentration up to one part per million seems to be the best way to decrease the percentage of tooth decay in the local population. This concentration makes the enamel more resistant without causing any excessive mottling of the tooth surfaces.

References

BODY FLUID DISTURBANCES

Dutcher, I., and Fielo, S. Water and Electrolytes. New York: Macmillan, 1967.

Hamit, H.F. Status of human plasma as a plasma volume expander. *JAMA*, 174:1617, 1960.

Howard, J.M. Fluid replacement in shock and hemorrhage. *JAMA*, 173:516, 1960.

Iseler, C. Blood—the age of components. *RN*, 36:31, 1973 (June).

Metheny, N., and Snively, W.D. Nurses' Handbook of Fluid Balance. Philadelphia: J. B. Lippincott, 1967.

Rasmussen, M.G., et al. Transfusion therapy. *New Eng. J. Med.*, 264:1034; 1038; 1961.

Rodman, M.J. Fluid and electrolyte balance. *RN*, 22:41, 1959 (May).

Snively, W.D. Jr., and Roberts, K. T. The clinical picture approach as an aid to understanding body fluid disturbances. *Nurs. Forum*, 12:132, 1973.

Wilson, J.S., et al. The use of dextran in the treatment of blood loss and shock. *Amer. J. Med. Sci.*, 223:364, 1952.

VITAMINS AND MINERALS

Council on Foods and Nutrition. Vitamin preparations as dietary supplements and as therapeutic agents. *JAMA*, 169:41, 1959.

DiPalma, J.R. Vitamins: facts and fancies. *RN*, 35:57, 1972 (July).

Griffith, W.H. The physiological role of vitamins. *Amer. J. Med.*, 25:666, 1958.

National Research Council. Recommended Dietary Allowances, ed. 7, Publication 1694. Washington, D.C.: Food and Nutrition Board, National Acad. of Sciences, 1968.

Pauling, L. Vitamin C and the common cold. San Francisco: W.H. Freeman, 1970.

Rodman, M.J. Blood-building B vitamins and how they work. *RN*, 22:33, 1959 (Nov.).

50

Drugs Used for Diagnosis

Drugs are sometimes administered to diagnose disease rather than to treat it. The basis for their use is the fact that diseased organs respond differently to some drugs than do normally functioning organs. For example, patients with myasthenia gravis respond to low doses of *edrophonium*+ (Tensilon) and *tubocurarine*+ in a manner different from patients in whom neuromuscular transmission is normal. This is the basis for the use of these muscle stimulants and relaxants for the differential diagnosis of myasthenia gravis from other disorders marked by muscle weakness (Chapter 21).

In this chapter, we shall consider some other drugs that evoke unusual responses in the presence of pathology. We shall also discuss drugs that are used to aid in visualizing internal organs by x-ray—radiographic agents (Table 50-1)—and we shall mention the general uses of radioactive isotopes for diagnosis.

Not taken up in this text are various materials of biological origin such as the skin test antigens used in testing for tuberculosis, diphtheria, and other infectious diseases. We shall also omit reference to chemical aids in diagnosing diabetes abnormalities in blood sugar, acetone, and so forth, as this subject lies beyond the scope of a pharmacology textbook. The details of diagnostic tests of all kinds may best be found in various excellent books that deal with clinical laboratory tests and their interpretation.

Tests of Gastric Acid Secretion

Drugs are sometimes employed to determine whether a patient's stomach has the ability to secrete gastric acid. Patients with pernicious anemia (Chapter 34) lack this capacity. Alcohol and caffeine are among the many chemicals capable of provoking increased secretion of gastric acid. However, histamine and its analogue, betazole, are more commonly employed for this purpose clinically.

Histamine phosphate strongly stimulates the gastric glands to secrete increased quantities of acid. If the stomach fails to respond to a subcutaneously administered dose of this drug, the presence of pernicious anemia or of stomach cancer may be suspected. This must, of course, be confirmed by other kinds of diagnostic tests.

The effects of histamine may not be limited to the gastric glands but can also affect the smooth muscle of blood vessels, the bronchioles, and other sites. Overdosage, accidental injection into a vein, or hypersensitivity may result in severe headache, breathing difficulties, or cardiovascular collapse. The use of histamine is contraindicated in patients with a history of bronchial asthma.

Betazole hydrochloride (Histalog) also stimulates gastric acid secretion and is used for the same purpose as histamine. However, it does not cause side effects as often or a severe as those seen with histamine. Headache, urticarial skin reactions, and bronchoconstriction are relatively rare, but caution is still required in asthmatic patients and others with a history of hypersensitivity. The most common side effects are sweating, flushing of the face and a feeling of warmth.

Azuresin (Diagnex Blue) is a substance also used for determining whether acid is present in the stomach or absent (achlorhydria). Its use eliminates the need to collect gastric acid with a stomach tube, as is the case when histamine or betazole are employed. Instead, the patient's urine is examined for the presence of this dye exactly two hours after the oral administration of the granules.

The presence of free hydrochloric acid in the stomach liberates a blue dye from the resin with which it is combined. This dye is then absorbed into the bloodstream and carried to the kidneys for excretion. The collected urine specimen is then examined visually and its color is compared with a standard. Side effects rarely occur, but the results of this test are less accurate than those obtained by gastric intubation and direct collection of stomach acid following administration of a gastric gland stimulant. False results are most likely to occur in the presence of kidney disease, impaired gastrointestinal absorption, and other pathological states.

Diagnosis of Glandular Function

Drugs of various kinds are employed to test the functioning of such endocrine glands as the anterior pituitary, pancreas, thyroid, and the adrenal medulla and cortex.

Metyrapone (Metopirone) is employed to test pituitary gland function. Ordinarily, when a person is subjected to stress, his anterior pituitary gland responds by increasing its output of the hormone corticotropin, as discussed in Chapter 35. This, in turn, stimulates the adrenal cortex to secrete its steroid hormones (Chapter 17).

In individuals with a normally functioning pituitary gland, metyrapone impedes corticosteroid production and secretion, resulting in an outpouring of corticotropin by the pituitary gland. In patients with poor pituitary gland function, this response to the administration of metyrapone is markedly reduced. This leads to a diagnosis of *hypopituitarism*.

Corticotropin (ACTH) is itself employed for testing adrenocortical function. Normally, the intramuscular injection of this pituitary hormone is followed by a marked increase in the blood level of adrenal corticosteroids. This does *not* occur in patients with *adrenal insufficiency*. In a similar test, corticotropin is infused slowly by vein, and the patient's urine is tested for increased adrenocorticosteroid levels. If *no* increase occurs the patient may be tentatively diagnosed as suffering from *Addison's disease*.

Pheochromocytoma, a tumor of the adrenal medulla and other chromaffin cell tissues, causes a form of secondary hypertension. The presence of this tumor may be detected by the patient's response to various diagnostic drugs. Injection of histamine, for example, stimulates chromaffin cell tumors to secrete a mixture of epinephrine and norepinephrine. This release of catecholamines in large quantities provokes a steep rise in blood pressure in patients with this tumor.

Phentolamine mesylate (Regitine), an alpha adrenergic blocking agent, is also used in testing for pheochromocytoma. However, unlike histamine, it does not cause a rise in blood pressure. Instead, patients with this condition respond to administration of this drug with a drop in blood pressure.

In patients with essential hypertension, however, the person's high blood pressure fails to fall significantly following injection of phentolamine. Thus, this drug aids the physician in differentiating between primary hypertension and high blood pressure that is the result of the presence of this tumor—a type of secondary hypertension (Chapters 24 and 26).

Thyrotropin and *radioactive sodium iodide* are employed in diagnosing thyroid gland malfunction in hypothyroidism and hyperthyroidism. The sodium salt of the hypoglycemic agent, *tolbutamide* (Orinase), is used in a diagnostic test for diabetes (Chapters 35 and 39).

Diagnosis of Kidney Function

Phenolsulfonphthalein (Phenol Red) is the chemical most commonly employed in studies of renal function. Although the test gives only a rough measure of the extent to which kidney function is reduced, its simplicity makes it useful for quick screening to determine whether the patient's excretory function is severely impaired. Poor elimination of the dye indicates that serious renal insufficiency may be present.

The patient forces fluids for about an hour before the test and then empties his bladder just before the dye is injected intravenously or into a muscle. Urine samples are collected at specified intervals and the amount of dye that appears in each sample is measured colorimetrically. Occasional allergic reactions are the only adverse effects reported.

Sodium aminohippurate, a substance secreted by the kidney tubules, is used to determine the capacity of the tubules to perform their excretory function. It is also employed to measure plasma flow through the kidneys. The drug is administered by vein in doses intended to raise the amount in the plasma to certain predetermined levels. The infusion is made slowly to avoid various side effects that occur when the plasma level rises too rapidly. These include a sudden sensation of skin warmth, and nausea or vomiting.

Liver Function Tests

Tests of hepatic function do not always detect the presence of gross damage that may be seen in a biopsy sample. Liver function, as determined by these tests, may seem more or less normal despite the presence of gross pathology.

Nevertheless, by the use of a battery of such tests, it is often possible to rule out some diseases or to determine the degree of their severity.

The ability of the liver to remove from the blood such dyes as *indocyanine green* (below) and sulfobromophthalein sodium is an index of functional capacity and of the extent to which it may have been reduced in such diseases as cirrhosis of the liver, or in hepatic and metastatic carcinoma.

Sulfobromophthalein sodium (Bromsulphalein) is the drug most commonly used for testing liver function. Healthy liver cells remove BSP from the blood and excrete it into the bile soon after the dye is injected intravenously. The damaged liver does not do so as readily. As a result, the dye stays in the bloodstream at higher levels for a longer time after injection.

The drug is injected slowly into a vein in one arm, and a blood sample is drawn from a vein in the other arm 45 minutes later. Colorimetric tests indicating the presence of less than 5 percent of the injected material are in the normal range. Care is required to avoid leakage into the tissues surrounding the vein. This is true not only because of the local irritation that follows, but also because allergic reactions occur more commonly when extravasation of the drug has occurred.

Diagnosis of Circulatory Function

Dyes and other drugs are sometimes injected directly into the bloodstream to help determine such aspects of circulatory function as blood volume and cardiac output. Their use sometimes produces data that aid the doctor in the management of shock and other disorders of circulatory function. These drugs rarely cause adverse effects.

Evans Blue is injected intravenously as a means of *determining the plasma volume* of patients who may be suffering from shock, heart failure, or other disorders leading to development of circulatory abnormalities. The degree to which the dye is diluted in the patient's plasma is measured colorimetrically from a blood sample withdrawn ten minutes after the injection is begun. This is compared with a sample taken before the dye was injected. The result of such studies sometimes helps the doctor decide on the type of treatment to be employed in cases of cardiovascular collapse, dehydration, and other disorders.

Indocyanine green (Cardio-Green) is a dye

used mainly for determining cardiac output, but it is also used to determine blood flow through the liver and hepatic function. A freshly prepared solution is injected intravenously, and the extent to which the dye is diluted in blood is measured in blood withdrawn from arteries. Adverse reactions have not been reported, but because of the presence of small amounts of iodide, caution is required in patients allergic to iodides. Radioactive iodine uptake tests cannot be performed for at least one week after the use of iodocyanine green.

Fluorescein and its salts are used to determine *circulation time,* the extent to which blood vessels are open or blocked, and for other purposes not involving circulatory function. The time required for the dye to move from the arm vein into which it is injected to various other blood vessels is measured by detecting fluorescence at the second site under ultraviolet light. This drug, which is excreted in the bile, is also used for outlining the bile ducts and gall bladder. Occasional nausea and vomiting is the only adverse effect. This dye is also used topically in the eye to detect defects in the conjunctival and corneal surfaces.

Sodium dehydrocholate (Decholin sodium), a bile salt, is used for determining circulation time as well as in the diagnosis and treatment of biliary tract disorders. This drug is not a dye; instead, the time it takes for the substance to travel from arm to tongue is measured by having the patient report the detection of a bitter taste. Unfortunately, nausea, vomiting, epigastric distress, and diarrhea may follow. More serious adverse effects, including fatal anaphylactoid reactions, have also been reported following rapid intravenous administration. Thus, its routine use in cardiovascular diagnosis is not recommended.

Radiopaque Media for Radiographic Diagnosis (Table 50-1)

Radiopaque substances are chemicals that cannot be penetrated by x-rays. They are employed as contrast media in order to make visible various internal structures, including the gallbladder and gastrointestinal tract, kidneys, lungs, and other organs. Except for barium sulfate, all the contrast media are iodinated organic chemicals.

Some of these substances are taken by mouth either for local radiopaque effects in the intestinal tract or for their effects after they are absorbed and excreted into organs such as the gallbladder. Other contrast media are instilled directly into the organ that is to be visualized—the bronchial tree, uterus, or spinal tract, for example. The most recently developed contrast media are safe enough to be injected intravenously, or even intraarterially.

However, safety is not always assured, and while the contrast media seem to be substances of low direct tissue toxicity, reactions of several kinds are common and sometimes prove serious or even fatal. Thus, the nurse who assists in such diagnostic procedures watches the patient closely for early signs of drug reactions, so that treatment measures can be instituted immediately. The patient is also observed for delayed reactions after he returns to the ward. If the patient is treated in a clinic or a physician's office, it is important to ask him to wait in the reception area, for a period mutually agreed upon by the nurse and the doctor, so that he can be observed immediately following the test. Often such an observation period can be combined with an offer of a cup of coffee, which is usually most welcome to the patient who has arrived in a fasting state for his diagnostic tests. The waiting period and offer of light refreshment also serve to lessen the anxiety usually engendered by such tests, before the patient resumes such activity as driving a car.

Barium sulfate is the most commonly used substance for outlining the viscera of the gastrointestinal tract. It is administered orally as a thick paste for esophageal studies or as a dilute suspension prior to searching for peptic ulcerations or upper gastrointestinal tract lesions. Lower bowel lesions are looked for following a cleansing enema and instillation of a large amount of a warmed barium sulfate retention enema.

Barium that is not completely expelled from the gastrointestinal tract may be constipating. Thus, the doctor often orders a cleansing enema after completing the procedure. In any case, it is important for the nurse to note the state of bowel motility and report this to the doctor. Other than its tendency to cause constipation, barium sulfate itself is an entirely safe substance pharmacologically. It does not irritate the gastrointestinal mucosa and is not absorbed into the systemic circulation.

Cholecystography, a procedure used in the diagnosis of gall bladder disease, is carried out with two types of radiopaque compounds: (1)

T A B L E   5 0 - 1   *Radiographic Diagnostic Agents (Radiopaque Media)*

Nonproprietary or Official Name	Proprietary or Trade Name	Dosage and Administration
Barium sulfate U.S.P.	. . . .	300 g orally or 400 g rectally in suitable suspension
Calcium ipodate N.F.	Oragraffin calcium	3 g
Ethiodized oil U.S.P.	Ethiodol	0.5 to 20 ml intracavitary
Iodized oil N.F.	Lipiodol	10 ml by special injection
Iodoalphionic acid	Priodax	3 g
Iodopyracet injection N.F.	Diodrast	20 ml I.M. or I.V.
Iopanoic acid U.S.P.	Telepaque	3 g
Iophendylate injection U.S.P.	Pantopaque	6 ml by special injection or intrathecally
Meglumine diatrizoate injection U.S.P.	Cardiografin; Gastrografin; Renografin	25 ml I.V. of a 60% solution
Meglumine iodipamide injection U.S.P.	Cholografin meglumine	20 ml of a 52% solution
Meglumine iothalamate injection U.S.P.	Conray	30 ml of a 60% solution I.V.
Propyliodone, sterile suspension U.S.P.	Dionosil	0.2 ml/kg of body weight intratracheal to a maximum of 18 ml
Sodium diatrizoate injection U.S.P.	Hypaque sodium	30 ml of a 50% solution I.V.
Sodium iodomethamate injection N.F.	Neo-Iopax	10 g I.V. and by special injection
Sodium iodipamide injection U.S.P.	Cholografin sodium	20 ml I.V. of a 20% solution
Sodium iothalamate injection U.S.P.	Angio-Conray; Conray-400	0.5 ml of a 66.8 or 80% solution per kg of body weight I.V. or intraarterial
Sodium ipodate N.F.	Oragraffin sodium	3 g
Sodium methiodal injection N.F.	Skiodan	20 g I.V. in 50 ml

those that are administered by mouth; and (2) those that are given intravenously.

The oral iodinated contrast media include *iopanoic acid* and the calcium and sodium salts of *ipodate*, which act quite quickly to make the gall bladder opaque to x-rays. These substances are taken a couple of hours after a fat-free evening meal. Nothing other than small amounts of water is taken by mouth before the x-ray examination on the next morning.

The intravenously administered substances, such as the sodium and meglumine salts of *iodipamide*, are used for better visualization of the gall bladder and bile ducts of patients in whom results were poor with the orally taken agents. Adverse reactions are much more likely with drugs that are administered by this route.

These adverse effects are especially likely to occur in patients with liver and kidney disease, for these organs do not readily excrete the injected dose of the drug when damaged by disease. Thus, procedures employing iodinated radiopaque compounds are contraindicated in patients with a history of hepatic or renal insufficiency resulting from acute injury of these organs. Patients whose history reveals hypersensitivity to iodine are also not good candidates for diagnostic procedures employing these agents.

During the first 15 to 30 minutes after injection of an iodinated diagnostic agent, the nurse should watch the patient carefully for signs of histamine-release reactions and other possible ill effects. Sneezing, wheezing, and skin swellings may be the first indications of even more severe anaphylactoid reactions. Thus, the nurse sees to it that the drugs and equipment for dealing with this dangerous emergency are always readily available during radiographic procedures employing parenterally administered radiographic drugs.

Some patients seem to be especially susceptible to cardiovascular effects that do not occur in the majority of people who receive ordinary injectable diagnostic doses. These reactions are often manifested by a fall in blood pressure and reflex tachycardia. Thus, it is desirable to check the patient's blood pressure periodically. Failure to detect and treat severe hypotension has been followed by myocardial infarction, renal failure, and other complications.

Urography—x-ray visualization of the urinary tract—is carried out shortly after intravenous injection of one of the water-soluble organic iodine contrast media, such as *meglumine diatrizoate* (Renografin) or *sodium diatrizoate* (Hypaque sodium). Soon after these materials are slowly infused, they are carried to the kidneys and begin to appear in the urine. Serial x-rays are taken beginning about five minutes after the contrast medium has been injected completely, when dense shadows develop in the urinary collecting system.

Retrograde urography. In this procedure the contrast medium is instilled into the kidneys through catheters placed by cystoscopy. Thus, the kidneys and the urinary collecting system are outlined without spreading the chemical throughout the body via the circulation. In both this and the above procedures, it is customary to administer a laxative about 12 hours before the administration of the contrast medium. This, and the subsequent withholding of food, empties the bowel and thus minimizes development of abdominal shadows that might make it difficult to interpret the urographic roentgenograms.

Renal arteriography delivers the contrast medium solution directly into the kidney arteries through rapid injection into the abdominal aorta. Although this procedure often reveals defects in the renal circulation better than any other test, it is relatively hazardous. Two new agents, *meglumine* and *sodium iothalamate*, are said to be safer than earlier contrast media for carrying out this test and such other angiographic procedures as cardiac, aortic, and cerebral circulatory x-ray studies. In such studies, the solutions are injected swiftly into the vessels of the organ that is to be visualized. For example, dilute solutions are injected directly into the carotid and vertebral arteries before x-rays of brain blood circulation are taken.

Instillation of oily or viscous iodized contrast media directly into hollow organs, rather than via the blood, is often employed for visualizing certain areas. For example, the uterine cavity and fallopian tubes are visualized by introducing *iodized oil* (Lipiodol), *ethiodized oil* (Ethiodol), or one of the water-soluble iodine preparations made suitably viscous by the addition of a thickening agent. This procedure, *hysterosalpingography*, is used in sterility studies to determine the patency of the tubes and in the diagnosis of other gynecological conditions.

Bronchography is carried out by introducing similar agents, including *propyliodone* (Dionosil), directly into the trachea, from which they spread down the tracheobronchial tree along the walls of this tract. After the roentgenograms are made, most of the material is removed by having the patient sit up and cough forcibly. Most of the rest of the chemical is apparently absorbed slowly and eliminated from the respiratory tract by other routes. However, some may remain in the lower lungs for long periods and cause chronic inflammatory reactions.

Myelography, visualization of the spinal cord, is carried out by instillation of an iodinated contrast medium into the subarachnoid space. This procedure is widely used for finding evidence of herniated intervertebral discs and other sources of spinal cord compression. Iophendylate, the agent most often used for myelography, is said to be better tolerated than the agents previously employed. Like the others, however, it is aspirated from the spinal fluid immediately after the fluoroscopic or roentgenographic examination.

RADIOACTIVE ISOTOPES

Radioactive isotopes are often given for diagnostic purposes because of the ease of detecting them even when widely distributed throughout the body. Even extremely low concentrations of isotopically labeled chemicals can be detected externally by instruments that pick up gamma rays emitted from organs in which the isotope is concentrated. For example, we have seen how radioactive iodine is used to diagnose thyroid gland disorders. Radioactive phosphorus is similarly employed for localizing brain tumors.

Other isotopes are sometimes used to trace the absorption of tiny amounts of vitamin B_{12}, to measure blood flow through the heart, kidneys, and elsewhere, and to visualize internal organs by holding a scintillation scanner over the body and determining the distribution of gamma ray-emitting radio isotopes. However, x-rays are often preferred for this, because they give clearer pictures of organ contours and motility and because the use of radiopharmaceuticals for diagnosis poses many pharmaceutical problems and requires considerable care to avoid exposure of patients and personnel to radiation.

When the nurse works with a patient undergoing diagnostic tests, an important part of her role involves supporting him as he waits for the results of tests. Someimes several days elapse before the patient learns these results, and this period can be one of mounting tension both for him and for his family. By promoting diversion and encouraging the patient to continue his usual activities as fully as possible, the nurse helps to lessen his anxiety and to combat feelings of helplessness.

References

Crocker, D., and Vandam, L.D. Untoward reactions to radiopaque contrast media. *Clin. Pharmacol. Ther.*, 4:654, 1963.

Elking, M.P., and Kabat, H.F. Drug induced modification of laboratory test values. *Amer. J. Hosp. Pharm.*, 25:485, 1968.

Hoppe, J.O. Some pharmacological aspects of radiopaque compounds. *Ann. N.Y. Acad. Sci.*, 78:727, 1959.

Rodman, M.J. Drugs used for diagnosis. *RN*, 22:43, 1959 (Dec.).

Wagner, H.N., Jr. Radioactive pharmaceuticals. *Clin. Pharmacol. Ther.*, 4:351, 1963.

Index

Please note: Each drug appears in the Index under its proprietary name or names, where applicable, as well as under its official or generic name. Thus the proprietary entry may be used to determine the official name under which all page references to the drug are given. The following abbreviations are used: *d* indicates a reference to one of the Drug Digest sections which follow most chapters; *n* is a reference to a footnote; *s* is a reference to one or more of the Summary sections found at the end of most chapters; *t* is a reference to a Table. In most cases *t* references will provide drug type and dosage range information.